SAUNDERS MANUAL OF
Medical Transcription

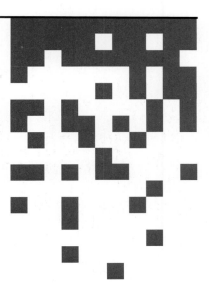

SAUNDERS MANUAL OF
Medical Transcription

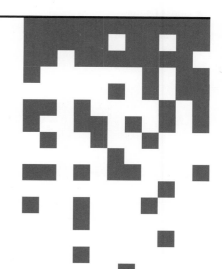

Sheila B. Sloane, C.M.T.
Formerly President, Medi-Phone, Inc.
Villanova, Pennsylvania

Marilyn Takahashi Fordney, C.M.A.-A.C., C.M.T.
Formerly Instructor of Medical Insurance,
Medical Terminology, Medical Machine Transcription,
and Medical Office Procedures,
Ventura College, Ventura, California

W.B. SAUNDERS COMPANY *A Division of Harcourt Brace & Company*
Philadelphia ■ London ■ Toronto ■ Montreal ■ Sydney ■ Tokyo

W.B. Saunders Company
A Division of Harcourt Brace & Company

The Curtis Center
Independence Square West
Philadelphia, Pennsylvania 19106

Library of Congress Cataloging-in-Publication Data

Saunders manual of medical transcription / [edited by] Sheila B. Sloane,
  Marilyn Takahashi Fordney.
      p.   cm.
    Includes index.
    ISBN 0-7216-3675-6
    1. Medical transcription.   I. Sloane, Sheila B.
  II. Fordney, Marilyn Takahashi.
    [DNLM: 1. Medical Records.   W 80 S2573 1994]
  R728.8.S277   1994
  653'.18 — dc20
  DNLM/DLC   93-25871

Saunders Manual of Medical Transcription   ISBN 0-7216-3675-6

Printed in the United States of America.

Last digit is the print number: 9   8   7   6   5   4   3   2   1

To the
transcriptionist,
whose care and accuracy
serve the well-being of
physician and patient alike

and

to our husbands, John and Alan,
for their continuous encouragement,
patience, and support

Contributors

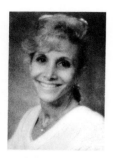

JACKIE ABERN, B.A., C.M.T.
Formerly Instructor in Medical Transcription, Oakton Community College, Des Plaines; Harper Community College, Palatine; Director, American Association for Medical Transcription; President, HSS Transcription, Inc., Northbrook, Illinois

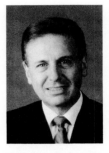

JOSEPH A. BELLANTI, M.D.
Professor of Pediatrics and Microbiology and Director of the International Center for Interdisciplinary Studies of Immunology, Georgetown University Medical Center; Director, Division of Immunology and Virology, Department of Laboratory Medicine, Georgetown University Hospital, Washington, D.C.; Past President of the American College of Allergy and Immunology

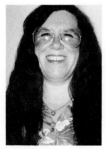

INGE BARTH, C.M.T.
Past President, American Association for Medical Transcription; Member, Medical Advisory Board, Medical Transcription Program, Denver Technical College; President, High Country Transcription, Inc., Colorado Springs, Colorado

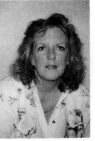

JANICE BLACKBURN, C.M.T.
Owner/Manager, MedScription, Glen Cove, New York; founder and first president of the Southern New York Chapter of American Association for Medical Transcription; Member of the National Board of Directors of American Association for Medical Transcription, 1981–1985; North Shore University Hospital, Glen Cove, New York

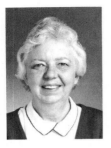

JULIA WATTS BUCHANAN, B.S.
Research Associate, The Johns Hopkins Medical Institutions, Division of Nuclear Medicine and Radiation Health Sciences, Baltimore, Maryland

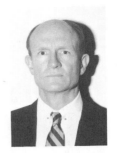

CHALMERS E. CORNELIUS, III, M.D.
Assistant Clinical Professor, Department of Dermatology, Thomas Jefferson Medical School, Philadelphia; Chief of Dermatology Service, Bryn Mawr Hospital, Bryn Mawr, Pennsylvania

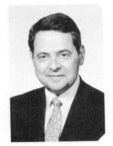

MICHAEL A. BUSH, M.D.
Clinical Associate Professor of Medicine, Cedars-Sinai Medical Center, UCLA School of Medicine, and Director, Diabetes Outpatient Training and Education Center, Division of Endocrinology, Cedars-Sinai Medical Center, Los Angeles, California

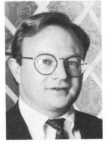

GARY WALTER CROOKS, M.D.
Assistant Professor of Medicine, University of Pennsylvania School of Medicine, and Assistant Director, Medical Consult Service, Hospital of the University of Pennsylvania, Philadelphia, Pennsylvania

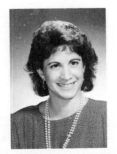

VICTORIA A. CIRILLO-HYLAND, M.D.
Clinical Associate, Hospital of the University of Pennsylvania, Philadelphia; Attending Physician, Dermatology Department, Bryn Mawr Hospital, Bryn Mawr, Pennsylvania

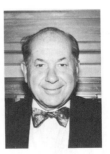

RAYMOND L. DEL FAVA, M.D.
Associate Clinical Professor of Radiology, Stritch School of Medicine, Loyola University, Maywood, and President, Medical/Dental Staff, St. Francis Hospital, Evanston, Illinois

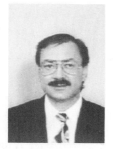

MICHAEL A. DiGIACOMO, D.P.M.
Clinical Professor, California College of Podiatric Medicine; Clinical Professor, Highland Hospital; Chief of Podiatry, Summit Medical Center, Oakland; Staff Podiatrist, Alta Bates Hospital, Berkeley, California

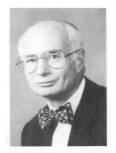

LESLIE P. DORNFELD, M.D.
Clinical Professor of Medicine and Attending Physician in Nephrology and Rheumatology, Medical Center of the University of California, Los Angeles; Attending Physician, Wadsworth VA Hospital, Los Angeles, California

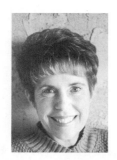

DEBORAH LYNCH EMMONS, C.M.A.
Recording Secretary, Ventura County Professional Women's Network; President, S.T.A.T. Transcription Service, Oxnard, California

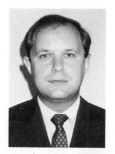

STEPHEN LLOYD FEDDER, M.D.
Attending Neurosurgeon, The Lankenau Hospital, Wynnewood, Pennsylvania

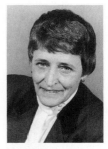

PATRICIA A. FENN, M.D.
Senior Attending Rheumatologist and Chief of Service, Bryn Mawr Hospital; Medical Director, Bryn Mawr Hospital Arthritis and Orthopaedic Center, Bryn Mawr; Clinical Assistant Professor of Medicine, the Medical College of Thomas Jefferson University, Philadelphia, Pennsylvania

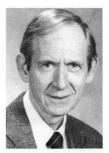

WILLIAM G. FIGUEROA, M.D.
Clinical Professor of Medicine, the Medical College of Thomas Jefferson University, Philadelphia; Chief of Pulmonary Medicine and Critical Care, The Lankenau Hospital, Wynnewood; Consultant, Paoli Memorial Hospital, Paoli; Consultant, Bryn Mawr Hospital and Bryn Mawr Rehabilitation Hospital, Bryn Mawr, Pennsylvania

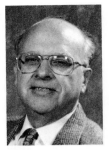

THOMAS G. GABUZDA, M.D.
Associate Member of the Cardeza Foundation for Hematologic Research and Professor of Medicine at the Medical College of Thomas Jefferson University, Philadelphia; Chief of Hematology, The Lankenau Hospital, Wynnewood, Pennsylvania

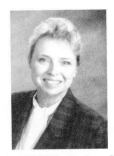

SONDRA SUE HEIN, B.A., C.M.T.
Instructor of Medical Terminology, Saddleback College, and President, Medical Transcription Service, Mission Viejo, California

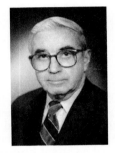

JOHN J. GARTLAND, M.D.
James Edwards Professor Emeritus of Orthopaedic Surgery and Chairman Emeritus of the Department of Orthopaedic Surgery, the Medical College of Thomas Jefferson University; Medical Editor, Thomas Jefferson University, Philadelphia, Pennsylvania

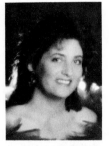

ELIZABETH ANN HUBEN, B.S., M.T.
President, Mineral King Chapter of the American Association for Medical Transcription; President, Medicus Scriptor, Tulare, California

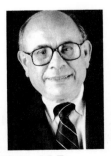

MORRIS GREEN, M.D.
Perry W. Lesh Professor of Pediatrics, Indiana University School of Medicine, Indianapolis; Attending Pediatrician, James Whitcomb Riley Hospital for Children, Indianapolis, Indiana

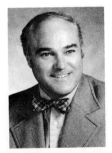

FRANK L. HUSSEY, Jr., M.D.
Attending Physician, Lutheran General Hospital, Chicago; Consulting Radiotherapist, Rush-North Shore Hospital, Skokie, and Alexian Brothers Regional Cancer Care Center, Elk Grove Village, Illinois

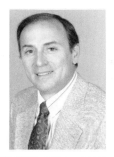

ROBERT S. IMPROTA, M.D.
Attending Physician and Clinical Instructor in Plastic Surgery, Ventura County Medical Center, Ventura; Attending Physician, Plastic Surgery, Pleasant Valley Hospital, Camarillo; Attending Physician, Plastic Surgery, St. John's Regional Medical Center, Oxnard, California; Formerly Clinical Assistant Professor in Plastic Surgery at Cornell Medical Center, New York Hospital, New York, New York

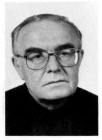

JOSEF V. KADLEC, S.J., M.D.
Associate Professor of Pediatrics and Microbiology and Member, International Center for Interdisciplinary Studies of Immunology, Georgetown University Medical Center, Washington, D.C.

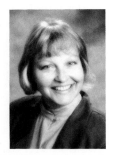

LYNN C. KEENE, B.S., M.S.
Instructor in Advanced Medical Transcription and Member of the Advisory Board, Orange Coast College, Costa Mesa, California

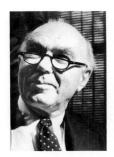

ZIGMOND M. LEBENSOHN, M.D.
Chief Emeritus, Department of Psychiatry, Sibley Memorial Hospital; Clinical Professor of Psychiatry, Georgetown University School of Medicine, Washington, D.C.

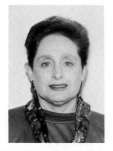

SANDRA LEVINE, C.M.T.
President, Secretary, Newsletter Editor, Membership Chairman, San Fernando Valley Chapter, American Association for Medical Transcription, San Fernando, California

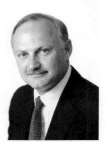

WILLIAM J. LEWIS, III, M.D.
Chief of the Division of Otolaryngology and President of the Medical Staff at The Lankenau Hospital, Wynnewood; Assistant Professor of Otolaryngology, the Medical College of Thomas Jefferson University, Philadelphia, Pennsylvania

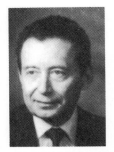

RAYMOND E. LIGUORI, M.D.
Medical Director, Cardiac Care Unit, St. John's Regional Medical Center, Oxnard, California

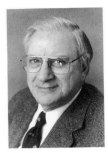

PHILIP R. NAST, M.D., F.A.C.P.
Senior Attending Gastroenterologist, Bryn Mawr Hospital, Bryn Mawr; Associate Clinical Professor of Gastroenterology, University of Pennsylvania School of Medicine, Philadelphia; Consulting Gastroenterologist, Coatesville Veterans Hospital, Coatesville, Pennsylvania

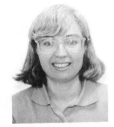

MARIE D. LOW, M.S., Ph.D.
Vice President, Business Development and Marketing, Marketing Services Division, R.L. Polk & Company, Toronto, Ontario, Canada

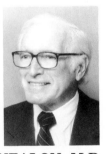

THOMAS F. NEALON, M.D.
Chairman Emeritus of Surgery, St. Vincent's Hospital and Medical Center, New York; Professor Emeritus of Surgery, New York Medical College, Valhalla, New York

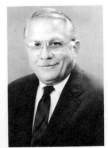

MORGAN L. MORGAN, M.D.
Active Staff, Hoag Memorial Hospital Presbyterian, Newport Beach; Emeritus Staff, Valley Presbyterian Hospital, Van Nuys; Chief Emeritus, Department of Obstetrics and Gynecology, Cedars-Sinai Medical Center, Los Angeles; Associate Clinical Professor Emeritus, University of Southern California Medical School, Los Angeles, California

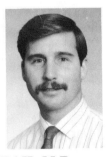

MARTY L. PRAH, M.D.
Active Staff, Kaweah Delta District Hospital, Visalia Community Hospital, Visalia, and Hanford Community Hospital, Hanford, California

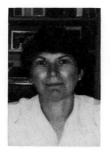

CAROLYN FOWLER SIDOR, M.D.
Clinical Instructor in Medicine, the Medical College of Thomas Jefferson University, Philadelphia; Assistant in the Division of Hematology-Oncology, The Lankenau Hospital, Wynnewood, Pennsylvania

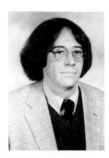

RONALD W. STUNZ, M.D.
Director, Emergency Services, and Chief of Service, Emergency Medicine, Bryn Mawr Hospital, Bryn Mawr, Pennsylvania

KERANO J. SPERRY
Media specialist, American College of Radiology, Reston, Virginia

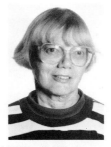

HAZEL L. TANK, C.M.T.
Quality Assurance Manager, AlphaScribe Express; Writer; Charter Member, San Diego Chapter of the American Association for Medical Transcription, San Diego, California

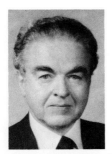

CHARLES G. STEINMETZ, III, M.D.
Attending Ophthalmologist, Bryn Mawr Hospital, Bryn Mawr; Ophthalmologist, Presbyterian Hospital and Scheie Eye Institute, and Attending Surgeon and Consultant in Pathology, Wills Eye Hospital, Philadelphia, Pennsylvania

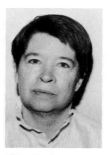

BRON TAYLOR, B.A.
Member, Phi Alpha Theta (Honor Society for Graduate Students of History); Transcriptionist and Writer, San Francisco, California

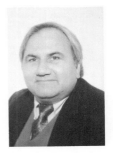

LOUIS T. VERARDO, M.D.
Associate Director, Family Practice Residency Program; Director, Continuing Medical Education; Physician-in-Charge, Employee Health Service; and Attending Physician, Family Practice, North Shore University Hospital, Glen Cove, New York; Clinical Assistant Professor of Family Medicine, Medical School of the State University of New York, Stony Brook Health Center, Stony Brook, New York

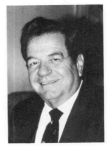

HENRY N. WAGNER, Jr., M.D.
Professor of Medicine and Radiology, Johns Hopkins University School of Medicine; Professor of Environmental Health Sciences, Johns Hopkins School of Hygiene and Public Health, Baltimore, Maryland

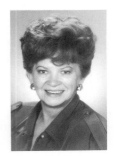

MEG WALSH
Vice-President of Marketing, Medical Transcription Service, Minneapolis, Minnesota; Member of the American Association of Medical Transcription

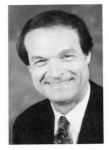

PAUL T. WERTLAKE, M.D.
Medical Director and Chief Pathologist, Metwest/Unilab Clinical Laboratories, Tarzana; Adjunct Faculty, Department of Clinical Sciences, California State University, Carson, California

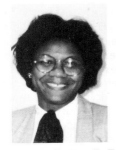

ETHEL L. WISE, R.R.T., R.P.F.T.
Director of Respiratory Care and Pulmonary Diagnostic Services, The Lankenau Hospital, Wynnewood; Adjunct Faculty, Hahnemann University, School of Allied Health Professions, Philadelphia; Adjunct Faculty, Gwynedd Mercy College, Gwynedd Valley, Pennsylvania

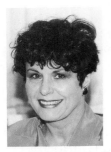

ADRIENNE C. YAZIJIAN, C.M.T.
Former President and Member of Board of Directors, American Association for Medical Transcription; Writer: President, MEDI-TRANScription, Ltd., San Diego, California

Appreciation

The heart of any reference book is its expert substance, and this is provided by our contributing writers. The very scope of our work made single-handed authorship impossible. Hence a wide variety of experts in medicine and medical transcription were called upon to share their knowledge and experience, and to them we owe an immense debt of gratitude. They all worked within rough guidelines we provided, but each was free to work in his or her own way. The result, we believe, is a book of uniform objectives but individual ways to their achievement. This is not a work of stereotyped attitudes but of views as diverse as those of our profession.

But contributors and editors working alone do not quite make a book; there are others to whom we are deeply indebted. We wish to thank our husbands, John and Alan, who offered support and encouragement throughout the preparation of the work and understanding of the priority it had on our time.

We are indebted to many individuals on the staff of the W.B. Saunders Company for their assistance in production of the book, especially Margaret Biblis, who provided skillful help and guidance.

A special thanks to PRODIGY Interactive Personal Service, which made daily communication easier, and to the authors, publishers, and manufacturers of equipment who have been generous in granting permission to reproduce illustrations.

Lastly, we express our heartfelt thanks to the reviewers and consultants who enthusiastically read each chapter and provided valuable suggestions and criticism. Without their help, the goal of keeping the manual current and well-informed might never have been achieved. We take great pride in naming here those who gave so unstintingly of their time and knowledge:

Ella M. Barnum, C.M.T.
Medical Transcriptionist and Instructor, Citrus Community College, Glendora, California

Patricia A. Bienvenue
Mental Health Clinic, Manchester, New Hampshire

Linda O. Cutcher
Mount Olive, Alabama

Jose Davies-Toll, C.M.T.
JDTS Medical Transcription, Arroyo Grande, California

Marcy O. Diehl, C.M.A.-A., C.M.T.
Instructor, Grossmont Community College, El Cajon, California

Ruth Ann Dill
Medical Transcriptionist, Mercy Hospital, San Diego, California

John L. Dusseau
Author and Former Editor, W.B. Saunders Company, Villanova, Pennsylvania

Deborah Emmons, C.M.A.
President, S.T.A.T. Transcription Service, Oxnard, California

Sheryl G. Evans, C.M.T.
Medical Transcription Services, Orangevale, California

Mary Fish, C.M.T.
Administrator, Channel Islands Surgicenter, Oxnard, California

Katherine Gerwien, C.M.T.
Accurate Medical Transcription, San Diego, California

Helene Golemon
Medical Transcriptionist, Oxnard, California

Judy Hinickle, C.M.T.
President, TransCom Resources, Menomonee Falls, Wisconsin

Patricia A. Ireland, C.M.T.
National Transcription Technologies, Inc., Orlando, Florida

Barbro R. Jensen
Medical Transcription, La Mesa, California

Dorothy L. Johnston, B.A.
Johnston Transcription Services, Birmingham, Alabama

Shelly Lesse
President, MediScribe, Conshohocken, Pennsylvania

Sandra Levine, C.M.T.
Medical Transcriptionist, North Hollywood, California

Claudia K. March, C.M.T.
Medical Transcriptionist, Summit Medical Center, Oakland, California

Patricia E. Marsden, C.M.T.
Bellflower, California

Barbara Moore-Giacalone
Medical Transcriptionist
La Mesa, California

Joyce Nakano, C.M.A.-A.
Instructor, Pasadena City College, Pasadena, California

C. Christie Nute, C.M.T.
Radiology Medical Group, Inc., San Diego, California

Kathryn A. Rambo, C.M.T.
Brea, California

Kimberly H. Rubsene, M.A.
Median School of Allied Health Careers, Pittsburgh, Pennsylvania

Janet Stiles
Dallas, Texas

Clare J. Terrill, C.M.T.
Santa Rosa Associates, San Luis Obispo, California

Jane Thomas
Thomas' Transcription Service, Santa Maria, California

Emilie Kogan Ulibarri, C.M.T.
Whittier, California

Cheryl E. Wade, C.M.T.
Typographics, Fillmore, California

Adrienne C. Yazijian, C.M.T.
President, MEDI-TRANScription, Ltd., San Diego, California

Foreword

The scribe who is skilled in his office, he is found worthy to be a courtier.*

It is an honor to have been asked to provide the Foreword for the *Saunders Manual of Medical Transcription*. It seems unfair that my small contribution should come first when the authors have done all the work. Nevertheless, I am happy to have been chosen to set the stage for the action that follows.

The quotation with which I begin this Foreword dates from the 11th century B.C. Its inclusion is not intended to be sexist, but rather to highlight the fact that for at least 3000 years of recorded history the talents of the transcriptionist have been held in high esteem.

My medical background has provided me with a profound respect for medical transcriptionsts and their importance on the health care team. The medical transcriptionist plays an integral role in building the all-important descriptive portion of the medical record, which includes history and physical examination, operative reports, progress notes, pathology and radiology reports, and discharge summaries. Medical transcription is an essential service to the field of medicine with no other options in sight. Would-be competitors lack the medical transcriptionist's knowledge of human anatomy and physiology and extensive medical vocabulary; automation of medical transcription remains firmly in the realm of science fiction.

As one who has done both medical writing and editing, I appreciate only too well the vast amount of work that goes into planning and writing a book. However, hard work and good intentions are not enough to justify a book's existence. A text worth buying and taking the time to study must adequately fill a need. The *Saunders Manual of Medical Transcription* does just that.

Sheila B. Sloane and Marilyn Fordney, well known for their publications and as leaders in the field of medical transcription, have created a unique and important manual and reference for medical transcriptionists. Reading this book, indeed memorizing it, is not a guarantee of becoming a great medical transcriptionist, but it is a good start.

The Instructions of Amenemope, Ancient Egyptian Literature. Vol II: The New Kingdom, translation by Miriam Lichtheim. University of California Press, Berkeley, 1974.

JAMES L. BENNINGTON, M.D.

Preface

This book seeks to answer a question easily put but difficult to answer: How much background information in medicine and in the basic tools of the profession must a transcriptionist have in order to do effective work and pursue career goals intelligently? The question arises because the transcriptionist must not only transcribe with accuracy but also must edit and even revise medical reports. This she can do only if she understands the essential nature of each specialty within which she works and if she has command of the principles and resources of her profession, which, like medicine itself, has its basis in science, skill, and technology. This, then, is the background information we hope to provide in this manual. It goes without saying that there is no clear consensus of precisely what should constitute this information; but a glance at the table of contents will disclose the scope of our concept of what it should be.

The reader will notice that we, perhaps lightheartedly, give the word "transcriptionist" a feminine gender. This is simply to avoid constant use of the awkward "he/she" or "s/he" and is not intended to neglect the interests of that able group of transcriptionists who are men.

The book is divided into three major parts. The first provides a background in the general principles and specific technologies of transcription. From consideration of medical ethics to advice in the techniques of writing, it is intended to offer to both seasoned and beginning transcriptionists information useful in the day-to-day practice of their profession and helpful in the advance of both their technical knowledge and their careers.

Part II offers both overview and detailed information about the individual specialties that constitute the broad panorama of medicine. Each offers insight into major modalities of diagnosis and therapy and provides specific examples of medical reports with graphs, charts, tables, and illustrations that illumine the nature of the specialty and of the transcriptionist's role in it.

Part III is a compendium of specific data that may not be found in standard reference books but should be useful in the daily work of transcription. The table of reference sources, for example, is a comprehensive listing of books relevant to the whole field of the principles and techniques of medical transcription. Models of letters and medical reports in current approved style are also shown with some of the variations that arise from their day-to-day use. Health agencies are listed in the event there is need to contact an association for a guest speaker or to request information useful in teaching a course in terminology or health science. Forms of address are included because one often has difficulty remembering the proper salutation for an official or dignitary. From acronyms to laboratory values, the appendices provide flesh for the bones of generalities.

Under our heading *Appreciation* we pay tribute to the many people who have assisted in the preparation of this manual; but in the end the value of any book must rest with those responsible for its plan and the fulfillment of its purposes. The path to publication of any book is never a straight line and in its tortuous following we hope we have succeeded in our objectives without notable error or omission. In the course of our work we have come to think highly of each other and of our emerging book. We bid it a fond farewell and hope that its place will be secure on the reader's desktop along with the personal computer, for this is your personal manual.

SHEILA B. SLOANE
MARILYN T. FORDNEY

Contents

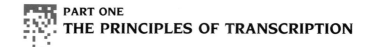

PART ONE
THE PRINCIPLES OF TRANSCRIPTION

CHAPTER 1
Medical Transcription: A Profession — 3
Janice Blackburn
    INTRODUCTION, 3
    TRANSCRIPTION SKILLS, 4
    EDUCATION, 5
    EMPLOYMENT OPPORTUNITIES, 5
    PROFESSIONALISM, 10
    CONTINUING EDUCATION, 10

CHAPTER 2
Medical Ethics —— 13
Deborah Lynch Emmons, C.M.A.
    ETHICS OF THE MEDICAL PROFESSION, 13
    MEDICAL ETHICS AND THE MEDICAL TRAN-
      SCRIPTIONIST, 13
    ACCURACY OF WORK, 20
    CONFIDENTIALITY, 22
    BIOETHICS, 24

CHAPTER 3
The Medical Record and the Law —— 27
Inge Barth, C.M.T.
    INTRODUCTION, 27
    MEDICAL REPORTS AND RECORDS, 27
    FAXING MEDICAL DOCUMENTS, 37
    LEGALITIES OF PSYCHIATRIC DOCUMENTS, 38
    RETENTION OF RECORDS, 38
    SUBPOENA, 38

CHAPTER 4
Building a Transcription Service —— 43
Jackie Abern, C.M.T.
Adrienne C. Yazijian, C.M.T.
    INTRODUCTION—A SCENARIO, 43
    SELF-EMPLOYMENT, 44
    HOME-BASED MEDICAL TRANSCRIPTION, 45
    EQUIPMENT, 45
    FINANCIAL MANAGEMENT, 51
    FEDERAL, STATE, COUNTY, AND CITY LAWS, 54
    NEGOTIATION AND CONTRACT, 55
    BUSINESS FORM, 57
    BILLING STATEMENTS, 57
    BOOKKEEPING, 58
    COLLECTING OVERDUE ACCOUNTS, 60
    OBTAINING CREDIT, 60
    BANKING, 60
    RETIREMENT ACCOUNTS, 61
    MARKETING, PROMOTION, AND PUBLIC RELA-
      TIONS, 61
    ADVERTISING, 62

CHAPTER 5
Equipment —— 67
Sandra Levine, C.M.T.
    INTRODUCTION, 67
    DICTATION AND TRANSCRIPTION SYSTEMS, 67
    COMPUTER SYSTEM, 68
    MEDIA AND DATA STORAGE, 68
    COMPUTER PRINTERS, 68
    TYPEWRITER, 69
    PURCHASING VERSUS LEASING EQUIPMENT, 69
    SETTING UP THE SYSTEM, 69

EQUIPMENT MAINTENANCE AND SUPPLIES, 69
EQUIPMENT FOR THE PHYSICALLY CHAL-
   LENGED, 70
ERGONOMICS, 71
FAX MACHINES, 72
PHOTOCOPY EQUIPMENT, 72
PAPER SHREDDERS, 72
PROBLEM SOLVING, 72

CHAPTER 6
**Marketing of Medical Transcription
Services** ——————————— 77
Inge Barth, C.M.T.
   INTRODUCTION, 77
   MARKET RESEARCH AND ANALYSIS, 77
   MARKET SEGMENTATION, 77
   TARGET MARKETING, 78
   SETTING PRICES, 79
   CHANNELS OF DISTRIBUTION, 80
   PUBLICITY AND PROMOTION, 80

CHAPTER 7
Management and Supervision ——— 83
Hazel L. Tank, C.M.T.
   INTRODUCTION, 83
   DELEGATING, 83
   QUALITY ASSURANCE, 86
   DELIVERING CRITICISM OR DISCIPLINE, 86
   INCENTIVE PROGRAMS, 87
   WORD PROCESSING, 88
   EMPLOYEE EVALUATION, 88
   TRAINING NEW EMPLOYEES, 90
   SALARIES, 90
   WORK STANDARDS, 90
   PERSONNEL, 91
   JOB DESCRIPTIONS, 93
   INVESTIGATION OF NEW TECHNOLOGIES, 94
   REFERENCE BOOKS, 94
   SUMMARY, 95

CHAPTER 8
**Editing and Phonetic Problem
Solving** ——————————————— 97
Bron Taylor, B.A.
   INTRODUCTION, 97
   TYPES OF ERRORS, 99
   EDITING, 101
   FOREIGN DICTATION, 101
   PROOFREADING, 102
   CORRECTING ERRORS, 102
   REFERENCE SOURCES, 104

CHAPTER 9
Writing for Publication ——————— 107
Marie D. Low, Ph.D.
   INTRODUCTION, 107
   SELECTING A BOOK TOPIC, 107
   SELECTING A PUBLISHING COMPANY, 108
   SUBMITTING A PROPOSAL, 110
   CONTRACTS AND NEGOTIATION, 111
   MANUSCRIPT PREPARATION, 112
   ILLUSTRATIONS, 114
   REFERENCES, BIBLIOGRAPHIES, AND FOOT-
      NOTES, 115
   OTHER MANUSCRIPT ITEMS, 115
   MANUSCRIPT PRODUCTION, 115
   MARKETING, 116
   COPYRIGHT, 118
   COAUTHORSHIP, 119
   SUMMARY, 119

CHAPTER 10
**Preparing to Teach Medical
Transcription** ——————————— 121
Sondra Sue Hein, B.A., C.M.T.
Lynn C. Keene, B.S., M.S.
   INTRODUCTION, 121
   COMMUNITY SURVEY AND ASSESSMENT, 122
   DEVELOPING A COURSE DESCRIPTION, 123
   COURSE OBJECTIVES, 127
   INTEGRATING COURSES INTO A COMPREHEN-
      SIVE CURRICULUM, 131
   MATERIALS AND EQUIPMENT, 131
   TEXTBOOKS, 131
   AUDIOVISUAL AIDS, 131
   GRADING AND CORRECTING, 132
   TESTING, 133
   EVALUATION, 137
   PROBLEM SOLVING, 137
   TEACHING TIPS AND TRAPS, 141

CHAPTER 11
**Building a Medical Reference
Library** ——————————————— 143
Meg Walsh, A.A.
   INTRODUCTION, 143
   USE OF THE ENGLISH DICTIONARY, 144
   USE OF THE MEDICAL DICTIONARY, 145
   MEDICAL WORD BOOKS, 146
   SPELLING, 147

PART TWO
THE MEDICAL BASIS OF TRANSCRIPTION

CHAPTER 12
Cardiology ——————— 151
Raymond E. Liguori, M.D.
   INTRODUCTION, 151
   ANATOMY AND PHYSIOLOGY, 151
   REPRESENTATIVE CARDIAC DISORDERS AND
      DISEASES, 155
   DIAGNOSIS OF CARDIOVASCULAR DISEASES,
      158
   CARDIOVASCULAR SURGERY, 169
   FORMATS, 171

CHAPTER 13
Dermatology ——————— 179
Victoria A. Cirillo-Hyland, M.D.
Chalmers E. Cornelius, III, M.D.
   INTRODUCTION, 179
   BASIC STRUCTURE AND FUNCTION OF THE SKIN,
      179
   ILLUSTRATED GLOSSARY OF DERMATOLOGIC
      TERMS, 181
   REPRESENTATIVE DERMATOLOGIC DISEASES,
      181
   DERMATOLOGIC DIAGNOSTIC PROCEDURES,
      199
   DERMATOLOGIC SURGERY, 200
   DERMATOLOGIC MODALITIES OF TREATMENT,
      200
   FORMATS, 206

CHAPTER 14
Emergency Medicine ——————— 207
Ronald W. Stunz, M.D.
   INTRODUCTION, 207
   EMERGENCY MEDICINE TRANSCRIPTION, 207
   GENERAL CHARACTERISTICS OF THE EMER-
      GENCY MEDICAL RECORD, 208
   PROCEDURES, 208
   DOCUMENTATION OF PREHOSPITAL TREAT-
      MENT, 209
   INTERPRETATION OF ANCILLARY STUDIES, 209
   ACCURATE TIMING, 209
   DISCHARGE INSTRUCTIONS, 209
   REFERRALS/CHART COPIES, 209
   EMERGENCY MEDICINE CHARTS, 209
   THE IDEAL TRANSCRIPTION SERVICE, 209

CHAPTER 15
Endocrinology ——————— 219
Michael A. Bush, M.D.
   INTRODUCTION, 219
   ANATOMY AND PHYSIOLOGY, 219
   REPRESENTATIVE DISEASES, 221
   SUMMARY, 228

CHAPTER 16
Family Medicine ——————— 229
Louis T. Verardo, M.D.
   INTRODUCTION, 229
   THE PRACTICE OF FAMILY MEDICINE, 231
   FORMATS, 233

CHAPTER 17
Gastroenterology ——————— 241
Philip R. Nast, M.D., F.A.C.P.
   INTRODUCTION, 241
   REPRESENTATIVE DISEASES, 242
   SURGICAL PROCEDURES, 248
   FORMATS, 250

CHAPTER 18
General Surgery ——————— 259
Thomas F. Nealon, M.D.
   INTRODUCTION, 259
   ANESTHESIA, 259
   SUTURES, 260
   REPRESENTATIVE DISEASES, 260

CHAPTER 19
Immunology and AIDS ——————— 287
Joseph A. Bellanti, M.D.
Josef V. Kadlec, S.J., M.D.
   INTRODUCTION, 287
   ANATOMY AND PHYSIOLOGY OF THE IMMUNE
      SYSTEM, 287
   OVERVIEW, 287
   PHYSIOLOGY, 290
   HIV AND AIDS, 291
   FORMATS, 291

CHAPTER 20
Internal Medicine ——————— 299
Gary W. Crooks, M.D.
   PERSPECTIVE, 299
   HISTORY, 299
   THE PRACTICE OF INTERNAL MEDICINE, 300
   EXAMINATION OF THE PATIENT, 301
   REPRESENTATIVE DISEASES, 302

CHAPTER 21
Laboratory Medicine ——————— 307
Paul T. Wertlake, M.D., M.S., M.B.A.
   INTRODUCTION, 307
   CHEMISTRY TESTS, 307
   HEMATOLOGY TESTS, 311
   SERODIAGNOSIS OF HEPATITIS A, B, C, D, AND
     E, 317
   TUMOR MARKERS, 321
   URINALYSIS, 326
   IMMUNOHEMATOLOGY: BLOOD GROUP AND
     TYPE, ANTIBODY SCREENING AND IDENTIFI-
     CATION, 337
   MEDICAL BACTERIOLOGY, 344
   MEDICAL MYCOBACTERIOLOGY, 351
   MEDICAL MYCOLOGY, 351
   MEDICAL PARASITOLOGY, 351
   MEDICAL ENTOMOLOGY, 352
   MEDICAL VIROLOGY, 352
   SEROLOGIC TESTING FOR AUTOIMMUNE DIS-
     ORDERS, 356
   ORGAN-DIRECTED AUTOIMMUNE DISORDERS,
     358
   THERAPEUTIC DRUG MONITORING (TDM), 359
   CRITICAL AND ALERT LABORATORY VALUES,
     359

CHAPTER 22
Nephrology ——————— 371
Leslie P. Dornfeld, M.D.
   INTRODUCTION, 371
   ANATOMY OF THE KIDNEY, 371
   EVALUATION OF RENAL DISEASE, 373
   REPRESENTATIVE DISEASES, 374
   RENAL REPLACEMENT THERAPY, 381
   CONGENITAL ABNORMALITIES OF THE KIDNEY,
     381
   SIGNS AND SYMPTOMS, 382
   TREATMENT OF RENAL DISEASE, 389

CHAPTER 23
Neurology and Neurosurgery —— 391
Stephen L. Fedder, M.D., F.A.C.S.
   INTRODUCTION, 391
   ANATOMY, 391

   REPRESENTATIVE DISEASES, 394
   NEUROLOGIC SIGNS AND SYMPTOMS, 396
   DIAGNOSTIC PROCEDURES AND TESTS, 396
   SURGICAL PROCEDURES, 397
   GLOSSARY, 398
   FORMATS, 403

CHAPTER 24
Nuclear Medicine ——————— 413
Henry N. Wagner, Jr., M.D.
Julia W. Buchanan, B.S.
   INTRODUCTION, 413
   REQUISITIONS AND REPORTS, 413
   THE DIAGNOSTIC PROCESS, 414
   HOW NUCLEAR MEDICINE STUDIES ARE PER-
     FORMED, 415
   DETECTION OF RADIOACTIVITY, 418
   TYPES OF NUCLEAR MEDICINE STUDIES, 419

CHAPTER 25
Obstetrics and Gynecology ——— 423
Morgan L. Morgan, M.D.
   INTRODUCTION, 423
   OBSTETRICS, 423
   DISORDERS OF PREGNANCY, 426
   OPERATIVE OBSTETRICS, 430
   GYNECOLOGY, 431
   GYNECOLOGIC SURGERY, 442
   DISEASES OF THE BREAST, 449
   OVERVIEW, 449

CHAPTER 26
Oncology-Hematology ——————— 453
Thomas G. Gabuzda, M.D.
Carolyn F. Sidor, M.D.
   INTRODUCTION, 453
   THE NATURE OF CANCER, 453
   DIAGNOSIS AND EVALUATION OF THE CANCER
     PATIENT, 454
   TREATMENTS, 462
   FORMATS, 477

CHAPTER 27
Ophthalmology ——————— 479
Charles G. Steinmetz, III, M.D.
   INTRODUCTION, 479
   OPHTHALMOLOGIC SUBSPECIALTIES, 479
   ANATOMY, 480
   REPRESENTATIVE DISEASES, 482
   SURGICAL PROCEDURES, 483
   INSTRUMENTS, 485
   FORMATS, 485

CHAPTER 28
Orthopaedics ——————— 491
John J. Gartland, M.D.
    INTRODUCTION, 491
    ORTHOPAEDIC DISORDERS OF CHILDREN, 491
    ORTHOPAEDIC DISORDERS OF ADULTS, 492
    MUSCULOSKELETAL TRAUMA, 492
    ANATOMY, 492
    REPRESENTATIVE DISEASES AND DISORDERS, 499
    REPRESENTATIVE INJURIES, 504
    GLOSSARY OF SURGICAL TERMS, 510
    SURGICAL INSTRUMENTS, 511
    FORMATS, 513

CHAPTER 29
Otorhinolaryngology ——————— 521
William J. Lewis, M.D.
    INTRODUCTION, 521
    ANATOMY, 521
    REPRESENTATIVE DISEASES, 526
    SURGICAL PROCEDURES, 541
    INSTRUMENTS, 546
    FORMATS, 546

CHAPTER 30
Anatomic Pathology ——————— 555
Paul T. Wertlake, M.D.
    WORK FLOW FOR INFORMATION GENERATION AND REPORTING, 555
    PATIENT CARE REPORTS, 555
    WORD PROCESSING AND COMPUTERIZED REPORTING, 566
    QUALITY ASSURANCE REPORTS, 569
    ADMINISTRATIVE REPORTS AND RECORDS, 569
    POSITION DESCRIPTION OF A PATHOLOGY SECRETARY, 571

CHAPTER 31
Pediatrics ——————— 573
Morris Green, M.D.
    INTRODUCTION, 573
    NEONATOLOGY, 573
    REPRESENTATIVE DISEASES, 579
    FORMATS, 591

CHAPTER 32
Plastic Surgery ——————— 595
Robert S. Improta, M.D.
    INTRODUCTION, 595
    GENERAL PRINCIPLES OF RECONSTRUCTION, 595

    IMPLANT MATERIALS, 597
    GRAFTS, 597
    FLAPS, 598
    RECONSTRUCTION OF CONGENITAL DEFORMITIES, 608
    BURN RECONSTRUCTION, 610
    BREAST SURGERY, 610
    COSMETIC SURGERY, 614
    INSTRUMENTS USED IN PLASTIC SURGERY, 622

CHAPTER 33
Podiatry ——————— 623
Michael A. DiGiacomo, D.P.M.
    INTRODUCTION, 623
    ANATOMY, 624
    REPRESENTATIVE DISEASES, 625
    TREATMENT, 636
    INSTRUMENTS, 643
    FORMATS, 645

CHAPTER 34
Psychiatry ——————— 649
Zigmond M. Lebensohn, M.D.
    INTRODUCTION, 649
    REPRESENTATIVE DISEASES, 650
    DIAGNOSTIC PROCEDURES AND TESTS, 652
    TREATMENTS, 653
    FORMATS, 654

CHAPTER 35
Radiology ——————— 661
Raymond L. Del Fava, M.D.
Frank L. Hussey, Jr., M.D.
Keri J. Sperry, M.D.
    INTRODUCTION, 661
    DIAGNOSTIC RADIOLOGY, 661
    RADIOLOGY REPORTS, 664
    RADIATION ONCOLOGY, 682
    RADIATION ONCOLOGY TEAM, 684
    FUTURE THERAPIES, 686

CHAPTER 36
Respiratory and Pulmonary Medicine ——————— 689
William G. Figueroa, M.D.
Ethel L. Wise, B.S., R.R.T., R.P.F.T.
    INTRODUCTION, 689
    ANATOMY, 689
    PHYSIOLOGY, 691
    REPRESENTATIVE DISEASES, 691
    SIGNS AND SYMPTOMS, 692
    DIAGNOSTIC PROCEDURES AND TESTS, 693

MEDICAL AND SURGICAL TREATMENTS, 694
SURGICAL PROCEDURES, 696
INSTRUMENTS, 697
FORMATS, 697

CHAPTER 37

Rheumatology ——————— 715
Patricia A. Fenn, M.D., F.A.C.R.
INTRODUCTION, 715
REPRESENTATIVE DISEASES IN RHEUMATOL-
OGY, 715
SURGICAL PROCEDURES AND INSTRUMENTS,
721
FORMATS, 721

CHAPTER 38

Urology ——————————— 731
Marty L. Prah, M.D.
Elizabeth Ann Huben, M.T.
INTRODUCTION, 731
ANATOMY OF THE URINARY TRACT SYSTEM,
731
ANATOMY OF THE MALE REPRODUCTIVE SYS-
TEM, 734
REPRESENTATIVE DISEASES AND DISORDERS,
734
PROCEDURES, 734
FORMATS, 745

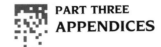

PART THREE
APPENDICES

APPENDIX 1

Table of Reference Sources, 755
ABBREVIATIONS DICTIONARY/GENERAL, 755
ABBREVIATIONS DICTIONARY/MEDICAL, 755
AIDS, 756
ANATOMY AND PHYSIOLOGY, 756
ANTONYMS, EPONYMS, HOMONYMS, SYN-
DROMES, AND SYNONYMS, 756
CAREER DEVELOPMENT, 756
CERTIFICATION, 757
COMPOSITION, 757
COMPUTERIZED DICTIONARIES/MEDICAL
SPELL CHECKERS, 757
DIAGNOSTIC AND PROCEDURE HANDBOOKS,
757
DICTIONARIES, ENGLISH, 757
DICTIONARIES, FOREIGN, 757
DICTIONARIES, MEDICAL, 758
DRUG REFERENCES, 758
EDITING, 758
EPONYMS, 758
EQUIPMENT, 758
HANDBOOKS (GRAMMAR, PUNCTUATION, AND
GENERAL CLERICAL INFORMATION), 759
HOMONYMS, 759
HUMOR AND GAMES FOR MEDICAL TYPISTS
AND TRANSCRIPTIONISTS, 759
INSTRUCTION, 759
INSURANCE, 759
LAW AND ETHICS, 759
MEDICAL RECORDS, 760
MEDICAL TERMINOLOGY, 760
MEDICAL TERMINOLOGY GUIDES, 761
PHARMACEUTICAL, 761
PROFESSIONAL IMAGE, 762
PROOFREADING, 762
REFERENCES FOR THE PHYSICALLY CHAL-
LENGED, 762
SELF-EMPLOYMENT AND FREELANCING, 763
SPECIALTY REFERENCES, 764
SPELLING BOOKS, ENGLISH, 768
SPELLING BOOKS, MEDICAL, 768
STYLE MANUALS/MEDICAL AND GENERAL, 769
TYPING AND TRANSCRIPTION, 770
VIDEO TAPES, 770
WORD DIVISION, 770
WORKING AT HOME/INDEPENDENT MEDICAL
TRANSCRIPTIONISTS, 771
WRITING SCIENTIFIC/TECHNICAL, 771

APPENDIX 2

Typing Styles for Letters and Reports, 772

APPENDIX 3

Combining Forms in Medical Terminology, 778

APPENDIX 4

Medically Significant Prefixes and Suffixes, 788

APPENDIX 5

Laboratory Values of Clinical Importance, 792

APPENDIX 6

Tables of Weights and Measures, 802

APPENDIX 7

Table of Chemical Elements, 808

APPENDIX 8

Acronyms for Selected Health Care Organizations, Associations, and Agencies, 814

APPENDIX 9

Voluntary Health and Welfare Agencies and Associations, 817

APPENDIX 10

Forms of Address, 821

APPENDIX 11

Postal Abbreviations for States, 832

APPENDIX 12

Common Prescription Abbreviations, 833

APPENDIX 13

Symbols and Metric Prefixes, 835

APPENDIX 14

The Greek Alphabet, 838

Index ————————————————— 839

PART ONE

The Principles of Transcription

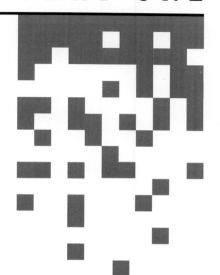

Janice Blackburn, C.M.T.

Medical Transcription: A Profession

INTRODUCTION

Medical transcriptionists, like other workers of technical competence, call themselves "professionals" and like to believe that the term is justly applied. Before believing, however, perhaps we should examine the meaning of "professional." In general, there is agreement that, for example, the ministry, medicine, law, and architecture are professions, but there is no general agreement about what a profession is. The characteristics defining a profession include (but are not limited to):

1. Possession of useful knowledge and skills, based on special training or education.

2. An orientation of work toward selfless service in the interest of a client.

3. Autonomy of action; that is to say, the professional must feel free to be guided by principles of action rather than directions from the client.

4. The existence of organizations to serve the internal and external needs of the profession and to set and enforce proper standards of conduct by their members.

Of these criteria, the most delicate is the second, for the implication is that a person working in a profession is motivated not primarily by considerations of personal gain but by a commitment to service and dedication to the work in which the professional is engaged. However, it must also frankly be admitted that the American Medical Association, the American Bar Association, and the American Association for Medical Transcription, responding to the needs of their members, have not least among their objectives raising the rewards for the professional service they represent. Perhaps it may be conceded that the professional person represents the high ideals of disinterested service but is not without a human interest in its recompense.

To explore the meaning and status of medical transcription, one must take several steps back in time to understand the value and importance placed on record keeping. The Latin prefix *trans* means "across," "beyond," or "through," and the Latin *scribere* means "to write." Hence, *transcribere* means "to copy over."

Scribes were especially important in ancient societies in which few people could read or write. They acted not only as copyists but were viewed as editors and interpreters of sacred writing and of the law. Many scribes in ancient times worked for kings or merchants and eventually may have become town clerks or even secretaries of state.

The Random House Dictionary of the English Language describes a scribe as "a professional copyist, especially one who made copies of manuscripts before the invention of printing; also called sopher, sofer (Hebrew), one of a group of Palestinian scholars and teachers of Jewish law and tradition, active from the 5th century B.C. to the 1st century A.D., who transcribed, edited and interpreted the Bible."

Understanding the importance of the ancient scribe brings an added sense of appreciation for the professional status of the medical transcriptionist today.

TRANSCRIPTION SKILLS

The career of medical transcription has gone through a period of evolution. The medical secretary of 20 or 30 years ago may have taken dictation while following the physician through hospital corridors. The medical transcriptionist of the 1990s may never have the opportunity to put a face to the name of the physician dictator. The equipment used by today's medical transcriptionist has also evolved, most particularly with the introduction of the computer (see Chapter 5 on equipment). State-of-the-art dictating equipment requires the physician to enter a personal identification number along with a specific code for the type of report to be dictated. This system also protects the confidentiality of the medical record.

These technologic advances have eliminated many menial tasks for medical transcriptionists, but technology has also brought about changes that may add further responsibilities and burdens for them.

The average dictation for an operative report of the early 1970s was less complicated than a similar dictation today. Additional procedures, the introduction of new equipment, and concern over medical malpractice have lengthened dictations in many cases. Reports have become more specific and fine-tuned.

Dictations for a cholecystectomy by way of the laparoscope are often twice as long as those used for the abdominal approach. Although these procedures have, indeed, been beneficial to the patient and the hospital, allowing shorter hospital stays and greater availability of hospital beds, they have increased the workload for the transcriptionist. They have further highlighted the need for up-to-date awareness of new approaches.

Health-care cost containment is the goal of the federal government, and one of the areas being looked at in order to cut costs is medical documentation. Many physicians and hospital facilities are looking at creative methods to simplify the process. Systems consisting of dataforms and computer software have been developed by many specialists in private practice. The dataform is custom-designed to the physician's practice: items are checked off and brief information either handwritten or dictated. The input is more data entry rather than actual transcription. The data are held in a database, so when a patient returns for future appointments a compilation of medications with patient comments, tests with results, diagnoses with diagnostic codes, and other data can be generated with the touch of a few keystrokes. The information is given in a series of lists or tables that take up less written space than sentences. Hospital facilities have developed dataforms that can be scanned, and the software prints a narrative report that looks just like a physician-dictated report. Such systems eliminate transcription, reduce manpower requirements, save time, reduce costs, improve accuracy, facilitate reports, and decrease the number of incomplete charts. Because of the large number of foreign physicians practicing in the United States and the variety of words used to express the same results, sometimes sentences can be interpreted differently. Thus, such systems improve communications because standardized terminology is used.

The introduction of acquired immunodeficiency syndrome (AIDS) into our society has made it necessary for the transcriptionist to master additional terminology. The new terms concerning the diagnosis and pharmacologic aspects of this disease have not lessened the never-ending and challenging problems the transcriptionist must face on a day-to-day basis. The word "challenge" may, indeed, be the operative word in defining the entire profession of medical transcription. The ability to face the ongoing challenge is a talent that has frequently been compared to artistic or musical ability. A patient referred to a transcriptionist at work in a physician's office as the "piano player." The general population is unaware of the skills required to participate in this profession—if they are even aware of the profession at all.

The primary responsibility of medical transcriptionists is to transfer a physician's knowledge regarding the patient into a legible legal document. Their knowledge of medical terminology must be precise, correct, and current. They must produce the required document on time and complete it with educated pride. They must possess fine-tuned auditory skills with the capability of interpreting different dialects, as well as the ability to edit dictation when necessary. The transcriptionists' editing skills should improve the clarity of the final document, without drastically changing it.

Medical transcriptionists must be on intimate

terms with reference material, exhausting all possibilities in the quest for accuracy. They must be familiar with and able to use appropriately all facets of medical terminology. Once a physician completes medical school and enters into a specialty, he or she may not be as familiar with medical terms from other specialties. However, medical transcriptionists are required to be fluent with all specialized medical terms. They must be proficient in English pronunciation, spelling, grammar, and punctuation. A general understanding of anatomy and physiology and of the legal implications of the practice of medicine is vitally important.

Above all, medical transcriptionists must have total respect for the medical record. Those dedicated to this profession will recognize the legal aspects of their work as well as the importance of confidentiality. Medical transcriptionists must never discuss a patient's record with any unauthorized person. They, like the physician, must never forget the portion of the Oath of Hippocrates that says, "Whatever, in connection with my professional practice, or not in connection with it, I may see or hear in the lives of men which ought not to be spoken abroad, I will not divulge, as reckoning that all such should be kept secret." (For more information on confidentiality, see Chapter 2.)

Dictation may be received in many forms. Dictators from a foreign country may have poor command of the English language, thus making transcription of their dictation extremely tedious. Nonetheless, it still remains the duty of the transcriptionist to produce an accurate medical document, and this requires patience and knowledge.

Information may be missing from a dictation for various reasons, sometimes because of equipment failure and sometimes because the physician may be tired or frustrated. At these times, it is the transcriptionist's responsibility to research, with accuracy, the missing information. A derogatory remark may sometimes appear within the dictation, and the transcriptionist faces an additional challenge and responsibility. Derogatory remarks have no place in a permanent medical record; should this occur, it must immediately be brought to the attention of the supervisor.

Since the role of a transcriptionist requires knowledge, skills, abilities, good working conditions, physical demands, many job responsibili-

ties, and certain performance standards, the American Association for Medical Transcription developed a model job description in 1990 (Figure 1–1). This is not intended as a complete list of duties and responsibilities but can assist a transcriptionist as a guideline in developing a job description for an employer.

EDUCATION

To perform the required tasks in this demanding profession, education is of prime importance. A personal survey was made of approximately fifty medical transcriptionists with a minimum of 10 years' experience in the field. Seventy-five per cent of those surveyed received their training on the job. The remainder received minimal education through trade schools and technical colleges.

Those entering the field will find that vocational/technical institutions offer a 3- to 6-month training program. Many 2-year colleges offer an Associate Degree from the Medical Secretarial Science Division. The 2-year programs often include such subjects as medical terminology, medicolegal topics, medical insurance, procedural and diagnostic coding, medical office procedures, business English, medical transcription, and keyboarding and word processing, as well as anatomy and physiology. Some colleges may include as part of the required curriculum an internship program in which the student will gain hands-on experience in a hospital or physician's office. This experience may prove to be a valuable asset when the graduate student seeks employment.

In addition to the technical knowledge that can be obtained from a formal education, patience and an inquisitive mind are also of prime importance. Personal integrity and dedication to the profession are a transcriptionist's most valuable assets.

EMPLOYMENT OPPORTUNITIES

The variety of employment opportunities for the medical transcriptionist are vast and include many areas of specialization. Within the hospital setting, one may find transcriptionists not only in the medical records department but also in radiology, surgical pathology, psychiatry, car-

American Association for Medical Transcription

AAMT Model Job Description:

Medical Transcriptionist

The *AAMT Model Job Description* is a practical, useful compilation of the basic job responsibilities of a medical transcriptionist. It is designed to assist human resource managers, department managers, supervisors, and others in recruiting, supervising, and evaluating individuals in medical transcription positions.

The *AAMT Model Job Description* is not intended as a complete list of specific duties and responsibilities. Nor is it intended to limit or modify the right of any supervisor to assign, direct, and control the work of employees under supervision. The use of a particular expression or illustration describing duties shall not be held to exclude other duties not mentioned that are of a similar kind or level of difficulty.

AAMT gratefully acknowledges Lanier Voice Products Division, Atlanta, Georgia, for funding the development of the *AAMT Model Job Description: Medical Transcriptionist*.

For additional information, contact AAMT, P.O. Box 576187, Modesto, California 95357. Telephone 209-551-0883 or 800-982-2182. FAX 209-551-9317.

Figure 1–1
AAMT Model Job Description: Medical Transcriptionist. Note the two paragraphs on the first page. The first gives the purpose of the job description, and the second paragraph outlines the latitude in the wordings of the descriptions. (From the American Association for Medical Transcription, Modesto, California, copyright 1990.)

AAMT MODEL JOB DESCRIPTION: MEDICAL TRANSCRIPTIONIST

Position Summary: Medical language specialist who interprets and transcribes dictation by physicians and other healthcare professionals regarding patient assessment, workup, therapeutic procedures, clinical course, diagnosis, prognosis, etc., in order to document patient care and facilitate delivery of healthcare services.

Knowledge, skills, and abilities:

1. Minimum education level of associate degree or equivalent in work experience and continuing education.
2. Knowledge of medical terminology, anatomy and physiology, clinical medicine, surgery, diagnostic tests, radiology, pathology, pharmacology, and the various medical specialties as required in areas of responsibility.
3. Knowledge of medical transcription guidelines and practices.
4. Excellent written and oral communication skills, including English usage, grammar, punctuation, and style.
5. Ability to understand diverse accents and dialects and varying dictation styles.
6. Ability to use designated reference materials.
7. Ability to operate designated word processing, dictation, and transcription equipment, and other equipment as specified.
8. Ability to work independently with minimal supervision.
9. Ability to work under pressure with time constraints.
10. Ability to concentrate.
11. Excellent listening skills.
12. Excellent eye, hand, and auditory coordination.
13. Certified medical transcriptionist (CMT) status preferred.

Working conditions:
General office environment. Quiet surroundings. Adequate lighting.

Physical demands:
Primarily sedentary work, with continuous use of earphones, keyboard, foot control, and where applicable, video display terminal.

Figure 1–1 *Continued*   *Figure continued*   **7**

AAMT MODEL JOB DESCRIPTION: MEDICAL TRANSCRIPTIONIST

Job responsibilities:	Performance standards:
1. Transcribes medical dictation to provide a permanent record of patient care.	1.1 Applies knowledge of medical terminology, anatomy and physiology, and English language rules to the transcription and proofreading of medical dictation from originators with various accents, dialects, and dictation styles. 1.2 Recognizes, interprets, and evaluates inconsistencies, discrepancies, and inaccuracies in medical dictation, and appropriately edits, revises, and clarifies them without altering the meaning of the dictation or changing the dictator's style. 1.3 Clarifies dictation which is unclear or incomplete, seeking assistance as necessary. 1.4 Flags reports requiring the attention of the supervisor or dictator. 1.5 Uses reference materials appropriately and efficiently to facilitate the accuracy, clarity, and completeness of reports. 1.6 Meets quality and productivity standards and deadlines established by employer. 1.7 Verifies patient information for accuracy and completeness. 1.8 Formats reports according to established guidelines.
2. Demonstrates an understanding of the medicolegal implications and responsibilities related to the transcription of patient records to protect the patient and the business/institution.	2.1 Understands and complies with policies and procedures related to medicolegal matters, including confidentiality, amendment of medical records, release of information, patients' rights, medical records as legal evidence, informed consent, etc. 2.2 Meets standards of professional and ethical conduct. 2.3 Recognizes and reports unusual circumstances and/or information with possible risk factors to appropriate risk management personnel. 2.4 Recognizes and reports problems, errors, and discrepancies in dictation and patient records to appropriate manager. 2.5 Consults appropriate personnel regarding dictation which may be regarded as unprofessional, frivolous, insulting, inflammatory, or inappropriate.
3. Operates designated word processing, dictation, and transcription equipment as directed to complete assignments.	3.1 Uses designated equipment effectively, skillfully, and efficiently. 3.2 Maintains equipment and work area as directed. 3.3 Assesses condition of equipment and furnishings, and reports need for replacement or repair.

Figure 1–1 Continued

AAMT MODEL JOB DESCRIPTION: MEDICAL TRANSCRIPTIONIST

Job responsibilities:	Performance standards:
4. Follows policies and procedures to contribute to the efficiency of the medical transcription department	4.1 Demonstrates an understanding of policies, procedures, and priorities, seeking clarification as needed. 4.2 Reports to work on time, as scheduled, and is dependable and cooperative. 4.3 Organizes and prioritizes assigned work, and schedules time to accommodate work demands, turnaround-time requirements, and commitments. 4.4 Maintains required records, providing reports as scheduled and upon request. 4.5 Participates in quality assurance programs. 4.6 Participates in evaluation and selection of equipment and furnishings. 4.7 Provides administrative/clerical/technical support as needed and as assigned.
5. Expands job-related knowledge and skills to improve performance and adjust to change.	5.1 Participates in inservice and continuing education activities. 5.2 Provides documentation of inservice and continuing education activities. 5.3 Reviews trends and developments in medicine, English usage, technology, and transcription practices, and shares knowledge with colleagues. 5.4 Documents new and revised terminology, definitions, styles, and practices for reference and application. 5.5 Participates in the evaluation and selection of books, publications, and other reference materials.
6. Uses interpersonal skills effectively to build and maintain cooperative working relationships.	6.1 Works and communicates in a positive and cooperative manner with management and supervisory staff, medical staff, co-workers and other healthcare personnel, and patients and their families when providing information and services, seeking assistance and clarification, and resolving problems. 6.2 Contributes to team efforts. 6.3 Carries out assignments responsibly. 6.4 Participates in a positive and cooperative manner during staff meetings. 6.5 Handles difficult and sensitive situations tactfully. 6.6 Responds well to supervision. 6.7 Shares information with co-workers. 6.8 Assists with training of new employees as needed.

Figure 1–1 *Continued*

diology, and so forth. Each of these departments requires terminology specific to its particular medical specialty. Some hospitals have transcription pools in which a transcriptionist may have the opportunity to transcribe a variety of reports from all departments within the hospital.

The medical transcriptionist may also be employed in a physician's office, medical clinic, nursing home, research center, insurance company, or medical publishing company, or by a medical transcription service. Some medical transcription services offer the medical transcriptionist the opportunity to work at home and will provide equipment and delivery service. Flexibility of work schedule may be ideal for the transcriptionist with young children. However, a transcriptionist working alone at home must have at hand the necessary medical reference material required to work independently.

A transcriptionist may choose to "moonlight," working full-time for a hospital and part-time in a physician's office, or freelance at home, transcribing for private clients. The opportunities are endless.

When applying for a position, it is important for medical transcriptionists to state the types of equipment with which they are familiar, such as computer and software programs. It is also important that they be specific about the types of reports they have transcribed and that they mention any subspecialty with which they are extremely familiar. If asked to take a test, they should become familiar with the surroundings, locate any reference material that might be needed, and have it close at hand. Also, they should take a few moments to listen to the dictation until they feel comfortable with the physician's voice before beginning to transcribe.

PROFESSIONALISM

In applying for a position, it is advantageous for the transcriptionist to note affiliation with a professional association and to state any certification acquired. A transcriptionist might be eligible to apply to three associations to take a certification examination: the American Association of Medical Assistants, Inc. (AAMA) offers

certification as a medical assistant administrative and/or clinical (CMA, CMA-A, CMA-C); the American Association for Medical Transcription (AAMT) gives certification as a medical transcriptionist (CMT); the American Medical Technologists (AMT) organization awards the registered medical assistant (RMA) for successfully passing an examination.

AAMA, AAMT, and AMT members have opportunities to attend local, state, and regional meetings and national conventions where they can participate in workshops, learn of educational advances in the field, visit exhibits showing new equipment, obtain up-to-date reference material, hear lectures, and establish a networking system with other medical transcriptionists and medical assistants.

For more information on AAMA, AAMT, and AMT and their certification programs, contact them at the following addresses:

American Association of Medical Assistants, Inc.
20 North Wacker Street, Suite 1575
Chicago, IL 60606

American Association for Medical Transcription
P.O. Box 57617
Modesto, CA 95357-6187

Registered Medical Assistant of AMT
710 Higgins Road
Park Ridge, IL 60068

Networking is vitally important to medical transcriptionists. In meeting other medical transcriptionists, they will be able to share thoughts regarding the work environment, receive ideas on how to deal with particularly difficult dictations, and receive input about any situation that may arise on a daily basis.

CONTINUING EDUCATION

In the field of medical transcription, it is vital to keep abreast of new procedures, drugs, and equipment. If transcriptionists have the opportunity to discuss new techniques or medications with physicians, pharmacists, and others on a medical staff, they may constantly update their education. The sources are plentiful. Literature is available through pharmaceutical companies, medical libraries, the public library, and the professional organizations discussed earlier (refer to Chapter 11 on building a medical reference library), as well as Appendix 1 featuring a list of references. Television programs are an additional source of obtaining current information; for example, the Lifetime (LIF) channel offers medical programs daily or on the weekends in many regions. It remains the responsibility of the professional transcriptionist to keep informed and constantly expand that "mind behind the machine."

Reference Sources

Finegan, Edward. *Attitudes Toward English Usage — The History of a War of Words.* Teachers College, Columbia University, New York/London, 1980.

Funk and Wagnall's *New Encyclopedia,* Vol. 23, 1985.

The Random House Dictionary of the English Language, 2nd edition, unabridged. Random House, Inc., New York, 1987.

Webster's *New World Secretarial Handbook,* 4th edition. Simon and Schuster, Inc., New York, 1989.

Deborah Lynch Emmons, C.M.A.

Medical Ethics

Medical transcriptionists come from all parts of the world and with them come many varied personal and professional ethical standards.

To get a sense of continuity and unity for the medical transcriptionist, it is essential that a code of ethical standards be followed that may or may not be separate from personal ethical standards.

ETHICS OF THE MEDICAL PROFESSION

Each segment of the medical profession has a code of ethics that pertains to that particular field. Several are relevant to this chapter. The Oath of Hippocrates (Figure 2–1) basically governs the ethics of physicians; a modern version for physicians, called the Lasagna Professional Oath, appears in Figure 2–2. The American Medical Association's Principles of Medical Ethics are given in Figure 2–3. There is a Code of Ethics and Standards of Medical Transcription Service Owners (MTSO) (Figure 2–4) and a Code of Ethics of the American Health Information Management Association (AHIMA), formerly the American Medical Record Association (Figure 2–5), for those associated with medical record keeping.

The American Association for Medical Transcription also has a code of ethics, which is discussed in the next section.

MEDICAL ETHICS AND THE MEDICAL TRANSCRIPTIONIST

The American Association for Medical Transcription Code of Ethics (Figure 2–6) provides the medical transcriptionist with a specific code of ethics which is the counterpart to the physician's Oath of Hippocrates.

Each section of the Code of Ethics of the American Association of Medical Transcription is quoted verbatim in the following pages with suggestions on how to observe and put into practice ethical conduct while accepting the ongoing challenge of this exciting and ever-changing profession.*

1. "Be aware that it is by our standards of conduct and professionalism that the entire Association is evaluated, for the conduct of one individual can be the vertex upon which the future of the Association may depend." Because all medical transcriptionists have different cultural backgrounds and belief systems, the difference between right and wrong is often a "gray" area. One unreasonable act may greatly influence another person or an entire group of professionals. For example, a seemingly innocent comment about a patient to another transcriptionist or other health-care professional ultimately may

---

*Interpretation and application of the AAMT Code of Ethics are the author's own and do not represent the official interpretation of the AAMT.

THE OATH OF HIPPOCRATES

I swear by Apollo, the physician, and Aesculapius and health and all-heal and all the Gods and Goddesses that, according to my ability and judgment, I will keep this oath and stipulation:

TO RECKON him who taught me this art equally dear to me as my parents, to share my substance with him and relieve his necessities if required; to regard his offspring as on the same footing with my own brothers, and to teach them this art if they should wish to learn it, without fee or stipulation, and that by precept, lecture and every other mode of instruction, I will impart a knowledge of the art to my own sons and to those of my teachers, and to disciples bound by a stipulation and oath, according to the law of medicine, but to none others.

I WILL FOLLOW that method of treatment which, according to my ability and judgment, I consider for the benefit of my patients, and abstain from whatever is deleterious and mischievous. I will give no deadly medicine to anyone if asked, nor suggest any such counsel; furthermore, I will not give to a woman an instrument to produce abortion.

WITH PURITY AND WITH HOLINESS I will pass my life and practice my art. I will not cut a person who is suffering from a stone, but will leave this to be done by practitioners of this work. Into whatever houses I enter I will go into them for the benefit of the sick and will abstain from every voluntary act of mischief and corruption; and further from the seduction of females or males, bond or free.

WHATEVER, in connection with my professional practice, or not in connection with it, I may see or hear in the lives of men which ought not to be spoken abroad I will not divulge, as reckoning that all such should be kept secret.

WHILE I CONTINUE to keep this oath unviolated may it be granted to me to enjoy life and the practice of the art, represented by all men at all times but should I trespass and violate this oath, may the reverse be my lot.

Figure 2–1

The Oath of Hippocrates. (Reprinted with permission from the Judicial Council Opinions and Reports, American Medical Association, Chicago, 1977.)

create a negative impact on that patient. This could potentially lead to a domino effect with many people being affected. If the remark happened to be about an unmarried woman's pregnancy, this would affect not only the pregnant woman but also the unborn child, the immediate and extended family, and other parties involved. Depending on the words used in making the remark, this could also be construed, in a medicolegal sense, as defamation of character.

2. "Conduct ourselves in the practice of our profession so as to bring dignity and honor to ourselves, the profession of medical transcription, and the American Association for Medical Transcription." In our professional and personal conduct, we are often judged by others, fairly or unfairly. In the professional description of a medical transcriptionist, not only are the technical skills addressed but also attitude, dress, and general appearance. As physicians are often

THE LASAGNA PROFESSIONAL OATH

I swear to fulfill, to the best of my ability and judgment, this covenant:

I will respect the hard-won scientific gains of those physicians in whose steps I walk, and gladly share such knowledge as is mine with those who are to follow.

I will apply, for the benefit of the sick, all measures which are required, avoiding those twin traps of overtreatment and therapeutic nihilism.

I will remember that there is art to medicine as well as science, and that warmth, sympathy and understanding may outweigh the surgeon's knife or the chemist's drug.

I will not be ashamed to say, "I know not," nor will I fail to call in my colleague when the skills of another are needed for a patient's recovery.

I will respect the privacy of my patients, for their problems are not disclosed to me that the world may know. Most especially must I tread with care in matters of life and death. If it is given me to save a life, all thanks. But it may also be within my power to take a life; this awesome responsibility must be faced with great humbleness and awareness of my own frailty. Above all, I must not play God.

I will remember that I do not treat a fever chart, or a cancerous growth, but a sick human being, whose illness may affect his family and his economic stability. My responsibility includes these related problems, if I am to care adequately for the sick.

I will prevent disease whenever I can, for prevention is preferable to cure.

I will remember that I remain a member of society, with special obligations to all my fellow men, those sound of mind and body, as well as the infirm.

If I do not violate this oath, may I enjoy life and art, respected while I live and remembered with affection thereafter. May I always act so as to preserve the finest traditions of my calling and may I long experience the joy of healing those who seek my help.

Figure 2–2
The Lasagna Professional Oath. (Reprinted with permission from Lasagna L: New York Times Magazine, 1964.)

judged by their mannerisms and dress, the medical transcriptionist is also judged in much the same way. For example, most people would hold little, if any, respect for a physician who was disheveled, unkempt, and used vulgar language. In keeping with that reasoning, the outward appearance of the medical transcriptionist should reflect a clean and professional appearance coupled with professional conduct. The medical transcriptionist is a highly trained professional whose outward appearance and manner of speaking should reflect that training and dedication. This is also expressed through the transcriptionist's attitude toward the profession, as well as the manner in which our peers and other professionals are spoken to.

3. "Place the goals and purposes of the Association above greed, personal gain, and interpersonal relationships by discouraging dissension and by working for the good of the majority." The medical transcriptionist will promote professionalism as well as be part of a supportive

PRINCIPLES OF MEDICAL ETHICS OF THE AMERICAN MEDICAL ASSOCIATION

Preamble:

The medical profession has long subscribed to a body of ethical statements developed primarily for the benefit of the patient. As a member of this profession, a physician must recognize responsibility not only to patients, but also to society, to other health professionals, and to self. The following Principles adopted by the American Medical Association are not laws, but standards of conduct which define the essentials of honorable behavior for the physician.

I. A physician shall be dedicated to providing competent medical service with compassion and respect for human dignity.

II. A physician shall deal honestly with patients and colleagues, and strive to expose those physicians deficient in character or competence, or who engage in fraud or deception.

III. A physician shall respect the law and also recognize a responsibility to seek changes in those requirements which are contrary to the best interests of the patient.

IV. A physician shall respect the rights of patients, of colleagues, and of other health professionals, and shall safeguard patient confidences within the constraints of the law.

V. A physician shall continue to study, apply and advance scientific knowledge, make relevant information available to patients, colleagues, and the public, obtain consultation, and use the talents of other health professionals when indicated.

VI. A physician shall, in the provision of appropriate patient care, except in emergencies, be free to choose whom to serve, with whom to associate, and the environment in which to provide medical services.

VII. A physician shall recognize a responsibility to participate in activities contributing to an improved community.

Figure 2–3
Principles of medical ethics. (Reprinted with permission from the 1992 Code of Medical Ethics, Current Opinions of the Council on Ethical and Judicial Affairs of the American Medical Association, Chicago, 1992.)

network to enhance the workplace, encourage and participate in continued education, and work toward the common goal of growth in the medical field. To assist the medical transcriptionist in working toward these goals, the American Association of Medical Transcription provides professional support, ongoing education, and a support network. For example, when working in an environment in which new transcriptionists are coming into the medical field, they can be a role model by stressing the positive aspects of being a medical transcriptionist and refusing to be a part of any dissension that may arise in the workplace. A veteran in this field might volunteer to help acquaint newcomers to the profession with the opportunities available to medical transcriptionists. Volunteer to speak at high school career days and local college classes about careers in medical transcription.

Professional standing is achieved through one's own merits and not by undermining another transcriptionist. Never diminish another transcriptionist, personally or professionally, because this undermines the credibility of the person speaking and creates ill-will in the workplace. For example, a transcriptionist working for a facility that subcontracts overflow work to a medical transcription service who goes directly to her employer and offers to provide better transcription services for a lesser charge is "undercutting" another transcriptionist. This greed in wanting to obtain an account in this manner is unethical and undermines the profession.

4. "Refuse to participate in or conceal unethical procedures or practices in relationships with other associations and individuals." The temptation to "gossip" or share privileged information with other individuals will always be

CODE OF ETHICS AND STANDARDS
OF MEDICAL TRANSCRIPTION SERVICE OWNERS

The goal of the alliance of medical transcription service owners (MTSOs) is to promote superior performance standards for MTSOs and to provide a forum for industry representatives to exchange information. Members of the alliance ascribe to the following Code of Ethics and Standards.

1. We pledge to provide medical transcription service of the highest professional standards to our clients in order to contribute to the quality and efficiency of the healthcare industry.

2. We pledge to conduct ourselves and our businesses in such a way as to bring dignity and honor to the medical transcription profession and industry.

3. We pledge to deal with our clients with the highest standards for integrity and honesty, and to communicate clearly our standards for protection of confidentiality, quality of transcription, turnaround time, and billing practices which include definable and verifiable units of measurement.

4. We pledge to protect and promote the dignity of our employees, to show respect for them as individuals, to honor their right to privacy, to encourage and reward continuing education, to uphold the highest professional standards for confidentiality and quality work, and to respect their employment rights as reflected in federal, state, and local laws.

5. We pledge to follow the highest ethical principles and procedures in relationships with colleagues in the medical transcription industry.

6. We pledge to achieve and maintain the highest attainable levels of professional competence in owners of medical transcription businesses.

Figure 2–4
Code of Ethics and Standards of Medical Transcription Service Owners, Health Professions Institute, Modesto, California, approved May 2, 1992.

present, when overhearing other transcriptionists speaking about another employee's medical record. This is intentional gossip, and it is the medical transcriptionist's responsibility to mention it to the supervisor. It is the responsibility of the medical transcriptionist to uphold the profession's principles and the principles of the employer, and to keep private what is heard. When meeting with other transcriptionists from different areas and in different situations, it is imperative that good medical ethics be practiced. For example, a transcriptionist may not be able to correct all the unethical practices but should adhere to the ethical standards put forth not

only in the MTSO Code of Ethics but also in the AAMT Code of Ethics (see Figures 2–4 and 2–6).

5. "Recognize the source of authority and powers delegated to us as individuals and observe the limitations and confinements of said authority and powers." It is the legal and ethical duty of the transcriptionist to be accurate—the foundation for an excellent medical transcriptionist. Do *not*, under any circumstance, randomly omit or change information that has been dictated. For example, a physician dictates "normal" blood chemistry results. Because it is "normal" does not mean that it can be left out ran-

---

CODE OF ETHICS OF THE AMERICAN HEALTH INFORMATION MANAGEMENT ASSOCIATION

PREAMBLE

The medical record professional abides by a set of ethical principles developed to safeguard the public and to contribute within the scope of the profession to quality and efficiency in healthcare. This code of ethics, adopted by the members of the American Health Information Management Association, defines the standards of behavior which promote ethical conduct.

1. The Medical Record Professional demonstrates behavior that reflects integrity, supports objectivity, and fosters trust in professional activities.

2. The Medical Record Professional respects the dignity of each human being.

3. The Medical Record Professional strives to improve personal competence and quality of services.

4. The Medical Record Professional represents truthfully and accurately professional credentials, education, and experience.

5. The Medical Record Professional refuses to participate in illegal or unethical acts and also refuses to conceal the illegal, incompetent, or unethical acts of others.

6. The Medical Record Professional protects the confidentiality of primary and secondary health records as mandated by law, professional standards, and the employer's policies.

7. The Medical Record Professional promotes to others the tenets of confidentiality.

8. The Medical Record Professional adheres to pertinent laws and regulations while advocating changes which serve the best interest of the public.

9. The Medical Record Professional encourages appropriate use of health record information and advocates policies and systems that advance the management of health records and health information.

10. The Medical Record Professional recognizes and supports the Association's mission.

Figure 2–5

Code of Ethics of the American Health Information Management Association (AHIMA) (formerly known as the American Medical Record Association), Chicago, Illinois, 1985.

---

domly. It is the medical transcriptionist's job to produce an accurate legal document that includes all information that has been dictated. It is *not* the transcriptionist's job to omit information under any circumstance. Any question about whether certain information dictated should be part of the medical record should be referred to the dictator or the immediate supervisor.

6. "Discharge honorably the responsibility of any Association positions to which we are elected or appointed." When elected to any office in conjunction with the American Association for Medical Transcription, the medical transcriptionist must know the role of that post and carry out the duties of that position with the utmost professionalism. If one cannot fulfill these duties, one should not accept the elected office.

7. "Preserve the confidential nature of professional judgments and determinations made by the official committees of the Association." As with all confidential information, what is discussed in official committee meetings is not to be discussed elsewhere unless it has been decided by the committee that certain information may be disclosed.

8. "Represent truthfully and accurately all professional committees in any official transaction, whether that transaction be within the Association or in the form of representation of ourselves as members of the Association." As a

---

CODE OF ETHICS OF THE AMERICAN ASSOCIATION FOR MEDICAL TRANSCRIPTION

1. Be aware that it is by our standards of conduct and professionalism that the entire Association is evaluated, for the conduct of one individual can be the vertex upon which the future of the Association may depend.

2. Conduct ourselves in the practice of our profession so as to bring dignity and honor to ourselves, the profession of medical transcription, and the American Association for Medical Transcription.

3. Place the goals and purposes of the Association above greed, personal gain, and interpersonal relationships by discouraging dissension and by working for the good of the majority.

4. Refuse to participate in or conceal unethical procedures or practices in relationships with other associations or individuals.

5. Recognize the source of authority and powers delegated to us as individuals and observe the limitations and confinements of said authority and powers.

6. Discharge honorably the responsibility of any Association positions to which we are elected or appointed.

7. Preserve the confidential nature of professional judgments and determinations made by the official committees of the Association.

8. Represent truthfully and accurately all professional committees in any official transaction whether that transaction be within the Association or in the form of representation of ourselves as members of the Association.

9. Protect the privacy and confidentiality of the individual medical record to avoid disclosure of personally identifiable medical and social information and professional medical judgments.

10. Strive to increase the body of systematic knowledge and individual competence of the medical transcription professional through continued self-improvement and the constructive exchange of knowledge and concepts with others in our profession.

Figure 2–6

Code of Ethics of the American Association for Medical Transcription. (From American Association for Medical Transcription, Modesto, California, revised 1987.)

member of a committee, the medical transcriptionist must uphold that position with dignity and professionalism.

9. "Protect the privacy and confidentiality of the individual medical record to avoid disclosure of personally identifiable medical and social information and professional medical judgments." When a patient enters into a physician's care, it is automatically assumed that the physician conforms to the Oath of Hippocrates and that the records and all information about patient care will be held in strictest confidence. This confidence can be broken only if the patient chooses to disclose the information or signs a release for disclosure. For example, if the transcriptionist knows the person whose chart note is being transcribed, the information is not to be mentioned to that person or anyone else. Even "anonymous" gossip may be too easily connected to a specific individual. Some employers require new employees to sign a statement or agreement of confidentiality (Figures 2–7 and 2–8).

10. "Strive to increase the body of systematic knowledge and individual competence of the medical transcription professional through continued self-improvement and the constructive exchange of knowledge and concepts with others in our profession." Just as the Hippocratic Oath tells physicians "primum non nocere" (defer to those with more appropriate training), a transcriptionist should always seek help from other skilled transcriptionists when questioning a term that is unfamiliar and when standard reference materials have not produced an answer. Other experienced transcriptionists are usually more than willing to help out and can provide valuable information and assistance. For example, many words and phrases sound similar but are associated with entirely different parts of the

STATEMENT OF CONFIDENTIALITY

TRANSCRIPTION COMPANY understands and agrees that in the performance of our duties as a contractor to COMMUNITY HOSPITAL, we must hold medical information in confidence.

Further, we understand that violation of our contractor's confidentiality may result in legal remedies being sought by COMMUNITY HOSPITAL.

Additionally, TRANSCRIPTION COMPANY's service facilities located at 1234 Main Street, Smalltown, USA, are secure under lock and key.

Security measures to insure confidentiality include, but are not restricted to, shredding of all disposable confidential material not returned, and a statement of confidentiality signed by all employees.

The confidentiality statement signed by all employees reads as follows:

I understand that the services that TRANSCRIPTION COMPANY performs for its clients are confidential, and to enable TRANSCRIPTION COMPANY to perform those services, its clients furnish to TRANSCRIPTION COMPANY confidential information concerning their affairs. The legal responsibilities and good will of the clients and the people they serve depends, among other things, upon our keeping such services and information confidential.

The Employee recognizes that the disclosure of information by the Employee may give rise to irreparable injury to TRANSCRIPTION COMPANY, the owner, or the subject of such information, and that accordingly, TRANSCRIPTION COMPANY, the owner, or the subject of such information may seek any legal remedies against the Employee which may be available.

_____ _____
Date   TRANSCRIPTION COMPANY
                                  President

Figure 2–7
An example of a statement of confidentiality that can be used by a transcription service company when hiring a new employee. It was developed by the Health Professions Institute, Modesto, California.

human body (e.g., ilium and ileum). By "networking" with an experienced transcriptionist, many questions can be answered and the ongoing goal of continuing knowledge is accomplished. Belonging to a professional organization and networking with peers at monthly meetings and at annual conventions greatly enhance the medical transcriptionist's knowledge as well.

ACCURACY OF WORK

Medical notes, also known as chart or progress notes, are the heartbeat of a medical practice and hospital care of a patient. These typed or handwritten notes are the guide to knowing not only what has been done in a patient's care but also what cannot be done, and they provide the

CONFIDENTIALITY AGREEMENT

Agreement is entered into by _____ (herein known as EMPLOYEE) and _____ (herein known as FACILITY).

EMPLOYEE understands that, in the performance of duties as a medical transcriptionist, all patient and client information is to be held in strictest confidence, including but not limited to the transcription of medical documents. EMPLOYEE recognizes that the disclosure of such information shall result in immediate dismissal from FACILITY. EMPLOYEE also acknowledges that any such violation may give rise to irreparable damage to FACILITY, and that FACILITY and any injured party may seek legal remedies against EMPLOYEE.

This AGREEMENT is entered into on (date).

_____
Employee signature

_____
Witness signature

Figure 2–8
An example of a confidentiality agreement that can be used by a facility when hiring a new employee. It was developed by the Health Professions Institute, Modesto, California.

primary source of information for the future care of the patient. Deletion of information or inaccurate transcription may cause irreparable damage to a patient's health care, as well as inaccurately informing a physician of what has transpired. For example, the difference between hypothyroidism (deficiency in thyroid function) and hyperthyroidism (excessive functioning of the thyroid gland) can make a crucial difference in treating the patient. Not only do these medical notes communicate to in-office and hospital personnel about a patient, but they are used to relay information to other health-care professionals.

Do not hesitate to ask questions of the physician or person dictating the report. It is far better to question than to guess or omit information. The information put into a report by the transcriptionist should reflect what was dictated.

Dictated information should not be randomly omitted because it is not understandable or does not make sense. If at all possible, questions should be asked about anything that is not understood or is unfamiliar. If a question is not

possible, a blank should be left with a note to the dictator attached to the transcription, stating what the phrase or word sounded like and initialed by the transcriptionist. It is extremely helpful to request and receive these notes back from the dictator. Through this process, knowledge will be gained, and the transcription will be more accurate. The medical records need to reflect an exact and complete record of the patient's care. It is of vital importance that the medical transcriptionist put the utmost effort into making this happen.

It is also important to establish a guideline in each medical facility for highlighting, boldfacing, underlining, or in some other way making certain information stand out from the rest of the record. This format is used for notations of the patient's diagnosis, allergies, immunizations, "no code blue" status (resuscitation efforts), refusal of treatment that has been recommended, or any other data that are deemed other than normal and routine information by the physician. For example, if a patient has an allergy to penicillin the chart note would be typed **ALLERGY TO PENICILLIN**, be underlined, or have some distinguishing feature to alert the reader.

Capital letters or boldface type may be used to alert the reader of the chart to the patient's allergy to medications, foods, or other substances. This method may also provide a reference to immunizations administered. If a patient refuses or declines a physician-directed referral or test, this can also be noted in a special way. For example, if a patient refuses to have an x-ray examination that has been requested by the physician, the chart may read *patient refuses x-ray examination.*

State laws governing discrimination should be taken into account when emphasizing information in the chart, especially in reference to age, race, sex, religion, and AIDS.

Any discrepancy in dictated information always needs to be checked and verified to provide an accurate file. Be alert to any discrepancies in transcription. For example, if a dictator has referred to the injured hand as "the right hand" and then changes to "the left hand," this information must be questioned and the correct statement placed in the medical record. This will ultimately provide a more accurate legal document for the health-care professional. It is *not* the transcriptionist's job to omit information or "guess" which hand is the "right" hand but rather to question what has been dictated.

Corrections

In the event that an error is found in the transcription, it is necessary to discover how the error was made and how to prevent its recurrence. If an error is discovered in proofreading by the transcriptionist or by the physician, there are several ways to make a legal, documented correction. Correction fluid or other similar products are *never* to be used to correct a mistake after a physician has signed a report or chart note. An error should be lined through and the correction indicated and initialed by the person correcting the error. If a physician has signed an operative report and then discovers an error, a correct version of the page is retyped and appended to the original typed document. A notation is made on the original document to "see the corrected version." It is extremely important to correct information that has been transcribed incorrectly.

In many office settings, adhesive-backed paper is used for transcription of chart notes. Once it is placed in the correct chart it should never be taken off or tampered with. If a chart note is incorrectly placed, it is moved to the correct medical record and the change noted and initialed. If asked to replace a dictation with one that already exists in the chart, the transcriptionist should explain that this is altering medical information and should not be done. All attempts to destroy records already in place should be stopped.

It is vitally important to destroy any rough drafts, reprints, or other medical information that contains any information about a patient. Many facilities use a device that shreds documents into fine strips. This eliminates the possibility of a piece of paper "floating" into the wrong hands. If there is no such device, then all papers containing patients' names should be torn into strips so the information cannot be read. First destroy the portion that gives the patient's name and then rip or shred the rest of the document. Never, under any circumstances, throw a piece of paper that has a patient's name on it into a wastebasket. A good rule of thumb is to imagine your name on that piece of paper. Would you want it thrown into the wastebasket without being torn up?

Imagine a patient's dismay upon discovering a piece of paper lying on the street with her name and medical information (such as a laboratory test) on it for anyone to see. This can happen. Protect yourself, your employer, and the patient. Use good sense when destroying medical information that is no longer needed.

With the advent of computers, electronic mailing devices, photocopiers, and centralized insurance billing, the medical record may be available to many persons associated with the care of the patient. When information is dictated and transcribed, every effort should be taken to transcribe this information in an accurate manner.

CONFIDENTIALITY

The medical transcriptionist must be responsible for maintaining confidentiality and must never discuss patient information other than with the dictating physician or an insurance company that has been authorized by the patient.

As medical data are input into a patient's record, either by way of computer or typewriter, the code of medical ethics must always be upheld and remembered. What is input in today's record will become a permanent part of a patient's chart.

Any questions concerning a patient should be directed to the physician in private and out of the hearing range of other patients. All communication with the physician or other health-care professionals should be made in strictest confidence. No question should ever be asked about a patient in front of another patient. If necessary, the physician should be called from the room to discuss the matter in question. If this is not done, the patient's rights to confidentiality have been violated.

A patient's trust in a physician is directly related to all personnel involved. The medical transcriptionist has the unique position of knowing a great deal more about the patient than some other members on the medical team. Along with this position comes the added responsibility of protecting that knowledge and treating it as privileged information.

Right of Privacy

Medical transcriptionists have the moral and ethical obligation to protect the patient's right to privacy. Each patient who comes to a health-care facility deserves the right to privacy. It is important to be aware of this when an entire family is seen by the same physician. If the transcriptionist knows that a member of a family is scheduled for a surgical procedure, it is a breach of confidentiality to ask another family member if their brother, sister, father, or mother is nervous about the upcoming surgery. It may be a courteous and seemingly innocent question, but if that family member does not want anyone, including the family, to know about the surgery, the transcriptionist has committed a serious breach of confidentiality.

It is extremely important, in all situations, to listen but not comment. Medical transcriptionists are often called upon to do a variety of jobs and, in this connection, a great deal of information is communicated during working hours that

should never leave the office. More to the point, the information that is heard through a transcriptionist's earphones should never be discussed anywhere.

Computer Access/Modems/Electronic Transmission Devices ■ In protecting the patient's right to privacy, computer access should be monitored and accessible only to authorized personnel. All computers should be locked at night or when not in use to avoid access by unauthorized personnel. Computer screens containing patient information should not be within the sight of other patients or other persons not directly connected with the care of the patient. If computer screens are within the sight of others, they should be blanked out or scrolled up when anyone is within viewing distance of the screen. All data input into the computer should be coded in such a way that access is not easily obtainable by persons other than those authorized to access by use of passwords. Every necessary step should be taken to protect the patient's right to privacy.

All medical information transmitted via facsimile machines (fax), modems, or other electronic devices should be monitored by specific authorized personnel transmitting data. The transcriptionist using a modem or fax should know to whom and where the information is going. All necessary precautions must be taken to protect the data that are being put into the system. See Chapter 3 for the proper wording to insert on a cover sheet for fax transmission.

As electronic communication (E-mail) becomes more popular, ethical standards and etiquette guidelines will have to be developed. Users need to be careful about expressing emotion in a message. Choose words carefully and eliminate humor, sarcasm, and anger. These can easily be misinterpreted because the receiver cannot see a grin or hear a chuckle. Assume messages are forever. Emotional responses to messages should not be made immediately. Do not write anything racially or sexually offensive on E-mail. Misdirected messages should be ignored but followed through to the intended recipient.

Privileged Information ■ Privileged information cannot be divulged by the physician unless the patient gives permission. This permission should be in writing and must be given by the patient.

Medical personnel, including transcriptionists, are often questioned about particular patients and their illnesses. Anyone not specifically directed by the patient to receive information about that patient should be told that the information is confidential. The best rule is not to talk about a patient to anyone other than those involved in the care and only then when it concerns the well-being of the patient. Just as the physician is sworn to uphold a high moral code and not to gossip, so is a medical transcriptionist.

Nonprivileged Information ▪ The data regarding admission and discharge to and from a general health-care facility (not to include substance abuse facilities), dates of treatment, and general condition of a patient are considered nonprivileged information. Certain sexually transmitted diseases, such as gonorrhea and syphilis, are reportable to the health department. Gunshot wounds and suspected child abuse cases are reportable in most states. The state laws should always be known and complied with in order to protect the employer, the employees, and the patient.

Privileged Communication ▪ Any communication between the patient and physician is privileged and cannot be released without written consent from the patient. All communication related to the transcriptionist via headsets or communicated in any other way is privileged communication and should be treated as such.

Sexually Transmitted Diseases ▪ In general, venereal diseases are reportable to local health authorities. However, HIV testing and AIDS confidentiality are classified differently, and each state has its own laws concerning this test. Much controversy exists over who should and should not be routinely tested, who should know of an HIV-positive patient, and the ultimate reality of protecting the HIV-positive patient's records.

BIOETHICS

Death, dying, euthanasia, advanced directives (living wills), transplants, abortions, genetics, reproductive technology, and social and personal issues are the root of bioethics, and the impact bioethics has on each culture is directly related to the social and personal issues of that culture.

Medical transcriptionists are often asked to transcribe dictation about subjects or moral issues that they may disagree with or be in direct moral conflict with. This is an area that will not be dealt with in great detail here but is an issue that must be addressed personally by each transcriptionist. If transcriptionists' moral or cultural values prohibit them from certain types of transcription duties, then this must be discussed with the immediate supervisor or person in charge. Transcriptionists have the ethical duty to perform their job in the most professional manner possible. If this cannot be accomplished because of moral and cultural belief systems, this must be addressed and dealt with in a professional manner.

Ethics of Medical Transcription Service Owners

To address poor or unethical business practices in the medical transcription field has been one of the goals of the Medical Transcription Service Owners (MTSOs), which meets annually and is sponsored by the Health Professions Institute in Modesto, California. The journal *Perspectives*, published by HPI, presented an article by Sally C. Pitman stating,

> In almost every gathering of business owners, abusive practices of some MTSOs are recounted, illustrating the difficulties of operating a business ethically in competition with businesses where the owners are unscrupulous or fraudulent or poor managers. Complaints fall into several categories: billing practices, employment practices, pricing practices, and quality assurance issues. Some abusive practices cited include the business that consistently underbids the prevailing rates, and once getting a contract, overbills the client or pads the bill; the business that is so vague in its billing practices that the client cannot verify the accuracy of the charges, or even understand how the bills are calculated; the business that pays workers as employees in the morning and in cash in the afternoon, thus avoiding payroll taxes on half its payroll; the business that doesn't respect the confidentiality of the medical reports in its possession, and doesn't teach its medical transcriptionists or support staff the importance of confidentiality; the business that doesn't pay decent wages or give benefits; the business that misclassifies workers and thus avoids paying pay-

roll and other taxes and benefits, making it difficult for tax-paying businesses to compete; the business that sells medical transcription for half the prevailing rates without the client understanding that the lines are half the standard length; the business that consistently wins contracts by underbidding other vendors, and then repeatedly defaults for nonperformance or poor performance in quality and turnaround time; the business that gives cash bounties to entice medical transcriptionists away from competitors—without proper notice of termination; the business that subcontracts work in clear violation of contracts that forbid it; the business that does not set or maintain quality standards for medical transcriptionists, hires inexperienced, poorly trained, or inadequately trained workers, and has no quality assurance controls; the business that routinely fails to keep turnaround time commitments; the business that colludes with dishonest physicians in altering previously signed and permanent medical transcripts in order to cover up malfeasance or malpractice of physicians; and the business that advertises that all its workers are certified medical transcriptionists but makes no effort to ascertain the validity or the currency of the credentials, and indeed employs medical transcriptionists who are not certified.

Having a Code of Ethics and Standards will not end these and other poor business practices, but having *some* service owners subscribing to a Code of Ethics and Standards can make a difference—to clients, employees, colleagues, and the industry as a whole. Ethical business owners can then say to their clients, their employees, and their colleagues, our values are expressed in the Code of Ethics and Standards of Medical Transcription Service Owners, and we are willing to be held to those standards (see Figure 2–4).

Ethical Problem Solving

Problem ■ Does a medical transcriptionist mention a father's upcoming surgery to another family member?

Solution ■ This is privileged information and should not be discussed with another family member unless the transcriptionist has been specifically given permission to mention this surgery to a family member.

Problem ■ If in a clinic or hospital setting, what does a transcriptionist do when a patient asks to read the chart note after it has been transcribed?

Solution ■ Even though patients technically are entitled to know what is in their chart note, this information should be presented to them by their physician or after they have signed a record release to a designated party. A transcriptionist unclear about how to handle this situation should direct questions to the immediate supervisor. A self-employed transcriptionist handling privileged information observes the same precautions.

Problem ■ What if an employer or client asks the transcriptionist to destroy a note/letter that is already in the chart and replace it with a new one?

Solution ■ This is a difficult situation, but medical ethics dictates that a medical record should not be altered in such a way as to replace records already a part of a legal medical record. Furthermore, there could be legal ramifications from altering medical records. (Please refer to the section in this chapter and in Chapter 3 on the legal and ethical way to make corrections in a medical record.)

Problem ■ The transcriptionist types a chart note about her best friend's husband who comes in to be treated for a sexually transmitted disease. The best friend knows nothing about this. Is it the transcriptionist's "duty" as a friend to mention this?

Solution ■ As honorable as her intentions may be, it is unethical and illegal to divulge this information. Remember, the transcriptionist is an extension of her employer. What she says about any patient would directly reflect on the employer. Under no circumstances should any privileged information be divulged to casual acquaintances or other sources not authorized by the patient to obtain such information.

Problem ■ A physician dictates a derogatory remark about a patient that has no bearing on the care given. Is it the transcriptionist's "duty" to transcribe this or question it?

Solution ■ Comments that are defamatory or derogatory and have no bearing on the medical issues at hand should be questioned. It is not the responsibility of the transcriptionist to delete this from the record but rather to question the dictator about whether the remark is essential to the medical record. This can then be determined by the dictator and, at that point, either transcribed or eliminated before it goes into the medical record. Direct any questionable comments to the employer.

Problem ■ What should the transcriptionist do when an employer asks that the date dictated be changed on an operative report?

Solution ■ The date of dictation should never be changed. Some facilities have a policy of typing separate entries at the end of a report to designate the date dictated, date transcribed, and/or date received. For example, date dictated (DD: 1/02/94), date received (DR: 1/03/94), or date transcribed: (DT: 1/03/94).

Problem ■ What if the physician/employer goes on vacation and gives approval to have a letter sent out in her or his absence?

Solution ■ A brief note can be typed and attached to the letter or report stating that a copy is being sent and the signed original will arrive after the physician returns from vacation. The original can be sent with a disclaimer statement at the bottom of the letter to read "Dictated but not read, to expedite delivery. Signed in doctor's absence by D.E."

Reference Sources

American Association for Medical Transcription. *Code of Ethics of the American Association for Medical Transcription*. Modesto, California, 1987.

Council on Ethical and Judicial Affairs of the American Medical Association. *1992 Code of Medical Ethics, Current Opinions*. Chicago, 1992.

Diehl, Marcy O., and Marilyn T. Fordney. *Medical Typing and Transcribing Techniques and Procedures*. W.B. Saunders Company, Philadelphia, 1991.

Norton, Clark. Threats to privacy. Is there no confidentiality? *Current*, Issue 319, January, 1990, pp. 14–18.

Pitman, Sally C. Legislating morality. *Perspectives*, Winter 1991–1992, p. 2.

Reich, Warren T. *Encyclopedia of Bioethics*, Vol. 3. The Free Press, New York, 1978.

Veatch, Robert M. *Cross Cultural Perspectives in Medical Ethics: Readings*. Jones and Bartlett Publishers, Boston, 1989.

Inge Barth, C.M.T.

CHAPTER
3

The Medical Record and the Law

INTRODUCTION

In the United States, legislation exists in each of the fifty states that requires hospitals and other health-care institutions to maintain medical records. In addition to these laws, nongovernmental agencies, such as the Joint Commission on Accreditation of Healthcare Organizations (JCAHO), American Medical Association, and American Health Information Management Association (AHIMA) (formerly known as the American Medical Record Association), have instituted standards with regard to the maintenance of medical records. Even if these laws and standards did not exist, the medical record would still need to be kept in order to provide the patient with the best possible care. This chapter will discuss the medical record and several laws concerning it.

MEDICAL REPORTS AND RECORDS

Medical records are maintained to document information regarding patient care accurately. They aid in planning patient care and evaluating the continuous condition and treatment of the patient. In addition, they serve to document communication between all health-care professionals and the patient. By having accurate documentation of patient care in the hospital, patients are legally protected, as also are the hospital and health-care workers. Medical records also may serve in providing data for re-

search and continuing education (Joint Commission on Accreditation of Healthcare Organizations, 1990).

Four types of data concerning the patient are included in the medical record: personal, financial, social, and medical. The patient's name, birth date, sex, marital status, next of kin, occupation, identification of physicians, and other items needed for specific patient identification are considered to be personal data required in the record (Roach, 1985). Financial data allow the institution to bill correctly for its services and include the name of the patient's employer, the patient's health insurance company, types of insurance and policy number, and Medicare and Medicaid numbers, if any (Roach, 1985). Social data include information regarding the patient's position in society and encompass the patient's race and ethnic background, family relationships, life style, any court orders or other directions concerning the patient and community activities. The patient's clinical record is the basis of the medical data. This information is to include the following (Roach, 1985):

History and physical examination
Treatment administered
Progress reports
Physicians' orders
Clinical laboratory reports
X-ray reports
Consultation reports
Anesthesia record
Operative report
Signed consent forms

27

Nurses' notes
Other reports pertinent to the patient's treatment

Whether the medical record is handwritten, typed, or generated via the computer, it must be an accurate recording of the treatment received by the patient in the health-care institution. Examination of these records by risk managers and other administrative and clinical assessment programs aid the hospital in verifying whether its standards are being maintained (Roach, 1985). To maintain accreditation by the JCAHO, hospitals must comply with certain regulations concerning the medical record.

Abbreviations ▪ Although abbreviations may be used, the JCAHO contends that these must be approved by the medical staff of the hospital, and a legend on the medical record must be available to those making entries into the record and those who interpret them. In addition, each abbreviation should have only one meaning (Huffman, 1985).

Deadlines for Medical Reports ▪ The JCAHO requires that the medical history and physical examination be completed within 24 hours of the patient's admission. Operative reports are to be dictated immediately after the operation and placed in the medical record as soon as possible. All other reports, such as x-ray reports, pathology reports, and reports of other diagnostic or therapeutic procedures, are to be entered into the medical record within 24 hours of their completion. With regard to an autopsy report, the provisional anatomic diagnoses are to be included in the medical record within 72 hours, while the final report should be entered into the record within 60 days (Joint Commission on Accreditation of Healthcare Organizations, 1990).

Completeness of Medical Reports ▪ The medical record is considered complete by the JCAHO when all entries regarding the "medical history, diagnostic and therapeutic orders, all reports of consultation and tests, progress notes, and clinical resumés" have been made and the attending physician has signed them (Southwick, 1988). In addition, a method is to be established to identify the authors of these entries. This identification may include a written signature, initials, or computer key. Rubber stamps are allowed in the authentication process (such as in pathology and radiology departments), but a signed statement must be filed in the hospital administration office acknowledging the fact that only the individual represented by the stamp will use it. In other words, the physician cannot delegate another to use that stamp (Huffman, 1985).

Medical records are important legal documents as they "are essential to the defense of professional negligence actions" (Roach, 1985). Therefore, all individuals involved in providing care to the patient are permitted to document that care in the medical record. This includes all physicians, nurses, laboratory personnel, podiatrists, physicians' assistants, clinical psychologists, dentists, and other personnel involved in the care and treatment of the patient (Roach, 1985). For example, after an operation a patient is being observed by a nurse, who fails to make accurate entries regarding the patient's condition in the record in a timely manner. If a malpractice suit is brought against the hospital by the patient, the jury may respond with an adverse verdict for the defendant. Southwick (1988) cites a case in the state of New York in which a patient had an allergic reaction to the anesthetic halothane during foot surgery. A notation was not made in the medical record of the patient concerning this allergy. A month later, while undergoing surgery on the other foot, the patient was given the same anesthetic and died. In this case, the jury favored the plaintiff, basing its decision solely on the fact that the anesthetic allergy had not been listed in the medical record.

A classic example of an incomplete medical record can be found in the case *Carr v. St. Paul Fire and Marine Insurance Company*. Carlos Carr came to the Emergency Room of Washington General Hospital with severe abdominal pain and vomiting. Only a licensed practical nurse and two orderlies were on duty. Although they could not reach the patient's physician, they failed to call another physician. The patient went home and died several hours later. For unknown reasons, the Emergency Room record was destroyed after the patient died. In the lawsuit that followed, the court stated:

> The plaintiff was greatly hampered in proving just what was done by the employees and what their examination disclosed, and the jury had a right to consider the effect that such destruction

had in determining the actual facts. It seems highly unreasonable that the findings of the physical condition of a person examined by the emergency room employees would be destroyed (George, 1980).

The court commented further, stating:

> No one knows the effect that such action had on the jury, but the jury certainly had a right to infer that the record, had it been retained, would have shown that a medical emergency existed and that a doctor should have been called and that more attention should have been given [to Mr. Carr] than was given (George, 1980).

The jury responded in favor of the plaintiff, awarding Mrs. Carr $35,000 in damages and $40,000 for the minor children of the deceased (George, 1980; Southwick, 1988).

Corrections ▪ Both major and minor errors may exist in the medical record. Minor errors are spelling and transcription errors, whereas major errors include physician's orders, omitted information, and errors in test results. Generally, the person who made the error is required to correct it. Carelessly altering the record gives the appearance of tampering; therefore, guidelines for correcting errors have been established. A single line should be drawn through the inaccurate material, allowing it still to be legible. The error is then dated and initialed by the person correcting it. An explanation of why the entry is being replaced should be made in the margins. The correction is then made and initialed with the date and time the correction was made. If space is a limitation, then an amendment can be made to the record (Hayt, 1977; Huffman, 1985; Roach, 1985; Southwick, 1988).

Ownership ▪ The control and ownership of the medical record lies with the hospital or the private physician who treats the patient in the office. Rules of ownership of the medical record can be found in the hospital-licensing regulations of the states. For example, in Pennsylvania, the regulation states: "Medical records are the property of the hospital, and they shall not be removed from the hospital premises, except for court purposes" (Roach, 1985).

Although the hospital or physician may have ownership and controlling rights of the medical record, many states recognize that the patient does have legal rights to the information contained therein. In fact, the AHIMA supports the right of access to the medical record by the patient "unless there are specific contraindications" (Huffman, 1985). In general,

> . . . the medical record is a confidential document, access to which should be restricted to the patient, to the patient's authorized representative, and to the attending physician and hospital staff members with a legitimate need for such access (Roach, 1985).

However, access can be denied if it would not be in the best interests of a patient's health (Roach, 1985) — that is, in psychiatric cases. In *Gotkin v. Miller,* a former mental patient in New York was denied access to her medical records. She sued the hospital, claiming that her federal constitutional rights were violated. The court upheld that the hospital did not violate her rights of "free speech, privacy, and protection against unreasonable searches and seizures, or deprivation of property without due process" (Roach, 1985). In Colorado, however, a patient may request in writing a summary of the psychiatric treatment rendered upon conclusion of the treatment.

Also, the American Hospital Association, as a guide to physicians and hospitals, published *A Patient's Bill of Rights* in 1972, which was revised in 1992. This document establishes that patients shall receive complete information concerning their treatment in the hospital, but it does not specifically state that patients may inspect their charts (Roach, 1985). The patient and a patient's representative may have access to the medical record, but some statutes limit this access until after the patient has been discharged.

Confidentiality ▪ Confidentiality, or privileged communication, must be assured the patient. The patient must feel that all information given to health-care professionals will remain confidential; "otherwise, the patient may withhold critical information which could affect the quality of the care provided" (Huffman, 1985). The Supreme Court has ruled that a person has a "'right to privacy' to make certain personal decisions without interference by government or other third parties" (Southwick, 1988), but it does not recognize information about that person to be confidential. In addition, there are no federal laws dealing with confidentiality of medical or personal information (Southwick, 1988). State law governs the matter of confidentiality and should be consulted before releasing medical information.

Many states have regulations concerning physician/patient privilege. This privilege belongs to the patient (Lewis and Warden, 1988) and prevents a physician from testifying in court concerning the "diagnosis, care, or treatment that he rendered to the patient unless the patient consents to such testimony or waives the protection by his conduct" (Huffman, 1985). However, in certain cases, a hospital or physician has a duty to reveal confidential medical information to a third party whether the patient has consented or not.

If there is a court order for the medical records to be accessible to a third party, then the patient's consent is not required. Certain statutes may require medical facts to be a matter of public record, for example, vital statistics, i.e., births, abortions, and deaths. Also venereal diseases and knife wounds or gunshot wounds must be reported, as well as child abuse. In addition, a physician or hospital has a duty to disclose medical information if injury or death could result to a third party. In *Jablonski v. United States,* the Veterans Administration Hospital was liable when its staff did not warn the household companion of a patient who had homicidal tendencies. Also, in approximately one third of the states, lien laws have been enacted. This provides the hospital

> . . . a legal claim under which the cost of hospitalization is paid from damages which the patient recovers from a third party whose negligence or civil wrong caused the patient's hospitalization. In turn, the third party is entitled to access to the patient's medical chart without authorization by the patient (Southwick, 1988).

However, a patient may seek damages for disclosure of the medical record in the event consent was not given and there was no statute allowing for the disclosure. The patient may bring suit against a hospital or physician based upon common law tort or a theory of contract law. Three theories to consider are invasion of privacy, breach of contract, and defamation.

Invasion of privacy can result from the unauthorized use of a person's name, professional skills, photograph, or personality. In *Clayman v. Bernstein,* the court prohibited the physician from using photographs for medical education purposes without the consent of the patient (Figure 3–1). In addition, lay persons may not be present at the time of surgery unless the patient has consented to their presence (Roach, 1985; Southwick, 1988). Figure 3–2 provides the proper wording of a form for this purpose.

The liability for breach of the physician-patient contract has been upheld by the court system. In *Hammonds v. Aetna Casualty and Surety Company,* the physician was held liable "when he disclosed medical information to hospital's insurer without the patient's consent" (Roach, 1985). Figures 3–3 through 3–6 give the wording of authorizations to disclose information.

Defamation, either libel or slander, can be either written or oral communication of false statements which tend to injure the patient's character or reputation (Huffman, 1985). In *Berry v. Moench,* a physician inquired of a second physician concerning a former patient. This inquiry was on behalf of the parents of a girl who was about to marry the patient. Upon learning from the physician's letter that the man their daughter was to marry was mentally unfit, the parents tried to stop the marriage. However, the marriage proceeded and the daughter was disowned by her parents. The court ruled that the second physician was to be held liable for the statements in his letter.

Disclosure of Information ▪ The medical record is an important medicolegal documentation of the care and treatment of a patient in a hospital or physician's office. It includes personal, financial, social, and medical information about the patient. Those involved in the care of the patient must document that treatment in a timely fashion, since errors or omissions in the hospital or physician record could place the hospital and physician, who have ownership and control of the medical record, at risk. In addition, the information contained within the medical record must remain confidential and may not be released without the consent of the patient. Only under certain circumstances can any of the information be released without the patient's consent.

Patient_____ Place_____ Date_____

In connection with the medical services which I am receiving

from my physician, Dr._____, I consent that photographs may be taken of me or parts of my body, under the following conditions:

1. The photographs may be taken only with the consent of my physician and under such conditions and at such times as may be approved by him.

2. The photographs shall by taken by my physician or by a photographer approved by my physician.

3. The photographs shall be used for medical records and if in the judgment of my physician, medical research, education or science will be benefited by their use, such photographs and information relating to my case may be published and republished, either separately or in connection with each other, in professional journals or medical books, or used for any other purpose which the physician may deem proper in the interest of medical education, knowledge, or research; provided, however, that it is specifically understood that in any such publication or use I shall not be identified by name.

4. The aforementioned photographs may be modified or retouched in any way that my physician, in his discretion, may consider desirable.

Signed_____
(*Patient*)

Witness_____

Figure 3–1
Form for patient consent for the taking and publication of photographs. (From Medicolegal Forms with Legal Analysis, Form 18, p. 37, American Medical Association, Chicago. Copyright 1991, all rights reserved.)

Patient_____ Place_____ Date_____

I authorize Dr._____ and the _____
_____ Hospital to permit the presence of such observers as they may deem fit to admit in addition to physicians and hospital personnel, while I am undergoing (operative surgery) (childbirth), examination, and treatment.

Signed_____

Witness_____

Figure 3–2
Form for patient consent to admit observers. (From Medicolegal Forms with Legal Analysis, Form 17, p. 36, American Medical Association, Chicago, Copyright 1991, all rights reserved.)

1. I authorize Dr._____ to disclose complete information to _____ concerning the medical findings and treatment of the undersigned from on or about _____ _____, 19____ until date of the conclusion of such treatment.

2. Further, I authorize the doctor to testify, without limitation, as to all of the medical findings and the treatment administered to the undersigned, in any legal action, suit, or proceedings to which I am, or may become, a party; and I waive on behalf of myself and any persons who may have an interest in the matter, all provisions of law relating to the disclosure of confidential medical information.

Witness_____   Signed_____
                             Place _____
                             Date _____

Figure 3–3

Authorization for disclosure of information by the patient's physician. (From Medicolegal Forms with Legal Analysis, Form 11, p. 25, American Medical Association, Chicago. Copyright 1991, all rights reserved.)

Figure 3–4

Authorization for disclosure of information by the examining physician. (From Medicolegal Forms with Legal Analysis, Form 12, p. 26, American Medical Association, Chicago. Copyright 1991, all rights reserved.)

I authorize Dr._____ to disclose complete information to _____ concerning the results of a physical examination of the undersigned made or to be made on _____, 19____, and to testify, without limitation, as to all findings of said physical examination, in any legal action or judicial proceedings to which I am, or may become, a party; and I waive on behalf of myself and any persons who may have an interest in the matter, all provisions of law relating to the disclosure of information acquired through said examination.

Witness_____   Signed_____
                             Place _____
                             Date _____

The American Medical Association researched legal exceptions or required disclosures of medical records and published the results in *Medicolegal Forms with Legal Analysis.**

The exceptions usually cited are for disclosures pursuant to court or administrative orders,[1] court ordered examinations,[2] to procure a dangerous drug or controlled substance,[3] when

*Medicolegal Forms with Legal Analysis, pp. 20–22. © 1991, American Medical Association, Chicago, reprinted with permission; all rights reserved.

[1] *Cal. Civil Code §56.10(b)(1); 29 U.S.C. §669-671 applied in G.M.C. v. Director of National Institute for Occupational Safety, 636 F.2d 163 (6th Cir. 1980).*
[2] *Nev. Rev. Stat. §49.225.*
[3] *Fla. Stat. Ann. §455.241.*

Figure 3–5

Authorization for examination of physician's records. (From Medicolegal Forms with Legal Analysis, Form 13, p. 27, American Medical Association, Chicago. Copyright 1991, all rights reserved.)

To Dr._____:
I authorize you to furnish a copy of the medical records of
_____, covering the period from
(state name of patient or "myself")
_____, 19____ to _____, 19____ or to
allow those records to be inspected or copied by _____.
I release you from all legal responsibility or liability that may arise from this authorization.

Witness_____   Signed_____

Date _____

Date_____Time_____
A.M.
P.M.

I authorize and request the _____ Hospital, and the physicians who attended me while I was a patient in said hospital during the approximate period from _____, 19____ to
_____, 19____, to furnish to _____ all information concerning my case history and the treatment, examinations or hospitalizations which I received, including copies of hospital and medical records.

Witness_____   Signed_____

Figure 3–6

Authorization to furnish information. (From Medicolegal Forms with Legal Analysis, Form 14, p. 27, American Medical Association, Chicago. Copyright 1991, all rights reserved.)

the patient has made his or her own physical or mental condition the basis for lawsuit,[4] or to disclose the existence of a dangerous disease,[5] gunshot wounds,[6] or child abuse.[7] Several articles discuss child abuse statutes thoroughly.[8] In other situations, such as investigations by a board of medical examiners, disclosure may be required for that proceeding only.[9]

Other statutes allow disclosure without patient authorization in limited circumstances. For example, Montana law allows the physician to report to the Division of Motor Vehicles patients with conditions that impair their ability to safely operate a motor vehicle.[10] California law allows the physician to disclose information to an insurer, employer, and other specified groups, persons or entities responsible for paying for the patient's health care services, to the extent necessary to allow responsibility for payment to be determined and made.[11] Similarly,

[4] *Tex. Civil Stat. (Vernon) art. 4495b §5.08(g)(1983).*
[5] *N.Y. Pub. Health Law §2101 (McKinney).*
[6] *N.Y.P.L. 265.25.*
[7] *Almost all states have mandatory reporting requirements for physicians in cases of suspected child abuse.*
[8] *Katz, S. et al., 1977. Legal Research on child abuse and neglect: past and future. Fam. Law Quart. 11(2):151-1984; and Sussman, A. 1974. Reporting child abuse: A review of the literature. Fam. Law Quart. 11:245-313 (1984).*
[9] *Tex. Civil Stats. (Vernon) art. 4495B §5.08(g)(1983) (Patient identity is protected).*

[10] *Montana 1983 New Laws 353.*
[11] *Cal. Civil Code §56.109(c)(2) & §56.29; See, however, Felis v. Greenberg, 273 NYS 2d 288 (1966), holding that the furnishing of information by a physician to an insurance company, without the patient's authorization constituted a violation of the patient-physician privilege.*

information may be disclosed to other health care professionals for the patient's diagnosis or treatment.[12]

Cases have arisen that question whether release only of a patient's name violates the confidentiality privilege. Often these cases turn on the particular factual situation; the court decisions have not been uniform. If release of the patient's name would identify the type of treatment received, the physician is advised to obtain the patient's consent prior to disclosure.[13] In some states, the statutory privilege has been extended to nurses,[14] psychologists, psychotherapists, marriage counselors, sexual assault counselors, and others.[15]

The privilege also extends to hospital records insofar as they tend to disclose what the physician learned during the course of treatment.[16] Generally, it has been held that where a physician is employed by an adverse party to examine a claimant, with no contemplation of any treatment, the information thus acquired is not privileged and the physician may testify as to such information.[17] Some states have codified this requirement for physician[18] and hospital[19] records. Many states have judicial decisions to the same effect.[20]

Some information is considered to be nonprivileged information and is unrelated to the patient's treatment. Examples of nonprivileged information include treatment dates, admission and discharge dates, and the patient's name.

An authorization for disclosure of information must be signed by the patient in order for the hospital or physician to release "privileged" information or information related to the patient's treatment and progress (Figure 3–7). Healthcare institutions, therefore, must abide by state laws and regulations, as well as the standards of nongovernmental agencies, to maintain a low risk of lawsuits against them.

Confidentiality regarding acquired immune deficiency syndrome (AIDS) and the human immunodeficiency virus (HIV) test has become an important issue for all health-care workers and facilities. Patients must sign an informed consent form before receiving the HIV antibody test (Figure 3–8). In addition, a special authorization for disclosure of information should be completed by the patient. Whereas some states are very explicit in their confidentiality laws regarding HIV and AIDS, some states still have vague statutes.

In Colorado, however, the law has been quite explicit since June, 1987, when Governor Roy Romer signed into law House Bill 1177. This legislation declares that AIDS is an infectious and communicable disease that endangers the population. Ellen Stewart, in a 1988 lecture, noted that under the AIDS law, a physician is required to report the name, date of birth, sex, and address of the individual who has a diagnosis of AIDS or has an HIV-related illness. The statute gives physicians immunity and absolves the duty of such physician to a third party, if the physician completes a report. Stewart outlined

---

[12] Id.

[13] Rudnick v. Superior Court, *114 Cal. Rptr. 603 (1974);* Marcus v. Superior Court of Los Angeles, *95 Cal. Rptr. 545 (1971);* People v. Florendo, *447 N.E.2d 282 (Ill. 1983) (Release only to grand jury permitted);* Geisberger v. Willuhn, *390 N.E.2d 945 (Ill. 1979) (Release of name alone no violation).*

[14] *Colorado Revised Statutes 13-90-107(1).*

[15] *Utah Code Annotated 78-3C-4 (1984) (Limited disclosure only).*

[16] State Of Iowa v. Bedel, *193 N.W.2d 121 (Iowa 1971);* Unick v. Kessler Memorial Hospital, *257 A.2d 134 (N.J. 1969);* Koump v. Smith, *250 N.E.2d 857 (N.Y. 1969);* Toole v. Franklin Investment Co., *158 Wash. 696, 291 P. 1101 (1930);* Metropolitan Life Ins. Co. v. McSwain, *149 Miss. 455, 115 So. 555 (1928).* Contra: Sarrio v. Reliable Construction Company, Inc., *286 A.2d 183 (Md. 1972).*

[17] Hardy v. Riser, *309 F.Supp. 1234 (Miss. 1970);* Hanlon v. Woodhouse, *113 Colo. 504, 160 P.2d 998 (1945);* McMillen v. Industrial Commission of Ohio, *37 N.E.2d 632 (Ohio 1941);* Bouligny v. Metropolitan Life Ins. Co., *133 S.W.2d 1094 (Mo. App. 1939);* Metropolitan Life Ins. Col. v. Evans, *183 Miss. 859, 184 So. 426 (1938);* City of Cherokee v. Aetna Life Ins. Co., *215 Iowa 1000, 247 N.W. 495 (1933);* Moutzoukos v. Mutual Benefit Health & Accident Assn., *69 Utah 308, 254 P. 1005 (1927);* Cherpeski v. Great Northern R. Co., *128 Minn. 360, 150 N.W. 1091 (1915);* Arnold v. City of Maryville, *110 Mo. App. 254, 85 S.W. 107 (1905).* Contra: Kramer v. Policy Holders' Life Ins. Assn., *5 Cal. App.2d 380, 42 P.2d 665 (1935);* Webb v. Francis J. Lewald Coal Co., *215 Cal. 182, 4 P.2d 532 (1931).*

[18] See, e.g., *Cal. Welfare & Inst. Code §5152.1 (1983) (Mental Health Records); Fla. Stat. Ann. §455.241.*

[19] *Fla. Stat. Ann. §395.017(3) (1983 Supp.);* Head v. Colloton, *331 N.W.2d 870 (Iowa 1983).*

[20] *No privilege for court appointed physicians.* Massey v. State of Georgia, *177 S.E.2d 79 (Ga. 1970);* cert. den. *91 S.Ct. 984 (1971);* Illinois v. Lowe, *248 N.E.2d 530 (Ill. 1969);* New York v. Fuller, *248 N.E.2d 17 (N.Y. 1969).*

AUTHORIZATION TO RELEASE MEDICAL INFORMATION

(The execution of this form does not authorize the release of information other than that specifically described below)

TO: (Print/type name & address of doctor or health care facility)	PATIENT: Name: S. S. No.: Birth Date:	RELEASE TO: (Name & address of organization, agency, individual to whom information is to be released)

I request and authorize the above-named doctor or health care provider to release the information specified below to the organization, agency, or individual named on this request. I understand that the information to be released includes information regarding the following condition(s):

☐ Drug abuse, if any ☐ Sickle cell anemia, if any   ☐ Alcoholism or alcohol abuse, if any ☐ Psychological or psychiatric conditions, if any

Information Requested:
☐ Copy of history & physical, discharge summary & operative reports
☐ Copy of outpatient & E.R. admissions
☐ Copy of complete hospital chart
☐ Other (specify) _____

Dates Covered:
☐ All admissions or care at this facility or by this doctor
☐ Limited to treatment dates & for conditions described below:
_____
_____
_____

Purpose(s) or need for which information is to be used:
☐ Damage or claim evaluation and presentation
☐ Other _____

<u>AUTHORIZATION</u> - I certify that this request has been made voluntarily and that the information given above is accurate to the best of my knowledge. I understand that I may revoke this authorization at any time, except to the extent that action has already been taken to comply with it. Redisclosure of my medical records by those receiving the above authorized information may not be accomplished without my further written consent. Without my express revocation, this consent will automatically expire upon satisfaction of the need for disclosure, but in any event:
☐ on _____ (date supplied by patient); or ☐ if revoked in writing by patient; or ☐ 180 days from the date hereof; or ☐ under the following condition(s):
_____
_____
_____

☐ Copies of records to be supplied to opposing counsel
☐ Other

OTHER CONDITIONS - A copy of this authorization or my signature thereon: ☐ may, ☐ may <u>not</u> be utilized with the same effectiveness as an original.

DATE	SIGNATURE OF PATIENT	PERSON AUTHORIZED TO SIGN FOR PATIENT Print or type name State how authorized: _____

Figure 3-7
Authorization to release medical information. (From Lorman Business Center, Inc., Eau Claire, Wisconsin, 1992. Confidentiality of Medical Records in Colorado, p. 119. All rights reserved.)

I voluntarily give my consent to be tested for exposure to the Human Immunodeficiency Virus (HIV). HIV is the term used for the virus that is thought to cause AIDS. I understand that my blood will be drawn for the purpose of determining whether I have been exposed to this virus.

I understand that the exact meaning of an HIV antibody test result may not be clear in my case. A positive result does not mean that I will come down with AIDS. A negative result does not ensure that I do not have early HIV infection or that I cannot transmit the infection.

I understand that all reasonable efforts to provide confidentiality and/or anonymity to the extent provided by law will be made. However, I understand that the results of this test will be recorded in my medical record. As medical record information, these tests results will be regarded as confidential, and the Hospital will not disclose these test results to unauthorized third parties without my express written authorization. I understand, however, that confidentiality cannot be absolutely guaranteed, and that the results will be available to physicians and other health-care professionals responsible for my care and treatment.

I understand that Illinois law requires that if this test result in combination with other data leads my physician to make a presumptive diagnosis of AIDS, then my case must be reported to the public health authorities and may be investigated by them.

I have been informed that if this test is positive a physician will provide counseling for follow up care and for precautions against transmitting this infection.

I understand that if I refuse this test my exposure to the HIV will remain unknown. My ability to infect others with this virus will also remain unknown.

I warrant that I freely give my informed consent and that I have not been forced, coerced or subjected to any constraint or inducement. I understand that I may withdraw this consent anytime prior to having my blood drawn.

_____ I hereby give consent for the performance of the HIV antibody test.

_____ I refuse consent for the performance of the HIV antibody test. I understand that this refusal may limit the clinical data available to my physician. However, this refusal will not affect my access to further care.

_____ _____
Signature   Date

_____
Witness

Editor's Note: *This form is reproduced with permission of Northwestern Memorial Hospital, Chicago, Illinois.*

Figure 3–8
Form to obtain informed consent for the HIV antibody test. (From Medicolegal Forms with Legal Analysis, Form 82, p. 196, American Medical Association, Chicago. Copyright 1991, all rights reserved.)

the main points of the legislation, from which I quote:

B. Confidentiality of Information

1. Reports from the physicians "shall be strictly confidential medical information." Such information *shall not be released,* shared with any agency or institution, or made public, upon subpoena, search warrant, discovery proceedings, or otherwise . . ." (emphasis added). There are exceptions to the strictly confidential nature of the medical information and they are:
   a. Data may be released for statistical purposes (excluding individual names);
   b. Data can be released to assist public health officials in controlling HIV infections;
   c. Medical information may be released to medical personnel in a medical emergency but only as is necessary to protect the life of the AIDS patient.

2. The AIDS statute is absolutely clear regarding the protections afforded to patients with the disease. Further, the statute directs that "No physician, health worker, or any other person and no hospital, clinic, sanitarium, laboratory, or any other private or public institution shall test, or shall cause by any means to have tested, any specimen of any patient for HIV infection without *the knowledge and consent* of the patient." The only exceptions are:
   a. If health of a health-care provider or custodial employee of the Department of Corrections or the Department of Institutions is immediately threatened by exposure to HIV in blood or other bodily fluids;
   b. When, due to patient's medical condition, consent cannot be obtained;
   c. Testing for seroprevalence surveys;
   d. When patient is *sentenced to and in the custody of* the Department of Corrections or is committed to the state hospital and confined to the forensic ward or the minimum or maximum security ward of the hospital.

3. Penalties
   a. Failure to make a report to the Department of Health by a physician, health-

care provider, or clinical laboratory results in a class 2 petty offense—fine is a maximum of $300.
   b. Any person who releases confidential medical information or breaches the confidentiality requirements may be subject to a misdemeanor—fine is not less than $500 or more than $5,000 or imprisonment in a county jail for not less than 6 months or more than 24 months, or both fine and imprisonment.

C. Actions Which Can Be Taken by the Department of Health

1. The AIDS statute confers on the Executive Director of the Colorado Department of Health the power to require persons he "knows or has reason to believe" have an HIV infection to be tested, obtain counseling, and cease and desist from specified conduct that endangers the health of others.

2. If a cease and desist order is violated, then the Executive Director may put restrictions on the person necessary to prevent the specified conduct, an initial period of restriction not to exceed 3 months, which order may be challenged by the patient in closed hearings before the District Court (Stewart, 1988).

In 1990, some changes were made to the Colorado law. Those doing research in an approved research protocol approved by the State Board of Health are now exempted from reporting those with the diagnosis of AIDS, HIV infection, or HIV-related illness.

FAXING MEDICAL DOCUMENTS

Faxing (facsimile communications) is a method for speedily sending and receiving information over telephone lines and is used more and more for medical communication. This technology has made it necessary for health-care facilities to develop new policies and procedures concerning the transmittal of confidential information. In addition to following federal regulations and hospital licensure laws, health-care facilities must also be in compliance with state statutes and accreditation standards.

Certain guidelines should be followed in the

transmittal of confidential medical information, such as obtaining a signed release from the patient before faxing a patient's records. When faxing confidential medical documents, a transmittal cover sheet is routinely sent (Figure 3–9). It is important to telephone the authorized receiver of the documents before the transmission is begun to arrange a specific time for the transmission. Also ask the recipient whether that facility has a protected number or security code programmed into the fax unit. Confidential information should be transmitted only to and from fax machines located in secure or restricted access areas, preferably in medical record departments. Health information should be faxed only when it is absolutely necessary and not as a matter of convenience (Feste, 1992; Fordney and Follis, 1993).

Should the fax transmittal be sent to an incorrect number, a request is made to that number for the destruction of all confidential documents that may have been received. An incident report is then filed with the risk manager of the healthcare facility (Feste, 1992).

For reasons of confidentiality, psychiatric records should not be faxed, except in cases of emergency (Fordney and Follis, 1993).

LEGALITIES OF PSYCHIATRIC DOCUMENTS

Two issues are of main concern in regard to psychiatric documents. The right of privacy of a patient should not be violated, except in certain circumstances, and physicians are required to maintain the confidences of their patients. These highly confidential medical records are often referred to as "safe files" or "locked files." Generally they are locked up in a file cabinet to protect their confidentiality.

A number of states have mental health confidentiality statutes that outline comprehensively the legal requirements of confidentiality (American College of Legal Medicine, 1988). Therefore, hospitals must consider state laws and the JCAHO requirements when developing policies and procedures for releasing psychiatric confidential information (Huffman, 1985).

RETENTION OF RECORDS

In general, hospitals keep medical records as prescribed by law or for a time considered appropriate by them. Each state may have its own retention laws. However, most states have no specific retention requirements for medical records. The American Hospital Association and the American Medical Association recommend that patient records be kept for at least 10 years (American College of Legal Medicine, 1988).

SUBPOENA

A subpoena is a legal order to appear in court (Figures 3–10 and 3–11). The clerk of the court signs the subpoena at the request of an attorney (American College of Legal Medicine, 1988). Whereas a subpoena requires a witness to be present, a subpoena duces tecum requires that the witness comes to court with specific records (Huffman, 1985).

A subpoena may be legally challenged. Perhaps it is an improper subpoena demanding confidential information regarding a patient or other patients who are not involved in the litigation process (Kapp, 1985). Perhaps the attorney is working on a case concerning a hysterectomy. He or she may subpoena the patient's records and all the records of patients who have had hysterectomies by a certain physician. The attorney may try to determine whether all hysterectomies this physician has done have followed the same procedures. The information may or may not be relevant to the case. However, the information from all the other hysterectomy cases is confidential; therefore, this may be considered an improper subpoena and should be challenged.

In the case of a medical office receiving a subpoena regarding a patient's confidential medical records, the office staff will contact the patient regarding the subpoena. The patient then can assert the right to confidentiality and may ask the judge to quash, that is, eliminate the subpoena. If the judge then orders that the information should be produced, the physician must appear in court with the information. The physician is thus protected by the court order in releasing the information.

PRACTON MEDICAL GROUP, INC.
4567 Broad Avenue
Woodland Hills, XY 12345-4700
Tel. 013/486-9002
Fax No. 013/488-7815

FAX TRANSMITTAL SHEET

To: _____ Date _____

Fax Number: _____ Time _____

Number of Pages (including this one): _____

From: _____ Phone _____

Note: This transmittal is intended only for the use of the individual or entity to which it is addressed, and may contain information that is privileged, confidential, and exempt from disclosure under applicable law. If you are not the intended recipient, any dissemination, distribution, or photocopying of this communication is strictly prohibited. If you have received this communication in error, please notify this office immediately by telephone and return the original FAX to us at the address below by U. S. Postal Service. The recipient of this patient information is prohibited from disclosing the information to any other party and is required to destroy the information after the stated need has been fulfilled. Thank you.

Remarks:_____

_____

_____

Instructions to authorized receiver: If you cannot read this FAX or if pages are missing, please contact this office. Please complete this statement of receipt and return to sender via the fax number above.

I,_____, verify I have received_____pages
                                                    (# of pp. incl. cover)
From_____.
        (sending facility name)

Figure 3–9
Example of a facsimile transmittal (fax) or cover sheet.

DISTRICT COURT, EL PASO COUNTY, COLORADO

CASE NO. _____ DIV. NO. _____ _____

☐ SUBPOENA (Personal)
☐ SUBPOENA TO PRODUCE (Subpoena duces tecum)

The People of the State of Colorado

TO: _____

You are ordered to attend and give testimony in the District Court of _____ County

at _____ (location)

on _____ (date and time), as a witness for _____

_____ in an action between _____

_____ plaintiff and _____

_____ defendant and also to produce at this time and place (if applicable):

_____

_____

_____

_____ now in your custody or control.

Date: _____   _____

Signature of Attorney for Plaintiff or Clerk/Deputy Clerk of Court.

RETURN OF SERVICE

State of _____

_____ County _____

I declare under oath that I served this subpoena or subpoena to produce on _____

_____ in _____ County, _____ on _____ at _____
Date   Time

at the following location:

☐ by (State Manner of Service)

☐ I am over the age of 18 years and am not interested in nor a party to this case.

Signed under oath before me on _____

_____   Name   Date

Notary Public*   ☐ Private process server

     ☐ Sheriff, _____ County

     Fee $ _____

     Mileage $ _____

*Notary should include address and expiration date of commission.

Figure 3–10

Subpoena form used by District Court, El Paso County, Colorado. (From Lorman Business Center, Inc., Eau Claire, Wisconsin, 1992. Confidentiality of Medical Records in Colorado, p. 101. All rights reserved.)

SUBPOENA

United States District Court	DISTRICT COLORADO
	DOCKET NO
V.	TYPE OF CASE ☐ CIVIL ☐ CRIMINAL
	SUBPOENA FOR ☐ PERSON ☐ DOCUMENT(S) or OBJECT(S)

TO:

YOU ARE HEREBY COMMANDED to appear in the United States District Court at the place, date, and time specified below to testify in the above-entitled case.

PLACE UNITED STATES DISTRICT COURT 1929 STOUT ST. DENVER, COLORADO 80294	COURTROOM
	DATE AND TIME

YOU ARE ALSO COMMANDED to bring with you the following document(s) or object(s):[1]

☐ *See additional information on reverse*

This subpoena shall remain in effect until you are granted leave to depart by the court or by an officer acting on behalf of the court.

U.S. MAGISTRATE[2] OR CLERK OF COURT JAMES L. MANSPEAKER, CLERK	DATE
(BY) DEPUTY CLERK	

This subpoena is issued upon application of the: ☐ Plaintiff ☐ Defendant ☐ U.S. Attorney	ATTORNEY'S NAME AND ADDRESS

(1) If not applicable, enter "none."

(2) A subpoena shall be issued by a magistrate in a proceeding before him, but need not be under the seal of the court. (Rule 17(a), Federal Rules of Criminal Procedure.)

Figure 3–11

United States District Court subpoena. (From Lorman Business Center, Inc., Eau Claire, Wisconsin, 1992. Confidentiality of Medical Records in Colorado, p. 102. All rights reserved.)

Reference Sources

American College of Legal Medicine. *Legal Medicine: Legal Dynamics of Medical Encounters.* St. Louis, 1988.

Council on Ethical and Judicial Affairs of the American Medical Association. *1992 Code of Medical Ethics, Current Opinions.* Chicago, 1992.

Diehl, Marcy O., and Marilyn T. Fordney. *Medical Typing and Transcribing: Techniques and Procedures,* 3rd edition. W. B. Saunders Company, Philadelphia, 1991.

Feste, Laura. *Guidelines for Faxing.* Professional Medical Assistant (PMA), American Association of Medical Assistants, Chicago, May/June, 1992.

Fordney, Marilyn T., and Joan Follis. *Administrative Medical Assisting,* 3rd edition. Delmar Publishers, Inc., Albany, New York, 1993.

George, James E. *Law and Emergency Care.* C. V. Mosby, St. Louis, 1980.

Hayt, Emanuel. *Medicolegal Aspects of Hospital Records.* Physicians' Record Company, Berwyn, Illinois, 1977.

Huffman, Edna K. *Medical Record Management.* Physicians' Record Company, Berwyn, Illinois, 1985.

Joint Commission on Accreditation of Health-care Organizations. *The 1991 Joint Commission AMH Accreditation Manual for Hospitals; Volume I, Standards.* Oakbrook Terrace, Illinois, 1990.

Kapp, Marshall B. *Legal Guide for Medical Office Managers.* Health Administration Press, Chicago, 1985.

Lewis, Marcia A., and Carol D. Warden. *Law and Ethics in the Medical Office.* F. A. Davis, Philadelphia, 1988.

Richards, Edward P., III, and Katharine C. Rathbun. *Medical Risk Management.* Aspen Publishers, Inc., Rockville, Maryland, 1982.

Roach, William E., Jr., et al. *Medical Records and the Law.* Aspen Publishers, Inc., Rockville, Maryland, 1985.

Southwick, Arthur F. *The Law of Hospital and Health Care Administration.* Health Administration Press, Ann Arbor, Michigan, 1988.

Stewart, Ellen E. Legal Decisions Affecting Medical Ethics (lecture). College of St. Francis, Colorado Springs, Colorado, July 6, 1988.

Wills, Lee R., et al. Confidentiality of Medical Records in Colorado (seminar). Presented by Lorman Business Center Inc., Eau Claire, Wisconsin, in Colorado Springs, Colorado, November 6, 1992.

Jackie Abern, C.M.T.
Adrienne C. Yazijian, C.M.T.

Building a Transcription Service

INTRODUCTION—A SCENARIO

A superior medical transcriptionist is employed by a transcription service to work at home. The service has provided all her equipment. Work is delivered to her door and picked up by the service upon its completion. The service is responsible both for paying the transcriptionist regularly and withholding the appropriate taxes. The transcriptionist puts in a set number of hours, and she may even receive benefits. Because she is good, and the demand for transcriptionists is great, she may set her own hours and take time off as she desires. In most cases she can work as many hours as she wants, but anything over 40 hours qualifies for overtime pay. Monetary rewards are limited only by the amount of time spent transcribing.

This transcriptionist mentions to a physician she knows that she transcribes medical reports at home. He tells her he has some dictation he would like her to transcribe. She goes to his office, picks up a tape, takes it home, transcribes it, and brings it back for signature. The physician is happy. He pays the bill. The transcriptionist is happy.

Several more clients are acquired in the same manner, and soon our transcriptionist finds that the money she is earning from them exceeds that which she is receiving from the transcription service. She must make a decision whether to continue working for the service or to devote all her time and efforts going into business for herself.

She chooses the latter and begins to plan for the time that she can phase out the service. The transcriptionist must now decide how she is going to set up her business. She must purchase equipment, buy insurance, find and furnish an office, and familiarize herself with both the financial and legal considerations of becoming self-employed. Ultimately she must cut the cord between her and her employer, declaring her independence.

Soon there is more work than she can possibly handle! She is making more money than she ever imagined, but she's reached her limit. She works 7 days a week, 16 hours a day, no vacations, no sick days, no holidays. If equipment breaks down, it is her responsibility to have it fixed. Clients will not wait for their work!

Our transcriptionist realizes that with a helper, she could pass on some of the excess work, pay out a portion of the income, and keep what is left. She has now arrived back where she began, except on the other end of the checkbook. Her mission is to find qualified medical transcriptionists and hire them. The more people hired, the more money for our entrepreneur, *but* the fewer hours spent transcribing, the more time spent marketing, training, and proofreading.

Again a decision must be made whether to transcribe or to be a businessperson. This is not a decision to be made lightly. The need for power versus the need for satisfaction must be evaluated carefully. If the choice is made to transcribe, the money will be good, but there will be a limit to what can be produced. If the choice is made to manage, the opportunities (and grief) are limitless, but transcription will be cut to a minimum.

If our transcriptionist decides to manage, she jumps into the entrepreneurial circus. And here we begin an in-depth look into a fascinating, flexible career.

SELF-EMPLOYMENT

Education/Preparation

A 4-year college degree is not of particular importance in medical transcription. It is fairly certain that one who answers the call to the profession is an individual with a tremendous interest in language; great spelling skills; excellent editing, grammar, and punctuation skills; and fast and accurate typing ability.

With those basics, every course taken, every subject studied, will add to improvement of transcription skills. A medical transcription program at a local vo-tech center or junior college is an excellent start. It can provide a basic knowledge of the hospital medical record, the terminology, and the equipment and procedures necessary to transform spoken word to hard copy. Every science course will aid in understanding medical dictation. Every liberal arts course will add to the knowledge and comprehension of the spoken word. Every business administration course will assist in formulation of plans for growth. Every education course will help in training new employees. There is no "upper limit" of knowledge—one can never be over-qualified!

Knowledge of medical terminology, however, is not enough. Knowing the medical words without knowing their meanings is like trying to communicate in another language without the ability to translate! One must get into those dictionaries and learn prefixes, root words, and suffixes. Learning is an ongoing experience for the medical transcriptionist.

With the absorption of this knowledge, and all the reference material that can be acquired, on-the-job experience ideally is obtained before one considers working independently. Employment in the medical record department of a full-service hospital for a minimum of three years, or until comfortable with the basic four reports, i.e., history and physical examinations, consulta-

tions, operative reports, and discharge summaries, plus many types of accented dictation, is the best learning experience for a beginner.

At home, sources for information must be at the fingertips as it is not always possible to receive outside help. Transcriptionists must be certain they are correct. Networking with other professionals is helpful, especially for home-based MTs. This is when membership in your local, state, or national professional association really pays off.

The home transcriptionist must be organized. Even if the "office" is in the middle of the kitchen, the kids are screaming, and the dryer is buzzing, one must have that unusual ability to shut everything off and work. Some people call this being focally oriented rather than peripheral. The schedule reigns!

Auxiliary Personnel ■ When starting a transcription business, the home transcriptionist will fill all positions. As success grows, her time might be more profitably spent doing those things for which she is more aptly suited.

Picking up and delivering work is a great way to meet new and existing clients. There is no substitute for the personal touch. Eventually, however, you may choose to use other avenues for this aspect of the business. It becomes cost effective to hire and train auxiliary personnel, sometimes using independent contractors (Figure 4–1).

Delivery Service ■ Several types of delivery services are available. The one chosen must be determined by the amount of work, the direction of the work (pick-up at the same time as drop-off), and the time involved. The high charges for multiple deliveries and pick-ups can offset the advantage of not having to drive, park, or use gasoline.

When the number of clients increases, an alternative is to hire a courier. A student or retired person who owns a car with insurance can be given a per hour or per trip fee, in addition to a mileage charge mutually agreed upon. Should the necessity for a full-time driver arise, the purchase (or lease) of a delivery car might be a tax advantage, and the courier might then be considered an employee.

File Clerk ■ It might become cost effective to hire someone to print and make copies. Hiring a student, retiree, or someone from a temporary agency would free the transcriptionist's time to enjoy leisure activities or get new business. For couriers *or* file clerks, remember to try the local temporary agencies. Listed in the yellow pages, these companies are valuable, as the "temp" you use will already be screened and you will have no "employee" details to worry you.

The home-based transcriptionist will learn that some other business-associated activities, such as cleaning, bookkeeping, and billing, may be done at less cost by outside agencies.

HOME-BASED MEDICAL TRANSCRIPTION

Planning the Home Office

A quiet place, free from distraction, is the ideal location for the home office. An extra bedroom can be great; the kitchen, if it is a family gathering place, can be a disaster.

For esthetics and relaxation, a room with a window is desirable. The "hidden" professionals, medical transcriptionists, have spent so many years in basement offices that looking out a window is infinitely more cheerful and soothing, making work less a chore. The window can occupy the eyes while the mind is busy. It enables mother to view her children at play. Or plan next year's garden. Or watch the dog. It is important to rest the eyes from the LED screen every 15 minutes, and looking at the horizon helps the eyes accommodate as the mind relaxes.

Once an office site has been selected, it should be solely dedicated to medical transcription. Home transcription services have a way of growing out of control unless there are four walls devoted to containing them.

Operating Requirements

Work Hours ■ One of the positives about medical transcription is its flexibility. The home transcriptionist can select working hours best suited to her life style. The most productive hours can be in the early morning when the world is still asleep. The telephone should be accessible, however, either by answering machine or answering service, 24 hours a day, 7 days a week.

If an office away from home is desired, it should be accessible at off hours to conform to the needs of both the employees and the varying work load.

Equipment

There was a time when an IBM Correcting Selectric typewriter and a standard transcriber were all that were needed. Those days are gone. Doctors take for granted now that they can revise, edit, and call back two weeks later to retrieve another copy of a report. They expect it because technology has provided it for them, and consequently the transcription service must comply. For further information on equipment, refer to Chapter 5.

Computer ■ IBM compatibility is essential. A dual floppy system with a hard disk drive capable of storing information sufficient for the needs of the growing service is essential. Computers should be able to handle both $5\frac{1}{4}$- and $3\frac{1}{2}$-inch floppy disks. The smaller ones are more durable, as they are completely encased in plastic. The word processing package must be something with which the transcriptionist is completely comfortable. Learning multiple word processing programs is not necessary, because Word Perfect 5.1 can accept documents created in most other software packages, as can Word Star 7.0. The monitor should be easy to read and relaxing on the eyes.

Printer ■ The printer should be letter quality at minimum. Laser printers create beautiful reports but have their limitations. Not all stationery can be used in the laser, as the heat from the copying device may melt the paint of embossed stationery. Lasers are also incapable of printing NCR or carbon forms, and an alternative printer must be used that can perform these functions.

Transcriber ■ Three types of transcribers are essential for a full-service company. In order of preference, the microcassette is the most popular. The tone quality is the best, and most physicians today use it in their private dictation. The standard cassette has become slightly less popular in recent years, probably because of its size and the fact that most dictating systems are using the micros. The mini-cassette is notorious for poor tone quality, defective cassettes, and the

RELATIONSHIP OF PARTIES

1. The parties to this contract agree that SUBCONTRACTOR is a professional person conducting a business and that the relation created by this contract is that of PRINCIPAL and INDEPENDENT CONTRACTOR. The SUBCONTRACTOR is not an employee of CSN and is not entitled to benefits including, but not limited to, withholding of federal and state taxes. In accordance with this relationship, the following criteria are addressed:

   a) CSN does not instruct the SUBCONTRACTOR as to location, hours, methods, etc. for completion of job. However, as stated above, SUBCONTRACTOR must comply with trade requirements for completion of job as specified or be held financially responsible.
   b) CSN provides no training for SUBCONTRACTOR.
   c) SUBCONTRACTOR provides only temporary integration for CSN depending upon work overflow, sometimes none at all.
   d) SUBCONTRACTOR can delegate or subcontract out.
   e) SUBCONTRACTOR has the freedom to hire, supervise and pay assistants as necessary.
   f) Duration of relationship is limited in time or as to specific result by SUBCONTRACTOR.
   g) Hours of work are set by SUBCONTRACTOR.
   h) SUBCONTRACTOR is free to choose who and when work is completed; SUBCONTRACTOR is free to provide services for other businesses.
   i) SUBCONTRACTOR conducts business at place of own business, off-premises of CSN.
   j) Order or sequence of work is set by SUBCONTRACTOR not CSN.
   k) Methods of payment as above; non-time based.
   l) SUBCONTRACTOR does not provide oral or written reports for CSN.
   m) Any business or travel expenditures are not reimbursed by CSN. SUBCONTRACTOR provides for own business and travel expenses.
   n) All tools/material required for completion of job is provided by SUBCONTRACTOR; none supplied by CSN.
   o) SUBCONTRACTOR provides facilities, equipment, etc. required for job completion.
   p) SUBCONTRACTOR acknowledges investment/expenses, works for set price dependent upon outcome, or otherwise has risk of profit or loss.
   q) SUBCONTRACTOR has multiple clients.
   r) SUBCONTRACTOR advertises, has own office, liability insurance; provides business license number and sample business cards to CSN.
   s) SUBCONTRACTOR must complete a job which is contracted; is liable for damages if incomplete.

Any falsification and/or misrepresentation of the above criteria for SUBCONTRACTOR as defined by the Federal and State regulations,

Figure 4-1
An example of a subcontractor's agreement that is professionally written, comprehensive, and legally protects both the transcription business and subcontractor. Minor adjustments may be needed in wording depending on state laws.

will result in immediate termination of contract and reimbursement for any and all damages as a result of this falsification or misrepresentation.

2. CSN during the term of this contract may engage other independent contractors and/or employees to perform the same work that SUBCONTRACTOR performs hereunder.

DURATION

Either party may cancel this contract on thirty (30) days notice.

LIABILITY

The work to be performed under this contract will be performed entirely at SUBCONTRACTOR's risk, and SUBCONTRACTOR assumes all responsibility for all of his/her normal operating expenses necessary for the performance of this contract. SUBCONTRACTOR agrees to save and hold CSN free and harmless from any and all damages and liabilities occasioned by the acts, negligence or misfeasance of SUBCONTRACTOR while engaged in his/her duties pursuant to this contract. SUBCONTRACTOR acknowledges above criteria for independent contractor and states that in fact, s/he falls within such guidelines as to be called SUBCONTRACTOR.

In the performance of work herein contemplated, SUBCONTRACTOR is an independent contractor with the authority to control and direct the performance of the details of the work, CSN being only interested in the results obtained. Therefore, SUBCONTRACTOR agrees to comply with all federal, state and municipal laws, rules and regulations that are now or may in the future become applicable to SUBCONTRACTOR or his/her business. These shall include, but not be limited to, obtaining any necessary business licenses and paying his/her own federal, state and municipal taxes as a self-employed individual. SUBCONTRACTOR agrees to provide evidence to CSN that s/he is complying with this provision of the contract. Failure to make said evidence available will constitute a breach of this contract and result in CSN's right to immediately cancel this contract. The measure of damages for breach of this provision of the contract shall be the actual losses suffered by CSN as a result. These include, but are not limited to, any sums required to be paid to federal, state or municipal entities by CSN because of SUBCONTRACTOR's failure to comply with said laws.

DATE: _____

NAME OF COMPANY   SUBCONTRACTOR

_____   _____
Partner

Figure 4-1 Continued

SUBCONTRACTORS AGREEMENT

The following contract is made between _____
_____ hereinafter referred to
as CSN, and

_____
Name of Subcontractor

_____
Address

_____
City, State, Zip

CSN is engaged in the business of providing medical transcription services to various medical entities in the surrounding community. At times of increased work load, CSN requests the support services on a temporary or piece work basis and wishes to contract with SUBCONTRACTOR to provide this additional medical transcription service.

DESCRIPTION OF WORK

1. CSN will contact SUBCONTRACTOR when there is overflow work to be performed.
2. If SUBCONTRACTOR accepts the work, s/he agrees to complete the job accordingly or s/he will fall within the clause of Breach of Contract. The job is to be completed in a timely manner within the reasonable legal expectations of medical transcription documents.
3. If SUBCONTRACTOR cannot meet the requirements of #2, then CSN has the right to immediately cancel this contract and reissue job lot to another subcontractor. SUBCONTRACTOR also acknowledges risk of penalty fee of $_____ for noncompletion. (See completion clause).
4. Any work which is subcontracted out by SUBCONTRACTOR must also be reviewed by SUBCONTRACTOR for accuracy before submitting to CSN.

PAYMENT

CSN will pay SUBCONTRACTOR for the work performed under this contract, according to the following schedule:

1. All piece work performed for ___ will be paid at $0.00/line.
2. All piece work performed for ___ will be paid by lump sum for job lot.
3. All other payment schedules for various medical entities are paid at $0.00/line.
4. Payment will be made within 45 days or sooner of satisfactory completion of job.

Figure 4–1 *Continued*

inefficiency of transcribers. However, in order to be ready for anything, one must be prepared with at least one mini, or the opportunity of getting one if needed.

Once it has been determined which equipment will be used most frequently, quality equipment should be purchased. A service contract is usually offered upon purchase, and if the quantity of transcribers is small, it might be worthwhile to purchase a service contract. If the business is being set up for multiple transcribers, however, maintenance agreements on all of them might not be cost effective. New equipment does not break down often, and is usually covered under warranty for several months.

Regarding lease versus purchase, each company is different. With some companies a percentage of the original purchase price must be paid at the end of the lease in order to own the equipment. With others, ownership occurs at no charge at the end of the lease. Obviously there is a significant penalty for the ability to pay the balance over time.

Facsimile Machine ▪ This piece of equipment has rapidly become an essential to every office—especially in medical transcription where stat reports are becoming increasingly necessary. An automatic redial and the capability of stacking multiple copies are two options that should be considered when purchasing a fax machine.

Office Copy Machine ▪ This is another essential. Clients want a copy of everything sent to them for their files. A basic plain paper copier is sufficient, but it must be one that makes at least 15 copies a minute. Enlargement and reduction, previously expensive options, are now standard with nearly every copier.

Telephone Line ▪ One main phone line is essential, and a second line is necessary when the main line is busy ("call waiting" on a home phone line could work until profits allow expansion). The business line should be kept separate from the personal line and should be answered in a professional manner. An answering machine for calls that come in when the transcriptionist cannot answer the phone will keep her from missing business. Answering machines from which messages can be retrieved from an outside telephone are highly recommended.

The telephone must be located within "grabbing distance" of the transcriptionist's desk.

Cordless phones or phones with external speakers are useful, because often much time will be spent "holding" and the work pace should not have to be slowed while holding. Any time-saving device will be valuable.

Incoming Dictating Equipment ▪ Digital equipment is considered the equipment of the future. This enables the transcriptionist to work from home and "key" into a main source of dictation. However, it is very sophisticated for the small service, in addition to being cost-prohibitive and unnecessary.

Answering Machine ▪ A simple answering machine might be all that is needed. An outgoing message might inform the dictator of the name of the service and the instructions for dictation. A *short* message is all that is necessary—dictators will be calling repeatedly, and will tire quickly of a long message. Installation of another telephone line is required (the cheapest phone service available, because outgoing calls will not be necessary). Incoming cassettes of the 60- or 90-minute variety should be used, *not* the 120, as the tone quality is poor.

As business increases, the transcriptionist might soon find that she has become a slave to her answering machine. If she ever expects to leave her office, she will need more than one answering machine, or perhaps one of another type. Each new answering machine requires a new phone line, but the telephone company can put all phones on a "hunt circuit," so that if one line is busy, a second or third line will accept the call.

Multitape System ▪ An alternative to multiple answering machines is the multitape system. This type of equipment handles 12, 18, or 24 cassettes, which are stored in the unit until needed, then ejected. Various settings enable recording capacity to suit the needs of the transcriptionist.

There is a great difference in price between a simple answering machine and the multitape system. However, the major dictating equipment companies have lease options available, which bring the payments down to a reasonable level over time.

Postage Meter ▪ A postage meter has proved to be a big timesaver when multiple mailings, such as billing, are required. The fee for rental is nominal, and many trips to the post office are eliminated. Combined with a scale, accurate postage also assures delivery of your mail promptly.

Furniture ▪ A comfortable chair that properly supports the back is essential. Many hours will be spent sitting, and the chair must be large enough to accommodate a transcriptionist's backside, to enable her to lean back comfortably, and to change position when needed. An ergonomic or hydraulic chair is recommended.

A desk with a corner wrap will maximize usable writing and storage surface. The wrap must conform to the contour of the room, and a left-handed transcriptionist will require a reverse-L shape.

File cabinets are necessary to hold the stationery and forms for each client. Clutter can cause confusion. It is recommended that one start with more space than needed, rather than having to expand later. Single letter-size drawer file cabinets work very well for multiple clients, as each drawer can hold a good-sized stack of stationery and envelopes and can be labeled individually, so supplies can be located quickly. A bookcase for reference material should be close at hand.

Reference Material ▪ A current medical dictionary and drug book are absolute essentials, as is an English dictionary. Books with explanations and definitions are much better than word lists for a beginner, but word books are informative as well. In addition, telephone books from the areas covered by the transcriptionist are essential. If space is at a premium, the "Physicians" sections should be cut out of the yellow pages. A complete ZIP code directory is also a necessary purchase.

As a medical transcriptionist's business grows, so will the reference library. There are dozens of books considered essential by medical transcriptionists, and everyone's library reflects the specialties for which they transcribe and their personal taste. Again, networking with other professionals will help in the choice of reference material. For further information refer to Chapter 11. It is expensive to keep up with current editions, but this is a business expense and is vital to a medical transcriptionist's effectiveness.

Payroll ▪ Employees must be paid on a regular basis. Although the company may have to wait 60 to 90 days for payment, according to most state laws, this cannot affect the staff. It is best to let employees know what is required of them with regard to payroll, the frequency of payment, and what time of day their check will be available.

The person assigned to compute payroll must have some mathematics ability, a calculator, tax tables, and a thorough understanding of Circular E, the "Employer's Tax Guide." Withholding of Social Security (FICA) and state and federal taxes is based on tables provided by the Internal Revenue Service and each state.

If bills go out once a month, money will be received throughout the month, peaking around the 20th, dwindling toward the 1st. This peak has been seen to get later into the month during economic downtimes and moves back again as the economy improves (Figure 4–2).

A solution to this problem is to bill twice a month. For many clients, this may be difficult. However, once the clients become familiar with the billing system, they either write two checks a month, or pay every other bill. Very large clients (i.e., hospitals) have no problem with paying twice a month, thus the cash flow crisis can be lessened.

Some time should be allowed for receipt of money before trying to make payroll. If workers turn in payroll summary sheets on the 1st and 15th, then clients should be billed at that time, and a week should be allotted before producing payroll. The summary sheet (Figure 4–3), which tabulates all the figures on the daily log sheets, is used for checks and balances for payroll records. Payday could be on the 8th and the 22nd.

Tax deposits must be made periodically, depending on the amount withheld from employees' gross pay. Quarterly and annual information and tax returns must be filed. There may be a service bureau in the area that specializes in small employers, and it may be cost effective to retain the service even for less than five employees.

Payroll service bureaus are specialists that have the resources to keep up with the ever-changing laws and deposit requirements. Most will take the input over the phone, via courier, or by modem. Most offer 1- to 2-day turnaround. They can make sure that all employees are paid the federal minimum wage and overtime is calculated correctly. They can make tax deposits and file returns correctly and on time.

For the small business owner with more than five employees, this one service is almost a re-

ABC TRANSCRIPTION SERVICE, INC.
"Specialists in Medical Transcription"
123 Main Street
Woodland Hills, XY 12345-0000
Telephone (013) 458-0299
FAX (013) 548-0198

Statement date	12/16/9X
Client number	151

Neil D. Bullock, M. D.
890 Garfield Avenue, Suite 100
Woodland Hills, XY 12345-0000

11/30/9X	Balance forward	292.80
12/04/9X	12 lines	1.56
12/09/9X	22 lines	2.86
12/13/9X	Payment on account	-292.80
	Balance due	4.42

BAL FWD	CURR CHGS	PAYMENTS	NEW BALANCE
292.80	4.42	292.80	4.42

PLEASE PUT ACCOUNT NUMBERS ON CHECK.

Figure 4–2
An example of a billing statement to a client.

quirement. Especially when cash is tight, there is a temptation not to make that payroll tax deposit when it is due. Take the temptation away and have the service bureau debit the checking account and make the deposit. Although a little interest will be lost that would have been earned on the money for two or three days, the 10 to 100 per cent penalty imposed for not making the deposit on time adds up very fast. Check competing services in the area, talk to other clients of theirs, and learn what service is offered at what price.

FINANCIAL MANAGEMENT

The success of a business hinges, to a great degree, on how well managed that business is. Even a sole proprietorship with no employees requires management skills for both day-to-day decisions and long-term planning. Such decisions can be made intelligently only when the financial effect of them can be predicted with reasonable accuracy. The predictions in most cases are based on past performance. Therefore, it is critical for the small business owner to have

SEMI-MONTHLY SUMMARY SHEET
Please submit by the 1st or 16th of each month!

NAME: _____

1 through 15 or 16 through end of _____ , 199__

DATE	CLIENT	# LINES	# HOURS			DATE	CLIENT	# LINES	# HOURS

TOTAL # OF LINES _____ × $ _____ /line = Total Amount Due $ _____
TOTAL # OF HOURS _____ × $ _____ /hour = Total Amount Due $ _____
TOTAL AMOUNT TO BE PAID $ _____

Figure 4–3

An example of a summary sheet that tabulates all the figures on the daily log sheets. This is used for checks and balances for payroll records.

and understand accurate financial information. In addition, the prospective business owner must have a clear understanding of the amount of cash that will be required and the financial risks involved in starting a business. An accountant is an essential part of this process, especially if the business is new to the owner. The business owner not only will be more prepared for the future by knowing the risks but also will become aware much sooner when changes are necessary. Remember, "people don't plan to fail, they fail to plan."

One can go through several exercises to get an idea of what may be involved in the new venture. A projected Income Statement is an estimate of income and related expenses over a period of time. Usually calculated on the accrual basis, this matches sales and costs to generate the sales over time. A projected Balance Sheet will state the assets and liabilities of a company at a point in time — it is a snapshot of the financial position. A projected Cash Flow is an analysis of the checkbook. Deposits and disbursements are estimated, with no effort to match them with the time period in which they were incurred.

Depending on geographic location, the market for services, the prevailing wages in the area, state or local requirements, and so on may not apply. When projecting into the future, especially with a new venture, certain assumptions must be made. The assumptions made are:

- The business form is that of a Sole Proprietor. The owner performs some transcription.

- All expenses are paid as incurred. Vendors are not extending credit.

- The owner is not withdrawing funds from the business, other than those earned as a transcriptionist.

- The owner is in the 15 per cent federal income tax bracket, the 8 per cent state income tax bracket, and on the cash basis of accounting for tax purposes.

- Accounts receivable are collected within 45 days.

- Equipment is leased over 60 months.

- The owner has the ability to finance the first months of operation, interest free.

- Estimated tax payments are based on the current year income.

Insurance

In today's changing insurance market, many policies are available. As a business owner, it is necessary to protect both income and property from unexpected loss.

Property Insurance ■ To protect business property in the event of a physical catastrophe (fire, theft, or other disaster), property insurance is a necessity. If the business is run from the home, often this can be included in the homeowner's or renter's policy, but the amount of equipment covered is often limited; a separate rider may be required for extensive coverage of equipment. To assure a tax deduction for the increased expense, a separate check should be written for the additional amount that applies to the business equipment. Request that the policy include a replacement cost rider. Damaged or destroyed equipment will be replaced with new equipment of a similar type, style, quality, and capability. This is extremely important, since without it, the amount of loss is only the current value of the equipment *as determined by the insurance company*. The replacement cost rider is well worth the expense.

Disability Insurance ■ Disability insurance provides protection in the event of physical or mental disability that results in the inability to continue to produce income. Private plans are available, as are individual, group plans, and some state plans.

In California, State Disability Insurance (SDI) is required for all employees working within the state, unless the employer provides a voluntary plan.* The employee pays the premium for this insurance through a mandatory payroll deduction. In addition, a self-employed person may elect coverage under the plan by paying quarterly premiums based on maximum quarterly earnings. The coverage is then the same for all covered under the plan. SDI benefits

---

*State programs for nonindustrial disability insurance exist in five states (California, Hawaii, New Jersey, New York, Rhode Island) and Puerto Rico. In each area the law is known by a different name.

are paid after the covered individual has missed at least three continuous days of work due to a nonwork-related injury, as documented by a physician. Benefits are based on past earnings and are paid for as long as the individual is out of work, up to a maximum of 52 weeks.

Group plans are available, sometimes through professional organizations, but they may require a minimum group size of ten or more. Premiums, usually paid monthly, are based on the age of the employee and the amount of wages earned. The employer can structure the policy to be effective only after State Disability has been exhausted. The employer may also be able to select limits, time periods for coverage, and the date coverage is to take effect.

An individual disability policy is the most flexible and can be structured to meet the policyholder's specific needs and financial requirements. Obtained through an insurance agent, it is usually the most expensive way to get disability benefits but can provide the most comprehensive coverage for the longest time period. Premiums are based on earnings, age, occupation, and benefits chosen. Riders may be available that allow for increased coverage based on inflation and earning ability. In addition, a rider may be purchased to provide benefits based on the ability of the policyholder to perform a specific profession only—a valuable benefit for skilled professions, when the disability is not severe enough to prevent work other than at the time of the disability. Premiums can be reduced by making the policy effective only after a certain period of disability (usually between 30 and 180 days.) This is useful when an individual policy is combined with either a group or state plan.

Life Insurance ▪ In the event of the death of the policyholder, life insurance provides protection for a named beneficiary. For a business owner, the beneficiary may be the business (if not a sole proprietorship), a partner, a creditor, or any other interested party. There are three basic types of life insurance: term, whole, and universal; specific policies can be combined to make a hybrid of them.

Term life, available individually or through a group, is usually the most inexpensive form of life insurance. Many professional associations provide group term insurance at nominal cost as a membership benefit. The face amount of the policy is the amount that will be paid to the beneficiary in the event of the covered individual's death. Premiums are paid each year for that policy year. The policyholder may cancel the policy at any time, and, unless the policy is guaranteed renewable, the insurer may choose not to renew at any policy anniversary. Premiums can increase with the insured's age, thus at some point they may become prohibitive.

Traditionally, life insurance has been what is known as *whole life*. This type of policy builds up a cash value as premiums are paid over the years. This cash value may be borrowed against, usually at a low interest rate. Premiums may be higher than for term life coverage, especially when both policies are compared at a young age. They are purchased through an insurance agent. The choice of benefits is usually great, and professional advice on structuring the plan to a specific situation should be sought.

In the past ten years, *universal life* has been offered as a sort of hybrid life insurance policy. Combining the benefits of term and group with a savings plan, this type of policy may suit certain financial situations. Again, professional advice on structuring a plan to specific needs should be sought.

Professional Liability Insurance ▪ Providing protection in the event of error or omission that causes another harm, professional liability insurance is a necessity in many professions in today's litigious society, especially those professions associated with the medical field. Coverage may be available through professional associations at a discounted rate. Limits may be based on sales or a set amount per claim. Prior acts may be covered for an additional premium.

FEDERAL, STATE, COUNTY, AND CITY LAWS

Laws with which a business owner must comply are varied and numerous, too numerous to list or explain here. Four basic areas with which an owner needs to be concerned include:

- Labor laws
- Payroll tax
- Income tax
- Sales tax

Check with local and state authorities to determine how these would apply to your transcription business.

Labor laws concerning employees' rights have mushroomed in the past several years. These laws govern working conditions, payment of employees, and other required employee benefits, as well as defining employees and other terms. Local, state, and federal regulations require the employer to comply with whichever is the most restrictive of the three. In addition to requiring Workers' Compensation Insurance, which must be carried by every employer in most states, the posting of certain notices in a conspicuous place is also required. The State Labor Board will be able to help determine which notices apply to a transcription service.

Payroll tax laws regulate the amount of payroll taxes that must be withheld from each employee's pay and how and when those amounts must be remitted to the government. Amounts withheld from an employee are considered trust funds. Severe penalties are imposed for neglecting to submit these funds to the government on time. The Internal Revenue Service publishes Circular E-Employers Tax Guide, which states the rules for federal payroll tax deposits. Each state publishes a similar bulletin if state withholding and taxes are required. The employee pays federal income tax and social security (FICA) through payroll deductions. The employer pays FICA and Federal Unemployment. Some states also require income tax and disability or unemployment tax to be withheld. Other states require the employer to pay the unemployment tax.

Based on the net income of the business, either the business entity itself (if a corporation or partnership) or the business owner (if a sole proprietorship) will pay a tax. If a separate entity, a separate tax return is filed for that entity. The entity then pays the tax owed. A sole proprietor, on the other hand, includes the business income and expenses on her own personal tax return on Schedule C—Profit or Loss from a Business or Profession. From the net income, self-employment tax is figured (FICA for sole proprietors). The net income from the business is included with all other income and loss amounts for the year to determine the taxable income. There are income tax benefits and restrictions to all business forms, and they should be researched to determine which is right for a particular situation. An accountant or attorney can help with the specific benefits that apply in the situation.

State sales tax may be a factor to consider. Some states, in their never-ending search for revenues, are imposing sales taxes on services rendered, not just products sold. If this is the case where the business is established, this will require collection of tax from clients and remitting same to the state on a regular basis. The sales tax return usually requires a reconciliation of total sales with taxable sales for the period and how the tax is calculated. A local accountant can determine how to comply with the law.

NEGOTIATION AND CONTRACT

Negotiations and contracts may be the most important factor in the success of a transcription service. How good the owner is at win/win negotiating will affect contracts awarded and work profits. Each contract entered into with a customer should clearly state:

- Rate charged
- Unit of measure
- Turnaround and/or delivery time
- Payment terms
- Output format (including the number of revisions allowed and under what specific circumstances)

By agreeing on these terms up front, much discussion, misunderstanding, and grounds for disagreement will be eliminated. The agreement should always be in writing, contain a date for review and/or renegotiation, and be signed and dated by both parties and a witness. If uncomfortable with a formal contract, a letter to a new client stating the terms will create an understanding and give the business an air of professionalism.

Subcontractors may be of great help especially during busy times (see Auxiliary Personnel Section and Payroll Section). To be classified as an independent contractor, the person must meet several conditions, otherwise he or she will be classified as an employee for federal and state withholding purposes. Table 4-1 summarizes the 20-factor chart used to determine whether a

Table 4-1 ■ **Common Law Employment Test of the Internal Revenue Service**

Factor	Suggests Employment	Suggests Independent Contractor
1. Instructions	Firm instructs on location, hours, methods of service, or firm has the right to do so	Absence of firm's right to instruct on, for example, location, hours, methods
2. Training	Firm provides training	No training by firm
3. Integration	Worker's services are "integral" part of firm's operation and critical to firm's success	Worker's services are "incidental" to firm's operations
4. Services rendered personally	Worker must render services personally	Worker can delegate or subcontract
5. Hiring/supervising paying assistants	Worker may hire/supervise and pay assistants only with firm's approval	Worker has discretion to hire/supervise and pay assistants
6. Duration of relationship	Lengthy, indefinite, or otherwise open-ended	Limited in time or as to specific result
7. Hours of work	Set by firm or inflexible	Set by worker
8. Amount of time required	Substantially full-time	Less than full-time
9. Workplace	Firm's premises	Off-premises of firm (e.g., worker's office)
10. Order or sequence of work	Set by firm	Set by worker
11. Reports	Worker provides oral/or written progress reports	No reports provided by worker
12. Methods of payment	Hour, day, week, or other measure of time	Nontime-based, e.g., lump sum for result, piecework
13. Business/travel expense	Reimbursed by firm	Paid by worker without reimbursement
14. Tools/materials	Provided by firm	Provided by worker
15. Significant investment	Firm provides facilities/equipment	Worker provides facilities/equipment
16. Realization of profit or loss	Worker cannot realize profit or loss (risk of nonpayment not viewed by IRS as loss)	Worker has investment/expenses, works for set price dependent on outcome, or otherwise has risk of profit or loss
17. Work for multiple firms	Worker has exclusive relationship with firm	Worker has multiple clients
18. Making services available to public	Worker doesn't "hold self out" to public	Worker advertises, has own office, has business cards
19. Firm's right to fire	Firm can fire worker at will	Worker cannot be fired at will in middle of contract term/project without firm liability for breach of contract
20. Worker's right to quit	Worker may quit at will	Worker must complete contract term/project or else have liability for breach of contract

worker is an independent contractor or employee. As the employer, the business owner may then be liable for any amounts that should have been withheld (and were not) for the period the independent contractor was deemed to be employed. Be careful! The basic tests are as follows:

- The independent contractor (IC) is in the business of providing transcription services.

- The IC can provide this service to other transcription services.

- The IC determines the method of producing the transcription and the equipment used. She usually provides her own equipment and work space.

- The business contracting with an IC determines only what the IC produces, not how it is produced.

- The business provides Form 1099-MISC to any IC who provides more than $600 in services in a calendar year.

To further assure that the independent contractor is, indeed, independent and not an employee, obtain copies of the contractor's local business license, workers' compensation insurance certificate, and professional liability insurance certificate; also a signed statement outlining the understanding that the person is, in fact, an independent contractor. An attorney can help here.

BUSINESS FORMS

Sole Proprietor ■ The easiest and least expensive to create of all forms of business, the sole proprietor is simply that: one person who makes the decisions and keeps the net profit. All profits are taxed at individual rates and reported on the individual's tax return. In addition, the sole proprietor must pay Self-Employment Tax on the net profit of the business. The equivalent of Social Security Tax (FICA) withheld from employees' gross pay, Self-Employment Tax is both the employer's and employee's portion, since the sole proprietor is, in effect, both. The sole proprietor may be required to make quarterly estimated tax payments to cover the annual liability on the net income from the business.

The liability for the actions of the business and its representatives is unlimited for the sole proprietor, which may make this an undesirable business form for one with substantial assets.

Partnership ■ A partnership is a separate legal entity, formed for a specific purpose. Between the partners, of which there can be any number, there should be a written agreement stating duties, profit-sharing, payment arrangements, contributions, buy-out provisions, and any other terms agreed upon at formation of the business. The importance of this partnership agreement is in direct relationship to the number of partners involved. It should be constructed with extreme care following the advice of an attorney, as it is designed to answer many tax and financial questions.

Although the partnership is a separate legal entity, liability for its actions is unlimited to the general partner(s). All business profits, interest, and dividends are taxed at individual rates, but some states may have a minimum state tax which must be paid in advance each year. Since the income is taxed to each partner, they may be required to make quarterly estimated tax payments, depending on their personal tax situation.

Corporation ■ A legal and formally established separate legal entity, a corporation may be the most difficult and expensive business to create. Stock is issued to shareholders, and liability is limited to each shareholder's investment in the stock of the corporation. Tax laws and rates differ from those applied to individuals.

Business profits are taxed at the corporate rate (if a C-Corporation), or the individual rate (if an S-Corporation). A financial advisor or attorney can advise which form is better for the situation. Some states impose a minimum state tax, regardless of income, which must be paid in advance each year. Either the corporation (C-Corp) or the shareholders (S-Corp) may be required to make quarterly estimated tax payments, depending on income.

BILLING STATEMENTS

Pricing Your Work ■ Before setting fees, it is important to determine one's worth as a transcriptionist. Fifteen dollars an hour "should" be an absolute minimum.

To determine the fee schedule, the number of lines produced in an hour should be computed. Charge by line is currently the most popular method of billing. The dollar amount desired should be divided by the number of lines produced to determine the fee for services.

> *Example*: For a desired income of $20/hour, with a production of 250 lines/hour: $20 is divided by 250, which yields 8 cents. Therefore, 8 cents/line should be charged.

There are other ways to charge, however. Billing by the hour might be judged negatively in comparison with what a doctor might pay someone in the office, even though the home-based medical transcriptionist is an independent contractor for the doctor's office. In addition, if rates are on an hourly basis, there must be total discipline (i.e., one cannot get up during transcribing reports to wash clothes, change the baby, or make personal phone calls). It is sometimes better to charge by the piece.

Other methods of charging are by the character, the word, or the page. The first can become confusing, not only to the client but to the transcriptionist. An advantage of this, however, is that the computer can count it fairly accurately, and time does not have to be wasted counting individual reports. The word is similar to the character, and easily done by the computer. The page is easier to count; however, the page must be defined (as must any billing unit), otherwise the same amount of money would be charged for a fifty-line page as for a two-line page. Although the page count may sound great, it does not lend itself well to statistical analysis and is too easily disputed. With the line count, "what you see is what you get."

Revisions require a different measure of charging. First, it must be determined how client's errors versus transcriptionist's errors and/or omissions will be corrected and billed. One's time can vary with revisions (and copy typing), and the rate charged should be agreed upon in the contract. The hypothetical $20 can be divided into quarters, with 15 minutes being a minimum charge and each quarter hour an additional $5. Or use a 10-minute increment as the base in charging, with $3/10 minutes for an $18/hour fee, and so on. An accurate track of time must be kept and presented in writing with the bill.

BOOKKEEPING

An elaborate bookkeeping system is not necessary, but if the basics are adhered to, growth can be painless.

Accounts Receivable ■ This is the money billed out for work done. Billing may be once a month or twice a month, but the schedule should be addressed in the contract and remain consistent. If billing is done regularly, the payment is more likely to be received regularly.

At the end of each batch of work (for an individual client), a batch sheet (Figure 4–4) is created, in duplicate or triplicate, containing the necessary information for the client, the transcriptionist, and the business owner. The original is sent to the client, a copy goes to the transcriptionist, and a copy is kept by the service owner. The client is instructed to keep his or her copy as a double check when the statement is received. The service owner's copy is a double check on work done.

Accounts Payable ■ This is the money paid out to creditors: phone bill, supplies, computer service contract, and so on. Prompt payment of bills looks good on one's credit rating. A business-size check book, perhaps with a perforated sheet for payroll deductions, is helpful. Balancing one's checkbook is essential—if this cannot be done personally, an accountant should be found who understands the fact that the owner is just starting out and who can grow with the new business owner.

Tax Reports ■ Federal payroll taxes withheld must be deposited periodically. The amount and frequency of deposits vary, depending on the amount withheld from employee pay. State payroll taxes may also have to be deposited. Check Circular E-Employer's Tax Guide, published by the IRS, for specific details.

In addition, quarterly tax payments must be made for state income and unemployment taxes (quarters ending March, June, September, and December); taxes are due by the end of the following month.

ABC TRANSCRIPTION SERVICE, INC.

"Specialists in Medical Transcription"

123 Main Street
Woodland Hills, XY 12345-0000
Tel: 013/458-0299
Fax: 013/548-0198

_____

_____

_____

TOTAL LINES _____   DATE _____

TOTAL REPORTS _____   TRANSCRIPTIONIST _____

CASE NAME	# LINES	DATE	CASE NAME	# LINES	DATE

Figure 4–4
An example of a batch sheet containing information for the client, transcriptionist, and business owner.

COLLECTING OVERDUE ACCOUNTS

Thirty days is a reasonable amount of time for collection of monies due. However, the amount due may not be paid within a 30-day period. Consider this and the fact that the business will need adequate financial backing to withstand late payments when starting out and when negotiating contracts.

Hospitals generally take 45 to 90 days to pay. Large medical groups can take even longer. Most private physicians pay in 30 days or less (and can be "shaken down" more easily than hospitals and large medical groups).

On the letter of intent (contract), it should be stated that monies are due in full within 30 days of statement. It may be desired to charge interest (the going rate) for past due balances. If so, this must be stated on the statement. A discount might be offered for monies paid in less time. (All this complicates what is supposed to be a "simple" billing system, however.) It also should be stated in the contract that if payment is not received within (so many) days, work will be held until payment is received.

When the 30-day time period has passed, the client should be notified that the account is PAST DUE. At 45 days, phone calls should be made. The person in charge of the account should be contacted first, then the accounts payable department. The name of a responsible individual should be obtained. Ascertain that the person is familiar with the transcription service and knows that the service is small and cannot wait any longer for payment. Calls should be made again at 60 days, then at 70, then 80, then 90 days. The client should be pestered but not harassed. Any contact regarding billing should be documented, including who was contacted, the person's title, and what was said. Not only does this provide proof of collection attempts should it be necessary to sue, it also provides a future record of the client contacts and who can obtain results.

If the amount being billed continues to increase, the client should be terminated (for breach of contract) before further damage occurs. Small Claims court is an inexpensive way to enforce collection. Commercial collection agencies may be of use, but weigh the amount kept as commission by the agency before retaining one (usually up to 50 per cent of all amounts collected). Often the first payment is the hardest one to get. One should not wait past 45 days to announce one's presence. Perhaps no communication has been made between the contact person (office manager) and the bookkeeping department, and it is up to the service owner to establish this connection.

Remember—a good client may become a worthless client if he doesn't pay.

One should always have a slush fund of one month's billing in reserve, allowing for the 30- to 60-day lag. It is good if this can be set aside and forgotten. If not, some "creative financing" has to be devised.

OBTAINING CREDIT

From a Bank ■ A line of credit should be obtained for a month's worth of receivables (this line of credit should grow as receivables grow). The bank will need collateral. They prefer money. If this is available, so much the better. If not, they should be offered equipment, stocks/bonds, and if necessary, receivables—a guarantee on the money due the service—which they may take if loan payments cannot be made.

From Credit Cards ■ As many credit cards as possible that have check-writing capabilities should be obtained. They should be used only when absolutely necessary (because of higher interest rates), after bank borrowing is at the maximum.

There should be no need to go any further than this. All other expenditures should be budgeted for, and one should be able to live within one's budget. The only thing that cannot be budgeted for is an increase in business. This increase can be devastating, if room for growth is not predetermined.

BANKING

Establish a relationship with a banker before the need for one arises. The old adage is true: "Banks only lend you money when you can prove that you don't need it." Get to know the bank manager by name, stop in and say hello when making a deposit or cashing a check, keep her or him updated on how well the business is doing. People like to be around winners and bankers are no different.

Business Checking ▪ The business checking account must be just that, business. All business receipts are deposited to it. Only business expenses are paid from it. The owner's salary is an expense that should be paid regularly. This account is not a private slush fund. It is the best place to get an idea of how the business is faring, and that cannot be done if the account is confused with personal items. Even if there is a fee, have the cancelled checks returned with the statement monthly. This will assist in reconciling the account, and should the business be subject to an audit, the actual checks may help prove deductions taken.

Retirement Accounts ▪ One of the benefits of being in business is the ability to set up tax-deferred accounts specifically designed to allow individuals to save for their retirement. All funds accumulate tax-deferred until they are withdrawn between ages $59\frac{1}{2}$ and $70\frac{1}{2}$ years.

The Individual Retirement Account (IRA) is the simplest version of this account. Depending on the earned income, an individual can contribute up to $2000/year to this account. It can be set up at a bank, a mutual fund company, or a variety of other financial institutions. The paperwork is minimal and record keeping consists of maintaining a record of the amounts deferred from tax (the annual contribution).

For self-employed individuals, the Keogh Plan can be similar to an IRA, but the limits for contributions are much higher and vary with net income from the business and the type of plan chosen. When the plan value exceeds $25,000, there is some administrative work and tax filing, but for a single person (or husband and wife only) involved in the plan, the filing is simple and easily handled. Two types of Keogh Plan are available, a defined benefit plan and a profit-sharing plan. Check with a financial advisor to see which plan is right for the business.

For the business owner who wants to offer a retirement savings plan to employees, the Simplified Employee Pension (SEP) may be the answer. Both employees and owners may be eligible, depending on the plan document. The maximal contribution that can be made by each employee depends on that employee's income but will probably be higher than what can be

contributed to an IRA. The employer may or may not contribute to each employee's account. Each employee's account is administered separately; the employee gets periodic statements sent directly to the home, where the performance of the investment can be monitored. Since the contributions are made by the employee through payroll deduction, the money in the plan is always 100 per cent vested to the employee, who may withdraw it at any time (maybe with penalty) and take it on leaving the employer.

Other retirement and pension plans are available for the business owner, but most require complex administration and application of discrimination rules. A financial advisor can help determine what is right for the business.

MARKETING, PROMOTION, AND PUBLIC RELATIONS

Business Cards, Stationery, Logo ▪ Professional stationery, business cards, even forms do not have to be expensive (Figure 4–5). What is most important is that they be professionally printed, possibly in two or three colors, including a logo. Nothing is gained by sending a flyer for a "professional" medical transcription service that has been run off on a copier on its last legs, and worse still with typos, on cheap copy paper, with a typed-in heading. Even computer-generated stationery, which can look good, gives a less than professional overall appearance.

Everything that is sent out of the office should be proofread completely with a clear head (and that includes work!). Don't forget to do a final check on professionally printed items, too! No one is infallible. Nothing turns off a potential client faster than a letter of solicitation that is sloppily assembled on the page or has misspellings.

A large, expensive order is not necessary. An order of 100 sheets of stationery, 100 second (blank) pages, 100 envelopes, and 100 business cards should cost less than $100.

Designed with some degree of creativity, a logo can set one transcription service apart from all others. Common logos are typewriter keyboards, computer screens, telephones, or a graphic made from the company initials (Figure 4–5).

ABC TRANSCRIPTION SERVICE
"Specialists in Medical Transcription"

Jane Sutton, CMT
123 Main Street
Any City, XY 12345-0000

Office 013-438-0987
Fax   013-287-0945

S.T.A.T.

Typing and Transcription

Mary English, CMT   Lynn Keene, CMT
013-345-9088   013-459-0023

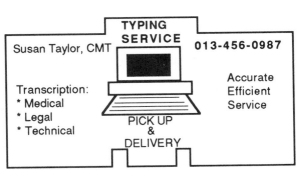

TYPING SERVICE

Susan Taylor, CMT   **013-456-0987**

Transcription: Accurate
* Medical   Efficient
* Legal   Service
* Technical

PICK UP
&
DELIVERY

Figure 4–5
Examples of several types of business cards illustrating logos and design layout.

ADVERTISING

The area in which one lives can contribute significantly to the success of advertising (Figure 4–6). A direct mail solicitation in a large metropolitan area may go unnoticed, whereas a friendly "Hi Neighbor" letter in a small rural area may command instant attention. The direct mail letter can be generated from a hospital staff list, a specialty directory, or the telephone book. Often a receptionist will file the letter away and will call if and when she needs transcription service.

A second type of letter, similar to the direct mail solicitation but more specifically intended, can be generated by reading the "Help Wanted" section in the Sunday paper. Such a letter might read, "This is in response to your recent ad in the Daily Herald. . . ."

A third letter can be generated upon receipt of an inquiry, usually by phone, from someone who has heard of the service and wants to know prices, turn-around time, and other details. A letter similar to the aforementioned can be used,

changing the opening sentences to read, "Thank you for your inquiry regarding our service. . . ." (Figure 4–7).

More useful than direct mail (especially with the cost of postage) is an advertisement in the journal of the county medical society and/or state medical association (see Figure 4–6). The cost of a display ad can be prohibitive, but the Classified Section, specifically under "Business Services" or even "Medical Transcription" (if one is lucky enough to encounter such a listing), can bring a number of inquiries each time the journal is published. Costs vary from journal to journal and from area to area. With this type of exposure, all phone calls received are positive ones, eliminating the personal "rejection factor" which is inherent in "cold calls." This method may provide personal contact with the physician, obviating the need to deal directly with the office staff and enabling establishment of a working relationship with the actual client.

If one ever has occasion to enter a medical office building, it might be wise to have on hand a handful of business cards or letters of intro-

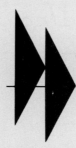

Hagedorn Secretarial Service, Inc.

"SPECIALISTS IN MEDICAL TRANSCRIPTION"

510 ZENITH DRIVE. GLENVIEW. IL 60025 (708) 296-0034

September 24, 1990

Illinois Medicine
Suite 700
20 N. Michigan
Chicago IL 60602

Please run the attached ad for the next 12 issues of Illinois
Medicine. Enclosed please find $53.00.

BOGGED DOWN WITH DICTATION? 24 hour phone in central dictation
system or your own cassettes. Will transcribe all your progress
notes, office correspondence and referral letters. Manuscript
preparation. Word processing. HSS, Inc., Specialists in Medical
Transcription. 708/296-0034. Toll free dictation.

Sincerely,

HAGEDORN SECRETARIAL SERVICE

Jackie Abern, President

Figure 4–6
Sample letter to a medical journal purchasing advertising space.

duction to distribute to each of the physicians' offices. This increases the likelihood of being remembered and called when the need arises. It is wise not to be pushy, just friendly and helpful, maintaining a low-key personality and promoting a high quality of professional work.

Listings in telephone books have been proved ineffectual in large metropolitan areas. First, very few Yellow Pages have a section for Medical Transcription, so that a medical transcription service will be listed under "secretarial services," resulting in requests to type résumés, or under "medical services," resulting in requests for laboratory work.

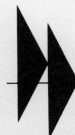

Hagedorn Secretarial Service, Inc.

"SPECIALISTS IN MEDICAL TRANSCRIPTION"

510 ZENITH DRIVE. GLENVIEW. IL 60025 (708) 296-0034

November 14, 1991

Phyllis Bellair
Vernon Hills Pediatrics
10 Phillip Road
Vernon Hills, IL 60061

Dear Ms. Bellair:

Thank you for your recent inquiry concerning HAGEDORN SECRETARIAL
SERVICE. We are one of the largest exclusively medical
transcription services in the Greater Chicago area, currently in
our third decade of service to the medical community. Our
transcriptionists are qualified in all branches of medical
dictation and our reputation is one of consistently accurate work,
fast turnaround time, and a delivery service which can provide you
with stat reports within an hour or two.

Our fee is based on the number of lines we transcribe (15
cents/line, standard sized stationery) and a photocopy of each
letter is provided at no extra cost. We pride ourselves in being
able to keep in personal contact with our clients at all times.
If there's anything you want us to do - just ask.

In addition to equipment for handling all types of dictation
(standard, mini- and microcassette), we have a phone-in service,
whereby you can dictate from any telephone, day or night. Our
work is done on word processing equipment and files kept
for two weeks, or longer if you like, in case you need to make
changes.

Feel free to give us a try; no account is too small or large for
us to handle. Please don't hesitate to contact me if there's
anything you'd like to discuss.

Again - thanks for your interest.

                            Sincerely,

                            HAGEDORN SECRETARIAL SERVICE, INC.

                            Jenny Hagedorn
                            Vice President

                            Jackie Abern, CMT
                            President

Figure 4-7
Sample letter to a prospective client, showing the professional stationery design and letter content.

Direct telephone solicitation can be compared with direct mail advertising in the results it generates—it will save time!

Networking has proved a reasonable source for potential clients. Meetings of a professional women's association or chamber of commerce, where people can get together after hours and exchange business cards and talk a bit about their business, can bring in many leads, and one may find some needed assistance too! The American Association for Medical Transcription is a great place to exchange information. Often a service with too much work will balance out another service that does not have enough. It can be done with a minimum of fuss.

Electronic networking is expanding the horizons for medical transcriptionists, especially those working at home. A basic understanding of electronic bulletin boards can be obtained from Melody Lee Gavigan's article ("Computer networking for medical transcriptionists") in the JAAMT, September-October, 1991, issue. Transcriptionists are eagerly lending a hand (via Prodigy, CompuServe, and other computer information services) to new and potential home workers. Many of the issues discussed in this chapter are discussed daily online, in personalized communications through the electronic network, and existing members are eager to respond to questions. (Bear in mind that communication may be read by prospective clients or contractors—and spell correctly!)

Reference Sources

References for books, journal articles, and miscellaneous publications can be found in Appendix 1.

Networking Organizations

American Association for Medical Transcription, P.O. Box 576187, Modesto, California 95357; (800) 982-2182

American Federation of Small Business, 407 South Dearborn Street, Chicago, Illinois 60605; (312) 427-0207

Internal Revenue Service Publications

Call 1-800-829-FORM (3676) to order
Publication 1—Your Rights as a Taxpayer
Publication 15—Your Federal Income Tax
Publication 334—Tax Guide for Small Business
Publication 541—Tax Information on Partnerships
Publication 910—Guide to Free Tax Services
Publication 937—Business Reporting
Circular E—Employer's Tax Guide
Form SS-8—Employee Work Status

Small Business Administration Service

Service Corps of Retired Executives (SCORE). Check the White Pages of your local phone book under U.S. Government for the local office; offers free and low cost business consulting, SBA guarantees on loans, and various other services

Local Library Resources

Periodicals, research materials, medical journals

The Accountant and/or Attorney and/or Insurance Agent

Advice on form of business
Guidance on bookkeeping system and tax compliance
Insurance advice

Equipment

INTRODUCTION

We are currently in the midst of an exciting time of growth in technology. This technologic growth has brought us the computer, which is the key piece of equipment for the medical transcriptionist. In the 1960s and 1970s the tools of the medical transcriptionist consisted of dictation disks or belts and a standard electric typewriter. Prior to that time, typists took shorthand and then transcribed on a manual typewriter.

In addition to the typewriter and the computer, there are dedicated word processors. Manual equipment is still in use in some facilities, but this appears to be rapidly changing.

DICTATION AND TRANSCRIPTION SYSTEMS

The process begins with dictation of the information to be transcribed. This is done by dictating into dictation equipment: either a desk model with microphone, a hand-held unit, or by way of telephone lines into a centralized unit. The dictation is recorded on cassettes or digitalized equipment.

Many transcriptionists working at home are currently using cassettes. However, this will change as more and more home transcriptionists switch to remote access digital systems. Cassettes come in two sizes, standard cassettes and microcassettes. Many physicians like the convenience of the smaller microcassette, but the tape is somewhat more fragile. The preference is for a good-quality standard C-60 cassette that is held together with screws. C-90 and C-120 tapes also

are available. These should be avoided as they are thinner and more susceptible to breakage.

Dictating equipment can be a combination of a dictating machine and a transcriber, or it may be simply a single unit. Medical transcriptionists are mainly concerned with the transcriber. A wide variety of machines are available with many features, such as variable backup, speed control, and one that allows the voice to remain normal when the speed is changed.

The type of machine purchased is determined by the type of work performed. If the initial clients use standard cassettes, it would be wise to purchase this type of machine first. A microcassette adapter or transcription unit can be purchased if it becomes necessary.

Most headsets are interchangeable. It is important to find the type that is most comfortable, as it will be worn many hours a day.

Many hospitals and large transcription services use dictation systems, the latest being digital systems. The physician dictates via the telephone. The dictation is recorded digitally and stored on a hard disk in a central processing unit. From this unit the transcriptionist may gain access to a given recording by her individual unit, which is like a touch-tone telephone. These systems allow for assignment of work to individual transcriptionists according to supervisory requirements, as well as monitoring of all activity on the system. Detailed database information is available for management reports. Dictation can also be re-recorded from these systems for distribution to transcriptionists using cassette transcribers.

A transcriptionist working at home may wish to have dictation equipment on site that is connected to a telephone line. Telephone call-in equipment can be as simple as a telephone answering machine for uncomplicated applications or as complex as a rotating cassette or digital system, such as those used in most hospitals. Transcriptionists should evaluate carefully this type of equipment and its expense to determine whether it would be beneficial and cost-effective for their particular operation.

COMPUTER SYSTEM

Today, computers are in standard use in transcription, although some facilities use dedicated word processors, a type of computer that is limited to word processing. Many types of equipment are available and have become less expensive as more products have appeared.

The two main types of personal computers on the market today are IBM-based and Macintosh systems. IBM systems are more widely used in certain applications but the Macintosh is also a very good system, offering easier manipulation of graphics. A consideration is that more generic parts are available and service can be more easily obtained for IBM or IBM-compatible equipment. Macintosh users will find that whatever they need has to be specifically designed for the Macintosh system, which generally pushes the cost higher.

MEDIA AND DATA STORAGE

It is no longer necessary for the medical transcriptionist to have paper copies of all transcribed material. The data can be stored on the hard drive for ready access, and then on floppy disks or streaming tape drives. For most word processing needs, a 386 computer with 1 megabyte of RAM and a 40-megabyte hard disk drive is usually adequate.

Floppy disks come in two sizes: $5\frac{1}{4}$ inch and $3\frac{1}{2}$ inch. The $5\frac{1}{4}$-inch size is more common, especially on lower-priced computers. The standard $5\frac{1}{4}$-inch diskettes, usually double-sided, can hold 360K of information. The newer high-density $5\frac{1}{4}$-inch diskettes hold 1.2 MB of data. The diskettes must be handled with care and stored in a diskette file box.

The $3\frac{1}{2}$-inch diskettes that are more rigid in construction and less vulnerable to damage with handling are preferred. These diskettes are also of two sizes: the standard, which holds 720K, and the high density, which holds 1.44 MB of data. Streaming tape drive cassettes are also available for high-volume, high-speed backups.

COMPUTER PRINTERS

The computer printer is an extremely important piece of equipment, because the document must have a professional appearance. As with computers, printer technology has come a long way. The four basic types of printers are:

- Daisy-wheel
- Dot-matrix
- Ink-jet
- Laser

Daisy-wheel printers give a clear, crisp copy. The work is neat and looks as though it were done on a typewriter. The main disadvantages to the daisy-wheel printer are its slow speed and its noise level. However, if these factors are not of primary importance, this type of printer can be purchased reasonably in the used market.

Dot-matrix printers, like daisy-wheel models, are impact printers and are widely available at the lower end of the price scale. The 24-pin dot-matrix printer provides good speed and acceptable letter quality printing, in addition to having a much faster draft mode that is excellent for rough work when applicable. The major drawback is that they are noisy. In the past the letter quality mode was not considered acceptable in certain situations, but the quality has improved and is now acceptable.

Ink-jet printers use an ink cartridge that fills a configuration of microscopic tubes with a heat element that, when energized, squirts a small droplet of ink onto the paper. While the unit cost may be initially less expensive than that of the laser, the ink cartridges are expensive, causing per page cost to become almost twice that of many laser and dot-matrix printers.

State of the art today is the laser printer. These printers range in speed from four to eleven pages per minute (these are not the industrial-type machines). They produce an ultra-clean copy at great speed and are extremely quiet. They work on the same principle as a photocopy machine. The initial cost is higher than that of most dot-matrix printers, but the difference in speed and quality may be worth it. The one drawback in regard to medical transcription is that they cannot handle multipart paper that is used in many hospitals. If not cost-prohibitive, it might be worth considering an additional impact printer for certain applications.

TYPEWRITER

A typewriter is still a piece of equipment to be considered. It can be very helpful for typing forms and is convenient for addressing envelopes. One can be purchased through a discount store.

PURCHASING VERSUS LEASING EQUIPMENT

There are many places to purchase equipment, such as retail or recycled office equipment stores, discount companies, and through reading newspaper classified advertisements for used equipment. As an independent self-employed or free-lancing transcriptionist, the equipment means one's livelihood. Therefore, it is important to purchase equipment to run the business in the most efficient and cost-effective ways possible.

It is possible to get used equipment, and for the transcriptionist just starting out, this is an economic way to begin. Many computers and printers become available as people upgrade their equipment. It is important to know who had the equipment originally and to be certain that there is a serial number on any used equipment as a guarantee that it is not of questionable origin.

New equipment can be leased. The greatest advantage of leasing is that it does not require an initial large cash output. One might consider leasing in order to avoid obsolescence in this time of booming technologic advances. There are two types of leases, operating leases and financing leases.

In an operating lease, the amount of payment and term of the lease are fixed, and at the end of the term the equipment is returned to the company. At the end of the financing lease, the lessee becomes the owner of the equipment. It is important to understand the terms of the lease. It is particularly important to know who is responsible for repair of the equipment.

If the equipment being considered is going to be used for a long period of time, then outright purchase or a financing lease should be seriously considered.

SETTING UP THE SYSTEM

When first setting up a system, it would be of value to have help from a computer consultant. However, a transcriptionist can have a "wizard" set up the system with many macros and complex adjuvants and not have a clear understanding of what has been done. This might make it difficult to connect other equipment or software to the system, thus necessitating further consulting costs.

First and foremost, the transcriptionist should learn the basics of the system and equipment to have some control of one's destiny. If someone is hired to set up the system, it is extremely important that the person comes well recommended and is someone whom the transcriptionist is able to work with. Then hire a consultant with reasonable support costs.

EQUIPMENT MAINTENANCE AND SUPPLIES

Most of the equipment needs relatively little maintenance. The number one rule is to keep it clean and dust-free. Dust covers for machines are an inexpensive form of insurance.

Keep food and drink away from equipment. If this is impossible, soft plastic keyboard covers are available that will protect debris from getting into the keyboard.

The computer is the foundation for the work performed and should not be used by children or others for game playing. Such activity could result in inadvertent loss or manipulation of data, as well as confidentiality risks.

Service contracts are available on almost any type of equipment. When medical transcriptionists worked on typewriters, it was almost essential to have a service contract because of a typewriter's mechanical nature. However, electronic equipment usually requires fewer repairs. The printer may be an exception to this as its many mechanical parts have a wear factor.

It is necessary to weigh the cost of a service call versus the cost of a service policy. Some transcriptionists do not find it cost-effective to maintain service policies and have paid for an occasional individual service call instead.

If using a Macintosh system, a service contract with the manufacturer may prove valuable, because Macintosh has its own specially trained service organization. Other computer repair services often do not handle Macintosh equipment.

The primary supplies required for a medical transcriptionist's equipment include: ink source for the printer—ribbons, toner, or multipart cartridges. It is also necessary to have a supply of floppy diskettes or streaming tape drive cassettes on hand. All these items are widely available on a discount basis, and many are also available through mail order. It pays to do a survey in cost comparison.

It is important to keep manuals for all equipment easily accessible. These manuals usually list guidelines for care and maintenance as well as directions for troubleshooting problems, which can often save the cost of a service call for repair.

EQUIPMENT FOR THE PHYSICALLY CHALLENGED

Technology in the nineties allows many more opportunities for the disabled than were previously possible. The Americans with Disabilities Act (ADA), signed in 1990, states that employers are required to make "reasonable accommodations" for disabled employees.

Standard computers present certain problems. Here are a few questions to think about: If unable to see the green LED light on the keyboard, how would a transcriptionist know whether the CAPS-LOCK key were turned on? If a person were unable to use both hands, how would one hit the CONTROL-ALT-DELETE to reboot the computer?

A number of obstacles have been addressed by the computer industry, including impairments of vision, hearing, speech, mobility, and learning. Some of the adaptive technologies available fall into the following categories: keyboard enhancement, optical scanners, speech synthesizers, and screen enlargers.

Some sources that attempt to address those issues as they apply to the physically disabled medical transcriptionist are listed here. Information may be obtained on equipment modification and special devices or assistance in the pursuit of a career as a medical transcriptionist.

The Alliance for Technology Access (ATA)
Contact: Foundation for Technology Access
1307 Solano Avenue
Albany, California 94706

Apple Computer, Inc.
Office of Special Education and
    Rehabilitation
20525 Mariani Avenue MS 43-S
Cupertino, California 95014

Closing the Gap
P.O. Box 68
Henderson, Minnesota 56044

The IBM National Support Center for
    Persons with Disabilities
P.O. Box 2150
Atlanta, Georgia 30301-2150

The Trace Research and Development Center
S-151 Waisman Center
1500 Highland Avenue
Madison, Wisconsin 53705

Health Professions Institute
P.O. Box 801
Modesto, California 95353

National Federation of the Blind (NFB)
1800 Johnson Street
Baltimore, Maryland 21230

American Foundation for the Blind (AFB)
15 West 16th Street
New York, New York 10011

LS & S Group, Inc.
P.O. Box 673
Northbrook, Illinois 60065

ERGONOMICS

Ergonomics is a buzz word of the 1990s. It is the science of arranging and designing the things with which people work in order to promote efficiency, comfort, convenience, and safety. Several important aspects to consider in relation to medical transcription are mentioned here.

The chair is of major importance in job performance. Improper height of the seat can cause stress on the spine. The thighs should be horizontal with feet elevated on a footrest to take strain off the back (be sure to allow for ankle movement with the foot pedal). If the seat is too high, make or purchase a foot stool, and if too low, obtain a cushion. In addition, there must be proper support of the spine, especially the lower back. A small pillow or cushion can be used if the chair is not adequate. Pillows can be purchased that are specially designed for lumbar support. Desks and chairs available with multiple adjustments might prove to be a wise purchase (Figure 5–1).

It is recommended that the keyboard height fall in the range of 23 to 28 inches high, and arms should be at about a 90-degree angle when the fingers are on the keyboard. Comfort of the hands and arms is very important because of

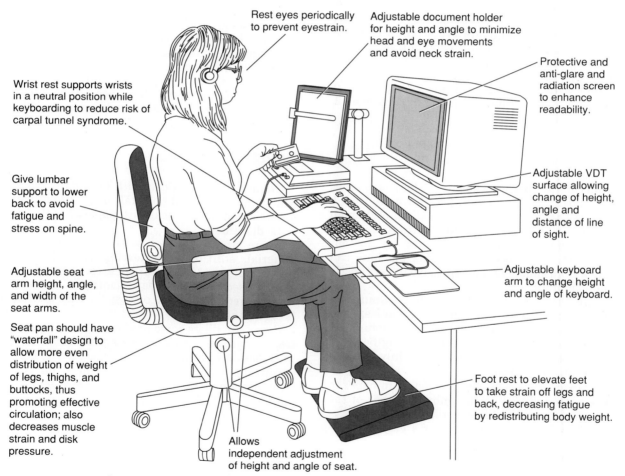

Rest eyes periodically to prevent eyestrain.

Adjustable document holder for height and angle to minimize head and eye movements and avoid neck strain.

Protective and anti-glare and radiation screen to enhance readability.

Wrist rest supports wrists in a neutral position while keyboarding to reduce risk of carpal tunnel syndrome.

Give lumbar support to lower back to avoid fatigue and stress on spine.

Adjustable seat arm height, angle, and width of the seat arms.

Seat pan should have "waterfall" design to allow more even distribution of weight of legs, thighs, and buttocks, thus promoting effective circulation; also decreases muscle strain and disk pressure.

Adjustable VDT surface allowing change of height, angle and distance of line of sight.

Adjustable keyboard arm to change height and angle of keyboard.

Foot rest to elevate feet to take strain off legs and back, decreasing fatigue by redistributing body weight.

Allows independent adjustment of height and angle of seat.

Figure 5–1
Adjustments that can be made at a work station to improve the system ergonomically.

problems of carpal tunnel syndrome experienced by those who use a keyboard extensively. Hand and arm supports are available. Elbow-armrests can be attached to the desk or chair; most importantly, a padded wrist support to keep the hands in the proper position is available.

The operator should not have to look up at the display screen. The top of the screen should not be above eye level. Glare on the screen can be reduced by rotating it or changing the angle. Brightness and contrast should be kept at a level that is comfortable to the eyes.

Eye strain is a common complaint, making proper lighting a key factor. The light source should be to one side or behind the keyboarder. A bright overhead light is difficult to deal with. Wearing dark clothing can help cut down glare. Antiglare screens are available that reduce glare and reflections, eliminate eye strain and headaches, and increase clarity and contrast.

Being aware of good working conditions and providing the proper equipment are essential to many years of medical transcribing without musculoskeletal problems and pain (Figure 5–2; Table 5–1).

FAX MACHINES

Facsimile (better known as fax) machines have been used in larger offices for more than a decade and are now seen in medium and small businesses. They enable transmitting of copies of information over phone lines for instant transferring of documents. A fax machine can range from simple and inexpensive to very costly and elaborate.

Physicians use the machines to communicate with pharmacies, insurance companies, and other physicians. A medical transcriptionist can fax a report to a physician for editing before a final report is printed, which certainly can improve final turnaround time.

Transmission is as easy as feeding in paper to be copied and dialing the phone number of the receiving machine. The transmitted copy can be typewritten, handwritten, or a graphic illustration.

The only cost of faxing a document is the expense of the phone charges plus the paper used in sending or receiving. Paper for fax machines is available at office supply stores.

Guidelines from the American Health Information Management Association (AHIMA) and the Joint Commission on Accreditation of Healthcare Organizations (JCAHO) need to be considered for the confidentiality and legality issues surrounding faxed reports as mentioned in Chapter 3.

PHOTOCOPY EQUIPMENT

The use of photocopy equipment is determined by the services one wishes to provide. With the use of a laser printer, an extra copy of a document can be provided easily and quickly. However, for an account that requires multiple copies, a photocopy machine should be available.

Many choices are available, ranging from a simple, desk-top model to a full feature model with automatic feeders and collators. The choice of a machine is determined by the volume of work expected and available funds.

The maintenance of desk-top machines requires periodic changing of the toner cartridge. The more elaborate machines need toner added and either a maintenance policy or periodic servicing.

PAPER SHREDDERS

Confidentiality is dealt with on a daily basis. Many physicians and hospitals make specific requests about how to deal with paperwork that is to be discarded.

There are a variety of ways to deal with this material, starting with tearing up the documents. Scissors (the least expensive "shredder") can be used, but if a great quantity of material needs shredding, the labor cost for that method is exceedingly high.

Paper shredders come in many sizes and range from small, inexpensive units that fit over a wastebasket to central units that are fed by conveyors for a large business. The need for this type of equipment depends on the size and requirements of a given operation.

PROBLEM SOLVING

Proper working equipment is essential for a medical transcriptionist. Therefore, if a problem does arise, here is a list of some steps to take toward remedying the situation.

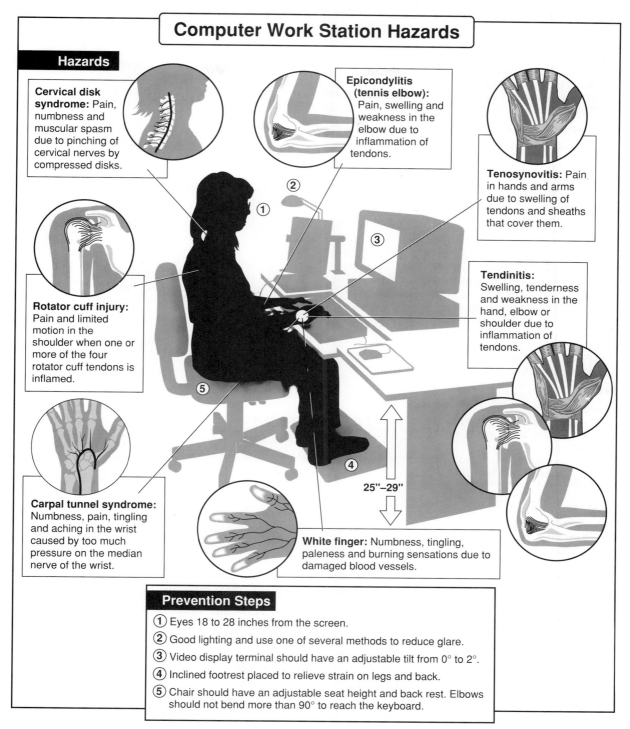

Computer Work Station Hazards

Hazards

Cervical disk syndrome: Pain, numbness and muscular spasm due to pinching of cervical nerves by compressed disks.

Epicondylitis (tennis elbow): Pain, swelling and weakness in the elbow due to inflammation of tendons.

Tenosynovitis: Pain in hands and arms due to swelling of tendons and sheaths that cover them.

Rotator cuff injury: Pain and limited motion in the shoulder when one or more of the four rotator cuff tendons is inflamed.

Tendinitis: Swelling, tenderness and weakness in the hand, elbow or shoulder due to inflammation of tendons.

Carpal tunnel syndrome: Numbness, pain, tingling and aching in the wrist caused by too much pressure on the median nerve of the wrist.

White finger: Numbness, tingling, paleness and burning sensations due to damaged blood vessels.

25"–29"

Prevention Steps

1 Eyes 18 to 28 inches from the screen.
2 Good lighting and use one of several methods to reduce glare.
3 Video display terminal should have an adjustable tilt from 0° to 2°.
4 Inclined footrest placed to relieve strain on legs and back.
5 Chair should have an adjustable seat height and back rest. Elbows should not bend more than 90° to reach the keyboard.

Figure 5–2
An illustration of hazards at a computer work station and the prevention and improvements that are possible.

***Table* 5–1 ▪ Ergonomic Guide for a Computer Work Station**

Table

Height	
Non-VDT tasks (fixed height)	29″
Non-VDT tasks (adjustable height)	26–30″
VDT screen and keyboard same surface (fixed height)	26–27″
VDT screen and keyboard same surface (adjustable height)	23–30″
Thickness	1.0–1.5″
Size (screen and keyboard on same surface)	Minimum 36″ wide by 30″ deep
Underside	
Minimum height	24″
Minimum depth:	
Knee level	16″
Foot level	26″
Minimum width	27″

Keyboard

Fixed support height	27″
Adjustable support height	23–30″
Fixed support slope	0°
Adjustable support slope	0–10°

Screen

Viewing angle (line of sight)	0° (to top of screen)
Viewing angle (line of sight)	40° (bottom of screen)
Viewing distance	13–28″

Reach

Near-reach distance	11.3″ radius
Fingertips of left hand to fingertips of right hand when hands in near or far-reach position	33.5″
Far-reach distance	22.4″
Fingertips of left hand to fingertips of right hand when hands in near or far-reach position	57.2″

1. Keep all manuals for equipment. Usually they contain troubleshooting guides to determine whether a call for a service person is needed. Many problems can be solved if one takes the time to check the manual.

2. Find other transcriptionists in the area who have similar equipment. They may have had similar difficulties and can offer suggestions.

3. Have some backup equipment, such as a printer or transcriber (these can sometimes be purchased inexpensively on the used market). This can avoid the need to have immediate service on costly equipment.

4. Have the name of a reliable person available if service is necessary, or check with others in the area to find someone who is dependable and easily accessible. Be sure to find out in advance whether this person knows the equipment in question. Always try to understand exactly what was done to remedy a problem situation, which will be valuable for possible future difficulties.

Reference Sources

Avila-Weil, D., and M. Glaccum. *The Independent Medical Transcriptionist.* Rayve Publications, Windsor, California, 1991.

Computer printers. *Consumer Reports,* 1992 Buying Guide Issue, pp. 303–305.

Human Factors Society, Inc. *American National Standard for Human Factors Engineering of Visual Display Terminal Work Stations.* Santa Monica, California.

Jones, Jeffrey R., et al. *Preventing Repetitive Strain at the Keyboard.* Krames Communications, San Bruno, California, 1991.

Norris, Michael. How to choose the right fax. *Business News,* January 1992.

Pons, Ted. Should you buy or lease your new office equipment? *Medical Economics,* March 19, 1990.

R & D Dictating Systems, 14618 Victory Boulevard, Van Nuys, California 91401; telephone 818/988-9110.

Unlocking the door: PCs and people with disabilities. *PC Today,* March 1991.

Marketing of Medical Transcription Services

INTRODUCTION

Medical transcription services vary in size and character. They range from the in-home, one-person medical transcription service to the large, office-oriented service, with many variations falling in between. While the service owner may have excellent skills in medical transcription, she often has little or no knowledge about marketing a medical transcription service. In a small service, the owner must do the planning and marketing herself, whereas in a larger service, a marketing representative might be hired to accomplish these tasks. This chapter will give a general overview of marketing strategies for both the small and large medical transcription service owner.

Even though the medical transcription service produces a specialized product, the following five marketing strategies must be considered: market analysis and market planning, planning and developing the service, pricing of services, channels of distribution for services, and promoting the service. Through these marketing strategies, the medical transcription service owner can develop a total marketing program.

MARKET RESEARCH AND ANALYSIS

In marketing analysis, research is necessary to determine the need for services, the location, and then to define the target audience before expending energy and money. First, determine the geographic distribution of your market. The focus could be the entire city and its suburbs, a particular neighborhood, or a small area around a medical center.

MARKET SEGMENTATION

Second, analyze the market segment to be served with medical transcription services. It can be divided between physician-based and hospital-based. The physician-based market segment can be divided into the various specialties which are listed in Table 6–1. In addition, the hospital-based market segment can be divided into specialty hospitals and general acute care centers. For instance, psychiatric and rehabilitative hospitals are considered specialty hospitals. General acute care hospitals are classified as the "traditional" hospital in which care for all specialties is offered. One can also segment each hospital according to departments utilizing medical transcription services:

Behavioral Medicine Department
Emergency Room and Trauma Center
Medical Records Transcription
Oncology Department
Pathology Department
Physical Medicine and Rehabilitation Department
Physical Therapy Department
Radiation Therapy Department
Radiology Department
Sleep Disorder Clinic

Table 6–1 ▪ **Medical Specialties Requiring Transcription**

Acupuncture	Nuclear medicine	Psychiatry, family
Adolescent medicine	Obstetrics and gynecology	Psychiatry, general
Allergy/immunology	Occupational medicine	Psychoanalysis
Anesthesiology	Oncology	Pulmonology
Arthritis	Ophthalmology	Radiology, diagnostic
Aviation medicine	Orthopaedics	Radiology, therapeutic
Bariatrics (weight control)	Otorhinolaryngology	Rheumatology
Cardiology	Pain control	Sleep disorders
Dermatology	Pathology	Sports medicine
Drug and alcohol abuse	Pediatrics	Surgery, abdominal
Emergency medicine	Pediatric allergy	Surgery, cardiovascular
Endocrinology	Pediatric cardiology	Surgery, colon and rectal
Environmental medicine	Pediatric endocrinology	Surgery, foot
Family practice	Pediatric gastroenterology	Surgery, general
Gastroenterology	Pediatric hematology/oncology	Surgery, gynecologic
Geriatrics	Pediatric neurology	Surgery, hand
Heart transplantation	Pediatric ophthalmology	Surgery, head and neck
Heart and lung transplantation	Pulmonary pediatrics	Surgery, neurologic
Hematology	Pediatric surgery	Surgery, ophthalmologic
Hypnosis	Physical medicine and rehabilitation	Surgery, orthopaedic
Infectious diseases	Plastic and reconstructive surgery	Surgery, thoracic
Infertility	Preventive medicine	Surgery, urologic
Internal medicine	Proctology	Surgery, vascular
Nephrology	Psychiatry, child	Urology

Sports Medicine and Rehabilitation Department

In this market research one must also determine the buying patterns of the market segments. In other words, either in the physician's office or the hospital, one needs to determine when, where, and how medical transcription services are purchased; who purchases them; and who makes the purchasing decision.

TARGET MARKETING

Opportunities for the transcription service can be gleaned from this data collection, and the service can decide which of the following strategies it wishes to follow. The first is *undifferentiated marketing,* in which the service can pursue the entire market and marketing mix and attract as many clients as possible. The service may wish to market its skills to both physicians' offices and hospitals, no matter what specialty. The second is *differentiated marketing,* in which several market segments are pursued and services are developed for each. In this manner, one

could either develop services for certain physician specialties or just hospitals. The third is *concentrated marketing,* in which the service attempts to acquire one market segment and develops one service for that market, selling either to physicians in one specialty or to a specialized hospital.

In addition to market segmenting, one must examine the market demand changes and trends. This may seem like a guessing game, but it challenges the medical transcription service owner to examine what changes might be expected in health care in the future. Over the past 10 years, reimbursement in health care has undergone drastic changes. The insurance industry has gone from paying hospitals 100 per cent for services to paying for diagnosis-related groups; in the future it will be going to relative value systems for paying physicians. In addition, health maintenance organizations (HMOs) and preferred provider organizations (PPOs) have changed the character of the insurance industry. These changes may have an impact on the target market.

Once the target market has been established,

the service needs to plan and develop the benefits it intends to offer. In addition, policies need to be established regarding the services and what types of guarantees will be offered, if any. A variety of services can be offered, including pick-up and delivery of dictation, phone-in dictation on tapes, phone-in dictation on a digital system (how large a system is required?), word processing (what type of computer/PC and what word processing program?), storage (how much, how long?), faxing, returning work by modem, and telecommunications. In addition, a medical transcription service can expand or contract any of the services at any time.

Comparisons of using in-house medical transcription services versus an outside medical transcription business can be made for the client. All costs in utilizing an employee can be included in the comparison. These include recruiting, hiring, training, equipment and supplies, maintenance, software enhancements, reference books, supervision, insurance, holidays, incentives, other benefits, and taxes.

An important goal to strive for, however, is standardization of quality. Physicians and hospitals want consistency in quality from the medical transcription service with which they contract. A quality assurance plan must be developed by the transcription service and adhered to at all times and be understood by the purchaser of those services.

SETTING PRICES

Managerial creativity, imagination, and skill are required in the pricing of medical transcription services, which has become an art considering the methods by which hospitals and physicians are being reimbursed. Pricing strategies tend to be cost-oriented, demand-oriented, or competition-oriented, according to Kotler and Clarke, 1987.

Setting prices on the basis of costs is referred to as *cost-oriented pricing*. Breakeven analysis is the most popular form of cost-oriented pricing. In breakeven analysis, one determines how many units of an item need to be sold to cover costs fully.

Demand-oriented pricing examines the demand for the service rather than the cost to set the price. In this pricing strategy, the price reflects the "perceived value" in the client's mind. Therefore, if the medical transcription service has a reputation for excellent quality and turn-around time, it can charge a higher fee for its services. Price discrimination is a form of demand-oriented pricing. The medical transcription service may offer several prices for a similar product. For this to work, the market must be segmentable and the segments must show different intensities of demand.

When a medical transcription service sets its prices based on what competitors are charging, this is called *competition-oriented pricing*. The service may charge the same price, a higher price, or a lower price.

> The organization does *not* seek to maintain a rigid relation between its price and its own costs or demand. Its own costs or demand may change, but the organization maintains its price because competitors maintain their prices. Conversely, the same organization will change its price when competitors change theirs, even if its own costs or demands have not altered (Kotler and Clarke, 1987).

The going rate, or imitative pricing, is the most popular type of competition-oriented pricing. The collective wisdom of the industry concerning the price that yields a fair return is felt to represent the going rate.

In addition to these pricing strategies, medical transcription services must consider whether they will base their fees by the word, by the line, by the page, by keystrokes, by bytes, or by characters. A word is considered to consist of five typed characters. A line is more difficult to define. It can be a 60-space PICA line of type, a 70-space ELITE line of type, or many variations in between. A page can also vary in length; it can be 60 lines, 55 lines, 33 lines, or whatever the medical transcription service deems appropriate to be charged by the page. Charging by the keystroke would include each instance in which there has been input on the keyboard. A byte is defined by Webster as "a group of adjacent binary digits often shorter than a word that a computer processes as a unit." Many computers provide information regarding the number of bytes that have been used in preparing documents. Also, software packages are available that will automatically give word or line counts.

CHANNELS OF DISTRIBUTION

Developing channels of distribution for the use of medical transcription services is also important. This part of the total marketing program involves decisions regarding how the organization will make its services available and accessible to the client. Physical access and time access should be considered. Physical access means the location of the business. For a small operation, one might begin transcribing in one's home or in a small office setting. On the other hand, a large office and many employees might be necessary to handle the requirements of the medical transcription service. Time access is the hours of operation and the turnaround time. Certainly, in a one-person operation, the medical transcriptionist does not want to be transcribing 24 hours a day. Therefore, a happy medium must be found regarding the hours one wishes to transcribe. In a larger operation, however, 24-hour coverage may be the ideal. Also, consider turnaround of the dictation — 24, 48, 72 hours; immediately; combinations of time depending on the reports; or continuously by modem.

PUBLICITY AND PROMOTION

Once the foregoing strategies have been determined, it will be necessary to promote the services. Personal selling, advertising, and indirect forms of promotion are methods that can be used. A promotional program in a service company has two major goals: to portray the service benefits in an appealing manner and to build a good reputation. With personal selling, there is a close relationship between the buyer and the seller.

Brochures can be effective in the marketing of a medical transcription service (Figure 6-1). As the brochure presents the image of the company, several issues must be carefully considered. These include copy content and style, layout, photography, art illustration, paper, inks, typography, art production, printer selection, and printing techniques and processes. It is also necessary to consider how the brochure will be used —direct mailing, field sales, and so forth. It is often helpful to have an advertising or design agency aid the medical transcription service in these very important decisions. While a professionally designed brochure is a significant investment, the cost/return ratio must be considered; however, a good brochure does not necessarily have to be an expensive brochure.

Advertising can take many forms. Brochures, ads in the Yellow Pages, ads in local medical society newsletters, and ads in the *Journal of the American Association for Medical Transcription* and *Perspectives on the Medical Transcription Profession* are several ways to advertise the services offered by the medical transcription service. Dependability of the service — "its consistent high quality" — and the courteous, friendly, efficient service can be promoted in an advertising campaign. Stationery, business cards, flyers, and logos are additional ways of promoting business. For further information, see the Marketing, Promotion, and Public Relations section and Figures 4-3, 4-4, and 4-5 in Chapter 4.

An indirect means of promotion is networking.

> Networking is a technique whereby individuals communicate and *connect* with each other to develop contacts, receive and give information, or obtain feedback; assurance that what we're doing is right (or wrong, in time to make adjustments) (Booras and Booras, 1986).

Networking is invaluable for ideas, referrals, information, or just moral support. Joining the Chamber of Commerce is one way of networking. Networking in this fashion can raise the level of awareness in the community by explaining what medical transcription is all about. Another way to network is to do so at the local chapter and state meetings of the American Association for Medical Transcription. Service owners must overcome the fear of sharing information with their competition in order for networking to be an effective marketing tool. Sharing information makes service owners stronger and more professional.

Setting up a display at meetings of the local medical society and American Health Information Management Association (AHIMA) (formerly known as the American Medical Record Association) can also be quite helpful in marketing your medical transcription service.

By following the five marketing strategies that have been discussed, the medical transcription

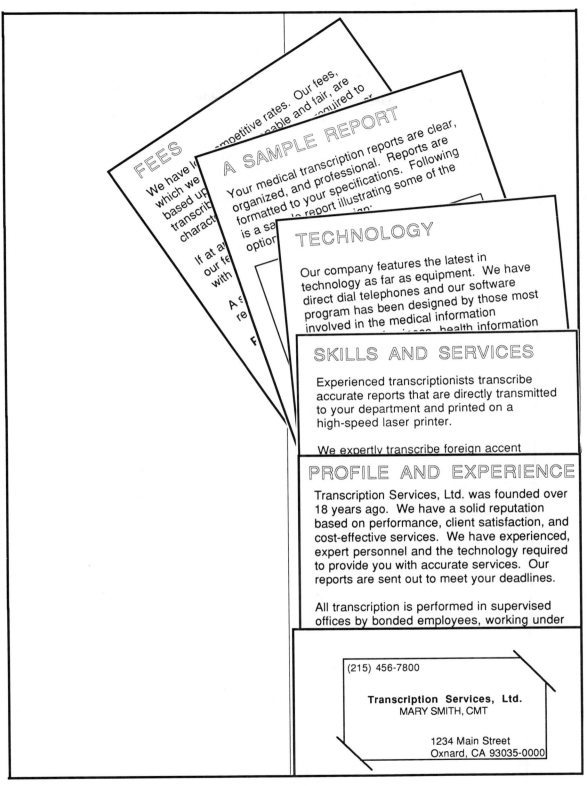

FEES

We have [c]ompetitive rates. Our fees, which we [reason]able and fair, are based up[on] [re]quired to transcrib[e] charact[er]

If at a[ny] our fe[e] with

A s[ample] re[port]

F[

A SAMPLE REPORT

Your medical transcription reports are clear, organized, and professional. Reports are formatted to your specifications. Following is a sa[mple] report illustrating some of the option[ ]

TECHNOLOGY

Our company features the latest in technology as far as equipment. We have direct dial telephones and our software program has been designed by those most involved in the medical information [ ] [busi]ness, health information

SKILLS AND SERVICES

Experienced transcriptionists transcribe accurate reports that are directly transmitted to your department and printed on a high-speed laser printer.

We expertly transcribe foreign accent

PROFILE AND EXPERIENCE

Transcription Services, Ltd. was founded over 18 years ago. We have a solid reputation based on performance, client satisfaction, and cost-effective services. We have experienced, expert personnel and the technology required to provide you with accurate services. Our reports are sent out to meet your deadlines.

All transcription is performed in supervised offices by bonded employees, working under

(215) 456-7800

Transcription Services, Ltd.
MARY SMITH, CMT

1234 Main Street
Oxnard, CA 93035-0000

Figure 6–1
Example of a brochure with an inserted business card to market a medical transcription service. This is a folded booklet with five inserts emphasizing important aspects of the business.

service owner can develop a total marketing program. This program will afford a comprehensive, systematic method of promoting medical transcription services and positioning the business as a viable alternative to in-house medical transcription services.

Reference Sources

Blough, Douglas. "It's not just your company's brochure, it's your business." *The Colorado Springs Business Journal,* November 15, 1991, p. 8.

Booras, Jane, and Alex Booras. *The Executive Suite Marketing Manual.* The National Association of Secretarial Services, St. Petersburg, Florida, 1986.

Health Professions Institute. Workshop for Medical Transcription Service Owners: Streamlining Operations in the Successful Medical Transcription Service. Chicago-O'Hare Marriott Hotel, Chicago, September 20, 1987.

Kotler, Philip, and Roberta N. Clarke. *Marketing for Health Care Organizations.* Prentice-Hall, Englewood Cliffs, New Jersey, 1987.

Stanton, William J. *Fundamentals of Marketing,* 4th edition. McGraw-Hill Book Company, New York, 1975.

Hazel L. Tank, C.M.T.

Management and Supervision

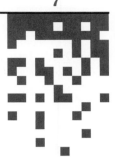

INTRODUCTION

If an expert medical transcriptionist stays in the field long enough, eventually she will probably come to the point of managing or supervising a transcription department in a hospital or service. It often comes as a surprise to a transcriptionist that the duties of supervisor can be quite different, and a new perspective is needed to handle the situations that arise. This is not to say that supervising is more difficult (albeit more challenging in some ways), but simply different. As one sage has put it, "Take the ball and run with it, but you have to catch it first."

In a hospital setting, the medical transcription supervisor will often find herself in the position of "in the middle." On the one hand she is the head of a "department within a department" — Medical Records, and on the other hand she has a certain amount of autonomy, finding herself on hospital planning committees, in an advisory position at local colleges, and serving in the capacity of supervisor of an intern program that services those colleges. She must often be available to give advice on many issues, such as whether or not to utilize a service to assist with production goals, how best to schedule vacations, and how to manage the various sections of her department, including the Printing/Modeming Department, Hardware/Software Department, and Quality Assurance.

Additionally, hospitals and services alike often have a Student Intern Program (SIP). The responsibility of managing this branch of the department falls to the medical transcription supervisor or the quality assurance manager. There must be coordination with the local col-leges regarding which students to accept into the program. Making space, equipment, tapes for transcription, and reference material available to the interns is also part of the job description of the person delegated to manage this community service program. This involves proofreading and correcting reports generated by the interns and usually comes under the Quality Assurance arm of the Medical Transcription Department. Local colleges who offer such programs usually prefer to have a working medical transcriptionist on the college advisory board to help coordinate the program. Figure 7–1 provides an example of how a Student Intern Program may be organized. The example uses WordPerfect software; however, it may easily be modified.

DELEGATING

The most difficult thing for a neophyte supervisor to do is delegate duties. The tendency is to do it one's self, since this has been the case in the past. A supervisor must evaluate the duties laid before her and make decisions about what can be accomplished in the time allocated, and act accordingly. Just how much delegation is possible will depend on the number of staff members available. If past policy was not to give employees individual responsibilities, perhaps it is time for a change. Most people learn best by doing and will rise to the occasion when given a measure of responsibility. The supervisor must determine how much responsibility each employee is capable of handling prior to making such assignments. This will take observation time; do not rush into making sweeping changes

---

STUDENT INTERN PROGRAM

Day One: Introduction to computers
        Verbal and written instructions

        Introduction to WordPerfect
         Verbal instruction leading into WP tutorial

        WordPerfect tutorial

Day Two: The "how to" day

        Magic Macros
         How macros work and how we use them
         Bodyworks — Other software that assists the transcriptionist
        Reference books, how to utilize
        Headers/footers, making, editing
        The spell checker
        Viewing the document

Day Three: Continue with Day Two program, if necessary.

        The working transcriptionist
         Transcribing actual, previously transcribed tapes

Balance of Week One or as Long as Deemed Necessary:

        Transcribing and honing skills in the profession, with transcription of actual, previously transcribed tapes until the intern feels comfortable with it

        Anatomy instruction as needed

Balance of Internship:

        Actual working transcribing of "live" tapes. All such transcriptions will be downloaded from the Student/Intern PC via floppy disk and transferred into the company network. These will be printed out and corrections noted on the hard copies. Nothing will be sent to any client unless the tapes are listened to by QA personnel and corrected. The hard copies with corrections will be returned to the intern.

NOTE: Interns will NOT use any macros except the client macros in order that they may learn how to save documents, spell check, view document, hyphenate, and transcribe "free hand."

Figure 7–1
An example of a Student Intern Program, incorporating the use of WordPerfect software.

until an evaluation of the situation and people involved can be done.

WORK SCHEDULES

Preparing work schedules can be a horrendous task. Everyone has a preferred time of day to work, a favorite work station, favorite dictation, and so forth. The supervisor must evaluate the amount and type of equipment available, the space available, and the most pressing needs of the company or hospital, while keeping in mind the needs and desires of the employees. If, for instance, there is only one transcriptionist who can transcribe neurology dictation, it would be wise to introduce another employee to this specialty. One method of achieving this is to have everyone submit a list of favorite specialty dictation, favorite dictator, and so forth, and make evaluations and assignments based on this information—but not too swiftly. Change, in order to be effective and nontraumatic to the personnel, must be introduced slowly and diplomatically. It is probably advisable to continue with the old regimen until all information is in regarding company requirements and employee desires before making changes.

COORDINATION OF WORK FLOW

Personal Relationships on the Job ■ It often comes as a shock to a newly appointed supervisor that relationships change with the promotion. People with whom the transcriptionist has worked for a long time, and with whom she had been close friends, are now subordinates; this situation can lead to strained relationships if not delicately handled. One should not be fooled into thinking it will not happen—it will. Perhaps an "old friend" will try to manipulate the supervisor with regard to work scheduling, equipment assignments, and the like. The supervisor might find herself engaged in prolonged social conversation on company time with such a person. The neophyte supervisor has to guard against falling into such a trap and yet not be aloof or out of the reach of the employees. Firm establishment of position with preservation of previously established friendships can be quite tricky, but it can be accomplished. Of greatest peril is the fellow employee who felt that she was the one qualified for the job. In such a situation, the supervisor needs to summon all the tact and wisdom at her command to win and retain the respect of the unhappy employee. A new supervisor cannot expect simply to take over a previously vacated position by storm or beg for the respect of her new employees. This is the time to "walk softly and carry a big stick."

Often, so-called personality problems that arise between employees turn out to be a simple matter. The supervisor should be aware of the "little things" that can offend, such as overpowering perfume, foul language, bigotry, body odor, and other things of this nature that might become uncomfortable situations. It would be easy to tell oneself that such matters are not the concern of the supervisor, but actually these are the things that can be disruptive, the "tempest in a teapot" that causes problems between employees. The "little things" are sometimes more problematic than salary differences or other events that might ordinarily be considered legitimate problems. A small situation often can erupt into a major one, and the supervisor must be diplomatic in dealing with these problems. Discussion of such considerations should be held in private and in strictest confidence, and the supervisor should NEVER engage in idle conversation with one employee about another, except in the most positive way. Accepting complaints from one employee about another is part of the job, but to comment one way or the other can show favoritism, which does not foster good employee relationships.

MEDICAL STAFF INTERACTION

Relationships in a hospital between the doctors/nurses and those in the Medical Record Department, and particularly the Transcription Department, can become a bit tense at times. Doctors may say they dictated a report, and may honestly feel that they did, but it is not there. Or perhaps the report in question *was* dictated but lost in some way. In such a situation, it is important never to assume the doctor, physician's assistant, or nurse is wrong; or assume that the Transcription Department is at fault. The supervisor cannot make any statement as to where a missing report might be until all the facts are available. The same is true for staff relations. If a doctor or nurse complains about one of the supervisor's employees, it is not fair to assume that either one is wrong, especially if there have been no previous complaints. It is necessary to keep an open mind and gather all the facts before making any decisions on how to deal with this situation.

MOTIVATING AND PRAISING

Medical transcriptionists, like everyone else, thrive on praise. The best work is usually done when only the best is expected. The transcriptionist always hears about the mistakes but seldom hears words of praise. A supervisor should take the time to reassure deserving employees by telling them they are doing a good job and that they are appreciated. When doctors or clients make positive remarks about a particular transcriptionist, this information should be passed along, or posted for all to read. Reinforcement of this kind can do wonders for the morale and productivity of the transcriptionist and can even act as a spur to encourage others to work toward receiving such recognition.

Motivation is a tricky subject. Money is a great motivator. Production workers who work on a line-count basis usually have enough motivation to produce a lot of lines. However, producing lines that are not up to quality standards will be counterproductive in the long run. Urging transcriptionists to produce better quality as well as quantity can also be augmented with tangible rewards.

QUALITY ASSURANCE

One way to encourage interest in quality transcribing is to initiate a program such as the Quality Assurance Score (QA Score) self-test shown in Table 7–1.

Another way is for the quality assurance manager to call up ten documents for each employee and grade them on the same ten points mentioned in the QA Score, giving a possible 100 points. Tangible reward is then given. Employees should be told that this type of scoring is taking place. One service company awarded ten cents per point for a score over 90, eight cents for a score between 80 and 90, and five cents for a score between 75 and 80. Although this was not a substantial financial reward, it *was* a reward and resulted in a significant improvement in the quality AND quantity of the reports generated. Production went up an average of 10 per cent within 3 weeks of implementing this program, and quality improved, with fewer errors found on proofreading. The transcriptionists seemed to enjoy the "silent" competition and in the long run benefited from the knowledge gained through better research, self-confidence, and pride in their work. Such a program is not for every department, naturally. Many large hospitals, especially teaching hospitals, have similar programs that are implemented on an as-needed basis, with the supervisor of the department in conjunction with the quality assurance manager making the determination as to which program is needed and when and how long to run it.

Table 7–1 ▪ What's Your QA (Quality Assurance) Score?

On a scale of 1 to 10, how do you measure up? Take this test using the following 10 points of quality transcription. Allow a point for each correct answer on a document.

1. Macro completed properly; i.e., name spelled correctly, number properly input, date and time correctly typed, date spelled in proper format.
2. Compound adjectives properly hyphenated, where appropriate.
3. Medications in prescription properly typed, e.g., Tylenol No. 3, 2 b.i.d., #20.
4. Headings in appropriate places.
5. Format faithfully followed.
6. Hyphenation appropriate, i.e., no two-letter hyphenation, no single-syllable words hyphenated, no proper names hyphenated.
7. Document properly routed with cc to whomever. Spell check done.
8. Complete sentences *that make sense.*
9. Standard abbreviations, when dictated, properly typed.
10. Word processing style proper, i.e., no hard returns except between paragraphs, at least two lines of text on final page, and so forth.

A SCORE OF 10 ON AT LEAST 10 DOCUMENTS DESERVES AN A!

DELIVERING CRITICISM OR DISCIPLINE

Criticism is hardly ever welcomed. However, constructive criticism is a necessary part of maintaining discipline, and it separates the excellent from the merely acceptable. If a supervisor allows errors to go unchecked, whether in transcribing or interpersonal relationships, the problem(s) will soon get out of hand. By dealing with each situation as it arises, the supervisor is less likely to encounter the same problem over and over.

Once employees realize that the supervisor is fair, yet firm, in her dealings with them, they will respect her decisions and will be more likely to abide by them cheerfully. An inoffensive way of delivering criticism can be in the form of a memo to all employees, outlining some problem and the solution for it. NEVER point out a problem that cannot be solved! Instruct people in proper procedures and reinforce these instructions if one or all of them seem to be slipping. Be consistent. One should not be "slipshod" or "wishy-washy" in dealings with employees or they are likely to think the supervisor is "blowing hot and cold." Enforce policies or eliminate them from the Procedure Manual.

Individual criticism can also be in the form of a memo. Using the system of proofreading outlined farther along in the chapter, a list can be kept of the errors encountered along with the correct method of spelling or word processing. Although these should be addressed to the employee in question, care must be taken not to single out an employee for personal attention, unless the goal is to motivate that person to higher standards. To be fair, review all employees' work and proofread to the same degree, giving comments individually. This can be done in a one-on-one conversation or via a personal memo. Make a duplicate copy of any memo sent to an employee, retaining it in the employee file for future reference.

When engaging in conversation with an employee regarding her errors, care must be taken to ensure that the tone is neither condescending nor accusatory. Some people would rather mull over a written commentary than engage in head-on confrontation. Ascertain how to handle each individual and proceed accordingly. In most LAN (local area network*) systems there is some form of electronic mail or communication system. By all means, utilize all the tools available to put across the point(s) needed to reach an errant employee.

INCENTIVE PROGRAMS

Many hospitals and transcription services have incentive programs. Transcriptionists are generally hard workers, and rewarding excep-

---

*A network of computer equipment that serves several users in a small area when connected by dedicated communications channels sharing disk storage and printers.

tional production with incentive programs is the most practical way to encourage diligence. This is usually done on a line-count or character count basis in which a target/goal of a certain number of lines or characters is set, and bonuses are paid for each additional increment of lines or characters. Table 7–2 gives an example of how this can be implemented. This is only one example of how an incentive program may be implemented and of course will not apply to new (under 90 days) employees, unless they are productive enough from the beginning to go on the incentive program. The industry standard minimum wage for the job must be established prior to instituting such a program, as there are times when poor dictation, equipment problems, interruptions, and so forth will slow down the best transcriptionist. This minimum wage would cover the times when the transcriptionist is not actually transcribing but doing other things in the department, such as monitoring the phones. Many services and hospitals allow transcriptionists an average wage to cover such periods. This wage is usually determined by calculating what the transcriptionist does in the way of line count (or whatever method of productive scale is in use) over a 2-week period and dividing by the number of hours worked in that amount of time (usually 80 hours), based on a 40-hour work week. Such a method could be considered fair and relate to the individual's capabilities.

Meeting Deadlines ▪ Hospitals usually have turnaround times tailored to the type of report, that is, history and physical examinations need to be in the medical record prior to the patient going to surgery, and operative reports must be on the chart within 24 hours of the event. Work should be assigned accordingly, keeping in mind that the fastest and most accurate transcriptionist will probably be the one assigned the most urgent work. It is not advisable to subject new employees to the pressure of rapid turnaround

Table 7–2 ▪ **Incentive Program Line Count**

Target line count	1200 lines at $0.05 per line
Bonus #1	1500 lines at $0.06 per line
Bonus #2	2000 lines at $0.07 per line
Bonus #3	above 2000 at $0.08 per line

time until they are well versed in the use of the equipment, formats, and doctors' methods of dictation.

Transcription services, on the other hand, usually have a contract with their clients to guarantee a certain turnaround time. In the case of emergency department reports, there is often a rapid turnaround—sometimes within an hour—in order to cover transfers, emergency admissions, direct admission to surgery, and such. When a service has this type of contract, these reports are sent immediately (stat) to the client via computer modem. Again, the most efficient transcriptionist(s) should be available on each shift to cover these rapid turnaround needs. It is up to the supervisor to ensure that such assignments are made.

WORD PROCESSING

Unfortunately, the Transcription Department does not always have the privilege of hiring employees. In a worst-case scenario, new employees are hired by the Personnel Department, and are never seen by the transcription supervisor until the day they report to work. Very often, skills they claim to possess are nonexistent. It is the responsibility of the supervisor to train the neophyte in word processing. No matter what system is in place, whether it be accessing a main frame, individual stand-alone personal computer (PC), or an LAN, it is inappropriate to leave a new person to "figure it out for herself." It is wrong to treat the computer as if it were a typewriter with a screen; there is much more to learn. Ideally, the department or company will have a training period of a week or so in order for new employees to familiarize themselves with the equipment, but this is not always possible. Learning should be gradual, with a "need-to-know" type of instruction, and rapidly progress to encompass all that the system is capable of doing. The more the transcriptionist knows with regard to the job, the easier it will be for the supervisor, as well as the transcriptionist. It is also the supervisor's responsibility to train the neophyte as well as the more experienced new employee in variations in style and format peculiar to the particular hospital.

EMPLOYEE EVALUATION

Performance Appraisal Systems ▪ When an employee is hired, a 90-day probation period is the best way to make an evaluation of how that employee is going to fit into the existing system. She should be notified of the 90-day probationary period, as well as when permanent employment will be instituted. If she has "failed" the 90-day trial and was made aware of this probationary period, there should be no qualms about notifying her that her services are terminated. Judgment should be based on quality and quantity of work produced, interaction with other employees, and adherence to the company rules. These conditions should be clearly outlined from the date of hire and reiterated at the time of becoming a permanent employee.

Usually, an annual appraisal of the employee will be required, most often at some time near the employee's anniversary date. The department head depends on the supervisor to provide information on how to make this appraisal. This is one reason it is necessary to keep a copy of all material regarding the employee's work, including any memo, complaint, or praise given, as these data can be reviewed and presented as evidence of the employee's progress. This appraisal will affect whatever pay changes or promotion is necessary.

Table 7–3 provides an example of how an employee appraisal may be made. In evaluating an employee, the supervisor must be sure that personal feelings do not enter into the overall evaluation of the employee's work standards. Personal friendships and animosities must be put aside—not always an easy thing to do, but necessary in order to be fair.

Documentation of Production ▪ Many word processing systems have a built-in line counter that prints out each day's work with totals for each transcriptionist plus a grand total. This is the ideal situation. Otherwise, an accountant (or the employee) must keep track of or tabulate the lines generated; however, relying on the employee to do this is not advisable. Implementation of some method of keeping track of individual and overall line counts is advisable. Investigation of various systems already in existence at other hospitals or services might be

Table 7-3 ■ **Employee Rating Scale**

Factor	1	2	3	4
Skill	Poor; often does unacceptable work; is careless; requires constant supervision	Fair; needs supervision and frequent checking	Generally good; makes only occasional mistakes; requires little supervision	Excellent; work A-1 all the time; makes few mistakes; needs very little supervision
Effort	Very slow; almost never completes job in time assigned for it	Erratic; sometimes fast and efficient, other times slow and unskillful	Steady worker; does job consistently, and sometimes does more	Exceptionally fast; does work well; does extra work to stay busy
Level of responsibility	Irresponsible in attendance; seldom carries out orders without being prodded	Some absences; sometimes needs a reminder to do work assigned	Attendance record good; reliable in work	Excellent attendance record; most reliable in doing work assigned; can always be depended on
Attitude	Uncooperative, often complains; is a disruptive force among other employees	Cooperates sometimes, but is often indifferent both to fellow workers and to quality of own work	Usually cooperative and attentive to work; gets along well with others	Exceptionally cooperative; very interested in work; always helpful to others and considerate of them

worthwhile if a workable system is not already in place. Publications of the American Association for Medical Transcription (AAMT) and the American Health Information Management Association (AHIMA) contain numerous articles by those who have had experience in the documentation of production, and the supervisor would do well to utilize these valuable resources.

Performance Problems

Slow Worker ■ The slow worker may be slow for a variety of reasons. It is the supervisor's responsibility to determine why the employee is not doing well and seek a viable solution to the problem. She may not be fully qualified to operate the equipment and perhaps needs more complete instruction. Perhaps she is not sufficiently motivated and needs some personalized attention in this regard. If an employee has "passed" the 90-day probationary period and has fallen behind in production from that period, perhaps a reevaluation and even a new probation period could be implemented. It may be that there are too many foreign dictators or too much terminology she has to reference. Determine the cause of the problem and offer solutions to the employee before taking more drastic action. Sometimes, just a little encouragement will help —but not always. One solution does not serve all situations. If an employee is slow because she is socializing rather than working, the supervisor needs to point this out.

The Untidy Worker ■ Every office seems to have at least one person who is physically untidy. This may be represented by unwashed coffee cups, paper clips scattered all over the work area, or wadded-up papers tossed carelessly onto the floor. In the most extreme cases, the person herself is untidy or perhaps has body odor. These problems require attention by the supervisor immediately. The Procedure Manual should certainly outline the standards of cleanliness expected from each employee. Leaving an untidy desk for the maintenance crew to handle shows a lack of professionalism and consideration. Body odor should be dealt with as soon as the supervisor is aware that it is a daily occurrence. Perhaps a diplomatic way to handle this latter problem is to take the employee aside and ask if she has a physical problem which might cause this symptom. In any case, the problem(s) must be dealt with quickly, because these situations affect all coworkers.

A similar problem is the employee who wears overpowering perfume or cologne. The Employee Manual should also offer guidelines for this problem.

Foul Language ■ Almost all adults (and even children) use a swear word now and then. In most hospitals and services, this is not tolerated. Infractions of whatever the rules may be should be dealt with on a one-to-one basis. A note will not suffice in this case; explanations are in order. The supervisor might say, "We don't do that here because it is offensive to the majority of our employees." Continuation of the infraction will have to be dealt with accordingly, based on the rules set forth in the Procedure Manual.

Socializing ■ It is imperative to allow time for employees to enjoy one another's company, such as scheduled break times and lunch periods. Hospitals routinely provide such periods. In many services, however, breaks and lunch periods are at the individual employee's discretion. Sometimes a problem arises regarding socializing between work stations, which can be disruptive to other workers. Such behavior is best discouraged as discreetly as possible. Smoking is rarely allowed in an office, and a place for coffee breaks and/or cigarette breaks and lunches should be available to the employees.

Grievances

No one likes to listen to grievances, but the supervisor gets them all. It is much better to have employees come to the supervisor with their grievances than to whisper among themselves. Perhaps a suggestion box would help curtail some of the problems that inevitably crop up in a workplace. If possible, an anonymous telephone help line can be of great advantage to both supervisor and employee.

The supervisor MUST listen to whatever grievances an employee has and do one of two things. (1) Sympathize, while pointing out that everyone has the same situation, and there is no solution at the present time. (2) Act to ameliorate the problem. This action may be a formal request to the employer or department head, in order to correct the problem. The supervisor should never take a bored or flippant attitude toward employee grievances, or she will lose the respect of that employee and the employee will assume an "It's us against them" attitude.

TRAINING NEW EMPLOYEES

A supervisor can designate someone to train new employees or have another person in the same job description available to answer questions and provide guidelines. Too often new employees are put in front of a word processor, given tapes to transcribe, and not even told where the restrooms are. DO NOT ALLOW THIS TO HAPPEN.

SALARIES

Pay scales vary from hospital to hospital and from service to service. In most cases, the supervisor does not set wages, or methods of incentive pay, if these are used. No system, whether straight production, hourly wage, or salary, should be less than ABOVE minimum wage. The medical transcriptionist is too valuable and too highly trained to be treated in a shabby manner. The setting of pay scales is not usually the supervisor's position. If there is a question, the employee may go to the Personnel Department, the employer, or accountant.

WORK STANDARDS

Evaluation of Quality

Quality assurance in medical transcription actually means proofreading. When proofing a document, the following points should be considered.

General Appearance ▪ Is the date in proper format (i.e., spelled out in a letter)?

Are all tabs aligned, particularly if there is a caption at the top of a letter or document?

Has proper format been followed regarding justification, paragraphing, subject headings, and so forth? In general, paragraphs should be no longer than approximately 16 lines. This not only enhances the appearance of the document but also makes reading and comprehension of the contents much easier.

Are words properly hyphenated, when needed? Words that should NOT be hyphenated include single-syllable words, two-letter word breaks, and proper names.

Too many hyphens at the ends of lines give a fencelike appearance to the right side of the document. In general, no more than two lines in a row should have hyphenated end words.

Is the text balanced? Keep *at least* two lines of text on every page of a document. Do not have a signature block alone on a page.

Spelling ▪ If the work is by a new employee, the document should be read word-for-word, looking for spelling errors and misused words. More experienced transcriptionists usually do not make such errors, especially since the advent of software spell checkers, and their work can be scanned more quickly.

Look for format errors. Most software systems have a "behind the screen" type of monitoring system, e.g., in WordPerfect it is <REVEAL CODES> which will show how the document was set up by the transcriptionist. There is usually a <VIEW DOCUMENT>, or "what you see is what you get" (WYSIWYG) screen on which to see how it will print out.

Search for "PRDisms" and Rapidtext (stenotype) errors. This applies to those transcriptionists using keyboard enhancement programs such as PRD+,* sophisticated macros, or court-reporting equipment as an adjunct to their transcribing skills. The most seasoned transcriptionist using these transcribing aids can make unwitting errors, or "finger faults," which may not be readily apparent, since this type of software can be inadvertently instructed to in-

*PRD+ Transcription Software is a computer software product by Productivity Software International, Inc., New York, New York 10017-4707.

sert words that are correctly spelled but are inappropriate. Many transcriptionists using Rapidtext have problems with punctuation as well, so this should be checked. Look for problems with parts of speech in work that has been generated utilizing these transcribing aids, as phonetically such things as the noun "follow-up" and the verb "follow up" are the same and do not always print out in correct form, especially if improperly stroked by the transcriptionist using Rapidtext.

Medical words that are sound-alikes also get "confused" in the sophisticated software, e.g., ilium versus ileum. If your establishment is following a certain style of spelling, such as using only preferred terms according to *Dorland's Illustrated Medical Dictionary,* look for deviations in words that may be spelled two ways. Consistency in transcribing is important, especially within a service where several different people are transcribing for the same doctor's clients.

Content ▪ Does it make sense? Simply because a transcriptionist is using sophisticated software, such as PRD+, this does not preclude errors. Often transcriptionists tend to rely on the software, including spell check, to do their work for them. This is not enough. Properly spelled words are not always appropriate or germane to the text.

Punctuation ▪ The tendency today is toward "open punctuation." However, certain rules of punctuation ALWAYS apply. A good grammar guide, such as *Medical Transcription Guide: Do's and Don'ts,* by Fordney and Diehl, can be of invaluable assistance.

Occupational Safety and Health Administration (OSHA)

See Labor Laws in Chapter 3.

PERSONNEL

Benefits Program Administration

Benefits are usually established by the employer; that is, the hospital or transcription service. Employees should be aware of the benefits available to them, which can be outlined either in the Procedure Manual (see later) or in a separate packet. The supervisor/manager should ensure that each employee has the information necessary at the time she becomes eligible for those benefits, which is generally after successful completion of the 90-day probationary period. Such benefits may or may not include vacation time, holidays, sick days, maternal leave, paternal leave, health insurance (covering the employee and/or dependents), life insurance programs, profit-sharing, and a 401-K retirement program.

Recruitment and Screening

If the method of hiring is through the classified section of the newspaper, the transcription supervisor should be the one to write the advertisement since she is qualified to state the requirements of the job. Screening may be done over the phone prior to the prospective employee's coming in to fill out an application. The supervisor can usually ascertain through conversation whether the applicant has been in the business for very long or is just out of school. It is too time consuming for the supervisor to have people drop in and fill out an application. An alternative or supplement to newspaper advertising is to recruit through the local AAMT chapter, since most chapters have a newsletter or make announcements of job opportunities at their monthly meetings. This could be a more reliable source for acquiring qualified personnel. However, AAMT does not endorse its members' qualifications as transcriptionists.

Hiring

When it has been determined that the applicant is qualified for the job offered (whether by résumé alone or testing), make it clear prior to hiring that the first 90 days are a probationary period, and that the new employee can be terminated at any time during that period without notice. Rules, such as those outlined in the Procedure Manual or Handbook, should be made clear from the outset so that there is no confusion about what will be expected of the new employee.

Dismissal

Firing an employee can be as traumatic for the supervisor as for the person being fired. No one should be fired without a fair trial. A 90-day probationary period gives the supervisor 3 months to determine whether the employee is qualified to fill the position. After 90 days, if there are reasons that necessitate firing someone, these reasons should have been discussed with the employee on at least one other occasion. Disrupting other employees, for instance, should have been a subject of discussion between supervisor and employee at an earlier time. If the practice continues, issue a warning, and if it persists, grounds will have been laid to justify the dismissal. Keep documentation of problems as they occur in the employee's file. This documentation will also be useful in the case of a disgruntled ex-employee applying to the Labor Board for wrongful termination. In the case of shoddy workmanship, the supervisor or quality assurance manager must keep documentation of the employee's progress or deterioration. Because an employee has "passed" the 90-day probationary period, it cannot be assumed that workmanship will continue at this level, which is one of the reasons that all employees' work be monitored periodically throughout employment. It is customary (and legally safer) to give 2 weeks' notice to a permanent employee.

Two week's notice is not necessary when an employee has caused a problem necessitating immediate dismissal. The cause can be insubordination, physical fighting, verbal abuse of another employee, obvious bigotry (first discussed with the employee at the outset to see whether the attitude changes), walking off the job, drug abuse, or stealing.

When there is not enough work to sustain the number of employees, document this information in a formal letter to the employee(s) being laid off. The employees will need this documentation to take with them to their next employer, and the supervisor will need a copy of it in the file to use in case of litigation, should this situation arise.

Management consulting firms have set up some guidelines for the painful procedure of termination. Some of the comments from these establishments include the following.

DO's	DON'Ts
▪ Give as much warning as possible for mass layoffs.	▪ Don't leave room for confusion when firing. Tell the employee in the first sentence that she is terminated.
▪ Sit down one-on-one with the individual in a private office.	
▪ Complete a firing session within 15 minutes.	▪ Don't allow time for debate during a firing session.
▪ Provide written explanations of severance benefits, if any.	▪ Don't make personal comments when firing someone. Keep the conversation professional.
▪ Provide outplacement services away from the hospital, if available.	▪ Don't rush a fired employee off-site unless security is really an issue.
▪ Be sure the employee hears about the termination from a manager, not from a coworker.	▪ Don't fire people on significant dates, such as Christmas Eve or the anniversary of their employment.
▪ Express appreciation for what the employee has contributed, if this is appropriate.	▪ Don't fire employees when they are on vacation or have just returned.

JOB DESCRIPTIONS

How to Write a Job Description

Every job should be clearly outlined. For medical transcriptionists, it would seem there should be no problem—one sits at the computer and transcribes, once the procedures are learned. Actually, there are degrees and ranks of employees in any office or facility, with lead transcriptionists, trainers, trainees, those assigned to handle staff requests, and so forth. Outline in numeric order. Clearly describe duties so there is no doubt concerning the responsibilities of each individual. If the supervisor is responsible for a printing section of the department, for instance, write a job description outlining the duties of those who do the printing. In the case of overlapping jobs, such as when a transcriptionist does her own printing or modeming, carefully document job duties so there is no confusion of responsibilities.

American Association of Medical Transcription Job Description

For an example of what might be considered in a job description, refer to the AAMT job description in Chapter 1, Figure 1–1.

Creation of a Procedural Manual

An employee should start on a new job knowing employer policies. Too often, new employees flounder, not knowing whom to go to for assignments, where to find reference books, and sometimes not even knowing restroom locations. Prior to beginning work, the supervisor can ascertain whether each employee has read the established Procedure Manual. This manual should be located in a conspicuous place for easy reference by new and established employees in the case of questions. In addition, each employee might be given her own copy. Once the supervisor has laid out the course of procedures of the office, it should be outlined in a manual and arranged in logical order with appropriate boldface headings for easy reference. Avoid situations in which employees wander around aimlessly trying to figure out how to do things. Refer the employee to the person to contact for situations such as the absence of a trainer or supervisor or the handling of doctor/nurse inquiries.

Outline company policies in the Procedure Manual (sometimes referred to as The Handbook), such as conditions of permanent hire, causes for termination, smoking areas, and general rules for employee deportment. Many establishments have the employee sign a paper stating she or he has read the manual and understands what it says. Wording of the manual can be important in case of litigation. For instance, the word "should" implies there is a choice for the employee, that she should do or should not do something. A better word is "will"—"The employee *will* be on time for her shift." Document guidelines and rules of employment that will be binding on both employee and employer, both of whom must be aware that this is a legal and binding document, admissible in a court of law.

INVESTIGATION OF NEW TECHNOLOGIES

The American Association for Medical Transcription (AAMT) and the American Health Information Management Association (AHIMA) constantly provide information about the latest techniques and equipment. Vendors at the exhibit halls of conventions and symposia are eager to provide information regarding their wares and willingly send sales representatives to the facility to demonstrate them. If the supervisor is on good terms with other establishments, it might be helpful to check them out, making sure to clear this method of investigation with the employer as well as the establishment in question. Once a hospital or service gets on a mailing list, a variety of information will come pouring in, so much so that it will often be as confusing as it is helpful.

Before making any recommendations about new equipment to the employer, it is wise to verify how well the technology works for someone else. It is not a good idea to be a pioneer when it comes to expensive equipment. Being "the first on the block to have one" is not advisable unless you actually can get a 90-day trial of the equipment. This is rarely possible, especially with the installation of an LAN.

REFERENCE BOOKS

The supervisor is responsible for maintaining up-to-date reference books so they are available to all transcriptionists. Aside from the obvious medical references (see Chapter 11 and Appendix 1, also include the local telephone directories, as well as telephone directories for out-of-town clients, the National ZIP code book, and when possible, hospital directories; a local medical society directory is a necessary reference. Almost all software companies publish a monthly or bimonthly magazine in addition to an operating manual. WordPerfect, WordStar, and Microsoft-Word, for instance, have monthly publications that contain updates, hints, useful articles, and answers to some of the software questions that are not covered in the operating manuals. Usually the supervisor can have the employer subscribe to these useful publications for the company, and it is to her advantage to have access to the information to be gleaned from monthly publications that deal with software, medical transcription, and office management in general.

Appendix 1 contains a comprehensive list of references considered essential to every medical transcription department. Often, seasoned transcriptionists will bring their own books to their work stations. Most medical transcription departments keep their own medical specialty lists that the supervisor should keep up-to-date or delegate someone to accomplish this.

For her own edification, the medical transcription supervisor might want to keep abreast of related articles in such publications as the *Journal of the American Association for Medical Transcription* (JAAMT), *Perspectives* (published by Health Professions Institute, or HPI), *Wall Street Journal, Business Magazine, Physician's Management Magazine, Medical Economics,* and the aforementioned software publications. All these publications have articles, hints, and suggestions that can be helpful and may possibly show the way to solving a particularly knotty problem the supervisor might be facing. It is important for the supervisor to remember that it really is not that "lonely at the top"—there is always someone out there who has gone through the same problem—and possibly has written an article about it. Symposia and seminars, which are relevant to many of the problems faced by the medical transcription supervisor, are constantly being offered by the professional medical transcription organizations.

Subscribing to JAAMT through the auspices of the American Association for Medical Transcription is certainly highly recommended. Suggested reading for the supervisor from this bimonthly magazine might be, for instance, *A do-it-yourself incentive plan,* Spring 1985, by Marilyn Craddock, C.M.T., R.R.A.; *The transcription circus,* Summer 1982, by Hazel Tank, C.M.T.; *Work standards you can live with,* Fall/

Winter 1987-1988, by Marilyn Craddock, C.M.T., R.R.A.; and *They are asking the wrong questions,* May-June 1991, by Claudia Tessier, C.M.T., R.R.A., to name but a few. There is always a section on style *(SOS: Standards of Style)* and at least one updated list of medical terms.

In the 1980s, a series of articles was published in JAAMT, titled *The Supervisor's Corner,* which had input from various supervisors around the country, and was edited by Mary Gallop, C.M.T. Back issues of JAAMT are available from the AAMT office in Modesto, California.

SUMMARY

The medical transcription supervisor has an awesome responsibility—not a job for the faint of heart. It means dealing with clients, subordinates, equipment, and employers. In most cases, the supervisor is categorized as "middle management" in hospitals and services alike. This means she is restrained from certain actions by those above her in rank and pressured to do many things by those subordinate to her. It means "keeping her cool" in the face of what may seem like unreasonable demands from the employer and equally unreasonable gripes from the employees. She must be sage and psychologist, a firm leader who does not dominate, yet a loyal follower as well. This is something like being a mother in a three-generation household, with the grandmother (employer) giving orders to mother (supervisor) and the children (employees) making their demands as well. Perhaps that is why most transcription supervisors are women. They have had the training and stamina for it.

Bron Taylor, B.A.

Editing and Phonetic Problem Solving

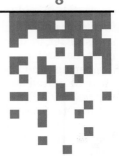

INTRODUCTION

> Every man's work, whether it be literature or music or pictures or architecture or anything else, is always a portrait of himself.
>
> SAMUEL BUTLER

Editing is a difficult challenge for both beginning and experienced transcriptionists. Most are very comfortable having one right way to do things: the proprietary name for the drug furosemide is spelled L-a-s-i-x and that's that; there's an undeniable satisfaction to that. There are no options or variations. Since most transcriptionists have put in long hours learning the right way to spell instruments, muscles, medications, and other medical terms, it can come as a shock to the beginner to discover that in the field of editing, there is often more than one acceptable way to type what has been dictated. In the Fall 1984 issue of *The Journal of the American Association for Medical Transcription (AAMT)*, Sally Pitman addressed this issue well. "Some medical transcriptionists," she wrote, "are uncomfortable with choices of alternate acceptable forms. To simplify their lives and reduce the number of uncertainties they face in their work, they would at times like to be told, 'there is only one right way'" (Pitman, 1984). Unfortunately, the only absolute in editing is that whatever choices one makes, one should be consistent.

Many hospitals have an "official" policy: "our transcriptionists never edit what a physician dictates." There is, however, an unofficial policy that advises transcriptionists to do their best, as quickly as possible, to "clean up" the reports. Some physicians feel they need no editing unless it is carefully done. Most dictate reasonably well although it is not their highest priority. They may be tired when they dictate and make errors, but they always appreciate careful editing. Others remember every comma they dictate and want each one left in the report, and the transcriptionist might be confronted with a red-faced desk-pounder when altering such an individual's work. What to do? Certainly, gender inconsistencies and noun/verb disagreements are corrected. As transcriptionists become more confident (that is, when they have heard a variant of the same report hundreds of times), more changes can be made.

The best guideline was that suggested by Vera Pyle in a 1981 AAMT workshop on editing. In discussing the medicolegal implications of letting obvious errors stay in the record, she described a case in which red cells in the urine were attributed by the dictator to menses in a patient whom he earlier had said was status posthysterectomy. Vera said that this was one of those cases in which the transcriptionist should not only edit but call the physician to advise him of the problem. Having reported her observation to the doctor, "I heard him suck in his breath and ask, 'And what did you do?' She replied, 'I checked the patient's chart and left out the part about its not being considered significant because the patient was menstruating.' He heaved a sigh of relief and said, 'Thank you'" (Pyle, 1981).

But what Vera did not feel it appropriate to say was, "You're going to have to find out what the red cells were all about." She said, "I was not there in the capacity of a consultant; I was simply there in the capacity of protecting the doctor, the hospital, and the patient." This is part of our function, and it is far removed from the passive transmitter of questionable information. A line must be drawn between editing discreetly and tampering, and there is a difference. Dictation must be edited subtly and carefully so the dictator responds favorably.

Most transcriptionists need to work very fast because of pressure from their supervisors or because they are working on a production basis. Clearly, editing is something that must be done quickly, thoughtfully, and carefully. Transcriptionists who work in hospitals are frequently on the receiving end of the somewhat adversarial relationship between physicians, who recognize the importance of having their charts current but do not make this their top priority, and directors of medical record departments, who can be critical and heavy-handed with doctors. The resulting discord is often heard through the earphones. Part of the transcriptionist's job is to factor out this irritation and help the physician produce the document that was intended, even if it is not exactly what was dictated.

Language in itself is peculiar. Note how quickly the meaning of the word "hopefully" has changed from "looking forward to with anticipation" to "I hope that." Within a decade or so other usage may seem archaic. All languages change. The Dutch formally simplify their syntax rules about every 5 years. In German, the dative case is disappearing; teachers tell their students to read the material but pay it no attention, as nobody uses it anymore. The French language changes, despite its formidable Academy, the purpose of which is to freeze the language into a pure form. English, a particularly strong and vigorous language, is able to incorporate words from every source effortlessly, and as many parts of speech. For instance, "angioplastiable" appeared almost as soon as angioplasty did, as did "arteriogrammed," as well as corrupted words such as the patient was "romied." Thus, English changes faster than most languages, giving it great power and making it today, as German was in the 19th century, the premier scientific language. Many excellent style guides are available to help in dealing with these shifting sands, but they are only guides and it is necessary to stay flexible, use common sense, and be consistent.

Spelling a drug incorrectly, confusing one drug with another, or leaving out a word such as "no" in front of "carcinoma" are major errors and could, if not caught, cause serious harm to a patient. However, spending a great deal of time over whether or not to use a hyphen is minor. One has to develop a sense of perspective. Indeed, there may not be a choice. If the transcriptionist owns a service, the dictators often set the style, which is followed except for English grammar or blatant medical errors. Therefore, it is necessary to recognize and learn each physician's style. The transcriptionist who works for a service must remember that the owner sets the style. Some hospitals have rigid styles and others do not care what the medical transcriptionists do as long as the work is turned out quickly. This gives the transcriptionist more freedom, and good style manuals can be consulted.

The worst thing a transcriptionist can do in a questionable situation is to guess. There is the temptation to try to make something one does not really hear correctly make sense, and some hair-raising errors have resulted from this process of rationalization. As Vera Pyle put it, "To me a blank is an honorable thing; it means you don't know." Sometimes, given the time constraints under which the transcriptionist works and the fact that it is not always possible to reach a doctor or obtain the chart, this may seem the only possible way out. However, some supervisors dislike blanks in reports, for any reason. At some hospitals, leaving blanks can result in a bad evaluation. In such situations, this encourages either guessing or omitting part of the dictation. Leaving a blank is working within the standards that professional scholars use; one never pretends to knowledge one does not have. When the document in question is someone's medical record, this becomes even more important. Leaving out the questionable material may seem to be the best choice, but what does that do to the physician who, in the worst scenario, may end up in court, questioned about why a particular test had not been done when in fact it had been completed but was unclearly dictated or omitted? Now, when most transcription is done on word processors, when changes can be called in and very quickly and conveniently changed, there is no excuse for guessing, but there never was, even in the days when transcriptionists had to erase three carbon copies whenever the dictators changed their minds.

There are style guides and beautifully written and edited journals to read and learn from, and there is the considerable satisfaction of having worked with a tired physician to produce the report that was intended and that can now be used for patient care, research, or other useful purposes. To contribute to making such a document as accurate as possible is no small matter.

TYPES OF ERRORS

Abbreviations ▪ Almost every hospital has an approved list of abbreviations so transcriptionists should try not to use an unapproved abbreviation even if the dictator did. If unorthodox abbreviations appear, transcriptionists should make a list of them for the dictator to be sure they are spelled correctly. Dictators seem overly fond of abbreviations; they save time and, to interns just out of training, they sound cryptic, important, and "medical." Medical transcriptionists dislike them, because the sound quality on many machines is such that many consonants sound alike, and a great deal of time can be wasted trying to ascertain what is really being dictated. The supervisor can be of help in getting physicians to adhere to the approved list; in the case of a service owner, the telephone can be of help.

Accuracy ▪ This is the goal of all transcriptionists at all times and in every setting. Accurate records contribute to good patient care. In the heat of actual transcription, often under physically suboptimal conditions and onerous speed constraints, careful attention should be paid to catching medical errors and to producing as much as possible as fast as possible. Grammatical errors should be changed automatically, but if a dictator favors a certain style which is not the transcriptionist's favorite, and the meaning is clear, give in.

Punctuation ▪ Errors occur from time to time regarding colons, commas, use of figures, symbols, periods, decimal points, capitalization, and the like. An experienced transcriptionist should always know the current rules of punctuation or have on hand a current reference book for grammar and punctuation (see Reference Sources at the end of this chapter and Appendix 1, List of References, under the heading Style Manuals, Medical and General).

There are subtle differences in punctuation and again, there is more than one correct way. If the transcriptionist works for one physician only, during the course of that employment the physician's way is the correct way. Most medical transcriptionists will work in many environments during their careers and must learn to be flexible. The thrust of knowledge for the medical transcriptionist is medicine, as well as correct style, and a whole armamentarium of correct styles needed to do the job right is necessary. "Right" does not mean according to one's favorite style manual; it means producing the most accurate document possible.

Electronic ▪ The transcriptionist should not depend on the spell checker in the word processor as a substitute for proofreading. Programming errors can be found in them, and they do not point out correctly spelled words used out of context. "The patient had tick douloureux" would pass, as would the incorrectly transcribed "eight-nerve damage" for "eighth nerve damage." A sentence like "The patient would benefit from an infection," when "injection" was meant would get through. Still, for catching the routine typos we all make, spell checking software is invaluable. Choosing to save a few minutes by not using the spell checker would be a serious mistake.

Hyphen and Word Division ▪ Hyphens are used mainly to aid the reader in clarity and pronunciation. Word processors and computers feature automatically justified margins thus taking word division at the end of a line out of a transcriptionist's hands. However, hyphenation is used when keyboarding some compound words and phrases. When using typing equipment, deciding when to hyphenate words at the end of a line can slow down production, so hyphenation might be avoided. Remember, a word divided in error is just as incorrect as a word misspelled. If in doubt about hyphenation, consult a good dictionary, English handbook, or word book that shows where words should be divided.

Technical Errors, Inconsistencies, and Redundancies ▪ Inconsistencies and redundancies should be discreetly edited out. Inconsistencies require considerable judgment and possible contact with the physician via a note or call. An obvious technical error ("potassium 136, sodium 3.9") may be a simple inversion but requires investigation unless one is positive that it is just an inversion. Catching this type of error is very satisfying, and if the dictator notices, even more so. Some hospitals have computers showing the laboratory data and current medications and all orders for every inpatient. Transcriptionists lucky enough to work in an institution with such a system should make good use of it. For outpatients, it is still necessary to use judgment and not simply omit unclear dictation.

Misspelling ▪ Good English and comprehensive medical dictionaries are the transcriptionist's best friends. In addition, many experienced transcriptionists keep a short list of difficult words for quick reference. This is an excellent resource. It is not uncommon for a transcriptionist to be able to spell the most difficult medical terms and then have problems with trying to remember how to spell some simple English words.

Possessives ▪ In *The Elements of Style* by Strunk and White (1979), words like Sachs are spelled "Sachs's" when possessive. Many other excellent style manuals disagree. This area poses a problem for many transcriptionists and many English-speaking people. Another issue related to possessives that has caused some debate in the transcription community is eponyms. Some prestigious journals and the American Medical Association's guide to *Current Medical Information and Terminology* favor the lack of the possessive for eponymic diseases. To many transcriptionists "Bell palsy" or "Kaposi sarcoma" sounds exceedingly odd now, but in 10 years it might be different. This is where Pyle's rule about not meddling applies. A physician who for 30 years has dictated "Parkinson's disease" is not going to accept the dictation if it is edited to "Parkinson disease." As the meaning is clear both ways, why offend the physician? Perhaps when everyone who learned that eponyms are possessives has retired, this change can be made painlessly, but upsetting the dictator when meaning is not enhanced is not the transcriptionist's function.

It is possible to persuade physicians to use words of which they may be unaware, such as "mitigate" for "militate" or "appraise" for "apprise," and if this is gently done, soon they will think they have been doing it correctly all along. A delicate touch is needed; diplomacy is everything. However, one should never type what is clearly wrong, because that will embarrass the physician and the institution and reflect badly on the transcriptionist. There are many physician personalities and many ways to handle them. Common sense is the guideline.

Semicolon ▪ Next to the use of the comma, the most common punctuation problem is when to use a semicolon. Some physicians dictate in one continuous sentence so it is up to the transcriptionist to decide when a period, comma, or semicolon is needed. The first rule is to use a semicolon to separate two or more closely related independent clauses when no conjunction is used.

Example: Ms. Doe will be unable to keep her appointment on July 6; her daughter is visiting for an extra 10 days. (This could also be made into two sentences.)

A second rule is to use a semicolon to separate independent clauses if either or both of them have been punctuated with two or more commas.

Example: About 10 days ago, she developed pain in the groin, which she ignored; and, finally, she came in for an examination on June 6 at the request of her gynecologist.

Use a semicolon between a series of phrases or clauses if any item in the series has internal commas.

Example: The patient received Cardizem CD 180 mg daily; Mevacor 20 mg orally with meals; and allopurinol, 1½ tablets daily.

When typing transitional expressions (however, furthermore, nevertheless, consequently, accordingly, anyhow, still, then) use a semicolon *before* when it is joining two independent clauses and use a comma *after* the expression when it is composed of two or more syllables.

Example: There is no evidence of fracture of the skull or facial bones; however, cloudiness of the sinuses is seen.

Spacing ▪ If one works for a service, where the amount of white paper on a page is important and physicians pay careful attention to it because it costs them money, do exactly what the supervisor wants. In a hospital setting, do not use huge block paragraphs, as they are hard to read. Use good judgment, follow the sense of the report, and put in paragraph breaks even if the dictator does not. In operative reports, begin a new paragraph when another step of the procedure is performed. An experienced transcriptionist will know all the different steps of the various operations: the preparation, the incision, the finding of the problem, dealing with other problems encountered, preparation for closure, closure itself, and the counts at the end. In very long narrative discharge summaries, when dates change, a new consultant comes in, or a new problem arises, a paragraph should be added. The transcriptionist has considerable leeway to improve the ease of reading of the report.

EDITING

The four levels of editing in medical transcription are:

- *Chart notes.* These are done in fragmented sentences, are intended for the physician's office record only, and receive the least attention (although here, as everywhere, scrupulous attention should be given to drug names).

- *Work done for a service.* Much of this is correspondence between physicians who know one another well and speak to each other often and who can write informally in private practice correspondence without losing precision.

- *Hospital work.* Most of this should be exquisitely formal (death summaries, autopsy reports) and done very carefully with attention to medical accuracy.

- *Journal editing.* This is professional editing in which highest accuracy and precision must be enforced. Hospital and service work, involving the needs of patients and often done at top speed, is not expected to attain the level of journal editing.

Grammar ■ Do the dictator a favor and fix errors in grammar.

Substandard Language ■ Slang and vulgar and inflammatory remarks have no place in a medical record. Physicians work under pressure and sometimes get angry and ventilate in this manner while dictating. Transcribing slang terms (such as referring to cancer as "mets" for metastases) is a very poor practice. If physicians stop to realize what they like in medical reports, usually they would want slang removed. If there is a question, one should write it on a separate piece of paper or let the supervisor hear the actual tape, if possible. Otherwise, this material is best discarded and carefully reworded by the transcriptionist.

FOREIGN DICTATION

One needs to be polite when contacting physicians whose English is a second language. They are well aware of their language problems; making the whole dictating and transcribing process adversarial will just make it worse.

Physicians who speak with an accent are not uneducated. Many of the best physicians speak English as a second language. It is necessary for the transcriptionist to learn to deal with difficult accents. The transcriptionist needs to transcribe as much "difficult" dictation as possible to overcome the beginner's initial fear of accents and develop an ear for understanding the variances of phonetic sounds. Those who grew up in a family with parents or grandparents from a foreign country often have an understanding ear. However, some may never develop the skill of transcribing for a foreign-born physician.

Tonality ■ One aspect of accents is their consistency. Once one has "cracked the code" for a given doctor's accent, it will begin to seem like fluent English. This needs to be taken on faith at first, but persistence pays off. A physician who pronounces a letter wrong by English standards will do it that way every time. The transcriptionist should listen and then consider the content of the typical report the physician has dictated. If a few telephone calls have to be made or notes written to supplement this, the transcriptionist should do that too.

Phrasing ■ Consistency applies here as well. Emphasizing the wrong syllable is frequent in people whose English is a second language, but they do it the same way every time. Keeping a list of phrases of very difficult dictators with accents may help until the physician's style has become familiar. (Sharing what one has learned with the other transcriptionists is beneficial.)

Inflection ▪ Persistence pays off here more than in any other area of transcription. Once one learns the rhythm, after an initial intimidating dictation or two, most accents are not so formidable, and one develops a reputation for having a fine ear. Sometimes it is necessary to ask (as in the case of one physician who baffled one transcriptionist after another with his constant use of the word "pegwaff." It was thought to be some obscure cardiology term. It turned out to be "paragraph").

Grammar ▪ This is where the experienced transcriptionist's excellent knowledge of English grammar comes to the forefront. Foreign physicians usually will translate from their native language into English with the grammar of the native language intact. This can mean adjectives following the nouns they modify and verbs coming at the end of the sentence. The ability to transcribe such dictation quickly, automatically transposing adjective/noun while placing the verb in a more appropriate position, and still listening through the heavy accent for medical accuracy, is the mark of an Olympic-grade transcriptionist!

PROOFREADING

The proofreader's function is something like that of a goalie in hockey. The transcriptionist as proofreader takes the final stand against errors appearing in the record. The first step is to look at the document as a whole. Are the dates correct? Is the name correct on page 2 and subsequent pages? Is the dictating physician listed as the signing physician? Is the patient's name correct and where it belongs? Is the report on the correct letterhead? If all this is correct, the report is read for its medical content. The transcriptionist very carefully checks reports that involve emotions, because that is when one is likely to miss errors. Production transcriptionists in a hurry should watch for errors such as repetitions ("a patient that that") which some spell checkers might not catch. Typos that are acceptable English words ("care" for "case") will get by the spell checker. Consistency of labora-

tory data should be noted. Any trick that works, that keeps the proofreader paying attention to the care with which the work has been put on the page, is useful (especially in these days of word processors, when work riddled with errors looks beautiful). Experienced transcriptionists have learned to listen to a little bell that goes off when there is an element of doubt. It is very important, in these days of required speedy production, to listen for that bell. If an experienced transcriptionist has doubts, it probably is wrong. The warning bell comes only with considerable experience and should be valued as the mark of skill that it is.

Also, there are machine glitches, when the information is simply not on the tape and the best transcriptionists in the world could not fill it in. This requires mandatory flagging.

Flagging or Tagging ▪ Supervisors who remove notes from transcriptionists to physicians are a nationwide problem, as reading through back issues of *The Journal of the AAMT* reveals. One has to be creative in getting around this problem. There are alternative ways either to mail documents or to telephone the physician. If these approaches do not work, direct discussion with the supervisor about the legal jeopardy into which the hospital and physicians are being placed, done politely and in a nonconfrontational manner, might produce results. If this is a continuing problem, maybe it is time to go to the supervisor's boss, to network at the next AAMT meeting, or to look at the want ads, as this is a dangerous practice for the hospital and the physicians and does not allow medical transcriptionists to use their skills. This is a lose/lose situation. A flagging or tagging note can be very simply produced if one's department does not already have a supply (Figure 8–1).

CORRECTING ERRORS

Because there are legal ramifications in regard to correcting medical documents, various acceptable methods will be stated here.

Hospital Reports ▪ In hospital transcription, retain the original transcript if it is necessary to retype a medical report. The physician should insert omitted words, correct all errors, and ini-

Dear Doctor:_____

Patient:_____

Number:_____

Date:_____

There is/are blanks in your report at the following locations:

_____
_____
_____

You can complete this by hand or dictate the missing part. If so doing, please call the Transcription Unit to say you are completing an incomplete dictation.

THANK YOU.

Transcription Unit

A

Dear Doctor _____ :

   RE: Patient name _____

        Report name _____

        Date dictated _____

☐ Please see blank on page ___ , paragraph _____ of this report. It sounded like _____

☐ Dictate more slowly and distinctly.

☐ Spell proper names.

☐ Spell unusual words in address.

☐ Spell patient names.

☐ Spell new and unusual surgical instruments.

☐ Spell new drug names.

☐ Spell new laboratory tests.

☐ Indicate unusual punctuation.

☐ Indicate closing salutation.

☐ Indicate your title.

☐ Indicate end of letter.

☐ Give dates of reports.

☐ Speak louder.

☐ Give patient's hospital number.

☐ Please read the area of this report indicated by the penciled checkmark for accuracy.

☐ Your dictation was cut off. Please fill in the rest of the report or redictate.

Thank you. Please return this note with corrections via hospital mail to:

Transcriptionist _____

Telephone No. _____ Date _____

B

Figure 8–1

Examples of flagging or tagging slips to be appended to a medical transcript for solving problem dictation. For emphasis, these forms may be printed on colored paper. A, This form requires fill-in by the transcriptionist to inquire about blanks on the transcript. B, A check-off form to cover many problems one might encounter when transcribing a document. (B reprinted with permission from Fordney, Marilyn T., and Marcy O. Diehl. *Medical Transcription Guide: Do's and Don'ts.* W. B. Saunders Co., Philadelphia, 1990.)

tial each correction directly on the original transcript. The second draft should contain the words "corrected for typing errors." The physician should sign both transcripts and they should be stapled together.

If the hospital transcription is paperless and the physician has electronically signed off the original dictation, an amendment stating the correct version of the report is transcribed. The original transcript should contain the statement "refer to the amendment."

Physician's Office Reports and Chart Notes ■ To make a correction on a chart note, draw a line through the error so as not to obliterate the words and type or write the correction above or below the error or make a separate correction entry. In the margin, write *correction* or *Corr.* and initial and date it. Never use self-adhesive typing strips to blot out an error.

Corrections on the Typewriter ■ Make corrections so the copy will not have to be retyped. Use good correction tools: a soft brush, correction fluid, correction tape, lift-off tape with correctable film ribbon. Realign material properly in the typewriter and use typewriter functions to make corrections (when available). Never attempt to cover up large mistakes with correction fluid unless it is a master for photocopy material. Correction fluid is best for punctuation errors. Never use an eraser over a keyboard or place paper with wet correction fluid back under the typewriter platen as these habits can cause equipment malfunction.

REFERENCE SOURCES

In this career field, there are wonderful reference sources, such as *Style Guide for Medical Transcription*, by Sally Pitman and Claudia Tessier, and *Medical Transcription Guide: Do's and Don'ts*, by Marilyn Fordney and Marcy Diehl. The latter is particularly good because it includes a twenty-page list of reference materials and publications with a section on style manuals, including thirteen references.

One of the joys of having learned medical transcription is that one can read and understand medical journals. This is a rewarding capability, because the more one reads good journals, the more one learns and sees excellent editing and transcription, and the more interesting one's job becomes—also, the more one realizes that there are many "correct" ways to use medical terminology. Journals are the cutting edge of science, and there is no better way to keep up to date than to read them. In this career field, there are two excellent journals, *The Journal of the American Association for Medical Transcription,* published six times annually and *Perspectives on the Medical Transcription Profession,* published quarterly by the Health Professions Institute in Modesto, California.

There are journals for every specialty. A visit to a medical library can be exciting. Where does one find journals? Most hospital transcriptionists are amazed to discover that they have access to the hospital library and even the MEDLINE search feature. At a service, the owner might ask the physicians to pass on journals they no longer need. A physician cannot keep all the journals that are received; there are simply too many.

Only a few clients have to agree for the office to accumulate a healthy pile of reading material.

Many physicians consider *The New England Journal of Medicine* the premier medical journal in the world. The *Journal of the American Medical Association* is also good and has a worldwide, multilingual readership. There are numerous others, from the fascinating *Emergency Medicine* to a number of nursing journals, which are full of articles about new instruments, tools, and procedures. If a particular journal is of special interest, one can subscribe to it.

Writing style manuals are abundant. The New York Times publishes one, *The New York Times Manual of Style and Usage,* as does The University of Chicago Press, *The Chicago Manual of Style.* William Zinsser wrote an excellent small book, *On Writing Well.* Another book small in size only is perhaps the most respected general book on good writing in American English. Written by William Strunk and E. B. White, it is called *The Elements of Style.* Charles Brusaw and associates produced a book called *The Handbook of Technical Writing,* which addresses scientific writers in general but is certainly appropriate to the needs of medical transcriptionists. Cambridge University Press has just issued David Crystal's *The Columbia Encyclopedia of Language* in paperback. All these can be read with great pleasure, as can the delightful book by John Dirckx, M.D., *The Language of Medicine.* The American journals themselves have style manuals, such as Edward Huth's *Medical Style & Format* (Huth is editor of the *Annals of Internal Medicine,* and the small but extraordinarily useful *Stylebook: Editorial Manual of the AMA*). Two intriguing books are Mimi Zeiger's *Essentials of Writing Biomedical Research Papers,* which could probably be used to win an argument or two, and Edith Schwager's *Medical English Usage and Abusage.* (In four of these books, one can find that one should write out numbers "one through eight," "one through nine," "one through ten," and "one through thirteen." Which is right? All of them, if the consistency rule is not violated.)

In summary, medical transcriptionists are an important part of the medical profession. An alert transcriptionist is in a position to be the last person to catch important medical errors dictated by a tired physician. Working with physicians to ensure accurate records is the heart of true professionalism.

Reference Sources

Fordney, Marilyn T., and Marcy O. Diehl. *Medical Transcription Guide: Do's and Don'ts.* W. B. Saunders Company, Philadelphia, 1990.

Pitman, Sally. *The Journal of the American Association for Medical Transcription.* Modesto, California, Fall, 1984.

Pyle, Vera. Editing. Paper presented to the American Association for Medical Transcription Workshop. Modesto, California, 1981.

Strunk, William, Jr., and E. B. White. *The Elements of Style: With Index.* Macmillan Publishing Company, New York, 1979.

Marie D. Low, Ph.D.

Writing for Publication

INTRODUCTION

The rapid expansion and increased professionalization of the medical transcription field during the past decade has brought a corresponding growth in the need for new educational and reference materials. Today, medical transcriptionist educators have at their disposal a wide range of textbooks on subjects from basic medical terminology to advanced medical-legal issues. If practicing in a clinic or hospital, transcriptionists have access to at least five medical dictionaries, innumerable word books on medicine, surgery, and the medical subspecialties, and a variety of style manuals. Nevertheless, the need for new ideas and fresh approaches continues to grow exponentially.

As their careers advance, medical transcriptionists may wish to join the growing group of those who have developed exciting (and sometimes profitable) second careers as text and reference book authors. Or, a transcriptionist may be invited by one of the field's professional journals (such as the *Journal of the American Association for Medical Transcription* or *Perspectives)* to submit an article for publication.

This chapter will help guide transcriptionists through the intricacies of the publishing process, with emphasis on book publishing.

SELECTING A BOOK TOPIC

To find a publisher, the book idea must:

1. Satisfy a *need* that is not currently being filled by available texts or references; and

2. Have a sufficiently large *audience* to offset the publisher's investment in production and marketing, while generating an acceptable profit.

The best book topics rarely arrive in sudden flashes of inspiration. They are much more likely to be the product of a continuous process of information-gathering and analysis. Chances of a favorable response from a publisher can be greatly increased if transcriptionists follow these guidelines before finalizing and submitting the proposal:

1. Review current medical transcription and other allied health journals. What subjects receive repeated attention? What issues appear to be increasing in importance?

2. Talk to practicing transcriptionists. Ask them for a "wish list" of hard-to-find information that would help them to do their jobs more effectively.

3. Talk to educators. Are new courses emerging in the medical transcription curriculum? Do the available textbooks provide the right instructional focus, sufficient practical exercises, and related materials such as interactive learning programs, sample examination questions, and teaching guides?

4. Identify the competition. Collect catalogs from allied health publishers at hospital or college book displays, and note the published titles in the selected fields. Read about new publications in journal announcements or promotions received in the mail. Check *Medical Books in Print* (published annually by R.R. Bowker and

Company, available in most libraries) for a current listing of books on related subjects.

When one is confident that a unique market niche for a book idea has been identified, prospective publishers can be considered.

SELECTING A PUBLISHING COMPANY

A decade ago, medical transcriptionist authors-to-be had a relatively straightforward choice of publishers, as only a handful were actively developing lists in the field. Today, most of the major health sciences publishers (and a host of smaller firms) regularly publish titles for transcriptionists (Table 9–1).

Selecting the right publisher can make a critical difference in the professional acceptance and financial success of the book. The goal is to sign with a publishing company that offers all the following services:

■ 1. *Knowledgeable acquisitions editors.* The editorial contact should be thoroughly familiar with the curriculum and core competencies of

Table 9–1 ■ **Publishers of Medical Transcription Books and Supplementary Materials**

American Association for Medical Transcription (AAMT) P.O. Box 576187 Modesto, CA 95357 (800) 982-2182 or (209) 551-0883	F.A. Davis Company 1915 Arch Street Philadelphia, PA 19103 (800) 523-4049
Appleton & Lange P.O. Box 5630 Norwalk, CT 06856 (800) 423-1359	Neil M. Davis Associates 1143 Wright Drive Huntingdon Valley, PA 19006 (215) 947-1752
Butterworth & Co. Publishers 80 Montvale Avenue Stoneham, MA 02180 (800) 544-1013	Carolyn Denny, CMT 5447 Capital Heights Avenue Baton Rouge, LA 70806-6007
Capitol Area Chapter of AAMT c/o Audrey Klocke Heintz, CMT 609 Hilltop Drive Milton, WI 53563	Facts and Comparisons, subs. of Wolters Kluwer U.S. Corp. 111 West Port Plaza, Suite 423 St. Louis, MO 63146-3098 (800) 223-0554
Churchill Livingstone 650 Avenue of the Americas New York, New York 10011 (808) 553-5426	FYI Book Company P.O. Box 1842 Santa Ana, CA 92702
CIBA-GEIGY 14 Henderson Drive West Caldwell, NJ 07006 (800) 631-1181	Health Professions Institute P.O. Box 801 Modesto, CA 95353 (209) 551-2112
Claremont Press Box 3434 Santa Monica, CA 90408 (213) 829-3238	Houghton Mifflin Company Two Park Street and One Beacon Street Boston, MA 02107 (800) 725-5000
CORE, division of Excerpta Medica Inc. 3131 Princeton Pike, Bldg. 2A Lawrenceville, NJ 08648 (609) 896-9450	William Kaufmann, Inc. 95 First Street Los Altos, CA 94022 (415) 948-5810
D & T Products P.O. Box 3501 Mission Viejo, CA 92690 (714) 458-3362	J.B. Lippincott 227 East Washington Square Philadelphia, PA 19106 (800) 441-4526

Table 9–1 ■ **Publishers of Medical Transcription Books and Supplementary Materials (*Continued*)**

McGraw-Hill Inc.
1221 Avenue of the Americas
New York, NY 10020
(800) 262-4729

Medical Arts Publishing
P.O. Box 36600
Grosse Pointe, MI 48236
(313) 886-5160

Merriam-Webster, Inc.
47 Federal Street
Springfield, MA 01102
(413) 734-3134

Mosby-Year Book
11830 Westline Industrial Drive
P.O. Box 46908
St. Louis, MO 63146-9934
(800) 633-6699

Omnimed, Inc.
P.O. Box 446
Maple Shade, NJ 08052
(800) 257-2326

Oryx Press
4041 North Central, Suite 700
Phoenix, AZ 85012-3397
(800) 279-6799

Oxford University Press
200 Madison Avenue
New York, NY 10016
(800) 334-4249

Parthenon Publishing Group Inc.
120 Mill Road
Park Ridge, NJ 07656
(201) 391-6796

Physicians' Desk Reference, div. of Medical
Economics Data
Five Paragon Drive
Montvale, NJ 07645
(800) 232-7379

PMIC
625 Plainfield Road, Suite 220
Willowbrook, IL 60521
(800) 633-7467

Prentice-Hall
15 Columbus Circle
New York, NY 10023
(800) 922-0579

Janet Christie Pugh, CMT
6158 Miller Road
Columbus, GA 31907

Random House, Inc.
201 E. 50th Street, 31st Floor
New York, NY 10022
(800) 726-0600

Rayve Productions Inc.
P.O. Box 726A
Windsor, CA 95492
(800) 852-4890

W.B. Saunders Company
Curtis Center, Independence Square West
Philadelphia, PA 19106
(215) 238-7800

South-Western Publishing Company
4770 Duke Drive, Suite 200
Mason, OH 45040
(800) 242-7972

Specialized Information Management
1443 E. 7th Street, Suite 204
Charlotte, NC 28204
(800) 248-4888

Springhouse Publishing Company
1111 Bethlehem Pike
Springhouse, PA 19477
(800) 346-7844

Sylvan Software
4521 Campus Drive #594
Irvine, CA 92715
(800) 235-9455

TransCom Resources
County Line Road
Menomenee Falls, WI 53051
(414) 251-1343

Triad Publishing Company
1110 N.W. 8th Avenue
Gainesville, FL 32601
(904) 373-5800

Williams & Wilkins
428 East Preston Street
Baltimore, MD 21202
(800) 638-0672

Based on a list compiled by the American Association for Medical Transcription, Modesto, California, © 1992. These addresses are for editorial use, not for book orders.

the medical transcription field and should have the necessary contacts to obtain helpful peer reviews of a manuscript. This person should also be an effective communicator, so that the transcriptionist will feel comfortable working together through the often stressful process of manuscript development and production.

■ 2. *Experienced designers.* The physical appearance of a book (cover and internal layout) is crucial to marketing it successfully. Publishers should have accomplished book designers on their staff, or access to knowledgeable freelancers.

■ 3. *Qualified copy editors.* Prior to production, a manuscript should be checked for grammatical accuracy, duplication, and internal consistency (spelling, citation of figures and tables). The publisher should provide these services at its expense.

■ 4. *Timely production.* Because most material in the medical and allied health sciences is time sensitive, a manuscript should be typeset and printed without lengthy delays. The average 250-page book requires 4 to 6 months to produce following submission of a final manuscript. The transcriptionist should ask for a detailed production schedule as part of the contract negotiation.

■ 5. *Effective marketing.* The publisher should have the resources and experience to reach a book's intended audience and generate sales. So that the book receives undivided attention, the publisher should not have a substantially similar work already on its list.

The best resource for information about publishers is authors who have worked with them previously. Transcriptionists can write or telephone authors whose books they have used in the field or in the classroom. Most authors will be happy to talk about their publishing experiences and provide referrals. It is recommended that a book proposal be submitted to three publishers. This will provide a range of editorial viewpoints and will permit the transcriptionist to evaluate different production and marketing plans.

SUBMITTING A PROPOSAL

When the three target publishers have been selected, it is time to prepare and submit a formal concept proposal. A proposal is always submitted in writing and must contain at least a cover letter and a preliminary table of contents or chapter outline. Additionally (particularly for a first-time author) the publisher may ask for a sample chapter of the manuscript, to demonstrate one's writing skill and understanding of the audience. A résumé is also helpful.

Cover Letter ■ Successful acquisitions editors receive many unsolicited proposals (called in the industry "over-the-transom" submissions). Hence, a brief and to-the-point submission package will have a better chance of attracting their attention.

Limit the text of the cover letter to a single page (single-spaced) if possible. Provide the following information, discussing each item in a separate paragraph.

1. *Identification of the need.* Explain why this idea is an important addition to the publisher's current book list and to the medical transcription field.

2. *Market analysis.* Identify the book's target audience. Will it be used primarily in the classroom, to train new transcriptionists? If so, for what standard courses could it be adopted? Or will it find its audience among practicing transcriptionists? In the hospital or clinic? In the physician's office? In both?

3. *Competitive analysis.* What published books are closest in audience and content? Why will this book contribute a unique point of view?

4. *Approximate number of pages,* and estimated number of tables, line drawings, and halftones (x-rays and photographs).

5. *Qualifications* of the transcriptionist-author. The transcriptionist shows why he or she is the right person to write on the chosen topic by providing a brief description of current professional position, education, affiliations and association memberships, and any articles, chapters, or books published previously.

Table of Contents ■ This should constitute a maximum of two pages. Include a listing of chapter titles and major subheadings.

Additional Tips ■ Editors are always more favorably impressed when they are addressed by name rather than by title only. Consult the *Literary Marketplace* (available at most libraries) to find the names and mailing addresses of the Allied Health Sciences editors at your target companies. To verify that the information is current, call each company's head office and check with the receptionist.

Editors also respond more positively to new authors who are recommended by authors whose books they have already published. If a colleague has worked with the publisher, the transcriptionist should by all means ask permission to use this person as a reference.

The Publishing Decision ■ Within 7 to 10 days after submitting the proposal package, a short acknowledgment from the editor will be received, either declining the idea or indicating that it is under active consideration. At this point, the transcriptionist may be asked for a sample chapter, if one was not submitted. The editor will probably obtain two or three reviews of the sample from medical transcription instructors or practitioners. The review process helps the editor forecast the potential sales and profits of the published book, which is information needed to prepare a proposal for the publisher's editorial board and obtain a publishing decision.

The review process generally requires another 2 to 4 weeks. After 4 weeks, it is appropriate to write or telephone to inquire about the status of the proposal, if a decision has not been received.

Handling Rejections ■ Transcriptionists should not be discouraged if one or more of the target publishers reject their ideas. It may simply be that the company has a similar work under development but not yet released, or that its production schedule is full and it cannot give the project sufficient attention. But if specific comments on the table of contents or sample chapter are received, they should be reviewed thoroughly before approaching other publishers.

CONTRACTS AND NEGOTIATION

Once a book proposal is accepted for publication, the transcriptionist-author will be asked to sign a contract outlining the responsibilities of both author and publisher. For consistency, most publishers in the health sciences have developed standard form agreements that can be changed via addenda to cover special circumstances.

Author's Responsibilities ■ In general, health sciences publishing contracts require the author to:

1. Prepare a manuscript that is acceptable to the publisher "in form and content." This means:
   a. Following the publisher's guidelines for manuscript submission; for example, correct margins, consistent citation of tables and figures, double spacing, typing on one side of the page only.
   b. Covering all the subjects in the final, approved table of contents.
   c. Responding to any suggestions made by the editors and reviewers.
2. Provide appropriate illustrations (photographs, line drawings and tables) at the author's expense.
3. Assume the costs of preparing final manuscript copy.
4. Obtain permissions to use previously published material and pay any permission fees.
5. Prepare a bibliography and index.
6. Submit the final manuscript by the agreed delivery date.

Publisher's Responsibilities ■ The publisher should assume responsibility for the following at its expense:

Design of the cover and internal pages.
Typesetting.
Printing.
Marketing and distribution.
Payment of author's royalty.
Filing for copyright protection.

Royalties ■ Because of their generally smaller audience, health sciences books pay royalties that may differ significantly from those paid for major "trade" publications (novels, biographies, and the like). The standard royalty rate in health sciences publishing is 10 per cent of the "list" price (that is, of the final selling price of the book to end users). Occasionally, however, contracts provide for the payment of royalties on "net" sales. In this case, the publisher will factor into the royalty calculation any discounts that must be provided to book wholesalers and retail bookstores to offset their cost of sales. The "net" sales number is nearly always lower than the "list" sales number. Hence, an author who is offered a "net" contract should determine whether the royalties being offered are actually lower, even if the royalty *rate* is higher.

A simple example demonstrates the preceding point:

	List Contract	Net Contract
Selling ("list") price	$30.00	$30.00
Trade discount (33⅓%)	10.00	10.00
"Net" price	20.00	20.00
Royalty rate	10%	12%
Author's royalty	$3.00	$2.40

Another clause seen in some health sciences publishing agreements is "escalating" royalties. Under a royalty escalation clause, the publisher minimizes the financial risks of publication by paying royalties at a lower rate until upfront investments in production and marketing have been recovered. Once the forecasted breakeven point is reached, however, the publisher makes the author a partner in the book's success by increasing the royalty rate at each of several agreed-upon sales milestones. Royalties might begin, for example, at 9 per cent of the list price for the first 25,000 copies of the first edition sold, increase to 11 per cent for 25,000 to 50,000 copies, to 12 per cent for 50,000 to 100,000 copies, and to 13 per cent for all copies sold after the 100,000 copy milestone is reached.

For authors with entrepreneurial instincts and confidence in their ideas, escalating royalty contracts can generate greater royalty compensation than standard 10 per cent of list agreements — provided, of course, that the book is successful. Remember, however, that royalty escalation is nearly always calculated *by edition*. If the publisher requests a second edition of the book, the royalty counter generally moves back to zero, even if over 100,000 copies of the first edition were sold.

Advances ▪ Sometimes a health sciences publisher will agree to support the author's costs in preparing a manuscript and illustrations. This financial assistance, which is frequently deducted from the royalties payable to the author after the book is published, is known as an *advance*.

An advance may be helpful to a transcriptionist if, for example, the project requires investment in new equipment, such as a computer or laser printer. But be prepared to be realistic. The million dollar advances paid to some highly visible novelists are unknown in health sciences publishing. Five hundred dollars to two thousand dollars is common.

Copyright ▪ To insure against unauthorized reproduction or usage, the book must be protected by copyright. (This subject is explained on page 118.)

Reviewing Publishing Contracts ▪ When the contract is received, the transcriptionist-author reviews it carefully before signing it. The advice of an attorney who is experienced in publishing and contract law is strongly recommended.

The contract should state the title of the work correctly and should specify accurately the proposed number of published pages, tables, and figures. The agreed-upon date for submission of the completed manuscript (as well as any interim dates, such as the date for submission of a final outline) also should be specified.

Royalty terms should be clearly stated, and any special provisions, such as escalating royalties or advances, that fall outside the publisher's standard terms should be covered in addenda. The contract also should differentiate clearly the responsibilities of the author and publisher in preparing and producing the manuscript.

Both an authorized representative of the publisher and the author must sign the final agreement, and each party should retain a fully executed copy as evidence of the agreement and the mutual commitment.

MANUSCRIPT PREPARATION

With a signed contract in hand, the transcriptionist-author is ready to embark on the exciting adventure of preparing the manuscript.

Getting Started ▪ Many authors (especially those writing books for the first time) assume that they must prepare their manuscripts in chronologic order, beginning with Chapter 1. Often, however, this is not the most efficient way to proceed. Because the first chapter is frequently an overview of subjects covered in the rest of the book, it might be written more effectively after the other chapters have been completed.

The best advice is to start with the chapter one feels the most comfortable with, regardless of where it falls in the table of contents. Getting even a few pages under an author's belt can provide the confidence needed to tackle the harder chapters.

Coherence ■ Whether the book is a textbook or a reference, the information in each chapter must flow logically and smoothly from one idea to the next. This process is known as *coherence*.

The best way to achieve coherence is to prepare a detailed outline for each chapter before beginning to write. First, list all the subjects it is desired to cover, in the order in which they are thought of. Do not worry about concept relationships at this stage; just try to be comprehensive and to get all the topics down on paper in random order.

After the random list is complete, patterns in the list are looked for. Items that deal with a similar theme are grouped together, and the notation on the list that expresses each theme most generally is identified. (If general themes were not included on the list, try to phrase them now.) After each idea on the list is associated with its best general theme, arrange the themes in an order that seems logical.

Two objectives are accomplished with this process. First, a detailed chapter outline is generated; second, the major headings and subheadings of the first draft are being set up.

Here is how the idea organization process worked to generate an outline for the present chapter. Note that in Stage 2, the major headings are organized to follow the publishing process in sequence, from finding an idea through manuscript preparation.

STAGE 1: IDEA GENERATION

Typing instructions
Figures
Tables
Royalties
Advances
Selecting a book topic
Selecting a publisher
Table of contents
Cover letter
Submitting a proposal

How publishing decisions are made
Responsibilities of author and publisher
Copyright

STAGE 2: IDEA ORGANIZATION

Selecting a book topic
Selecting a publishing company
Submitting a proposal
  Cover letter
  Table of contents
  The publishing decision
Contracts and negotiation*
  Author's responsibilities
  Publisher's responsibilities
  Royalties
  Advances
  Copyright
Manuscript preparation*
  Typing instructions
Illustrations*
  Figures
  Tables

Grammar and Style ■ A complete discussion of grammar and style is beyond the scope of this chapter. Suffice it to say that the publisher will expect a manuscript that follows the accepted rules of modern English usage, so that the task of the copy editor is limited to a final check for consistency. Many excellent references on grammar and style are available. For the names of a few, see Reference Sources at the end of the chapter.

Presentation ■ Every publishing company has its own requirements for submission of manuscript copy. The editor should include a style guide when the signed contract is returned. If a style guide is not received, the author should be sure to ask for one.

The following general guidelines are acceptable to most health sciences publishers:

1. Type the manuscript on $8\frac{1}{2}$-by-11-inch white bond paper, and use one side of each page only.

2. Double-space all copy, except tables.

3. Leave $1\frac{1}{2}$-inch margins at the top, bottom, and both sides of each page.

*New major headings added as part of Stage 2.

4. Number each page in the upper righthand corner with a composite number showing the chapter first and the page number within the chapter second, separated by a hyphen. (For example, 6–5 designates the fifth manuscript page of Chapter 6.) Do not number pages sequentially throughout the book unless specifically requested to do so.

5. Cite all figures and tables within the text, again using the composite numbering system. (Figure 9–4 designates the fourth figure in Chapter 9; Table 8–2 designates the second table in Chapter 8.)

6. Include a list of references at the end of each chapter, and/or a Bibliography at the end of the book.

7. Begin each new chapter on a fresh page, and center the chapter title on the page, capitalizing it and underscoring it.

8. Submit legends for all figures on a separate sheet. Include all required permissions.

Electronic Manuscript Submission ▪ The publisher may wish to copy edit and typeset the manuscript electronically, if it is prepared in machine-readable format. This strategy avoids repetitive keystroking and permits more rapid production, with less risk of typographic errors.

If the publisher has this capability, the editor will request a disk along with a hard copy of the manuscript.

ILLUSTRATIONS

Whether a book-length manuscript or simply an article or chapter is being prepared, illustrations will help reinforce the message. This section discusses the two principal types of illustrations: figures and tables.

Figures ▪ Figures include *line drawings* (artwork, graphs, and charts) and *halftones* (photographs and radiographs). The publisher will expect either type of figure to be submitted in a form ready for reproduction: generally as 5-by-7-inch glossy prints.

All line art should be rendered by an experienced illustrator. If the figures include anatomic drawings, these should be prepared by a trained medical illustrator. Authors who live near a university medical school can check to see whether the school has a medical illustration staff. Qualified medical artists also can be located by contacting the Association of Medical Illustrators, headquartered in Chicago, Illinois.

The author meets with the artist to discuss the requirements of the artwork. A price quotation should be obtained. The illustrator will appreciate any pencil sketches or background information for the figures. Remember: most publishing contracts specify that the cost of illustrations is the author's responsibility. This investment can be minimized by using figures only where they are necessary, and by stating the requirements clearly. An author can also save on the cost of preparing original figures by borrowing figures from previously published works. However, if this is done, the author must be sure to follow the instructions for obtaining permission.

If preprinted forms will be included among the illustrations, many publishers will permit authors to submit the original documents for photographing. Graphs and charts may be submitted as neatly prepared computer output.

Because of the high costs of color work (especially in halftones), many books include black and white illustrations only. (Check with the editor to determine whether the publisher has budgeted for color.) If photographs of patients are included, the editor will request the author to provide a written release from the patient or to mask out the eyes prior to preparing a 5-by-7-inch glossy print.

All figures should include a short *legend* or caption that briefly summarizes their content. Remember to submit all legends on a separate copy sheet. The publisher will match them to their illustrations during page makeup.

Tables ▪ Tables are arrays of numerical data arranged into columns and rows. If the author has access to a high-resolution laser printer, the publisher may ask for tables as camera-ready copy. Otherwise, type the manuscript for each table clearly and the publisher will typeset it.

Be sure to title each table, as well as its individual rows and columns. A short legend for each table could be provided, as done for figures, but this is not essential, since the table's title frequently defines its purpose.

REFERENCES, BIBLIOGRAPHIES, AND FOOTNOTES

When an author relies on previously published material, or on personal interviews, to obtain information for the manuscript, these sources must be credited in a reference list or bibliography. (Generally, source citations at the ends of chapters are called References. A Bibliography is a consolidated reference list at the end of the book.)

Although texts for the medical transcription field rarely require lengthy source citations, the copy editor's task can be simplified by following these formats:

For a book:

Smith, A.B.: *Teaching Medical Transcription.* MT Press, New York, 1992.

For a chapter within a book, or an article in a journal:

Jones, C.D.: The future of medical transcription. *Journal of the American Association for Medical Transcription,* Vol. I, No. 4 (Fall, 1992), pp. 6-18.

Both reference lists and bibliographies should be alphabetized by author.

Footnotes can be used either to add information that is too detailed for the manuscript itself, or to give immediate credit to important sources. We suggest keeping the number of footnotes to a minimum, especially in textbook writing, as they can be distracting to the reader.

OTHER MANUSCRIPT ITEMS

Index ■ If the author's work is lengthy, the publisher may wish to include an index. An index is like a very detailed table of contents, but with the entries constructed in reverse order, so that most are placed under the most general word in the entry. For example:

Phenomenon, Raynaud's
Cyst, ovarian
Joint, lumbosacral

The author may prepare the index, or the publisher may do it. (The latter instance may involve a small charge to royalties.) In our opinion, indexing is usually best left to the experts. The author who decides to prepare the index should ask the editor for a copy of the publisher's indexing instructions.

Teacher's Guide ■ Textbooks intended for college or vocational school adoption are usually published with accompanying Teacher's Guides, designed to assist instructors in developing successful classroom preparations and in testing students for core competencies. The Teacher's Guide should parallel the table of contents of the text, covering the following elements for each chapter:

■ Learning objectives

■ Instructional plans (different sequences for teaching chapter material, and so on)

■ Enrichment activities (role-playing exercises, case studies, possible field trips)

■ Examination questions (multiple choice, true/false, essay)

Because Teacher's Guides are often provided to instructors free of charge to encourage adoption of the text, they are prepared inexpensively, often from camera-ready copy. The author with desk-top publishing software for a personal computer will be able to prepare very professional-looking originals for the Guide, complete with headings in a variety of type sizes and fonts. If desk-top publishing software is not available, the editor can provide blue-margined sheets for use with standard word-processing programs.

MANUSCRIPT PRODUCTION

The long-awaited day has arrived, and the manuscript is complete. Now the exciting process of production is about to begin. The first production step, after the manuscript has been mailed to the editor, is peer review.

Peer Review ■ The author probably was introduced to the process of peer review when the table of contents or sample chapter was submitted. Because the decision to publish any book is a major financial investment, the editor must insure that the final manuscript is both technically accurate and marketable. The editor will therefore commission one or two full reviews before initiating copy editing and typesetting.

The peer review process requires 2 to 4 weeks, after which the editor will provide the author with anonymous summaries of the reviewers' suggestions, and sometimes even with reorganized or rewritten chapters. The author should try to consider the comments as objectively as possible, remembering that a fresh perspective can often pick up points that close involvement with the manuscript led the author to miss. However, if the author believes strongly that a recommended change is inappropriate, by all means she or he should consult with the editor.

Design ▪ The book's cover is the face it first presents to the world, and an appealing presentation can certainly enhance its marketability — whether it is displayed at a convention, photographed for an advertisement, or "comped" by a textbook sales representative. To ensure that their titles demonstrate the best design principles, publishers retain experienced designers on staff or work with qualified freelancers.

A successful cover design speaks immediately to the book's audience. A six-volume reference work in cardiovascular surgery, for example, must establish the authority and experience of the editors and contributors. Its cover will be classic and conservative, possibly burgundy with gold foil stamping. If an illustration is shown, it will be a simple schematic drawing.

In contrast, a textbook intended for new college students will manifest a brighter, more contemporary feel. Its cover might be silk-screened in several colors, and it may even show one or more photographs.

The publisher's Design Department will also select the book's internal typefaces: text, chapter titles, and headings. Here, the goals are easy readability and accessibility, but the type fonts chosen will depend on the audience.

Copy Editing, Proofs, and Proofreading ▪ As a final check on spelling, grammar, punctuation, and sentence structure, the manuscript will be reviewed by a copy editor. Copy editors (who often hold degrees in English) also check that all tables and figures are cited in the text, and that headings are utilized consistently. If the manuscript has many contributors, they will insure that all have followed the agreed-upon style. Finally, they mark the headings for the typesetter and check the references and bibliography.

After the copy editors complete their work, the production department typesets the manuscript into galley proofs. "Galleys" are long sheets of type that have not yet been made up into pages. Figure and table legends are usually set into a single galley sheet, and their correct position in the text is indicated in the margins.

The author will receive a set of galleys to proofread, along with the marked-up manuscript. Although the publisher's proofreaders review the galleys, it is also the author's responsibility to check them carefully. Look for typographic errors, missing words or paragraphs, and missing figure and table citations. The author should try to keep changes to corrections of outright errors. Changes to typeset copy are very expensive, and this is not the time for major adding and rewriting. All corrections should be marked on the galleys using standard proofreaders' marks (Figure 9–1).

Most publishers have a policy limiting proof corrections to 10 per cent of the original manuscript. An excess correction charge may be made to an author's royalties if changes exceed that amount. (Check the contract.) However, if facts have changed since the manuscript was submitted or a factual error is noted that was previously missed, the necessary corrections must be made.

After the marked galleys are returned to the publisher, the changes will be reviewed by the copy editor, then made by the production department prior to the preparation of page proofs. "Pages" are an author's last opportunity to review the manuscript before it goes to press. All tables and figures should now be in their correct positions, accompanied by their legends. At this stage, corrections should be limited to typos and other obvious mistakes, as any rewriting can affect the pagination of the entire chapter.

After page proofs are returned, all that remains between the author and publication day is printing and binding. Four to six weeks later, bound copies should be in the author's hands.

MARKETING

Books in the health sciences are promoted and sold through five channels:

▪ Convention exhibits

▪ Space advertising

▪ Direct mail

INFORMATION BULLETIN
Proofreaders' Marks

Use color (not red, not black) pen or pencil. Make two marks for every correction: one in text and one in the margin. A mark in text may be a caret (∧) or a line drawn through the character or word to be deleted. If there are several changes to be made in one line, arrange them in sequence left to right separated by a slash line. For the same correction repeated in one line, write the correction and a slash for each repetition (example: ∧// to add two commas). For number corrections, slash through the wrong digit(s) in text, write the correct digit(s) in the margin, and circle the complete correct number in the margin: 7/60 61 (7610).

MARGIN MARK	EXPLANATION	TEXT EXAMPLE	MARGIN MARK	EXPLANATION	TEXT EXAMPLE
ℐ	TAKE OUT CHARACTER INDICATED.	Your ℐ proofs	¶	START PARAGRAPH.	read.⌐ Your
⌃ ⌄	LEFT OUT, INSERT.	Yor proof. / Your prof.	no ¶	NO PARAGRAPH; RUN IN.	marked. / Your proof
#	INSERT SPACE.	You proof.	⌣	LOWER.	Your proof (3).
✕	BROKEN LETTER.	Your proof.	⌐	RAISE.	Your proof (3).
⌄⌄#	EVEN SPACE.	A good proof.	⊏	MOVE LEFT.	⊏ Your proof.
⊂⊃	CLOSE UP; NO SPACE. DELETE & CLOSE UP	Your prooOf. / maOnner.	⊐	MOVE RIGHT.	⊐ Your proof.
tr	TRANSPOSE.	A proof good.	‖⊏	ALIGN TYPE.	‖⊏ Three dogs. Two horses.
wf	WRONG FONT. (SIZE OR STYLE OF TYPE)	Your (proof)	⊙	INSERT PERIOD.	Your proof∧
lc	LOWER CASE.	Your Proof	⋏	INSERT COMMA.	Your proof∧
sc	SMALL CAPITALS.	Your proof.	⋏	INSERT COLON.	Your proof∧
c=sc	CAPITALS AND SMALL CAPITALS.	Your proof.	⋎	INSERT APOSTROPHE.	Your mans
caps	CAPITALS.	Your proof.	⋎	INSERT SUPERSCRIPT.	kg · gᵥ dayˉ¹
ital	ITALIC.	Your proof.	⋏	INSERT SUBSCRIPT.	H₂O
rom	ROMAN.	Your (proof)	⋎/⋎	INSERT QUOTATION MARKS.	Marked it∧ proof∧
bf	BOLD FACE.	Your proof.	⋏	INSERT HYPHEN.	A proofmark.
spell out	SPELL OUT.	Queen (Eliz)	?	INSERT QUESTION MARK.	Is it right∧
[/]	INSERT BRACKETS.	The∧ Smith∧ girl	are: was ⊘	QUERY FOR AUTHOR.	Your proof∧ read by
(/)	INSERT PARENTHESES.	Your proof∧1∧	⁻/ₙ	INSERT 1-EN DASH.	ad libitum∧ fed
▭	INDENT 1 EM.	∧ Your proof.	⁻/ₘ	INSERT 1-EM DASH.	Your proof∧
▭▭	INDENT 2 EMS.	∧ Your proof.	2/ₘ	INSERT 2-EM DASH.	Your proof∧
▭▭▭	INDENT 3 EMS.	∧ Your proof.	stet	LET IT STAND. (RESTORE ORIGINAL)	Your proof.

Figure 9–1

A sample of proofreaders' marks.

■ Textbook adoptions and bookstore sales

■ Field (direct) sales

For medical transcription titles, textbook adoptions and direct mail generally contribute the greatest proportion of sales.

Medical textbook publishers, maintain a staff of textbook sales personnel or "travelers," who visit instructors, discuss their course outlines, and suggest ways in which the publisher's textbooks can satisfy the instructor's teaching objectives. An instructor who "adopts" the text will ask the college bookstore to order sufficient copies for students. The publisher then distributes copies to the bookstore, applying the trade discount (generally about 30 per cent off the list price), so that the store can cover its overhead and selling expenses.

Direct mail promotes the sale of single copies for reference (rather than textbook) use, although it can also be used to support field activities for textbook sales.The publisher's marketing department rents lists from a professional organization or journal, then merges the lists by computer to eliminate duplicates. The mailing piece must generate immediate interest so that prospects have an incentive to open it and review the copy. Mailings addressing the recipient by name (through the use of laser personalization) usually perform the best.

A mailing may promote just one book, but those mailings offering a selection of related titles are the most cost-efficient. Response to mailings averages 2 to 3 per cent, but because books are sold at the list price (without a trade discount), such sales can be very profitable.

Although the publisher should assume the responsibility and expense of marketing the book, an author's experience and contacts can play a vital part in achieving sales success. Prior to publication, the author should be sure to provide the editor with lists of

1. Professional journals in which it is believed the book should be advertised;

2. Courses in which the book could be used as a required or supplementary text, and the names of instructors who should receive complimentary adoption copies;

3. Mailing lists that might be rented; and

4. Conventions at which the author believes the book should be displayed.

COPYRIGHT

The copyright in a work protects it from unauthorized use by others. Books are copyrighted in the name of either the author or the publisher; in medical publishing, the latter situation often pertains, because publishers wish to be able to publish a revision prepared by another author or editor in the event that the original author is unable to do so.

The present United States copyright law was enacted by Congress in 1976 and took effect on January 1, 1978. Under this law, copyright in a work exists from the moment the work is created, regardless of whether or not it is published and whether or not the author formally files for copyright protection. Copyright protection lasts for the life of the author, plus 50 years.

Because under most circumstances copyright is presumed to belong to the author, the author must explicitly transfer it to another individual or entity in order to forgo his or her rights in the work. (This situation will prevail, for example, if the publisher wishes to copyright the author's textbook in its name.)

An important exception to this general rule, however, is "works made for hire." Works made for hire are those specifically commissioned by a person other than the author. In this case, the law assumes that this third party, and not the author, induced the work's creation. Examples of works made for hire include:

1. Contributions to collective reference works, such as this chapter, or an article for a magazine;

2. Translations;

3. An adjunct to a work prepared by another author, such as a Foreword, Appendix, or illustrations; and

4. Works prepared by employees as part of their employment, such as user's guides for software.

Unless the work is deemed to have been prepared by an employee, the parties must agree in writing that the work is indeed a work made for hire. Generally, the writer is asked to sign a statement to this effect and to transfer explicitly any copyright.

The duration of copyright for works made for hire is shorter than for works copyrighted in the name of the author: 75 years from publication or 100 years from creation, whichever is less.

To understand how copyright law applies to an author, it is important to know what can be copyrighted and what cannot.

Titles cannot be copyrighted. Although the text of this reference book has copyright protection, its title could be used again by another author.

Facts are not themselves copyrightable. However, the *organization* of those facts can be protected by copyright, provided that the *arrangement* of the facts shows a modicum of originality. For example, in a work on biomedical history, the historical facts themselves are not protected by copyright, but the way in which a particular author organizes and presents those facts may be protected, provided the author does not use an organization previously copyrighted by another author.

Quotations are protected by copyright. In referencing another author's work, the author should not quote directly more than five lines in succession without utilizing quotation marks and acknowledging the source in the reference list or in a footnote. Written permission should be obtained from the copyright owner to quote more than 200 words in succession. The publisher can provide authors with forms to simplify the process of obtaining permissions.

The subject of copyright (especially the determination of whether or not a work is made for hire) is exceedingly complex. If an author is uncertain about the work's copyright status, we strongly recommend that the author obtain the counsel of an attorney experienced in copyright and intellectual property law. One can be located by checking the *Martindale-Hubbell Law Directory,* which lists lawyers in all fifty states and is available in most large public libraries.

COAUTHORSHIP

An author who enjoys the sense of personal accomplishment that authorship provides may wish to share the experience by coauthoring an article or book with a professional colleague. If so, the author should be sure to establish a clear plan for division of the work (preferably in writing) *before* beginning to write. Coauthorship is not unlike marriage. The author and the colleague will be working very closely together, perhaps for months, and disputes are inevitable in the absence of well-thought-out plans. Ideally, each author or editor should be responsible for the same number of chapters, and royalties should be shared equally.

Properly planned, coauthorship can be a very rewarding experience. It gives one the benefit of another person's expertise (which may be quite different), divides the work load, and often shortens the time to publication.

SUMMARY

Writing a book is a demanding but enormously gratifying experience. It is little wonder that the medical transcription field has so many repeat authors. We hope that the information in this chapter will inspire others to join their ranks and experience the thrill of publication.

Reference Sources

Associated Press Staff. *Associated Press Stylebook and Libel Manual.* Addison-Wesley, Boston, 1992.

Editorial Staff. *The Chicago Manual of Style,* 13th edition. University of Chicago Press, Chicago, 1982.

Scott, R. Who owns what: Freelancers, mailers and the 1976 copyright law. *Who's Mailing What!,* Special Report, 1988.

Strunk, W., Jr., and E. B. White. *Elements of Style,* 3rd edition. Macmillan, New York, 1979.

United Press International. *United Press International Stylebook,* 3rd edition. National Textbook Company, Lincolnwood, Illinois, 1992.

United States Government. *Copyright Law of the United States of America.* Washington, D.C., 1992.

Sondra Sue Hein, B.A., C.M.T.
Lynn C. Keene, B.S., M.S.

CHAPTER
10

Preparing to Teach Medical Transcription

INTRODUCTION

The field of medical transcription is both demanding and precise. Because of the wide scope of technical information and English fundamentals required to be a first-rate transcriptionist, the level of expertise in teaching medical transcription is crucial. Therefore, the question must first be asked, "Who is qualified?" Prospective teachers need to examine their own qualifications in terms of education, experience, and motivation. Indeed, compiling program prerequisites, designing a course description and outline, and stating course objectives sometimes appears easier to standardize than the task of defining the criteria for those who aspire to teach medical transcription. Furthermore, the integrity of the profession is directly related to the quality of instruction the students receive.

Originally, there were no formal courses offered in medical transcription. Those in the field could not rely on universally accepted standards and practices unique to medical typing. Instead, beginners simply learned from established veterans in the field. The flaw in this hands-on training was that erroneous information was passed on along with accurate information, simply because "that's the way we've always done it." However, certain guidelines had to be established to avoid perpetuating misconceptions and to ameliorate certain myths. Preparing students for the rigors of deciphering sometimes unintelligible, frequently ambiguous, and occasionally conflicting medical dictation is an extremely de-

manding role; but the hallmark of any outstanding teacher is diligent dedication.

Focusing on the goal of setting high standards, the following criteria can serve as a guide for the ideal medical transcription instructor:

- College level education in business administration, health sciences, education, English, biology, or related fields (e.g., computer science)

- A minimum of 3 years' experience in medical transcription (i.e., as a hospital transcriptionist, as a transcriptionist in a multispecialty group, as a supervisor transcriptionist, and as a home-based transcriptionist)

- Certification through the American Association for Medical Transcription (AAMT)

- Bachelor's degree

Admittedly, these are daunting credentials, but they could certainly serve as a benchmark to judge a candidate's ability to teach medical transcription and to ensure the caliber of instruction required to maintain a high level of consistency, competency, and professionalism that medical transcription courses deserve. In addition, a capable instructor must have both leadership and communication skills, as well as organizational ability. Also, one must be able to construct effective tests—one of the most difficult challenges in teaching. The ability to proofread accurately in correcting students' work is equally essential. Finally, knowledge of computer skills and medical terminology completes the profile of the ideal medical transcription instructor.

In addition to the qualifications in academics and experience, teachers need to be familiar with all aspects of the profession and the unique opportunities offered in each arena. Instructors must present a balanced lecture on the various work settings, such as employment in a medical office, in a hospital (medical records, pathology, or radiology departments), self-employed working at home, subcontracting, or transcribing for a service.

Students need to be exposed to the advantages and disadvantages of the different work environments in order to make informed decisions about where to begin their careers. Decisions are also dependent on what their skills are when they leave school. This knowledge enables students to shift from one work setting to another as they grow in their profession and as their lifestyles change. For example, a student without the responsibilities of family life with children might choose to enter the medical transcription field in a clinic that offers the stimulation and valuable assistance that other, more experienced medical transcriptionists can provide. Later, perhaps with small children, this student might choose to start a home-based business of her own as an independent contractor. Armed with the experience and knowledge acquired during previous employment in a clinic, this student can bring classroom education involving home businesses and job expertise together successfully. Conversely, a home-bound student might begin her career by becoming a self-employed medical transcriptionist in her home. Changes in family life over the years, such as being needed less by growing children or becoming divorced or widowed, might present the opportunity to elect a change in the work environment. Faced with a need for more comprehensive medical benefits, or a desire for the company of others, or even a desire for a new challenge in the medical transcription field, a move to a hospital or a clinic setting might be the appropriate career choice.

Not only can students choose their work locations, but also teachers can explore the different venues available to them.

Thus, preparing to teach medical transcription involves exploring a variety of options and decisions for the instructor as well as the student. These choices focus on evaluating teacher credentials, investigating teaching opportunities, and examining medical transcription programs.

COMMUNITY SURVEY AND ASSESSMENT

Before a school can begin to offer a course in medical transcription, attention must first focus on the community's needs. Local hospitals, clinics, and physicians' offices may be canvassed, either by mail or telephone, to determine whether there is a market for future graduates from the school. These medical facilities can also be evaluated for possible externships, as well as for potential job placement. With these objectives in mind, job descriptions, pay scale, minimum hiring requirements, length of probation period, and so forth, can also be obtained.

Investigate and research existing programs, if any, in the community and surrounding areas. If such programs, or partial programs, are already in place, academic articulation by talking with the administrators and instructors is strongly recommended. Overlap in fulfilling the community's requirements can be avoided if the courses offered at each learning site complement rather than compete with each other. For example, one institution may offer extensive preparatory course work in computer skills, English fundamentals, biology, or anatomy but no course in medical transcription is available. A second school, contemplating a course in medical transcription, may already be offering medical terminology in conjunction with a medical assisting program. This school can initiate a medical transcription course without also having to develop supplementary courses already organized in other educational settings. Thus, redundancies in time, effort, and money can be avoided. Ongoing communication and exchange of ideas will enhance the rapport between the various schools and benefit the community as a whole.

Although not ideal, medical transcription can be taught in environments that do not provide computers for each student. In some situations, there may be need for a class in computer instruction; however, the funding for equipment may be unavailable, at least in the beginning. In a regular classroom setting, students can review the essentials of English and learn the correct form for medical transcription of terms, abbreviations, drugs, and so forth. They can refine proofreading skills by reading their transcription exercises. They can also interact with the teacher regarding questions, inconsistencies, and special problems encountered during independent transcription when students use either their own or the school's equipment. When a school observes the value and the need for a medical transcription class, often it will allocate funds for the equipment necessary to provide first-rate instruction to the students.

The qualified instructor who is well grounded in the various aspects of the profession must also consider all the possible teaching environments. Some of these are:

- Adult education (high school students, high school graduates, and adults)

- Vocational education or trade technical schools

- Community colleges

- Regional occupational programs (ROP)

- State rehabilitation schools for those injured at work and being retrained in another field

- Proprietary (private) schools

- In-service training

- Private tutoring

- Welfare/work programs

DEVELOPING A COURSE DESCRIPTION

Just as one uses a map to travel by car, a course outline serves a similar purpose. Developing a specific, comprehensive, and thorough outline makes the journey from student to graduate more efficient, effective, and clear. The American Association for Medical Transcription has researched and developed a COMpentency PROfile for Medical Transcription Education Programs called COMPRO (Figure 10–1). This is an excellent reference source in developing a course description. It can also be used to evaluate any classes or courses that may already be available in the community.

One of the first issues to be addressed in a course outline is a statement of purpose. What is the goal for the course? State this clearly and concisely. Students need to know the destination of their educational journey and just how the proposed course will enable them to get there. Having established that goal, the next logical question to ask is what is needed. What specific skills are essential to begin the journey? The school catalog can list, depending on state policy, either prerequisites or suggestions for other associated courses to maintain a minimum standard for class eligibility. The school counselor or instructor can advise students regarding skills in typing speed, English skills, knowledge of medical terminology, computer literacy, and so forth. In developing a program module for medical transcription, it is imperative to recognize the limitations of a beginning course. Reviewing English grammar and punctuation, identifying the types of medical reports encountered in the field and their respective formats, and mastering the mechanics of transcription are primary focal points. These goals will be discussed in greater detail when we outline the basic core requirements.

The parameters of a beginning course in medical transcription must be flexible enough to meet the divergent needs of the students. However, by narrowing the scope of a beginning course and having specific goals in mind, certain areas can be covered in depth in order to give the student a more thorough and appropriate understanding of medical transcription in general. Ideally, all beginning medical transcription courses would have a basic core:

1. Learn the spelling and the meaning of medical terms (abbreviations, anatomic, disease, surgical, and drug terms).

2. Utilize correct English grammar, punctuation, and composition.

3. Learn various forms and styles of medical reports, documents, letters, and chart notes.

4. Learn specialized rules for correctly transcribing numbers, figures, and abbreviations.

5. Become skilled in operation of equipment (transcribers, word processors, and computers).

6. Become familiar with and efficient with reference materials.

COMPRO®

A COMpetency PROfile for Medical Transcription Education Programs

Introduction

COMPRO®, a competency profile for medical transcription education programs, is the foundation of *The Model Curriculum for Medical Transcription*™ developed by the American Association for Medical Transcription with the assistance of medical transcription practitioners, supervisors, and educators. These documents constitute the standards by which educators should develop and evaluate medical transcription programs.

COMPRO® is a comprehensive document consisting of a recommended program goal statement, program prerequisites, and competencies in four categories: English language usage, technology, medical knowledge, and discrimination and integration. It is designed to assist in preparing students for entry-level employment in medical transcription. Thus, AAMT recommends that educators incorporate all aspects of COMPRO® into their programs by following the guidelines of *The Model Curriculum for Medical Transcription*™.

COMPRO® also provides medical transcription supervisors and human resource managers essential information for developing job descriptions, assessing qualifications, and evaluating performance.

For more information on COMPRO®, *The Model Curriculum for Medical Transcription*™, and AAMT, write or call AAMT, P. O. Box 576187, Modesto, CA 95357; telephone: 209-551-0883 or 800-982-2181; FAX 209-551-9317.

Program Goal Statement

An educational program in medical transcription will prepare the student for entry-level employment as a medical transcriptionist, by providing the basic knowledge, understanding, and skills required to transcribe medical dictation with accuracy, clarity, and timeliness, applying the principles of professional and ethical conduct.

Program Prerequisites

As demonstrated by exam:
1. Minimum typing speed of 45 corrected words per minute (cwpm).
2. English usage competency equivalent to that of a high-school graduate.
3. Spelling competency equivalent to that of a high-school graduate.
4. Listening skills:
    a. Normal level of audiometric acuity.
    b. Ability to listen with comprehension at high-school graduate level.

Figure 10–1

A COMpetency PROfile for Medical Transcription Education Programs (COMPRO). (Reprinted with permission of the American Association for Medical Transcription, Modesto, California, 1987.)

English Language Usage Competencies (E)

E1. The student will demonstrate correct English usage, applying the rules of proper grammar, punctuation, and style and using correct spelling and logical sentence structure.

E2. The student will demonstrate the ability to use English grammar, spelling, and style references and other resources.

Technology Competencies (T)

T1. The student will demonstrate the ability to operate designated word processing, dictation, and transcription equipment.

T2. The student will demonstrate a general knowledge of the various kinds of word processing, dictation, and transcription equipment.

T3. The student will demonstrate a knowledge of trends and developments in word processing, dictation, and transcription equipment.

Medical Knowledge Competencies (M)

M1. The student will demonstrate knowledge of medical terminology including prefixes, suffixes, combining forms, root words, plurals, abbreviations, acronyms, eponyms, homonyms, antonyms, synonyms, foreign words/phrases, and colloquialisms.

M2. The student will demonstrate the ability to use medical references and other resources for research and practice.

M3. The student will correctly define, identify, pronounce, and spell medical terminology related to anatomy, physiology, laboratory tests, drugs, clinical medicine, surgery, pathology, and radiology.

M4. The student will demonstrate knowledge of human anatomy and physiology.

M5. The student will demonstrate knowledge of clinical medicine including the diagnosis and treatment of common diseases and conditions.

M6. The student will demonstrate knowledge of common laboratory tests including diagnostic indications, techniques, expressions of values, and significance of results.

M7. The student will demonstrate knowledge of common drugs and their indications, actions, dosages, and administration.

M8. The student will demonstrate knowledge of surgery including diagnoses, techniques, findings, equipment, instruments, and accessories.

M9. The student will demonstrate knowledge of basic procedures, techniques, and findings in radiology and pathology.

Figure 10–1 *Continued*   *Figure continued*

Discrimination and Integration Competencies (D)

D1. The student will meet progressively demanding medical transcription accuracy and productivity standards.

D2. The student will be able to recognize, evaluate, and interpret inconsistencies, discrepancies, and inaccuracies in medical dictation and appropriately edit, revise, and clarify them while transcribing, without altering the meaning of the document or changing the dictator's style.

D3. The student will demonstrate the ability to proofread and correct transcribed medical reports.

D4. The student will demonstrate a knowledge of the healthcare record and an understanding of the medicolegal aspects of medical transcription practices.

D5. The student will demonstrate an understanding and application of ethics in the medical transcription profession.

D6. The student will demonstrate an awareness of the dynamics of the work environment and the importance of professional development.

D7. The student will accurately transcribe original medical dictation through the application of the competencies specified in the categories of English Language Usage, Technology, Medical Knowledge, and Discrimination and Integration.

D8. The student will complete a clinical externship (recommended length, 240 hours) during the last semester/quarter of the program. A medical transcription work setting is required, with student duties limited to medical transcription emphasizing the basic four reports (histories and physicals, operative reports, consultations, and discharge summaries) and including various other medical reports. The student will be evaluated jointly by the instructor and employer/supervisor on transcription accuracy and productivity and professional and ethical conduct.

Figure 10–1 Continued

7. Develop excellent proofreading and editing skills.

8. Understand advantages and disadvantages of various work settings and opportunities.

9. Integrate effective performance expectations into the classroom to develop positive attitudes and to learn how to get along with and without people.

10. Learn the most effective method of working for physicians in an office, hospital, or in one's home.

Course outlines will differ based upon the diversity of division or department standards, equipment, textbook and materials preferences, and financial limitations of the respective institutions. Thus, preparing individual course outlines will reflect the previously suggested goals found in the basic core in order to satisfy as many requirements as possible in a beginning course.

COURSE OBJECTIVES

Upon completion of a working course outline, formulating a syllabus is next (Figure 10-2). It provides a guide for the student with regard to required materials and/or textbooks and also lists recommended reference sources. A good syllabus is a complete outline of what the instructor intends to cover in class each session, when work is expected to be completed, dates of evaluation, how evaluation is performed, procedures and tests, and special events (i.e., field trips, guest speakers, and so forth).

Although a syllabus should be fairly specific in its content and time frame, many instructors find it necessary to alter the actual class time spent on certain areas of study. In a class where the majority of students are especially deficient in English skills, it may be necessary to devote more time to reviewing proper punctuation than originally scheduled. To cover the essential goals of the class, it is equally important to recognize that some students may need to be referred to other classes for remedial work in areas such as English, speed typing, or word processing so that the entire class is not penalized for a few students' deficiencies. A good teacher is sensitive to and cognizant of the unique needs of each class.

Adhering to a rigid schedule should not take precedence over adequate comprehension and appropriate levels of performance. With experience, the time required to cover each objective will become more realistic and more efficient.

Evaluation policies can be explained in a syllabus so the students are able to judge the criteria being used by the instructor to determine grades. There is no universal method of grading, and each instructor usually devises a system that best suits the individual style of teaching. An example showing how errors can be weighted using a point system is seen in Figure 10-3.

No discussion of course objectives would be complete without some suggestions directed at those instructors who, either by design or demand, are fortunate enough to be able to guide their students through an advanced course in medical transcription. Advanced students generally have a defined career objective, such as wishing to work in a hospital, clinic, or office or as a self-employed independent contractor. An advanced course can be tailored to meet the needs of these students.

For the students seeking entry level employment at a hospital, clinic, or office, as well as the currently employed student on sabbatical from a hospital, an advanced class should have a library of "live" tapes (taken from actual dictation by physicians with patient information deleted) concentrating on at least five specialties. The best tapes are those that represent varying levels of difficulty in transcription. Students can proceed at their own pace. Students can be graded on their competency as the level of difficulty in transcription increases. (Refer to the list of suggested resources at the end of this chapter.)

Entry-level employment seekers in hospital transcription would also benefit a great deal from an externship program. Coordination between a school and local hospitals and clinics allows students to work in a hospital transcription department while being closely monitored by a transcription supervisor. The student's practical knowledge is enhanced through on-the-job training offered by the hospital in conjunction with the school. This on-site experience, coupled with additional transcription from tapes in the school laboratory, would give the advanced student invaluable experience and confidence to begin hospital transcription work.

Those advanced students on educational

COURSE SYLLABUS
MEDICAL TRANSCRIPTION I

Instructor: Semester:
Ticket #:   Time & Day:
Location: Phone:

COURSE DESCRIPTION:

This course is an introduction to medical transcription with emphasis on proper grammar, punctuation, and spelling; correct use of medical terms; proper formats used in a variety of reports and dictation; proofreading and editing transcription appropriately. Speed and accuracy are developed throughout the course.

COURSE OBJECTIVES

1. Operate transcribing equipment.

2. Transcribe basic medical reports, letters, and chart notes.

3. Recognize, pronounce, and spell basic medical terminology.

4. Proofread and correct a variety of medical documents.

5. Use standard medical references efficiently.

6. Transcribe histories and physicals, discharge summaries, and other medical reports.

7. Use correct, current, and competent language skills.

8. Recognize inconsistencies, discrepancies, and incorrect medical dictation.

9. Seek employment in a variety of medical settings: Independent contractor in an office, at home, or for a service; hospital medical record departments; clinics, urgent care facilities.

10. Utilize current technology in word processing and transcription.

TEXTBOOK: *Medical Typing and Transcribing* by Diehl and Fordney. Published by W. B. Saunders.

GRADING: Final grade with be based upon the total number of points accumulated in the following areas: Transcription assignments, textbook exercises, mid-term and final examinations.

CLASS PROCEDURES:

1) A timed typing test will be given during the first lab session in class. A minimum of 40 WPM is a prerequisite for the class.
2) Lab times will be predetermined at the time of enrollment.
3) Tapes may be duplicated only with the instructor's permission for independent transcription outside the lab.

Figure 10–2
Sample syllabus.

TRANSCRIPTION QUALITY EVALUATION ANALYSIS CHECK LIST

Problem	Point Value	No. of Errors	Solution
Word omission	1	_____	Proofread for content
Transcription blank(s)	1	_____	Flag document
Wrong word	1	_____	Relisten slowly to understand dictator
Spelling error			
Medical	.75	_____	Take time to find word in reference books
English	.75	_____	Do not guess at correct spelling
Inappropriate blanks	.50	_____	Try to understand voice of dictator
			Locate word(s) in reference books
Punctuation error(s)	.50		
_____colon			Take time to punctuate item(s)
_____comma			Do not guess at punctuation to save time
_____dash			Find rule in textbook
_____exclamation mark			Have reference books on hand
_____parentheses			Proofread twice—once for meaning and once for details
_____period			
_____quotation marks			
_____semicolon			
_____underscore			
English-usage error(s)	.50		
_____abbreviations			Take time to learn correct usage rule(s)
_____capitalization			Do not guess on correct usage to save time
_____compound words			Find usage rule in textbook
_____hyphenation			Have reference books on hand
_____numbers			Proofread twice—once for meaning and once for details
_____possessives			Correct redundancies and inconsistencies
_____plurals			Edit slang or inflammatory remarks
_____prepositions			
_____pronouns			
_____subject-verb agreement			
_____word usage			
Keyboarding error(s)	.25	_____	Proofread for details
			Get equipment malfunction fixed
Format or style error(s)	.25	_____	Know correct format(s)
			Do not guess on correct format to save time
			Find item(s) in texbook
			Have reference book(s) on hand
Incorrect method(s) or procedure(s)	?	_____	Listen carefully and follow instructions
			Write down instructions and keep in an accessible location
			Keep instructions given earlier for recurring jobs
Unfinished transcription	?	_____	Retype exercise(s), problem(s), letter(s), or report(s) because of uncorrectable errors
			Try to speed up time looking for data
			Handle materials efficiently
			Try not to make too many corrections
			Have tools, supplies, and/or reference books on hand

Total Error Value _____

Figure 10–3
An example of a transcription quality evaluation analysis checklist.

leaves from hospitals will be returning, in some cases, to a specific department, i.e., radiology or pathology. A series of tapes concentrating on a particular specialty is ideal for them. These students could be challenged by the increasing level of difficulty of the tapes and subsequently find their base of knowledge broadened significantly.

Occasionally, hospitals initiate their own on-the-job training program. Guidelines regarding hospital policies, work load expectations, and evaluations are clearly outlined. Actual hands-on transcription can be accomplished by the student under close direction of the training supervisor. More difficult and diversified dictation is gradually introduced as the student's level of mastery increases. Often, students are encouraged to take advantage of policies allowing tuition reimbursement and higher salary levels as reward for successful completion of continuing education classes. Both the hospital and the student gain with these incentives.

A school setting offering an advanced medical transcription course affords a unique opportunity to the student whose goal is self-employment. The objective can be approached through seminar/independent study rather than through a structured curriculum. An instructor who has first-hand experience as a self-employed medical transcriptionist brings additional credibility to the classroom. Each student is aware of the required number of tapes to be transcribed by the end of the semester. Time management, responsibility for turning in transcription assignments, and networking are left completely up to the student. The work load in an advanced class should consist entirely of transcribing progressively more difficult tapes in a variety of specialties, including more challenging dictation (e.g., dictators for whom English is a second language). A course replicating the working transcriptionist's emphasis on self-discipline, organization, and responsibility is the ideal.

By the end of the term, each student will have a much better understanding of both the advantages and pitfalls of working at home. This may enable the advanced student to make the transition from school to home-based work more smoothly. This transition from school to self-employment does not appear to be as intimidating a prospect as some have been led to believe.

In a class where a large percentage of students wish to transcribe at home, networking early in the course is strongly encouraged. By developing studying/working relationships with their classmates, the students can evaluate each other's progress in terms of possible future work partners, for vacation backups, or tandem jobs. Classmates who are home-based are also only a telephone call away for help with difficult or confusing dictation. In this manner, they can serve as resource persons for each other.

Networking advantages as a student member in a local chapter of the American Association for Medical Transcription can include information on potential jobs, as well as a reference for answers to transcription problems. Students are eligible to join the organization for a reduced fee and are entitled to full membership privileges: attending meetings, seminars, and conventions; discovering helpful transcription information; and receiving the national journal and chapter and state newsletters. Again, establishing and maintaining contact and forming a network with other experienced transcriptionists can be an invaluable asset to beginning students. This should definitely be encouraged in all medical transcription classes.

Often some students begin work with a client or two while enrolled in an advanced transcription class. These students can submit actual transcription (names and identifying data deleted) for course credit. Basically, this is a work/study program in which the instructor can help spot errors and answer questions, guiding the student during this critical learning period. Individual student evaluations for grading purposes can be based on a student's growing comprehension, accuracy, and speed gained during training with a new client.

In addition, an instructor whose class is focused primarily on home-based employment can offer the class current information about setting up a professional home office, including guidance regarding purchasing equipment and reference materials. The instructor who operates a home-based medical transcription service can serve as an invaluable source of practical knowledge with regard to marketing the service, cultivating clients, and billing procedures, as well as identifying the legal ramifications of implementing a home-based business.

INTEGRATING COURSES INTO A COMPREHENSIVE CURRICULUM

Although a beginning course encompasses a basic understanding of medical terminology, pharmacology, and human diseases, for example, these subjects are most often covered in ancillary classes. In fact, to further enhance a basic knowledge in medical transcription, there are several peripheral courses that should be included in a good program.

The courses recommended in the AAMT *Model Curriculum for Medical Transcription* are listed in Table 10–1.

Some schools offer a Certificate of Achievement upon completion of required courses. A graduate of this program has not only become well grounded in the fundamentals of transcription but also has gained a measure of confidence and pride upon completion of the Certificate requirements. Often medical transcription is a mandatory part of medical assisting programs at some community colleges throughout the country.

MATERIALS AND EQUIPMENT

See Chapter 5 for information on transcribers, word processors and typewriters, computers, and other transcription equipment.

TEXTBOOKS

Before selecting a textbook, evaluate all textbooks available very carefully. Books used in class become reference material for most students long after the class is completed, so it is imperative that the book chosen be as correct, current, and comprehensive as possible.

The first consideration is the author's qualifications as an authority in the medical transcription field. This involves the formal education, training, and experience of the author(s).

Examine the textbook for content and organization, keeping in mind the course objectives and goals. Cost, although a consideration, should not be the most important issue, since a good

Table 10–1 ■ The AAMT Model Curriculum for Medical Transcription

Semester I	Semester III
Applied English Usage	Disease Processes II
Fundamentals of Medical Terminology	Medicolegal Concepts and Ethics
Word Processing and Machine Transcription	Advanced Medical Transcription I
Semester II	**Semester IV**
Advanced Medical Terminology	Advanced Medical Transcription II
Disease Processes I	Professional Development
Fundamentals of Medical Transcription	Medical Transcription Practicum

textbook will serve as a reference resource for many years.

A good textbook will have a teacher's manual to help with sample questions and answers, projects, hints, additional resources, and so forth. This is especially important for the novice instructor.

One textbook for a beginning course in medical transcription is the latest edition of *Medical Typing and Transcribing Techniques and Procedures* by Diehl and Fordney (see Bibliography). Basics of grammar and punctuation as they apply to transcription practices are introduced to the students along with exercises throughout the book to reinforce the rules and increase learning retention.

A final word of advice when choosing a textbook or recommending reference books to students: Always ask for the *latest edition* of the book to be purchased.

AUDIOVISUAL AIDS

Audiovisual aids are tools used by instructors, generally during class, to enhance the learning process. Visuals can also be offered in the room, such as use of a bulletin board, to emphasize points that might not necessarily be touched upon during class time. Some of the most common visual aids will be mentioned here.

Overhead Transparencies ▪ One of the most popular teaching tools used during class to clarify student understanding is the overhead transparency. This is because class lighting can be left as is, and the equipment is easy to use. Overhead transparencies are especially effective in reinforcing English grammar and punctuation rules, as well as underscoring the importance of properly transcribed numbers and abbreviations in medical transcription. For example, an instructor gives a written handout as an exercise to be completed at home. At a subsequent class meeting, a transparency of the uncorrected exercise is projected for discussion. During the question-and-answer period, the transparency is corrected by the class with the instructor's help. Following this, each student compares his or her written assignment with that of the transparency, and any misunderstandings can be cleared up immediately.

35-mm Slides ▪ This form of audiovisual aid requires that class lights be turned off, thus making it difficult for students to take notes. It diminishes class interaction. The equipment takes a longer time to set up and use, cutting down valuable class time.

Video Tapes ▪ A number of video tapes are available on transcription as a career, punctuation and grammar, surgery, self-assessment, and so forth. Refer to this chapter's Reference Sources for further information.

Handouts ▪ Handouts can serve as learning tools as well as add interest and humor to a medical transcription class. These can be in the form of take-home quizzes, exercises to be discussed at the next class meeting, or simply new information to be added to reference materials. Since the field of medicine is constantly changing, with new terms, drugs, and procedures emerging each year, it is important to make students aware of the necessity to be vigilant in updating their references and to be sure that they have the latest information available. This is another reason to encourage students to become members of professional organizations so they will stay abreast of these changes. Lists of commonly misspelled medical and English words can be distributed in handouts, and these can serve as a source for spelling tests throughout the course.

Flashcards ▪ Flashcards are extremely useful in teaching word meanings, suffixes, and prefixes. All students should be encouraged to take a class in medical terminology for more in-depth study of the language of medicine, since this is the backbone of the profession.

Bulletin Boards ▪ To motivate and keep students interested in the career field, items can be posted on a class bulletin board as well as in a school display case to encourage students to join a transcription course. Items might be advertisements for transcription jobs, posters announcing Medical Transcription Week from the American Association for Medical Transcription, cartoons, dictation and/or transcription bloopers, and so forth.

GRADING AND CORRECTING

Grading is one of the most difficult parts of teaching any class, and transcription is no exception. In addition to teaching students the content of the course, a good instructor also equips students with tools to monitor their work after graduation. One of the key skills required in medical transcription is the ability to proofread. Toward this end, meticulous proofreading of the students' work is of paramount importance. If the instructor is lax in this important aspect of teaching, students might feel that proofreading their work is not critical; but if the instructor is consistently thorough when grading transcription work, marking each error in grammar, punctuation, and spelling, students learn early in the course that this is an essential part of their work as medical transcriptionists.

Students can be given the responsibility of proofreading their own transcription assignments and marking any "differences" they find in their work against a key provided by the teacher as a guideline.

A beginning student may have many marks on his or her work in the early stages of training; however, if the student finds and marks each deviation from the key, no points are deducted from the grade. For instance, if 10 points are assigned to each exercise, a student can achieve a perfect score of 10 in spite of having multiple marks indicating differences and/or errors. This helps students see their mistakes without being threatened with a bad grade before learning the basic elements of transcription. However, if the teacher finds a mistake/difference that the student misses, a point is deducted. Using this method, especially in the early weeks of class, students learn very quickly that careful proofreading is to their advantage. It reinforces the importance of continued vigilance in this vital aspect of transcription. Once this concept is firmly established, the key can be withheld and grading can be done entirely by the instructor.

Some instructors prefer to mark transcripts as either acceptable (A) or not acceptable (NA) rather than using point or percentage systems. Another option to mark papers is:

- P   Perfect
- M   Mailable
- C & M   Correctable and mailable
- NM   Not mailable
- C R & R   Correct, retype, and resubmit

One of the advantages of allowing beginning students to find their own mistakes is that they are able to see clearly and quickly the areas in which they are deficient. However, not all differences are necessarily mistakes, since some decisions are subjective judgments (e.g., paragraph breaks, or including or omitting commas; in certain circumstances this depends on whether the transcriptionist thinks the information is essential or nonessential, and both interpretations can be supported and be grammatically correct).

It is important to remind students that they are not taking a course in medical transcription to learn or improve their typing skills; therefore, redoing work from written copy does not accomplish the goal of transcribing from dictation. This involves listening, not copying. After students move past their initial apprehension about transcribing, more emphasis can be directed toward format, appearance, and style. Meanwhile, students can be challenged to continue transcribing new material that is progressively more complex, requiring a higher level of proofreading and terminology.

Another method that some instructors employ is giving each type of error a different weight. This presents grading in a more realistic light, because a document could be mailed with a punctuation error but could not be mailed if a word were misspelled or if there were omitted dictation (Figure 10–4).

Determining the final letter grade can be done by converting the total points possible into percentages (Figure 10–5A). Since some of the grading methods presented are more complex than others and involve mathematics and record keeping, a computer software program can make the job easier and more efficient for a beginning instructor. For further information on grading software, refer to this chapter's Reference Sources.

Progress reports can be printed out periodically on a routine basis or when a student questions his or her status in the class. Such reports serve as constructive and encouraging guidelines for students. On the other hand, if they are doing inferior work, reflected by poor scores, they can increase their study time and effort. For the teacher, periodic printouts of the students' cumulative scores minimizes problems with those who have a false sense of accomplishment (Figure 10–5B).

Progress reports serve another vital purpose for the teacher and student alike. Mistakes in the grade record are detected earlier and can be corrected promptly. Students are generally quick to point out any deviation in their record, especially if it is to their advantage. Being apprised of their status in the class throughout the course gives students confidence that their final grade is a fair and accurate measure of their medical transcription ability.

TESTING

The purpose of testing is to evaluate a student's expertise, knowledge, and skills before, during, and at the completion of the course. It is also a mechanism by which the instructor can measure the effectiveness of teaching techniques, materials, and approach. Essentially, a good test is a measurement of and for instruction. The form and content of any given test should be directly related to the specific objectives outlined in the course syllabus.

In the beginning session of a course, a pretest can be given to help determine the level of competency in such basic areas as English, typing speed and accuracy, and knowledge of medical terminology (Figure 10–6). This enables the in-

POINT SYSTEM OF GRADING TRANSCRIPTION ASSIGNMENTS

Because proofreading is of paramount importance in the medical transcription profession, emphasis is placed on refining this skill throughout the course, particularly in the early weeks. Keys are provided for the students to compare their transcription against that of the key. Grades are based on accuracy of proofreading rather than knowledge of skills not yet acquired relating to the rules of medical transcription. In this manner, students are rewarded for proofreading and not penalized for lack of technical knowledge.

Toward this end, no points are deducted for differences marked by the student. One point is deducted only when the instructor finds a difference between the student's work and the key. Thus, a student may make multiple "errors" on early dictation exercises, yet earn a perfect score--if all differences from the key are detected and marked.

After an appropriate time, the key is withheld and all subsequent grading is done by the instructor. At this point, a weighted system is adopted:

2 points deducted for: - omitted dictation
                         - incorrect or misspelled English or medical word

1 point deducted for: - punctuation errors
                         - grammatical errors
                         - typographical errors

Figure 10–4

An example of a point system of grading transcription assignments.

structor to focus on areas of weakness early in the course, possibly supplying appropriate additional assignments that would address needs specific to the class that might not be included in the syllabus.

Another benefit of an early diagnostic test is that it allows a student who is severely deficient in a critical area to make appropriate choices as to whether there would be any benefit in taking a remedial class either concurrently or before at-

POINT REPORT

Class   MEDICAL TRANSCRIPTION
Term   Spring Semester 1994
Entry Number   1
Description   Letters #1 and #2
Date   01-28-94
Points Possible   20

Roll #	Name or Number	Points	%	Grade	*	To Date	*
1	ALLEN, SHARON	19.0	95.0%	A	*	91.6%	*
2	BROOKS, CAROL	17.0	85.0%	B	*	98.7%	*
3	BURNS, SANDRA	14.0	70.0%	C	*	93.0%	*
4	CARPENTER, JACK	12.0	60.0%	D	*	87.8%	*
12	324590	17.0	85.0%	B	*	82.5%	*
13	343446	18.5	92.5%	A	*	75.0%	*
14	280471	16.0	80.0%	B	*	77.5%	*
15	500234	19.5	97.5%	A	*	95.0%	*

A

PROGRESS REPORT

Class   MEDICAL TRANSCRIPTION
Term   Spring Semester 1994
Student Roll Number 12
Student Name   STONE, JENNIFER
Permanent Number   324590
Date Processed   1-24-94

Entry#	Description	Possible	Received
1	Letters #1 and #2	20	18
2	Letter #3	10	9
3	Chart Note #4	10	7

B

Figure 10–5
A, An example of a point report showing conversion of points into percentages. For confidentiality, student numbers can be used instead of names with names to be used for the teacher's reference. (Printed with permission of Digital Concepts and Insights, Mission Viejo, California.) B, An example of a student's progress report showing possible points and received points for transcription exercises. (Printed with permission of Digital Concepts and Insights, Mission Viejo, California.)

MEDICAL TRANSCRIPTION

Name:_____ Date:_____

Address:_____ Phone:_____

Typing experience: approximate number of years and/or experience_____;

number of words per minute, if known:_____

Transcribing experience, if any (include name and type of equipment):_____

_____

Medical terminology background:_____

_____

Reason(s) for taking this course:_____

_____

Specific area(s) of interest in medical transcription:_____

_____

PRETEST

Directions: Correct errors in grammar, spelling, punctuation, and manner of expressing numbers in the following sentences.

1. Of 63 people who recieved questionaires only eleven responded before the designated date; December 16th.

2. While conclusions were based on highly subjective data; the students were not asked to repeat they're survey.

3. The 14-page document was prepaired by Helen and me, it was the most difficult report we had ever writen.

4. Only one of our employee's know the combination but he is on a three week vacation.

5. If I had began the task earlier I would have completed it today, but the new target date for completion has been set for February 2nd.

6. Shipments which were recieved last week have been tagged, shipments which were recieved this week will not be tagged until tomorrow.

7. Neither the office manager or his assistance has been invited to the party, this has had a negative effect on the morale of office personnel.

8. Did you read What Russia Wants in the last issue of "U. S. News and World Report.

9. The responsibility is ours, the authority is yours'.

10. Before we discuss this issue further lets invite our guests to sit their briefcases in the adjoining room.

11. Our principle reason for making this request is because the firm has revised its' position on reemployment.

12. The company has reversed their decision to meter 2nd, third, and 4th class mail.

13. Our methods were different than you's but, as you can see from the inclosed sheet our result's are similar to your's.

Figure 10-6

An example of a medical transcription pretest.

tempting medical transcription. At this point, some students might even decide to pursue a completely different course of study. Generally, if someone hates to type or finds spelling English words difficult, such a person would be better off finding out as early as possible that medical transcription is not the field to pursue.

Once instruction begins, tests become valuable tools for teacher and student alike. Not all tests need to be used as part of a student's final grade, however. Some serve as self-tests. Indeed, a good textbook includes an ample number of self-tests, giving the student many opportunities for immediate feedback.

In a medical transcription course, restricting tests to multiple choice quizzes, essay questions, or spelling tests, although helpful, is inappropriate. The medical transcription teacher needs to develop periodic tests of a student's ability to transcribe medical information accurately in an appropriate period of time. Administer transcription tests at least twice during an average course of study and more often if possible. Only through realistic transcription exercises and tests can an instructor evaluate a student's progress and speed.

If the class is in a setting where students exchange information, books, and/or tests, consider alternating test questions or dictation exercises and compose original test materials for each new group of students. Compose tests of original "live" dictation whenever possible and change them for each class. Although this requires more work on the teacher's part, the results reflect a more accurate picture of a student's progress and expertise in transcribing medical dictation.

Tests given for final grading purposes are critical to most students and serve as a true evaluation of students' mastery of medical transcription. Written tests are useful adjuncts to the transcription parts; however, there is only one sure test of a student's ability to transcribe a medical document and that is by doing it.

Whatever an instructor decides to use in the way of test material, it is important to realize that there are no shortcuts to evaluating a student's work in transcription. Every comma, every word, and every drug and dosage are critical in a medical document. The person grading a student's work must be dedicated to careful examination of everything turned in, especially in a test situation. This task requires scrupulous proofreading on the grader's part, and it can be very time consuming, demanding, repetitive, and, at times, boring. There is, however, no better way of confirming a student's ability to transcribe dictation at a level that is appropriate for an entry level transcriptionist.

EVALUATION

Ultimately, evaluating the results of a student's performance is crucial. This evaluation is important for several reasons. It makes students aware of areas that might need additional work, possibly in the form of more classes that are not necessarily required to complete the transcription program at their particular school. On the other hand, when students experience growth and success, evident by performing at a high level in a test situation, it reinforces the skills they have mastered and gives them more confidence in themselves. Equally as important is what the instructor learns from evaluating students. Discovering patterns of success or failure gives the teacher valuable insight into areas of instruction that should be improved, changed entirely, or expanded.

Besides evaluating the students' performances, it is equally important to obtain feedback from students about the course. This can be done with a handout to be completed anonymously by the students (Figure 10–7). This helps the instructor grow professionally and makes future classes better.

Finally, it is important to examine the failures, as well as the successes, periodically in terms of effectiveness as an instructor (Table 10–2). In this way, a dedicated instructor can concentrate on the areas that need improvement.

PROBLEM SOLVING

There is no classroom instruction that does not present problems of some type or another. In this section, some of the most common problems will be mentioned, along with suggestions for solving them.

COURSE EVALUATION

Do not put your name on this paper. Please read all of the questions through before answering them.

1. At the beginning of the course, did you feel that your knowledge of medical transcription was: (circle one)
   a. good   b. average   c. poor

2. At the end of the course, do you feel that your knowledge of medical transcription is: (circle one)
   a. worse   c. improved somewhat
   b. the same   d. improved a great deal

3. Do you feel that the amount of homework assigned was: (circle one)
   a. not enough   b. adequate   c. too much

4. Do you feel that tests have been:
   a. unfair and tricky
   b. usually fair and reasonable
   c. on material not covered sufficiently in class
   d. on material taught in the course
   e. too few
   f. too weighted (not enough short quizzes)

5. What did you like best about the course? (circle items) review sheets, handouts, textbook, bulletin board displays, overhead transparencies, guest speakers, flash cards, _____

6. What specific suggestions do you have for improving the course? (drill on more punctuation, spelling, oral participation, etc.)_____
   _____
   _____

7. What courses not on the schedule would you like to have offered?
   _____

8. Do I have any habits or characteristics that bother you, or that you particularly like? Explain.
   _____
   _____

9. Additional comments, criticisms, or suggestions:
   _____
   _____

Figure 10–7

An example of a student evaluation questionnaire of a course in medical transcription. (Reprinted with permission from Diehl, Marcy O., and Marilyn T. Fordney. *Medical Typing and Transcribing Techniques and Procedures*. Philadelphia, W. B. Saunders Co., 1991.)

Table 10–2 ▪ **Self-Evaluation Checklist for Teachers**

Failure Signs	Success Signs
_____ 1. Embarrass students unnecessarily (put students on the spot, commenting on dress, etc.).	_____ 1. Show concern for students' feelings and viewpoints. Invite students' opinions.
_____ 2. Spend class time discussing your own accomplishments or personal life.	_____ 2. Stay on the subject. Use practical examples to explain points.
_____ 3. Fail to compliment students when they do a good job.	_____ 3. Praise students often; try to provide chances for success.
_____ 4. Take the "easy way out" (fail to discipline when appropriate, start class late, etc.).	_____ 4. Conscientious in providing worthwhile learning activities, discipline, and use of class time.
_____ 5. Regularly borrow materials from other faculty members instead of creating your own.	_____ 5. Continually involved in preparing instructional materials to improve teaching.
_____ 6. Fail to teach actively (let students try to teach some units or do "homework" in class).	_____ 6. Well prepared for each class. Use class time for active teaching.
_____ 7. Provide no variation in teaching techniques and materials.	_____ 7. Maintain interest by varying methods and materials.
_____ 8. Grade tests unfairly. Test on material not covered in class.	_____ 8. Administer and grade tests freely. Review before a test.
_____ 9. Fail to return test papers and assignments promptly.	_____ 9. Provide students prompt feedback about their work.
_____ 10. Use guest lecturers and field trips as a substitute for teaching.	_____ 10. Bring in guest speakers only to augment assigned material.
_____ 11. Give little attention to supervising work of each student.	_____ 11. Help students singly and also teach them on a group basis.
_____ 12. Distract students by mispronouncing or misusing words.	_____ 12. Show mastery of the English language. Use correct grammar.
_____ 13. Become irritated or angry too easily—have no patience.	_____ 13. Show patience in working with students; rarely show anger.
_____ 14. Take everything too seriously (lack sense of humor).	_____ 14. Maintain a good sense of humor and sometimes joke with the class.
_____ 15. Give no attention to appearance—careless about cleanliness.	_____ 15. Dress appropriately and be careful about personal hygiene.
_____ 16. Appear to be unhappy and unfriendly most of the time.	_____ 16. Speak and act in a happy, positive manner.
_____ 17. Call in sick when you are not ill.	_____ 17. Be dependable in class attendance.
_____ 18. Fail to compliment other teachers on their accomplishments.	_____ 18. Provide positive reinforcement to colleagues for achievements.
_____ 19. Refuse to do anything extra (serve on committees, sponsor student activities).	_____ 19. Volunteer to direct student activities. Carry your share of committee assignments.
_____ 20. Do not keep up-to-date with profession by reading professional literature or attending professional meetings.	_____ 20. Read professional articles and research reports, take additional courses, and attend professional meetings.

Slow Learners ▪ An effective instructor strives to explain both lecture and laboratory material in several different ways, as well as using visual aids (e.g., overhead projector, handouts, and bulletin board) to clarify information. Still, some students may find it more difficult than others to learn medical transcription. If the struggle to comprehend the fundamentals of transcription is due to a weak foundation in English, the student can be referred to additional classes in basic English in conjunction with the medical transcription course. Supplemental drill work in the form of written exercises incorporating English grammar rules as they apply to medical typing can be assigned. The student can then self-correct the exercises from keys supplied by the instructor, thereby obtaining instant feedback on progress.

An open laboratory in basic keyboarding, as well as more comprehensive courses in specific computer programs, can help the student who has only a minimal grasp of the mechanical skills required in a laboratory setting.

However, even with the augmentation of other course work and extra written drills, some students may be unable to keep pace with the rest of the class. In these cases, the instructor is justified in suggesting that the students postpone continuing the class in medical transcription until all review classes in English, medical terminology, or computer literacy are completed. This is important for two reasons:

1. To forestall a sense of failure, or

2. To preserve self-esteem from being eroded by consistently falling behind the rest of the class.

This suggestion enables the class to continue on schedule without allowing one or more students' inability to keep up impede the progress of the class as a whole.

Learning Disadvantaged (Cultural Differences) ▪ In dealing with students for whom English is the second language, the biggest stumbling blocks encountered seem to be English grammar, sentence construction, subject/verb agreement, and syntax. The greatest help for these students is found in the English as a Second Language classes or laboratories within the English Department of most schools. If no language classes are available, recommendations are basic English composition and grammar courses, a Business English class, or a basic remedial English class.

Physically Challenged ▪ The best source of help for aspiring transcriptionists who are physically challenged is the Department of Rehabilitation in their respective schools and states. These departments supply financial aid in the form of acquisition of special equipment for schools and for individuals who require help to become self-sufficient and employable in the medical transcription field. For information on equipment for the physically challenged, see Chapter 5.

Inconsistencies in Instructional Materials ▪ Unfortunately, medical transcription is not "permanent and stationary," and it never will be. The medical realm of knowledge is constantly growing, changing, and expanding. New terms, procedures, diseases, names, and instruments are added to published literature yearly. Technology has given us new, faster, more efficient machines and methods of transcription. With all of this, guidelines and rules of transcription have undergone changes. In some cases, punctuation rules differ: e.g., some sources do not use a comma between a drug name and the dosage whereas others do. Inconsistencies cause confusion when trying to teach students the "right" way to transcribe information. Therefore, the instructor often has to indicate guidelines illustrating the "preferred" style of transcription, as well as pointing out the secondary options.

Students are quick to point out inconsistencies in class, whether they involve what is in a book, a dictionary, or what someone has told them. Although the instructor cannot ignore such interruptions, it is best to avoid expending too much time or effort trying to explain minor differences. Once a textbook has been chosen, it should serve as the guideline for class work and test material.

One authoritative source for settling disputes regarding inconsistencies of style, punctuation, spelling, and so forth, is the American Association for Medical Transcription (AAMT). Inform students that this is one more advantage of being a student member of AAMT. The association has access to the latest, most complete, and most accurate reference resources available, and staff members at the Association are always willing to answer questions.

Finally, when faced with inconsistencies in information, a teacher can always resort to common sense to resolve some problems and encourage students to do the same — as long as what they decide to do does not cause confusion.

TEACHING TIPS AND TRAPS

The following handy hints will help in becoming a better instructor:

1. Get involved in the school's advisory board meetings. These long-range planning sessions set the tone for the program's curriculum requirements.

2. Have advanced students help grade the beginning students' work. This reinforces proofreading skills, knowledge of terminology, and transcription practices. In addition, students find this enhances confidence and pride in the lessons learned.

3. Encourage students to help each other in the laboratory with computer software, terminology, and format, as this simulates a working transcriptionist's environment.

4. Suggest that students devote 20 minutes per day on reviewing past lessons or studying new material. Research has shown that shorter, more frequent study sessions are significantly more effective in comprehending and retaining knowledge than are single, long periods of attempted learning.

5. Avoid personal commentary. A brief introduction regarding qualifications and experience as a medical transcriptionist is sufficient.

6. Strive toward a friendly, professional atmosphere during class to help establish good work habits.

7. Be aware of changes in medical transcription; stay current.

8. Avoid becoming too rigid in teaching techniques, opinions, and ideas. Be willing to listen to new and different approaches to teaching students.

9. Make the class interesting by alternating lectures, exercises, and audiovisual aids and inviting guest speakers. For videos, booklets, and literature on specific diseases, contact some of the voluntary Health and Welfare agencies and associations shown in the appendices.

10. Use mnemonic devices liberally (e.g., il*i*um/h*i*p bone; not il*e*um). Be creative and encourage students to devise their own aids to help them remember difficult or confusing terms.

11. Be enthusiastic!

Reference Sources

Books for Teachers

American Association for Medical Transcription. *Techniques for Teaching in a Medical Transcription Program.* Modesto, California, 1988.

American Association for Medical Transcription. *Analysis: Civil Service Classification of Medical Transcriptionists.* Modesto, California, 1981.

Brookfield, Stephen. *The Skillful Teacher.* Jossey-Bass Publishers, San Francisco, 1990.

Diehl, Marcy O., and Marilyn T. Fordney. *Instructor's Manual for Medical Typing and Transcribing Techniques and Procedures.* W. B. Saunders Company, Philadelphia, 1992.

Ericksen, J. *The Essence of Good Teaching.* Jossey-Bass Publishers, San Francisco, 1984.

Fordney, Marilyn T., and Marcy O. Diehl. *Medical Transcription Guide: Do's and Don'ts.* W. B. Saunders Company, Philadelphia, 1990.

Hassel, Patricia L., and David R. Palmer. *Marketing Allied Health Educational Programs.* Eagle Publishing and Communications, Santa Clara, California, 1992.

Health Professions Institute. *The Teacher's Manual.* Modesto, California, 1992.

Johnson, Spencer, and Constance Johnson. *The One Minute Teacher.* William Morrow and Company, New York, 1986.

Turley, Susan M. All of the above (article on test construction). *Perspectives,* Fall 1990, pp. 8–10.

Video Tapes for Teachers

Punctuation and Grammar Video, Surgery Video, and Self-Assessment Video. American Association for Medical Transcription, P. O. Box 576187, Modesto, California 95357-6187; telephone 800/982-2182.

Radiology: The Big Picture Video and Radiation Oncology — Waging War Against Cancer video. Complimentary copies are available from Ms. Keri Sperry at the American College of Radiology, 1891 Preston White Drive, Reston, Virginia 22091; telephone 703/648-8900.

Grading Software for Teachers

Bobbing Software (Macintosh), 67 Country Oaks Drive, Buda, Texas 78610-9338; telephone 800/688-6812.

Digital Concepts and Insights (IBM and IBM-Compatible), 28032 Wentworth, Mission Viejo, California 92692; telephone 714/951-0657.

Chariot Software (Micro Grade) (Macintosh), 3659 India Street, San Diego, California 92103; telephone 619/298-0202.

Custom Business Software (Top Score) (IBM and IBM-Compatible), Rancho Cordova, California 95670; telephone 916/852-6030.

Excelsior Software Inc. (Grade 2 for Windows) (IBM and IBM-Compatible), P.O. Box 3416, Greeley, Colorado 80633; telephone 800/473-4572.

Transcription Tapes for Courses

American Association for Medical Transcription, P. O. Box 576187, Modesto, California 95357-6187; telephone 800/982-2182.
General Medicine Module, General Surgery Module, and Radiology Module.

Health Professions Institute, 2105 Lancey Drive, Suite 1, Modesto, California 95355; telephone 209/551-2112.
Beginning Medical Transcription (12 audiocassettes), Cardiology Transcription Unit (4 audiocassettes), GI Transcription Unit (4 audiocassettes), Orthopedic Transcription Unit (4 audiocassettes), Pathology Transcription Unit (4 audiocassettes), Radiology Transcription Unit (3 audiocassettes).

South-Western College Division, 5101 Madison Road, Cincinnati, Ohio 45227-1490; telephone 800/543-8440.
Conerly, Donna L., Forrest General Medical Center: Advanced Medical Terminology and Transcription Course (text-workbook, 16 audiocassettes and IBM/Tandy software).
Frensilli, Frederick J., Metropolitan Medical Center: Medical Terminology and Machine Transcription Course, (text-workbook, 12 audiocassettes and IBM/Tandy software).

W. B. Saunders Company, Independence Square West, Philadelphia, Pennsylvania 19106-3399; telephone 800/545-2522 or (in Florida) 800/433-0001.
Diehl, Marcy O., and Marilyn T. Fordney: Medical Typing and Transcribing Techniques and Procedures Audio Tapes (3 audiocassettes with letters, chart notes, H & Ps, operative reports, discharge summaries, pathology reports, radiology reports, and consultation reports).

Meg Walsh, A.A.

Building a Medical Reference Library

INTRODUCTION

A medical reference library is essential for the medical transcriptionist.* Because of the ever-increasing technical terminology of medicine, reference materials are numerous and constantly changing. New discoveries, new concepts, new theories — all must have, it seems, new words or new groupings of words to describe and define them in speech and in print. The advances of medicine, with changing procedures, new medications, and the creation of new specialties, require that the medical reference library for the transcriptionist be kept up-to-date.

Since transcription involves much more than medical terminology, a reference library must have a complete English language dictionary. This should contain names and addresses of colleges and universities; geographic names of towns, cities, states, and countries; rules regarding punctuation and capitalization (as well as examples of usage); and an appendix of foreign phrases.

It is understood that those using the medical reference library already have a basic introduction to medical terminology and require supplemental references to increase their knowledge. The references available vary from the most current edition of a comprehensive medical dictionary (with its tables, plates, subheadings, definitions, spellings, and pronunciation keys in an organized manner by alphabetic arrangement and cross-reference) to highly specialized word books either covering a variety of medical specialties or emphasizing one particular specialty. A comprehensive medical dictionary is the primary reference for a transcriptionist. However, word books that have an alphabetic listing of words or phrases without definitions allow for quicker searches.

In the last 10 years, word books have become more important to the transcriptionist as medicine has become increasingly more specialized. Word books often contain proper nouns and terms for procedures, solutions, and surgical instruments that are not available in a dictionary. Although medical word books have an important place in transcription, the entries without definitions must often be more precisely defined by use of a dictionary.

Medical word books have increased in number and scope. They may be simple alphabetic lists of words without definition, or an alphabetic listing of words and phrases. Each type of publication has advantages and disadvantages, and each will often require the use of a leading medical dictionary for clarification. Word books represent a great advance for the medical reference library. They should be carefully chosen, with consideration of the manner in which the author has compiled and arranged words. Some word books show where words may be properly divided if they fall at the end of a line.

There are several comprehensive references for pharmaceuticals. The major criteria for selecting a good drug book are the manner of al-

---

*For a complete listing of reference books, computer software, Braille books, and audiocassettes, see Appendix 1.

phabetic indexing, the thoroughness of description of the drug, and, most important for the transcriptionist, the differentiation between generic and brand names. Leading pharmaceutical references are updated monthly, quarterly, or annually. Some pharmaceutical references list the drug name without further description except for a clue to its medical specialty or other classification. These can serve as quick references differentiating between generic and brand names but are limiting in that they do not describe method of administration, dosage, or any other user information. In addition, if updated annually, their usefulness is further limited.

Another source for pharmaceutical reference is the formulary that each medical facility maintains. With the advent of computers, these formularies are now more complete and up-to-date.

The medical transcriptionist who is building a medical reference library should be guided by the type of transcription required, whether it be for a physician's office, a multispecialty clinic, a general hospital, or a medical research and teaching facility. Each encompasses its own terminology, and the selection of reference books requires a knowledge of available publications suited to the specialized skill involved. At least one reference source should include abbreviations and acronyms.

A medical reference library would not be complete without style guides. Style that conveys accuracy and clarity is essential. The style guides for medical writing and transcription hold that the style should conform to certain rules that characterize scientific writing. For scientific journals or hospital and physicians' office charts, the language must be clear, concise, and accurate. Though dictators have wide variations of style in their personal correspondence, it should be in agreement with accepted practice in large medical centers and small community hospitals. The transcriptionist, with the aid of recognized references of quality, assists both dictator and reader by rendering a technically accurate and unambiguous document.

Additional references that the transcriptionist will find useful are textbooks in anatomy and physiology, for they often provide the meaning of Latin terms not found in other standard reference sources. In addition, for the physically challenged, books are available on tape or in Braille. Software programs using voice synthe-

sizers have proved helpful for those who are visually impaired.

These and other reference sources can be found in Appendix 1.

USE OF THE ENGLISH DICTIONARY

English language dictionaries are indispensable for spelling, pronunciation, hyphenation, and definition of English words. Those entering the field of medical transcription must have a good command of English, since medical transcription requires accuracy in English as well as in medical terminology. In their desire to be concise, dictators in many specialties use English terms that reflect their advanced education, as well as the idiomatic expressions of their specialties.

A language dictionary is a tool used by students long before they pursue their chosen careers. Familiarity with this type of dictionary is essential prior to entering the professional field as a medical transcriptionist. The full meaning of a word, the shades of that meaning, and its context can be explored and used in conjunction with medical terminology. An English dictionary can also help determine such things as synonyms, antonyms, connotations, grammar, and idiom. These are all important features that increase the vocabulary of the transcriptionist and, thus, the quality of the transcription. As a general rule, dictionaries become outdated every 8 to 10 years. It is wise to purchase a current edition periodically. For the names of English language dictionaries that should be included in a medical reference library, see Appendix 1.

When transcribing for a specialty such as psychiatry, a good English language dictionary is an essential reference. Psychiatric and psychologic dictation is less likely to be as technical as the dictation of a neurologist or a pathologist. When a psychiatrist performs a mental status examination and tests the patient's fund of knowledge, she or he may also test the transcriptionist's fund of knowledge. The same is true with psychologic test reports. Although the correct spelling of psychologic tests and the description of a patient's medical history are technical, such is not the case when evaluating the patient. The terminology used in this instance is fundamental

English dictated by well-educated professionals wishing to define their impressions in a precise manner. Adjectives are unusual and coined phrases frequent. With the change in the ethnic mix of our population, psychiatry is evaluating many more patients with different cultural backgrounds. Dictators who speak unfamiliar languages, use unfamiliar currency, and have unusual birth places, all require the help of a comprehensive English dictionary.

Examination of *Webster's Ninth New Collegiate Dictionary* will reveal much more than spelling, pronunciation, hyphenation, and definitions. This dictionary contains an index of many features, including chemical elements, listing of languages, and money, as well as punctuation. Some of this information may be available in other references but is easily found in this one.

USE OF THE MEDICAL DICTIONARY

The medical dictionary is the transcriptionist's major reference and, in spite of one's education or experience, is usually consulted daily. Because terminology is constantly changing and many medical terms evolve annually, it is preferable that the dictionary be the latest edition. Debate over the use of terms, spelling, hyphenation, and capitalization should be authenticated by the medical dictionary.

Many esoteric subjects often contain terms that are adequately and clearly defined only to those who have at least a basic knowledge of medical terminology. Although the key words in a definition are expected to be defined elsewhere in the dictionary, the chase from one word to another often leads to confusion for the novice. Searching for a major word in a definition can uncover other words to be defined, resulting in uncertainty and, in many cases, the incorrect word.

A medical dictionary differs from a language dictionary in that entries are listed under the governing noun, with multiple word terms listed as subentries. This presents problems to the transcriptionist when confronted with a multiword term. "Look under the noun," represents a challenge for the inexperienced, further complicated by the dictator's use of an incorrect or indistinct noun. The ease with which a transcriptionist locates terminology in a major medical dictionary is enhanced by a working familiarity with it.

Most transcriptionists develop a thorough understanding of the organization of one major medical dictionary. Although this is sufficient, it is wise to have two principal medical dictionaries for reference. The medical dictionaries that most experienced medical transcriptionists prefer because of their large scope and ready acceptance will be discussed here.

Dorland's Illustrated Medical Dictionary, 27th edition, states it contains 30,000 more entries than other medical dictionaries, and it is comprehensive. This edition reflects some significant changes in the placement of certain entries (consult "Notes on the Use of This Dictionary"). Main entries are listed alphabetically, with subentries in the same boldface as the main entry and in the same paragraph.

The appendices are as follows:

- Temperature Conversion Chart
- Multiples and Submultiples of the Metric System
- Tables of Weights and Measures
- Tables of Metric Doses with Approximate Apothecary Equivalents
- Laboratory Values of Clinical Importance

Over the years, this dictionary has been accepted as a primary reference and is, therefore, a must for the medical reference library.

Dorland's Pocket Medical Dictionary is also available and can serve as a directory to the most used words. This is not meant to replace the comprehensive Dorland's medical dictionary but is intended as a quick reference.

The second major comprehensive dictionary is *Stedman's Medical Dictionary,* 25th edition, published by Williams & Wilkins Company, 1990. The style is an index-like, single-entry format, making it simple to scan for words. It has an additional feature—a Subentry Locator for multiword terms, listed by their modifying words. An example is the dictated phrase "biliary xanthomatosis." The uncertainty of the term is clarified by the noun entry "xanthomatosis," with the subentry locator word being "biliary."

However, if the noun is misunderstood, or perhaps not located, it may well be positioned under some other synonymous noun entry. In this instance, the Subentry Locator lists:

biliary: atresia; calculus; canaliculus; cirrhosis; . . . xanthomatosis.

The Appendix is unique to Stedman's and can be a valuable resource for the transcriptionist as a spelling checker. Appendices include

- Subentry Index
- Blood Groups
- Laboratory Analyses and Observations (Reference Values)
- Comparative Temperature Scales
- Weights and Measures
- Common Latin Terms Used in Prescription Writing

Stedman's also publishes *Stedman's Pocket Medical Dictionary* for fast and easy access. It is limited in scope and definition and is meant to be an adjunct to the comprehensive Stedman's medical dictionary.

Other medical dictionaries differ in style and size, length of definition, cross-referencing, illustrations, and appendices. Several are excellent "pocket dictionaries" for quick reference but are not extensive enough to serve as the medical transcriptionist's major medical dictionary. See Appendix 1 for a listing of medical dictionaries. The listing is not intended to be complete, but rather a guide to some of the more commonly used dictionaries. The medical transcriptionist should always review the Table of Contents before purchasing a dictionary. The color plates and tables as well as the appendices should be examined to evaluate which is appropriate for the given medical setting.

MEDICAL WORD BOOKS

In 1973, Sheila Sloane published *The Medical Word Book* as a vocabulary and spelling guide for medical transcriptionists. This word book was a new concept and was welcomed by the profession. The second edition added terms for Radiology and Nuclear Medicine and increased in size to over 900 pages. The third edition, published in 1991, added a category for Immunology and AIDS, reflecting the changing terminology of medicine. Currently, transcriptionists have an abundance of word books in almost all specialties from which to choose.

Word books evolved because of the increased demand for accurate documentation of medical records. They also make it easier and quicker to locate a term than trying to find it in a dictionary. Because hand-written documentation often is not legible and too brief, physicians began dictating more detailed reports and chart notes. Transcriptionists find they are always searching for a new surgical instrument, a new drug, the proper name of a procedure, or a newly discovered bacterium or virus. The progress in medicine and its complexities, the requirements of third parties for accurate documentation, and the advent of many new specialties make the transcriptionist a vital link in the chain of medical communications. The informal system of questioning the dictator for accuracy, or searching a medical journal for some documentation, proves too time consuming. Transcriptionists developed their own word books, but were limited by the terminology of their own experience. An incoming specialist with new instruments and procedures became a fresh challenge.

The medical dictionary did not fully serve the needs of the transcriptionist by virtue of its size, the fact that it was not timely enough, and, according to its policy, included only terms that were accepted and drugs that were of proven clinical value or historical importance. Word books filled the gap; even though terms were sometimes not totally accepted they could at least provide consistency for the sake of spelling.

Coined words and phrases, as well as medical slang or jargon, used within a medical specialty found their way into word books. These "words" were very hard to verify, and the dictator was not a reliable source. Many terms went against the accepted rules of forming English words.

With the surge in the volume of medical documentation, dictators started to develop a type of "medical shorthand." Words were shortened, verbs became nouns, and abbreviations or acronyms became common usage.

The burden of proof now lies with the transcriptionist, who needs guidelines for putting this "new terminology" on paper. The private physician's transcriptionist must submit documentation to insurance companies, hospital medical record rooms, and other physicians, and, most importantly, communications to patients. The style and concise terminology must conform to certain standards. The use of a word book may be the answer to words of a particular specialty, or medical terminology in general.

Through the use of word books, transcriptionists have been able to rely on an author who diligently collected words and, to the best of the author's knowledge, verified some form of consistency.

The available books vary in scope and design and may be a general medicine word book or dedicated to one medical specialty. They may be merely alphabetic word lists, word lists and phrases, or, as with *Current Medical Terminology* by Pyle, also may include definitions indicating usage.

In contrast, *Medical Word Book, A-Z,* by DeLorenzo and Fedun, is an alphabetic arrangement of words and phrases, without definition and without indication of medical specialty. As an example of the number of words in this book, the entry for "cell(s)" contains 67 subentries; many are obscure and, even for the experienced transcriptionist, need further clarification.

The general word book titled *The Medical Word Book,* third edition, by Sloane, has three divisions: General Terms, Systems and Specialties, and Guide to Terminology. The General Terms division includes medical terms in alphabetic order, which are repeated in the second division according to classifications. The second division contains 15 systems or specialties, cross-referenced to other specialties for further clarification. The third division lists abbreviations, combining forms, rules for plurals, a table of chemical elements, and a table of weights and measures.

It is not my intention to evaluate all available word books but to point out variations and to serve as a guide for finding the appropriate word books for a good reference library. Listing the word books by category, whether it be general or medical specialty, allows the transcriptionist to acquire them as the need arises. It is recognized that word books are just that, and that time often does not allow extensive searching. Selecting a complete word book with cross-referencing and distinctions as to where the word applies

(medical specialty, laboratory medicine, psychiatry) is very important.

SPELLING

Correct spelling is a fundamental requirement of effective transcription — correctness not only in the spelling of technical terms of medicine but also in the usual vocabulary of the English language. It is just as important to differentiate between *principal* and *principle* as it is to spell *psyche* correctly.

Building a strong vocabulary requires constant attention to individual problems, such as the use of double letters or word endings. Developing a broad English vocabulary is important in order to devote the time necessary for increasing one's medical vocabulary, the real heart of transcription. Difficulties with words (for example, *precede* and *proceed* and *reversible* or *changeable*) need to be conquered quickly. A personal listing for problem words may be necessary until frequent use commits them to memory. However, most transcriptionists admit that even after years of transcription, certain terms still present problems. Thus, a word book designed for the individual's own use may be the answer. Often, the mere act of putting the word on paper will serve to commit it to memory. Even with a dictionary and a medical word book at hand, misspellings will occur because of the volume of work or time constraints.

With the advent of computerized spell checkers, the spelling of many problem words can be verified. However, spell check does have its limitations and will not "think" for the transcriptionist. A spell checker will not highlight an accepted word; thus, in addition to spelling problems, the transcriptionist may have a word exchange problem (for example, the keying of "milk" when "mild" is dictated, and *midget* for *midgut* will sound right to the computer). Neither will trigger a spell checker, but the error is obvious. An individual's knowledge of spelling and transcribing idiosyncrasies is important, since a spelling mistake is often simply a reflex error.

Another spelling error is the incorrect transcription of the final letter of a word. Adding an "s" to "word" does not create an incorrect word, but the sentence, "The patient gave only one-words answers," obviously is incorrect. Only proofreading catches this error, and a list of common "errors" may assist the transcriptionist in what others may see as a spelling problem.

English Words ▪ In addition to acquiring an English language dictionary, the medical transcriptionist must also acquire a good command of the use of the dictionary. If spelling difficulties include word endings, the "ie or ei" difficulty, "-cede or -ceed" use, or double consonants, one of the texts on building skills will be helpful. *Medical Typing and Transcribing Techniques and Procedures,* by Diehl and Fordney, has a chapter on "Spelling, Word Division, and Using References" that outlines many spelling rules and their exceptions and lists difficult word endings, division of words, and use of prefixes. Although an English dictionary is the medical transcriptionist's best resource for spelling, this type of manual will bring to mind the basic rules and thus make it easier to commit these rules to memory.

Medical Terms ▪ The spelling of medical terms has changed over the years (e.g., annulus to anulus, chorioid to choroid, calyx to calix). A current medical dictionary demonstrates these changes, and transcriptionists note the new spellings as they appear in current editions. Some words are revised in their spelling to make them easier to read or pronounce. Although it is difficult at first to change old spelling habits, new spellings are readily accepted by transcriptionists who want to be in the mainstream and who welcome streamlined terms.

Combining forms are often not constant in their spelling. Many prefixes have variations, such as dermo- or dermato-, phaco- or phako-. Some prefixes can also be difficult to distinguish by sound (i., hypo- and hyper-, ad- and ab-, ecto- and endo-). When searching through a medical dictionary, both prefix forms as well as the definition must be checked to be sure that the word selected is the proper choice. Some dictionaries give a "see also" classification (e.g., Stedman's lists "dermato-: combining form relating to the skin. See also derm-, dermato-, and -dermo-").

Many prefixes that once were separated from the root word by a hyphen are now combined to make one word (e.g., nondiagnostic, antihypertensive, posttraumatic).

In summary, the discussion of these reference books is merely a guideline to building a useful medical library that must be kept current because of the constant changes in medical terminology. A thorough understanding of how the reference is organized and the intention of the author for its use is essential. Each medical dictionary has its own type of arrangement for tables, color plates, vocabulary, and appendices. It is necessary to become familiar with the organization by reading the introduction, which explains how it should be used. Although often overlooked by the user, the introduction gives the transcriptionist a more powerful tool, since the organization of entries and the information contained in the appendices can now be put to use. The same applies to pharmaceutical references and word books. Each author or editor conveys a sense of organization that must be understood in order for the publication to be useful.

PART TWO

The Medical Basis of Transcription

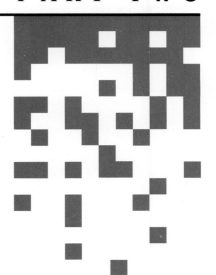

Raymond E. Liguori, M.D.

Cardiology

INTRODUCTION

Dramatic advances have occurred during recent decades in the fields of cardiology and cardiovascular surgery. Although cardiovascular diseases are the leading cause of death in Western societies, many afflicted patients may now benefit from such procedures as catheter balloon dilatation of diseased arteries or from a surgical bypass procedure. Improved diagnosis and treatment, a better understanding of underlying mechanisms, and a wider pursuit of preventive measures have led to a 40 per cent decline in the death rate from coronary heart disease.

ANATOMY AND PHYSIOLOGY

The heart is located in the midmediastinum, a cavity of the thoracic cage. It has four chambers, a right and a left ventricle and a right and a left atrium. The sole function of the cardiovascular system is to provide transportation of life-sustaining elements to the tissues and to remove or modify waste products. The left ventricle pumps blood into the systemic circulation through the aorta and its branches, and the right ventricle propels blood through the main pulmonary artery into the right and left branches to each lung (Figure 12–1).

The rich capillary network of the air sacs allows oxygenation of the blood in the lungs before it returns to the heart by way of the pulmonary veins. Except in the presence of a congenital anomaly, when additional or anomalous veins may be present, the upper and lower pulmonary veins drain the pulmonary venous bed into the heart.

The systemic venous circulation is drained by the superior vena cava above and the inferior vena cava below into the right atrium of the heart. Each of the heart chambers has an exit and an entrance valve, allowing efficient and unidirectional flow. The mitral valve separates the left atrium and ventricle, and the tricuspid valve, the right atrium and ventricle. Except for the mitral valve, which has an anterior and a posterior leaflet, the remaining three valves (tricuspid, pulmonary, and aortic) each have three cusps, or leaflets.

The myocardium, or heart muscle, is enclosed in a two-layered sac called the pericardium. One layer, intimately attached to the myocardial surface or epicardium, is called the visceral pericardium, and a second layer is known as the parietal pericardium. The interposed space normally contains about 0.5 ounce of clear fluid, allowing free movement of the heart against the pericardial sac. The inner surface of the heart or endocardium also covers the heart valves. The fibrous skeleton, or supportive structure of the heart, includes four rings called annuli. Each valve has a supporting annulus. The valves are tethered to the inner walls of the ventricles by chordae tendineae at the papillary muscles.

The atrial septum divides the atrial chambers, and the interventricular septum divides the ventricles. In the fetus, an alternative path for blood flow is a hole between the upper cardiac chambers. It is called the foramen ovale. If it is larger than normal and persists after birth, it is called an atrial septal defect. Ventricular septal defects and other variations of birth defects may

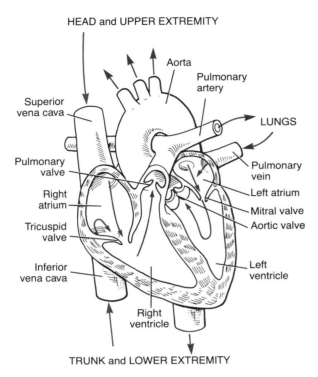

HEAD and UPPER EXTREMITY

Aorta

Pulmonary artery

Superior vena cava

LUNGS

Pulmonary valve

Pulmonary vein

Right atrium

Left atrium

Mitral valve

Aortic valve

Tricuspid valve

Inferior vena cava

Left ventricle

Right ventricle

TRUNK and LOWER EXTREMITY

Figure 12–1

Flow of blood through the heart. (From Guyton, A. C. *Textbook of Medical Physiology*, 6th ed. W. B. Saunders Company, Philadelphia, 1981.)

blood supply of the right and left ventricles, including the septum. Variations, called dominant right, balanced, or dominant left coronary artery circulations, may be seen. A left intermedius or intermediate artery may also be present in some, as may an obtuse marginal vessel. Atrial circumflex and sinus nodal arteries lie in the upper portion of the heart. The venous drainage is provided by the coronary sinus, in the heart's crux along the atrioventricular sulcus (groove), and also by the middle and great cardiac veins that drain other regions of the heart.

The innervation of the heart is briefly described since arrhythmias and the therapies used to treat them frequently invoke these terms. Clusters of nerve cells that carry or give rise to the heart's electrical impulse are called the sinus node and atrioventricular or A-V node. The cardiac impulse travels by way of atrial internodal branches and below the A-V node over the common bundle, the right and left bundle branches terminating at the Purkinje fibers innervating individual muscle fibers. The autonomic nervous system, namely both the sympathetic and para-

be seen. These include valve deformities, abnormal communications, incompletely developed or absent structures, at times in complex combinations, and other anomalies.

Coronary anatomy has assumed more importance with the growth of arteriography and coronary artery surgery (Figure 12–2). Derived from the Latin word *corona,* or crown, the coronary artery network supplies the heart in an inverted crownlike fashion. Three arteries feed the heart muscle (myocardium). The left coronary artery is the source of two, the left anterior descending, coursing down the front and the left circumflex coronary artery, which flexes around the left posterior aspect of the left ventricle. It also gives rise to marginal branches. The left anterior descending (LAD) artery has diagonal and septal perforator branches.

The right coronary artery contributes to the

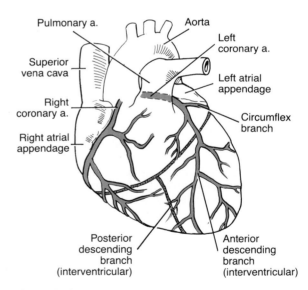

Pulmonary a.

Aorta

Left coronary a.

Superior vena cava

Left atrial appendage

Right coronary a.

Circumflex branch

Right atrial appendage

Posterior descending branch (interventricular)

Anterior descending branch (interventricular)

Figure 12–2

Coronary arteries supplying the heart. a = artery. (From Jacob, S. W., C. A. Francone, and W. J. Lossow, *Structure and Function in Man*, 5th ed. W. B. Saunders Company, Philadelphia, 1982.)

sympathetic nerves, also has representation in the heart, richly supplying the blood vessels with fibers. The immediate origins of these nerves are from the thoracic and cervical sympathetic and parasympathetic nerves and ganglia (nerve cell clusters), which in turn are connected to the brain by way of tracts and cranial nerves (Figure 12–3).

History and Physical Examination ▪ A history and physical examination by the physician forms the foundation of a workup (see Figure 12–14). This is usually followed by various tests, such as blood studies, radiographs, radioisotope tests, electrocardiography, echocardiography, and other more invasive methods, such as heart catheterization and coronary arteriography.

Of special importance in the patient's history is the occurrence of prior cardiovascular disease episodes, or the presence of various risk factors for heart disease. The history and physical examination reports often will include references to drugs commonly used to treat cardiovascular

disease (Table 12–1). The risk factors include hypertension, rheumatic fever, metabolic disorders, smoking, and lipid disorders. In the bloodstream, the lipids are carried by complex molecules of protein, carbohydrates, and fats in solution or suspension. They are called lipoproteins, triglycerides, and phospholipids, and abbreviated references are made to low density lipoproteins (LDL) and high density forms (HDL). In good health, high HDL and low LDL levels are desirable with a high HDL/LDL ratio. Individuals with an elevated serum cholesterol along with a low HDL and an elevated LDL are at higher risk for coronary artery disease in the form of atherosclerosis.

The recorded history should include details of symptoms, such as dyspnea (shortness of breath), tachypnea (rapid breathing), or erratic breathing characterized by periods of apnea (absent breathing), and Cheyne-Stokes respiration (a slow crescendo of increasing breathing rate and depth). The dyspneic patient may be unable to lie flat and is thereby orthopneic, having to

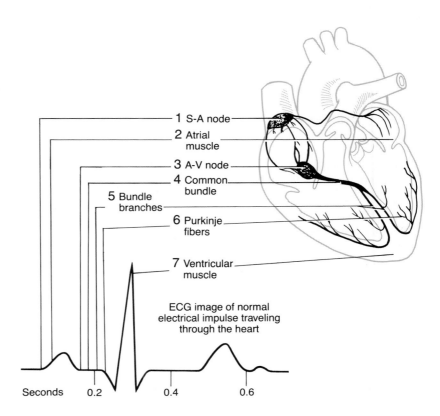

Figure 12–3
Conduction system of the heart. (From Chabner, D. E. *The Language of Medicine.* W. B. Saunders Company, Philadelphia, 1991.)

1 S-A node
2 Atrial muscle
3 A-V node
4 Common bundle
5 Bundle branches
6 Purkinje fibers
7 Ventricular muscle

ECG image of normal electrical impulse traveling through the heart

Seconds   0.2   0.4   0.6

Table 12–1 ▪ Drugs Commonly Used in Treatment of Cardiovascular Disease

Cardiotonics

digoxin
digitalis
dobutamine
dopamine
glycosides
Lanoxin

Coronary Vasodilators

Cardilate isosorbide dinitrate (Isordil)
nitroglycerin (Nitro-Bid, Nitro-Dur, Nitrostat,
    Transderm-Nitro)
papaverine HCl (Pavabid)
Peritrate

Vasopressors

Aramine
dobutamine (Dobutrex)
dopamine HCl (Intropin)
epinephrine (Adrenalin)
isoproterenol (Isuprel)
Neo-Synephrine
norepinephrine (Levophed)
Vasoxyl

**Antihypertensives or Used in Combination
with Diuretics**

beta-blockers
calcium blockers
hydralazine (Apresoline)
Diupres
Esimil
methyldopa (Aldomet)
Minizide
prazosin (Minipress)

Beta-Blockers

atenolol (Tenormin)
esmolol (Brevibloc)
labetalol (Sectral, Normodyne)
metoprolol (Lopressor)
nadolol (Corgard)
pindolol (Visken)
propranolol (Inderal)
timolol (Blocadren)

Calcium Channel Blockers

diltiazem (Cardizem)
nicardipine (Cardene)
nifedipine (Adalat, Procardia)
verapamil (Calan, Isoptin)

Antiarrhythmics

adenosine (Adeno-card)
amiodarone
bretylium

disopyramide (Norpace)
ethmozine (Enkaid)
flecainide (Tambocor)
lidocaine
mexilitine (Mexitil)
procainamide (Pronestyl)
quinidine (Quinidex, Quinaglute Dura-Tabs)
tocainide HCl (Tonocard)
Xylocaine

Antihypertensives with Diuretics

Aldactone
Aldactazide
chlorothiazide
Diuril
Dyrenium
Esidrix
ethacrynic acid (Edecrin)
hydrochlorothiazide
indapamide (Lozol)
Lasix
metolazone (Diulo)
triamterene (Dyazide)

Angiotensin-Converting Enzyme Inhibitors

Altace
captopril (Capoten)
enalapril (Vasotec)
lisinopril (Prinivil, Zestril)

**Hypolipemics (Cholesterol and Other
Lipid-Reducing Agents)**

Atromid-S
cholestyramine (Cholybar, Questran)
colestipol (Colestid)
gemfibrozil (Lopid)
lovastatin, an HMG-CoA reductase inhibitor
    (Mevacor)
niacin, nicotinic acid (Nicobid)
pravastatin (Pravachol)
probucol (Lorelco)

Anticoagulants

Coumadin
dicumarol
heparin
Panwarfin
protamine sulfate

Thrombolytics (Clot-Dissolving Agents)

Abbokinase
Activase
Eminase
Streptase
streptokinase
tissue plasminogen activator (TPA or t-PA)
urokinase

stand or sit up to breathe. Paroxysms of dyspnea during the night are commonly noted in left ventricular failure. Right heart failure is more apt to be associated with peripheral edema — pitting and swelling of the feet, ankles, and legs. If it is extreme, it may cause ascites (abdominal fluid accumulation) or, if more generalized, a worse form called anasarca.

Myocardial ischemia (myocardial deficiency of blood flow) may produce pain in the upper torso and upper extremities and less often in the upper epigastrium. It is called angina pectoris. It has an oppressive, vicelike quality and variably may radiate to the arms, shoulders, jaws, back, or even the skull. More often it is in the midanterior chest, spreading to the left arm and shoulder or bilaterally. Weakness and sweating, or diaphoresis, and at times nausea, faintness, or overt syncope may occur. Palpitations and tachycardia may signify an arrhythmia, or stressed heart.

Physical examination reveals many useful signs in most patients. Inspection may show cyanosis of the nail beds and lips, skin pallor, diaphoresis, and cervical or jugular venous distention (distended neck veins). Abnormal chest wall movements may be palpated, and stethoscopic examination may reveal murmurs, clicks, rubs, whoops, honks, or bruits. The murmurs or bruits may be continuous, systolic, or diastolic in timing. Systole represents the heart's contraction phase followed by diastole, or the rest phase. Careful examination of the pulses of the arteries of the feet, dorsalis pedis, and of the femoral arteries of the groin, posterior tibial, may indicate the character of lower extremity blood flow. The brachial, radial, and ulnar arteries are the peripheral vessels of the upper extremities. The carotid pulses may be felt, and pulsations sometimes are visualized in the neck. Table 12–2 lists common physical signs demonstrated during examination of the chest and extremities.

Crackling sounds (rales) at the lung bases may signify fluid in the air sacs, or congestive heart failure. In more severe forms of congestive failure, wheezes may be audible, and hemoptysis (coughing of blood) may be detected by the history or observation. Retinal examination often reveals changes of the optic fundus that mirror the effects of blood vessel disease, such as A-V nicking, widened luminous reflex, tortuosity of arterioles, hemorrhages, or exudates.

Table 12–2 ▪ Common Physical Signs of the Chest and Extremities

Chest Examination

auscultatory sounds: S1, S2, S3, and S4
blowing
bruit
crescendo
decrescendo
diastole
ejection click
gallops
grades 1, 2, 3, or 4 murmur
holosystolic
midsystolic click
musical murmurs
opening snap
pansystolic
paradoxic or physiologic splitting of S2, attenuated A2, fixed S2
pulmonary sounds: P1, P2
rasping
rumbling
systolic click
thrill(s)

Extremity Examination

clubbing
cyanosis
erythema
pitting edema
positive Homan's sign
pretibial edema
pulses: dorsalis pedis, femoral, popliteal, posterior tibial, radial, ulnar
spooning of the nails

REPRESENTATIVE CARDIAC DISORDERS AND DISEASES

This section presents representative disorders and diseases of the heart. A more extensive list of these is given in Table 12–3.

Heart Failure ▪ Heart failure is the term used to describe the abnormal function of the heart, resulting in its failure to meet the body's needs. It is often, but not always, due to a disorder of heart contraction or relaxation. It is distinguished from circulatory failure in which the problem involves the circulatory system outside the heart, such as the volume of blood, the

***Table* 12–3 ▪ Classifications of Cardiovascular Disorders**

Abnormalities of Circulatory Function

cardiac arrhythmias
cardiovascular collapse and sudden death
heart failure
high cardiac output states
hypotension and syncope
noncardiac forms of acute circulatory failure
pacemaker disorders
pulmonary hypertension; systemic hypertension*

Diseases of the Heart, Pericardium, Aorta, and Pulmonary Vascular Bed

acute myocardial infarction
atherosclerosis, generalized
cardiomyopathy and myocarditis
congenital heart disease
coronary atherosclerosis and other coronary heart disease
cor pulmonale and pulmonary thromboembolism
diseases of the aorta
infective endocarditis
pericardial disease
primary tumors of the heart
renal disorders related to heart disease
traumatic heart disease
valvular heart disease

---

*Hypertension is no longer referred to as "mild," "moderate," "severe," or "very severe." A patient can be normal (less than 130/less than 85) or high-normal (130–139/85–89), or can have hypertension stage 1 (140–159/90–99), stage 2 (160–179/100–109), stage 3 (180–209/110–119), or stage 4 (210 or higher/120 or higher).

---

amount of hemoglobin that carries oxygen, or the state of the peripheral vessels. Heart function may be normal in cases of circulatory system overload with salt and fluids, but pulmonary congestion and edema may occur. Circulatory failure may occur in hemorrhagic states and in severe anemia, extreme fluid depletion, or high heart output states, such as beri beri and hyperthyroidism. More commonly, heart failure is seen in clinical practice as a manifestation of a heart muscle disorder, such as ischemic (coronary) heart disease or myocarditis.

Heart Valvular Disorders ▪ Heart valvular disorders are also often implicated. The most common forms of congenital heart disease are congenital aortic valve disease, including bicuspid aortic valve, atrial and ventricular septal defects, and patent ductus arteriosus. Less common, more complex forms are seen, such as tetralogy of Fallot, endocardial cushion defects, persistent truncus arteriosus, tricuspid atresia, and Ebstein's anomaly of the tricuspid valve.

Valvular heart disease, in which the valve either is incompetent, with leakage or insufficiency, or is tight (stenotic), with obstruction to flow, is another disorder. Valve dysfunction may lead to heart failure and myocardial damage. Mitral stenosis is a common complication of rheumatic heart disease, whereas mitral insufficiency is seen in myxomatous degeneration of the valve with mitral valve prolapse, severe cardiomyopathies, coronary heart disease, and rheumatic heart disease. Aortic stenosis and insufficiency may be acquired and have numerous causes. Infective endocartitis may cause disruption, deformity, or perforation of any of the cardiac valves. Abscesses of the myocardium and sinus of Valsalva or septal perforation may occur in endocarditis.

Myocardial Infarction ▪ Unstable angina is a complication of coronary heart disease and may be followed by myocardial infarction. Ulceration or plaque disruption at the intimal surface of the coronary artery is often implicated. A partially or fully obstructive thrombus may occur. Spontaneous lysis or dissolution of the thrombus may produce relief. Thrombolytic agents, such as streptokinase or TPA (t-PA), are used acutely in selected patients presenting with an acute myocardial infarction. If given early enough, before necrosis develops, some myocardial salvage may be obtained.

Percutaneous transluminal coronary angioplasty (PTCA) or catheter-mounted balloon dilatation is a commonly applied invasive technique for the relief of disabling coronary artery stenosis or obstruction. When used in the setting of unstable angina or recent infarction, it may be described as "rescue angioplasty."

Severe infarction may produce cardiogenic shock and pulmonary edema. Intra-aortic balloon augmentation of the heart output may save patients, some of whom are helped by follow-up emergency angioplasty or surgery. Cardiotonic agents, such as dobutamine, dopamine, and diuretics and other supportive measures are often used. Elective application of angioplasty in the symptomatic patient may require balloon dilation of the obstructed coronary artery. Less commonly, a low profile rotating blade (Rotablator) mounted in a catheter is used by an innovative method called coronary atherectomy. Excimer laser ablation of the lesions is currently being applied as an experimental technique.

Cardiomyopathies ■ Cardiomyopathies are divided into those associated with hypertrophy of the heart (hypertrophic cardiomyopathy) and restrictive and dilated forms. Angina, dyspnea, fatigue, and syncope characterize the hypertrophic form. This is usually first seen in young adults or children. Restrictive or infiltrative forms are described in sarcoidosis, amyloidosis, and hemochromatosis. More often one sees the dilated form, as after toxin or alcohol exposure, or an idiopathic form. Viral infections are incriminated in many cases of myocarditis. Rickettsial organisms, as in Rocky Mountain spotted fever and Q fever, spirochetes, and various fungi and bacteria are other causes. These include syphilis, Legionnaires' disease, coccidioidomycosis, diphtheria, and streptococcus. Noninfectious causes include the following, which is only a partial list:

- arsenic
- carbon monoxide
- chloroquine
- daunorubicin and Adriamycin
- disopyramide
- emetine
- 5-fluorouracil (5-FU)
- heat stroke
- hypersensitivity reactions
- hypothermia
- lead
- lithium
- mercury
- phenothiazines
- phosphorus
- radiation
- rejection of transplant
- scorpion sting
- snake bite
- thyroid hormone
- tricyclic antidepressants
- wasp and spider stings

Cardiac Tumors ■ Cardiac tumors include the following:

- angioma
- atrial myxoma
- leukemia
- lymphoma
- melanoma
- metastatic carcinoma
- myeloma
- rhabdomyoma
- rhabdomyosarcoma
- sarcoma

For further information on cardiac tumors, see Chapter 26 on oncology-hematology.

Pericarditis ■ Heart sac inflammation usually presents with characteristic pain and is most often seen with viral infections, with myocardial infarction, or in an idiopathic form. It is a common complication of myocardial infarction (postmyocardial infarction syndrome, or Dressler's syndrome), postcardiotomy syndrome, and chronic renal failure. A typical classification can be outlined as follows:

1. Acute nonspecific or idiopathic
2. Acute myocardial infarction
3. Postmyocardial infarction syndrome
4. Postcardiotomy syndrome
5. Connective tissue disorders, as rheumatic fever, rheumatoid disease, disseminated lupus, scleroderma
6. Infections: bacterial, including tuberculosis; fungi; viral, as Coxsackie B; and others
7. Malignancy
8. Trauma, penetrating and nonpenetrating
9. Rupture of great vessels, as dissection of the aorta
10. Postoperative bleeding after cardiothoracic surgery

Pericardial tamponade, or fluid accumulation with compression of the heart, is most often seen with tuberculosis, the aforementioned mechanisms 7 to 10, and chronic renal failure. It may be accompanied by pulsus paradoxus, Kussmaul's sign, and an electrocardiographic finding called electrical alternans. Constrictive forms of pericarditis are differentiated from restrictive cardiomyopathies.

Diseases of the Aorta and Major Arteries ■ Diseases of the aorta and major arteries include the following:

1. Buerger's disease (thromboangiitis obliterans)
2. Atherosclerosis
3. Aneurysms, including dissecting forms
4. Marfan's syndrome, characterized by dilatation and weakness of walls of major arteries and valves of the heart, especially aortic aneurysm and aortic valve disease in combination
5. Leriche's syndrome
6. Takayasu's arteritis
7. Coarctation of the aorta

Cor Pulmonale ▪ Cor pulmonale describes pulmonary artery hypertension in the presence of some combination of right ventricular dilatation or hypertrophy. Chronic bronchitis and pulmonary emphysema are the most common causes. Seven to ten per cent of all heart disease in the United States is due to cor pulmonale. It may accompany bronchiectasis, pneumoconiosis (induced by environmental dust exposure), chest deformities (congenital and acquired), and recurrent pulmonary emboli.

Related Renal Diseases ▪ Renal diseases attended by heart disease include glomerulonephritis, chronic parenchymal renal disease, pyelonephritis, polycystic kidneys, and collagen vascular diseases, such as lupus and polyarteritis. Chronic renal disease, especially in combination with diabetes, commonly results in accelerated atherosclerosis and aortic valve disease.

DIAGNOSIS OF CARDIOVASCULAR DISEASES

Noninvasive Diagnostic Procedures ▪ Procedures that are normally pain-free and do not involve the passage of catheters into blood vessels are called noninvasive. Such tests include, but are not restricted to, the following:

1. Electrocardiogram
2. Echocardiogram
3. Echo-Doppler studies
4. Radiologic or x-ray
5. Nuclear imaging
6. Vectocardiography and phonocardiography (rarely used methods)
7. Blood studies, including blood lipids, cardiac enzymes, and others
8. Exercise testing, including treadmill stress test, bicycle ergometry, thallium stress test, and exercise echocardiography
9. Pharmacologic stress tests: dobutamine, adenosine, and dipyridamole stress
10. Holter or dynamic electrocardiographic monitoring
11. Pacemaker analysis

Some of these procedures are discussed in more detail later.

Electrocardiography ▪ Electrocardiography remains the most commonly applied tool in cardiac diagnosis, but it is followed in frequency and often overshadowed in diagnostic value by echocardiography. The electrocardiogram, usually referred to as the ECG, is obtained by a method that uses a wire lead system composed of five or eleven electrodes, one on each of the four extremities, and one or six on the precordium on the six sites of the chest wall chosen to record the heart's electrical activity. The ECG provides important information about cardiac rhythm, anatomy and pathophysiology. The minute current generated is amplified and recorded. The wave contours have been assigned letter designations, referred to as the P, Q, R, S, and T components, or combinations thereof, as P-R, QRS, ST, or QT. A U wave may be described (Figure 12–4). Cardiac arrhythmias, although detected clinically on physical examination, are usually confirmed by the ECG. For an abbreviated classification of cardiac arrhythmias, see Table 12–4. Left or right ventricular hypertrophy, combined hypertrophy, and left, right or bi-atrial enlargement may be described. Electrolyte disturbances, such as hypokalemia, hyperkalemia, hypercalcemia, and hypocalcemia, are detected on the electrocardiogram (Figure 12–5). Myocardial infarction and ischemia are common indications for the ECG (Figure 12–6). Infarctions

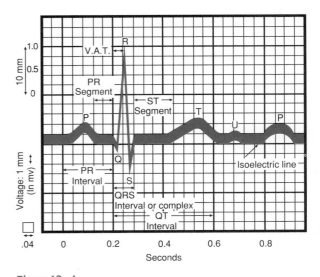

Figure 12–4

A diagram of electrocardiographic complexes, intervals, and segments. P wave = spread of excitation wave over the atria; QRS wave = spread of excitation wave over the ventricle; T wave = electrical recovery and relaxation of the ventricles.

Table 12–4 ▪ Classification of Cardiac Arrhythmias

Sinus Node Disturbances

Sinus rhythm represents the normal state, and sinus bradycardia (rate less than 60 per minute) may occur normally, as well as sinus arrhythmia. Sinus tachycardia also is normal with activity increase, adrenaline stimulation, fever, excitement, or in the normal fetus or neonate. Other varieties classified as abnormal are

    sinus pause or sinus arrest
    sinoatrial (SA) exit block
    wandering pacemaker
    sick sinus node with sinus pause, SA block, and
      tachycardia-bradycardia syndrome
    sinus nodal re-entry

Atrial Rhythm Disturbances

    premature atrial complexes (PACs)
    atrial tachycardia
    atrial flutter
    atrial fibrillation
    atrial tachycardia with block
    automatic atrial tachycardia
    multiform or chaotic atrial tachycardia
    atrial tachycardia due to re-entry

AV Junctional Rhythm Disturbances (Involving AV Node or Nearby Tissue)

    premature AV junctional complexes
    AV junctional rhythm
    nonparoxysmal AV junctional tachycardia
    AV nodal re-entrant tachycardia
    re-entry over a retrograde conducting (concealed) pathway

Pre-Excitation Syndromes (Wolff-Parkinson-White)

    Lown-Ganong-Levine syndrome
    short PR syndrome
    other accessory bundle syndromes (Kent's,
      Mahaim's fibers)
    reciprocating tachycardias
    orthodromic, antidromic tachycardia

Ventricular Rhythm Disturbances

    premature ventricular complexes (PVCs)
    idioventricular rhythm
    atrioventricular dissociation
    ventricular tachycardia
    ventricular fibrillation
    bigeminy, trigeminy, quadrigeminy
    Torsades de pointes
    bidirectional ventricular tachycardia
    electrical alternans
    nonparoxysmal and paroxysmal ventricular tachycardia

Other Arrhythmias

    long QT syndrome
    ventricular flutter
    heart block, including first, second, and third degree or complete heart block
    Wenckebach's conduction, 2:1, 3:1, 4:1 AV block
    fascicular block and hemiblock, as left anterior or posterior fascicular block
    pacemaker arrhythmias

---

may be described as anterior, posterior, inferior, lateral, anteroseptal, or in combination, as anterolateral, inferoseptal, inferoposterior, posterolateral, and so forth. At times the word *diaphragmatic* is substituted for inferior in describing an infarct or segment of the heart. Pericarditis may also be reflected by pattern changes that involve T waves and the ST segments of the electrocardiogram.

Stress electrocardiography, or the stress test, is commonly employed in the diagnosis of disorders of heart function and ischemic heart disease (Figure 12–7).

Echocardiogram and Echo-Doppler Studies ▪ Echocardiography and cardiac echo-Doppler studies have been among the most dramatic and important adjuncts in cardiac diagnosis during the last few decades (Figure 12–8). Anatomic and pathophysiologic information can be obtained quickly, at the bedside or on an ambulatory patient, in an efficient and relatively inexpensive manner compared with invasive or radionuclide techniques. Information can be stored on videotape and a strip chart recorder. Exercise stress echocardiography utilizes digitized computer techniques and a supine bicycle or treadmill or, alternatively, pharmacologic stress with dobutamine or other agents may be used. Conventional echocardiography has proved very useful in pericarditis, myocardial infarction, congenital heart disease, and valve dysfunction. The addition of the Doppler technol-

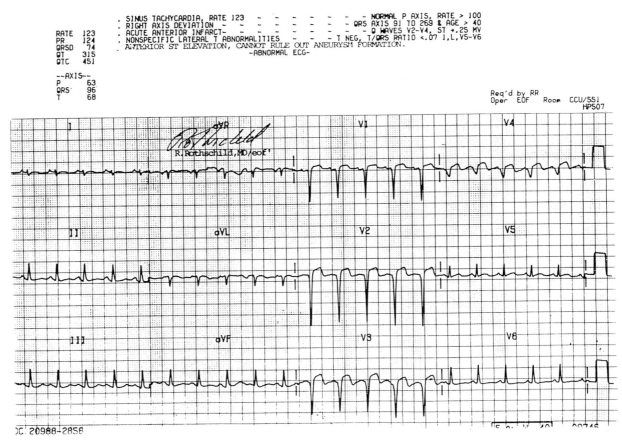

Figure 12-5
An abnormal electrocardiogram (ECG).

ogy has enabled measurement of valve gradients and orifice size by indirect methods (modified Bernoulli's equation), and the detection of small shunts. Cardiac catheterization may be averted, especially in young children and infants with congenital heart disease or in adults with mitral stenosis or cardiac tumor. Valve prolapse is readily demonstrated on the echocardiogram, as are cardiac hypertrophy and chamber dilatation.

Nuclear Imaging ▪ Nuclear imaging in the assessment of heart disease may utilize such function assessments as first-pass radionuclide angiography and equilibrium gated blood pool imaging. More common uses include thallium-201 for myocardial perfusion imaging or exercise thallium studies. The recent application of Cardiolite, or imaging with single photon emission tomography (SPECT), has enhanced diagnostic sensitivity (Figure 12-9). A more elaborate method requiring positron emission tomography is labeled PET scanning and is not widely available. Occasionally one encounters the use of myocardial infarct avid agents, which accumulate in the area of necrosis of the myocardium as technetium-99m or stannous pyrophosphate. On the horizon, and in the experimental mode, is the use of magnetic resonance imaging (MRI) in heart disease diagnosis. High strength static magnetic fields, low strength changing magnetic fields, and radiofrequency pulse sequences are employed to generate tomographic images. This allows one to obtain dynamic cine images, and it is a three-dimensional technique. Aortic dissection can be diagnosed by these methods, but,

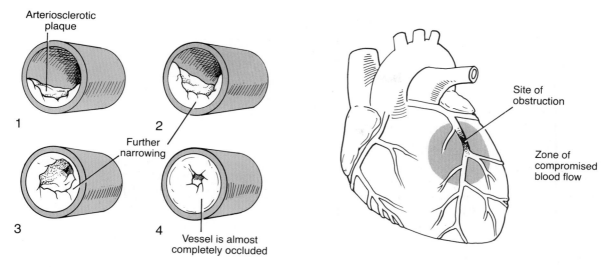

Figure 12-6

Ischemia and infarction produced by coronary artery occlusion. *Left,* An arteriosclerotic plaque forms on the intima of the vessel and projects into the lumen. As the plaque enlarges it provides a rough surface that can lead to the formation of a thrombus that further narrows the vessel lumen. Eventually the opening is too narrow to supply the heart's oxygen needs, and the surrounding tissue becomes ischemic or dies (*right*).

in such acutely ill patients, the use of bedside transesophageal echocardiography may be preferable in certain circumstances.

Holter Monitoring ▪ Prolonged ECG recording (Holter monitoring, ambulatory monitoring) in patients engaged in regular activity allows the documentation of cardiac arrhythmias while correlating with symptoms. Some instruments permit accurate detection of pattern changes, such as ST segment shifts, and may lead to the diagnosis of silent myocardial ischemia, or activity- and stress-induced ST changes (Figure 12-10)

Invasive Diagnostic Studies ▪ These are studies in which the passage of catheters into blood vessels or other invasive techniques are performed. Some of these tests include the following:

1. Angiography
2. Cardiac catheterization
3. Coronary arteriography
4. Aortography and run-off studies
5. Pulmonary angiography
6. Electrophysiologic studies

Cardiac catheterization and coronary arteriography are discussed in more detail next.

Cardiac Catheterization and Coronary Arteriography ▪ Since its introduction more than 60 years ago, catheterization with small-diameter tubes of blood vessels leading to or from the heart has achieved widespread use (Figure 12-11). Initially utilized primarily for the diagnosis of congenital heart disease, this method provides physiologic information by enabling pressure and oxygen saturation analysis. The addition of dye injections for dye dilution curve studies and hydrogen electrodes led to detection of intracardiac shunts. Fluoroscopy, a video camera and monitor, and a 35-mm cine camera permitted the recording of injections of radiopaque dyes for anatomic information (Figure 12-12).

The technique of coronary arteriography has subsequently come into widespread use and provides detailed anatomic information about coronary artery anatomy. When it is coupled with radiopaque dye injections into the left ventricle (ventriculogram), important functional and anatomic information can be obtained.

The detailed parameters of study at cardiac catheterization are designated on the catheterization forms (Figure 12-13), which vary with

Text continued on page 169

UNIVERSITY HOSPITAL
1234 Main Street
Oxnard, CA 93030-0000

STRESS TEST SUMMARY

Date: December 2, 1994
Time: 10:09 A. M.

Patient: Makena W. Lee   Attending: William Fish, M. D.
ID: 320945   Referring: Raymond Blue, M. D.
Age: 30   DOB: 9-20-63

                                    Max Predicted HR: 191
                    % of Max Predicted HR achieved: 105%

Weight: 140
                                    STANDING HR: 82
Sex: F   Max HR: 201 @ 14:10

Medications: STANDING BP: 117/67
                                    Max systolic BP: 224 @ 11:50
                                    Max diastolic BP: 92 @ 16:10

                                    METS achieved: 15.0

Interpretation:

The patient exercised for 14 minutes on the Bruce protocol, peak heart rate achieved was 200 BPM, or 105% of maximum predicted for age. The blood pressure response to exercise was normal. No chest pain was noted.

The resting ECG was normal. The electrocardiographic response to exercise was nonischemic and no arrhythmias were induced.

IMPRESSION:

1. Good functional capacity for age.
2. Clinically and electrocardiographically negative for ischemia.
3. No arrhythmias.

_____
WILLIAM FISH, M. D.

mtf

Figure 12–7
An example of a stress electrocardiography report.

UNIVERSITY HOSPITAL
1234 Main Street
Oxnard, CA 93030-0000

ECHOCARDIOGRAM REPORT

Name: Karen H. Card
DOB: 12/02-03   Age: 90   MR: 1029967   Sex: F   Date: 12-28-94
Ht: 5' 3"   Wt: 120   BP: 180/96   Doctor: Hui Chan, M. D.
Reason for test:

Pericardial effusion:	Absent	Small (20-100 ml)	Moderate (100-500 ml)	Large (> 500 ml)
Mitral valve:	Normal	Abnormal	Not recorded	
Tricuspid valve:	Normal	Abnormal	Not recorded	
Aortic valve:	Normal	Abnormal	Not recorded	
Pulmonary valve:	Normal	Abnormal	Not recorded	

Echocardiogram dimensions:

M-Mode	Normals	Pat.	2-D	Normal	Pat.
LVEDD	2.5-5.6 cm	4.3	LVEDD	3.6-5.2 cm	
LVESD		2.4	LVESD	2.3-3.9 cm	
Minor diam short	25-50%		Minor diam. short	18-42%	
RV diam (sup)	0.7-2.3 cm		Left atrium	2.1-3.7 cm	
RV diam (LL)	1.0-2.6 cm	0.9			
IVS thickness	0.5-1.1 cm	1.9	Other 2D		
IVS amplitude	0.5-1.1 cm	0.9	Observations	Normal	Abnormal
LVPW thickness	0.7-1.1 cm	1.1			
LVPW amplitude	0.5-1.2 cm	1.0	LV wall motion		
Left atrium	1.9-4.0 cm	3.6	RV wall motion		
Aortic root	2.0-3.7 cm	3.2	Pericardium		
Aortic valve	1.6-2.6 cm	1.6			
E pt.-Sep. S.	< 0.5 cm		Comments:		

Interpretation: X M-Mode X 2D Doppler

CONCLUSIONS:

1. Technically difficult study with moderate signal scatter.
2. Chamber dimensions: Within normal limits with left atrial size being borderline prominent.
3. Ventricular function: Moderate concentric left ventricular hypertrophy with normal systolic function. LV ejection fraction and wall motion are normal. Right ventricular wall motion also normal.
4. Valves: Moderate sclerosis of the aortic and mitral annulus with mild aortic valve leaflet sclerosis. Valve motion appears normal. Doppler color flow screen reveals trace to mild aortic insufficiency and trace pulmonic insufficiency.

1/3/94 mtf   Hui Chan, M. D.

Figure 12–8
An example of an echocardiogram report.

UNIVERSITY HOSPITAL
1234 Main Street
Oxnard, CA 93030-0000

CARDIOLITE
STRESS ELECTROCARDIOGRAM

ATTAINED MAXIMAL RATE: 150   AMR /PMR x 100 = 89%
PREDICTED MAXIMAL RATE: 168

Resting EKG

During Exercise	Post	TIME Speed MPH	% Grade	Heart Rate	Blood Pressure	METS	
0	ERECT @ REST			61	184/110		Sinus rhythm with non-specific low to diphasic T waves in leads I, II, aVL, V5-V6
I	3'	1.7	10	98	190/110		
II	6'	2.5	12	130	220/106		
III	9'	3.4	14	150	210/100		
IV	30			148	210/100		
V	1			112	210/98		
VI	2			100	212/96		
VII	3			98	212/96		
VIII	5			90			

OTHER OBSERVATIONS: Functional Aerobic Impairment: +5%
The patient exercised for 9 minutes stopping with fatigue, dyspnea, and a burning discomfort across the anterior chest which appeared to be related to inspiration and was noted after 7 minutes of walking. It cleared approximately 5 minutes post exercise.

Modified 12 lead ECGs reveal no significant change in the ST segment during or after exercise. There is J point depression but no significant ST depression at the 80 msec. At rest, intermittent inversion of the P wave is noted in leads II, III, aVF suggesting an intermittent ectopic atrial rhythm. No other arrhythmia observed. Elevated blood pressure readings noted.

IMPRESSION:
1. TREADMILL EXERCISE ELECTROCARDIOGRAM: NEGATIVE FOR ISCHEMIA; symptom limited study with a submaximal level of myocardial stress.
2. Average effort tolerance for age, with exertional chest discomfort of equivocal significance and possibly of pulmonic origin.

NAME: Ronald O. Simpson   SEX/AGE M/52   DOB 2/20/39
PT NO. 2390399   MR NO. 2388996 OP
PHYSICIAN: B. Elliott, M. D.   DATE 11/30/94

_____
Bernard Elliott, M. D.

12/3/94 mtf

Figure 12–9
An example of a Cardiolite (imaging with SPECT—single photon emission tomography) stress electrocardiogram report.

UNIVERSITY HOSPITAL
1234 Main Street
Oxnard, CA 93030-0000

HOLTER REPORT

Patient: Evelyn T. Stevens
ID No.: 12098765
Age: 60   Sex: F
Referred by: Carol Smith, M. D.
      from:

Date:	12/30/94
Hook-up date:	11/30/94
Time:	14:20:00
Duration:	23:46:12

Indications: IRREG HB
Medications: Theo-Dur, Calan, Lanoxin, Tofranil, Coumadin

SUMMARY

105648   QRS complexes
12   Ventricular   ectopics which represent <1% of total QRS complexes
184   Supraventricular   ectopics which represent < 1% of total QRS complexes
        Paced QRS complexes   which represent   % of total QRS complexes

VENTRICULAR ECTOPY
10 Isolated
 0 Bigeminal Cycles
 1 Couplets
 0 Runs
 0 Beats in Runs
 0 Beats LONGEST at 0 BPM at

SUPRAVENTRICULAR ECTOPY
155 Isolated
 8 Couplets
 4 Runs
13 Beats in Runs
 4 Beats LONGEST at 147 BPM at 17:06:16 26-DEC-9X
 4 Beats FASTEST at 147 BPM at 17:06:16 26-DEC-9X

HEART RATES
 58 MIN at 23:33:15 26-DEC-9X
 75 AVG
109 MAX at 12:44:45 27-DEC-9X

S-T LEVELS Channel 1
+1.0 mm at 18:56:55 26-DEC-9X
-1.0 mm at 19:53:25 26-DEC-9X

INTERPRETATION:
1. Patient monitored for 24 hours using a full disclosure system (repeat study due to technical difficulties with original study).
   Patient's basic rhythm is of sinus origin with rates varying from 58-109 per minute, averaging approximately 75 per minute.
2. Supraventricular arrhythmias: Rare to occasional isolated APC's with 3-4 brief runs of atrial tachycardia of 3-4 beats duration. No sustained ectopic tachy- or brady-arrhythmia or A-V block.
3. Ventricular arrhythmias: Rare isolated VPC's, total of 12, with one couplet; no ventricular tachycardia.
4. ST segments: No significant variation.
5. Symptoms: No significant change noted in relation to notations of "shortness of breath" or "strong palpitations."

Signed_____Date: 12/30/94 mtf

Figure 12–10

An example of a Holter monitor report.

UNIVERSITY HOSPITAL
1234 Main Street
Oxnard, CA 93030-0000

CARDIAC CATHETERIZATION AND ANGIOGRAPHY REPORT

Name: Hugo F. Slaney   Angiogram Number: 94-870
DOB: 9-04-30   MR: 1987802   Sex: M   Study Date: 10-2-94

HEMODYNAMICS: At rest in sinus rhythm, the left ventricular end diastolic pressure is at the upper limits of normal. No aortic valve gradient.

CINEANGIOGRAMS:

LEFT VENTRICLE: RAO projection. Large area of calcification involving the posterior wall. This probably represents a large aneurysm. An LAO projection was not done. The aneurysm is confirmed by 2D echo. Probable mural thrombus noted. In this projection, the wall motion is generally poor. The anterolateral wall appears to be hypokinetic but the inferior wall is akinetic. Estimated ejection fraction 15-20%.

LEFT MAIN CORONARY ARTERY: Mildly narrowed at its orifice to about 25%.

LEFT CIRCUMFLEX ARTERY: Completely occluded after a small first marginal branch. Distal vessel fills by adjacent collaterals.

LEFT ANTERIOR DESCENDING ARTERY: 60% irregular mid stenosis followed by an eccentric plaque which protrudes into the lumen. The narrowing at the eccentric plaque is about 50%. First diagonal artery is small. Second diagonal artery is moderately large and has several branches. The distal LAD is normal.

RIGHT CORONARY ARTERY: Subtotally occluded proximally with post stenotic dilatation. It is a moderately small vessel distally giving rise to a small posterior descending and moderately small posterolateral branch.

CONCLUSIONS:
I. Atherosclerotic coronary artery disease.
    A. Complete occlusion of the left circumflex artery.
    B. Subtotal occlusion of the right coronary artery.
    C. 60% stenosis of the mid LAD.

II. Poor LV function with severe global hypokinesis and inferior akinesis. There is evidence of calcified inferoposterior ventricular aneurysm with probable old thrombus.

COMMENT: Continued medical therapy was advised.

10/02/94 mtf   Kevin T. McCarthy, M. D.

Figure 12–11
An example of a cardiac catheterization and angiography report.

B. Surf. Area: Ht: Wt:

	Normal mmHg Rest	Baseline	O2 Sat
Peripheral Artery	$\frac{100-140}{60-90}$ $\overline{70-105}$		
Aorta	$\frac{100-140}{60-90}$ $\overline{70-105}$		
Left Ventricle	$\frac{100-140}{3-12}$		
Left Atrium	$\overline{2-12}$		
Pulmonary Capillary	$\overline{2-12}$		
Pulmonary Artery	$\frac{15-30}{4-12}$ $\overline{9-18}$		
Right Ventricle	$\frac{15-30}{2-8}$		
Right Atrium	$\overline{2-8}$		
Superior Vena Cava			
Inferior Vena Cava			

	NORMAL	
Cardiac Output	Varies with Size	
Cardiac Index	2.6 - 4.2 L/min/M^2	
Pulse Rate		
Stroke Volume	Varies with Size	
SV Index	30-65 cc/bt/M^2	
Stroke Work		
Stroke Work Index		
Ejection Fraction	59-75%	
LV DP/DT		
Pulm Vasc Res	100 dynesec cm. -5	
Sys Vasc Res	1300 dynesec cm. -5	
Pulm Flow		
Shunt Flow		
A-V O-2 Difference	30-50 mL/L	

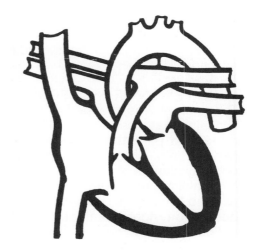

VALVE	GRADIENT	INSUFFICIENCY	Ca++	AREA
Aortic		0 [ ] 1+ [ ] 2+ [ ] 3+ [ ] 4+ [ ]		
Mitral		0 [ ] 1+ [ ] 2+ [ ] 3+ [ ] 4+ [ ]		
Tricuspid		0 [ ] 1+ [ ] 2+ [ ] 3+ [ ] 4+ [ ]		
Pulmonic		0 [ ] 1+ [ ] 2+ [ ] 3+ [ ] 4+ [ ]		

Name: _____

H_2 - Platinum Electrode Study:

     [ ] Negative   [ ] Positive

     Level: _____

O_2 - Shunt Study:

     [ ] Negative   [ ] Positive

     Level: _____

Date: _____

Figure 12–12

An example of a form accompanying a cardiac catheterization and angiography report.

UNIVERSITY HOSPITAL
1234 Main Street
Oxnard, CA 93030-0000

CARDIAC CATHETERIZATION PROCEDURE NOTE

RE: Theresa Lopez
DOB: 11-12-36
MR #: 450-99-22
CATH #: 93-3400
CATH DATE: 12-02-94

OPERATORS: Frank M. Jasper, M. D.
                            Jerome K. Lesser, M. D.

PROCEDURE: Right ventricular biopsy and right heart catheterization.

BRIEF HISTORY:
The patient is a 55-year-old white female with a history of idiopathic dilated cardiomyopathy who underwent cardiac transplant in May, 1993. Her most recent biopsy was done in January, 1993 and showed moderate acute rejection and, since that time, she has had symptoms of shortness of breath and dyspnea on exertion. Her medications, including cyclosporine and prednisone, were increased and she was started on methotrexate and is now admitted to undergo repeat right ventricular biopsy and right heart catheterization for followup of acute rejection.

DESCRIPTION OF PROCEDURE:
The patient was prepped and draped in the usual sterile technique and 2% lidocaine was used to anesthetize the right neck. Right ventricular biopsy was performed percutaneously via a #9F short sheath placed in the right internal jugular vein. Stanford bioptomes were used to obtain six right ventricular endomyocardial biopsy specimens. The first bioptome used was successful only in obtaining one biopsy specimen as the bite of the forceps was not sharp and a second bioptome was needed. Following successful biopsy specimen acquisition, right heart catheterization was performed using a wedge pressure balloon catheter passed from the right internal jugular vein to the pulmonary capillary wedge pressure position with simultaneous ECG and pressure monitoring. After these data were recorded, the catheter was removed and the sheath was pulled with pressure applied to the right neck and hemostasis was achieved. Biopsy specimens were sent to pathology.

MEDICATIONS:
Versed 0.5 mg IV.

COMPLICATIONS:
None.   (continued)

Figure 12–13
An example of a cardiac catheterization procedure note typed in full block format.

RE: Theresa Lopez
DOB: 11-12-36
MR #: 450-99-22
CATH #: 93-3400
CATH DATE: 12-02-94
Page Two (Cath)

ESTIMATED BLOOD LOSS:
Less than 10 ml.

HEMODYNAMIC RESULTS:
Right atrial pressure mean of 10. Right ventricular pressure of 35/8. Right pulmonary artery pressure of 35/17 with a mean of 27. Pulmonary artery wedge pressure mean of 20. Aortic cuff pressure of 113/80, mean of 91.

CONCLUSIONS:
1. Successful right ventricular endomyocardial biopsy.
2. Mild elevation of right heart pressure and pulmonary cath wedge pressure.

_____   _____
Frank M. Jasper, M. D.   Jerome K. Lesser, M. D.

mtf

D: 12-02-94
R: 12-05-94
T: 12-06-94

cc: James T. Carson, M. D.
       Martin G. Gamble, M. D.

Figure 12–13 *Continued*

each laboratory and are often computer processed and printed. Nuclear laboratory studies most often used are the thallium-201 scintigram, Persantine-thallium scintigraphy, first-pass radionuclide angiography, and the technetium pyrophosphate study.

Echocardiography and cardiac echo–Doppler studies may replace the need for cardiac catheterization in many patients, especially those with congenital heart disease, mitral stenosis, and cardiac tumors.

CARDIOVASCULAR SURGERY

Cardiovascular surgery has made dramatic and substantial contributions to the management of heart disease during the past four decades. Complete cures have been achieved in several forms of congenital disorders and extraordinary palliation in others. Of special importance have been coronary bypass surgery, valve repair and replacement, and aneurysm repair. Peripheral bypass vessel procedures, such as femoral-popliteal, and endarterectomies of atherosclerotic plugs or plaques have been used frequently. Newer techniques include laser ablation of lesions of peripheral vessels.

Other procedures include pacemaker implantations and automatic defibrillators and antitachycardia devices implanted transvenously and surgically to treat so-called "sudden death" or catastrophic arrhythmias. Cutting of tracts or catheter-guided ablation of accessory bypass tracts of the heart, as in Wolff-Parkinson-White syndrome, has been used with success. More recently, catheter-guided radiofrequency ablation has been employed.

Median sternotomy incisions are now the rule in most open heart surgery procedures, as is the use of cardiopulmonary bypass, myocardial protection measures, and ventilatory assistance. Postoperatively, supportive measures may include the use of intermittent positive pressure breathing (IPPB) and intermittent mandatory ventilation (IMV).

Anesthetic methods have improved dramatically in recent decades with better supportive measures, drugs, and an enhanced understanding of drug application. Invasive monitoring, postoperative ventilatory support, and early extubation, along with the judicious use of positive inotropic agents that increase myocardial tone and other vasoactive drugs, have played major roles.

Both inhalation anesthetic agents and intravenous drugs are being used with the gaseous agents, including ethrane, halothane, isoflurane, and nitrous oxide. Intravenous agents include diazepam (Valium), fentanyl, ketamine, morphine, and pentothal. Muscle relaxants used intravenously are D-tubocurare, pancuronium, succinylcholine, and vecuronium.

Surgery for Congenital or Acquired Heart Disease* ▪ Congenital heart disease, seen largely in pediatric surgery programs, may require any one or more of the following procedures: pulmonary artery banding, ligation or li-

gation-excision of anomalous pulmonary veins, baffles, patches such as Dacron or Teflon, Mustard's, Senning's, or Rastelli's operations—the latter for transposition of the great vessels, arterial switch procedure, partial correction of Ebstein's anomaly, cardiac transplantation, Damus-Fontan operation, and Damus-Rastelli operation. For further information on pediatric cardiology, see the pediatric specialty section, Chapter 31.

Surgery for congenital or acquired heart disease often involves the use of myocardial protection during the operation. The viability of the vulnerable myocardial tissue and the nervous system is protected in this manner. These measures include extracorporeal circulation with cardiopulmonary bypass and the perfusion of the coronary circulation with myocardial protective solution. By the balanced use of drugs, fluid, blood, or colloid volume replacement, the patient is protected against hypotension, hypertension, and myocardial necrosis. Pharmacologic cardioplegia (heart arrest) is achieved by administering intravenous potassium, magnesium, and procaine, along with other stabilizing agents. Cross-clamping of the aorta is often needed as well, especially with valve repair or replacement procedures. Topical cooling with ice ("slush") is a useful adjunct, especially in patients with hypertrophied ventricle. Distal graft perfusion with warm noncardioplegic flow after unclamping of the aorta warms the heart and washes out the cardioplegic solution. Intra-aortic balloon counterpulsation or ventricular assisted pumping is used on patients with severe left ventricular dysfunction.

Orthotopic Cardiac Transplantation ▪ Orthotopic cardiac transplantation is reserved for patients with end-stage congestive heart failure. Since the late 1980s, greater survival and reduced morbidity have resulted from safer cardiopulmonary bypass, improved myocardial preservation techniques, and prevention and treatment of cardiac rejection. Over 2000 pa-

---

*When dictating about congenital heart defects, cardiologists may refer to S,D,D and S,L,L transposition (note no spaces after the commas). The "S" in both instances refers to situs solitus. The second letter in each set refers to the way the heart loops, "D" representing the heart being on the right with the ventricle on the right and "L" representing the heart being on the left with the ventricle on the left. The third letter refers to the pulmonary arteries, "D" representing the pulmonary arteries being located on the right and "L" representing the pulmonary arteries being located on the left. This abbreviated format is used by physicians when describing the anatomy of transposition to another physician; it is readily understood by the doctors but often not by the transcriptionist.

tients received cardiac transplantation worldwide in 1987. Immunosuppressive therapeutic agents include cyclosporin-A, steroids, azathioprine, and OKT3. Combined heart and lung transplantation is offered in the presence of severe pulmonary and heart disease. The workup of these patients is extensive and includes not only the standard heart and lung function studies but also determinations of stool guaiac and creatinine clearance, blood and tissue typing, antileukocyte antibody screening, HIV antigen status, and viral antibody titers.

Cardiac Surgery for Infective Endocarditis ■ Cardiac surgery is used for infective endocarditis in cases of

- major embolism
- progressive heart failure
- heart block
- relapse of infection on therapy
- flail leaflet(s)
- large vegetations
- persistent bacteremia on therapy
- fungal endocarditis
- prosthetic valve dehiscence or obstruction
- new regurgitant murmur in aortic valve prosthetic endocarditis

False aneurysms and intramyocardial abscesses may occur in endocarditis. Intravenous antibiotic drugs that are used include cephalosporin agents, gentamicin, methicillin, penicillin, vancomycin, and others.

Heart Valve Surgery ■ Valve surgery procedure selection is based upon many factors and may involve a closed commissurotomy, open commissurotomy, reconstructive surgery, or valve replacement. Bioprostheses employed include those made from human tissue, such as homograft valves, or porcine valves preserved with glutaraldehyde. Pericardial tissue prostheses are used infrequently. The most common prosthetic valves utilized in recent years include:

- Björk-Shiley convexo-concave
- Björk-Shiley spherical
- Carpentier-Edwards
- Edwards-Duromedics
- Hancock's
- Ionescu-Shiley
- Lillehei-Kaster
- Omniscience
- St. Jude's medical
- Smeloff-Cutter
- Starr-Edwards

Relative freedom from thrombogenicity (clot-forming potential) is achieved with bioprosthetic valves, which result in a higher actuarial survival and more favorable hemodynamics when compared with the alternative prosthetic valves.

Some valve and coronary bypass procedures are done with hypothermia and potassium cardioplegia for myocardial preservation, whereas others are performed with hypothermic fibrillatory arrest.

Aneurysmectomy or aneurysmorrhaphy is used for large ventricular aneurysms that cause congestive heart failure or severe ventricular arrhythmias. Pericardial constriction and tamponade may require resection, and recurrent tamponade may justify surgical "window" drainage after an echocardiographically guided pericardiocentesis or ECG-guided drainage has failed.

FORMATS

History and Physical ■ The cardiologist's history and physical examination report includes the following (Figure 12–14):

- Reason for admission
- History of present illness
- Past medical history
- Review of systems
- Physical examination
- Diagnosis
- Discussion

Record of Operation ■ The record of operation (Figure 12–15) includes the following information:

- Patient information
- Name of anesthesiologist
- Date of operation
- Preoperative diagnosis
- Postoperative diagnosis

Text continued on page 178

UNIVERSITY HOSPITAL
1234 Main Street
Oxnard, CA 93030-0000

HISTORY AND PHYSICAL

NAME: FABER, PAUL   DOCTOR: J. JAMESON, M. D.

MR#: 0309677   ADMISSION DATE: 07/24/94

REASON FOR ADMISSION:
Abdominal pain, nausea, inability to take food orally, malaise and fatigue.

HISTORY OF PRESENT ILLNESS:
The patient is 81 years old, known to this hospital since 1990. He has a history
of coronary artery disease and has undergone CABG. He has impaired left
ventricular function, CHF and intractable atrial arrhythmias. He also has
moderate aortic stenosis with an aortic valve area of 1 cm squared at last
determination. His most recent admission here was for permanent pacemaker
implantation which was done by Dr. B. McClintock in September, 1990. The
patient was discharged on September 15, 1990, with a new dual chamber
pacemaker. This pacemaker was placed because of symptomatic bradycardia
while receiving amiodarone for control of refactory atrial arrhythmias.

The patient complains of inability to eat food. This has been going on since his
discharge from the hospital. He notes that everything he puts in his mouth tastes
sweet, causes some nausea with the sensation of wanting to vomit. Vomiting
does not occur; however, he cannot eat food. For the last day or two, he has had
some abdominal pain, which is described as a sensation of something sticking in
his lower chest and upper abdomen in the epigastric area. No chest pain.

PAST MEDICAL HISTORY:
CABG in 1990, performed because of angina. At that time, left ventricular
function was normal. Vein grafts were placed at the first diagonal, the LAD and
the second obtuse marginal branch of the circumflex, along with the
posterolateral branch of the distal right coronary artery. In April, 1990, the patient
was admitted to the hospital with shortness of breath, which was abrupt in onset,
with some associated chest discomfort. He was treated medically for CHF. At
that time, he was on flecainide for atrial arrhythmias. In June, 1990, the patient
was admitted with CHF, felt to be secondary to discontinuation of medications. In
October, 1990, the patient underwent TURP for benign prostatism. I have no
documentation of the tissue diagnosis, however. On October 16, 1990, the
patient was again admitted to the hospital with symptoms of shortness of breath
and atypical chest pain. Also noted was progressive deterioration in weight and
energy, which was felt to be secondary to left ventricular dysfunction. An
echocardiogram was performed and demonstrated poor left ventricular function
with global hypokinesis, of at least moderate degree; severe hypokinesis to

Figure 12–14
An example of a history and physical consultation report dictated by a cardiologist and typed in full block report format.

172

akinesis involving the anteroseptal and apical segments of the left ventricle and the apical segments of the inferior wall. The lower septum was also hypokinetic. The estimated ejection fraction was 20 to 25%. There was aortic sclerosis of moderate severity with a gradient of 28 mmHg and an aortic valve area of 1.0 cm squared by continuity calculation. There was aortic insufficiency which was thought to be mild and mitral regurgitation which was felt to be moderate. Mild tricuspid regurgitation was also felt to be present. The left ventricle was enlarged at 7.2 cm, and there was bi-atrial enlargement and right ventricular enlargement. On May 20, 1990, he was admitted to the hospital with diagnoses of ischemic cardiomyopathy, supraventricular tachycardia, aortic stenosis and CHF. Heart catheterization was performed, which was interpreted as ischemia and not felt to be the major problem. The patient's symptoms were secondary to left ventricular dysfunction. The resting heart rate at that time, during cardiac catheterization, was sinus tachycardia at 100 beats per minute, the systemic BP was 85 systolic/diastolic 48. Left ventricular systolic pressure was 140. His pulmonary artery pressure was elevated at 50 systolic/28 diastolic with a wedge pressure of 24 mmHg and a V wave of 40. The aortic valve area was 1.1 cm squared by Gorlin formula. The mitral valve area was 2.3 cm squared; the cardiac output by thermodilution technique was said to be 8 L/min. Coronary and vein graft angiography demonstrated severe three-vessel coronary disease with patent vein grafts to the right coronary artery, the obtuse marginal branch of the circumflex artery, and to the diagonal branch of the LAD artery.

Left ventriculography demonstrated an ejection fraction of approximately 33% by visual inspection. Severe mitral regurgitation was present. Interpretation of this study by Dr. D. Dornfeld was, as noted; 1) Triple-vessel coronary disease with patent vein grafts. 2) Severely depressed left ventricular systolic function with severe mitral regurgitation. 3) Moderately severe, but not critical, aortic stenosis. 4) Elevated left ventricular filling pressures consistent with CHF.

It was during this admission that the patient did develop significant problems with atrial tachycardias; the mechanism, apparently, was an automatic atrial arrhythmia or an intra-atrial reentrant tachycardia. Aberrant conduction to the ventricle caused some confusion with ventricular tachycardia, and the tachycardia was poorly tolerated hemodynamically. Conventional anti-arrhythmic drugs did not suppress the tachycardia. The patient was started on amiodarone. I am unsure of the date the medication was started.

As noted previously, the patient's most recent admission was for a pacemaker secondary to episodes of bradycardia caused by his heart disease in association with the amiodarone medication.
(continued)

Figure 12–14 *Continued*   *Figure continued*

FABER, PAUL
0309677
J. JAMESON, M. D.
07/24/94
H & P CONTINUED 3

REVIEW OF SYSTEMS:
As noted above. Otherwise, significant for some episodic dizziness without frank syncope. No palpitations. Shortness of breath is unchanged in severity from previous admissions and is not a major component of the patient's complaints. The patient does have abdominal distress, but has had normal bowel movements as of yesterday. There is no history of recent GI bleeding. No hematemesis or melena. No bright red blood per rectum. The abdomen was distended one or two days ago, but this has resolved. The patient does not have any history of recent jaundice or change in urine color. There is no history of recent cough. No chest pain is noted. The patient denies any change in peripheral edema. No weakness or numbness in the extremities. No visual disturbances. No paralysis. No seizures.

PHYSICAL EXAMINATION

GENERAL:
The patient is mildly cachectic, pleasant, awake, alert, oriented times four and cooperative.

VITAL SIGNS:
BP 92/60. P 90 paced rhythm. R 24 unlabored. T 95.3⁰.

SKIN:
Decreased skin turgor. No jaundice. No skin lesions.

NECK:
No evidence of JVD.

CHEST:
Clear to A&P.

CARDIAC:
Distant heart sounds. The PMI is diffuse. A 2/6 systolic murmur at the apex and a 2/6 systolic murmur at the base. No diastolic murmur is heard. No pericardial rub.

ABDOMEN:
Normoactive bowel sounds. Soft, nontender and not distended. Deep palpation causes no discomfort. Liver and spleen are not felt.

EXTREMITIES:
Good quality pulses. No clubbing or cyanosis. There is mild edema of the lower extremities.
(continued)

Figure 12–14 *Continued*

FABER, PAUL
0309677
J. JAMESON, M. D.
07/24/94
H & P CONTINUED 4

NEUROLOGIC:
Grossly normal.

RECTAL:
Mild diffuse prostatic enlargement is noted.

LABORATORY:
WBC 6.600, hgb 13.1, hct 38.8%, platelet count normal 146,000. Differential
within normal limits. Biochemical panel, amylase, chest x-ray, and ECG are all
pending at the time of this dictation.

DIAGNOSIS:
1. Coronary atherosclerotic heart disease.
2. Status post pacemaker.
3. Amiodarone toxicity.
4. Possible gastric malignancy.

DISCUSSION:
The patient has peculiar symptoms with unclear etiology at this time. The
gastrointestinal complaints and change in taste may be attributable to
amiodarone toxicity. His hemodynamic status at the present time does not
appear to be any different than previously recorded on recent admissions to the
hospital. The possibility of GI disease of an occult nature, specifically a
carcinoma, cannot be totally excluded at this time and the history of food sticking
in the esophagus is somewhat suggestive of this. Also to be considered are
biochemical abnormalities, specifically hypercalcemia, hypothyroidism, and
hyponatremia.

I feel the patient should be admitted to the hospital for observation. In addition to
the above noted tests which have been ordered, formal complete thyroid panel
will be obtained. I am also planning an upper GI barium study and the possibility
of an ultrasound of the liver to evaluate the patient's biliary and hepatic system.
Amiodarone will be withheld, in lieu of the patient's previous problems with
tachycardias. If amiodarone is the culprit in the patient's symptoms, catheter
ablation of the A-V node could be a consideration in attempts to control the
patient's previous rapid atrial tachycardias. A pacemaker is already in situ and is
not a contraindication to attempting this procedure, if indicated.

_____
JAMES JAMESON, M. D.

mtf

D&T 09/25/94

Figure 12-14 Continued

UNIVERSITY HOSPITAL
1234 Main Street
Oxnard, CA 93030-0000

RECORD OF OPERATION

NAME: DOBBS, CHARLES F.   SURGEON: B. CANTOLLONI, M. D.

MR#: 8902352

DATE: 1/20/94

cc: Dr. Davis, Dr. Jeffers, Dr. Kenneth McDaniels, Dr. Tim Savers

ASSISTANT: J. GOLDSTONE, M. D.

ANESTHESIOLOGIST: P. PEARL, M. D.

OPERATION BEGAN: 0745
OPERATION ENDED: 1340

PREOPERATIVE DIAGNOSIS: Aortic insufficiency.

POSTOPERATIVE DIAGNOSIS: Aortic insufficiency due to perforation of noncoronary leaflet.

OPERATION PERFORMED: Aortic valve replacement using a #24 aortic homograft from the American Red Cross donor #06-T-00718. EBO Rh 0 positive. Size #24 mm. Aortic valve allograft tissue identify number 05-T-0051672.

FINDINGS: Pericardium: Pericardium was normal. There were no adhesions. Ascending aorta: Ascending aorta was moderately dilated, although normal with normal orientation. Myocardium: The patient's myocardium showed evidence of biventricular enlargement. Valves: The patient's aortic valve was a typical tricuspid valve with vegetations present on the noncoronary leaflet with a perforation just about in the middle.

DESCRIPTION OF OPERATION: After good general anesthesia had been obtained, the patient was prepped and draped in the usual sterile manner. Mediastinotomy was performed. Thymus was split in the midline. Pericardium was opened and pericardial sutures were placed. The patient was then systemically heparinized and cannulated in the usual fashion, placed on cardiopulmonary bypass, and cooled to 30° C. A left ventricular vent was then placed in the right superior pulmonary vein, left atrial groove and also connected to the cardiopulmonary bypass unit.

(continued)

Figure 12–15

An example of an operative report for a patient with aortic insufficiency. It is typed in indented style format.

DOBBS, CHARLES F.
8902352
B. CANTOLLONI, M. D.
1/20/94
RECORD OF OPERATION CONTINUED 2

At 30°C, the aorta was cross clamped, the route opened in a hockey-stick incision, and then 1250 cc of blood cardioplegic solution infused into the right and left coronary ostia with good electromechanical standstill. The heart was then packed in ice after placement of an isolation pad posteriorly. Stay sutures were placed in the aorta of #4-0 Tevdek. The valve was debrided. The noncoronary leaflet was sent for cultures since that was the leaflet involved.

The patient's aortic annulus sized to a #25 St. Jude sizer, a #24 homograft was available and that was thawed per protocol according to the American Red Cross. It was then trimmed and then, using interrupted technique of #4-0 Prolene, one was placed below the left coronary ostia in the native aorta and then below the right coronary ostia in the native aorta and then halfway in between towards the noncoronary sinus. These were then placed through corresponding segments of the aortic homograft and then again, as noted, using the interrupted technique #4-0 Prolene sutures were placed entirely around the native aortic annulus and finally through the aortic annulus.

At the level of the left and right coronary commissures, the sutures were placed straight across at the level of the right and noncoronary commissure. They followed the annulus to avoid the conduction tissue. The valve was then seated and sutures were tied and cut. Cardioplegia was then reinfused into each coronary ostia every 10 minutes and the heart continued to be packed in ice. The valve was then scalloped. No. 4-0 Tevdeks with pledgets were placed on each commissural post. The posts were placed at normal anatomic position and retracted fully in order to suspend them adequately.

At that point, #4-0 Prolene sutures were placed through the top of the native commissure and then through the midpoint of the homograft commissure and tied. Then using running #4-0 Prolene sutures, starting at the left main, the scalloped native aorta was sutured to homografted aorta. At the level of each commissure, the running #4-0 Prolene was brought out through the native aorta and through a pledget which was then tied. The noncoronary commissure was closed using horizontal mattress suture of #3-0 Prolene followed by its over-and-over stitch and then bringing that above the level of the noncoronary commissure on the homograft.

The noncoronary commissure was run to complete the closure. The aorta was then closed in the usual fashion, as noted above. At that point, the aorta was unclamped and a #21 gauge needle was placed into the root and the patient was rewarmed. Removal of the vent from suction showed the valve to be completely competent. After adequate payback timing and rewarming and after de-entering

(continued)

Figure 12–15 Continued

Figure continued

DOBBS, CHARLES F.
8902352
B. CANTOLLONI, M. D.
1/20/94
RECORD OF OPERATION CONTINUED. 3

the heart, we came off bypass quickly with the head down and the carotids clamped and then went back on bypass again.

We then stayed on bypass for about 5 more minutes and then again came off bypass slowly. After coming off of bypass, epicardial echo Doppler was performed using colorflow which showed no evidence at all of aortic insufficiency. At that point, the patient was decannulated and Protamine was given. Temporary right ventricular and right atrial pacing wires were placed. A #4 Argyle chest tube was placed in the anterior mediastinum. Then after making sure adequate hemostasis had been obtained, the sternum was closed with wire, fascia with Dexon, subcutaneous tissue with Dexon, and skin with an automatic stapling device. The patient tolerated the procedure well and left the operating room in satisfactory condition.

BERNARD CANTOLLONI, M. D.

mtf
D&T 1/21/94

Figure 12–15 Continued

- Operation performed
- Procedure
- Findings
- Description of operation

Reference Sources

Baue, Arthur, et al. *Glenn's Thoracic and Cardiovascular Surgery,* 5th edition. Appleton and Lange, Norwalk, Connecticut, 1991.

Braunwald, Eugene. *Heart Disease,* 4th edition. W. B. Saunders Company, Philadelphia, 1992.

Hurst, J. Willis. *The Heart,* 6th edition. McGraw-Hill Book Company, New York, 1986.

For references of specific application to medical transcription, see Appendix 1.

Victoria A. Cirillo-Hyland, M.D.
Chalmers E. Cornelius, III, M.D.

CHAPTER
13

Dermatology

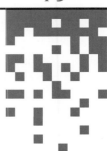

INTRODUCTION

A dermatologist is a doctor of medicine who subspecializes in the medical and surgical management of diseases of the skin. The successful practice of dermatology employs knowledge of pediatrics, internal medicine, allergy and immunology, endocrinology, and geriatrics.

After 4 years of college and 4 years of medical school, training for certification in dermatology requires 1 year of internal medicine training followed by 3 years of dermatology residency. To receive Board certification, one must pass the American Board of Dermatology examination at the completion of residency training. Two advanced fellowships in dermatology require an additional 1 to 2 years of training. The first, dermatopathology, involves extensive microscopic study of the skin. The second, dermatologic surgery, involves advanced training in skin surgery.

BASIC STRUCTURE AND FUNCTION OF THE SKIN

The skin is the largest organ of the body, weighing an average of 4 kilograms and covering an area of 2 square meters. It functions to protect us from the stresses of the surrounding environment.

The skin is composed of two layers, the epidermis and the dermis. The subcutaneous tissue, also referred to as the subcutis or panniculus, is located beneath the dermis.

The epidermis is primarily composed of cells called keratinocytes. It is divided into four layers:

- Basal layer
- Stratum spinosum
- Stratum granulosum
- Stratum corneum

The basal layer is composed of undifferentiated proliferating stem cells. Newly formed cells from this layer migrate upward and begin the process of differentiation.

The stratum spinosum lies above the basal layer and is composed of keratinocytes, also known as squamous cells. These cells produce keratin, which is a fibrous protein. This stratum spinosum derives its name from the "spines" or intercellular bridges that extend between cells.

The stratum granulosum, or granular layer, is composed of cells that contain keratohyaline granules, which are visible with light microscopy.

The stratum corneum is composed of large, flat, keratin-filled cells. They are vertically stacked in layers that range in thickness from 15 layers on most surfaces, to as many as 100 layers on the palms and soles (Figure 13–1).

In summary, the epidermis is composed of cells that divide in the basal layer, keratinize in the stratum spinosum and granular cell layers, and ultimately differentiate into "dead" cells in the stratum corneum. It takes approximately 4 weeks for migration of a cell from the basal layer to the stratum corneum, where it will be shed.

In addition to basal cells and keratinocytes, the following four cells are also located in the epidermis:

- Melanocyte
- Langerhans' cell

179

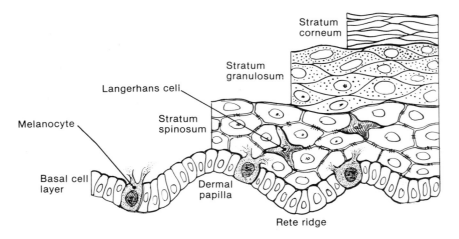

Figure 13–1
Stratum corneum. (From Lookingbill, Donald P. *Principles of Dermatology*. W. B. Saunders Co.,
Philadelphia, 1986, p. 3.)

▪ Indeterminate dendritic cell

▪ Merkel's cell

Melanocytes are pigment-producing cells with
long, squidlike extensions called dendrites. They
are located in the basal cell layer. The dendrites
facilitate the transfer of pigment granules, called
melanosomes, to neighboring keratinocytes. The
number of melanocytes in the epidermis is the
same regardless of race or color. The number
and size of the melanosomes account for racial differences in skin color. Sunlight stimulates
melanocytic activity and transfer of melanosomes.

Langerhans' cells are also dendritic cells that
have an immunologic function. They are located
between keratinocytes. On electron microscopy,
diagnostic tennis racket-shaped organelles,
called Birbeck's granules, can be seen.

Indeterminate dendritic cells lack melanosomes and Birbeck's granules. In some ways
they are similar to Langerhans' cells; however,
their exact function is unknown.

Merkel's cells are located directly above the
basement membrane. They probably enhance
touch sensation.

The junction between the epidermis and
dermis is referred to as the basement membrane
zone. It permits selective exchange of cells and
fluid between the epidermis and dermis. Furthermore, it provides structural support for the
epidermis and "glues" the epidermis to the
dermis.

The dermis contains blood vessels, nerves, and
cutaneous appendages. It is much thicker than
the epidermis. The principal components of the
dermis are collagen and elastic fibers and ground
substance, which are synthesized by dermal fibroblast cells. Collagen and elastic fibers are fibrous proteins that provide structural support to
the dermis. The ground substance fills the
spaces between fibers.

Beneath the dermis is the subcutaneous tissue. It is composed of fat cells or lipocytes, which
are separated by islands (septa) of collagen and
blood vessels.

The skin appendages include the eccrine and
apocrine sweat glands, hair follicles, sebaceous
glands, and nails.

Eccrine sweat glands help regulate body temperature by releasing sweat onto the surface of
the skin. The sweat evaporates, thereby facilitat-
ing the cooling process. There are 2 to 3 million
eccrine sweat glands on the body, which can
secrete 10 liters of sweat per day.

Apocrine sweat glands are responsible for
body odor. The odor results when bacteria act on
odorless apocrine sweat. Apocrine glands are
most numerous in the axillae (armpits) and anogenital region.

Hair follicles are located over the entire body
surface, with the exception of the palms and
soles. Similar to skin and nails, actively dividing
matrix cells differentiate and ultimately form a
keratinous structure, the hair shaft. Hair growth
is cyclic and is composed of three phases:

- Anagen (growing)
- Catagen (transition)
- Telogen (resting)

The length of the phases varies from one site to another. The hair follicles are attached to thin muscles called arrector pili. When they contract, they pull the hair straight up, thereby producing "goose bumps"!

Sebaceous glands form as an outgrowth from the upper portion of the hair follicle. Together they form the pilosebaceous unit. They are most abundant on the face and scalp and produce an oily substance called sebum. Their secretory activity is under the influence of androgens (male hormones).

Nails, similar to skin and hair, are made of keratin that is produced by a matrix of dividing and differentiating cells. The nail unit has four components:

- Proximal nail fold
- Matrix
- Nail bed
- Hyponychium

The proximal nail fold protects the matrix and forms the cuticle. The matrix produces the cells that will ultimately become the nail plate. The nail bed is the surface on which the nail plate lies. The pink color of the nail bed is due to blood vessels in the dermis. The hyponychium is located just beneath the distal free edge of the nail (Figure 13-2).

ILLUSTRATED GLOSSARY OF DERMATOLOGIC TERMS

See Figure 13-3.

REPRESENTATIVE DERMATOLOGIC DISEASES

Papulosquamous Disorders

The characteristic lesions are red, scaling macules, papules, or plaques

Psoriasis ■ Psoriasis is a common dermatologic disease affecting 1 to 2 per cent of the population. It is an inflammatory condition of unknown etiology in which increased proliferation of the epidermis results in excessive accumulation of abnormal stratum corneum, called scale. The average age of onset is 21 years.

Clinically, psoriasis is characterized by sharply demarcated, erythematous (red) papules and plaques with overlying silvery scales typically located on the knees, elbows, intergluteal cleft, and scalp. However, psoriasis can affect

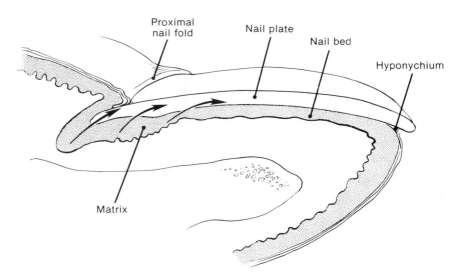

Figure 13–2
Hyponychium. (From Lookingbill, Donald P. *Principles of Dermatology*. W. B. Saunders Co., Philadelphia, 1986, p. 7.)

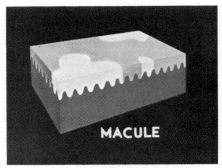

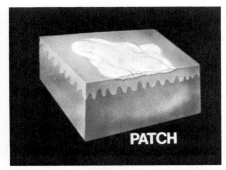

A. A flat skin lesion, recognizable by virtue of its color being different from that of the surrounding normal skin. The most common color changes are white (hypopigmented), brown (hyperpigmented), and red (erythematous and purpuric).

B. A macule with some surface change—either slight scale or fine wrinkling.

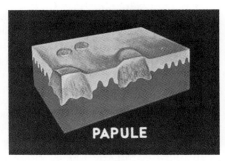

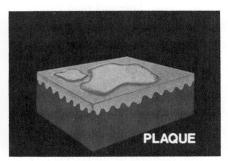

C. A small elevated skin lesion, less than 1 cm. in diameter.

D. An elevated, "plateau-like" lesion greater than 1 cm. in diameter but without substantial depth.

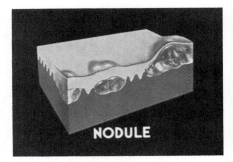

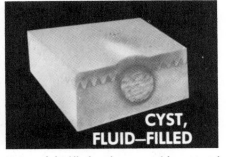

E. An elevated, "marble-like" lesion greater than 0.5 cm. in both width and depth.

F. A nodule filled with expressible material that is either liquid or semisolid.

Figure 13–3
Illustrated glossary of dermatologic terms. (From Lookingbill, Donald P. *Principles of Dermatology*. W. B. Saunders Co., Philadelphia, 1986.)

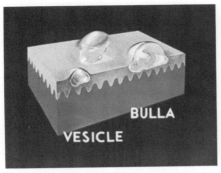

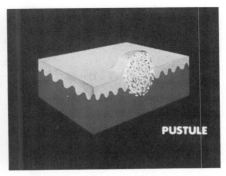

G. Blisters filled with clear fluid. Vesicles are less than, and bullae greater than, 1 cm. in diameter.

H. A vesicle filled with cloudy or purulent fluid.

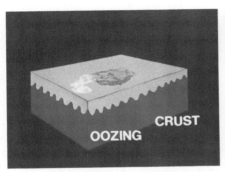

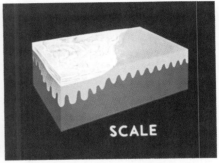

I. Liquid debris (e.g., serum or pus) that has dried on the surface of the skin. Most frequently crusts result from breakage of vesicles, pustules, or bullae.

J. Visibly thickened stratum corneum. Scales are dry and usually whitish in color. These features help distinguish scales from crusts, which are often moist and usually yellowish or brown.

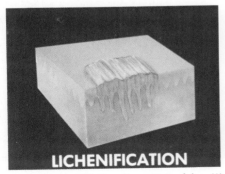

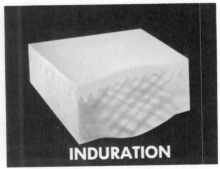

K. *Epidermal thickening* characterized by: (1) visible and palpable thickening of the skin with (2) accentuated skin markings.

L. *Dermal thickening* resulting in skin that *feels* thicker and firmer than normal.

Figure 13–3 Continued

Figure continued

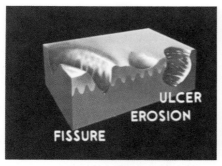

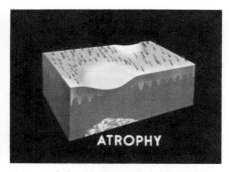

M. A fissure is a thin, linear tear in the epidermis. An erosion is wider but is limited in depth, being confined to the epidermis. An ulcer is a defect devoid of epidermis as well as part or all of the dermis.

N. Loss of skin tissue. With epidermal atrophy, the surface appears thin and wrinkled. Atrophy of the much thicker dermal layer results in a clinically detectable depression in the skin.

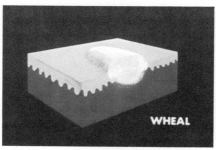

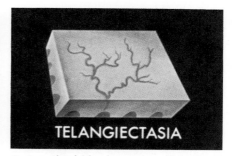

O. A papule or plaque of dermal edema. Wheals (or *hives*) often have central pallor and irregular borders.

P. Superficial blood vessels sufficiently enlarged as to be clinically visible.

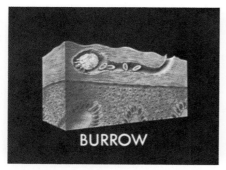

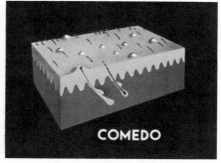

Q. Serpiginous tunnel or streak, caused by a burrowing organism.

R. Plural, *comedones*. The noninflammatory lesions of acne, which result from keratin impaction in the outlet of the pilosebaceous canal.

Figure 13–3 *Continued*

any body surface. In 10 per cent of cases it is associated with arthritis. The following nail abnormalities are frequently seen: pitting (small circular depressions in the nail plate), onycholysis (distal separation of the nail plate from the nail bed), discoloration of the nail bed, and subungual debris. Forty per cent of cases have a familial tendency. Psoriasis usually lasts a lifetime, with a tendency to flare in the winter and improve in the summer. Remissions of varying periods of time, however, occasionally occur.

The diagnosis is usually based on clinical appearance; a skin biopsy specimen provides confirmatory data.

Therapy consists of topical (external) and systemic (internal) medications. Topical steroids are the agents most commonly used to treat psoriasis. They have both antimitotic (inhibit cell division) and anti-inflammatory activity. Intralesional steroids can be used for localized disease. Topical tars and anthralin are hydrocarbons that also have antimitotic and anti-inflammatory properties. Ultraviolet light can be used alone or in conjunction with other modalities of treatment. It, too, has antimitotic and anti-inflammatory activity. Patients can be treated with natural sunlight or with artificially produced UVB light, a midrange sunbeam spectrum ultraviolet light. The combination of UVB and coal tar therapy is known as the Goeckerman regimen. Agents used to decrease the amount of scale include salicylic and lactic acid preparations.

Systemic therapy is reserved for those patients who have extensive skin involvement or incapacitating arthritis. Methotrexate is the most common and most effective antiproliferative drug used in psoriasis. Careful monitoring of blood studies is essential while using this potentially dangerous medication. Bone marrow suppression and liver toxicity are the major concerns. Intermittent liver biopsies are thus required. Etretinate (Tegison) is a vitamin A derivative reserved for treatment of pustular psoriasis and erythrodermic (total body involvement) psoriasis. Due to potential liver and lipid abnormalities, blood studies must be followed. PUVA is a combination of the photosensitizing medication psoralen (P) and long-wave ultraviolet A light (UVA). Unlike UVB light, UVA is not effective when used alone. Psoralen interferes with cell division when photoactivated by UVA light, thus slowing epidermal proliferation.

Seborrheic Dermatitis ▪ This is a chronic, scaling, erythematous, inflammatory eruption of unknown etiology. The hairy regions of the body, especially the scalp, eyebrows, ears, central face, chest, groin, and axillae are affected. Seborrheic dermatitis may present initially in the neonatal and prepubertal periods of life when sebaceous gland activity is increased.

Although the exact cause of seborrheic dermatitis is unknown, excessive epidermal proliferation and the overgrowth of normal yeast flora (*Pityrosporum*) have been described.

The diagnosis is a clinical one. Therapy consists of topical steroids, antifungals, tar preparations, and medicated shampoos. For unusually resistant cases, systemic tetracycline (antibiotic) can be used.

Lichen Planus ▪ Lichen planus is an idiopathic skin disorder characterized by severely itchy, flat-topped, purple polygonal papules with fine scales and white lines (Wickham's striae). The lesions are typically located over flexor surfaces (wrists, forearms, ankles), oral mucosa, genitalia, scalp, and nails. Most cases resolve after 6 to 18 months. However, some cases persist for years. Permanent scarring alopecia (loss of hair) as well as permanent destruction of the nails may occur. Ulcerative lesions in the mouth can degenerate into squamous cell cancer.

Drug-induced lichen planus has been described most often with thiazide diuretics. However, other drugs can also induce lichen planus.

The diagnosis is usually a clinical one; however, a skin biopsy specimen may be needed to diagnose lichen planus of the scalp and oral cavity.

The treatment of lichen planus is difficult. If drugs are possible inciting agents, they should be discontinued. Therapy consists of topical, intralesional, and systemic steroids. Empiric trials with vitamin A, dapsone, griseofulvin, UVB light, and PUVA have been described.

Pityriasis Rosea ▪ This acute, mild, self-limiting idiopathic skin disorder is characterized by oval erythematous macules, papules, and plaques with fine, "cigarette-paper"–thin scales peripherally. Pityriasis rosea begins with a solitary larger plaque called the herald patch. Lesions are characteristically located on the trunk and proximal extremities.

Since numerous cases occur in young adults in the spring and fall, pityriasis rosea is thought to be secondary to an as yet unidentified viral agent.

When pityriasis rosea is suspected, a serologic test for syphilis (RPR, VDRL) should always be performed, as secondary syphilis can closely mimic this disease.

Lesions usually spontaneously resolve in 6 to 8 weeks. However, topical and systemic steroids, sunlight, or UVB light may be used as needed.

Atopic Dermatitis ▪ This idiopathic skin disorder frequently occurs in patients with asthma, allergies, and hay fever. In the acute phase, it is characterized by erythematous weeping plaques. In the chronic phase, it is characterized by xerotic (dry), lichenified (exaggerated skin markings), scaling plaques.

The distribution of the lesions depends on the age of the patient. In infancy, involvement of the face and groin is most common. In early childhood, involvement of the flexor surfaces begins, and in adulthood the hands and feet are frequently affected. Severe itching is a constant feature of all stages.

Intermittent bacterial (*Staphylococcus aureus*, group A beta-hemolytic *Streptococcus*) and viral (molluscum contagiosum, warts, herpes simplex) infections are common.

No studies are diagnostic for atopic dermatitis. Thus, a detailed personal and family history of asthma, allergies, hay fever, and the location of the lesions is crucial in the evaluation of patients with atopic dermatitis. A skin biopsy specimen is not diagnostic but can be helpful in ruling out other papulosquamous disorders.

Treatment consists of "good skin care," topical and systemic steroids, and antihistamines. Good skin care includes infrequent bathing with a mild soap, frequent moisturization, and removal of irritants from the environment (stuffed animals, feather pillows). Food elimination diets can be tried empirically in an effort to eliminate triggering factors. Secondary infection with bacteria and viruses should be treated accordingly. Severe atopic dermatitis may require ultraviolet radiation (UVB light) treatment.

Vesiculobullous Disorders*

Vesiculobullous (blistering) disorders are characterized by the formation of vesicles (less than 1 cm in diameter) and bullae (more than 1 cm in diameter). When the lesions form in the basement membrane zone they are tense and more difficult to rupture than the flaccid lesions that form within the epidermis.

Pemphigus Vulgaris ▪ Pemphigus vulgaris is a chronic, autoimmune-mediated skin disorder characterized by the formation of blisters and erosions on the skin and mucous membranes. In its most severe form it can be life-threatening. The superficial blisters are flaccid and thus rupture easily. Large, denuded crusted erosions are typically seen. Nikolsky's sign refers to peripheral extension of the blister when pressure is applied to the roof of the lesion.

A skin biopsy is the definitive diagnostic procedure. The blister of pemphigus vulgaris occurs within the epidermis. There is loss of cohesion between keratinocytes, referred to as acantholysis. Direct and indirect immunofluorescence studies reveal deposition of immunoglobulins (IgG) and complement (C3) between the epidermal cells. The binding of immunoglobulin induces the release of mediators of inflammation which leads to acantholysis.

Systemic therapy consists of steroids, immunosuppressive agents (azathioprine, cyclophosphamide, gold, methotrexate), and antibiotics as needed for secondary infection. Local care includes soaks, topical steroids, and antibiotics as needed.

Bullous Pemphigoid ▪ This chronic, autoimmune-mediated skin disorder is characterized by subepidermal blisters. The groin, axillae, and flexure surfaces are frequently affected. Approximately 29 per cent of patients have oral involvement. The blisters are tense (form in basement membrane zone) and occur on erythematous or normal skin. They do not rupture as easily as pemphigus vulgaris blisters. Older lesions may be crusted and eroded.

A skin biopsy is the definitive diagnostic procedure. The blister of bullous pemphigoid occurs subepidermally. Direct and indirect immunofluorescence studies reveal deposition of a linear band of immunoglobulin (IgG) and/or complement (C3) along the basement membrane zone.

Systemic therapy consists of steroids, immun-

---

*Herpes simplex, herpes zoster, and varicella will be discussed with viral infections.

osuppressive agents, and antibiotics as needed for secondary infection. Local care includes soaks, topical antibiotics, and steroids as needed.

Dermatitis Herpetiformis ▪ This is a chronic, intensely itchy, blistering skin disorder characterized by grouped papules, vesicles, and hivelike plaques (urticaria) symmetrically distributed on the elbows, knees, upper back, and buttocks. Excoriations and erosions may be all that are seen secondary to frequent scratching. Patients have a hypersensitivity to dietary gluten (wheat protein).

A skin biopsy is diagnostic. Direct immunofluorescence studies of perilesional skin reveal deposition of immunoglobulin (IgA) in the upper dermis.

Systemic therapy consists of dapsone, sulfapyridine, and antihistamines. Dietary control with avoidance of all gluten-containing products can be most efficacious. Local care includes topical steroids.

Porphyria Cutanea Tarda ▪ The porphyrias are a group of diseases characterized by abnormalities in the synthesis of the protein heme, leading to excessive accumulations of various intermediate proteins. Porphyria cutanea tarda is the most common porphyria, and involvement is limited to the skin. It is characterized by vesicles, bullae, erosions, crusts, scars, and milia (small white papules) on sun-exposed skin, especially the dorsa of the hands. Excessive hair growth is noted on the temples and upper cheeks. Hyperpigmentation in sun-exposed areas is common. Porphyria cutanea tarda can be precipitated by alcohol, estrogen, high doses of antimalarials (chloroquine, hydroxychloroquine), and antiseizure medications (phenobarbital).

A skin biopsy reveals a subepidermal blister. A 24-hour urine collection shows elevated levels of uroporphyrins and coproporphyrins. The urine is dark brown and fluoresces red with Wood's light examination. Liver enzymes and iron levels are typically elevated.

Therapy consists of stopping any exacerbating factor and limiting sun exposure. Furthermore, weekly phlebotomy (blood draws) are usually performed until urine porphyrin levels fall to an acceptable level. Other therapies include treatment with antimalarial medications, which at low doses will cause porphyrins to be slowly released from the liver and subsequently excreted into the urine.

Allergic Contact Dermatitis ▪ This blistering skin disorder occurs from contact with a substance to which the patient has previously been sensitized. Common offending agents include poison ivy, nickel, and rubber chemicals. Initial exposure to the causative agent initiates an immunologic reaction, which on subsequent exposure culminates in the itchy skin eruption. Contrariwise, an irritant contact dermatitis requires no prior exposure to the substance as it is directly toxic to the skin (acids, alkalis). Allergic and irritant contact dermatitis lesions consist of erythematous papules, plaques, vesicles, and bullae. In the acute phase, the lesions are "weepy" and drain clear fluid. The geometric arrangements of the lesions typically have sharp cut-offs.

The diagnosis is usually based on clinical history and examination. A patch test (discussed in Dermatologic Diagnostic Procedures) can be performed if the offending agent is unknown once the acute event has resolved.

Therapy consists of removing the offending agent. Topical therapy includes soaks and steroids. Antihistamines help reduce the itching. Systemic steroids are indicated in severe cases of contact dermatitis.

Urticaria and Erythema

In urticaria, the characteristic lesion is a wheal, which is a papule or plaque of edema (swelling) in the dermis. Erythema is a red appearance of the skin, which occurs secondary to increased blood flow through superficially dilated blood vessels.

Urticaria (Hives) ▪ Urticaria is a common condition affecting approximately 20 per cent of the population at some point in their lives. Transient (lasting less than 24 hours) wheals of dermal edema develop in the skin. They may be red or pale compared with the surrounding skin. The size, shape, and location of the wheals can change rapidly. The etiologic agent is often not identified, and practically any physical (cold) or chemical (cat dander) agent may produce hives. However, the most common causes include drugs, infections, food, and emotional stress.

The diagnosis is a clinical one. A history of difficulty in breathing may alert one to the onset of anaphylactic shock (sudden onset of urticaria, respiratory distress, and decreased blood pressure).

Therapy consists of stopping any suspected agent. Most urticarial eruptions will resolve spontaneously without therapy. Cool water compresses, topical steroids, and antihistamines are used to provide symptomatic relief. Systemic steroids may be required for severe cases. Anaphylactic shock requires IMMEDIATE emergency attention.

Erythema Multiforme ▪ This acute, self-limiting, immunologic reaction pattern in the skin is characterized by the "target" or "iris" lesion. The most common offending agents are drugs and infection, especially recurrent herpes simplex. In many cases a cause is never identified. The eruption is characterized by symmetrically arranged erythematous papules and plaques, target lesions, and occasionally bullae. The target lesion has three zones of color:

▪ Dark red center or blister

▪ Pale zone around the center

▪ Red periphery around the pale zone.

Acute attacks will normally resolve in approximately 2 to 4 weeks.

Severe clinical variants of erythema multiforme include Stevens-Johnson syndrome and toxic epidermal necrolysis (TEN). Stevens-Johnson syndrome is characterized by mucous membrane lesions, severe blistering of the skin, and high fevers. This can be a life-threatening process lasting from 4 to 6 weeks. Toxic epidermal necrolysis is a rare, life-threatening dermatologic emergency. It may begin with areas of erythema but quickly progresses to bullae and sloughing of the skin. Toxic epidermal necrolysis is most commonly caused by drugs and is fatal in approximately 30 per cent of cases.

Mild erythema multiforme often requires no treatment as it spontaneously resolves. However, antihistamines, topical steroids, and systemic steroids are used as needed. The antiviral medication acyclovir is used to treat recurrent herpes simplex–induced erythema multiforme. Stevens-Johnson syndrome and toxic epidermal necrolysis require hospitalization for treatment and management.

Viral Exanthems ▪ Many viral infections are accompanied by urticaria and erythema. These exanthems are self-limiting and require only symptomatic therapy.

Bacterial Infections

Folliculitis, Furuncles, and Carbuncles ▪ Folliculitis is an inflammatory reaction that develops around hair follicles. It is caused by friction, drugs, and infection. The most common cause is a perifollicular infection with the bacterium *Staphylococcus aureus*. The lesions consist of erythematous papules and pustules. A furuncle (boil) is a large, tender, well-circumscribed perifollicular abscess. A carbuncle is composed of two or more confluent furuncles. Folliculitis, furuncles, and carbuncles begin in a hair follicle. Folliculitis is typically asymptomatic whereas furuncles and carbuncles are painful.

A bacterial Gram stain and culture of the pustular material will guide antibiotic selection. Therapy of localized lesions consists of antibacterial soaps, topical antibiotics, and topical steroids if the lesions are itchy. Systemic antibiotics are reserved for more severe cases of folliculitis, furuncles, and carbuncles. Furthermore, furuncles and carbuncles often need surgical incision and drainage to expedite their resolution.

Impetigo Contagiosa ▪ This common superficial infection of the skin is caused by the bacterium *Staphylococcus* or *Streptococcus*. It occurs more commonly in warm climates and most frequently in children. Bullous impetigo is caused by *Staphylococcus,* which produces subcorneal vesicles or bullae. The bullae rupture rapidly, leaving honey-colored crusts. Nonbullous impetigo is caused by *Streptococcus* and forms superficial pustules with surrounding erythema. They also rupture readily, leaving honey-colored crusts. Removal of the crusts reveals a superficial, shiny base. The face, neck, and extremities are the most common sites of involvement. The lesions are very contagious.

A bacterial culture is helpful in guiding antibiotic therapy. Treatment consists of antibacterial soaps and topical and systemic antibiotics.

Ecthyma ▪ Ecthyma is a deep streptococcal skin infection. An ulcer often develops with marked surrounding erythema. Ecthyma most commonly occurs on the lower extremities following an insect bite or other trauma to the skin. Treatment is similar to that for impetigo contagiosa.

Ecthyma gangrenosum is a severe skin infection with the bacterium *Pseudomonas aeruginosa*. The initial lesion consists of grouped vesicles surrounded by purple halos. The vesicles rapidly rupture, forming ulcers with black necrotic centers. They are usually located on the buttocks and extremities in gravely ill patients. Bacterial culture of the lesion and blood cultures will identify the causative organism. Therapy consists of intravenous antibiotics and acetic acid soaks.

Cellulitis and Erysipelas ▪ Cellulitis is an infection of skin that causes a warm, tender, mildly indurated plaque. The most common etiologic agents are the bacteria *Staphylococcus* and *Streptococcus*. The portal of entry is often a fissure in the skin or an insect bite. Cellulitis most frequently occurs on the lower extremities.

Erysipelas is a type of cellulitis caused by group A beta-hemolytic streptococcus. The involved area characteristically has an "orange peel" appearance (very indurated). Erysipelas is classically located on the face. Constitutional symptoms (fever, chills, fatigue) may be present.

If drainage is present, a bacterial Gram stain and culture should be done. Furthermore, blood cultures should be performed with febrile episodes.

Therapy consists of topical soaks and systemic antibiotics.

Staphylococcal Scalded Skin Syndrome ▪ This uncommon skin disorder is characterized by diffuse, painful erythema and superficial shedding of large sheets of skin. It occurs most frequently in neonates and young children. Staphylococcal scalded skin syndrome can be clinically indistinguishable from toxic epidermal necrolysis. The etiologic agent is *Staphylococcus,* which commonly infects the throat or eye conjunctiva. The *Staphylococcus* produces an exfoliative toxin that binds to the granular zone of the epidermis, causing the split. A bacterial culture of the skin, therefore, would not identify the organism.

One must distinguish staphylococcal scalded skin syndrome from toxic epidermal necrolysis. A frozen-section microscopic examination, as well as a skin biopsy, can distinguish between the two. In staphylococcal scalded skin syndrome the split is very superficial in the epidermis, whereas in toxic epidermal necrolysis the split is deeper in the epidermis (basement membrane zone).

Therapy consists of systemic antibiotics.

Toxic Shock Syndrome ▪ Toxic shock syndrome is an acute, febrile multisystem illness that causes a diffuse macular erythematous eruption. It is most commonly caused by a toxin producing staphylococcus bacteria, which has been isolated from the cervix in menstruating women. Therapy requires immediate hospitalization for intravenous antibiotics and further medical management.

Erythrasma ▪ Erythrasma is a superficial bacterial infection caused by the diphtheroid bacteria *Corynebacterium minutissimum*. It is characterized by sharply demarcated, brown, slightly scaling plaques in the axillae, groin, and fourth toe web spaces.

The Wood's light examination is diagnostic. It reveals coral red fluorescence, which results from the presence of porphyrin. The treatment of choice is topical or systemic erythromycin.

Intertrigo ▪ Intertrigo is a superficial inflammatory skin disorder that occurs where two skin surfaces oppose each other (beneath the breasts, groin). Friction, heat, and moisture in the affected fold favor the growth of bacteria, yeast, and fungi. The area becomes eroded and fissured, and patients complain of itching and burning. Intertrigo is commonly seen in warm climates and in obese patients.

Treatment is directed toward elimination of the friction and moisture. Topical antibiotics and antifungals are the major agents used to treat intertrigo.

Meningococcemia ▪ Meningococcal infection caused by the bacteria *Neisseria meningitidis* most frequently infects the upper respiratory system and is asymptomatic. Occasionally, infection of the upper respiratory system is followed by meningococcemia (bacteria spread to the blood) which may be acutely mild, acutely life-threatening, or chronic.

In the acute, mild form of meningococcemia, a maculopapular eruption is seen most commonly on the trunk and is associated with constitutional symptoms. On occasion, purpuric (nonblanching erythema since blood has leaked outside the blood vessel) lesions may be seen.

In the acute, life-threatening form of meningococcemia, a diffuse purpuric eruption occurs most prominently on the trunk and lower extremities. The lesions typically begin on the hands and feet. The mucous membranes and internal organs are also affected with the hemorrhagic process. It is abrupt in onset and fatal within hours. Emergency medical management is needed. Intravenous penicillin must be started IMMEDIATELY.

In the chronic form of meningococcemia, a macule, papule, or nodule with a central purpuric area may be present. The lesions are frequently seen on the trunk and extremities. Recurrent attacks (for weeks to months) with constitutional symptoms may last up to 3 days.

Bacterial Gram stain and culture of the nasal cavity, blood, and cerebrospinal fluid reveal the causative organism, *Neisseria meningitidis*. Bacterial Gram stain and culture of the skin lesions are usually negative.

The treatment of choice for all forms of meningococcemia is intravenous penicillin.

Gonococcemia ▪ Caused by the bacteria *Neisseria gonorrhea,* gonococcal infection is a sexually transmitted disease most commonly affecting the mucous membranes. Males typically have urethritis and females, cervicitis. However, the bacteria may spread via the blood (gonococcemia) to involve the skin and other organs. Painful hemorrhagic vesiculopustules occurring in crops of a few lesions are quite characteristic. They frequently occur on the joints of the hands and feet. These lesions occur 2 to 21 days after exposure.

Bacterial Gram stain and cultures from the blood, genitalia, rectum, and throat should be performed. The skin rarely yields the causative organisms.

Treatment consists of systemic penicillin. Hospitalization is required for gonococcemia.

Rocky Mountain Spotted Fever ▪ This fever is endemic to areas of North and South America where the tick vectors are found. The bacteria *Rickettsia rickettsii* invade blood vessels of the skin and internal organs, causing a true vasculitis (inflammation of blood vessels). The skin eruption begins as small, red macules that become purpuric as the disease progresses. They usually begin on the wrists and ankles and move centrally to the trunk and face and distally to the palms and soles. Constitutional symptoms precede the skin eruption by 3 to 7 days.

Direct immunofluorescence studies of a skin biopsy identify the causative organisms. Treatment involves removing all ticks, ideally within 2 hours of attachment. Systemic oral tetracycline or chloramphenicol is the drug of choice. Intravenous administration may be required for severe cases.

Lyme Disease ▪ The tickborne spirochete (bacteria) *Borrelia burgdorferi* is the causative agent in Lyme disease. It occurs primarily in the northeast, midwest, and western parts of the United States between June and August. Erythema chronicum migrans is the early skin manifestation of the disease. A later skin sequela of chronic infection is acrodermatitis chronica atrophicans. Erythema chronicum migrans begins with a small, red papule. Approximately 3 to 32 days after the tick bite, there is expansion of erythema around the papule.

Constitutional symptoms frequently accompany erythema chronicum migrans. If untreated, Lyme disease can permanently affect the cardiac, neurologic, and musculoskeletal systems.

A skin biopsy stained with a special silver stain reveals the causative organisms.

The treatment of choice for early Lyme disease is the oral antibiotic doxycycline. In advanced disease, intravenous therapy is required.

Acrodermatitis chronica atrophicans is characterized by diffuse blue/red, paper-thin skin on the extremities. It occurs almost exclusively in Europe and is believed to result as a late sequela of *Borrelia burgdorferi* infection.

Viral Infections

Herpes Simplex ▪ Herpes simplex is an acute, self-limited, usually recurrent, intraepidermal, vesicular eruption that is caused by infection with herpes simplex virus. The oral form, commonly known as "fever blisters," is most often caused by herpes simplex virus type 1 (HSV-1). The genital form is usually caused by herpes simplex type 2 (HSV-2). However, HSV-2 may cause oral lesions and HSV-1 may cause genital lesions secondary to oral-genital contact. The characteristic lesions are grouped vesicles on an erythematous base. The vesicles may have a central depression (umbilication).

Primary infection with herpes simplex is more severe and lasts longer than recurrent infections. Furthermore, constitutional symptoms accompany primary infections.

Recurrent attacks occur in the same location and are often preceded by localized burning, itching, or pain. Reactivation of the virus may be precipitated by fatigue, stress, fever, and sunlight exposure.

The diagnosis can be confirmed with a viral culture or Tzanck's preparation (defined in the section on diagnostic procedures), which reveals multinucleated giant cells, indicative of viral infection. Acyclovir is the drug of choice for herpes simplex infections.

Varicella ▪ Varicella (chickenpox) is an acute, highly contagious, itchy, intraepidermal, vesicular eruption caused by the varicella-zoster virus (a member of the herpes virus family). It is most commonly seen in childhood and is mild and self-limited. Infection typically occurs via respiratory droplets, although it can occur via contact with the skin lesions. The vesicle has been described classically as a "dewdrop on a rose petal." Lesions can be seen in all stages of evolution (papules, vesicles, crusts). They typically occur in crops over the trunk, face, scalp, and mucous membranes. Constitutional symptoms are always present. The disease is more severe in adults, and varicella pneumonia can be a fatal complication.

The diagnosis is usually a clinical one; however, confirmatory data can be obtained with a viral culture.

Treatment is directed toward symptomatic relief: cool soaks, antihistamines, and topical antibiotics as needed. Acyclovir, according to recent reports, can shorten the duration of the disease. In severe cases, intravenous acyclovir is needed.

Herpes Zoster ▪ Herpes zoster (shingles) is an intraepidermal, vesicular eruption resulting from reactivation of the varicella-zoster virus that has been dormant in the dorsal nerve root after varicella infection. A decrease in immune function probably has a role in the reactivation, as most cases occur in the elderly or in immunocompromised patients. The classic eruption of grouped vesicles on an erythematous base occurs in a dermatomal distribution (bandlike, following the anatomic pathway of the nerve). The outbreak is often preceded by itching, burning, pain, and tingling in the involved dermatome. A complication, postherpetic neuralgia, may occur in patients over the age of 50 years. Postherpetic neuralgia is defined as pain persisting at least 4 weeks after healing of the lesions and may be a debilitating long-term problem.

The diagnosis is usually a clinical one; however, confirmatory data can be obtained with a viral culture or Tzanck's preparation. Treatment includes topical soaks, antihistamines, analgesics, and oral acyclovir in uncomplicated cases. Intravenous acyclovir is needed for more severe disseminated disease. An ophthalmologist should be consulted if the eye is affected. Unfortunately, there are no consistently effective medications for the prevention of postherpetic neuralgia. When given early in the course of the eruption, systemic steroids can decrease the acute pain. Antidepressants, narcotics, intralesional steroids, and nerve blocks have been tried with varying success to treat postherpetic neuralgia.

Molluscum Contagiosum ▪ Molluscum contagiosum is caused by cutaneous infection with a pox virus. The lesions typically occur in children and are firm, dome-shaped papules with a central umbilication. A "cheesy" core can be expressed from them. They are typically located on the face, trunk, and extremities in children and on the genitalia in sexually active adults. They are spread via close physical contact.

The diagnosis is a clinical one; however, confirmatory data can be obtained by microscopic evaluation of the cheesy core. Characteristic molluscum bodies are seen.

Treatment consists of Retin-A cream, acetic acid, surgical curettage, or liquid nitrogen. Spontaneous resolution may also occur.

Measles ▪ Measles, caused by the measles virus, is characterized by a maculopapular (morbilliform) eruption, conjunctivitis, and an upper respiratory infection. It is primarily seen in children. Koplik's spots, white papules on an erythematous base on the buccal mucosa (cheek) near the upper molars, are pathognomonic for measles. The eruption usually begins on the scalp and face and progresses down to involve the trunk and extremities. Complications include otitis media (infection of the ear), pneumonia, and encephalomyelitis (inflammation of the brain and spinal cord).

The diagnosis is a clinical one; however, confirmatory measles antibody titers can be obtained. Treatment consists of supportive care with analgesics and bed rest. A routine measles vaccination is given at 15 months of age.

Rubella ▪ Rubella (German measles), caused by the rubella virus, is characterized by a pale pink maculopapular eruption (smaller lesions than in measles) and posterior cervical, suboccipital, and postauricular lymphadenopathy.

The diagnosis is a clinical one; however, confirmatory rubella antibody titers can be obtained. Treatment consists of supportive care. A vaccination is available and all women should receive one prior to becoming pregnant. Infants born to mothers who have had rubella during the first trimester of pregnancy may have fatal complications.

Verrucae ▪ Verrucae (warts) are intraepidermal lesions caused by local infection with the human papilloma virus. They can occur at any age but are frequently seen in children. The clinical appearance is often determined by the location site. The common wart, known as verrucae vulgaris, is a dome-shaped, flesh-colored, rough-surfaced papule. Black dots (occluded blood vessels) are seen on its surface. The usual sites of involvement are the hands and fingers. The filiform wart has finger-like projections and typically occurs on the face and neck. The flat wart is often subtle in appearance. It is flesh colored, slightly raised, and frequently located on the face and hands. The plantar wart occurs on the sole of the foot (plantar surface). It is usually covered by a thick callus. Condyloma accuminata are venereal warts and thus located on the genitalia or perianal area. They have a cauli-flower-like appearance.

Warts are usually not biopsied unless a diagnosis of squamous cell carcinoma is being considered.

Therapy consists of the following destructive modalities: surgical excision; liquid nitrogen; salicylic, lactic, and acetic acids; podophyllin (cytotoxic agent used for condyloma accuminata); electrodesiccation; canthardin (blistering agent); Retin-A; topical 5-fluorouracil (cytotoxic agent); and intralesional bleomycin (cytotoxic agent). Sensitization with DNCB (dinitrochlorobenzene) has also been used to initiate an immune response in patients with numerous warts.

Fungal and Yeast Infections

Dermatophytosis ▪ Dermatophyte infections, often referred to as "ringworm," are caused by a group of related fungi that invade the stratum corneum of the skin, nails, and hair. Inflammation of the deeper layers of skin is a secondary reaction to the fungal organism. All dermatophyte infections are contagious.

Tinea corporis (ringworm of the body) occurs on nonhair-bearing skin. The lesions are typically erythematous, ring-shaped, scaling plaques with central clearing and raised borders.

Tinea pedis (athlete's foot) is a dermatophyte infection of the feet. It can have the clinical appearances of

- Interdigital fissuring, maceration, and scaling
- Dry scaling hyperkeratosis of the soles
- Inflammatory vesicles and bullae.

Tinea manus is a dermatophyte infection of the hands. It occurs as a mildly erythematous, hyperkeratotic scaling eruption on the palms. Vesicular lesions on the palms may represent an id reaction, which is a secondary allergic reaction that results from a fungal infection elsewhere.

Tinea cruris ("jock itch") is a dermatophyte infection of the groin, most commonly seen in males. Chronic moisture and friction of two opposing skin surfaces predispose to this condition. A typical lesion consists of a scaly, erythematous plaque with an advancing border on the inner thigh.

Tinea capitis (ringworm of the scalp) is a highly contagious dermatophyte infection of hair. Scaly, erythematous areas with patchy hair loss are common. This is most frequently seen in children.

Tinea unguium (onychomycosis) is a dermatophyte infection of the nails. Flaky debris beneath the nail, discoloration, crumbling, and thickening of the nail are common.

A KOH examination (potassium hydroxide preparation — see diagnostic procedures later) of the scaling lesions reveals the diagnostic fungal hyphae. A fungal culture will identify the specific fungi positively.

Treatment of minor disease consists of topical antifungal medications. More severe cases, as well as tinea capitis and tinea unguium, require the systemic antifungal agent griseofulvin. Systemic steroids in conjunction with antifungal medication are recommended for extensive inflammatory cases.

Candida ▪ This yeastlike fungus usually produces a beefy red skin eruption surrounded by satellite pustules. Heat, moisture, diabetes, obesity, antibiotic therapy, and immunocompromised states promote its growth. *Candida* skin infections are most commonly seen in areas where two skin surfaces meet (groin, beneath the breasts, between the fingers). Oral candidiasis is referred to as thrush. Perleche, a common inflammatory eruption occurring at the corners of the mouth, is frequently infected with *Candida*. Paronychia, an inflammatory condition of the skin surrounding the nail, is caused by invading bacteria, fungi, and/or yeast.

A KOH examination reveals the diagnostic pseudohyphae of *Candida*. A fungal culture will identify the causative organism positively.

General therapeutic considerations include reducing moisture and friction in the involved areas. Topical therapy with antifungals and steroids will eliminate *Candida* and help reduce the secondary inflammation. In severe cases, systemic antifungal treatment may be required.

Tinea Versicolor ▪ Tinea versicolor is a common superficial fungal infection of the stratum corneum with the yeastlike fungus *Malassezia furfur*. Clinically, the lesions consist of fine, scaling patches that can be of varying color (versicolor), including white, pink, or tan. Tinea versicolor is exacerbated in warm weather and most frequently involves the chest and back.

A KOH examination reveals the diagnostic hyphae and spores ("spaghetti and meatballs") pattern of *Malassezia furfur*.

Treatment with topical antifungals is effective for most cases. However, extensive disease may require systemic antifungals.

Deep Mycoses ▪ Most of the deep or systemic fungal infections result from inhalation of dust particles contaminated with fungi. Secondary infection of the skin with nodules, abscesses, and ulcerations is common to all types of deep mycoses. Primary infection into the skin may occur with trauma (puncture wound).

The deep mycoses include

- Sporotrichosis
- Coccidioidomycosis
- Histoplasmosis
- North American and South American blastomycosis
- Chromoblastomycosis
- Mucormycosis
- Aspergillosis
- Cryptococcosis
- Actinomycosis
- Nocardiosis
- Mycetoma
- Rhinosporidiosis
- Alternariosis

Identification of the causative agent can be made via special stains and fungal culture of a skin biopsy. Therapy consists of appropriate systemic antifungal medications. Surgical excision of involved areas may also be needed.

Venereal Infections

Herpes simplex has already been discussed (see p. 190).

Syphilis ▪ Syphilis is an infectious venereal disease caused by the spirochete *Treponema pallidum*. The primary stage is characterized by a painless chancre (ulcer) at the site of infection. The secondary stage consists of a papulosquamous eruption of red/brown scaling macules and papules, lymphadenopathy, flesh-colored mucous patches in the oral cavity, and flesh-colored moist papules, condyloma lata, in the anogenital region. The tertiary stage is characterized by nodular ulcers (gummas). Approximately 33 per cent of untreated syphilis cases will develop complications of the neurologic and cardiovascular systems.

The diagnosis of primary syphilis can be made with dark field microscopic examination of fluid obtained from the base of the chancre. Within several weeks of infection, blood studies (rapid plasma reagin [RPR], Venereal Disease Research Laboratory [VDRL], fluorescent treponemal antibody-absorption test [FTA-ABS], micro-hemagglutination–*Treponema pallidum* [MHA-TP]) will reveal results consistent with infection. A skin biopsy prepared with silver stain will identify the causative organism, *Treponema pallidum*.

Therapy varies according to the stage of the disease. Systemic penicillin is the treatment of choice for syphilis.

Chancroid ▪ Chancroid is an infectious venereal disease caused by the bacterium *Haemophilus ducreyi*. The disease is more common in males. The chancre begins as a papule, which becomes a pustule and ultimately a painful ulcer. Without treatment, approximately 30 to 50 per cent of patients develop painful lymphadenopathy (buboes) that may drain pus.

The diagnosis is a clinical one. A smear of the fluid from an ulcer or draining lymph node may reveal the causative organism. A bacterial culture may also identify the organism.

Therapy consists of topical care with soaks

and antibiotics as needed for secondary infection. Oral erythromycin and Bactrim are the drugs of choice for treatment of chancroid.

Lymphogranuloma Venereum ▪ This infectious venereal disease is caused by *Chlamydia trachomatis,* an intracellular obligatory parasite. The primary stage lesion is a painless papule, vesicle, or ulcer that often goes unnoticed since it resolves rapidly. The second stage consists of constitutional symptoms and lymphadenopathy (groove sign), which may drain pus. The tertiary stage develops in untreated patients and is characterized by the formation of strictures, fistulas, and abscesses in the anorectal region.

The diagnosis is a clinical one. However, specific confirmatory laboratory studies include the lymphogranuloma venereum complement fixation test (LGV-CF), enzyme-linked immunosorbent assay (ELISA), and direct immunofluorescence. A culture of exudate may also identify the causative organism.

Treatment with the oral antibiotics tetracycline, erythromycin, sulfamethoxazole, and doxycycline is effective. Suppurative nodes should be drained via needle aspiration.

Granuloma Inguinale ▪ This is a mildly contagious, chronic granulomatous disease that involves the groin and genital and perineal areas. The causative organism is the bacterium *Calymmatobacterium granulomatis.* The initial painless lesion is a beefy red, soft papule that subsequently forms an ulcer. Multiple lesions combine to form large plaques with pebble-like bases. Subcutaneous nodules form in the groin (pseudobuboes).

The diagnosis is a clinical one. However, confirmatory studies include microscopic examination of a touch preparation from an ulcer or biopsy, which reveals the diagnostic Donovan's bodies.

Treatment with the oral antibiotics tetracycline, doxycycline, or Bactrim is recommended.

Pediculosis Pubis ▪ Pubic lice, *Phthirus pubis,* are commonly transmitted via sexual contact. Female lice lay approximately eight to twelve eggs per day. Clinical lesions consist of red papules and numerous excoriations (scratch marks). Pubic lice infest the hair in the genital area and may migrate to the lower abdomen, thighs, chest, and occasionally the axillae, eyelashes, and eyebrows. Patients typically complain of itching.

The diagnosis is made by physical examination and microscopic evaluation of an involved hair, which reveals eggs (nits) firmly attached to the shaft.

Treatment with Kwell shampoo or Nix rinse is recommended. Topical steroids and antihistamines will reduce the itching and inflammation. White petrolatum is used to treat eyelash involvement. Recently worn clothes, sheets, and towels should be laundered.

Collagen Vascular Disease

The collagen vascular diseases are a group of poorly understood autoimmune disorders that often involve the skin.

Discoid Lupus Erythematosus ▪ This form of lupus erythematosus is characterized by chronic skin lesions, which consist of five characteristic features: (1) atrophy, (2) telangiectasias, (3) erythema, (4) scaling, and (5) follicular plugging. The face, ears, neck, and scalp are most frequently involved. Approximately 5 per cent of cases will progress to systemic lupus.

Systemic lupus is a multisystem inflammatory disease most commonly affecting young to middle-aged women. The diagnosis is based on the American Rheumatism Association criteria. The most characteristic cutaneous lesion is the "butterfly" rash, which is an erythematous plaque extending from one cheek across the nose to the other cheek. Other skin findings include a generalized maculopapular eruption, discoid lupus–type lesions, purpuric papules, bullae, ulcers, scarring alopecia, and palmar telangiectasias ("lupus palms"). Signs and symptoms involving any organ system can also be seen in systemic lupus.

Subacute cutaneous lupus consists of photosensitivity and erythematous scaling lesions in sun-exposed areas. The cutaneous lesions have a psoriasiform or annular appearance. They are most commonly seen on the face, neck, shoulders, and extensor surfaces of the arms. Constitutional symptoms are usually present.

Establishing a diagnosis of discoid, subacute, and systemic lupus can be difficult. A thorough clinical history and physical examination are needed. A skin biopsy can also be helpful. Specialized studies include blood antibody assays (ANA, antinuclear antibody) and immunofluorescence testing (lupus band test). Routine screening blood studies, urinalysis, and chest x-ray film should be obtained if systemic lupus is suspected.

Treatment ■ Discoid lupus: Sunblock, topical and intralesional steroids, camouflage cosmetics, and antimalarial medications. Subacute cutaneous lupus: Sunblock, antimalarial medications, nonsteroidal anti-inflammatory drugs, and systemic steroids. Systemic lupus: Strict avoidance of sun and sunblock, antimalarial medications, systemic steroids, and immunosuppressive agents. Bullous lupus: Dapsone.

Dermatomyositis ■ This is an inflammatory disorder primarily affecting the skin and muscles. The disease is more common in women. The skin lesions consist of inflammatory, erythematous, flat-topped papules on the knuckles and fingers (Gottron's papules), periorbital swelling and redness (heliotrope), diffuse erythema, telangiectasias, and atrophy. Weakness of the shoulder and pelvic muscles is characteristic, and patients will have difficulty combing their hair and climbing stairs.

The diagnosis involves a thorough clinical history and physical examination. Other helpful diagnostic studies include blood muscle enzyme levels, electromyography, muscle biopsy, and skin biopsy.

Therapy consists of systemic steroids, immunosuppressive agents, and antimalarials.

Scleroderma ■ This multisystem disease causes the skin to become hard, atrophic, smooth, and ivory-colored (hidebound skin). The disease is more common in middle-aged women. Sclerodactyly (tapering of the fingers) is a common finding, which may ultimately lead to clawlike hands. Findings secondary to sclerosis include a small, pursed mouth and a beaklike nose. Abnormalities in pigmentation, telangiectasias, ulcers, and calcification of the skin may also be seen. Morphea is a localized form of scleroderma that is limited to the skin.

The diagnosis involves a thorough clinical history and physical examination. Other helpful diagnostic studies include blood antibody levels, skin biopsy, x-ray films, pulmonary function tests, and esophageal pressure measurements.

Therapy for systemic scleroderma is difficult, and D-penicillamine is the drug of choice.

Rheumatoid Arthritis ■ This is a multisystem disorder primarily affecting the joints. In-

volvement of the skin may occur; it consists of rheumatoid nodules over bony prominences, purpuric lesions, and lower extremity ulcers.

The diagnosis involves a thorough clinical history and physical examination. Other helpful diagnostic studies include blood rheumatoid factor antibody levels, antinuclear antibody levels, and skin biopsy.

Treatment of rheumatoid nodules is not recommended as it may precipitate ulceration. The vasculitic lesions are treated with systemic steroids and antimalarials.

Acne and Acneiform Dermatoses

Acne ■ Acne is a common disorder affecting the pilosebaceous unit. It occurs most frequently in adolescents but can occur at any age. Acne can be quite mild or can be grossly disfiguring. The lesions consist of open comedones ("blackheads"), closed comedones ("whiteheads"), or inflamed papules, pustules, nodules, and cysts. The face, chest, neck, and back are most commonly involved. Scarring is a frequent complication of inflammatory lesions. The exact etiology of acne is unknown; however, excessive production of sebum by the sebaceous glands, abnormal shedding of cells that line the hair follicles, and the bacteria *Propionibacterium acnes* have been identified as contributing pathogenic factors.

Clinical examination is diagnostic. Treatment consists of topical medications for mild acne. These include Retin-A, benzoyl peroxide, and antibiotics. For more severe disease, systemic antibiotics are the mainstay of therapy. For the most severe form, nodulocystic acne, Accutane, estrogens, and systemic steroids may be used.

Rosacea ■ Rosacea is a chronic inflammatory eruption of unknown etiology primarily affecting the central face. It is characterized by erythema, papules, pustules, telangiectasias, and enlargement of the sebaceous glands. Rhinophyma (pronounced thickening of the nose with sebaceous gland enlargement) may occur. The lack of comedones helps distinguish rosacea from acne.

Treatment consists of topical and systemic antibiotics. Surgical revision of rhinophyma may also be performed.

Acne Keloidalis ■ Acne keloidalis is an acneiform eruption in which inflammation and secondary bacterial infection in a pilosebaceous unit lead to scarring and keloid formation. Acne keloidalis nuchae (back of neck) is commonly seen in black men whose curly hair induces a chronic folliculitis as it re-enters the skin (ingrown hairs).

Treatment consists of topical and systemic antibiotics as needed for secondary infection. Topical and intralesional steroids are the mainstay of therapy for the keloid component.

Hidradenitis Suppurativa ▪ This chronic inflammatory nodulocystic disease of unknown etiology involves the apocrine areas of the skin (axillae, groin, perianal). It begins with painful inflamed pustules and cystic lesions that rupture and coalesce to form sinus tracts.

The diagnosis is a clinical one. Bacterial cultures of draining lesions can help guide antibiotic therapy.

Therapy consists of systemic antibiotics, intralesional steroids, surgical therapy, and Accutane.

Benign Epidermal, Dermal, and Subcutaneous Growths

Milia ▪ Milia are small, white, keratinous cysts that occur primarily on the face, especially under the eyes. They may also develop in early scars. They are thought to occur as a result of occlusion of the pilosebaceous unit.

Treatment includes incision and expression of the material with electrodesiccation of the cyst wall, and Retin-A.

Skin Tags ▪ Skin tags (papillomas, acrochordons) are small, flesh-colored to dark brown papules most frequently seen in middle age. There is a familial tendency, and they typically occur on the neck, axillae, groin, and eyelids.

Skin tags can be removed by scissor excision, electrodesiccation, or cryosurgery.

Neurofibroma ▪ These are benign growths of the nerve sheath. They may occur as solitary lesions or as multiple lesions (von Recklinghausen's disease). A neurofibroma is a soft, white/pink lesion that will invaginate into the subcutaneous tissue with downward pressure ("button-hole response"). They can occur on any skin surface.

A skin biopsy may be needed to confirm the diagnosis. Treatment is surgical excision.

Seborrheic Keratosis ▪ Seborrheic keratoses are benign, wart-like growths of the epidermis seen most commonly with advancing age. They are typically brown/black, well-circumscribed papules or plaques with a "pasted on" appearance. There is a predilection for the trunk, face, and inframammary area. The etiology of seborrheic keratosis is unknown, but a familial tendency is noted.

Therapy is not required; however, removal is often desired for cosmetic purposes. A curettage or cryosurgery is the preferred method of treatment.

Xanthomas ▪ These focal collections of lipid (fat)-laden cells frequently involve the dermis or tendons. They may be occult markers of underlying systemic disease (atherosclerosis). They appear as yellowish papules, plaques, and nodules.

The diagnosis can be confirmed with a skin biopsy.

Therapy consists of treating any underlying lipid abnormality, trichloroacetic acid applications, and surgical excision.

Lipomas ▪ Lipomas are benign growths of the subcutaneous fat. They are characteristically mobile, rubbery nodules that occur in the fourth and fifth decades of life. They are usually solitary lesions located on the thighs, buttocks, abdomen, trunk, forearms, and posterior neck.

A therapeutic excisional biopsy is diagnostic. Liposuction is also a treatment option.

Epidermal (Keratinous) Inclusion Cyst ▪ An epidermal inclusion cyst is a dermal cyst lined by the epidermis. It is typically a flesh-colored, mobile, firm nodule. A central opening may be evident, from which foul-smelling, cheesy material can be expressed. There is a predilection for the face, neck, upper chest, and back.

A therapeutic excisional biopsy is diagnostic. If a cyst has ruptured, systemic antibiotics and intralesional steroids can be used for several weeks prior to excision.

Pilar Cyst ▪ A pilar cyst (wen) is a dermal cyst that arises from the pilosebaceous structure and occurs most frequently on the scalp. Surgical excision is the treatment of choice.

Hypertrophic Scars and Keloids ▪ These result from excessive scar formation following cutaneous injury. Hypertrophic scars are limited to the area of injury whereas keloids outgrow the area of injury. Increased metabolic activity of the dermal fibroblast has been observed. Hypertrophic scars and keloids are firm, thickened, fibrous papules, nodules, and plaques. Hypertrophic scars typically occur on the jaw, chest, and shoulders. Keloids are commonly located on the ears, chin, shoulders, neck, back, and upper chest and occur more frequently in blacks.

The hypertrophic scar will usually resolve spontaneously. Intralesional steroids are the treatment of choice for keloids and can accelerate the resolution of hypertrophic scars. Surgical excision of keloids followed by intralesional steroids is also a treatment option.

Dermatofibroma ▪ A dermatofibroma (histiocytoma) is a benign, raised, firm nodule of focal dermal fibrosis. The overlying epidermis is often hyperpigmented and thickened. Application of lateral pressure will lead to dimple formation. They are more commonly seen on the legs of women. The etiology is unknown.

Treatment consists of surgical excision for diagnostic and cosmetic purposes. Cryosurgery is occasionally effective.

Cherry Angiomas ▪ Cherry angiomas are benign growths of capillaries. They are bright red, dome-shaped, small papules that typically occur on the arms and trunk with advancing age. The etiology is unknown.

Therapy is not necessary; however, electrodesiccation or laser ablation can be done for cosmetic purposes.

Premalignant and Malignant Tumors

Actinic Keratosis ▪ Actinic keratoses are very common premalignant growths of the epidermis caused by sunlight exposure. The lesions are typically rough, scaly erythematous macules or papules. They are most commonly located on sun-exposed areas of the body, including the face, neck, ears, and dorsal hands. The transition to squamous cell carcinoma occurs in less than 1 per cent per year per actinic keratosis.

The definitive diagnostic procedure is a skin biopsy.

Therapy consists of cryosurgery, curettage, dermabrasion, or chemical peels for extensive involvement; topical 5-fluorouracil inhibits DNA synthesis in lesional skin.

Squamous Cell Carcinoma ▪ These are malignant growths of keratinocytes. They are most frequently located on sun-exposed areas of the body with advancing age. Squamous cell carcinoma is locally invasive and has the potential to metastasize. Clinically, an indurated, scaling plaque, nodule, or ulceration is seen. Causes include sunlight, x-rays, and chemicals (arsenic, soot). Furthermore, a squamous cell carcinoma can occur in sites of chronic injury, such as a burn scar or ulcer.

A skin biopsy is required for definitive diagnosis.

Therapy will vary depending on tumor size and location. Curettage and electrodesiccation, surgical excision, cryosurgery, and radiation therapy are often performed. Mohs' surgery (described in the section on dermatologic surgery) is reserved for recurrent or large tumors, tumors with poorly defined margins, and those occurring at sites with high post-treatment recurrence rates (eyelid).

Basal Cell Carcinoma ▪ These are the most common form of skin cancer. They arise from the epidermal basal cells. They rarely metastasize but can be locally very destructive. Sunlight is the most frequent cause of basal cell carcinoma and thus sun-exposed parts of the body are usually affected. Clinically, pink pearly nodules or plaques, with a central umbilication or ulcer, rolled margins, and surface telangiectasias, are seen in many cases.

A skin biopsy is required for definitive diagnosis.

Treatment will vary, depending on tumor size and location. Therapeutic considerations are similar to those for squamous cell carcinoma.

Malignant Melanoma ▪ This is a cancerous growth of the epidermal melanocyte. Sunlight probably plays a role in its development. The incidence is rising rapidly. Four types of melanoma are recognized:

▪ Lentigo maligna (elderly patients with excessive sun damage)

▪ Superficial spreading (approximately 70 per cent of all melanomas)

- Acral lentiginous (most common in blacks, on the hands and feet)
- Nodular (progresses rapidly to metastatic disease)

The clinical hallmarks of melanoma consist of the "ABCDs": *a*symmetry of the lesion, *b*order irregularity, *c*olor variation (blue, black, white, red), and *d*iameter greater than a pencil eraser.

The diagnosis often can be made on clinical examination. However, a skin biopsy is needed for definitive diagnosis. A complete excisional biopsy is preferred for adequate prognostic staging of the disease.

Therapy varies according to thickness and the presence of metastasis. Complete surgical excision is the treatment of choice. Clinically enlarged lymph nodes should be excised and examined by a pathologist for evidence of metastasis. Unfortunately, available therapy for metastatic disease is not curative but may offer palliation.

Cutaneous T-Cell Lymphoma (CTCL) (Mycosis Fungoides) ▪ This uncommon lymphoma of the skin is caused by the malignant growth of T cells (type of white blood cell) in the dermis, which often migrate into the epidermis. The lesions vary from asymptomatic, erythematous, thin, scaling plaques in early disease to intensely itchy, indurated plaques, nodules, and ulcers in advanced disease. The typical distribution of early lesions includes the trunk, thighs, and buttocks. Sézary's syndrome is a systemic variant in which the abnormal T cells circulate in the blood and a generalized erythroderma is present.

A skin biopsy can be consistent with or diagnostic of CTCL. Thus, specialized studies, including T-cell subtyping and T-cell gene rearrangements, may provide further diagnostic information.

Treatment of disease limited to the skin consists of topical nitrogen mustard (toxic to the tumor), electron beam therapy, and PUVA. Photophoresis (see page 200) is recommended for more extensive disease.

Kaposi's Sarcoma ▪ Kaposi's sarcoma is a malignant tumor of endothelial cells (cells lining blood vessels). The clinical lesions consist of red/blue macules, papules, plaques, and nodules. Two types have been described: (1) a classic form, seen in elderly Mediterranean men, that progresses slowly and is characteristically local-

ized to the lower extremity, and (2) an AIDS-associated form that is often very extensive and fatal as vital organs are affected. The etiology is unknown.

The diagnosis is suggested by clinical appearance; however, a skin biopsy will be diagnostic.

Treatment is indicated in the classic form if the lesions are symptomatic. Unfortunately, no current form of therapy is very successful in treating the AIDS-associated form. Radiation therapy and chemotherapy are currently being used.

Ulcers

An ulcer is a lesion in which the epidermis and part of the dermis are lost. Although the gross appearance of various ulcers is similar, there are numerous specific causes. For all types of non-healing chronic ulcers, periodic biopsies should be performed to rule out underlying malignancy or infection.

Venous Stasis Ulcers ▪ These usually occur on the medial aspect of the lower leg, just above the medial malleolus (ankle). The surrounding skin characteristically reveals "stasis" changes: brownish discoloration, edema, mild scaling, and inflammation. Varicose (enlarged) veins may be present. It is the most common type of chronic ulceration affecting the leg.

Any condition that increases venous pressure —for example, prolonged recumbency, thrombophlebitis (inflammation of the vein), and pregnancy—can predispose to thrombosis (clotting) and ulceration.

Venous stasis ulcerations will heal within a few weeks if the predisposing condition can be eliminated. However, in most instances the predisposing condition is chronic. Therapeutic measures include leg elevation to improve the circulation, debridement of ulcers with soaks and whirlpool, topical antibiotics, specialized dressings, Unna paste boots (zinc oxide paste supportive boot), and topical benzoyl peroxide (antibacterial, antifungal, promotes development of granulation tissue). Skin grafts are reserved for very large ulcers or those that have failed to heal spontaneously after several months of therapy.

Ischemic Ulcers ▪ An ischemic (arterial) ulcer usually occurs just above the lateral malleolus (ankle) secondary to a compromise in the arterial blood supply. The ulcers are characteristically painful and well demarcated ("punched-out"). Predisposing conditions include arteriosclerosis, diabetes, high blood pressure, collagen vascular disease, and embolic phenomena (bacterial, cholesterol emboli).

The diagnosis requires a thorough clinical history and physical examination. Decreased skin temperature and hair growth on an involved extremity are common physical findings. Diagnostic studies include noninvasive Doppler ultrasound or, if needed, invasive arteriography (arterial dye study) to visualize the vessel.

Therapy consists of identifying and treating the underlying cause of arterial compromise. Local care is the same as that for venous stasis ulcers. Surgical correction may be required to restore adequate blood flow. Hyperbaric oxygen therapy is also used (see page 200). Skin grafting will be successful only if the underlying blood supply is restored.

Neuropathic Ulcers ■ These ulcers are anesthetic and occur in patients with neurologic disorders. Predisposing diseases include diabetes, polyneuropathy, syphilis, and leprosy. The ulcer results secondary to persistent trauma as the patient does not experience pain. The soles of the feet are most frequently affected.

Diagnosis requires a thorough clinical history and physical examination, with special attention to the neurologic system. An x-ray study of underlying bone to rule out osteomyelitis (infection of the bone) should be performed.

Therapy consists of identifying the underlying neurologic disorder. If not reversible, efforts should be directed at preventing further trauma by protective dressings and shoes. Topical care is the same as that mentioned for venous and arterial ulcers.

Decubitus Ulcers ■ A decubitus ulcer (bed sore) is seen in chronically ill patients who are confined to bed. The ulcer forms when continuous pressure interferes with the blood supply to the skin. Secondary infection is common and can lead to further deterioration of the ulcer. Osteomyelitis is a frequent complication. Clinically, it begins as an erythematous macule that rapidly ulcerates. The ulcer typically spreads beneath its skin borders, which is referred to as undermining. The most commonly affected sites include the heels and sacral area.

The goal of therapy is prevention. Frequent position changes and specialized dressings and mattresses are helpful. Topical care is the same as previously discussed for venous, arterial, and neuropathic ulcers.

Pyoderma Gangrenosum ■ This is an uncommon, recurrent ulcerative disorder. It is commonly associated with systemic diseases, such as ulcerative colitis, Crohn's disease, arthritis, paraproteinemia (abnormal immunoglobulin production), hepatitis, and malignancy. The etiology is unknown. Trauma is believed to play a role, as 30 per cent of patients develop pathergy (lesion develops at site of minor skin trauma). Clinically, the initial lesion is a tender, erythematous papule that evolves into a pustule and rapidly ulcerates. The ulcers are well demarcated, with irregular outlines. Elevated purple borders with surrounding erythema, undermining, and necrotic bases are very characteristic of pyoderma gangrenosum. The lower extremities are most commonly involved; however, any part of the body can be affected.

The diagnosis requires a thorough clinical history and physical examination. Bacterial and fungal cultures to rule out underlying infection, x-ray studies to rule out osteomyelitis, skin biopsy, and screening tests for underlying disease should be performed.

Local therapy consists of whirlpool baths, soaks, and topical antibiotics. Early lesions should be treated with intralesional steroids. For extensive disease, systemic steroids and immunosuppressive agents are used.

DERMATOLOGIC DIAGNOSTIC PROCEDURES

Potassium Hydroxide (KOH) Examination ■ A KOH examination is used to evaluate for a yeast or fungal infection. Scales are scraped from a lesion with a scalpel blade and are placed on a glass microscope slide. One to two drops of 15 per cent potassium hydroxide are placed on the slide, then covered with a coverslip. The KOH dissolves the proteins of cells, nails, and hair but has no affect on yeast or fungal elements. The slide is gently heated with a match, then evaluated microscopically for the presence of hyphae and spores, which are fungal and yeast elements.

Tzanck's Preparation ▪ This is used to evaluate for a viral skin infection. A fresh vesicle is unroofed with a scalpel blade, and the base of the lesion is scraped. The material is placed on a glass microscope slide, which is air-dried. The specimen is stained with Giemsa or Wright's stain and a drop of immersion oil is placed on the slide. The specimen is then microscopically evaluated for the presence of multinucleated giant cells, which are indicative of viral infection.

Patch Testing ▪ Patch testing is a useful tool for identifying responsible agents in patients with allergic contact dermatitis. Suspected materials obtained from a patch kit are applied to the skin under a patch for 48 hours. The patches are then removed and the sites are evaluated for positive reactions (redness, vesicle formation). A final reading of the sites is performed at 96 hours.

Wood's Light Examination ▪ A Wood's light is a long-wavelength ultraviolet black light. This examination is done in a dark room, and the lamp is held approximately 6 inches from the area to be examined. A positive test is noted when fluorescence is produced (coral-red in erythrasma secondary to *Corynebacterium minutissimum* infection).

DERMATOLOGIC SURGERY

Currettage ▪ A curet (also curette) is a round knife that can be used to remove a lesion for diagnostic or therapeutic purposes.

Shave Biopsy ▪ This is performed by using a scalpel or razor blade to shave a lesion off the skin. The depth of the biopsy is determined by the angle of the blade and amount of pressure applied.

Punch Biopsy ▪ A punch biopsy is performed by using a sharp, circular "cookie-cutter"–like tool to remove a cylindric piece of tissue. A suture may be used to close the round defect in the skin.

Elliptic Scalpel Excision ▪ This is performed by using a blade to excise a piece of tissue in the shape of an ellipse. Sutures are required to close the defect.

Mohs' Surgery ▪ In this specialized surgical technique, each horizontal section of tissue removed by a scalpel is immediately examined via frozen sections under the microscope to be sure the lesion is totally removed. Thus, at the time of operation the surgeon can be certain that all the lesion is removed.

Cryosurgery ▪ Cryosurgery involves the destruction of tissue by using liquid nitrogen (−196 degrees), which causes cell death through conversion of a cell's water into ice. Most of the destruction occurs during the thawing phase.

Electrosurgery ▪ This involves the destruction of tissue by using electric current.

Laser Surgery ▪ Laser (*l*ight *a*mplification by *s*timulated *e*mission of *r*adiation) is a means of destroying tissue. The heat generated following the light beam's absorption by various tissue components causes the damage.

DERMATOLOGIC MODALITIES OF TREATMENT

Ultraviolet Light ▪ The cheapest source of ultraviolet is the sun. However, artificial sources of light have been developed to treat several dermatologic conditions (psoriasis). Fluorescent bulbs that can emit ultraviolet radiation (UVB or UVA wavelengths of light) are placed in a light box. PUVA therapy involves administration of an oral photosensitizing medication called psoralen prior to UVA exposure.

Hyperbaric Oxygen ▪ In this therapy, the patient breathes 100 per cent oxygen at increased atmospheres of pressure in a specialized chamber. This procedure can increase the oxygen saturation of the blood, thereby aiding the healing of ulcers.

Radiation ▪ Radiation therapy utilizes ionizing radiation (short wavelengths) as a means of destroying tissue (tumors).

Photophoresis ▪ This specialized process is used to treat cutaneous T-cell lymphoma. Patients take the oral ultraviolet-enhancing medication psoralen. The patient's blood is withdrawn and delivered through a machine that emits UVA light and then returns the blood to the patient. The exact therapeutic mechanism of action of UVA light on the blood cells is unknown.

Text continued on page 206

BRYN MAWR HOSPITAL
130 South Bryn Mawr Avenue
Bryn Mawr, PA 19010-0000

HISTORY AND PHYSICAL

NAME: Shirley Blaine   DOCTOR: Chalmers E. Cornelius, M.D.

MEDICAL RECORD # 0388-556   ADMISSION DATE: 4/24/94

HISTORY: A 21-year-old female presents complaining of a very itchy rash
which developed approximately twelve hours after working in the garden. The
lesions first appeared on her hands and forearms but have continued to
spread to her legs, face and abdomen. She recalls having a similar episode as
a child. Current therapy consists of calamine lotion.

PAST MEDICAL HISTORY: Asthma.

MEDICATIONS: None.

ALLERGIES: Penicillin leads to hives.

PHYSICAL EXAMINATION: Numerous linear vesicles ranging from one to three
millimeters are scattered on the extremities, abdomen, and face. Periorbital
edema is noted.

ASSESSMENT AND PLAN: Allergic contact dermatitis most likely secondary to
poison ivy. Recommended a short tapering course of prednisone over two
weeks. Atarax 25 mg. every six hours as needed for itching. Temovate
ointment to involved areas twice a day for two weeks.

_____
CHALMERS E. CORNELIUS, M.D.

CEC:ssb
D: 4/25/94
T: 4/26/94

Figure 13–4
An example of a history and physical examination.

BRYN MAWR HOSPITAL
130 South Bryn Mawr Avenue
Bryn Mawr, PA 19010-0000

OPERATIVE REPORT

PATIENT: Sally Brownley   DATE: 2/3/94
SURGEON: Chalmers E. Cornelius, M.D.   RECORD # 29876-02
ASSISTANT SURGEON: James Black, M.D.
CIRCULATOR: Elizabeth Ebert, R.N.

PREOPERATIVE DIAGNOSIS: Basal cell carcinoma on left cheek.

POSTOPERATIVE DIAGNOSIS: Same.

OPERATION: Removal of tumor, left cheek.

CONSENT: Written consent was obtained by Drs.
                               Smith and White.

PROCEDURE: The left cheek was prepped and draped in a sterile fashion. A total of 10 ccs. of Lidocaine 1% with epinephrine was injected into the left cheek. Once anesthesia was obtained, a 3 x 1 cm. elliptical incision was made. The tumor was removed. Electrocautery was used for hemostasis. Three 5-0 vicryl subcutaneous sutures were placed. Three 6-0 ethilon vertical mattress sutures were placed to close the primary defect. The patient tolerated the procedure well.

INSTRUCTIONS: The patient was instructed to cleanse the area twice a day with hydrogen peroxide followed by Polysporin ointment. She was shown how to place a Telfa dressing over the surgery site.

FOLLOW-UP: The patient will return in five days for suture removal.

_____
CHALMERS E. CORNELIUS, M.D.

CEC:ssb
D: 2/4/94
T: 2/4/94

Figure 13-5
An operative report on the removal of a basal cell carcinoma of the left cheek.

BRYN MAWR HOSPITAL
130 South Bryn Mawr Avenue
Bryn Mawr, PA 19010-0000

CONSULTATION

NAME: Sharon Crooks   MEDICAL RECORD # 36598
CONSULTANT: V. A. Cirillo-Hyland, M.D.   DATE: 6/3/94
ATTENDING PHYSICIAN: John Drake, M.D.

REASON FOR CONSULTATION: Please evaluate "rash" on back.

HISTORY: The patient is a 25-year-old white female who was admitted to the hospital on June 2, 1994 with relapsing Hodgkin's lymphoma for further chemotherapy. The patient noticed a painful, itchy "rash" which started on her back and spread around to her abdomen within a day. She had varicella as a child.

PHYSICAL EXAMINATION: Temperature, 101 degrees. There are grouped vesicles, ranging in size from 2 mm. to 6 mm. in a T10 dermatomal distribution on an erythematous base.

LABORATORY DATA: A Tzanck preparation was performed and revealed multinucleated giant cells.

DIAGNOSIS: Herpes Zoster.

PLAN: The plan is to begin intravenous acyclovir on this immunocompromised patient for 10 to 14 days. I will also use Atarax 25 mg. every six hours as needed for itching, the topical antibiotic Bactroban to prevent secondary infection, and warm saline soaks every shift for 20 minutes.

Thank you for the courtesy of this consultation.

_____
                    VICTORIA A. CIRILLO-HYLAND, M.D.

VAC:ssb
D: 6/4/94
T: 6/5/94

Figure 13-6
A consultation report for a patient with herpes zoster.

BRYN MAWR HOSPITAL
130 South Bryn Mawr Avenue
Bryn Mawr, PA 19010-0000

DISCHARGE SUMMARY

NAME: Jean Gordon

DOCTOR: Chalmers E. Cornelius, M.D.

MEDICAL RECORD # 336790

DATE OF ADMISSION: 1/11/94

DATE OF DISCHARGE: 1/16/94

DISCHARGE DIAGNOSIS: Cellulitis.

HISTORY OF PRESENT ILLNESS: The patient is a 40-year-old white female with no significant past medical history, who closed a car door on her left ankle three days prior to admission. Within twenty-four hours she noticed a zone of redness around the abrasion which continued to spread up her leg over the next day. The area was exquisitely tender to touch. She is currently treating the area with hydrogen peroxide twice a day.

PAST MEDICAL HISTORY: None.

MEDICATIONS: None.

ALLERGIES: None.

SOCIAL HISTORY: The patient works at the post office and is single.

PHYSICAL EXAMINATION: General: Well appearing middle aged female in no acute distress.

Vitals: BP=160/60, T=100, R=12.

Skin: Left lateral malleolus with 1 x 2 cm. ulceration surrounded by a 3 cm. erythematous, indurated tender plaque.

Nodes: No lymphadenopathy noted.

HEENT: Head: Normocephalic, atraumatic; Eyes: pupils equally round and react to light; Ears: Tympanic membranes with cone of light reflex; Nose: Without lesions; Throat Without lesions.

Neck: Supple, carotids 2+.

Back: No costovertebral angle tenderness.

(continued)

Figure 13–7
A discharge summary for a patient with cellulitis.

NAME: Jean Gordon   Page two
MEDICAL RECORD   #336790

        Lungs: Clear to auscultation.

        Cardiac: Regular rate and rhythm. No murmurs.

        Abdomen: Bowel sounds heard. No hepatosplenomegaly.

        Extremities: Pulses 2+ throughout. No cyanosis, clubbing
        or edema.

        Neurologic: Non-focal.

LABORATORY DATA: Notable for WBC 14.6 with 60% polys and 8% bands.

HOSPITAL COURSE: The patient was admitted to the Dermatology Service and received four days of intravenous Ancef. Her fever and WBC returned to normal. She received warm saline soaks twice per day.

DISCHARGE MEDICATIONS: Keflex 500 mg. q.i.d., topical Bactroban to ulceration twice a day.

FOLLOW-UP: The patient will see Dr. Jones in two weeks.

                                                                _____

                                                 CHALMERS E. CORNELIUS, M.D.

CEC:ssd
D: 1/16/94
T: 1/18/94

Figure 13–7 Continued

FORMATS

Samples of a dermatologic history and physical examination report, an operative report, a consultation report, and a discharge summary are presented in Figures 13–4, 13–5, 13–6, and 13–7.

Reference Sources

Arnold, Harry L., et al. *Andrews' Diseases of the Skin,* 8th edition. W. B. Saunders Company, Philadelphia, 1990.

Bondi, Edward E., et al. *Dermatology Diagnosis and Therapy.* Appleton & Lange, Norwalk, Connecticut, 1991.

Fisher, Alexander A. *Contact Dermatitis,* 3rd edition. Lea & Febiger, Philadelphia, 1986.

Fitzpatrick, Thomas B., et al. *Dermatology in General Medicine,* 3rd edition. McGraw-Hill, New York, 1987.

Habif, Thomas P. *Clinical Dermatology,* 2nd edition. C. V. Mosby, St. Louis, 1990.

Lever, Walter F., et al. *Histopathology of the Skin,* 7th edition. J. B. Lippincott, Philadelphia, 1990.

Lookingbill, Donald P., et al. *Principles of Dermatology.* W. B. Saunders Company, Philadelphia, 1986.

For references of specific application to medical transcription, see Appendix 1.

Ronald W. Stunz, M.D.

Emergency Medicine

INTRODUCTION

Emergency medicine was granted official status as a specialty field in 1979 and is practiced nationwide by over 23,000 physicians. The dictated chart in emergency medicine has been a relatively recent development, and in fact, many hospitals still rely on handwritten Emergency Department records. However, several factors contribute to the trend of increased reliance on transcribed records:

1. Pressure from insurance carriers to have a more complete and legible record from which to determine appropriate reimbursement.

2. Recognition on the part of the hospital risk-management officers that dictated records are inherently complete and thus more reliable as a medical-legal document.

3. Recognition by emergency physicians that, in addition to the convenience factor associated with dictated records, such records can enhance capture of billable procedures, facilitate quality assurance, and improve their risk management profile.

The American College of Emergency Physicians, in a 1985 resolution, gave its official support to "the provision by hospitals of services for dictation and immediate transcription of emergency patient records."

EMERGENCY MEDICINE TRANSCRIPTION

Although there is a body of knowledge, vast in scope and applied precisely within a narrow time frame, required for the practice of emergency medicine, there is little that is unique to the field. Emergency medicine is a specialty of breadth, involving the treatment of nearly the entire spectrum of medical problems. It has been said that a good emergency medicine specialist is one who is skilled in the management of the first 30 minutes of any medical problem imaginable. Thus, in committing to paper the record of a visit to the Emergency Department, the transcriptionist must draw upon the vocabulary, techniques, and procedures of nearly every branch of medicine.

The initial stabilization of patients with traumatic injuries ranks high on the necessary skill list of emergency physicians. In keeping with recommendations by the American College of Surgeons Committee on Trauma, many states have established trauma systems that mandate the transport of critically injured people to designated hospital emergency departments functioning as trauma centers. These specialized centers are characterized by enhanced levels of skilled staffing and specialized equipment and services designed to afford the patient with life-threatening traumatic injuries the best possible chance of survival.

Emergency medicine transcription carries a particular set of problems that the transcriptionist must be prepared for.

Turn-around Time of Transcribed Records ▪ The medical evaluation and treatment record of patients seen in the Emergency Department must be rapidly transcribed and available to other physicians and nurses who will subsequently care for the patient. This requirement is especially acute for patients admitted to the hospital. On average, 35 to 45 per cent of all patients admitted to hospitals are first seen in the Emergency Department. In many practices, admitted patients constitute between 10 and 20 per cent of overall patient volume. Ideally, the dictated and transcribed Emergency Department record should be completed and on the patient's hospital chart within 1 hour of dictation. In some cases, a "stat" transcription may be required within several minutes of dictation.

For nonadmitted patients, there is still a premium on rapid turn-around time for transcribed records, since a significant number of discharged patients will return for further treatment (or, in some institutions, for follow-up care) within days, or sometimes even hours of their initial visit. Availability of the previous record is essential to sound patient management.

Interrupted/Incomplete Dictation ▪ To understand why some of the dictations received by the transcriptionist are interrupted or incomplete, it is necessary to understand the mind-set and working environment of the emergency physician. It is not uncommon for the emergency physician to have ten or more active cases reverberating in the mind. In the space of several minutes, the emergency physician may have to communicate with three or four nurses and one or more private physicians, as well as patients and their families. Then, in the midst of this juggling act, a new and critically ill patient arrives by ambulance. An Emergency Department is not an island of tranquility, and some dictated records will reflect this fact. An interrupted dictation can be frustrating for the transcriptionist and the physician alike, and it may be necessary for the transcriptionist to leave a message reminding the physician where to resume dictating. Similarly, the physician may not include information that the experienced transcriptionist knows should be a part of the record; a written or phone message to this effect would be greatly appreciated by the busy physician.

Inconsistent Records ▪ For the aforementioned reasons, it is not uncommon for the physician to make mistakes within the body of the dictation. A common example of this would be the confusion of right and left in the record of a patient with an extremity injury. The physician may give a detailed description of injury to the left ankle, but when referring to the radiology report, dictates a report relating to the right ankle. Here, the transcriptionist can provide an invaluable service by making the physician

aware of this inconsistency. As another example, the physician may document a codeine allergy as part of the history and then prescribe codeine as part of the treatment. This may represent an honest mistake, or the patient's report of a codeine allergy may simply have been a statement of previously experienced side effects to the medication (a common circumstance). In either case, it is appropriate for the transcriptionist to make the physician aware of a potentially critical contradiction.

GENERAL CHARACTERISTICS OF THE EMERGENCY MEDICAL RECORD

Reliance on Physical Findings

More than most specialists, emergency physicians rely on physical findings to sustain their diagnosis. There are two principal reasons for this:

1. It is good medicine. Never do we learn so much about a patient as through careful history taking and a detailed attention to clinical findings.

2. It is often the only means available of gathering information in the shortest amount of time. In this regard, it is helpful for the transcriptionist to have access to a complete medical dictionary as well as a textbook of physical diagnosis. Emergency physicians often will refer to a finding using a proper name to indicate it — e.g., Rovsing's sign, Brudzinski's sign, Tinel's sign.

Limited Examinations ▪ Minor problems such as a finger laceration or a knee sprain will involve detailed examination of only the affected part. In these cases, details of past medical history, social history, and examination of other parts of the body will usually not be included unless they have some specific importance to the disposition or treatment of the patient.

PROCEDURES

Emergency medicine mandates the performance of a number of procedures. In extreme, life-threatening circumstances, several physicians may be performing procedures simultaneously on the same patient whereas the dictated note covering all these procedures may be completed only by the physician in charge. The physician usually will be quite specific about the material used (size of catheters, type of suture material), anesthetic agents, specific techniques, and the results of the intervention and how the patient tolerated it. Examples of common procedures in emergency medicine include wound closure, insertion of nasogastric tubes, catheterization of the bladder, placement of central venous catheters, endotracheal intubation, insertion of chest tubes, and placement of catheters for peritoneal lavage.

DOCUMENTATION OF PREHOSPITAL TREATMENT

Many patients arriving in the Emergency Department will have received care from prehospital transport personnel (emergency medical technicians [EMTs] or paramedics). Although most hospitals keep a separate log to document prehospital orders given by emergency physicians, the physician often will dictate details of care given prior to arrival of the patient. These orders may range from immobilization techniques (hard cervical collar; long spinal immobilization board), to establishing venous access, to specific medication orders.

INTERPRETATION OF ANCILLARY STUDIES

As part of the emergency evaluation of patients, the emergency physician may be obliged to interpret and dictate into the record the results of laboratory studies, x-ray films, and electrocardiograms (ECGs). For radiologic and electrocardiographic interpretation, the physician usually will note whether the reading is his own, or that of a radiologist or cardiologist. In the case of laboratory studies, the physician may dictate the specific numerical values of each test or simply state that it is within normal limits.

ACCURATE TIMING

The Joint Commission on Accreditation of Hospitals (JCAH) requires emergency physicians to keep an accurate account of the time of patient arrival, time seen by the physician, and time of discharge or transfer. These may be included in other portions of the patient record, but the physician may choose to dictate them into the record of the patient encounter.

DISCHARGE INSTRUCTIONS

In most hospitals, a copy of the written instructions given to the patient is usually included on the permanent chart, and the physician may not include specific discharge instructions in the dictation. On the other hand, the physician may wish to record in the dictation details of verbal instructions given to the patient that may not appear on the written instruction form.

REFERRALS/CHART COPIES

Most patients seen in Emergency Departments have private physicians who need to be kept informed of the nature and outcome of their patient's visit. Thus, the emergency physician often will request that a copy of the dictated record be forwarded to the private physician. Additionally, patients often will be referred for specialty care, either while still in the Emergency Department, or for follow-up as outpatients. These referral physicians also will require a copy of the emergency physician's findings. As with all patient records, confidentiality must be respected in handling and forwarding emergency medicine transcriptions.

EMERGENCY MEDICINE CHART

The accompanying charts represent several types of Emergency Department records (Figures 14–1 to 14–4). It is important to note that the amount of documentation increases proportionally to the complexity of the case.

THE IDEAL TRANSCRIPTION SERVICE

To be maximally effective, a transcription service for emergency medicine records should be

Text continued on page 218

BRYN MAWR HOSPITAL
130 South Bryn Mawr Avenue
Bryn Mawr, PA 19010-0000

PATIENT: Charles Cranston DATE: 06/07/94

MR # 17-67-23 DOB:: 09/28/35 ARRIVED: 0804 EXAMINED: 0840

CHIEF COMPLAINT: Lower abdominal pain.

HISTORY\HISTORY OF PRESENT ILLNESS: The patient is a 59-year-old white male who began experiencing left flank and left lower quadrant abdominal discomfort last night while attending a party. The patient stated that the pain did wax and wane and was associated with a full feeling in his lower abdomen. The patient did get some relief last night from the pain and was able to sleep for several hours but awakened with a similar discomfort early this morning. The patient has had some nausea but no vomiting. The patient has been urinating somewhat more frequently than usual but denies any urinary tract discomfort.

There is no prior history of any abdominal problems or kidney stones. He does have a past medical history of hypertension for which the patient takes Loniten and Tenormin.

PERSONAL PHYSICIAN:
ALLERGIES: No known allergies.
MEDICATIONS: Loniten and Tenormin.
TETANUS STATUS:

EXAMINATION: Vital signs: Temperature 98.8, pulse 72, respiratory rate 12, blood pressure 142/92. General appearance: The patient is a somewhat heavyset 59-year-old white male complaining of severe flank and abdominal pain.

PHYSICAL EXAMINATION:
HEENT: Normocephalic, atraumatic. Pupils equal, round, reactive to light. Extraocular movements are intact. Sclerae nonicteric. Mucosa pink. His throat is clear. His tongue is moist, mobile and midline.
NECK: Supple without nodes or masses. His carotids are full and there is no jugular venous distention.
LUNGS: Clear to auscultation. There is tenderness over the left costovertebral angle area to percussion.
HEART: Regular rhythm without murmur, gallop or rub.

Continued on page 2

Figure 14–1

An example of an Emergency Department record for a patient with lower abdominal pain who was admitted to the hospital with a diagnosis of renal colic with left ureteral calculus. This report is typed in the style used in the Emergency Department at Bryn Mawr Hospital, Bryn Mawr, Pennsylvania.

Page 2

ABDOMEN: Soft with minimal left lower quadrant tenderness without guarding, rebound or masses. There is no palpable hepatosplenomegaly and his bowel sounds are hypoactive.
GENITALIA: There is no testicular swelling or tenderness to palpation.
RECTAL: Examination was deferred.
EXTREMITIES: No evidence of skin rash and there is no clubbing, cyanosis or edema.

INTERPRETATIONS:

ONE VIEW X-RAY OF THE ABDOMEN: Read by the Emergency Physician reveals normal gas pattern, no evidence of any free air and no sign of any radiopaque stone.

LABORATORY: Urinalysis was positive for occult blood and occasional red cells. The patient was sent to x-ray for an intravenous pyelogram.

IVP X-RAY: Read by the radiology resident as compatible with an obstructing area in the distal left ureter. No stone could be identified on KUB and there was no sign of significant hydronephrosis.

I discussed the patient's care with Dr. Smithson of the Urology Service. It was determined that the patient should be admitted to a hospital bed for pain control.

HOSPITAL COURSE: While in the Emergency Department the patient was treated with Toradol which gave him only partial relief. This was followed with Demerol and Phenergan which made the patient significantly more comfortable.

MEDICAL DECISION MAKING:

DIAGNOSIS:
1. Renal colic with left ureteral calculus.

PLAN:
1. The patient was transferred to the Urology Service at approximately 1400 hours.

CONDITION AT DISCHARGE: Stable.
Time Out: 1400

_____
Ronald W. Stunz, M.D.

RWS:sbs
DOD: 06/07/94
DOT: 06/07/94

Figure 14-1 *Continued*

BRYN MAWR HOSPITAL
130 South Bryn Mawr Avenue
Bryn Mawr, PA 19010-0000

PATIENT: Sarah Fenton   DATE: 08/09/94

MR # 20-84-32   DOB: 6/23/77   ARRIVED: 1433   EXAMINED: 1500

CHIEF COMPLAINT: Laceration right thumb.

HISTORY\HISTORY OF PRESENT ILLNESS: The patient states that she was slicing lettuce with a slicer and cut her right thumb. She denies any other injury or complaint. She denies numbness or tingling in the finger. She is right hand dominant. She is a college student.

PAST MEDICAL HISTORY: None.

PAST SURGICAL HISTORY: Noncontributory.

PERSONAL PHYSICIAN:
ALLERGIES: Ceclor.
MEDICATIONS: Seldane.
TETANUS STATUS: Less than five years ago.

EXAMINATION: Vital signs: Temperature 98.4, pulse 80, respiratory rate 18, blood pressure 120/80. General appearance: The patient is a 17-year-old female in no acute distress. Alert and oriented times three. The patient is cooperative and responsive to examination.

PHYSICAL EXAMINATION:
RIGHT HAND: Reveals a 1 cm flap-type laceration on the distal pad aspect of her right thumb. This goes right up to the end of the nail, but does not involve the nail bed at all. There is no foreign body with inspection. Neurovascularly intact distally. There is no evidence of any other injury. There is no subungual hematoma.

HOSPITAL COURSE: The wound is anesthetized by digital block with 1.5 cc of 2% Lidocaine, as well as some local infiltration 0.2 cc. The wound is irrigated with 500 cc of sterile and normal saline. It is sutured with two 5-0 simple interrupted Ethilon sutures and then three Steri-Strips with benzoin to approximate the wound edges. Sterile dressing.

Continued on page 2

Figure 14–2
A report on a young woman seen in the Emergency Department with a laceration of her right thumb. This report is typed in the style used in the Emergency Department at Bryn Mawr Hospital, Bryn Mawr, Pennsylvania.

MEDICAL DECISION MAKING:

DIAGNOSIS
1. Laceration right thumb 1 cm.

PLAN:
1. Suture sheet is given to patient.
2. Stitches out in 10 days.

CONDITION AT DISCHARGE: Stable.
Time out: 1545

Gregory W. Higbee, D.O.

GWH/rlw
DOD: 08/09/94
DOT: 08/09/92

Dictate, Inc. 525-5678 for the Bryn Mawr Hospital.

Figure 14–2 Continued

BRYN MAWR HOSPITAL
130 South Bryn Mawr Avenue
Bryn Mawr, PA 19010-0000

PATIENT: Thomas Kennedy   DATE: 08/09/94

MR # 18-43-22   DOB: 02/23/88   ARRIVED: 2221   EXAMINED: 2319

CHIEF COMPLAINT: Laceration to chin.

HISTORY\HISTORY OF PRESENT ILLNESS: The patient is a 6-year-old white male who was horsing around at home, fell and hit the anterior symphysis of his chin on the ground without any loss of consciousness. He denies any visual or speech changes. He has not been nauseous and appears his normal self to his parents. There is no neck pain. He denies any injuries to his teeth or tongue and states his jaw moves normal. He denies any injuries to his chest, spine, abdomen, pelvis or extremities. Mother states he has no medical problems and is currently on his tetanus, having received a preschool booster.

PAST MEDICAL HISTORY: There are no medical problems.

PERSONAL PHYSICIAN:
ALLERGIES: No known allergies.
MEDICATIONS:
TETANUS STATUS: As above.

EXAMINATION: Vital signs are fine.

PHYSICAL EXAMINATION:
HEENT: He has a 2.0 cm gentle curvilinear laceration on the anterior portion of the chin. The mandible moves normally. There is no temporomandibular joint crepitus.   There is no intraoral sign of trauma. The mandible is stable and the teeth are atraumatic.
NECK: Nontender and there is full range of motion.

HOSPITAL COURSE/PROCEDURES: The area was cleansed with Betadine times two. It was then numbed with a total of 1.5 cc of 2% Xylocaine locally with an additional .5 during the procedure. The area was then irrigated with 120 cc of normal saline. The wound was explored. Its depth was through the subcutaneous fat. There was no foreign body seen. It was then closed in the usual sterile manner using seven simple interrupted 6-0 nylon sutures and dressed with Neosporin and a Band-Aid.

Continued on page 2

Figure 14–3
An example of an Emergency Department report of a child with a chin laceration. This report is typed in the style used in the Emergency Department at Bryn Mawr Hospital, Bryn Mawr, Pennsylvania.

Page 2

MEDICAL DECISION MAKING:

DIAGNOSIS:
1. Chin laceration, repaired.

PLAN:
1. He was given the usual head and wound precautions.
2. They were told to follow-up with a physician of their choice.

CONDITION AT DISCHARGE:
Time out: 2325

_____

Christopher X. Daly, M.D.

CXD/sbs
DOD: 08/10/94
DOT: 08/101/94

Dictate, Inc. 525-5678 for the Bryn Mawr Hospital

Figure 14–3 Continued

BRYN MAWR HOSPITAL
130 South Bryn Mawr Avenue
Bryn Mawr, PA 19010-0000

PATIENT: Patricia Colbert   DATE: 7/11/94

MR# 16-93-12   DOB: 06/13/36   ARRIVED: 0946   EXAMINED: 1100

CHIEF COMPLAINT: Injured back.

HISTORY\HISTORY OF PRESENT ILLNESS: The patient is a 58-year-old white female who slipped several hours prior to admission on wet grass, landing on her buttocks. She sustained immediate pain in her mid-back. She denies any injury to her pelvis or lower extremity. She denies any neurologic symptomatology or paresthesias of the extremities. She denies any shortness of breath. She denies striking her head, she denies any neck pain.

PAST MEDICAL HISTORY: Positive for lower back problems for which she has seen a chiropractor. She has environmental allergies.

PERSONAL PHYSICIAN:
ALLERGIES: No known drug allergies.
MEDICATIONS: Premarin and Provera.
TETANUS STATUS:

EXAMINATION: Vital signs: Temperature 97.6, pulse 82, respiratory rate 20, blood pressure 130/80. General appearance: The patient is a well-developed, well-nourished 58-year-old white female who is present and in no acute distress.

PHYSICAL EXAMINATION:
HEENT: Head is normocephalic, atraumatic. Her ears, nose and throat are unremarkable.
NECK: Supple without any spinous tenderness and a full range of motion.
BACK: Her thoracic spine reveals tenderness in the mid portion to lower portions of the thoracic spine in the mid-line. There is no palpable bony deformity or step-off. There is no rib tenderness.
LUNGS: Clear. No costovertebral angle tenderness.
HEART: Regular sinus rhythm without murmurs, rubs or gallops.
ABDOMEN: Soft and nontender without active bowel sounds.
PELVIS: Stable.
EXTREMITIES: Atraumatic.
NEUROLOGIC: Grossly intact.

Continued on page 2

Figure 14–4

A report of a 58-year-old woman seen in the Emergency Department with a back injury and admitted to the Orthopedic Surgery Service. This report is typed in the style used in the Emergency Department at Bryn Mawr Hospital, Bryn Mawr, Pennsylvania.

Page 2

DIAGNOSTIC TESTS REVIEWED: THORACIC SPINE X-RAY: Three views, read by Emergency Physician reveals a compression fracture of the eighth thoracic vertebrae.

HOSPITAL COURSE/PROCEDURES: She was medicated here with Toradol 60 mg intramuscularly, which gave her considerable pain relief, but still left her unable to effectively ambulate. Given the patient's inability to ambulate without a great deal of pain, it was thought advisable to admit her to the hospital. I discussed her case with Dr. Brown, of the Orthopedic Surgery Service, who will take her on his service.

MEDICAL DECISION MAKING:

DIAGNOSIS:
1. Fracture of the eighth thoracic vertebrae

PLAN:
1. Transfer to the Orthopedic Surgery Service

DISPOSITION: Care of patient transferred.
CONDITION: Stable.
Time Out:

_____
Ronald W. Stunz, M.D.

RWS:sbs
DOD: 7/11/94
DOT: 7/11/94

Dictate, Inc. 525-5678 for the Bryn Mawr Hospital

Figure 14–4 Continued

computerized. For storage and retrieval of documents, taking advantage of the capacities of modern computers is almost mandatory. Electronic storage of dictated records allows substantial quality assurance tracking to be done, using key words and programmed default settings. Rapid review of old records, without endless paper shuffling, is possible in such a system, with the number of records available limited only by disk space.

An efficient system used by an Emergency Department may involve phoned dictations, taped, transcribed, and returned via computer modem. The charts may be printed in triplicate on a laser printer and electronically stored on the computer's hard disk. Turn-around time may average over 2 hours per chart, but the transcription service might place a premium on having all charts returned prior to the end of the physician's working shift. Charts requested "stat" are generally transcribed and received within an hour of dictation.

It is a good policy to have the physician responsible for its dictation, *but only this physician,* make dictated alterations or corrections to its content after reviewing the transcribed chart. This important safeguard prevents unauthorized alteration of a critical medical-legal document. Transcriptionists should accurately time any addenda or significant alterations to the medical record.

In conclusion, the challenge of emergency medicine felt by all who labor at it daily is shared by the transcriptionist in the accurate transcription of its records. The constantly changing variety of cases and the opportunity to participate in the creation of the definitive documentation of these encounters offer significant satisfaction to the transcriptionist.

Reference Sources

Butaka, W. R. *Emergency Department Medical Record in Emergency Medicine Risk Management.* American College of Emergency Physicians, Dallas, Texas, 1991.

DeGowin, Richard L. *DeGowin and DeGowin's Bedside Diagnostic Examination.* Macmillan, New York, 1987.

Tintinelli, J., et al. *Emergency Medicine: A Comprehensive Study Guide,* 3rd edition. American College of Emergency Physicians. McGraw-Hill, New York, 1991.

For references of specific application to medical transcription, see Appendix 1.

Endocrinology

INTRODUCTION

Endocrinology is a subspecialty of internal medicine. Like other internists, endocrinologists receive specialized training after medical school, generally 3 years of internal medicine internship and residency followed by a 1- to 3-year fellowship in endocrinology. To be fully qualified as an endocrinologist, the doctor then sits for board examinations given by the American Board of Internal Medicine in "Internal Medicine" (at the end of residency) and in "Endocrinology and Metabolism" (at the end of the fellowship).

Most newly trained endocrinologists today sit for their endocrine boards and have practices dealing with all aspects of endocrinology. Years ago it was more common to have a practice that might be devoted only to a limited aspect of the endocrine system, such as thyroid disease, or might focus completely on diabetes. The term *diabetologist* is sometimes used to designate these latter physicians.

ANATOMY AND PHYSIOLOGY

Endocrinology is concerned with the actions of special chemicals, called hormones, in the body. A hormone, which comes from the Greek word meaning a distant messenger, is a biologically active chemical secreted by a specialized organ in the body (called a gland) which circulates in the bloodstream and has effect on a distant target organ in the body. Hormones are secreted by the so-called ductless glands to distinguish them from glands that put their products not into the bloodstream but into a duct, such as a sweat gland or digestive glands. The lay public often call lymph nodes glands, but this is a misnomer, and these organs play no current role in the endocrine system.

There are several ductless glands, including the thyroid, parathyroids, thymus, suprarenal glands or adrenals, pituitary body or hypophysis, pineal body, gonads (ovaries and testes), and pancreatic islets (Figure 15–1). The thyroid gland is a butterfly-shaped gland that wraps around the windpipe. When signaled by the pituitary the thyroid produces hormones that speed up or slow down metabolism. The four parathyroid glands, situated around (or sometimes within) the thyroid, regulate calcium levels in the blood. The thymus gland is situated below the thyroid and is believed to play a major role in the functioning of the immune system. Two adrenal glands sitting on top of each kidney produce hormones controlling our response to stress. The hormones made in the adrenal cortex fight inflammation and help control blood-sugar and mineral levels. A gland located in the central lower portion of the brain is called the pituitary. It is known as the "master gland" because it signals other endocrine glands to turn on and off. Another small gland in the brain is called the pineal gland; it may work with the pituitary in regulating body temperature, motor activity, sleep, and mood.

The gonads consist of the ovaries in the female and the testes in the male. The ovaries produce estrogen and progesterone, whereas the testes produce testosterone and other androgens. All these hormones are responsible for sexual characteristics and reproduction. The pancreas is about 4 to 6 inches long; it lies behind the stomach and extends transversely from the concavity of the duodenum to the spleen. In addi-

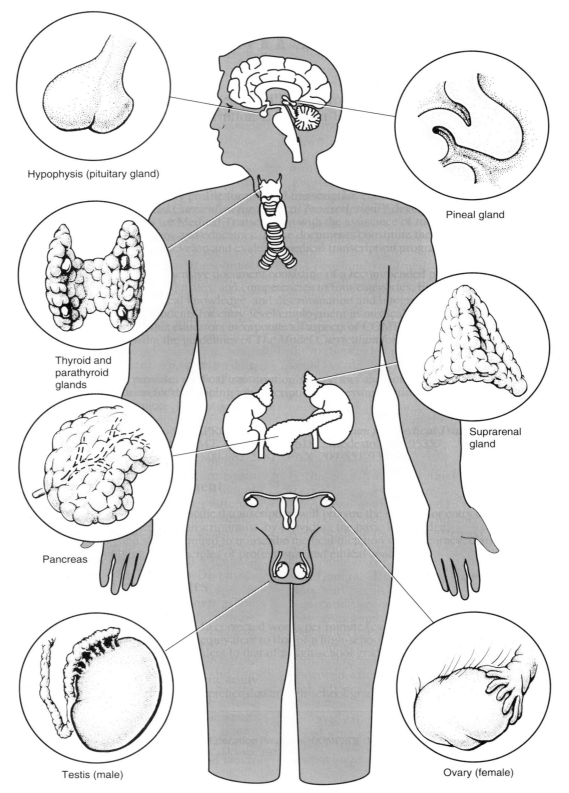

Hypophysis (pituitary gland)

Pineal gland

Thyroid and parathyroid glands

Suprarenal gland

Pancreas

Testis (male)

Ovary (female)

220

Figure 15–1

The endocrine glands and their locations in the body.

tion to secreting digestive enzymes, it produces such hormones as insulin and glucagon, which regulate blood-glucose levels. Specialized cells in the kidney, the intestines, and other organs also secrete hormones. The kidneys produce hormones that maintain normal blood pressure and regulate production of red blood cells. For quick reference, Table 15–1 lists the major endocrine glands, their hormones, and the actions they produce.

REPRESENTATIVE DISEASES

Many syndromes, diseases, and congenital conditions are due to hypo- or hypersecretion of

Table 15–1 ▪ **Hormone Production and Function of Endocrine Glands**

Gland	Hormone	Function
Thyroid	Thyroxine, triiodothyronine	Regulates metabolism in body cells Stimulates passage of calcium into bones from blood
Parathyroids	Parathyroid hormone	Regulates calcium in the blood
Adrenals		
▪ Cortex	Aldosterone (mineralocorticoid)	Regulates the amount of salts in the body
	Cortisol (glucocorticoid)	Regulates the quantities of sugars, fats, and proteins in cells
	Androgens, estrogens, and progestins	Maintains secondary sex characteristics
▪ Medulla	Epinephrine (adrenaline)	Sympathomimetic
	Norepinephrine (noradrenaline)	Sympathomimetic
Pancreas		
▪ Islet cells	Insulin	Regulates the transport of glucose to the body cells
	Glucagon	Increases blood sugar by causing conversion of glycogen to glucose
Pituitary		
▪ Anterior lobe	Growth hormone (GH; somatotropin)	Increases bone and tissue growth
	Thyroid-stimulating hormone (TSH)	Stimulates production of thyroxine and growth of the thyroid gland
	Adrenocorticotropic hormone (ACTH)	Stimulates secretion of hormones from the adrenal cortex, especially cortisol
	Gonadotropins	
	▪ Follicle-stimulating hormone (FSH)	Stimulates growth of eggs and ovarian hormone secretion
	▪ Luteinizing hormone (LH)	Promotes ovulation; male hormone secretion (ICSH)
	Prolactin (PRL)	Promotes growth of breast tissue and milk secretion.
	Melanocyte-stimulating hormone (MSH)	Increases pigmentation of the skin
▪ Posterior lobe	Antidiuretic hormone (ADH; vasopressin)	Stimulates reabsorption of water by kidney tubules
	Oxytocin	Stimulates contraction of the uterus during labor and childbirth
Ovaries	Estradiol	Develops and maintains female secondary sex characteristics
	Progesterone	Prepares and maintains the uterus in pregnancy
Testes	Testosterone	Promotes growth and maintenance of male secondary sex characteristics

Adapted from Chabner, Davi-Ellen. *The Language of Medicine*, 3rd edition. W. B. Saunders Company, Philadelphia, 1984.

the endocrine glands, as shown in Table 15–2. However, this chapter includes a broad discussion only of diabetes, the most common endocrine disease.

Diabetes Mellitus ▪ Diabetes is the most common endocrine disorder encountered in clinical practice. Between 10 and 15 million Americans have diabetes, and approximately half of them do not even know they have it! This occurs because early changes in diabetes may occur without any symptoms or may raise the blood sugar only to a minimal extent, making it difficult to diagnose without careful attention to normal values. In addition, there is sometimes a reluctance on the part of the physician and the patient to call mild blood sugar changes "diabetes" because of the fearful implications of this disease.

Diabetes is a condition in which there is inadequate insulin in the body for the patient's metabolic needs. *Metabolism* is a term that describes the means by which the body handles the variety of nutrients taken in from a dietary source. Fats, proteins, and sugars are absorbed and transported to the liver for initial processing. In that organ, these nutrients are either stored, broken down, shipped out for use by other organs, or changed in some way to meet later nutritional needs. This factory-like process is controlled by the availability of the nutrients and by the hormones bathing the liver, including insulin, glucagon, and epinephrine.* In addition, these hormones have effects on the manner in which distant organs, such as muscle tissue and fat tissue, handle the available nutrients.

An inadequacy of insulin can come about for at least two important reasons. First, there simply may be very low levels of insulin circulating in the bloodstream. This occurs when the pancreas has been damaged, since the islet cells of the pancreas are responsible for secretion of insulin. However, another mechanism that may lead to insulin inadequacy is *insulin resistance*. This occurs when, despite adequate circulating levels of insulin, the target organs for insulin's action (liver, muscle, fat) are not responsive to the circulating insulin levels. Since insulin (and other hormones) works by binding to a specific receptor on the surface of its target organs, attention has been given to receptor number in diabetes. It has now been well determined that in obesity insulin receptor number decreases, leading to a certain degree of insulin resistance. However, binding to the receptor is only the first step in insulin action, and it has now been determined that a so-called "postreceptor" defect is also present in diabetes, further reducing the cell's ability to respond to insulin's signals.

In the face of either inadequate circulating

---

*Also referred to as adrenaline.

Table 15–2 ▪ **Abnormal Conditions of Endocrine Glands**

Gland	Hypersecretion	Hyposecretion
Adrenal cortex	Adrenal virilism Cushing's disease	Addison's disease
Adrenal medulla	Pheochromocytoma	
Pancreas	Hyperinsulinism	Diabetes mellitus
Parathyroid glands	Hyperparathyroidism (osteitis fibrosa cystica)	Hypoparathyroidism (tetany, hypocalcemia)
Pituitary (anterior lobe)	Acromegaly Gigantism	Dwarfism Panhypopituitarism
Pituitary (posterior lobe)	Syndrome of inappropriate antidiuretic hormone	Diabetes insipidus
Thyroid gland	Exophthalmic goiter (Graves' disease, thyrotoxicosis) Nodular (adenomatous) goiter	Cretinism (children) Endemic goiter Myxedema (adults)

insulin levels or insulin resistance (or both), the body's metabolic pathways are not well controlled. This generally leads to increased production of glucose by the liver and decreased utilization of glucose by fat and muscle tissue. The net effect of these changes is elevated sugar in the bloodstream. In addition, diabetic patients have abnormal fat metabolism (see the discussion on diabetic ketoacidosis on page 225) and protein metabolism. The latter becomes obvious when a child with poorly controlled diabetes fails to grow properly, despite adequate calorie intake, until enough insulin is given to normalize protein-handling and bodily growth.

The Clinical Picture of Diabetes ■ As diabetes develops, blood sugar may rise from its normal levels of 70 to 110 mg/dl fasting and 150 mg/dl or so following meals. Early rises in glucose level may be unnoticed by the patient and the physician, but by the time the sugar rises to greater than 180 mg/dl, symptoms may occur. At blood levels higher than this, the so-called renal threshold is exceeded, and sugar excretion in the urine is seen. Increased urine sugar (called glycosuria), works like a sponge, drawing increased amounts of water into urine production, leading to excessive urination. This finding, called *polyuria,* is the cardinal and classic sign of poorly controlled diabetes. Continued excess urination leads to progressive dehydration and often a dry mouth. These symptoms compel the patient to drink increased fluids, a symptom called *polydipsia.* Although the patient may think that the increased drinking is causing the urinating, the situation is really happening the other way around!

Further dehydration can lead to complaints of blurry vision as fluid shifts from the lens of the eye. Fatigue may ensue, as does weight loss—initially to the joy of the patient but eventually clearly out of proportion to the degree of patient need. This weight loss is largely because of excessive loss of fluid, salt, potassium, and other essential minerals. Weight loss may continue despite increased eating, called *polyphagia.* The classic "polys" of uncontrolled diabetes (polyuria, polydipsia, and polyphagia) were described by the Greeks 3000 years ago and are still taught to interns and patients today.

These manifestations of diabetes are acute symptoms; that is, they will occur after a short time of elevated blood sugar. This is especially true if the sugar has risen relatively quickly. Conversely, the patient may have very high levels of blood sugar and still report very few symptoms if the sugar has risen very slowly. Other symptoms may occur after a number of months of poorly controlled diabetes, including infectious complications of diabetes. This can present as recurrent vaginitis (usually from yeast infections) or "boils," which are subcutaneous abscesses usually caused by *Staphylococcus* bacteria. After decades of poorly controlled diabetes, chronic diabetic complications may occur. These are shown in Table 15–3 and involve vascular and neurologic changes in the body.

Types of Diabetes ■ Diabetes is divided into two clinical types: Type I and Type II. Type I diabetes is insulin-dependent diabetes. These patients *must* be treated with insulin to preserve life. The problem in metabolism is secondary to very low circulating insulin levels caused by an essentially nonfunctioning pancreas. The cause of pancreatic damage is currently the object of considerable diabetes research. Some attention has been given to the possibility of a virus damaging the pancreas, but most current theories suggest that autoimmunity, that is, the body's attack on its own organs by the immune system, is the cause of this form of diabetes.

The typical patient with Type I diabetes is young, hence its former term *juvenile-onset diabetes.* The patient is often thin and may present to the physician in diabetic ketoacidosis (see next section). This patient usually is given multiple shots of insulin to control the metabolism.

Type II diabetes is by far the more common form. This is noninsulin-dependent diabetes, implying that the patient has some internal insulin. Some of these patients have, in fact, high levels of insulin, but because of their profound insulin resistance the insulin is unable to do its job in controlling their metabolism. These patients may be treated with weight loss, diet, exercise, pills (oral hypoglycemic agents) and, if necessary, insulin. However, treatment with insulin does not make them Type I or truly insulin-dependent, a concept that is sometimes confusing to the general physician. Eighty per cent of Type II patients are overweight, and they often have a strong family history of diabetes. The two types of diabetes are compared in Table 15–4.

Table 15–3 ■ **Complications of Diabetes**

Type	Tissue Changes	Clinical Syndromes	Signs and Symptoms
Macrovascular	Arteriosclerosis	Peripheral vascular disease Coronary artery disease Cerebrovascular disease	Intermittent claudication Angina/myocardial infarction Transient ischemic attack/stroke
Microvascular	Basement membrane thickening Microaneurysm formation Increased capillary "leakiness"	Retinopathy: background or proliferative Nephropathy: first sign is proteinuria	Visual changes Hypertension Kidney failure
Neuropathic	Demyelination Decreased nerve conduction velocity	Symmetric sensory peripheral neuropathy Mononeuropathy: peripheral or cranial nerve Autonomic neuropathy	Numbness and tingling in fingers and toes

Diabetic Emergencies ■ Blood sugars that go out of control slowly may be associated with very few symptoms. However, a few situations in diabetes lead to rather severe symptoms and may present as true emergencies. The first diabetic emergency, *hypoglycemia,* occurs when the blood sugar goes too low. This is seen only in patients who are known to be diabetic and are undergoing treatment. Maintenance of normal blood sugar requires a balance of the proper amount of insulin to balance the patient's calorie intake. If too much insulin (or oral agents) is taken, the blood sugar falls to low levels. This causes the body to secret epinephrine, a hormone that can raise the blood sugar. The epinephrine discharge gives the patient symptoms of heart palpitations, sweats, lightheadedness, and nervousness. If this discharge is inadequate to raise the blood sugar, or if the sugar falls extremely fast, the patient may also have symptoms related to a decrease in glucose to the brain, including mental dullness, sleepiness, and even coma. This form of diabetic coma is treated by the addition of glucose, orally in the early stages or by intravenous injection by paramedics if the patient is comatose. It can also be treated by a simple subcutaneous injection of glucagon, a pancreatic hormone that raises blood sugar. This is commonly done by the patient's parents or spouse at home.

Another diabetic emergency can occur in patients with Type I diabetes, either at initial presentation or during a period of markedly inadequate insulin care. In this circumstance, there is inadequate insulin to control fat metabolism, and the increased burning of fat leads to production of excess ketones. Ketones are normal products of fat metabolism, but since they are acids in the body, they can cause problems if they are present to a high degree. The acidosis that may come from increased ketone production leads to

Table 15–4 ■ **Clinical Features Important in the Classification of Diabetes**

Type I Diabetes	Type II Diabetes
Insulin-dependent diabetes	Noninsulin-dependent diabetes
Patients *must* be treated with insulin	Patients *may* be treated with insulin
Insulin levels are very low	Insulin levels may be high, "normal," or low
Ketosis-prone	Nonketosis-prone
Patients are usually lean	Patients are usually obese
Usually "juvenile onset" (peak onset at early puberty)	Usually "adult onset," although occasionally seen in children
Often little family history of diabetes mellitus	Often strong family history of diabetes mellitus

nausea, vomiting, abdominal pain, and a peculiar form of hyperventilation called Kussmaul's respirations. Patients with symptoms of abnormal fat metabolism also have marked signs of abnormal glucose metabolism and complain of extreme thirst, dehydration, and the "polys" of uncontrolled diabetes. This patient, often a child, is in *diabetic ketoacidosis,* the classic presentation of Type I diabetes.

A less common diabetic emergency, but one with even greater significance, is so-called hyperosmolar coma, or hyperosmolar hyperglycemic nonketotic diabetic coma (HHNK). This can occur in patients with Type II diabetes who have some insulin circulating in their body. The maintenance of some small level of insulin prevents these patients from making excess ketones when their diabetes is uncontrolled, but, if they are in a setting where they cannot adequately hydrate themselves (such as in a nursing home), slow, progressive, and profound dehydration may occur. After weeks to months of continued dehydration, such patients' blood sugars may be as high as 1000 mg/dl. Prompt treatment of this condition is imperative, but it may still be associated with a mortality rate of up to 50 per cent. This is especially significant compared with a mortality rate of less than 5 per cent in diabetic ketoacidosis.

Treatment of Diabetes

DIET ■ Diet is the cornerstone of diabetes treatment. In the preinsulin era, before 1922, extreme carbohydrate-restricted diets were the only means of diabetic control. This was generally inadequate to control Type I diabetes but did lead to some prolongation of life, albeit at the risk of chronic malnutrition. With the advent of insulin, liberalization of the diet became possible, although the standard was still to treat people with diabetes with low-carbohydrate intake. In the 1950s and 1960s, it was increasingly recognized that low-carbohydrate diets were generally high-fat diets, and increased fat intake might be especially detrimental in patients who were at risk of developing chronic circulatory complications, such as arteriosclerosis. In the past 20 to 30 years, there has been increasing interest in high-carbohydrate, low-fat diets in diabetes, but with carbohydrate that is present in complex form, such as starches and grains. The current diet recommended by the American Diabetes Association is 60 to 70 per cent complex carbohydrates, compared with the standard American diet that is no more than 40 per cent carbohydrate.

ORAL HYPOGLYCEMIC AGENTS ■ These agents are commonly used in the treatment of Type II diabetes. These medications, related to the sulfa compounds used as antibiotics, have effects both on increasing insulin secretion by the pancreas and on overcoming the insulin resistance of the target cells. A list of commonly used oral agents is seen in Table 15–5. Physicians may prescribe these by either generic or brand names. New oral agents are being developed each year; one, metformin, is likely to be introduced soon. This medication has a different chemical structure than the other oral agents and may prove to be useful in treatment, either alone or in combination with the older drugs. Metformin is available now in Europe, Canada, and Mexico but not in the United States.

INSULIN ■ Insulin has been used in the treatment of diabetes since Banting and Best isolated it in 1922. There are short-acting, intermediate-acting, and long-acting insulins; the style of usage has varied over the years and may still vary considerably among physicians of different training and expertise. Of those listed in Table 15–6, the schedules most commonly used today involve mixtures of intermediate-acting and short-acting insulin (usually NPH and regular), given twice a day, before breakfast and before dinner. Some physicians may still attempt to treat diabetes with one shot of insulin a day, but that is usually less successful. More aggressive schedules of insulin use try to imitate the insulin

Table 15–5 ■ Oral Hypoglycemic Agents

Brand Name	Chemical Name	Maximum Daily Dose (Mg)
First-Generation Agents		
Orinase	tolbutamide	2000
Diabinese	chlorpropramide	500
Tolinase	tolazamide	1000
Dymelor	acetohexamide	1500
Second-Generation Agents		
Micronase	glyburide	20
Diabeta	glyburide	20
Glynase	micronized glyburide	12
Glucotrol	glipizide	40

Table 15-6 ▪ **Differentiating Features of Insulins Used Today**

Source of Insulin

> Human (the standard of the future)
> Mixed beef/pork (most common in United States)
> Pure pork
> Pure beef

Concentration ("units per ml")

> U-100 (standard in United States)
> U-80 (not currently sold in United States)
> U-40 (not currently sold in United States)

Length of Action

> Short-acting:
>> Regular
>> Semi-lente
>
> Intermediate-acting:
>> NPH
>> Lente
>
> Long-acting:
>> Protamine zinc (PZI)
>> Ultralente

secretion pattern in the normal body. Thus, patients are given regular insulin before each meal (to give a little squirt of insulin similar to that which comes internally from a normal pancreas). In addition, a very long-acting insulin may be used to give a base of insulin working 24 hours a day and to carry the patient through the night. Alternatively, patients on three shots of regular insulin before meals may be treated with a bedtime shot of intermediate-acting insulin in order to give them adequate insulin action while they sleep.

SELF-BLOOD GLUCOSE MONITORING ▪ This is probably the most important change in diabetes care since the introduction of insulin. It was introduced in the early 1980s. Patients have measured sugar in their urine since the early part of this century, but this is an inefficient means of judging overall metabolism. Self-blood glucose monitoring, sometimes called home glucose monitoring, occurs when patients use a plastic finger sticker with a lancet (penlet, autolet, or other forms) to obtain a drop of blood from the finger. This blood is then placed on a plastic strip impregnated with a chemical system that changes color or density depending on the glucose level in the blood. Patients may read their glucose level by comparing the color change to a visual chart, as in visual Chemstrips, or by placing the strip in a machine to get a somewhat more accurate reading. The most commonly used machines for self-blood glucose monitoring are the One-Touch, Accucheck, Exac-Tec, and Glucometer. However, new machines are developed annually.

Complications of Diabetes ▪ The ultimate challenge in diabetes care is to prevent the long-term problems that may affect the health of the diabetic patient dramatically. These complications fall into three major categories, as shown in Table 15-3. Macrovascular complications involve large blood vessels that carry blood to the major organs of the body. These vessels are lined by layer upon layer of cells, and deposits in this layer that are indistinguishable from the arteriosclerosis seen in the general population occur in diabetic patients. The diabetic patient may develop this arteriosclerosis at an earlier age and may have more diffuse problems in the body, but the pathologic changes appear to be the same.

The clinical problems associated with macrovascular disease in diabetes depend on which blood vessels are involved and how much deposit is seen there. The most common problems involve the peripheral vascular system, that is, the vessels that carry blood to the arms and legs. As the circulation to the legs is progressively impaired, patients may develop a symptom complex known as intermittent claudication. In this syndrome, the patient has no pain at rest because the blood supply to the legs at rest is so minimal and easily provided by even diseased arteries. But when the patient begins to exercise, the increased blood flow cannot be provided to peripheral muscles. The patient then complains of pain in the legs with exercise and pain that disappears at rest but returns with further exercise. If this peripheral vascular disease progresses further, pain may occur at rest and may compromise the blood supply to distal areas of the feet. Ultimately, gangrene of the toes may set in, leading to the risk of amputation.

Other macrovascular problems in diabetes involve deposits in the coronary arteries, the arteries that supply blood to the heart muscle itself. This may lead to angina or myocardial infarction. Similarly, arteriosclerotic deposits in the cerebrovascular system can lead to strokes and transient ischemic attacks (TIAs).

Unlike *macro*vascular changes, which occur in the general population as well as in people with diabetes, the *micro*vascular (or small blood vessel) changes are seen only in the diabetic population. These changes occur in very small arterioles and capillaries and involve thickening of the membranes in the walls of the capillaries, loss of some of the capillary-supporting cells, and outpouchings (microaneurysms) of the capillary wall. Although these microvascular changes may be found in many places in the body under the microscope, they are likely to cause clinical disease in only two organs, the eye and the kidney.

Diabetic Retinopathy ■ The retinal circulation located at the back of the eye is prone to microvascular changes leading to diabetic retinopathy. Two forms of this complication occur. The most common is *background retinopathy,* associated with leakage of blood (hemorrhage) or fat (exudates) in the retina at the back of the eye. Further changes lead to retinal edema (more serious when it involves the macula, the area of the retina providing our most precise vision) and microaneurysms, which may be seen by the physician as red dots on the back of the eye. Patients are usually unaware of background retinopathy changes. Although background retinopathy is very common, it is less likely to lead to visual loss than the severe stage called *proliferative retinopathy.* In this situation, new blood vessels grow (proliferate) in the back of the eye and may grow out of the plane of the retina into the body or vitreous of the eye. These new blood vessels are fragile and may bleed into the body of the eye (vitreous hemorrhage), which obstructs the patient's vision to a considerable degree. Following bleeding, vitreous scar tissue may form and, if this is attached to the retina, the retraction of the scar will lead to a retinal detachment, seriously worsening the vision. To treat retinopathy, a laser can be used to coagulate new blood vessels effectively when they are seen or to prevent growth of new blood vessels. Prevention, however, is still the best means of control.

DIABETIC NEPHROPATHY ■ Another microvascular manifestation of diabetes is diabetic nephropathy, or kidney disease. Due to the apparent leakiness of renal capillaries, one of the earliest findings in diabetic kidney disease is protein in the urine. (This manifestation, called proteinuria, may be seen in other kidney disorders as well.) Proteinuria can be measured in a random urinalysis or in a 24-hour quantitative urine specimen. In recent years, new methods of measuring very small amounts of protein in the urine have been introduced into clinical practice. One test, called microalbuminuria, allows measurement of protein leakage some 10 years before the standard tests can do so. Microalbuminuria may be expressed as a concentration, milligram per gram of creatinine, or as an excretion rate, micrograms per minute. The latter may be obtained either from a 24-hour urine specimen or a timed overnight specimen.

Microalbuminuria or other measures of mild protein excretion may be seen in up to a third of patients with diabetes in the first decade of the disease. Some patients progress to *macro*albuminuria in the second decade and are then at risk of significant decrease in renal function. By this stage, hypertension is commonly seen, and control of blood pressure is an important factor in overall diabetes care. (Certain blood pressure medicines, such as the ACE [angiotension-converting enzyme] inhibitors and some calcium channel blockers, appear to be especially effective in reducing kidney damage in patients with diabetes. It has been proposed they be used even in diabetics who show proteinuria without hypertension.) As kidney function starts to fail, creatinine clearance shows a progressive decrease, leading to chronic renal failure. Because of overall problems with circulation, diabetic patients are often not good candidates for hemodialysis. However, chronic ambulatory peritoneal dialysis (CAPD) and kidney transplantation are very effective in treating kidney failure in diabetic subjects.

NEUROPATHY ■ The remaining important complication that can be seen in patients with diabetes is diabetic neuropathy. Effects on nerve function in patients with diabetes may occur because of changes in cellular metabolism and buildup of toxic substances derived from intracellular glucose. The most common manifestation of diabetic neuropathy is a symmetric sensory polyneuropathy. This condition can give the patient numbness and tingling in fingers and toes and may even proceed to increasing discomfort with burning and pain or a progressive diminution in nerve sensation over time. A complete absence of sensation in a patient with diabetes is dangerous because patients may not recognize damage to their feet that comes from minor trauma, tight shoes, or hot baths. Damage the patient cannot feel, if associated with poor circulation, often leads to foot infections and puts the patient at risk of serious diabetic amputations.

Other manifestations of neuropathy include so-called mononeuropathies, which can lead to isolated painful nerves or to decreased function in certain cranial nerves. This can lead to difficulty in eye movements or in a Bell's palsy picture with a partially droopy face. The remaining form of neuropathy is autonomic neuropathy. The autonomic nervous system controls a variety of relatively automatic functions, including dilation of the pupil of the eye, proper control of sweat glands, proper swallowing and digestive movements, and orgasms and erections. All these systems have the potential to go wrong with diabetic neuropathy, but fortunately this is a relatively unusual finding in diabetes. Postural hypotension, with decreased blood pressure on arising, is another manifestation of autonomic neuropathy and may be associated with increased risk of cardiac problems and sudden death.

SUMMARY

Ongoing treatment of a patient with diabetes remains a challenge for the patient, the physician, and the entire medical care team. Patient education is an important factor in care, and lifestyle changes involving diet, exercise, and weight loss are crucial factors for regularizing the patient's overall metabolism. Current concepts support the fact that excellent control of blood sugar can prevent the majority of diabetic complications. Normalizing the blood sugar remains the primary goal of diabetic care.

Reference Sources

DeGroot, Leslie J., et al. *Endocrinology,* 2nd edition (3 volumes). W. B. Saunders Company, Philadelphia, 1989.

Wyngaarden, James W. *Cecil Textbook of Medicine,* 18th edition. W. B. Saunders Company, Philadelphia, 1988.

For references of specific application in medical transcription, see Appendix 1.

Louis T. Verardo, M.D.

Family Medicine

INTRODUCTION

Family practice, a relatively new specialty, has evolved from an older tradition of general practice. Prior to World War II, the majority of physicians in the United States (and probably in other countries as well) were considered generalists, all sharing a common background in training, the 1-year rotating internship. The "rotating" portion of this description referred to the different areas of the hospital (or service) to which the newly graduated doctor would be assigned on a monthly basis. The typical schedule included several months each on medicine, surgery, obstetrics and gynecology, and pediatrics, plus specific time devoted to the Emergency Department (or Accident Room, as it was sometimes called). At the conclusion of the year, all interns would be eligible to take the state licensing examination, and those who passed had one of two choices. They could apply for an extension of their in-hospital training, usually in a particular specialty area, which was called a *residency*. Salaries being pretty low for this kind of work, and without the possibility of living at the hospital (as he did when he was an intern), it usually helped if the doctor had access to another source of income, usually from his family (note: I use "he" deliberately, since it was rare at that time for significant numbers of women to be educated as physicians).

Another option after internship, and probably the one more typical at that time, was to go into practice, i.e., "hang out one's shingle." With a license, the doctor was authorized to practice the full range of medicine and surgery, including pediatrics and obstetrics/gynecology, in his office, and frequently in the hospital as well, provided he had the proper "privileges." *Privileges* refers to the various medical activities (including specific surgical procedures) performed for patients in the course of their hospitalization. Well-trained interns generally had little difficulty getting most of the usual clinical privileges, including the opportunity to deliver babies and to perform certain basic operations, such as tonsillectomies and appendectomies. More senior physicians (sometimes a specialist, sometimes another general practitioner) would regularly review each doctor's case records and performance, and a decision would be made as to whether that doctor's privileges should continue, be canceled, or be modified in some way.

This system began to change rapidly after World War II. Spurred on by technology, there was an explosive growth in medical research. Social and political factors led to the proliferation of large medical centers. Medical knowledge appeared to increase exponentially, beyond the capacity of a single individual to absorb all that information. It became clear to many medical students that success meant focusing on one discipline within medicine (and here I am using the term to include all the specialties) and becoming expert in that area. As they graduated, these students took the same internship training as their predecessors had taken, but with a major difference: after that year, rather than go into practice, many of them decided to remain in training and obtain a residency in a specialty (internal medicine and its subdivisions, or subspecialties, was a particularly popular choice). With increased governmental funding in the form of grants, residents could even remain in training to become fellows, and this group of trained physicians became the backbone of clinical research and medical education.

Against this backdrop, the role of the general physician in an increasingly complex medical world was coming into question. Some people argued that it was simply impossible to expect a medical school graduate to learn all that he needed to know about treating patients after a 1-year internship, especially if he also wanted to treat those same patients in the hospital. Others were inclined to restrict all hospital work to a select group of specialized physicians based in or near the hospital; the justification for such a restriction often was based on a mixture of motives. Some generalists had been perceived as not keeping up educationally with the changes in medical knowledge; their therapies appeared dated and based on concepts that had been challenged by the newer information available. An increasingly sophisticated American public wanted the newer technologies incorporated into their regular medical care. Finally, the rotating internship began to be phased out; in its place arose the straight internship: a year of training in a single specialty, usually the initial year in a continuum of training in that same specialty. (A few years later, the requirement for a separate internship was dropped for most disciplines within medicine, and those specialties that did require a prior year of training usually accepted a straight internship.)

Interest in general practice among medical students declined precipitously, and even some established general practitioners acknowledged what they thought was the inevitable by leaving their practices and applying for training in a specialty. Medical school faculty, who had always seemed to favor clinical research over clinical practice anyway, directed many of their medical students into specialty and subspecialty careers. Group practice, with its teams of specialists working in partnership on behalf of a designated patient population, appeared to be the wave of the future; the solo generalist was perceived as an anachronism.

The American Board of Family Practice ▪ General practice did *not* die, however; a remarkable transformation took place instead. In 1966, all the interested parties in this national debate came to a similar conclusion, viz., that the American public would be well served by a new type of physician, one with more (and better) training than the general practitioner; one dedicated to incorporating preventive medicine and health maintenance into the care of patients with acute and chronic illness; and one willing to interact (and intercede) with other physicians on behalf of his or her patients (I include "her" at this point, because an increasing number of medical school graduates were now women). This consensus culminated in the creation of a new specialty, the American Board of Family Practice, in February, 1969. (Boards of medical specialties offer a certification that doctors achieve after demonstrating practical skills and after taking a special examination; although voluntary, this certification is often required by hospitals when a doctor requests staff privileges.)

Residency programs in family practice were created all across the country, and a significant percentage of American medical school graduates took training in this new discipline. Many of the programs retained the rotating internship format for the first year of training, since it had proved quite successful in quickly giving new graduates exposure to a wide variety of clinical disciplines. The remaining three years of residency involved hospital work in some subspecialty areas of internal medicine and pediatrics (including the cardiac care and intensive care units), formal training in an area called "behavioral sciences" (an incorporation of psychiatric principles into general patient care), and exposure to specific surgical disciplines, such as orthopedics, urology, otolaryngology, and ophthalmology—some of these latter disciplines were taught primarily in an outpatient setting.

This type of broad training, coupled with the requirement that residents in family practice had to care for a group (or panel) of patients, including pregnant women, whom they would see in a simulated office setting, represented a significant departure from traditional postgraduate medical education. Although some decried what was felt to be watered-down training in some of the disciplines (especially surgery and obstetrics/gynecology), others acknowledged that these new physicians would probably tailor their activities to reflect those clinical entities seen most frequently in a particular practice. Elective time was left in the third year of training to pursue particular areas of interest, as well as to secure more in-depth exposure to areas of anticipated future practice needs.

More than 20 years have passed since the Board of Family Practice was approved. In numbers of residency programs throughout the country, family practice is the second largest specialty (internal medicine is first, surgery is third, obstetrics/gynecology is fourth, and pediatrics is fifth). In terms of numbers of residents in training, over 7000 physicians are on duty annually in this discipline. Increasing numbers of graduates from these programs have helped reverse the decline in generalism described earlier, with an estimated 95 per cent of the communities in the United States having access to a family physician. While most family practitioners provide direct patient care, a few graduates have pursued careers in public health or have obtained positions of leadership within medical organizations such as the American Medical Association and the National Institutes of Health. The American Board of Family Practice has provided an innovative alternative to continued specialty and subspecialty fragmentation by championing the use of "Certificates of Added Qualifications," such as in geriatrics (this was cosponsored with the American Board of Internal Medicine). These certificates represent an opportunity to recognize additional expertise within a particular general discipline, while preserving that discipline's primary importance (these certificates lose their validity if the original board certification is not maintained).

Out of the shadow of the general practitioner, then, has stepped the family physician: qualified by complete (and better) hospital training; formal training in office-based practice, especially in areas relative to the psychosocial aspects of patient care; an awareness of the interdependence of all physicians, with training on how to "co-manage" patients with other colleagues; and *still* with the broad training necessary to serve as the physician of first contact for a particular patient population. Such a physician seems uniquely qualified to respond to the further changes anticipated in both society and the medical profession.

THE PRACTICE OF FAMILY MEDICINE

With the broad scope of practice just discussed, it appears that almost any disease can be seen by a family physician. Actually, the range of conditions encountered falls into some fairly predictable patterns, once a few variables are factored in, such as:

- The physician's practice (rural, suburban, urban)
- Office and hospital setting
- Residency training
- Obstetric services

Each of these variables has an impact on the types of patient problems seen by the family physician; some representative (but not exclusive) examples of some of the ways practices may vary among family physicians, based on these variables, are discussed next.

The Physician's Practice (Rural, Suburban, Urban) ■ Physicians in a rural area tend to utilize the broad training of family medicine to treat a wider variety of ages and ills than their counterparts elsewhere (and often without ready access to consultants). These doctors may provide prenatal care to pregnant women, and deliver and care for the newborn babies. They often perform minor surgical procedures (such as repair of simple lacerations) in a local hospital's Emergency Department (to which they also provide on call coverage for medical emergencies), and assist surgeons in the operating room (in general, only when the surgeon is operating on a family physician's personal patient). In the office, in addition to performing procedures such as sigmoidoscopy and simple casting, rural doctors tend to treat both children and adults for acute illnesses, such as infections, and chronic disease—hypertension, diabetes mellitus, and arthritis. They try to incorporate preventive measures such as immunizations and screening tests into their practice routinely; family physicians, in fact, by virtue of the broad age range of patients seen, are in a unique position both to provide and maintain the currently recommended schedule of vaccines. Finally, they provide a measure of counseling and informal psychotherapy to patients struggling with a primary psychiatric diagnosis or coping with personal and social stresses of a medical illness.

It is interesting that many serious illnesses can initially appear to a physician in a very undramatic fashion. A prime example is hypertension, or high blood pressure, which is often first brought to the patient's attention when the blood pressure is checked serendipitously and found to be elevated, while the patient feels quite well. On the other hand, some self-limited illnesses can be quite dramatic when they first manifest themselves; a good example is infectious mononucleosis, which can make the patient feel quite sick (and ironically, this is "just a virus"). Depression, which can be both common in practice and dramatic in onset, can be managed in most cases by the family physician in an office setting.

Suburban and urban family physicians, although generally similar to their rural counterparts, tend to incorporate less surgical and obstetric care into their daily routines. There may be instances when the family physician in a more populated area may not be the personal doctor for everyone in a particular family. Some of these differences are due to greater availability of specialty colleagues in the city and its surrounding suburbs.

Office and Hospital Settings ■ Family doctors working primarily in an outpatient or ambulatory setting will tend to see certain basic categories of patients. The pediatric age group tends to be either infants for well-baby care or children with acute illnesses, especially of an infectious nature, e.g., sore throats, gastroenteritis, and croup. Sicker children may be seen by the family doctor, but those children are typically cared for by pediatricians. Young adults usually are seen for infectious diseases or for acute injuries such as sprains, strains, minor lacerations, and nondisplaced fractures of the hands, feet, and ribs. The doctor's ability to take care of these problems in the office may depend on the availability of imaging and surgical equipment in that setting. Frequently, young adults are seen for problems that are not strictly medical but which fall into that area called "behavioral medicine" alluded to earlier; these problems include stress on the job, marital discord and difficulties related to sexual functioning. The elderly living outside of nursing homes, either alone or with relatives are seen for both acute and chronic illnesses, particularly arthritis, hypertension, and diabetes mellitus.

Family doctors caring for hospitalized patients will have obtained specific privileges to manage such patients. For younger patients, this means that the family doctor will take care of children with simple infectious conditions, re-serving consultation with a pediatrician or pediatric subspecialist for those patients with serious, life-threatening conditions. In a similar fashion, adults with pneumonias, or out-of-control diabetes, or drug overdoses are generally managed by their family physician alone, with consultation on a case-by-case basis. Patients requiring critical care in an intensive care or cardiac care unit are frequently admitted by the family doctor and then co-managed with the appropriate specialist, e.g., cardiologist, neurologist, throughout the duration of the hospital stay.

Residency Training ■ The major family medicine difference here is reflected in the hospital. As a general rule, the younger, residency-trained family doctors are more active in the care of their patients in the critical care units than their older counterparts who did not obtain formal residency training in family medicine. The previous unwillingness to grant critical care privileges to general practitioners reflected, in part, the time constraints of the 1-year rotating internship; there simply was not time enough to provide sufficient training in the care of these patients. It also reflected the increasing complexity of the care and the need to manage them in a multidisciplinary way.

Obstetrical Services ■ The organization of the practice, both from a logistic and a demographic standpoint, reflects the major difference in family medicine. Family physicians incorporating obstetrics into their practice tend to form groups so that they can "build in" some coverage for nights and weekends and for those days when they have to cancel all office appointments because of attending someone in labor. They also tend to have a practice more oriented toward the pediatric population, since they are often asked to provide ongoing care for the children they deliver. Many of these physicians provide their female patients with gynecologic and obstetric care (regular pelvic examinations and Papanicolaou smears, as well as contraceptive information). Patients requiring additional diagnostic evaluations and treatment modalities outside the scope of primary care are referred to a gynecologist for consultation.

Surgical Procedures ■ Surgical technique is a part of the training of every family doctor; however, the extent to which a family physician performs surgical procedures depends on the geography of the practice. One major procedure not specific to a particular practice location is flexible sigmoidoscopy. A fiberoptic endoscope, 65 cm. in length (there are shorter lengths of 35 cm.), can be used both to examine and biopsy the lower portion of the colon, and this technique is taught to existing practitioners and trainees. This procedure has added significantly to the ability of primary care physicians to discover early colon cancers, thus complementing the already-established routines of digital rectal examinations and the test of stool for occult blood (the guaiac test).

Instruments ▪ In addition to the surgical instruments used by some family physicians to perform selected procedures, one may find some nonsurgical instruments in a family doctor's office. One example is the spirometer, a device used to measure pulmonary function. Basically a bellows connected to a tube that looks like a vacuum cleaner hose, this device allows physicians to obtain a reading on several parameters, or measurements, of lung activity. These measurements become helpful in assessing patients who smoke or who may have chronic lung diseases, such as asthma or emphysema. The newer models of these machines are hooked up to computers and can provide very sophisticated printouts for the patient's chart.

Another machine utilized in the office is the electrocardiograph, or the ECG machine. This instrument allows the physician to obtain a tracing of the electrical activity of the heart, which enables diagnosis of any of the following conditions: cardiac arrhythmias (irregular heart beats); cardiac ischemia (diminished blood flow through the coronary arteries); past or current myocardial infarction (actual damage sustained during a "heart attack"); or hypertrophy (a muscular enlargement of one of the chambers of the heart, usually the left ventricle, which is different from enlargement of the heart seen in congestive heart failure).

Some family physicians include an x-ray machine in their offices. Both from the point of view of their training and from a medical-legal standpoint, these physicians usually restrict themselves to obtaining simple x-ray films of the chest, abdomen, skull, and the extremities. Some family doctors have set up laboratory equipment in their offices, for performing a few simple tests that are done mostly for patient convenience (e.g., throat and urine cultures, complete blood counts, and blood sugars).

Certain specialized equipment for screening a patient's hearing and sight may also be seen in the family practitioner's office. An audiometer is used to screen for unsuspected hearing loss and to document the extent of such a loss when it is found. A tympanometer is used to assess hearing loss indirectly by measuring the extent to which the tympanic membrane moves when the ear is stimulated with sound; typically, this technique is used with infants and younger children in whom ear problems such as otitis media are suspected, and from whom one is unable to obtain a history directly. Vision can be tested either on the standard Snellen visual acuity charts, which come in several versions, including one for preschoolers and another for older children and adults who cannot read, or with a more complicated vision tester, which will test for additional functions, including depth perception and color vision, and which can be programmed to screen for amblyopia and strabismus.

Many family physicians are beginning to get training and experience in the use of several instruments for the diagnosis and treatment of selected problems in office gynecology. The colposcope, a type of low-power microscope mounted on a special stand, is used during the pelvic examination to diagnose cellular changes in the cervix that may not be seen on a standard Papanicolaou smear. Treatment for such changes may sometimes be cryosurgery—the use of a special probe that freezes the cervix and subsequently causes the surface cells to return to normal. Because this represents a relatively new area of clinical expertise for many family physicians, a gynecologist may be asked to provide consultation in the comanagement of patients requiring these procedures.

FORMATS

Letters generated by a family physician's office generally involve the following:

▪ Notification of patients regarding upcoming or missed appointments;

▪ Reports to patients of laboratory results (although many physicians would prefer to do this face-to-face in the office);

NORTH SHORE UNIVERSITY HOSPITAL
at Glen Cove
St. Andrew Lane
Glen Cove, NY 11524-0000

HISTORY AND PHYSICAL

NAME: GUIDO ALVEREZ   MEDICAL RECORD # 38-87-33
DOCTOR: DR. LOUIS VERARDO   DATE OF ADMISSION: 3/26/94

HISTORY: The patient is a 32-year-old Hispanic male who was admitted through the emergency room on the evening of 3/26/94, with the diagnosis of acute diverticulitis. The patient was in his usual state of health, which is self-described as good, when he began experiencing abdominal pain earlier this morning. The patient states he had a large meal the day prior to his admission at a local restaurant. He stated he was fine until he awoke in the morning with some lower abdominal discomfort which persisted throughout the day. The patient states he had a bowel movement yesterday evening which was described as slightly loose, but had neither diarrhea nor his usual movement. The patient came to the emergency room, where he was initially evaluated by Dr. Swain. The patient is usually followed by Dr. Morris and he is away on vacation this week. I am covering for him. Dr. Swain contacted me several hours after the patient was first seen here in the emergency room. He gave me a status report on his condition and reviewed the results of the laboratory work. He had an elevated white blood cell count on his CBC done in the emergency room and this count was reported as 15,600 with a differential demonstrating a marked shift to the left (84 segs., 3 bands, 8 lymphs, 4 monos., and 1 eos.)

Additional evaluation included a three position of the abdomen x-ray, amylase, electrolytes, BUN, glucose, creatinine, and urinalysis; these studies were all unremarkable.

Since I was delayed in the office, I requested that an IV be started with D5 half normal saline to run at 125 cc. an hour and I evaluated the patient when I arrived at the hospital shortly after 8:30 p.m. By the time I saw the patient, he clearly had mild rebound noted earlier by Dr. Swain, as well as some

(continued)

Figure 16–1
An example of a transcribed history and physical examination in the style preferred at the North Shore University Hospital.

GUIDO ALVEREZ   Page two
MEDICAL RECORD # 38-87-33

tenderness on palpation in the left lower quadrant. Rectal examination had
been done earlier by Dr. Swain and was found to be unremarkable. The
remainder of the physical examination was unchanged from that of Dr. Swain,
specifically, HEENT was unremarkable. The neck was supple and nontender.
The thyroid was within normal limits. The chest examination revealed the
lungs to be clear to percussion and auscultation. The heart was within
normal limits. Abdominal examination, as noted above. The right lower
quadrant revealed prior appendectomy scar, the patient having sustained an
appendectomy by Dr. Brown in the past. The extremity examination was
unremarkable (note specifically, the straight leg raising test was negative
bilaterally). Rectal examination was as noted above, neurological examination
was grossly intact.

IMPRESSION: LEFT LOWER QUADRANT PAIN OF SUDDEN ONSET IN
                 THIS 33-YEAR-OLD HISPANIC MALE WITH THE MOST
                 LIKELY DIAGNOSIS BEING ACUTE DIVERTICULITIS.

PLAN: Add intravenous antibiotics, specifically Ampicillin 1 gm. q 6 h. The
patient will be kept NPO, will be re-evaluated by me in the morning, and a
repeat CBC will be done at that time.

_____

                    LOUIS VERARDO, M.D.

LV:bp
D: 3/27/94
T: 3/27/94

Figure 16–1 *Continued*

- Correspondence with colleagues;
- Correspondence with official medical agencies, e.g., the Health Department;
- Varied correspondence typical of a small business, such as supply requisitions or purchase orders.

Many family physicians still use a handwritten entry in the patient's record for the bulk of their charting, but this is changing. The availability of transcription services is now sufficient to make the typewritten note both affordable and expected. Typically, the entry is written either freeform or in the S-O-A-P format: Subjective (the patient's reason for the visit); Objective (the findings on examination plus any pertinent test data); Assessment (what is the diagnosis?); and Plan (what action is planned in response to the clinical problem). Generally, these entries will be

NORTH SHORE UNIVERSITY HOSPITAL
At Glen Cove
St. Andrew Lane
Glen Cove, NY 11524-0000

CONSULTATION

NAME: EVELYN BARKER   MEDICAL RECORD# 46-79-22
CONSULTANT: LOUIS VERARDO, M.D.   DATE: 6/13/94
ATTENDING PHYSICIAN: R. SMITH, M.D.

REASON FOR CONSULTATION: Medical evaluation of abdominal pain.

HISTORY: The patient is a 75-year-old white female who has been here on the unit for less than a week having been transferred from St. Francis Hospital after a vascular procedure (aortofemoral bypass for significant peripheral vascular disease). The patient was doing well until several days ago when she articulated to the nursing staff and to her physicians that she was experiencing some belly pain. She has a prior history in the remote past of having sustained diverticulosis and diverticulitis. She also has a prior history of hypertension which is mild and is well managed on a regimen she is undergoing currently which includes Lopressor. She did not experience any diarrhea, nor any nausea and vomiting. She had no fever. She has had a prior history of constipation when she has sustained various moves to an unfamiliar location and she also apparently had some dyspepsia during her previous hospitalization because she was transferred over from St. Francis on Pepcid on b.i.d. dosage. The patient had initial evaluation by Dr. Jensen on an emergent basis and a WBC that was available for my review showed no evidence of elevation, only a slight decrease in hemoglobin and hematocrit, but this is not significant compared to her admission hemoglobin and hematocrit. She also had a flat plate and upright of the abdomen . These were reviewed and aside from questionable small air fluid level in one loop of small bowel on the upright film, there were no significant findings.

I saw the patient on the afternoon of 6/13/94. She was resting comfortably in her bed. In fact, she had just recently returned from the dining room and she was able to eat her noon time meal. The patient is a pleasant, talkative, 75-year-old white female, alert and oriented times three. Color was good. She did not appear diaphoretic. The skin was warm and dry to touch. Gross examination of the head, eyes, ears, nose and throat was within normal limits. The neck was supple, nontender. The chest revealed the heart to have a regular rhythm, no murmurs, rubs or gallops. The lungs were clear to percussion and auscultation. On abdominal examination, first finding was the presence of a suture line in the mid-abdomen which was intact and appeared to be healing well.
(continued)

Figure 16-2
An example of a consultation report, discussing a medical evaluation of a patient with abdominal pain.

EVELYN BARKER   Page two
MEDICAL RECORD#: 46-79-22

Her belly was soft. There was tenderness to deep palpation, particularly in the left lower quadrant, although it was very minimal in the right lower quadrant and there was some slight rebound noted on the left. Rectal examination was performed. There was some tenderness on manipulation of my finger in her rectal ampulla. The stool was noted in the ampulla and it was found to be guaiac negative. There were bilateral external skin tags noted at the anus. The extremities were within normal limits. The neurological and mental status examination was grossly intact.

LABORATORY DATA: The laboratory work and the x-rays are as described above.

IMPRESSION: I believe the patient's abdominal pain is due to mild diverticulitis.

PLAN: The plan is to offer Bactrim double strength 1 tablet q. 12 hours for the next ten days. She should also have some increased fiber in her diet, particularly Metamucil one teaspoon p.o. t.i.d. I will follow her clinically with you and I will continue
 observation and plan further evaluation including surgical consult should her abdominal pain not resolve.

Thank you for the courtesy of this consultation.

                                            LOUIS VERARDO, M.D.

LV:bp
D: 6/13/94
T: 6/15/94

Figure 16–2 *Continued*

modest in length, since many of the patients will be well known to the doctor from previous evaluations. New patients require extensive notation, especially if the visit is for an initial comprehensive history and complete physical examination; this forms part of the database suggested for each patient in this type of problem-oriented medical record. Another component of this record is the problem list, which indicates all the medical and nonmedical diagnoses made in treating a particular patient.

Most medical reports a family physician needs to create fall into the aforementioned categories, with the exception of those reports pertaining to

NORTH SHORE UNIVERSITY HOSPITAL
At Glen Cove
St. Andrew Lane
Glen Cove, NY 11524-0000

DISCHARGE SUMMARY

NAME: FRANK DIAZ
PHYSICIAN: LOUIS VERARDO, M.D.

MEDICAL RECORD #: 80-12-34
DATE OF ADMISSION: 3/26/94
DATE OF DISCHARGE: 3/29/94

HISTORY: The patient is a 43-year-old Hispanic male. On the evening of 3/26/94, following an initial evaluation in the emergency department for gradual onset, left lower quadrant discomfort, fever, and elevated white count he was admitted to the hospital. The patient had eaten a large dinner the night before and initially thought he may have experienced some food poisoning. However, he only had one slightly loose stool on the evening of 3/25/94, otherwise he experienced no vomiting, nausea or any significant diarrheal illness.

In the emergency department the patient's initial clinical picture suggested acute diverticulitis and he was admitted for further evaluation and treatment. (X-ray studies that had been obtained in the emergency department failed to reveal any pulmonary pathology or any sign of intestinal obstruction. There was, however, significant fecal material located throughout the colon).

HOSPITAL COURSE: The patient's hospital course was uneventful. He was initially placed on an NPO status with intravenous hydration and intravenous antibiotics, specifically ampicillin one gram q.i.d. Within 24 hours the patient experienced approximately 40-50% reduction in his left lower quadrant tenderness and white count went down from approximately 16,000 to 13,000. Electrolytes and other renal studies were normal at the time of his admission and remained normal throughout his hospitalization.

On the second hospital day, following no significant change in his white count and an apparent temperature spike to 101 degrees throughout the evening, gentamicin 80 mg. intravenous piggyback q. 8 hours was added to the therapeutic regimen.

The patient's diet was gradually progressed to clear liquids and then to a regular diet and he tolerated this well. Additional therapy in the form of Metamucil one teaspoon b.i.d. was added on the third hospital day.

(continued)

Figure 16–3
An example of a discharge summary for a patient with acute diverticulitis.

FRANK DIAZ   Page Two
MEDICAL RECORD #: 80-12-34

As the patient's condition continued to improve with almost a 90% diminution of this abdominal discomfort, with loss of rebound and a decrease of his white blood cell count to the 8,000 range with a normal differential, a decision was made to discharge the patient on the morning of 3/29/94, with the following medications: ampicillin 500 mg. p.o. q.i.d. times one week, Flagyl 250 mg. p.o. t.i.d. times one week, Metamucil one teaspoon b.i.d. indefinitely until follow-up is obtained with Dr. Alverez, the patient's usual physician. Finally, the patient was instructed that in about one month's time from discharge, he would be sent for barium enema study to document the anatomic status of his colon, particularly the presence of any significant diverticulosis.

The patient was advised to keep his physical activity light and he was particularly advised to avoid any activity which would cause him to sustain any blunt trauma to the abdomen. He was further advised that he could return to work on Monday, April 1, 1994, if his physical condition warranted it. The patient was instructed to contact Dr. Alverez in about one week's time from discharge for a follow-up appointment and for coordination of the follow-up barium study noted above.

The patient's condition on discharge was good with significant improvement having been noted in his condition from his admission several days prior.

FINAL DIAGNOSIS: 1. ACUTE DIVERTICULITIS (Resolving)

Both the discharge instructions and my personal instructions to the patient reflected a warning about having him consume any alcohol for the time period he is on the Flagyl medication, so he may avoid an Antabuse-like effect. The patient appeared to understand this and indicated that he would not consume any alcohol during the time he was under this treatment.

_____

LOUIS VERARDO, M.D.

LV:bp
D: 3/29/94
T: 4/2/94

Figure 16–3 Continued

hospitalized patients. These include the history and physical; the consultation report; and the discharge summary. Family physicians do not provide operative reports as a general rule, unless they are privileged to perform general surgical procedures as the surgeon-of-record. The availability of in-house or contract transcription services, with computerized word processing capability and sometimes even remote access, has made it possible for family doctors to dictate almost all the medical information necessary for the care of a hospitalized patient (the daily note still is generally handwritten in most institutions). A brief description of each of these medical reports follows.

History and Physical Examination (H & P) (Figure 16–1) ▪ This is subdivided into

- The chief complaint, a narrative description of the events that brought the patient to the hospital,

- The past medical and surgical history,

- The family and social history (social history in this context means occupational history and health habits such as smoking and drinking),

- The review of systems, a comprehensive listing of both general symptoms (such as weight loss and fatigue) and those symptoms associated with a specific organ or group of organs (such as the presence of nausea or vomiting, or difficulties with constipation or diarrhea).

- The physical examination at the time of admission, which is the record of the objective evidence obtained from the patient by using the techniques of inspection, palpation, percussion, and auscultation,

- The impression of the diagnosis or diagnoses, including those one expects to eliminate (or rule out) and those one expects to confirm,

- The treatment plan, including an overview of the orders, that is, requests for specific intravenous fluids, drug therapy, and further diagnostic testing.

Consultation Report (Figure 16–2) ▪ A consultation is a request for specific diagnostic or therapeutic information from one physician to another. This usually reflects the need for some special expertise on the part of the physician being consulted. It can also reflect a personal physician's increased knowledge of a particular patient. Although family physicians are generalists by trade, they frequently may answer consultations from colleagues regarding a patient's fitness for emergency or elective surgery; this is called a medical clearance.

Discharge Summary (Figure 16–3) ▪ At the conclusion of a hospitalization, the attending family physician will dictate a narrative outline of the hospital stay. This will include

- An abbreviated version of the admission, history and physical examination,

- A description of the hospital course, including any complications,

- Documentation of any procedures done to the patient,

- Names and specialties of any consultants called in to see the patient,

- The final diagnosis or diagnoses, which may differ significantly from the original impression, and

- Specific discharge instructions to the patient detailing what medications to take, what activities are permitted, when the patient is to return for follow-up in the physician's or consultant's office.

Reference Sources

McWhinney, I. R. *A Textbook of Family Medicine.* Oxford University Press, New York, 1989.

Medley, E. Scott. *Common Health Problems in Medical Practice.* Williams & Wilkins, Baltimore, 1982.

Rakel, Robert E. *Textbook of Family Practice,* 4th edition. W. B. Saunders Company, Philadelphia, 1990.

Taylor, Robert B. *Family Medicine: Principles and Practice,* 3rd edition. Springer-Verlag, New York, 1988.

For references of specific application to medical transcription, see Appendix 1.

Philip R. Nast, M.D., F.A.C.P.

Gastroenterology

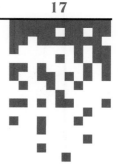

INTRODUCTION

Gastroenterology is the study of the structure, function, disorders, and diseases of the digestive organs. The gastrointestinal tract consists anatomically of everything from the mouth to the anal canal. Its parts are the mouth, pharynx, esophagus, stomach, duodenum, and small intestinal tract, which is divided into the jejunum and the ileum. The colon is divided into the cecum with the appendix, ascending colon, hepatic flexure, transverse colon, splenic flexure, descending colon, sigmoid colon, and rectum. In addition, the digestive system utilizes the liver, the gallbladder and its ductal system, the pancreas and its ductal system, as well as the peritoneum (Figure 17–1).

Gastroenterology, like other specialties of medicine, is divided into subspecialties such as hepatology, endoscopy, and nutrition. Some gastroenterologists specialize primarily in diseases of the stomach or gallbladder or inflammatory diseases of the intestinal tract.

Nutrition

The nutritionist is often not a physician but a highly qualified registered dietitian who has specialized in the practical application of diet in the prophylaxis and treatment of disease. Patients with ulcer disease once were treated with hourly cream and milk and very little else in the way of food; but as years went by, it was discovered that this therapy was not needed to heal ulcers and, indeed, might cause elevation of cholesterol with consequent cardiovascular damage.

The nutritional needs of the body are now better understood, especially in relation to conditions that require special diets. For instance, nontropical sprue or gluten enteropathy is caused by hypersensitivity to gluten, and diets of such patients have to be gluten-free. To make the diet palatable and nutritious, dietitians have devised a host of special foods, formulas, and supplements that are gluten-free and allow the patient to live a normal life even on a restricted diet.

It has also been learned that the human body fares better on a high-fiber diet. The American diet for years was inadequate in fiber, so that many of the common disorders, such as irritable bowel syndrome, diverticulosis, and possibly colon cancer, were aggravated by diet. Nutritionists now play an active role in the management of diet, utilizing their knowledge of the needs of the body and advising patients in the best ways to control caloric intake and to maintain good nutrition and good bowel function.

Endoscopy

One of the most revolutionary advances in the specialty of gastroenterology occurred through the introduction of endoscopy. Endoscopy is a method by which the physician can look inside the intestinal tract through the endoscope and diagnose and treat conditions. For years this was accomplished simply by looking into the mouth or anal canal through a hollow tube with a light; but through sophisticated technology many new instruments were developed. A lens system was used to magnify the images. The light sources were improved. A fiberoptic bundle was developed that allowed light and images to be trans-

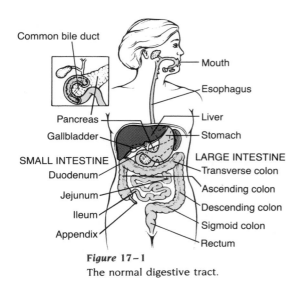

Figure 17-1
The normal digestive tract.

mitted through instruments that could be curved in any direction. More recently a computer chip was developed that can transmit video pictures to monitoring screens in color. By utilizing these systems one can record the endoscopic images on video tapes, laser disks, photographic pictures, and so forth.

REPRESENTATIVE DISEASES

So many disease processes affect the gastrointestinal system that we will describe representative diseases from each of the areas of the intestinal tract and explain their signs and symptoms, diagnostic procedures, and common therapeutic modalities (Figure 17-2).

The Mouth and Pharynx ■ The mouth and pharynx are part of the gastrointestinal system but commonly fall into the care of the otylaryngologist for treatment. There is some cross-over in the management. Conditions such as stomatitis, which is caused by *Monilia* or herpes, are frequently treated by someone other than a gastroenterologist.

Esophagus ■ Increasingly the diagnosis and treatment of diseases of the esophagus fall into the care of the gastroenterologist. The esophagus is the tube that carries the food from the pharynx to the stomach. This organ can be burned, torn, and inflamed. Ulcers, infections, varicose veins, and fistulas can develop in its

walls. Foreign bodies can get stuck in it. Hiatal hernia may occur at the distal end of the esophagus, associated with reflux of stomach acid into the esophagus with development of strictures, ulcers, stenosis, and Schatzke's rings. Anemia may cause webs to develop. There can be diverticula, acquired or congenital, that interfere with swallowing of food. The esophagus may be studied by radiology with barium or by endoscopy. Ultrasound of the esophagus is used either intraluminally or externally. Cytologic studies are done to determine the presence of tumor cells. Many older tests are still performed, such as the string test for checking bleeding sources. Manometry studies are made measuring the pressures and the waves going through the esophagus.

What do patients complain about when they have a problem with the esophagus? One of the most common symptoms is heartburn, or pyrosis. This occurs when acid from the stomach regurgitates upward into the esophagus, causing the esophagus to contract and burn. There can be pain, especially pain on swallowing, when there are lesions of the esophagus, such as an ulcer, or inflammatory disease. The patient may complain of dysphagia when there is a hiatal hernia, stricture, esophageal spasm, or cancer of

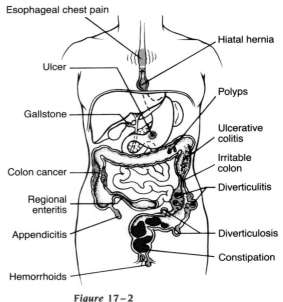

Figure 17-2
The diseased digestive tract.

the esophagus. These symptoms must be investigated and the cause diagnosed in order to determine what is taking place and how to treat it.

A patient with a hiatal hernia and gastroesophageal reflux disease (GERD) usually presents with distress in the lower chest and upper stomach. This is often associated with heartburn, with a sour brash coming back into the throat, or with difficulty in swallowing. The pain and discomfort are associated with belching after large meals and may occur even when the patient lies down to sleep. A sphincter between the esophagus and stomach normally is closed except upon swallowing. When one swallows, food passes through the sphincter into the stomach, but when the stomach contracts, the sphincter keeps gastric contents from regurgitating back into the esophagus. When the sphincter becomes incompetent, either with or without hiatal hernia, the gastric contents can regurgitate into the lower portion of the esophagus. The lining of the stomach is covered with protective mucus. The cells are columnar and somewhat protected against the acid and the contents inside the lumen of the stomach, but the lining of the esophagus is without any such mucous protection and is very susceptible to the acid of the stomach. The acid regurgitates into the lower end of the esophagus and can inflame and burn these cells. The esophagus contracts in trying to empty itself of these foreign elements, and this may cause pain, heartburn, and what is described at dyspepsia.

Inflammation of the distal end of the esophagus can also occur, and the cells actually can be damaged enough so that frank ulcers will form. Recurrent ulcers may lead to strictures. Sometimes a Schatzke's ring forms, or a tight, scarred stricture may occur. When this takes place, the patient has difficulty getting food to pass through the area. Meat not well chewed may actually stick in that area and obstruct and may require removal before the patient is able to swallow again. Sometimes it is necessary to dilate the patient's esophagus after the food has been removed to enlarge the interior of the esophagus enough to allow food to pass through. It may be necessary to repeat this procedure several times to avoid recurrent problems with obstruction.

When upper gastrointestinal endoscopy is performed, the lining of the esophagus can be examined through the scope. The diameter of the lumen can be determined, as well as the presence of a hiatal hernia, inflammation, or ulcer. Cytology brushings for malignancy and biopsies to determine the extent and depth of inflammation can be performed through the scope. Also, a foreign body in the esophagus can be removed through the endoscope. Bougies of various kinds can be used to dilate the lumen of the esophagus that has been scarred enough to inhibit the proper passage of food.

An upper gastrointestinal (GI) series can be performed to show how the barium administered to the patient passes through the tract: whether it refluxes back into the esophagus, how narrow a stricture might be, or how large a hiatal hernia might be. This study enables the physician to recognize an ulcer or cancer. Manometry studies measuring the peristaltic waves in the esophagus determine if and how they are impaired. They also measure the lower esophageal sphincter tone and demonstrate whether the sphincter is incompetent, allowing excess regurgitation of gastric contents into the esophagus. Any or all of these diagnostic procedures may be used to study such presenting problems.

Treatment of gastroesophageal reflux disease can be effected simply by changing one's habits; that is, decreasing the size of meals, decreasing irritants such as chocolate and alcohol, and elevating the head of the bed at night. Other preventive measures include not lying down after large meals and using antacids to neutralize acid that has been regurgitated to the esophagus. The use of antacids helps neutralize the acid produced by the stomach. H_2 antagonists such as Tagamet, Zantac, Axid, or Pepcid are also used. Prilosec is a medication that shuts off the pump that produces acid in the stomach; it is very effective in decreasing gastric acid production.

Teaching a patient better habits about food intake, avoiding irritants, and using common sense frequently bring these symptoms under control. However, if the patient already has strictures from scarring, it may be necessary to initiate more radical treatment. This will involve frequent dilatations of the esophagus with bougies to enlarge the lumen. Surgical correction of a hiatal hernia may also be necessary. The creation of a new sphincter to stop the persistent regurgitation of the contents of the stomach into the esophagus may be required.

There is a condition called Barrett's esophagus; in a severe exaggeration of this disorder the lining of the distal end of the esophagus is changed and becomes more like the lining of the stomach. This transition predisposes the patient to additional ulcerations of the esophagus, and in this case, there is a very high incidence of cancer developing. This condition requires aggressive follow-up and treatment to prevent such a complication.

One of the complications of a hiatal hernia and stricture is a foreign body obstruction. This occurs frequently as people get older. The obstruction develops when they eat too fast or try to swallow a piece of meat or other food that is too large to pass through the narrowed area at the end of the esophagus. Under these conditions, patients present with a great deal of distress because they are unable even to swallow saliva. The foreign body must be removed. This can be done by using the endoscope and special extractors that can be passed through the various lumens to grab the impacted piece of food, lift it out of the area of obstruction, and remove it, piece by piece, until the esophagus is cleared. Then an evaluation must be made as to whether or not this patient is a candidate for dilatation.

One of the most distressing problems is cancer of the esophagus. In such cases, biopsy specimens should be taken through the gastroscope (an extremely important diagnostic tool) to make the diagnosis. If cancer is found, a decision will have to be made as to whether it should be surgically removed or treated with chemotherapy or x-ray therapy, or a combination of all three modalities. Lasers can be used by passing a laser bundle down through the gastroscope to treat the tumor that is obstructing the esophagus by burning it away and making the lumen adequate enough for food to pass. There are many other treatments, such as putting stents through tumors, too numerous to mention here.

Stomach ▪ The stomach is the next largest organ. The most difficult problem with the stomach is determining whether or not the patient has an ulcer, a tumor, or a hemorrhage. Gastric ulcers are common and are frequently caused by stress, by medications such as aspirin or nonsteroidal anti-inflammatory drugs (NSAIDs), or by inherited ulcer diathesis. The common symptom is pain (Figure 17–3). Complications are perforation, bleeding, and obstruction with vomiting. The physician can make the diagnosis by looking through the upper gastrointestinal endoscope and biopsying through the scope. X-ray studies are frequently made, but the advantage of the endoscope is the ability to biopsy the lesion. One must differentiate between benign and malignant gastric ulcers, because benign ulcers can be treated medically with such drugs as antacids, the H_2 antagonists, Carafate, and Prilosec, whereas carcinoma most often must be treated with surgery, x-ray treatments, and/or chemotherapy. Gastric ulcers that do not heal ultimately might have to be treated by surgical removal to avoid the complication of carcinoma. Further studies, such as measuring acid content and hormone analysis of gastrin levels, should be done to determine whether or not there might be tumor-producing hormones that enhance acid secretion. The nutritionist, at this point, can give the patient a good, well-balanced, nonirritating diet. The patient should be asked to avoid alcohol, caffeine, black pepper, and drugs that would irritate the stomach. If the patient has cancer or if the patient's ulcer does not heal, or if there is the complication of bleeding that will not stop, a surgeon may be needed to perform a subtotal gastrectomy, vagotomy, pyloroplasty, or other surgical procedure for treatment of ulcers and cancers of the stomach.

The stomach may bleed from drugs that irritate it and cause gastritis. It may bleed from varicose veins associated with cirrhosis of the liver or from ulcers. The bleeding can sometimes be controlled by use of a heater probe or laser through the gastroscope. Bleeding from the stomach is a medical emergency; if it cannot be stopped medically, a surgeon must enter the abdomen, tie off the blood vessel that is bleeding, and then treat the underlying cause.

Duodenum ▪ The duodenum is similar to the stomach in that it ulcerates and may bleed, perforate, and obstruct. Carcinomas of the duodenum do exist, but they are not as common as in the stomach. The management of a duodenal ulcer is similar to that of the gastric ulcer, but the likelihood of malignancy is not as great.

Small Intestine ▪ Diseases of the small intestinal tract are not as common as those of the stomach and the colon, but they do occur, especially tumors such as lymphomas. Inflammatory bowel disease, sometimes called Crohn's disease,

A Right upper quadrant (RUQ):
   Hepatitis
   Cholecystitis, biliary colic
   Duodenal ulcer
   Pyelonephritis
   Pancreatitis (bilateral)
   Myocardial infarction, ischemia
   Pneumonia with pleural reaction
B Left upper quadrant (LUQ):
   Ruptured spleen
   Gastric ulcer
   Duodenal ulcer
   Pancreatitis
   Pyelonephritis
   Gastritis
   Splenic enlargement
   Myocardial infarction,
   ischemia
   Pneumonia with pleural
   reaction
   Ruptured aortic aneurysm
   Perforated colon
   (tumor, foreign body)
   Renal pain
C Right lower quadrant (RLQ):
   Appendicitis
   Ectopic pregnancy
   Diverticulitis
   Kidney stone
   Intestinal obstruction
   Leaking aneurysm
   Twisted ovarian cyst
   Pelvic inflammatory disease
   Incarcerated hernia
   Renal pain
D Left lower quadrant (LLQ):
   Ectopic pregnancy
   Diverticulitis
   Kidney stone
   Appendicitis
   Leaking aneurysm
   Renal pain
   Incarcerated hernia
   Perforated colon
   Pelvic inflammatory disease
   Intestinal obstruction
E Epigastric:
   Duodenal and gastric ulcer
   Esophagitis
   Myocardial infarction
   Gallbladder

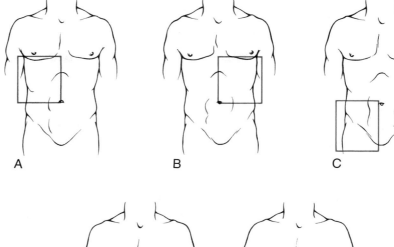

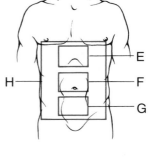

F Periumbilical:
   Intestinal obstruction
   Appendicitis
   Pancreatitis
   Abdominal aortic aneurysm
   Diverticulitis
G Suprapubic:
   Urinary tract infection
   Pelvic inflammatory disease
   Acute urinary retention
H Diffuse pain:
   Peritonitis

Acute pancreatitis
Early appendicitis
Sickle cell crisis
Mesenteric thrombosis
Gastroenteritis
Dissecting or rupturing aneurysm
Colitis
Intestinal obstruction
Uremia, diabetes mellitus
Diverticulitis
Strangulated groin hernia

Figure 17–3

Abdominal pain by location, showing medical terms associated with each quadrant. (Redrawn from Schwartz, G.R., Safar, P., Stone, J.H., et al. Principles and Practice of Emergency Medicine, 2nd ed. Philadelphia, W.B. Saunders Company, 1986, p. 725.)

regional enteritis, or terminal ileitis, is a devastating disease and its cause is unknown. It is a disease process in which ulcerations and granulomas occur in various portions of the small intestinal tract. There may be obstruction and bleeding that interfere with absorption and digestion. It may cause severe pain, weight loss, and a whole host of debilitating problems. The diagnosis of this condition is made by x-ray, gastroscope, or colonoscope. Sometimes laparoscopic examination is done. In this procedure, a small scope is inserted through the abdominal wall and the intestinal tract visualized by looking through the instrument. Biopsy specimens can be taken and the diagnosis made. This disease process is a lifetime problem, characterized by exacerbations and remissions. It is treated with a host of medications, including Azulfidine, Dipentum, steroids, antibiotics, and immunosuppressant drugs. Operation is frequently needed, but it is not a cure in all cases because there may be recurrence elsewhere in the intestinal tract. The disease can involve any part of the intestinal tract, including the esophagus, stomach, and colon.

When the physician studies the small intestinal tract in a patient with gluten enteropathy (caused by an allergy to gluten, which is found mostly in wheat), characteristic signs and symptoms are seen on x-ray films. Biopsies may be done through upper gastrointestinal endoscopy of the duodenum and upper small intestinal tract. The villi of the intestines may be so flattened that they cannot absorb sufficient digested materials to maintain nutrition. This condition is treated simply by avoiding gluten, and though it sounds simple, it may be quite difficult to do when people so frequently dine out. Avoiding gluten returns the villi to normal and allows the patient to absorb food properly. The small bowel is studied by utilizing fecal analysis of undigested and unabsorbed fat and protein. Radioactive-labeled fats are used to see whether they are absorbed; and special sugar tests such as xylose and glucose tolerance tests are also utilized.

Colon ▪ The colon can have multiple diseases. By far the most important ones are carcinoma, polyps, and diverticular disease. Other conditions, such as bleeding telangiectasia, are important as well. The colon is studied with x-rays, as in barium enema, and endoscopy, such as sigmoidoscopy, flexible sigmoidoscopy, and colonoscopy. Sometimes the colonoscopist cannot reach the cecum and x-ray films must be made, but by and large, the aforementioned studies are effective in making the diagnosis of colon disease.

Polyps are important because it is believed that as they grow they may become cancerous and, therefore, should be removed when found. With the use of colonoscopy and such techniques as hot biopsies and snares, the polyps can be removed without major surgery before they become cancerous. Cancer of the colon leads to obstruction, bleeding, and anemia, and it should be removed by surgery if at all possible. Polyps can be handled by the endoscopist through colonoscopy, as well as by the use of laser through the colonoscope. Biopsy can be performed through the colonoscope, and bleeding sometimes can be controlled by using heater probes and lasers. Colonoscopy is used primarily for the diagnosis and treatment of polyps but also in the diagnosis of cancer and other conditions of the colon, such as ulcerative colitis and Crohn's disease.

Ulcerative colitis is an inflammatory disease of the colon that does not spread into the other portions of the intestinal tract, whereas inflammatory bowel disease, such as Crohn's disease, can develop in the small intestinal tract as well as the large intestinal tract. Colonoscopy permits biopsy and diagnosis of diseases of the intestinal tract. If inflammatory disease of the colon does exist, it can be treated with Azulfidine, Dipentum, topical steroids, topical sulfa, systemic steroids, and antibiotics. The intestinal tract must be watched closely in the instance of ulcerative colitis, because carcinoma of the colon is often a complication in patients who suffer from this disease.

Another important problem in the United States is that of diverticulitis and diverticulosis. These disorders do not exist in many other societies; but in the United States, with our low-fiber diets, it is believed that people are more prone to develop diverticulosis. In this condition, small pockets develop along the side of the intestinal tract. Although the pockets themselves do not cause any trouble, they may become infected, bleed, or perforate.

Eveyone has an appendix but not everyone gets appendicitis. Many people have diverticula but not everyone gets diverticulitis. Diverticulitis (inflammation of a diverticulum, especially in the wall of the colon) can be a devastating problem with obstruction, bleeding, and perforation. Frequently it can be treated by the use of antibiotics and diet, but at times surgical removal of the segment of the intestinal tract that has diverticula is necessary.

Rectum ▪ Diseases of the gastrointestinal tract cannot be discussed without also mentioning hemorrhoids. Hemorrhoids are varicose veins around the anal canal. If they are above the so-called dentate line, they are internal hemorrhoids; below that line, they are external hemorrhoids. Bleeding is a complication that must be evaluated to make certain that it is not coming from a polyp or carcinoma. Hemorrhoids can be painful and often their surgical removal is the only treatment.

Liver ▪ Associated with the gastrointestinal tract are the liver, gallbladder, and pancreas.

The liver can harbor many diseases, such as hepatitis, syphilis, tuberculosis, fungal infections, leptospirosis, and abscesses. Tumors of the liver, malignant and benign, primary and metastatic, are frequently a problem. Parasites such as amoebae and *Schistosomiasis* may appear, and metabolic abnormalities such as those associated with carbohydrate metabolism and alcoholism may occur.

Hepatitis takes the form of hepatitis-A, hepatitis-B, hepatitis-C, and also hepatitis non-A, non-B, non-C. Hepatitis-A is common; the patient may have an infectious disease process that lasts only for a number of weeks and nearly everyone recovers without complications. Hepatitis-B and hepatitis-C and non-A and non-B are different. Hepatitis-C is spread by blood transfusions, and hepatitis-B is spread in the same way that AIDS is spread, through blood transfusions, dirty needles used for drug injections, and sexual contact. Not all cases of hepatitis-B and hepatitis-C are curable. A large percentage, perhaps 20 per cent of such patients, develop chronic hepatitis, which then goes on to cirrhosis of the liver, carcinoma, bleeding, encephalopathy, or total liver failure.

Cirrhosis means hardening of the liver, and it is an end-stage disease. It has many causes, such as primary biliary cirrhosis or alcoholic or Laennec's cirrhosis, or it may be secondary to postnecrotic changes of hepatitis. It is complicated by portal hypertension that may lead to esophageal and gastric varices and bleeding from these varices. Hepatic encephalopathy with high blood ammonias causing the patient to become confused and incapacitated may occur. Large amounts of ascites, or fluid, may collect in the belly and may go on to damage the kidneys; this is the so-called hepatorenal syndrome for which there is no therapy so that death usually ensues. Cirrhosis can develop from high iron content, called hemochromatosis. This should be treated, before cirrhosis develops, by recognizing high iron in the liver and bleeding the patient periodically to remove the iron and decrease its toxic effect upon the liver.

When the liver becomes diseased, the most recognizable sign is jaundice. Bilirubin cannot be handled by the liver and it backs up into the bloodstream and tissues. The whites of the eyes and the skin turn yellow. Many other abnormalities take place when the liver fails. Coagulation defects occur, so that bleeding and bruising are more common since blood platelets are low when the spleen is involved. Proteins are not made, and toxic products of metabolism are not disposed of. Treatment consists of making the diagnosis and then trying to correct the defect. Diagnosis can be made by examination of liver biopsy specimens, as well as by a host of blood tests.

Gallbladder ■ The liver disposes of byproducts of metabolism through the gallbladder system, then down the hepatic ducts into the common duct and the duodenum. The bile is eliminated from the body, and the byproducts pass out through the body via the stool. The bile contains compounds that emulsify fats, allowing them to be digested properly. On the side of the common duct is a storage tank called the gallbladder. When the sphincters are closed and the body does not require the bile, it is stored in the gallbladder; when the body needs it, the gallbladder and ductal system contract and the sphincters open, allowing the bile to pass into the intestinal tract. While the bile is stored in the gallbladder, it may become concentrated and stones may form. These stones can lead to obstruction of the gallbladder system, causing cholecystitis, and they may pass into and obstruct the common duct. However, these are benign conditions that require effective diagnostic measures to determine the course of necessary care and therapy.

Ultrasound can be used to tell whether the gallbladder is inflamed or contains stones. Computed tomography (CT) scans of the gallbladder and liver can be done. X-rays and endoscopic retrograde cholangiopancreatography (ERCP) can sometimes be used. ERCP is an endoscopic examination utilizing a special instrument through which a catheter is placed into the biliary duct system. After the catheter is placed in the duct, dye is injected into both the gallbladder and pancreatic ductal systems to help make a diagnosis. A needle can be guided into the liver and dye injected into the ducts to visualize that system as well. The physician can look through new, tiny scopes that can be passed into the ductal system, enabling the physician to determine whether or not there are stones and whether the process is benign. Stones can be treated surgically or medically. Some of the new therapies for gallstones are lithotripsy, laparoscopic cholecystectomy, cannulation of the common duct with sphincterotomy, and papillotomy. Standard surgical removal of the stones and gallbladder is also a common treatment. Medically, drugs have been developed that are effective in dissolving gallstones; however, many stones do recur after the drugs are discontinued.

Pancreas ▪ The pancreas is an organ that sits deep in the abdomen, behind the duodenum and stomach; it is associated with the gallbladder system. It produces insulin, which takes care of the digestion of carbohydrates and enzymes, such as amylase and lipase, that pass through the ductal system of the duodenum. These enzymes digest fats, proteins, and carbohydrates. The pancreas is studied by means of ultrasonography, CT scans, ERCP, and blood tests. Diseases of the pancreas include acute and chronic pancreatitis, benign pseudocysts, and malignant tumors. Unfortunately, carcinoma of the pancreas often does not show symptoms until it is too late to cure the patient. Insufficient digestion of proteins, fats, and carbohydrates results in steatorrhea, weight loss, and poor nutrition. These problems can be studied by measuring fecal fats and proteins that are undigested.

Irritable Bowel Syndrome ▪ The most frequent disorder that a gastroenterologist treats is a functional one not associated with any organic disease like ulcers or tumors. It is very common in the population of the United States, almost 70 per cent of whom will suffer from functional irritable bowel syndrome at one time or another. It is characterized by a change in bowel habits, with intermittent diarrhea or constipation or a combination of both. In addition, it may be associated with abdominal pain and cramps, nausea and vomiting, belching, and increased flatulence.

It is not clear why this happens; but the normal digestive process of eating food, digesting it in the stomach and duodenum, and absorbing it in the small intestinal tract with fluid resorption in the large colon is somehow altered. A patient may have diarrhea that allows the contents entering the large intestinal tract to pass through the colon so rapidly that water is not resorbed, or constipation because of spasm of the circular muscles of the colon that allows too much water to be resorbed and results in smaller, hard bowel movements.

In the normal course of events, what should happen is that the waste products of digestion collect in the left side of the colon; as the day progresses, the water is absorbed and the material lingers in the distal left colon. The following morning, usually after breakfast, there should be a gastric colic reflex that moves the material into the rectum, causing a distention of the rectum and the urge to have a bowel movement. Defecation should follow.

Unfortunately, in the United States, many children never learn this pattern. Either they do not eat breakfast or, if they do, they then rush to the school bus or arrive at school just when they feel the urge to have a bowel movement and it is suppressed. This allows the stool to remain in the colon for a long period of time, and the normal urge is lost.

The diagnosis of this disease process is often made by elimination of possible alternatives. First, ulcers, tumors, and cancer must be ruled out to be certain that the symptoms are, indeed, due to a functional problem and not an organic one. Thus, diagnostic studies through radiology, blood analysis, and endoscopy are performed. The characteristic history, physical examination, and negative diagnostic studies will allow the physician comfortably to make the determination of irritable bowel syndrome.

The therapy, however, is not quite so simple. The physician must understand the patient's emotional problems, if there are any. The physician must make the patient understand the symptoms and what causes them, and a program of diet and medication that the patient can tolerate must be developed. It often takes many months to bring this functional disorder under control, and sometimes it is a lifetime problem. Symptoms may switch from constipation to diarrhea and vice versa. Making the patient understand how this wide variety of symptoms is part of the same syndrome can be difficult. Antispasmodic drugs, bulk agents, and diet are used to treat this disorder. No one medication program works for everyone, and there are multitudes of different medications and approaches to its handling.

SURGICAL PROCEDURES

Various surgical procedures have been developed in the treatment of gastrointestinal disease, many of these consisting of removal of the portions of the intestinal tract that are diseased. The surgeon may want to remove a carcinoma of the esophagus, stomach, small bowel, or colon. An ulcer of the stomach with bleeding and complications also may have to be operated upon. Many operations are used for treatment of an ulcer, including removal of the segment of the intestinal tract containing it. But there are also operations like vagotomy, which cuts the vagus nerve that is believed to be the source of stimuli for production of ulcer-promoting acid. When a vagotomy is performed, it is also necessary to do a pyloroplasty — an incision at the distal end of the stomach through the sphincter that allows the stomach to empty properly. Other operations for ulcers include selective vagotomies in which only the fibers that go to the stomach are cut, and gastroenterostomies of two types: Billroth I and Billroth II. The former is a direct anastomosis of the stomach and the intestinal tract in line; the Billroth II operation is a modification through which a portion of the small intestinal tract is swung up and anastomosed to the stomach so that the stomach can empty into the intestinal tract and skip the duodenum.

Multiple operations are also associated with the pancreas. Cysts of the pancreas may be marsupialized and drained into the stomach. In Whipple's operation (pancreatoduodenectomy), excision is performed of all or part of the pancreas, together with the duodenum, and a multitude of anastomoses have to be done to reconnect the gallbladder system and the stomach to the small intestinal tract. Another operation of the pancreas is the Roux-en-Y procedure in which the tail of the pancreas is removed and an anastomosis is made to a loop of the small intestinal tract.

For diverticular disease or cancer, segments of the colon may be removed. More recently, the laparoscope is being used by surgeons to remove such segments. Ulcerative colitis is a specific problem in which the colon may be removed and an ileostomy may be created. More recent procedures allow the surgeon to remove the mucosal lining of the rectum, bring down a loop of the small intestinal tract, and make a very large pouch. Removing the entire colon allows the contents of the small intestinal tract to empty into that pouch and allows the patient to have bowel movements through the rectum using the normal sphincter.

A dramatic change has taken place in surgery of the gallbladder. The old-fashioned cholecystectomy is now largely replaced by laser laparoscopic cholecystectomy, utilizing the laparoscope and laser rather than large incisions, thus allowing the patient to have a more rapid recovery. At times, when stones are found in the common duct that cannot be removed with this technique, an ERCP (endoscopic retrograde cholangiopancreatography) instrument is passed, utilizing sphincterotomy to remove stones from the common duct after the gallbladder has previously been removed by laparoscopic techniques.

Other specific operations have been developed over the years, including those done on the sphincter between the esophagus and the stomach to control gastroesophageal reflux disease and hiatal hernias, and the so-called wraparound surgical procedure that creates a new sphincter and stops the patient from regurgitating material into the esophagus.

At the other end of the GI tract, hemorrhoids have always been a problem. Old-fashioned hemorrhoidectomies cut out these hemorrhoids. More recently, internal hemorrhoids have been removed using a special laser-controlled instrument. Also, rubber bands have been placed around the base of the hemorrhoids, allowing their removal with less morbidity and more rapid recovery.

Instruments ■ By far the most important instrument used in gastroenterology is the endoscope and variations of it. The original endoscopes were hollow tubes that one looked through, and they were quite difficult for the patient to tolerate. Tubes that went down the esophagus required the patient to be in a straight line, much like the circus sword swallower, in order for the physician to see and operate through them. The advent of fiberoptic instruments allows the scope to get around corners and to pass through the mouth or rectum and go up or down the intestinal tract. These instruments allow the physician to put air or water into the intestinal tract and to remove fluid and contents through channels by suction. They also allow passage through the channels of biopsy instruments, retractors and retrievers, lasers, and sphincterotomy tools.

These instruments allow the gastroenterologist to look inside the esophagus, stomach, duodenum, proximal small bowel, ducts of the gallbladder and pancreas, and colon. They allow the physician to inject dye into the duct systems, utilizing the ERCP instruments to visualize the whole ductal system of the gallbladder and the pancreas.

The instruments used in the colon are primarily of three types: the old-fashioned rigid sigmoidoscope, a straight tube through which the examiner looks and which is usually between 25 and 30 cm. long; a flexible sigmoidoscope that is between 35 and 60 cm. long and allows visualization of the left colon where most lesions occur, particularly diverticulitis; and the colonoscope, which is approximately 185 cm. long and allows visualization of the entire colon. Through these instruments, bleeding can be controlled with the use of laser, heater probes, or bipolar probes. The most recent endoscope is the video system. The colored chip picks up an image and transmits it to a processor that allows visualization on a monitor screen, recording on a video tape recorder, photography, or a floppy disk record with preservation of the material for future review. Figure 17–4 is a photograph of the Olympus Evis 100 videoscope with its various components.

Various instruments are used in gastroenterology. Biopsy of the liver uses either needles that go through the skin into the liver or a laparoscope. Peritoneoscopes are also being used for surgical procedures.

Other instruments are the manometer, which measures both the pressure waves going through the esophagus and the lower esophageal sphincter tone, and mercury dilating bougies and brisk dilators of various kinds, which permit the break-up of strictures from inside the esophagus, thus opening it up. Almost every day, new instruments and new variations of the old instruments are being developed to reach specific areas of the intestinal tract.

FORMATS

Letters ▪ As in any practice, one of the most important tools of gastroenterology is the letter written to a referring physician. The letter must review the reason the patient was referred and the examinations that are going to be or have

been performed, the initial impression and diagnosis, and the proposed plan of treatment.

Chart Notes ▪ For many years, chart notes were written by hand, but with recent changes in documentation requirements by Medicare, more physicians are dictating their notes. These notes must always be dated. They summarize the chief complaint, the past medical history, the social history, and the family history. The physical examination is divided into general findings and specific findings of the head, eyes, ears, nose and throat, neck, chest, abdomen, and nervous system. Any special examination done, such as an endoscopy, is noted. Medicines prescribed are listed, as well as responses to previous medications. An impression of the presenting problem is given and a future discharge plan included.

Medical Reports

The History and Physical Examination (Figure 17–5) ▪ The initial history and physical taken by a gastroenterologist is quite extensive. It includes the main facts about the present illness, the history of previous operations and illnesses, a review of systems, records of allergy, and a social and personal history. The patient's gastroenterologic history is more detailed and includes dietary habits. Such items as pain, nausea and vomiting, gas and bloating, diarrhea, and constipation, and any evidence of bleeding are emphasized. The physical examination includes a statement of general appearance and a complete record of examination of the patient's head, eyes, ears, nose and throat, neck, chest, heart, breasts, abdomen, extremities, and rectum and the result of endoscopic and neurologic examinations.

The Operative Report ▪ A typical operative report is seen in Figure 17–6. This is a very important document. It includes the location of the operation, the patient's name, hospital number (if one is available), date, indication for the procedure, and the preoperative and postoperative diagnosis. The operation performed, the surgeon, and the assistants all must be listed. The type of anesthesia used and a summary of the operative findings must be noted, as well as a description of the procedure. This is followed by the surgeon's signature.

Discharge Summary ▪ The format of the discharge summary is dictated by the policy of the hospital from which the patient is being dis-

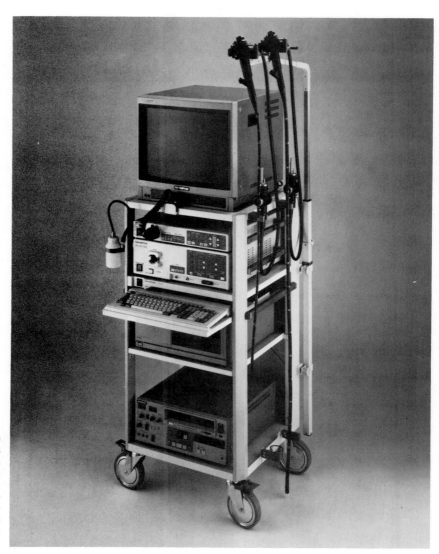

Figure 17-4
The Olympus Evis 100 videoscope with its various components. This video system allows visualization on a monitor screen, and recording via a video tape recorder, photography, or floppy disk record, with preservation of the material for future review. (Courtesy of Bryn Mawr Medical Specialists Associated, Bryn Mawr, Pennsylvania.)

charged. It usually contains the patient's hospital number, name, and admission and discharge dates. The diagnoses and surgical procedures performed are listed. The names of all consultants are recorded. A summary briefly outlines why the patient was admitted to the hospital, what the patient's course was in the hospital, and what the conclusion was. It includes whether or not the patient was discharged improved or otherwise. It notes what follow-up care has been recommended and the discharge plan, drugs, and diet.

HISTORY AND PHYSICAL EXAMINATION

DATE   7/27/94

NAME   Janice Darwin   OCCUPATION   Secretary   AGE   40

ADDRESS   555 North 3rd Street   HOME PHONE   215/525-1111   S Ⓜ W D
          Bryn Mawr, PA 19010-0000

REFERRED BY   James Brown, M.D.   OFFICE PHONE 215/527-1234

PAST HISTORY

Surgical

     T & A - Age two.
     Appendectomy - Age 20.
     D & C - Age 27.

Medical

Jaundice   -0-

Other   No serious illness except
       Infectious mononucleosis
       in high school.

EENT System

Headache   - Occasional migraine

Cardio-resp. System

Pain in chest	- 0
Cough	- 0
Shortness of breath	- 0
Palpitation	- 0
Swelling of feet	- 0
Date of Last Chest X-Ray	- 10 years ago
Date of Last EKG	- Never

Musculo-Skeletal System   - None

Endocrine System   - None

G.U. System

Burning	- 0
Frequency	- 0
Blood in Urine	- 0
Kidney Stones	- 0

Menstrual History

Date of Last Pelvic Examination   - Dr. Jones - two
                              months ago

General

Allergies or Reactions to Medicines	- 0
Exposure to Chemicals	- 0
Fever	- 0
Insomnia - Sleep Habits	- No problem
Nervous Tension	- Unaware of any

Family History

             L & W

Father	67 - L & W
Mother	63 - L & W

Brothers

     One brother L & W

Sisters

     - 0

Children

     Two - ages 10 & 12
     Both girls - L & W

Spouse

     44 - L & W

Diabetes	- 0
Cancer	- 0
Ulcer	- 0
High Blood Pressure	Father on treatment
Tuberculosis	- 0
Arthritis	- 0
Other	- 0

Figure 17-5
A completed History and Physical form generated by the gastroenterology group at Bryn Mawr Medical Specialists
Associated.

PAIN OR DISTRESS

Location — Occasional cramps

First Noted

Frequency

Duration of Each Episode

Type and Severity

Radiation

RELATION TO	RELIEVED BY		AGGRAVATED BY	
	YES	NO	YES	NO
Food			X	
Medication	N/A			
Vomiting		X		X
B.M.	X		X	
Position		X		X
Tension		X		X
Other				

Appetite	— Good
Weight gain or loss	— None
Trouble Swallowing	— None
Heartburn	— Very rare
Nausea	— 0
Vomiting	— 0
Foods Which Disagree	— Spicy foods and "junk foods"
Belching	— 0
Excessive Flatus	— 2+
Distension of Abdomen	— 2+

Bowel Habit	Usual Habit	Present Time
Frequency	Daily	Diarrhea 3 to 4 times each A.M.
Consistency	Formed	
Mucus in Stool	— 0	
Red Blood in Stool	— 0	No blood
Black Stools	— 0	

Use of { Laxatives / Enemas / Suppositories

Breakfast — Orange juice, bagel, banana   Coffee — Two cups A.M.

Lunch — At work - anything - fast foods   Alcohol — 2 to 3 times a week

Dinner — Normal - meat, vegetables, salad and dessert   Smoking — None

Bedtime — None

Figure 17-5 Continued

Figure continued

Past Studies   – None

Medications During Past 6 Months
        – Tried Maalox on her own
        – Uses multivitamins and Vitamin C, 500 and Vitamin E 400

History   Two to three week history of change in her bowel habits. Some stress with economy problems. Works as a secretary requiring more time than usual and less time to take care of home and her two girls. Life becoming a rat race on weekends. Must work to supplement family income.

Husband in new construction and work slow. Diarrhea past two to three weeks. First bowel movement associated with cramps which go away with BM. First BM semi-soft. Two to three hours later she has watery diarrhea, yellow in color without blood. Occasionally urgent call but no incontinence. Tried Maalox on her own. When she eats lunch and sometimes after supper she gets urgent loose stool also. No BM's after retiring.

Figure 17–5 *Continued*

PHYSICAL EXAMINATION

Height 5'4"   Weight 120#   Blood Pressure 120/80   Pulse 80   Temperature 98.6

Skin   - Neg.
Ears   - Neg.
Eyes   - Neg.
Mouth   - Neg.
Thyroid   - Neg.
Lymphatic System - Neg.
Breasts   - Unremarkable
Heart   - Regular sinus rhythm. No murmur
Lungs   - Clear
Abdomen   - Flat
 Liver   - Not palpated
 Spleen   - Not palpated
 Masses   - None
 Tenderness   - Left lower quadrant
 Distension   - None
 Hernia   - None
 Scars   - Appendectomy scar
Musculoskeletal - Neg.
Peripheral Pulses - Normal
Neurological   - Normal
Rectal Examination - Neg.
Sigmoidoscopy - Prepare for flexible sigmoidoscopy

Working Diagnosis   Final Diagnosis
     Irritable colon

Interim Therapy   Letter sent to referring M.D. DATE: _____
       - Bentyl 10 mg. 4 X day

Studies   - CBC
                 SMAC
                 Urine
                 Flexible sigmoidoscopy

_____ M.D.
              Philip R. Nast, M.D.

Figure 17-5 Continued

BRYN MAWR HOSPITAL
130 South Bryn Mawr Avenue
Bryn Mawr, PA 19010-0000

OPERATIVE REPORT

PATIENT: THOMAS CLARK   UNIT # 22-56-74-77   DATE: 2/5/94

INDICATION: Persistent vomiting and difficulty swallowing.

PREOPERATIVE DIAGNOSIS: Same. Rule out esophagitis, esophageal
stricture, and ulcer.

POSTOPERATIVE DIAGNOSIS: Gastritis, hiatal hernia, esophagitis.

OPERATION PERFORMED: Upper endoscopy with biopsy.

SURGEON: Philip R. Nast, M.D.

ASSISTANT: H. Smith, R.N.

ANESTHESIA: Versed 2 mg. IV. Demerol 50 mg. IV.

OPERATIVE FINDINGS AND DESCRIPTION OF PROCEDURE:

The proper informed consent was obtained from the patient. The patient's throat was sprayed with 10% Xylocaine. Sedation was 2 mg. of IV Versed. The procedure was done in the lateral Simms position. The Olympus GIF-Q20 scope was passed without difficulty. The scope was passed into the patient's duodenum. The duodenum was normal. As the scope was withdrawn from the patient's stomach, the pylorus was examined and it was also normal . The distal end of the stomach was inflamed and showed clinical gastritis. Three biopsies were taken for histology, electron microscopy, and CLO test with minimal associated bleeding. The remainder of the patient's examination was unremarkable except for a hiatal hernia and evidence of reflux esophagitis noted in the distal end of the patient's esophagus. Cytologies were taken and sent to the laboratory as well. The patient tolerated the procedure well and had no postoperative complications. Future plan will depend on the results of the biopsies.

PHILIP R. NAST, M.D.

PRN:ssb
D: 2/6/94
T: 2/7/94

Figure 17–6
An example of an operative report, discussing an upper endoscopy with biopsy to rule out esophagitis, esophageal stricture, and ulcer.

Reference Sources

Berk, J. Edward (Ed.). *Bockus Gastroenterology,* 4th edition. W. B. Saunders Company, Philadelphia, 1985.

Siegel, Jerome H. *Endoscopic Retrograde Cholangeopancreatography.* Raven Press, New York, 1992.

Sivak, Michael V., Jr. *Gastroenterologic Endoscopy.* W. B. Saunders Company, Philadelphia, 1987.

Sleisinger, Marvin, and John S. Fordtran. *Gastrointestinal Diseases: Pathology, Diagnosis, Management,* 4th edition. W. B. Saunders Company, Philadelphia, 1989.

Weihnauch, Thomas R. *Esophageal Manometry.* Urban and Schwarzenberg, Baltimore, 1981.

For references of specific application to medical transcription, see Appendix 1.

General Surgery

INTRODUCTION

The word "surgery" comes from the Greek *chirurgia,* meaning work with the hands. It is the branch of medicine dealing with trauma and disease that require operative intervention. Surgery is a vast field, in which the surgeon is called on to treat or repair trauma, infections, physical disorders, developmental anomalies, and tumors (either benign or malignant).

There are thousands of possible surgical procedures, and many of these are carried out in variations that are the subject of endless discussion and controversy. The literature of surgical research and surgical practice is immense, with single organs of the body often requiring multivolume operative monographs.

Many years ago the physician handled all the medical needs of a family (delivering babies, performing operations, treating illnesses, and caring for accident victims). Today most physicians specialize, and modern surgery has separated into many branches, such as

- Cardiovascular surgery
- Colon and rectal surgery
- Gastrointestinal surgery
- General surgery
- Neurologic surgery
- Obstetric-gynecologic surgery
- Ophthalmologic surgery
- Orthopedic surgery
- Pediatric surgery
- Plastic surgery
- Surgical oncology
- Thoracic surgery
- Trauma surgery
- Urologic surgery

The general surgeon diagnoses and surgically treats diseases and disorders of any body system, especially those unclaimed by other surgical specialists. All surgeons have had some training in general surgery before beginning residency training in a specific surgical specialty. Some general surgeons subspecialize in abdominal, breast, endocrine, vascular, and pediatric general surgery.

This chapter will touch on five of the most common surgical conditions and diseases: cancer of the lung, cancer of the breast, congenital pyloric stenosis, cancer of the colon and rectum, and appendicitis. Special surgical procedures are discussed in other chapters.

A word about differentiating the words cancer and carcinoma. A cancer is a cellular tumor, the natural course of which is fatal. Cancer cells, unlike benign tumor cells, exhibit the properties of invasion and metastasis and are highly anaplastic. Cancers are divided into two broad categories of carcinoma and sarcoma — the first any malignant neoplasm deriving from epithelial tissue and the latter a connective tissue neoplasm.

ANESTHESIA

For major surgery, a general anesthetic is often used. A drug can be administered intravenously or gas can be given that produces unconsciousness and analgesia (Table 18–1). In certain circumstances, a general anesthetic is contraindicated and spinal anesthesia is used. A drug is given by intrathecal injections and provides nerve blockage (Table 18–2) so the patient can feel no pain below a controlled level. The usual anesthesia in these situations is spinal or epidural. Epidural block is used primarily for

259

Table 18–1 ▪ **General Anesthetic Drugs and Gases Commonly Used in Surgical Procedures**

Drug or Gas	Administered by	Some Characteristics and Uses
Nitrous oxide (N₂O)	Inhalation	Nonflammable but supports combustion; rapid induction and recovery; good for brief anesthesia when muscle relaxation is unimportant
Halothane (Fluothane)	Inhalation	Nonexplosive; potent; rapid induction of anesthesia; incomplete muscle relaxation; potentially toxic to liver
Enflurane (Ethrane)	Inhalation	Nonflammable halogenated ether; rapid induction and recovery; supplementary muscle relaxants may be needed
Isoflurane (Forane)	Inhalation	Nonflammable; rapid induction and recovery with minimal aftereffects; profound respiratory depressant
Thiopental sodium (Pentothal sodium)	Intravenous	Used for initial induction prior to gas and for very brief procedures; rapid uptake from circulatory system
Methohexital sodium (Brevital)	Intravenous, rectum	Rapidity, duration, and potency vary; used for induction and brief anesthesia; circulatory and respiratory depressant
Sodium thiamylal (Surital)	Intravenous	Used for induction and for brief anesthesia; ultrashort-acting barbiturate
Ketamine hydrochloride (Ketaject, Ketalar)	Intravenous, intramuscular	Dissociative agent for brief or, with additional doses, for prolonged operations; rapid induction agent; produces amnesia and analgesia; may cause psychologic reactions
Fentanyl and droperidol (Innovar)	Intravenous	Combination narcotic analgesic and tranquilizer used for neuroleptoanesthesia

From Fuller, Joanna. *Surgical Technology; Principles and Practice*, 2nd edition. W. B. Saunders Company, Philadelphia, 1986, p. 63.

obstetric, rectal, and perineal surgery. Spinal block is used to block the nerve roots to the abdomen, pelvis, or lower extremities. For superficial or minor surgical procedures, local anesthesia is used. The drug is injected directly into the tissues at the incision site.

SUTURES (Figure 18–1)

Sutures are associated with sewing tissues but can be used to ligate (tie) bleeding vessels. Table 18–3 lists some of the commonly used suture materials with specific trade names.

Stainless steel sutures come in various sizes, as shown in Table 18–4, and these numbers are dictated for operative reports.

The suture used must be as strong as the tissue it approximates, so different suture materials are used for different parts of the body (Table 18–5).

Various surgical needles are used, depending on the type and depth of the tissue involved.

Many of them are named for the person who invented them. Some traditional names of needles are listed in Table 18–6.

REPRESENTATIVE DISEASES

In 1992, it was estimated that cancer will develop in 870,000 Americans, and that 450,000 will die of the disease.*

Cancer of the Lung

Cancer of the lung is the predominant cause of death from cancer in both men and women. It had always been the prevailing cause of death from cancer among men, but in recent years it has also become the commonest cause of death

*From American Cancer Society. *Facts and Figures, 1992.* New York, 1992.

Table 18–2 ■ **Some Agents and Drugs Often Used by the Anesthesiologist**

For Spinal Anesthesia

Bupivacaine hydrochloride (Marcaine)
Procaine hydrochloride (Novocain)
Tetracaine hydrochloride (Pontocaine)
(These drugs may be weighted with glucose to make them heavier than spinal fluid.)

For Local Anesthesia

Chloroprocaine hydrochloride (Nesacaine)
Procaine hydrochloride (Novocain)
Tetracaine hydrochloride (Pontocaine)
Lidocaine hydrochloride (Xylocaine)
Mepivacaine hydrochloride (Carbocaine)
Bupivacaine hydrochloride (Marcaine)

For Analgesia

Fentanyl
Meperidine hydrochloride (Demerol)
Morphine sulfate
Sufentanil

To Treat Shock and/or Hemorrhage

Whole blood
Human plasma
Plasma or serum albumin
Plasma expander (Dextran)
Vasopressor agents
Electrolyte fluids
Crystalloid solution (Ringer's lactate)

To Raise Blood Pressure

Methoxamine hydrochloride (Vasoxyl)
Ephedrine sulfate
Mephentermine sulfate (Wyamine)
Phenylephrine hydrochloride (Neo-Synephrine)
Levarterenol bitartrate (norepinephrine, Levophed)
Metaraminol bitartrate (Aramine)
Isoproterenol hydrochloride (Isuprel)
Dopamine hydrochloride (Intropin)

To Relax Muscles

Succinylcholine chloride (Anectine, Qualicin)
Decamethonium bromide (Syncurine)
Gallamine triethiodide (Flaxedil)
Tubocurarine chloride, curare
Pancuronium bromide (Pavulon)

From Fuller, Joanna. *Surgical Technology; Principles and Practice*, 2nd edition. W. B. Saunders Company, Philadelphia, 1986, p. 64.

from cancer in women as well. In the past, more men than women smoked and the men smoked heavily. In recent years, however, the gap between the numbers of male and female smokers has narrowed, as has the death rate.

The American Cancer Society estimates that cigarette smoking is responsible for 83 per cent of the cases of cancer of the lung among men and 43 per cent of the cases among women (more than 75 per cent overall.) Those who smoke two or more packs a day have cancer of the lung mortality rates 15 to 25 times greater than those of nonsmokers.

The cancer death rate for male smokers is double that for nonsmokers, and the rate for female smokers is 30 per cent higher than for nonsmokers.

Cell Types ■ The cell types most commonly seen are

1. Epidermoid carcinoma

2. Anaplastic small cell carcinoma

3. Adenocarcinoma

4. Anaplastic undifferentiated large cell carcinoma

5. Bronchoalveolar papillary carcinoma

1. Epidermoid or squamous cell carcinoma accounts for 34 per cent of all proven bronchogenic carcinomas.

This tumor commonly originates in the first bronchus. It grows slowly and has a tendency to form a nodular mass. Proximally, the extension is usually peribronchial so that the lumen of the bronchus is constricted. The tumor metastasizes to the regional lymph nodes later and less extensively than in anaplastic carcinoma or adenocarcinoma.

Central necrosis and cavitation are usually found only in epidermoid carcinoma. If central necrosis occurs, the radiograph shows a thick-walled, shaggy cavity with an air-fluid level. Patients with a necrotizing carcinoma rarely show the toxic clinical picture of patients with pyogenic lung abscess. Epidermoid carcinoma is the most common cavitating tumor of the lung. Since the tumor extends mainly by peribronchial infiltration, the bronchial mucosa does not seem to be invaded as early as in other types of tumors. Consequently, on bronchoscopic examination, the bronchus is seen to be contracted,

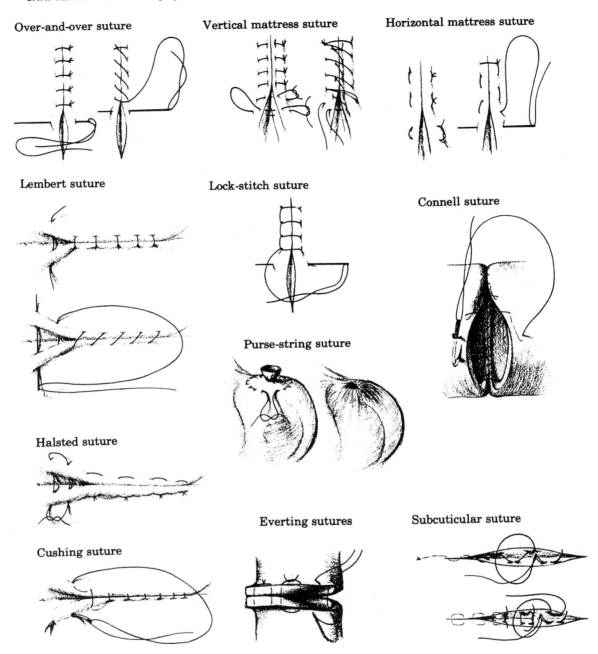

Over-and-over suture

Vertical mattress suture

Horizontal mattress suture

Lembert suture

Lock-stitch suture

Connell suture

Purse-string suture

Halsted suture

Everting sutures

Subcuticular suture

Cushing suture

Figure 18–1
Various types of sutures and knots. (From Nealon, Thomas F. *Fundamental Skills in Surgery*, 3rd ed. W. B. Saunders Company, Philadelphia, 1979.)

Table 18–3 ■ **Suture Materials**

Suture	Absorbable	Material	Manufacturer
Cotton	No	Cotton	Ethicon, Inc.; Davis & Geck
Dacron	No	Polyester fiber	Davis & Geck
Dermalon	No	Nylon	Davis & Geck
Dermalene	No	Linear polyethylene	Davis & Geck
Dexon	Yes	Polyglycolic acid	Davis & Geck
Ethibond	No	Braided polyester	Ethicon, Inc.
Ethiflex	No	Polyester fiber	Ethicon, Inc.
Ethilon	No	Monofilment nylon	Ethicon, Inc.
Flexon	No	Twisted stainless steel	Davis & Geck
Gut, plain	Yes	Collagen	Ethicon, Inc.; Davis & Geck
Gut, chromic	Yes	Collagen, chromic salts	Ethicon, Inc.; Davis & Geck
Mersilene	No	Braided polyethylene fiber	Ethicon, Inc.
Neurolon	No	Monofilament nylon	Ethicon, Inc.
Perma-Hand	No	Silk	Ethicon, Inc.
Polydek	No	Braided polyester	Deknatel
Prolene	No	Polypropylene	Ethicon, Inc.
Stainless Steel	No	Stainless steel	Ethicon, Inc.
Surgilene	No	Polypropylene	Davis & Geck
Surgilon	No	Braided nylon	Davis & Geck
Tevdek	No	Polyester fiber	Deknatel
Ti-Cron	No	Polyester fiber	Davis & Geck
Vicryl	Yes	Polyglactin 910	Ethicon, Inc.

From Fuller, Joanna. *Surgical Technology; Principles and Practice*, 2nd edition. W. B. Saunders Company, Philadelphia, 1986, p. 124.

Table 18–4 ■ **Stainless Steel Suture Sizing**

	Gauge										
B & S	#40	#35	#32	#30	#28	#26	#25	#24	#23	#22	#20
U.S.P.	6-0	5-0	4-0	3-0	2-0	0	1	2	3	4	5

From Fuller, Joanna. *Surgical Technology; Principles and Practice*, 2nd edition. W. B. Saunders Company, Philadelphia, 1986, p. 125.

Table 18–5 ▪ **Recommended Suture Uses and Sizes**

Location/Use	Material	Size	Location/Use	Material	Size
Blood vessels/ ligation	Chromic gut Cotton Silk Polyester	3-0 to 0 3-0 to 0 3-0 to 1 5-0 to 0	Hernia repair	Chromic gut Cotton Silk Polyester Stainless steel	3-0 to 1 2-0 to 1 3-0 to 0 3-0 to 0 5-0 to 3-0
Blood vessels/ anastomosis	Silk Polyester Polyethylene	7-0 to 2-0 6-0 to 2-0 6-0 to 4-0	Intestine	Chromic gut Silk Cotton	5-0 to 2-0 5-0 to 2-0 2-0
Biliary system	Chromic gut Cotton Silk Polyester	3-0 to 0 3-0 to 0 3-0 to 0 4-0 to 0	Joint capsule	Chromic gut Cotton Silk Stainless steel Polyester	4-0 to 0 2-0 3-0 5-0 4-0 to 1
Bone/approximate	Stainless steel Polyester Polyethylene	3-0 to 0 3-0 to 0 4-0 to 0	Kidney	Chromic gut Plain gut	4-0 4-0
Breast	Chromic gut Silk Polyester	3-0 to 0 3-0 to 0 3-0 to 0	Lip	Chromic gut Plain gut	5-0 5-0
Bronchus/ligation	Chromic gut Silk Polyester	0 to 1 3-0 to 0 3-0 to 0	Liver	Silk Chromic gut	2-0, 0 2-0, 0
Cleft palate	Nylon Silk Polyester	3-0 to 2-0 3-0 3-0, 4-0	Muscle	Plain gut Chromic gut Cotton Silk Polyester	3-0 to 0 3-0 to 0 3-0 to 0 3-0 to 0 3-0 to 0
Dura mater	Silk Polyester	6-0 to 4-0 6-0 to 4-0	Nerve/repair	Silk Nylon Polyethylene Stainless steel Polyester	9-0 to 4-0 9-0 to 4-0 6-0 to 4-0 9-0, 6-0 7-0 to 5-0
Eye/cataract	Chromic gut Silk Nylon	7-0, 6-0 9-0 to 4-0 10-0 to 9-0	Pancreas	Cotton Silk	3-0 3-0
Eye/muscle repair	Dacron Chromic gut Plain gut Polyester	5-0 6-0 to 4-0 6-0 to 4-0 5-0	Perineum	Chromic gut	4-0 to 3-0
Eye/lid	Silk Polyester	6-0 to 4-0 6-0, 5-0	Peritoneum	Chromic gut Silk Cotton Plain gut Polyester	3-0 to 0 4-0 to 1 3-0 to 0 0 3-0 to 2-0
Fascia	Chromic gut Silk Stainless steel Polyester Cotton	2-0 to 1 2-0 to 0 4-0 to 3-0 2-0 to 0 2-0, 0	Rectum	Chromic gut	4-0 to 0
Heart	Silk Polyester	6-0 to 2 5-0 to 0			

Table 18–5 ■ **Recommended Suture Uses and Sizes** *Continued*

Location/Use	Material	Size	Location/Use	Material	Size
Skin	Nylon	6-0 to 2-0	Tendon	Polyethylene	5-0 to 3-0
	Polyethylene	5-0 to 3-0	(*Continued*)	Nylon	5-0 to 3-0
	Silk	6-0 to 2-0			
	Polyester	6-0 to 3-0	Thyroid	Chromic gut	3-0 to 0
	Stainless steel	5-0 to 2-0		Cotton	3-0 to 0
				Silk	3-0 to 0
Skull	Stainless steel	5-0 to 4-0		Polyester	3-0 to 0
Stomach/	Chromic gut	5-0 to 2-0	Tonsil	Plain gut	3-0 to 0
anastomosis	Cotton	3-0 to 0			
	Silk	3-0 to 0	Ureter	Chromic gut	4-0
	Polyester	4-0 to 2-0	Urethra	Chromic gut	4-0
Tendon	Stainless steel	5-0 to 3-0	Uterus	Chromic gut	2-0 to 0
	Polyester	5-0 to 3-0			

From Fuller, Joanna. *Surgical Technology; Principles and Practice*, 2nd edition. W. B. Saunders Company, Philadelphia, 1986, p. 127.

and the normal longitudinal folds of the bronchus are accentuated but intact.

2. Undifferentiated small cell carcinoma occurs in approximately 25 per cent of tumors of the lung. The majority of carcinomas begin in the main bronchus. This centrally located, rapidly growing tumor soon forms an irregular mediastinal mass. While spread is in all directions, it is most rapid and most pronounced into the mediastinum and to adjacent regional and distal lymph nodes. This type of tumor is very often inoperable. Even though the lesion can be resected surgically without apparent involvement of lesion or mediastinal nodes, distant metastasis has usually already occurred.

Radiographs of an anaplastic small cell carcinoma demonstrate an irregular mass, either adjacent to or already blending in with the mediastinal shadow.

3. Adenocarcinoma occurs in approximately 25 per cent of tumors of the lung. The incidence of adenocarcinoma is rising faster than that of the other types. The tumor develops more commonly in the peripheral portions of the lung and presents as a well-differentiated mass. Its growth rate is intermediate between that of the

Table 18–6 ■ **Traditional Needle Types**

Name	Description
Ferguson ("Fergie")	Half-circle; delicate tapered shaft
Keith	Straight; medium weight; cutting point
Mayo	Half-circle; heavy; tapered shaft and point
Milner	Straight; delicate; tapered shaft and point
Surgeon's regular (Martin)	Half-circle; medium weight; cutting point, tapered shaft
Trocar	Half-circle; heavy; spear-shaped point, tapered shaft

From Fuller, Joanna. *Surgical Technology: Principles and Practice*, 2nd edition. W. B. Saunders Company, Philadelphia, 1986, p. 128.

rapid-growing anaplastic carcinoma and that of the slow-growing epidermoid carcinoma. Its central growth is less pronounced than its peripheral growth. Heterogeneous spread is more common with this histologic type than with the other two because of the excellent vasculature of the bed in which it originates.

There is a tendency to consider adenocarcinoma of the lung as metastatic carcinoma and either to abandon treatment or to spend a considerable amount of the patient's time and money attempting to find a nonexistent primary. Generally, it is felt that it is not worthwhile to look for a primary lesion unless there is some positive reason to suspect its presence.

4. Undifferentiated large cell carcinoma makes up 16 per cent of tumors of the lung. This cannot be classified readily as either squamous cell carcinoma or adenocarcinoma. The undifferentiated large cell carcinomas are considered anaplastic carcinomas that show no apparent evidence of differentiation. The diagnosis of large cell carcinoma is made primarily on the basis of exclusion of other cell types. The 5-year relative survival rate is only 13 per cent in all patients, regardless of stage at diagnosis. The rate is 41 per cent for cases detected when the disease is still localized, but only 18 per cent of lung cancers are discovered early.

5. Bronchoalveolar carcinoma, also known as alveolar cell carcinoma, occurs infrequently.

Signs and Symptoms ▪ Cancer of the lung can mimic almost any other pulmonary disease. In the majority of patients, when symptoms appear they are referable to the respiratory system. However, the symptoms do not always appear early in the course of the disease. Cough is the first symptom in half the patients in whom cancer of the lung is present and in 90 per cent by the time they consult a physician. The cough is at first nonproductive, but after it becomes productive, it may become sufficiently bothersome to interfere with eating and sleeping, and as a result the patient will begin to lose weight. If the cough worsens, the patient may think it is a cigarette cough and may decide to stop smoking; this will improve the cough temporarily, but after a time the cough will again worsen. The patient may develop some discomfort in the chest, but this should be differentiated from severe pleuritic pain that requires narcotics for relief. The latter symptom has a bad prognosis

because it suggests tumor extension into the chest wall, whereas vague discomfort is more likely due to atelectasis.

The cough will ultimately result in some hemoptysis. The hemoptysis is not massive but merely streaking of the sputum with blood. It is unfortunate that this is an early symptom in only about 8 per cent of patients, for it appears in more than one half of patients before they consult a physician. No other symptom galvanizes the referring physician or the patient into action so readily as the appearance of blood-stained sputum. All adults who have hemoptysis should be examined by bronchoscopy.

In a similar symptom complex, first symptoms are due to pneumonitis. The patient complains of a high temperature and a cough. This is commonly diagnosed as viral pneumonia and antibiotic drugs are prescribed. This respiratory infection persists longer than 2 weeks, within which time ordinary infections should clear. The disease often has barely cleared before it recurs. Consequently, patients who have respiratory infections that persist for an inordinately long period of time, or that seem to recur with unusual frequency, should be suspected of having carcinoma of the lung. As the disease progresses, dyspnea that is probably a result of interference with the function of a portion of the lung will develop.

Wheezing is of variable importance. It can occur when a tumor has partially occluded a bronchus.

Far less common but of more importance is the occasional finding of unilateral wheeze caused by the tumor compressing the bronchus to one lung. Surprisingly, in such a situation, the patient can identify the side of the thorax from which the wheezing emanates. This is confirmed by auscultation.

Hoarseness is noted in a significant number of individuals. This is a distinctive symptom because it is usually evidence that a carcinoma of the left upper lobe has become incurable. The hoarseness is caused by invasion by the tumor of the left recurrent laryngeal nerve as it winds under the arch of the aorta.

The best outlook is for the individual who has no symptoms and in whom the lesion has been picked up either on a routine chest radiograph or as a coincidental finding during some other radiographic examination. The lack of symptoms is usually due to the small size of the lesion. Overholt and associates were able to excise the cancer in all of a group of patients whose lesions were discovered by radiographic survey; in more than two thirds of these, the tumor had not extended beyond the lung.* In the findings of the Pulmonary Neoplasm Research Project, the 70-mm. photofluorogram has proved an equal and in several instances a superior method to radiographs in screening asymptomatic patients for evidence of carcinoma of the lung. On the other hand, 14×17 conventional radiographic films are useful for study of specific problems and for comparison with earlier films.

Surgeons and physicians who have treated cancer of the lung understand that early recognition of the disease offers a better chance of being cured.

In 1980, the American Cancer Society organized a study to recommend to the public what could be done to detect cancer earlier and in a more curable state. The Society had four main concerns. First, there must be good evidence that each test or procedure is medically effective in reducing morbidity or mortality; second, the medical benefits must outweigh the risk; third, the cost of each procedure must be reasonable compared with expected benefits; and finally, the recommended actions must be practical and feasible. A careful review of all well-known programs failed to demonstrate that early detection, with a combination of chest radiographs and sputum cytology, had a beneficial effect on mortality for lung cancer, even in high-risk populations.

The American Cancer Society has changed its policy and does not recommend any tests for the early detection of cancer of the lung in asymptomatic patients. Instead, it urges a focus on primary prevention; helping smokers to stop (or to switch to low tar and nicotine cigarettes) and keeping nonsmokers from starting. People with signs and symptoms of cancer of the lung should consult their physician.

Diagnostic Procedures and Tests

Physical Examination ■ Carcinoma of the lung produces few physical findings unless the disease is in an advanced state. The rare unilat-

*Cited in American Cancer Society. *Facts and Figures, 1992.* New York, 1992.

eral wheeze is important. Attention should be paid to the usual sites of metastasis. Involved nodes may be palpated most commonly in the supraclavicular fossa, with those in the axilla palpated next in frequency. Questioning the patient about whether any new lumps have been noticed may disclose some metastases in areas not usually involved. Liver and complete neurologic examinations should be carried out.

Radiographs ■ A radiograph of the chest is the most important diagnostic test available for the detection of cancer of the lung. Any abnormality of the chest radiograph that might possibly indicate a bronchogenic carcinoma should be followed without delay to a definite diagnosis. The practice of observing these lesions over a period of time has, happily, nearly disappeared. It is an extremely dangerous practice, because all too often the choice of taking periodic films of a patient delays treatment while the lesion goes from a curable to an incurable situation. In the light of our present knowledge, it is unjustifiable to use periodic examination of the chest to evaluate a lesion if there is any reasonable likelihood that the diagnosis might be bronchogenic carcinoma. Administration of radiation therapy to determine whether a lesion is radiosensitive has no place as a diagnostic procedure. Tomography and, to a lesser extent, angiography have assumed a much more important position in the diagnosis and staging of carcinoma of the lung. Furthermore, for opportunities to treat more carcinomas of the lung in a localized stage, more lesions must be seen that are only suggested on a screening plain film and are firmly identifiable by tomography, both PA and lateral. Some surgeons have found tomography and angiography helpful in determining the presence or absence of mediastinal disease preoperatively.

Bronchoscopy ■ Any patient suspected of having a bronchogenic carcinoma should have a pulmonary workup, including both chest radiograph and bronchoscopy. The chest radiograph will not reveal lesions within the mediastinal and hilar shadows. The flexible fiberoptic bronchoscope extends the accessibility of the bronchial tree to the bronchoscopist. Cytology examinations of secretions collected at bronchoscopy have yielded positive results in 40 per cent of patients over and beyond the 25 per cent in whom it was possible to get a positive bronchoscopic biopsy. These results have been improved with the addition of endobronchial brushing.

Mediastinoscopy ■ After bronchoscopy, the next most important diagnostic procedure is mediastinoscopy. Cervical mediastinoscopy is best accomplished by anterior cervical mediastinotomy via a collar incision and a mediastinoscope for the right lung lesions and a second left interspace mediastinotomy for lesions of the left upper lobe or left hilum.

Exploratory Thoracotomy ■ When radiographs, bronchoscopic cytology, and mediastinoscopy fail to establish a definite diagnosis, an exploratory thoracotomy must be undertaken.

Treatment

Resection ■ Surgery remains the most effective therapy for cancer of the lung. Although pneumonectomy was once considered the treatment of choice, it provides no advantage over lobectomy if the tumor can be encompassed with the lesser procedure. Since the survival of patients with Stage I disease is favorable, the risk of these patients developing a second primary tumor is very real. Because the 5-year survival rate after second operations for metachronous lung lesions is 36 per cent, many surgeons are advocating conservative resections for Stage I lung cancer. For further information see Figures 18–2 and 18–3.

Cancer of the Breast

Incidence ■ Since the decline in the death rate due to cancer of the uterus beginning in 1944, cancer of the breast has been the most common cause of death from cancer in women.

In spite of extensive efforts by the medical profession, there has been very little change in the death rate from breast cancer. Recent figures in the General Accounting Office report on breast cancer, 1971–1991, show an increased *incidence* of breast cancer in this 20-year period.

Only 10 years ago National Cancer Institute officials were setting the goal of a 50 per cent reduction rate in death from carcinoma of the breast; but the death rate is in fact increasing. In 1991, an American woman's chances of having a malignant tumor of the breast were double what they were in 1940.

Those women with a history of the following are at high risk for developing cancer of the breast.

1. Delivery of first full-term child after age 30 years. The risk of developing cancer of the breast increases with the age at which a woman bears her first full-term child. Women who are first parous before age 18 years have a risk of developing breast cancer that is approximately 0.3 times the risk of those whose first delivery of a full-term child is age 35 years or older.

2. Cancer of the breast in other family members.

3. Repeated exposure to ionizing radiation, including atomic explosions.

4. Chronic mastitis.

5. Long-term treatment with estrogen.

Thus, the etiologic background of breast cancer may be thought of as having a triangular configuration, a three-sided aspect. On the one side are the genetic factors of race, ethnic background, and family history. On the second side are endocrine factors including the presence of ovaries, the adverse effects of late pregnancy or multigravidity, and the increased incidence of the disease at menopause. Finally, on the third side of this etiologic triangle are the carcinogenic factors, including such things as external ionizing radiation. Probably the most important in local carcinogenesis is the distinct possibility that a virus is involved.

Classification ■ Nuclei of tumor cells have been characterized according to their differentiation into three nuclear grades. Contrary to conventional methods of grading, Grade I represents the most anaplastic nuclear appearance and Grade III the most well-differentiated. In 1000 cases of the National Surgical Adjuvant Breast Program (NSABP), only 8.5 per cent of tumors exhibited well-differentiated nuclei (Grade III), and about one third were considered to be poorly differentiated. Different investigators found varying degrees of tumor necrosis in 60 per cent of 1539 National Surgical Adjuvant Breast Program patients, which correlated with increased rates of treatment failure.

Spread ■ The spread of cancer through the breast has been summarized by Haagensen as the following:

1. Direct infiltration into the breast parenchyma

2. Along mammary ducts

3. By breast lymphatics

Direct infiltration tends to occur by ramifying projections, which give a characteristic stellate appearance on gross examination (lack of circumscription). If allowed to continue, direct involvement of the overlying skin or deep pectoral fascia may occur.

In regional spread, tumors spread via the lymphatics to the axillary, internal mammary, and supraclavicular lymph nodes. In approximately 40 to 50 per cent of patients with cancer of the breast, the cancer spreads to axillary lymph nodes, with axillary nodal involvement directly related to the size of the primary tumor.

Patients with histologically negative axillary nodes have a markedly improved survival rate compared with patients with histologically positive nodal involvement. Furthermore, patients with one to three positive axillary nodes do better than patients with four or more positive nodes. Haagensen reported a 76 per cent 10-year survival with histologically negative axillary lymph nodes and a 48 per cent 10-year survival if the nodes were positive. In those patients who had one to three positive nodes, there was a 63 per cent 10-year survival, which fell to 27 per cent when four or more nodes were positive. At the current level of our understanding, the presence of spread to the axillary nodes represents the single most important prognostic factor for patients with cancer of the breast.

Even larger-sized lesions have a relatively good prognosis if the axillary nodes are negative. The incidence of axillary nodal involvement is followed at a distance by internal maxillary, supraclavicular, and intercostal nodal involvement.

Age has been found to be the only good correlation with prognosis in patients in the National Surgical Adjuvant Breast Program.

Factors in Recurrence ■ In a prospective study of factors that might be helpful in predicting early (2-year) recurrence of breast cancer, the Breast Cancer Group found degrees of differentiation of tumor, blood vessel invasion, patient age, tumor size, and axillary lymph node status to be of value.

In an effort to identify the 20 to 30 per cent of patients with early cancer of the breast whose disease recurs in the decade after operation, my colleagues and I classified the risk of cancer group of T1N0M0* tumors on the basis of four histologic characteristics:

■ Poor cytologic differentiation

■ Lymphatic permeation

■ Blood vessel invasion

■ Invasion of the tumor into the surrounding soft tissues (poor circumscription)

Tumors were considered high-grade (poor cytologic differentiation) when there were variations in nuclear size and chromatic clumping, a high rate of mitotic activity, irregular nuclear membranes, and a single cell pattern of invasion (except in cases of lobular carcinoma). This was present in 22 per cent of patients. Four of the recurrences occurred in the 18 T1N0M0 and in the 14 T2N0M0 tumors with that isolated marker. The diagnosis of lymphatic permeation based on the presence of nests of tumor cells within lymphatic spaces was the most common characteristic present in 36 per cent of the tumors. It occurred in 34 patients as an isolated marker; four of these tumors recurred. Special stains were not used to determine blood vessel invasion. The pathologist made this diagnosis on the basis of tumor thrombi within the lumen or invasion of the walls of the blood vessel by malignant cells. It was present in 14 per cent of cases. Blood vessel invasion usually occurred in combination with one or more of the other characteristics in the more malignant tumors and was found as an isolated marker in only one T2 tumor that recurred.

Tumors were considered poorly circumscribed when there was an irregular pattern of invasion of the carcinoma into adjacent tissues. The evaluation was based on both gross and microscopic appearances of the tumor. This was present in 36 per cent. It was an isolated marker in 57 tumors, 12 of which recurred.

Each of these determinants has equal prog-

---

*In the TNM classification, tumor is T, N is nodes, and M is metastasis.

ST. VINCENT'S HOSPITAL
153 West 11th Street
New York, NY 10011-0000

OPERATIVE REPORT

PATIENT: George Grayson   DATE: March 5, 1994

HOSPITAL NO: 93-12-85   ROOM NO: Star 4

SURGEON: Thomas F. Nealon, M.D.

ASSISTANT: Howard Smithson, M.D.

ANESTHESIOLOGIST: Robert Green, M.D.

PREOPERATIVE DIAGNOSIS: Carcinoma of the right lung.

POSTOPERATIVE DIAGNOSIS: Same.

OPERATION: Right pneumonectomy.

PROCEDURE: The patient was placed on the operating table in a supine
position. He was anesthetized with intravenous sodium Pentothal. An
endotracheal tube was inserted, attached to the anesthesia machine and
anesthesia was continued with endotracheal general anesthesia. The patient
was turned on his left side. The skin of the thorax was prepared with Betadine
and draped with sterile linen. The chest was opened by way of a right
posterolateral skin incision over the course of the right fifth rib. The rib was
removed subperiosteally and the chest was entered through the periosteal bed.
The ribs were retracted with a Finochietto self retaining rib retractor. The lung
was fully expanded. There was no free fluid in the chest. The lung was
palpated. There was a 2 cm. mass in the right main bronchus, 2 cm. beyond
the carina. This was not adherent to the chest wall or any of the mediastinal
structures. Careful examination of the lung and the mediastinal structures
showed no evidence of malignancy in the lungs. Since we already had a tissue
diagnosis from the preoperative bronchoscopy, it was not necessary to do
another bronchoscopy. We, therefore, decided that the patient could tolerate
an operation and that operation could and should remove all the tumor in the
chest.

(continued)

Figure 18–2
An example of an operative report on a patient having a right pneumonectomy for carcinoma of the right lung.

There were no adhesions from the lung to the chest wall. There were six normal appearing lymph nodes in the mediastinum, near the main bronchus. These were swept out onto the lung. The superior branch of the right pulmonary vein was clamped and ligated with 2-0 ligatures and divided. This allowed full access to the right pulmonary artery which was, ligated and divided proximal to the tumor.

The tumor involved the right main bronchus and extended into the adjacent lung. It was decided to divide the right main bronchus at the level of the carina. The remaining right pulmonary vein was then ligated and divided. Lung clamps were attached to the right lung tissue and traction cleared this from the carina. The extraneous tissue, six lymph nodes and the bronchial vessels were clamped, ligated, and divided. A 3-0 silk suture was placed in the trachea above the point of division. A small incision was made and the bronchus further divided with intermittent cutting and suturing of the bronchus until it was fully divided. This made it possible to lift the lung free of the chest. Any oozing points were clamped and ligated with interrupted silk sutures. The mediastinum was examined for any oozing. The closure of the bronchus was checked by filling the chest cavity with sterile physiological saline and having the anesthesiologist exert pressure on the anesthesia circuit. No bubbles came from the bronchial stump, indicating the closure was air tight.

A flap of pleura was raised and sutured over the bronchial closure to reinforce it. The entire empty hemithorax was examined for residual tumor or persistent bleeding. There was none.

A rib approximator was inserted and attached to the ribs on either side of the thoracotomy, above and below the remaining ribs adjacent to the thoracotomy. The ratchet attachment was closed until the edges of the wound were brought together and the ribs sutured together. Hemostasis was established and the chest wound was closed with interrupted silk sutures after the self-retaining retractor had been removed from the chest.

_____

THOMAS F. NEALON, M.D.

TFN:bp
D: 3/5/94
T: 3/6/94

Figure 18–2 *Continued*

ST. VINCENT'S HOSPITAL
153 West 11th Street
New York, NY 10011-0000

PATHOLOGY REPORT

PATIENT: George Grayson   DATE: March 5, 1994

HOSPITAL NO: 93-12-85   ROOM NO: Star 4

PHYSICIAN: Thomas F. Nealon, M.D.   PATHOLOGY NO: 14-58-34

SPECIMEN SUBMITTED: Right lung tissue.

GROSS DESCRIPTION: The specimen consists of the right lung. The entire right lung is intact. All major vessels have been ligated with interrupted silk sutures and are intact. The main bronchus showed evidence of being cross clamped by a crushing clamp. This has been removed two cuts below the division of bronchus.

This is a malignant tumor, 0.5 cm. in diameter emerging from the bronchus from lung. There were no other masses in the lung. The overall tumor was 4 cm. Six normal appearing lymph nodes are attached to the bronchus. The point of the division of the tumor by the bronchoscopic biopsy was evident. The point of section looked malignant.

1.   The tumor was made up of squamous cell carcinoma of the lung, intermediate grade. The tumor was well encapsulated. There was no evidence of blood vessel invasion.

2.   Six lymph nodes without evidence of tumor.

3.   The tumor was totally removed.

THOMAS TALBOT, M.D.
PATHOLOGIST

TT:bp
D: 3/5/94
T: 3/6/94

Figure 18-3
An example of a pathology report typed in the format used by St. Vincent's Hospital.

nostic impact, which was cumulative, as they occurred together. This analysis made it possible to subdivide the node-negative T1N0M0 and T2N0M0 lesions into (a) a low-risk group with none of these characteristics and a 99 per cent 10-year, disease-free survival rate, (b) an intermediate risk group (T1N0M0 +, T2N0M0, and T2N0M0 ++, +++, and ++++) with only a 30 per cent disease-free survival at 10 years. Those tumors with more markers recurred earlier, and the patients died sooner than in the other two groups. This group of tumors is obviously more virulent than other early cancers of the breast.

The 5-year survival rate for localized breast cancer has risen from 78 per cent in the 1940s to 92 per cent today. If the breast cancer is in situ (not invasive), survival rate approaches 100 per cent. If the cancer has spread regionally, however, the survival rate is 71 per cent. For persons with distant metastasis, the survival rate is 18 per cent.

Diagnosis

Signs and Symptoms ▪ The first indication that a woman might have cancer of the breast is a *lump* in the breast. Usually, this is found by the woman herself. It may be found as part of a routine breast self-examination or felt by the patient while bathing or dressing. Pain is not common and rarely severe.

Nipple discharge is the second most common sign. Retraction or distortion of the nipple and dimpling of the skin are rare complaints but can be indicative of cancer. Skin lesions — ulcers, peau d'orange, dimpling, or redness — are symptoms of late disease.

History ▪ A careful history of the patient and her complaint is taken, beginning with her age. It includes any previous problems with her breasts, menstrual problems, and family history of breast disease and cancer as well as the reason for the examination. The complaint is discussed in detail. The patient may have noted enlarged axillary or supraclavicular nodes, edema of the skin, redness or ulceration — all indicative of more advanced disease. Pain may be due to metastasis to the spinal column.

Examination of the Breast ▪ Careful examination of the breast is done on every patient. The breasts are carefully examined with the patient sitting facing the physician in the following positions: (1) with her arms at her side; (2) with her arms elevated; (3) with her hands pressed firmly against her hips; (4) bending forward.

The physician then palpates the breast by pressing the breast against the chest wall, palpates the more protuberant part of the breast by pressing it between the flat of the fingers using both hands, and palpates for supraclavicular nodes and axillary nodes. To examine the axillae, the physician pushes the fingers into the axilla and has the patient drop her arm by her side while palpating high in the axilla, pressing anything suspicious against her chest wall. The patient is then examined in a supine position on the examining table, a pillow placed under the shoulder of the side to be examined. The patient is asked to place her hand on that side, under her head, and the breast is examined against the firm pectoralis major muscle. Using the balls of the fingers, the physician carefully and lightly presses the breast tissue against the chest wall. Using this technique, the entire breast can be carefully examined, a small portion at a time, in a clockwise direction. Next, the nipple is gently palpated and then squeezed to see whether there is any discharge. The process is repeated on the other breast. Finally, a search is made for any palpable supraclavicular nodes, axillary nodes, or an enlarged liver.

Breast Self-Examination ▪ When there is no evidence of disease, the physician should instruct the patient in the technique of breast self-examination, which the patient should perform *monthly*. In the menstruating patient, the examination should be done immediately after completion of her period. If she has ceased to menstruate, it should be done on approximately the same day each month. The American Cancer Society has developed a pamphlet to help women examine their breasts.

Differential Diagnosis ▪ The malignant lump is usually solitary, unilateral, solid to hard, irregular, poorly delineated, nonmobile, painless, and nontender. When the tumor is seen at an early stage, it frequently will not have grown enough to have characteristic findings. If the tumor has grown enough to have these findings, it probably has already spread. In its early stages, it is firm and barely palpable. As it grows, it is hard and somewhat irregular and may involve the overlying skin or underlying muscle and fascia. With progression, hard lymph nodes appear in the axilla. The nipple may retract, distend, or produce a bloody discharge. The overlying skin may dimple. Eczema on the nipple may really be Paget's disease, carcinoma, or inflammatory carcinoma in which the skin edema is not really an infection but carcinoma in the lymphatics of the skin.

Mammography ▪ This is a radiographic technique that has made it possible to identify malignant lesions that cannot be felt. If the lesion is malignant, the mammogram will reveal masses that show some of the following characteristics:

▪ Concave or scalloped edges

▪ Very fine calcification within the tumor

▪ Thickening of the skin over the tumor

Mammography is able to identify lesions that are too small to palpate. This is resolved by marking the tumor with needles under radioscopic guidance prior to operation. Cancer of the breast detected by mammography tends to be at an extremely early stage and affords the possibility of high cure rates.

There has been concern on the part of some physicians that regular mammograms are dangerous owing to radiation. Because of this, the American Cancer Society has made the following recommendations:

1. All women over 20 years of age should perform breast self-examination monthly.
2. Women aged 20 to 40 years should have a breast physical examination every 3 years, and women over 40 years of age should have a breast physical examination every year.
3. Women should have a baseline mammogram between ages 35 and 40 years.
4. Women under 50 years of age should consult their personal physicians about the need for mammography in their individual cases.
5. Women over age 50 years should have a mammogram every year (low base, 0.5 rad total).
6. Women with personal or family histories of breast cancer should consult their physicians about the value of more frequent examinations or about the need to begin mammography before the age of 50 years.
7. Women should have a mammogram any time it is needed for better diagnosis.

Treatment
Localized Cancer of the Breast ▪ Surgical excision is the treatment of choice for localized cancer of the breast. This was not always the case. The outlook was considered hopeless until 1894 when good results were reported in the treatment of cancer of the breast by radical mastectomy. This consisted of removal of the entire breast, the pectoralis major muscle, the pectoralis minor muscle, and all the axillary contents. All these cases were incurable, but the operation lowered the high (82 per cent) local recurrence rate and decreased the morbidity. This encouraged other surgeons to use radical mastectomy to treat breast cancer. As more patients were treated with radical mastectomy, they began to arrive with earlier and more curable lesions. This operation was considered standard initial therapy for "primary operable breast cancer" for 8 decades.

For further information on breast cancer, see Figures 18–4 and 18–5.

Pyloric Stenosis

Infantile Hypertrophic Pyloric Stenosis ▪ This is an abnormality of the pyloric musculature that causes gastric outlet obstruction in infancy. It is characterized by projectile vomiting and a demonstrable pyloric thickening. It is the most common surgical disorder producing vomiting in infancy. The incidence is approximately 3 per 1000 live births in the United States. Known predisposing factors include male sex, firstborn child, susceptible rate, and known family history.

Signs and Symptoms ▪ Progressive vomiting, gastric waves, and a palpable pyloric tumor constitute the diagnostic triad of pyloric stenosis. The vomiting may begin insidiously in the newborn period, increasing gradually to almost complete obstruction at the second to the fifth week of life. In the "textbook course," vomiting begins at 2 to 3 weeks of age and becomes progressively more severe.

The vomiting is forceful and projectile, fluid often being forced through the infant's nose and mouth. The infant becomes malnourished and the weight becomes stationary and then decreases, often below birth weight.

As one watches the abdomen after a feeding, when the stomach is full, contractions of the stomach proceed across the abdomen from left to right. These gastric contractions finally termi-

ST. VINCENT'S HOSPITAL
153 West 11th Street
New York, NY 10011-0000

OPERATIVE REPORT

PATIENT: Gloria Breen   DATE: 3/3/94

HOSPITAL NO: 94-36-31   ROOM NO: 1024

SURGEON: Thomas F. Nealon, M.D.

ASSISTANT: John Haines, M.D.

ANESTHESIOLOGIST: Richard Ives, M.D.

PREOPERATIVE DIAGNOSIS: Breast biopsy on 3/1/94
                                 reported as adenocarcinoma
                                 of the left breast, low grade.

POSTOPERATIVE DIAGNOSIS: Adenocarcinoma of the
                                 breast, low grade.

OPERATION: Quadrantectomy of left
                                 breast.
                                 Left axillary node dissection.

PROCEDURE: The patient was placed on the operating table with her left arm extended on an arm board. Anesthesia was induced with intravenous sodium Pentothal. An endotracheal tube was inserted and anesthesia was continued with endotracheal inhalation anesthesia. The chest, the left shoulder, and arm were prepared with Betadine and draped with sterile linen.

The incision was transverse which excised the scar of the biopsy incision as well as the operative field of the biopsy operation and extended into the incision laterally into the axilla. The skin overlying the breast was raised with subcutaneous dissection. This main incision was carried down to the pectoralis major and then swept laterally at the level of the pectoralis major muscle. When this reached the lateral edge of the pectoralis major, the muscle was raised and the under surface of the pectoralis major exposed. The dissection was carried over the under surface of the pectoralis major muscle

(continued)

Figure 18–4
An example of an operative report on a patient undergoing quadrantectomy of the left breast, typed in the format used by St. Vincent's Hospital.

Gloria Breen   Page two
94-36-31

until the pectoralis minor muscle was exposed. This was dissected laterally and retracted medially. All of the tissue in the exposed axilla was dissected free and excised after retraction to open the axilla.

We found nothing that could be considered malignant. There were no lymph nodes which could be identified. The area was dissected free up to the apex of the axilla and was removed en masse.

Hemostasis was established. A Jackson-Pratt suction apparatus was led from the site of the removed breast through the axilla and through a hole in the lateral flap of the closure. The wound was closed with interrupted silk sutures. The Jackson-Pratt drain was attached to the bulb which created continuous suction. This was taped to the skin of the thorax. The operative incision was covered with sterile gauze.

The patient tolerated the operation well and left the operating room in good condition. The operative specimen was sent to the pathology laboratory.

_____
THOMAS F. NEALON, M.D.

TFN:bp
D: 3/3/94
T: 3/4/94

Figure 18–4 *Continued*

nate with a burst of vomiting, and at that time palpation of the epigastrium above the umbilicus and slightly to the right will most likely disclose an abdominal mass that can be moved up and down and is the thickened pyloric musculature. This so-called tumor is described as an "olive" and may measure 2 cm. in length and 1.5 cm. in diameter. It is easiest felt with the stomach emptied either by earlier vomiting or by placing a gastric tube into the stomach to evacuate its contents. Palpation of the tumor when the infant is anesthetized prior to laparotomy verifies the clinical finding and improves the ability to palpate the "olive" in the future.

Diagnostic Procedures and Tests ■ Radiographic examination, while not often necessary, is indicated in those infants in whom pyloric stenosis is suspected but in whom the tumor cannot be palpated. The diagnostic features of the radiograph are an enlarged stomach, which may or may not empty easily and quickly, but which upon emptying discloses an elongated, slightly curved, narrowed pyloric channel with the so-called shoulder sign. The lack of emptying does not guarantee the diagnosis of pyloric stenosis, and the stomach may not always be enlarged. The narrowed, curved pyloric channel, the "string" sign, is essential.

Nonoperative Treatment ■ It has been known for many years that certain infants with mild vomiting and proven pyloric stenosis will improve over a period of time with the adminis-

ST. VINCENT'S HOSPITAL
153 West 11th Street
New York, NY 10011-0000

PATHOLOGY REPORT

PATIENT: Gloria Breen   DATE: 3/3/94

HOSPITAL NO: 94-36-31   ROOM NO: 1024

PHYSICIAN: Thomas F. Nealon, M. D.   PATHOLOGY NO: 13-23-16

SPECIMEN SUBMITTED: Tissue from quadrantectomy and axillary node dissection.

GROSS DESCRIPTION: The specimen consisted of a partial mastectomy specimen. The areola was not included. There is a sutured incision which was the site of an earlier biopsy. This is encompassed in the specimen. The cavity of that opening does not extend to the surface. The excision encompassed the entire biopsy operative field as well as the incision.

There is normal appearing breast tissue adherent to the skin. Fibrous tissue is adherent to the major specimen and represents the dissection from the axilla.

 Six normal appearing lymph nodes were included. There is no residual carcinoma in this specimen or the six nodes.

IMPRESSION: Quadrantectomy specimen including six normal lymph nodes.

_____
JOSEPH MILLER, M.D.
PATHOLOGIST

JM:bp
D: 3/3/94
T: 3/4/94

Figure 18–5
An example of a pathology report on tissue obtained from a partial mastectomy.

tration of antispasmodics such as atropine methylonitrate (Eumydrin) or scopolamine methylonitrate (Skopyl). The prolonged course and high failure rate of nonsurgical treatment and the side effects of drugs, which may include ileus with overdosage, make the surgical treatment of pyloric stenosis preferable when adequate facilities are available.

Surgical Procedures ▪ Pyloromyotomy (Figures 18–6 and 18–7) is usually done through a

ST. VINCENT'S HOSPITAL
153 West 11th Street
New York, NY 10011-0000

OPERATIVE REPORT

PATIENT: Frank Chasen   DATE: March 12, 1994

HOSPITAL NO: 93-23-56   ROOM NO: 493

SURGEON: Thomas F. Nealon, M. D.

ASSISTANT: James Gray, M.D.

ANESTHESIOLOGIST: Jonathan Wager, M.D.

PREOPERATIVE DIAGNOSIS: Infantile hypertrophic pyloric
                                   stenosis.

POSTOPERATIVE DIAGNOSIS: Same.

OPERATION DIAGNOSIS: Pyloromyotomy.

PROCEDURE: The baby was placed in the supine position on the operating
table. A nasogastric tube was passed and with gentle suction, the gastric
contents were evacuated. An endotracheal tube was passed and anesthesia
carried out with endotracheal anesthesia. The abdomen was opened through a
transverse abdominal incision and made to the rectus muscle which was split
vertically. The anesthesiologist inflated the stomach with the nasogastric tube.
That made it easy to palpate and adjust the position of the pylorus. The
pylorus was held between the thumb and third finger allowing the index to
adjust the position of the pylorus. The aim was to divide the hypertrophied
gastric wall down to the mucosa; the avasculature area of the pyloric tumor.

The anterior superior surface was identified and the serosal incision begun
just proximal to the pyloric vein. The incision was extended back beyond
hypertrophy to the normal gastric wall. Care was taken to go no deeper than

(continued)

Figure 18–6

An example of an operative report on an infant with infantile hypertrophic pyloric stenosis undergoing a pyloromyotomy.

Frank Chasen   Page two
Hospital No: 93-23-56

the muscularis. Some of the air in the stomach was forced into the duodenum by sewing the stomach. Air readily passed into the duodenum. There was no evidence of perforation. The stomach was returned to the peritoneal cavity, pylorus first.

Hemostasis was established and the abdominal wound was closed with interrupted 5-0 silk sutures.

                                    THOMAS F. NEALON, M.D.

TM:sb
D: 3/12/94
T: 3/13/94

Figure 18-6 *Continued*

transverse skin incision followed by vertical splitting of the right rectus muscle and fascia. Of the various instruments devised to separate the muscle fibers without perforating the duodenum, the Benson pyloric forceps is widely used. A superficial V extension at the duodenal end of the myotomy incision to prevent duodenal perforation has been suggested. If perforation occurs during the myectomy, it is usually recognized and can be repaired in a number of ways. The preference is to close the perforation transversely with interrupted 5-0 silk sutures and rely upon gastric suction for 2 hours postoperatively to decompress the stomach. In the past, the perforation has been closed by suturing the omentum over it. Pyloromyotomy for infantile hypertrophic pyloric stenosis has proved to be an efficient, safe treatment with minimal mortality and morbidity and lasting relief of symptoms.

Cancer of the Colon and Rectum

After skin cancer, malignant tumors of the colon and rectum are currently the most common malignancy in the United States.

Carcinoma of the colon varies considerably in size, radiographic appearance, and malignant potential. Although the usual adenocarcinoma of the large bowel is a bulky tumor with well-defined edges surrounding a central ulcerated area, some adenocarcinomas may develop as pedunculated polypoid lesions that may be interpreted as benign polyps on radiographic evaluation. The usual carcinoma of the large bowel is well differentiated. The poorly differentiated, anaplastic tumors generally are more malignant and more invasive. Some pathologists believe that anaplastic tumors showing colloid or mucinous change are more malignant in their behavior, particularly in young people. These growths spread by direct invasion of the bowel wall through lymphatic and venous channels with direct extension to other organs and transperitoneally. Histologic evidence indicates that spread of carcinoma cells in the bowel wall infrequently extends beyond 2.5 cm. on either side of the growth.

Carcinoma of the colon limited to the bowel wall without lymph node metastasis bears a good prognosis when adequately excised. When lymph nodes are involved in the immediate area

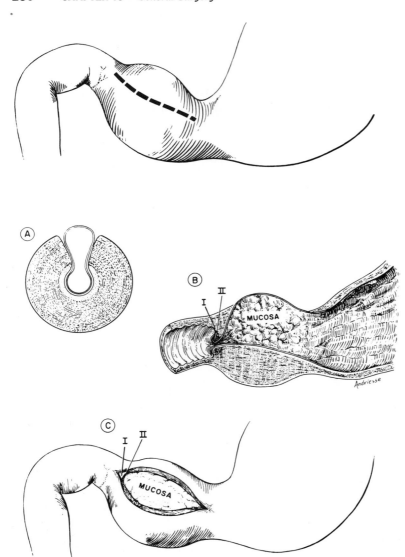

Figure 18–7
Pyloromyotomy, the operation that divides the muscle fibers down to the mucosa, relieving the obstruction. (From Holder, Thomas, and M. W. Keith Ashcraft. *Pediatric Surgery*. W. B. Saunders Company, Philadelphia, 1980.)

of the tumor, prognosis is only fair. Extensive node involvement, especially to distant sites, generally indicates a very poor prognosis.

Extension beyond the serosa of the bowel wall is of prognostic significance, since it may lead to the implantation of tumor cells in the periosteum and in adjacent structures. Perforation of the wall of the bowel with abscess formation further increases the likelihood of incurability. Carcinomas of the cecum tend to be less invasive and have a lower percentage of lymph node metastasis. Carcinomas of the rectum and rectosig-

moid areas infiltrate the bowel wall more rapidly and frequently metastasize.

In the past 30 years, the location of colorectal cancer seems to be shifting from the distal 25 cm. of the colon to more proximal locations, such as the right colon. This could call for more frequent surveillance by barium enema and colonoscopy of the large bowel proximal to the rectosigmoid area. Fiberoptic sigmoidoscopy has replaced the rigid 25-cm. scope for evaluation of the distal 6 cm. of the small bowel.

Predisposing Factors ■ Abundant evidence

strongly supports the theory that familial multiple polyposis, villous polyps, adenomatous polyps, and ulcerative colitis predispose people to the development of carcinoma of the colon. In all four conditions, epithelial proliferation is marked.

Decompression and Staged Operations ▪ Carcinoma of the colon causing complete intestinal obstruction, with an occasional exception, requires immediate operative decompression of the colon. Malignancy of the large bowel usually affects the elderly. Acute obstruction tremendously increases morbidity and mortality. Statistics indicate that if patients with carcinoma of the large bowel become obstructed and require emergency treatment, the mortality rate is more than doubled compared with that for elective surgery before obstruction. Carcinoma of the left colon accounts for at least 90 per cent of the cases of acute intestinal obstruction of the colon from malignancy. This is because carcinoma in this part of the large bowel is common, the bowel contents are more solid, and the tumors tend to encircle the bowel.

Diagnostic Procedures and Tests ▪ Preoperative radiographic examination may give valuable information. A plain survey film of the abdomen taken in the supine, erect, and decubitus positions will usually indicate the location of the obstruction in the colon. Other valuable information concerning the competency of the ileocecal valve, the presence or absence of a massively distended cecum, and the size of the small bowel may also be gained. In certain selected cases, the judicious use of a careful barium enema may be needed to confirm the diagnosis. Barium should not be allowed to flow along the constricting lesion, nor should it be given by mouth.

The appropriate corrections of fluid and electrolyte imbalances and blood volume deficiency should be undertaken before subjecting the patient to anesthesia and operation. This can be done in a relatively short time — if necessary, in a matter of several hours.

Some form of proximal intubation should be used, and the stomach is emptied of its contents before anesthesia is begun. The presence of a Miller-Abbott tube in the intestinal tract is desirable and useful. However, laparotomy and decompression should not be unduly delayed while attempts are made to maneuver the tube through the pylorus. If the tube is in the stomach at the time of laparotomy, occasionally it may be directed by the surgeon into the small bowel.

Once the patient is anesthetized, the surgeon's obligation is to release the acute obstruction while learning as much about the offending lesion as possible. Exploration of the abdomen may be unwise in terms of the patient's condition and postoperative course. These patients are best treated by preliminary colostomy or cecostomy and sometimes by both colostomy and cecostomy, to be followed later by resection of the growth.

Resection ▪ Barring evident blood-borne metastasis to the lung, the absence of lymphatic metastasis is generally the best index of prolonged survival. Statistical evidence indicates that blood vessel invasion is less important as a prediction of death from carcinoma than lymph node metastasis.

When colorectal cancer is detected in an early localized stage, the 5-year survival rates are 90 per cent for colon cancer and 83 per cent for rectal cancer. After the cancer has spread regionally to involve adjacent organs or lymph nodes, the survival rates drop to 60 per cent and 50 per cent, respectively. Survival rates for persons with distant metastases are less than 7 per cent.

In selecting the appropriate operation for malignant lesions of the colon and rectum, a procedure should be planned that will remove as much of the important lymphatic drainage as possible. As in other operations, the magnitude of the procedure must be compatible with the patient's ability to tolerate it. Radical resections of two or three of the main arteries of the colon may not be well tolerated by the older patient and a compromise must be reached (Figure 18–8).

Risks and Prognosis ▪ Mortality figures for colon operations vary according to the type of patients treated. Operative mortality tends to be higher in the older, poor-risk patients, particularly when they present with an intestinal obstruction. At one center, operative mortality for colostomy and polypectomy was 0 to 3 per cent. If the colon was resected (Figure 18–9) for benign adenomas, operative mortality was 2 per cent. If the resection was done for fibroadenocarcinoma, mortality has been 3 per cent.

Survival for 5 years following resection of the colon for carcinoma is variously reported from 34 per cent with lymph node metastasis to 68 per

ST. VINCENT'S HOSPITAL
153 West 11th Street
New York, NY 10011-0000

OPERATIVE REPORT

PATIENT: Sharon Crawford   DATE: May 18, 1994

HOSPITAL NO: 74-34-65   ROOM NO: Star 9

SURGEON: Thomas F. Nealon, M.D.

ASSISTANT: John Keller, M.D.

ANESTHESIOLOGIST: Sherman Howell, M.D.

PREOPERATIVE DIAGNOSIS: Carcinoma of the transverse colon.
Two weeks ago the patient was
operated on at this hospital for an
intestinal obstruction which was
due to a carcinoma of the transverse
colon. A bar colostomy was
performed. In the interim period,
the colon was cleaned out
proximally and distally. No other
lesions were found.

POSTOPERATIVE DIAGNOSIS: Same.

OPERATION: Colectomy.
Colocolostomy.

PROCEDURE: The patient was placed on the
operating table in a supine position.
Anesthesia was begun with intravenous sodium Pentothal. An endotracheal
tube was inserted and inhalation endotracheal anesthesia was continued
throughout the operation.
(continued)

Figure 18–8
An example of an operative report on a patient having a colectomy and a colocolostomy.

Sharon Crawford   Page two
Hospital No: 74-34-65

There was a functioning transverse colostomy in the right upper quadrant.
The abdomen was doubly prepped and draped. Using sharp dissection the
colostomy was freed from the skin of the abdomen. This merely freed the
colostomy from the adhered abdominal skin. The abdomen was not entered.
The colostomy wall was closed with interrupted silk sutures. Drapes were
removed and a full new abdominal prep carried out.

The colon was freed with sharp dissection from the abdominal wall opening in
the peritoneal cavity. This allowed the closed colostomy to drop into the
peritoneal cavity

The entire peritoneal cavity was examined. The liver was free of any tumor.
The entire large and small bowel was examined. There was a 4 cm. irregular
tumor in the mid-portion of the transverse colon encircling the colon. There
was no evidence of any more tumor in the abdomen. The mesenteries were all
clear of tumor. It was decided to resect en masse the tumor, the hepatic and
splenic flexures, the transverse mesocolon and the omentum.

 The omentum was freed, the midcolic artery was divided within 1 cm. of the
superior mesenteric artery. The arcade of the hepatic flexure was divided
where it came off the right colic artery. On the left side the arcade was divided
at the left colic artery. Hemostasis was established. It was possible to bring
the remaining right colon and left colon together in an end-to-end
anastomosis. A very adequate anastomosis was made.

The rents in the mesentery were closed. Hemostasis was established. The
wound was closed with interrupted silk sutures. The specimen was examined.
There was an adequate margin. No lymph nodes were noted.

The patient tolerated the procedure well and left the operating room in good
condition. Patient discharged from the hospital with wound well healed and
bowels moving satisfactorily.

                              THOMAS F. NEALON, M.D.

TFN:ssb
D: 5/18/94
T: 5/19/94

Figure **18–8** *Continued*

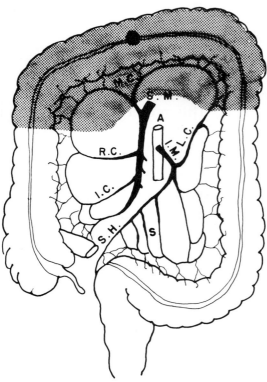

Figure 18-9
The extent of a colon resection for centrally located lesions of the transverse colon. (From Nealon, Thomas F. *Management of the Patient with Cancer.* W. B. Saunders Company, Philadelphia, 1986.)

cent without lymph node metastasis. Survival is slightly higher following right colon resection than after resection of the left colon. The closer to the anal sphincter the tumor is situated, the lower the survival rate following abdominoperineal resection. If the lesion is situated just inside the anal sphincter, the survival rate at the end of 5 years is about 40 per cent.

Appendicitis

Acute appendicitis is one of the commonest abdominal and gastrointestinal operations for all ages. It reaches its peak occurrence in the second and third decades and rarely occurs before the age of 2 years. The majority of patients are between 5 and 30 years of age. Although the frequency of the disease decreases after 40 years, between the ages of 17 and 64 the annual incidence for men is 1.5 per thousand and for women, 1.9 per thousand. For further information on this condition, see Figure 18-10.

Reference Sources

American Cancer Society. *Facts and Figures, 1992.* New York, 1992.

Haagensen, C. D. *Diseases of the Breast,* 3rd edition. W. B. Saunders Company, Philadelphia, 1986.

Holder, M. Thomas, and W. Keith Ashcraft. *Pediatric Surgery.* W. B. Saunders Company, Philadelphia, 1980.

Nealon, Thomas F. *Fundamental Skills in Surgery,* 3rd edition. W. B. Saunders Company, Philadelphia, 1979.

Nealon, Thomas F. *Management of the Patient with Cancer,* 3rd edition. W. B. Saunders Company, Philadelphia, 1986.

Sabiston, C. David, and C. Frank Spencer. *Gibbons Surgery of the Chest,* 3rd edition. W. B. Saunders Company, Philadelphia, 1976.

Silverberg, E. Cancer statistics. *CA* 40:9-28, 1990.

For references of specific application to medical transcription, see Appendix 1.

ST. VINCENT'S HOSPITAL
153 West 11th Street
New York, NY 10011-0000

HISTORY AND PHYSICAL

PATIENT: Gregory Williams   DATE: July 9, 1994

HOSPITAL NO: 86-90-14   ROOM NO: 856

PHYSICIAN: Thomas F. Nealon, M.D.

CHIEF COMPLAINT: Gregory Williams, a 17-year-old white male, presented himself to the emergency room at 7:45 a.m. complaining that he had a pain in his abdomen which started last evening and has persisted and worsened throughout the night.

DETAILS OF PRESENT ILLNESS: The pain was originally in the mid portion of his abdomen, but it gradually shifted and is mainly in his right lower quadrant. He had no nausea or vomiting. He ate a normal dinner, but has had nothing by mouth since he awakened at 6:00 a.m. He did not sleep well during the night because of the discomfort. He has never had an attack like this before. His bowels have not moved. He has urinated twice without discomfort and with no effect on the abdominal pain.

PAST HISTORY: His only previous illnesses were tonsillitis, measles, and chickenpox with no complications or sequelae.

PHYSICAL EXAMINATION: Physical examination reveals a tall, thin, well-developed white male in obvious discomfort who is more uncomfortable when he moves. He is alert and answers all questions intelligently. His temperature was 99.4° F., pulse 100, blood pressure 110/78. Examination of his nose and throat were all normal. Physical examination of his chest failed to show any abnormalities. Abnormal findings were primarily in the abdomen, without contact. His abdominal musculature seemed tense and he was holding himself tense. He was not breathing deeply. Excursions were flat. On abdominal palpation, his abdominal muscles were tense in the epigastrium and in the right lower quadrant. On palpation, he had severe tenderness and board-like

(continued)

Figure 18–10

An example of a history and physical examination on a patient admitted to the hospital through the emergency room with acute appendicitis.

Gregory Williams   Page two
86-90-14

rigidity in the right lower quadrant. Rebound tenderness was most pronounced in the right lower quadrant. Bowel sounds were not remarkable. On rectal examination, his rectum was clear and there was marked tenderness in his rectum, high on the right side. There were no hernias.

LABORATORY RESULTS: A blood count revealed a WBC of 16,000 with an increase in his differential. Urinalysis was normal.

IMPRESSION: On the basis of the blood count, history, and physical examination, a diagnosis of acute appendicitis was made and immediate operation was recommended. He agreed. Prior to operation he had a physical examination by the surgical resident who found no contraindications to spinal anesthesia or an appendectomy.

PLAN: Gregory was admitted to the hospital and immediate appendectomy was performed.

_____
THOMAS F. NEALON, M.D.

TFN:bp
D: 9/9/94
T: 9/10/94

Figure 18–10 *Continued*

Joseph A. Bellanti, M.D.
Josef V. Kadlec, S.J., M.D.

Immunology and AIDS

INTRODUCTION

Broadly speaking, immunology is the study of the mechanisms enabling a host organism to protect itself from foreign invaders and to maintain its own identity by differentiating "self" from "nonself." Although the field of immunology traces its origins to antiquity, the major growth of the field as a science occurred over the past century, culminating within the past 20 years with discoveries of the molecular and genetic bases that govern immunologic responses. The occurrence of the acquired immune deficiency syndrome (AIDS) in the early 1980s catapulted immunology into the public domain. This chapter presents an overview of immunologic principles and their applications to human disease, including AIDS, that will assist the medical transcriptionist in an understanding of material presented for transcribing, editing, and communication.

ANATOMY AND PHYSIOLOGY OF THE IMMUNE SYSTEM

Unlike other organ systems, such as the cardiovascular and gastrointestinal systems, which are neatly packaged in discrete anatomic sites, the immunologic system is diffusely and strategically found in all sites and throughout cell tissues of the body. Furthermore, the cells and cell products that carry out immunologic functions are connected, interrelated, and interdependent through communication systems that involve a neurologic, endocrinologic, and immunologic network (Figure 19–1).

OVERVIEW

For ease of discussion, we may speak of five components of the immune system and its response to foreignness: (1) environment, (2) target cells, (3) phagocytic cells, (4) mediator cells, and (5) B and T cells and their products.

Environment

Most substances that confront and stimulate the immune system are in the exterior world. Shown in Figure 19–2 is an "Alice in Wonderland" view of the myriad of foreign substances we encounter in our daily lives. These range from the simplest of chemicals, food products, and plant and animal products to a whole host of biologic and chemical products that have become available as a result of our ever-expanding biotechnology and biomedicine. Foreign substances that evoke immune responses are called *antigens*. Specialized antigens that give rise to allergic disease are called *allergens*.

Target Cells

A foreign substance may be introduced into the host by any of the natural portals of entry, —inhalation, ingestion, or contact—or may arise within the host as a result of mutation, infection, or malignancy. Once introduced, the foreign substance has an impact on a variety of target cells that may be injured or destroyed, giving rise to disease (Figure 19–3). The signs and symptoms of disease will depend upon the

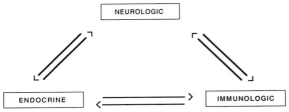

Figure 19-1

Network illustrating the interrelationships among the neurologic, endocrine, and immunologic systems.

location of the target cells. Shown in Table 19–1 are some examples of the effects of environmental agents on various target cells and the resultant diseases.

Phagocytic Cells

Certain cells of the immune system are capable of ingesting and destroying foreign substances that invade or arise within the host. The process of ingestion by cells is called phagocytosis, and the cells that carry out these functions are called phagocytic cells (Figure 19–4). In the

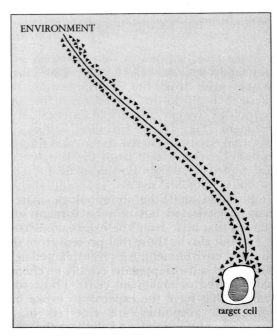

Figure 19-3

Effects of environmental agents on target cells. (From Bellanti, Joseph A. *Immunology* III. W. B. Saunders Company, Philadelphia, 1985.)

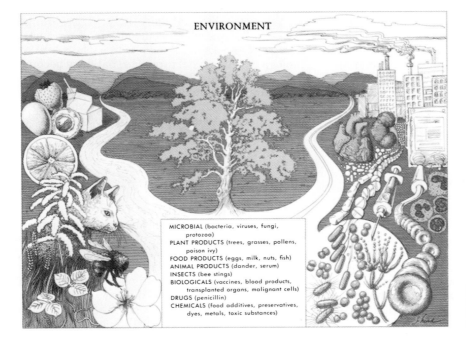

MICROBIAL (bacteria, viruses, fungi, protozoa)
PLANT PRODUCTS (trees, grasses, pollens, poison ivy)
FOOD PRODUCTS (eggs, milk, nuts, fish)
ANIMAL PRODUCTS (dander, serum)
INSECTS (bee stings)
BIOLOGICALS (vaccines, blood products, transplanted organs, malignant cells)
DRUGS (penicillin)
CHEMICALS (food additives, preservatives, dyes, metals, toxic substances)

Figure 19-2

Examples of environmental agents. (From Bellanti, Joseph A. *Immunology* III. W. B. Saunders Company, Philadelphia, 1985.)

***Table* 19–1 ▪ Effects of Environmental Agents on Various Target Cells**

Location of Target Cell	Example of Effect	Resultant Disease
Skin	Disruption of skin cells	Dermatitis
Respiratory tract	Destruction of mucous cells or muscle cells	Asthma
Gastrointestinal tract	Increased inhalation and secretion	Vomiting
Circulatory system		Anemia

human there are three types of phagocytic cells: (1) macrophages (in tissues) or their circulating counterparts, monocytes; (2) neutrophils or polymorphonuclear (PMN) cells; and (3) eosinophils. The measurement of these cells is helpful in the diagnosis of certain diseases. For example,

an elevation of the number of neutrophils or PMNs is commonly seen in bacterial infections; an elevation of eosinophils may be an indicator of allergic disease.

Mediator Cells

Certain cells of the immune system contain potent chemical substances (mediators), which, when released following contact with the foreign substance, can affect target cells or other cells of the body and augment response to injury, a set of responses referred to as *inflammation*. These cells are called mediator cells (Figure 19–5). The molecular basis of these reactions has been identified with the specific mediator substances, such as histamine, that are released from the mediator cells. Clinically, these responses are characterized by increased blood flow with resultant redness (erythema) and warmth, and leakage of fluid from blood vessels with swelling (edema); upon stimulation of nerve endings, they provoke pain. Usually the inflammatory re-

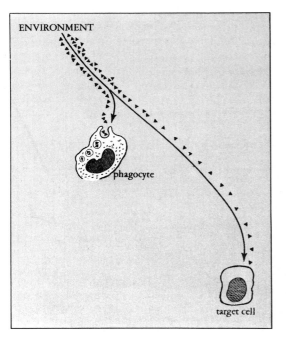

Figure 19–4
Phagocytic cells: mobilization factors and functions. (From Bellanti, Joseph A. *Immunology* III. W. B. Saunders Company, Philadelphia, 1985.)

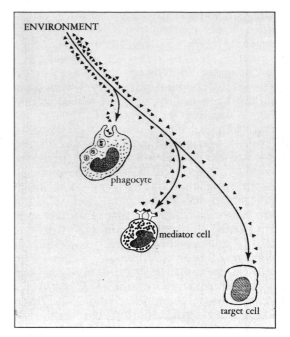

Figure 19–5
Mediator products and their effects on target cells (e.g., allergy) or phagocytic cells. (From Bellanti, Joseph A. *Immunology* III. W. B. Saunders Company, Philadelphia, 1985.)

sponses are mild and give rise to limited symptoms. Occasionally, however, they may be severe and life threatening, as in the case of severe allergic reactions.

B and T Cells

The cells at the heart of the immune system are the B cells and T cells (Figure 19–6). The terms B and T refer to the embryologic origin of these cells in either the bone marrow (B) or thymus (T) gland. These cells form the two arms of the immune system. B cells react with antigen to form specific products referred to as *antibody,* which form the immunoglobulins or gammaglobulins found in the serum and tissues. In the human, there are five major classes: IgG, IgM, IgA, IgD, and IgE. This is the humoral or circulating arm of the immune response, which can neutralize circulating antigens, such as bacteria or viruses.

The T cells react with antigen through a T cell receptor that is made up of structures similar to immunoglobulin (Ig). The T cells are designed to react with antigen presented on other cell surfaces and are particularly well suited for antigens that are inside cells.

PHYSIOLOGY

Immunologic responses serve three functions: defense, homeostasis, and surveillance (Table 19–2). The first function, defense against invasion by microorganisms, is the classic function of the immune response and has been studied by immunologists for more than a hundred years. When the cellular elements of defense are successfully deployed, the host will emerge victorious in the struggle with microorganisms. However, when these elements are *hyperactive,* certain undesirable features occur, such as allergy or hypersensitivity. Conversely, when these elements are *hypoactive,* there may be an increased susceptibility to repeated infections, as seen in the immunologic deficiency disorders.

The second function, homeostasis, fulfills the universal requirement of all organisms to preserve the uniformity of their cell type. It is concerned with the recognition of self versus nonself and with the normal degradative or catabolic functions of the body that are charged with the removal of damaged cellular elements, such as circulating red cells or white cells. These may be damaged during the course of a normal life span or may arise as a consequence of injury. Aberrations of homeostasis are seen in the autoimmune

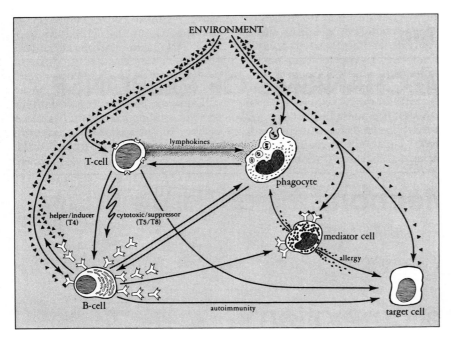

Figure 19–6
Total array of immunologic responses to the environment. (From Bellanti, Joseph A. *Immunology* III. W. B. Saunders Company, Philadelphia, 1985.)

Table 19–2 ▪ **Functions of the Immune System**

Function	Nature of Immunologic Stimulus	Example	Aberrations Hyper-	Hypo-
Defense	Exogenous	Micro-organisms	Allergy	Immunologic deficiency disorders
Homeostasis	Endogenous or exogenous	Removal of effete and damaged cells	Autoimmune disease	—
Surveillance	Endogenous or exogenous	Removal of cell mutants	—	Malignant disease

diseases, in which these mechanisms are unduly enhanced.

The third function of the immune system is the most recently recognized and concerns itself with surveillance against cancer. This function monitors the recognition of abnormal cell types that constantly arise within the body. These mutants may occur spontaneously or may be induced by certain viruses and chemicals. Failure of removal of these mutant cells has recently been assigned a causal role in the development of cancer.

From what has been described, it is clear that the cells and cell products of the immune system are uniquely poised to react to virtually all kinds of foreign substances that may enter the host or arise within it.

The efficiency with which the foreignness is eliminated determines whether the outcome will be successful. If the foreign substance can be removed, the host remains in a protected state called immunity. If the foreign substance cannot be removed, the encounter may be deleterious and lead to injury of the host, as seen in allergy, autoimmune disease, or cancer. Shown in Table 19–3 are clinical examples of disorders of the immune system, together with the signs and symptoms of proposed mechanisms that are involved in their development.

HIV AND AIDS

A special type of viral infection is that of the human immunodeficiency virus (HIV). Unlike other viruses, HIV has the propensity to infect the T lymphocytes as well as macrophages and B cells and the neurologic system. This results in

a severe acquired immune deficiency characterized by opportunistic infection caused by organisms such as *Candida,* by malignancy, and by CNS degeneration. HIV infection can range from an asymptomatic type of infection to mildly symptomatic to severe, full-blown symptomatic disease referred to as acquired immune deficiency syndrome (AIDS). Although many believe that all cases of HIV symptomatic infection lead to AIDS and death, this is not known with certainty.

FORMATS

Consultation Letters ▪ A review of Table 19–3 reveals that a wide variety of medical and surgical specialists may be involved in immunologic consultations. Therefore, a consultation letter may originate with the infectious disease specialist, hematologist-oncologist, rheumatologist, allergist, pulmonologist, nephrologist, or surgeon.

In each case the letter serves the following purposes: (1) It informs the referring physician that the patient has been examined; (2) it describes the initial presenting chief complaint, history of present illness, past history, serial history, and review of systems, together with a description of the findings detected on physical examination; (3) it gives the initial differential diagnoses, with a proposed plan for diagnostic procedures; (4) it gives a recommended plan of management or treatment and acknowledges the referral as a courtesy of the referring physician.

A typical referral letter from an allergist-immunologist is seen in Figure 19–7. The physi-

Table 19–3 ▪ **Representative Diseases of the Immune System**

Disease Type	Type of Medical Specialist	Example	Signs and Symptoms	Diagnostic Procedures	Treatment
Infections	Infectious diseases, pulmonologist	Staph, Tbc, flu, HIV	Fever	WBC, immune function tests	Antibiotics, gamma-globulin
Allergies	Allergist	Allergies, asthma, eczema	Conjunctivitis, sinusitis, wheezing	Elevated IgE tests, high eosinophil	Symptomatic antihistamine, bronchodilator, steroids
Auto-immune	Rheumatologist	Arthritis, SLE	Swollen joints, fever, rash	High WBC, + serology	ASA, steroids, NSAIDs
Transplant	Surgeon, nephrologist, hematologist	Kidney or bone marrow transplant	Graft rejection, fever, rash	High WBC, immune function test, kidney function test	Immuno-suppressive agents, steroids
Malignancy	Internist, pathologist, hematologist-oncologist	Various tumors	Weight loss, cachexia	CBC, tumor-specific antigens	Cytotoxic chemicals, irradiation, surgery

cian was asked to evaluate a two-year-old child with recurrent infections who was suspected of having an immune deficiency.

Discharge Summary ▪ Another important document is the summary of a patient's hospital course. This is usually prepared by the attending physician, but a discharge form also can be prepared by the consulting physician. Figure 19–8 is a typical discharge summary for a patient with AIDS.

Reference Sources

Abbas, Abul K., et al. *Cellular and Molecular Immunology.* W. B. Saunders Company, Philadelphia, 1991.

Bellanti, Joseph A. *Immunology III.* W. B. Saunders Company, Philadelphia, 1985.

Bryant, Neville J. *Laboratory Immunology and Serology,* 2nd edition. W. B. Saunders Company, Philadelphia, 1986.

Gorbach, S. L., J. G. Bartlett, and N. R. Blacklow (Eds.). *Infectious Diseases.* W. B. Saunders Company, Philadelphia, 1992, pp. 1005–1020.

JOSEPH A. BELLANTI, M.D.
GEORGETOWN UNIVERSITY MEDICAL CENTER
3800 Reservoir Road
Washington, DC 20007
202-687-8227

December 21, 1994

James M. Smith, M.D.
1234 Green Street
Washington, DC 20004

RE: Robert Brown Doe
Date of Birth (DOB): 12/21/92

Dear Dr. Smith:

Thank you for referring the above patient for evaluation of recurrent infections. Robert is a 2-year-old white male who was the product of a full-term uncomplicated gestation born to a healthy G1 P1 AbO 28-year-old mother. Birth was uneventful and the infant was discharged at 4 days of age. He was breast fed for the first 6 months at which time a cow's milk formula was begun. At about 8 months of age the infant developed a respiratory infection and otitis media and was treated with amoxicillin. Although he improved, recovery was not complete and following this he has had at least twelve bouts of recurrent upper respiratory infections with otitis media over the past 2 years.

Significant is a history that Robert has a 5-year-old brother who also develops respiratory infections presumably from exposure to other children in school. There is a strong family history of allergic disease on the paternal side of the family.

There are no smokers at home but the family has a dog.

(continued)

Figure 19–7
An example of a referral letter.

Figure continued

James M. Smith, M.D.   Page two

Physical examination revealed a well-developed, well-nourished 2-year-old child in no distress. Vital signs were normal. There was good skin color and no rashes. Examination of the ear drums revealed dull membranes bilaterally with evidence of extensive scarring. There was good tonsillar development and several cervical nodes were palpable, measuring about 2 x 2 cm.

The differential diagnoses in this case include several possibilities. The most likely diagnosis is that of allergic disease, given the family history, exposure to a dog, and repeated infections which commonly accompany allergic disease. Also to be considered is the possibility of underlying immune deficiency, particularly B-cell deficiency with agammaglobulinemia which, although rare, is known to be associated with this clinical picture of recurrent otitis media.

The following diagnostic procedures were obtained:

1.   A complete blood count revealed

      Hemoglobin = 12 gm/dl
      Hematocrit = 38
      WBC = 12,800/mm^3
      PMN = 48 per cent
      Lymphocytes = 40 per cent
      Eosinophils = 10 per cent
      Monocytes = 2 per cent

2. Quantitative Immunoglobulins

      IgG = 500 mg/dl (normal 520-1080 mg/dl)
      IgA = 240 mg/dl (normal 36-165 mg/dl)
      IgM = 260 mg/dl (normal 72-160 mg/dl)
      IgE = 240 U/ml (normal 0-100 U/ml)

3. RAST testing to certain foods were:

      milk = 3+
      egg = 0
      wheat = 1+

(continued)

Figure **19–7** *Continued*

James M. Smith, M.D.   Page three

The finding of high eosinophil count, high IgE and positive RAST testing to milk strongly support a diagnosis of milk allergy. The normal quantitative immunoglobulins exclude a diagnosis of agammaglobulinemia. We would recommend a course of environmental control, elimination of milk products and appropriate antibiotics and decongestants when attacks occur.

These attacks of recurrent infection should lessen and gradually disappear over the next year. Attention should be given to other factors which could contribute to blockage of eustachian tubes, such as enlarged adenoids and if found might warrant evaluation by an otolaryngologist and consideration of adenoidectomy.

Thank you for referring this interesting patient.

Sincerely,

Joseph A. Bellanti, M.D.
Attending allergist/immunologist

JAB:ssb

Figure 19–7 *Continued*

GEORGETOWN UNIVERSITY MEDICAL CENTER
3800 Reservoir Road
Washington, DC 20007

DISCHARGE SUMMARY

PATIENT'S NAME: Edwin Walton
MEDICAL RECORD NO: 122-3450
ADMISSION DATE: 10/21/94
DISCHARGE DATE: 12/1/94

ATTENDING PHYSICIAN: Joseph A. Bellanti, M.D.

FINAL DIAGNOSIS: AIDS

Edwin Walton is a 37-year-old black male who presented to the emergency room with a 9-month history of recurrent oral candidiasis, cough, low-grade fever and a twenty-pound weight loss. He is an unemployed laborer who for the past year has felt progressively ill and has received episodic care at various emergency rooms. He was married and is now divorced and denies a history of homosexuality. He admits to intravenous drug use on at least 3 occasions. Because of recurrent oral candidiasis and cough he was admitted to the inpatient service.

On physical examination his vital signs included: P = 100/min, R = 80/min, BP = 110/70. He appeared thin, emaciated and in acute respiratory distress. Examination of his oral cavity revealed extensive whitish exudates on his tongue, buccal mucosae, and pharynx. Several fine rales were detected throughout all lung fields particularly at the bases posteriorly.

CBC revealed a WBC = 10,800 with 87 per cent PMN, 5 per cent lymphocytes, 6 per cent eosinophils, 2 per cent basophils. Quantitative immunoglobulins were normal. A profound decrease in CD4 cells was observed (< 100 cells/mm^3) with normal number of CD8 cells (800 cells/mm^3). HIV antibody test was positive; P24 antigen was positive

A chest x-ray revealed diffuse interstitial pneumonia with hyperexpansion of lung fields.

(continued)

Figure 19–8
An example of a discharge summary for a patient with a typical case of HIV infection with full-blown AIDS.

RE: Edwin Walton   Page two
Medical Record Number 122-3450

Initial impression was candidiasis and pneumonitis, possibly a **Pneumocystis carinii** pneumonitis (PCP). Bronchial lavage confirmed the diagnosis of PCP and the organism was identified by silver-methenamine staining.

The patient was treated with Ketoconazole, trimethoprim-sulfa and amoxicillin and gradually improved. Following discharge he was placed on azathioprine (AZT) and will be followed in ambulatory clinic.

JOSEPH A. BELLANTI, M.D.

JAB:ssb
D: 12/1/94
T: 12/2/94

Figure 19–8 *Continued*

Gary W. Crooks, M.D.

Internal Medicine

PERSPECTIVE

Internal medicine is the largest of the formally recognized and governed specialties of medicine. But in a real sense it is scarcely a specialty, for it embraces the whole spectrum of disease and disorder. The difficulties of childbirth and the diseases of childhood are sometimes reflected in the maladies of adulthood that the internist sees and cares for, and the complex, devastating diseases of old age are also the province of the physician. Internists must recognize too the role that emotional disturbance plays in the ongoing course of illness; and, although they may not perform surgery, they must be aware in prognosis of the promise, the limitations, and the hazards of surgical intervention in a thousand different medical situations.

This diverse character of internal medicine is reflected in its division into subspecialties, some of which — for example, gastroenterology and cardiology — are of greater scope and numbers than many independently organized specialties such as plastic surgery or nuclear medicine. Still, internists may be thought of as specialists in the sense that through the referral system their area of expert knowledge has become that of the management of more difficult and complex diseases. The family physician, however well qualified, is more likely to refer a case of complex ongoing rheumatoid arthritis to the internist/rheumatologist than to manage it alone. Hence the internist will see many instances of despotic or intractable disease and in their management will call upon special knowledge and special experience.

It is often said that medicine is both art and science and that the enormous expansion of its scientific underpinning has dramatically changed the nature of medical care. And this is true because, largely in the 20th century, bioscience has become more solid, more precise, and more immediately useful, as in the discovery of insulin and the antibiotics and in the development of the Salk and Sabin vaccines. However, the biochemist can deal in hard facts and the biophysicist in solid theories, but the internist must often deal with uncertain facts and conflicting theories. Especially in care of the terminally ill and the desperately disturbed patient, the physician will find art more useful than science and must often heed the ancient admonition to become the treatment itself.

HISTORY

The roots of specialization lie deep in the past. Herodotus, writing in the 5th century B.C. of his visit to Egypt, mused over the nature of medicine:

> The practice of medicine they split up into several parts, each doctor being responsible for the treatment of only one disease. There are, in consequence, innumerable doctors, some specializing in diseases of the eyes, others of the head, others of the teeth, others of the stomach, and so on; while others again deal with the sort of troubles which cannot be exactly localized.

Perhaps we may ascribe this division and diffusion of medicine to a plethora of physicians

The author gratefully acknowledges the editorial assistance of John L. Dusseau in preparation of this chapter.

rather than to an abundance of knowledge, for Herodotus says,"Doctors are all over the place."

In America internal medicine achieved identity in the early 20th century when many general physicians began to limit their practice to care of adults so that they might offer their patients treatment informed by a growing body of special knowledge. The discovery of new diagnostic tools (radiology, electrocardiography, and clinical chemistry) created a distinction between general practitioner and internist that was sharpened by the foundation of the American College of Physicians in 1915. However, the College decided not to offer a certifying examination for competence in internal medicine similar to that of the British College of Physicians but to establish in 1936 a separate American Board of Internal Medicine as the examining body. The Board retains an informal connection with the College, as it does with the American Medical Association, but examines and certifies candidates independently and, through its requirements, has had a profound influence on postgraduate training in medicine both here and throughout the world.

At the end of World War II the American government began to make available through the National Institutes of Health huge sums of money for medical research. With the advances in research came major new technical modalities of both diagnosis and treatment (endoscopy, computed tomography, dialysis, organ transplantation, nuclear radiotherapy, and radioimmunoassay), and these too served not only to set off internal medicine as a specialty but also to establish within its framework important subspecialties. With continued funding of basic research, some of the subspecialties have developed autonomous powers and focus their attention on challenging problems of bioscience that are sometimes narrow in their implications.

THE PRACTICE OF INTERNAL MEDICINE

Within the academic departments of internal medicine there are now sections responsible for teaching comprehensive care that differs from training in family practice — mainly in exclusion of pediatrics, obstetrics, and minor surgery and in an emphasis on complex illnesses and the scientific bases of medical practice.

The exciting advances in medicine have themselves created problems. Therapy now makes use of powerful new drug agents, many of which can be harmful and some lethal. In addition to their intrinsic toxicity, these agents may interact with each other to produce unwanted effects. Few hospital patients today receive less than a half dozen medications, so that a substantial part of hospital medicine is devoted to overcoming the untoward effects of therapy. There are risks too in present sophisticated diagnostic procedures — notably a 1 per cent incidence of death or serious complication from coronary or cerebral angiography. Knowing when to stop has become as important as knowing where to begin.

The internist will continue to pursue a path bold in possibility but cautious in change. Internists must deal with such commonplace problems as nausea and pain that offer innumerable etiologic possibilities. They cannot control the environment from which their patients come nor the ill effects of habits they cannot control. They know that the recollections of patients are faulty and their complaints sometimes exaggerated or misplaced. Internists cannot reduce their cases to subcellular fractions in order to determine what is happening. They must question their own judgment and the opinions of their colleagues. They work, therefore, in an atmosphere of doubt and uncertainty and make their decisions on the basis not of fixed rules but of probabilities. They will make mistakes and, if they are good physicians, they will learn from them. They are the gatekeepers to other medical and surgical specialties and coordinate the wide-ranging care of internal medicine with that of more narrow and intensely developed disciplines.

It will be seen from the foregoing that much of the substance of internal medicine is already covered in the subspecialty chapters of this book and that their models of charts and reports are applicable to all of internal medicine. In any event, to present a detailed map of its whole domain would be impossible in a brief space. Therefore, what follows offers a general commentary on examination of the patient and terse descriptions of a few representative diseases significant to the medical population as a whole.

EXAMINATION OF THE PATIENT

It is recommended that the average healthy individual over the age of 40 years and with no active medical problems be examined once a year. Opinions vary among internists as to the recommended schedule for a physical examination for those under 40 years of age, but most agree that after the age of 30 years the patient should be examined every 2 years. The female patient should be seen annually for a gynecologic examination, and at age 35 years she should have a screening mammogram and one every 2 years after the age of 40 years. Women over 50 years of age should have a mammogram annually.

After the age of 50 years, men should have a prostate examination every year and the examination should be accompanied by a specific blood test for prostatic cancer known as prostate-specific antigen (PSA).

Both men and women should have a rectal examination, and the stool should be examined for hidden or occult blood by means of a guaiac or Hemoccult kit. Everyone over the age of 50 years should have a sigmoidoscopy or proctoscopy every 3 to 4 years to screen for colonic polyps that can be precancerous.

However, the physical examination is always preceded by a dialogue (the interview) between patient and physician in which the patient usually presents a problem and looks to the internist with expectation and hope that whatever fears and questions he or she may have will be discussed and answered in an attentive and sympathetic manner. The patient expects to be heard and understood, and it is incumbent upon the physician to be a good listener, for often the way in which the patient expresses symptoms and concerns offers the key to important medical conclusions.

Indeed, the most powerful tool in the diagnostic process is the interview. The physician listens carefully to the patient's account of the chronology and symptoms of the illness and so forms diagnostic hypotheses that are tested in the patient's unfolding story and later by the physical examination and laboratory studies. In a sense the physical examination begins at the very moment the doctor first sees the patient, for he is then immediately aware of the patient's appearance, of signs of his emotional state, and of his physical and mental limitations. Not only is close attention paid to what is said but the interviewer is also alert to nonverbal clues, often sensing the existence of subtle symptoms and interrelationships that are unrecognized by the patient.

After the interview a screening physical examination is begun. It is in part influenced by hypotheses developed during the interview but is carried out sequentially and completely regardless of any presumed diagnosis, because, especially in the aged, presenting symptoms and abnormalities are often the result of more than one disorder. Efficient physical examination rests on two underlying principles: The examination is done by regions and is carried out in an organized sequence. The following is an outline of procedure followed by many internists:

- Skin (noting long-standing dermatoses).
- HEENT (head, ears, eyes, nose, and throat, noting soreness).
- Neck (particularly noting thyromegaly, carotid bruits, or adenopathy).
- Chest (auscultation and percussion, noting egophony, tactile fremitus, rales, or rhonchi).
- Back (costovertebral angle tenderness, kyphoscoliosis).
- Heart (S1, S2, S3, S4, point of maximal impulse [PMI]).
- Abdomen (hepatosplenomegaly, normoactive bowel sounds, epigastric tenderness, suprapubic tenderness and right upper quadrant [RUQ] or left lower quadrant [LLQ] tenderness).
- Genitourinary tract (evidence of hernia, scrotal masses, epididymitis).
- Rectum (prostatic nodularity, rectal masses, hemorrhoids, often described by their position on an imaginary clock).
- Lower extremities (noting pulse and presence of edema).

Laboratory tests, as deemed necessary, are instituted after the physical examination. A few initial tests are usually carried out to detect unsuspected common entities such as anemia, diabetes, or chronic renal disease. Other studies are done to confirm or rule out diagnostic first impressions. Simple tests often yield decisive information, and hazardous tests are undertaken only if there is no alternative for them. The key words in modern interpretation of diagnostic laboratory studies are *sensitivity* and *specificity*. Sensitivity is the probability that a given test will be positive when a specific disease is present, and specificity is the probability that a given test will be negative when a specific disease is not present. To exclude the possibility of lupus erythematosus, a sensitive test is chosen such as the antinuclear antibody test, and to confirm the diagnosis the specific double-stranded DNA antibody test is employed.

REPRESENTATIVE DISEASES

Diabetes Mellitus ■ Diabetes mellitus is a disorder of carbohydrate metabolism characterized by hyperglycemia and glycosuria and resulting from inadequate production or utilization of insulin, a hormonal substance produced by the endocrine glands of the pancreas. The exact cause of such metabolic failure is unknown, but heredity and obesity both seem to be causal factors. Environmental factors too play their role; alcohol abuse and excessive intake of sweets are causative agents. But the disease is a complex constellation of anatomic and biochemical abnormalities in which lack of insulin results in an inability to metabolize glucose and in which the capacity to store glycogen in the liver and the active transport of glucose across cell membranes is impaired. Its signs and symptoms are sugar in the urine, an increase of blood sugar, thirst, hunger, weakness, and weight loss. Prolonged hyperglycemia can cause premature vascular degeneration and atherosclerosis, and uncontrolled diabetes can lead to diabetic acidosis and death. For fuller details of the causes, diagnosis, and management of diabetes, see Chapter 15 on Endocrinology.

Osteoarthritis ■ Osteoarthritis is a chronic disease affecting the joints, especially those bearing weight. It is a complex response of the joint tissues to genetic and environmental factors, characterized by degeneration of cartilage and overgrowth of bone. Idiopathic osteoarthritis is a common variety encountered in the process of aging but unrelated to systemic or local disease. Secondary osteoarthritis is more clearly provoked by antecedent factors, such as inflammatory, metabolic, endocrine, or developmental disorders.

But environmental factors play a role in either form of osteoarthritis. The simple wear and tear of daily life or the undue exposure of joints to the trauma of difficult physical labor or prolonged sports activity affects the synovium of the joints and may produce severe pain, inflammation, and decreased range of motion. The hands especially will show a number of deformities, such as Heberden's nodes and swollen metacarpophalangeal or distal interphalangeal joints. The knees too may show fluid collection, bursitis, patellar subluxation, and crepitus. For a fuller account of osteoarthritis, its physical findings, its modes of therapy, and examples of its reports, see Chapter 37 on Rheumatology and Chapter 28 on Orthopaedics.

Hypercholesterolemia ■ Public interest in high cholesterol levels has been dramatic in the last 4 or 5 years, although many people fail to realize that the reason to treat cholesterol is to decrease the risk of cardiac and cerebrovascular disease, particularly strokes or cerebrovascular accidents (CVAs). Other risk factors for atherosclerotic disease include smoking, diabetes, family predisposition, hypertension, obesity, sedentary life style, and perhaps Type A personality.

Total cholesterol is the sum of low-density lipoprotein (LDL) cholesterol, high-density lipoprotein (HDL) or good cholesterol, and triglycerides. It is important to have the total less than 200 mg/dl, and to have the HDL over 35, preferably in the 50 to 60 mg/dl range. If the HDL value is very low, that is an independent risk factor for coronary artery disease (CAD). Much of our knowledge of the natural history of hypercholesterolemia comes from the *Framingham Study,* which demonstrated the correlation between chronic hypercholesterolemia and increased incidence of ischemic heart disease. Although elevated LDL levels may occur in individuals in response to high saturated fat and cholesterol, the significant presence of hypercholesterolemia in the population remains unexplained. Its cause has been called "multifactorial," suggesting interaction of genes with environmental factors.

Hypertension ■ Elevated blood pressure, or hypertension, is one of the most prevalent illnesses in our society. Up to one third of adult Americans may suffer from it. Risk factors are family predisposition, smoking, obesity, lack of exercise, alcohol use, and salt intake. Hypertension is called "the silent killer," because most patients exhibit no symptoms even though elevated blood pressure is damaging vital organs, particularly the heart, kidneys, and eyes.

Malignant hypertension is the syndrome of markedly elevated blood pressure (diastolic blood pressure more than 140 mm Hg) associated with papilledema. Accelerated hypertension is the syndrome of markedly elevated blood pressure associated with hemorrhages and exudates. Untreated accelerated hypertension usually progresses to a malignant state, and both malignant and accelerated hypertension are the cause of widespread degenerative damage in the walls of resistance vessels, including retinopathy, hypertensive encephalopathy, hematuria, and renal dysfunction. Malignant hypertension is usually fatal unless treated promptly and vigorously.

Edema ■ In its consideration we should think of edema as a commonly presenting symptom rather than a disease. Once called dropsy, it is the abnormal accumulation of fluid in the body tissues or cavities and causes swelling or distention of the affected parts. It is often characteristic of congestive heart failure but it can accompany many other diseases and conditions, including obesity, venous insufficiency, renal disease or failure, cirrhosis of the liver, anemia, and severe malnutrition. Accumulation of fluid within the lungs is a serious complication of cardiac failure, whereas abnormal collection of fluid in the pleural space can be a symptom of any of many infectious diseases and circulatory disorders. Since edema is a symptom, its alleviation can be effected only by treatment of its underlying cause.

Bilateral edema is the accumulation of fluid in the lower extremities. In its analysis the physician must determine the bilaterality of the process, for if the edema is bilateral it can be caused by any of the edematous diseases, whereas unilateral edema of the extremities may have a localized cause such as a clot in the deep venous system of the leg, which is termed deep venous thrombosis (DVT) and which requires emergency treatment. Studies should be done, including Doppler studies, impedance plethysmography, and perhaps venography. If there is concern that the clot may have broken off from the leg and traveled to the lung, a ventilation-perfusion scan (V/Q scan) may be obtained, followed by a pulmonary arteriogram or pulmonary angiogram. If the presence of a clot is confirmed, then the patient must be treated with heparin intravenously, followed by several months of Coumadin, an oral anticoagulant. If the cause of unilateral edema is not a clot, then other causes such as local trauma or a tumor obstruction to the return of lymph fluid need to be considered.

Most edema is bilateral and can be described as pitting in nature. If one presses against the skin of the edematous area, a dent is left that can be graded on a scale from trace to 4+. It can further be graded as to the extent of the body it encompasses: ankle edema, pretibial, or extending into the thighs or even the abdomen. If the entire body including the face is edematous, this is known as anasarca. A common cause for edema that is nonpitting is hypothyroidism.

The treatment for edema is directed at the etiology and then elevation of the edematous extremities. Diuretics such as Lasix (or furosemide), Bumex, hydrochlorothiazide or Dyazide are used to mobilize fluid. Attempts are made to estimate the patient's so-called dry weight and initiate a regimen that will maintain it.

Upper Respiratory Infections and Bronchitis ■ Upper respiratory infections are infections of the nose and throat, usually viral in nature. As the common cold and influenza viruses have no known effective antidote, their treatment is supportive with the use of fluids and antipyretics. Patients may present with symptoms of low-grade fever, rhinorrhea, sore throat, or pharyngitis. In some cases these are the first signs of more serious bacterial infections that will need more intensive therapy. If a cough becomes productive of yellow, green, or brown as opposed to clear mucus, this is suggestive of a bacterial process either anew or following a viral infection. Such a process requires treatment by antibiotics such as erythromycin, penicillin, ampicillin, amoxicillin, cephalosporins, or Cipro.

A patient who seems gravely ill may, in fact, have an infection not involving the airways or bronchioles, such as one sees in bronchitis or tracheobronchitis, but may have pneumonia. Pneumonia involves the air spaces of the lung and, on physical examination, is manifested by the lack of breath sounds in a particular area of the chest. Findings may include dullness to percussion, tactile fremitus, egophony, rhonchi, and rales. The patient may have a very high fever, lack appetite, and, in severe cases, be dyspneic or short of breath (SOB), and also have decreased mental function because the lung cannot supply enough oxygen to the blood, which in turn cannot deliver enough to supply the brain's needs.

Pneumonia will often require hospitalization, particularly when it occurs in a patient over the age of 65 years or in one with chronic cardiopulmonary conditions such as asthma, emphysema, chronic obstructive pulmonary disease (COPD), or congestive heart failure. Similarly, pneumonia in the diabetic patient, in the patient with a lymphoproliferative disorder or in one with AIDS is a very serious condition. For further information and examples of reports, refer to Chapter 36 on Pulmonary and Respiratory Medicine.

Cellulitis ■ Cellulitis is an infection of the skin that occurs because of a break in the natural barrier the skin provides to the external world. Its most common cause is dryness or cracking of the skin, but it can come from a break in the skin caused by a dog bite, a cat scratch, an intravenous catheter, or a thorn.

On examination, the area will be red or erythematous, swollen, and indurated (filled with extra fluid as the body responds by delivering extra white blood cells to fight off infection). The infection can spread by entering the lymphatic system, with resulting red streaks or lymphangitis. This can then deliver bacteria into the blood stream, resulting in bacteremia. If enough bacteria enter the system the result is termed septicemia, colloquially known as blood poisoning. This can result in seeding of multiple organ systems and thus diffuse infection. Perhaps the most serious of these disseminated infections is the involvement of the heart valves in a condition known as endocarditis. Although cellulitis resembles urticaria, its inflammatory skin lesions are readily distinguished from hives by their persistent enlarging nature and by their pain and warmth. Group A streptococci and *Staphylococcus aureus* are the most common responsible organisms.

Cellulitis is treated locally with warm compresses and elevation and a variety of antibiotics such as dicloxacillin, Keflex, Bactrim, Septra, and ciprofloxacin.

Peptic Ulcer Disease and Reflux Esophagitis ■ A common complaint of peptic ulcer is a history of heartburn or nonspecific chest pain. The leading cause of this discomfort is an irritation in the stomach from the production of too much acid, so-called acid indigestion. In its earliest and least dangerous form, the distress is well treated with antacids. If it goes on for a period of time, the patient can develop a frank gastric or peptic ulcer. Ulcers not only can cause pain but also can bleed, resulting in a life-threatening situation.

Patients with a bleeding ulcer will usually have abdominal pain and will often pass a dark or black and tarry stool or bloody stools known medically as hematochezia. Because they are anemic, these patients may eventually suffer from fatigue.

Instead of forming an ulcer in the lining of the stomach or in the duodenum, the constant overproduction of acid can result in an irritation of the esophagus, a condition known as reflux esophagitis. This is particularly common in association with another entity known as a hiatal hernia. Though often dismissed by patients as only "heartburn," it can, in fact, lead to a serious change in the lining of the esophagus, a condition termed Barrett's esophagus. This in turn can lead to malignant changes in the lining of the esophagus and to esophageal carcinoma.

The symptoms separating these benign and serious conditions are often hard to differentiate. Therefore, studies such as upper endoscopy, a barium swallow, or an upper gastrointestinal (UGI) series may be performed. Once the entity is diagnosed, the treatment is with a family of drugs known as H_2 antagonists, such as Tagamet, Zantac, or Pepcid. A newer drug that eliminates acid production entirely is Prilosec. For further information and illustrations or examples of reports, refer to Chapter 17 on Gastroenterology.

Anemia ■ Anemia is a condition in which the concentration of hemoglobin in the circulatory blood is less than normal. It is caused by an insufficient number of erythrocytes (red blood cells), an abnormal level of hemoglobin in the individual blood cells, or by both these factors operating simultaneously. Whatever the cause of anemia, it causes similar signs and symptoms because of the reduced capacity of the blood to carry oxygen. The symptoms include pallor, weakness, dizziness, and fatigue. In severe cases breathing is difficult and abnormalities of heart and digestive action appear, especially exacerbation of existing heart disease. Iron deficiency anemia, a common type of anemia, is caused by insufficient iron in the body, essential for the formation of hemoglobin in the erythrocytes. However, in the adult the most common cause of anemia is chronic blood loss. Pernicious anemia is caused by inability of the body to absorb vitamin B_{12}. Also any disease or injury to bone marrow can cause anemia, especially bone marrow destruction by irradiation or chemical agents. Several inherited anemias seem to have an unusual ethnic distribution. Among them are sickle cell anemia and thalassemia major, a disease usually fatal before adulthood.

Once a patient is found to be anemic, an evaluation is begun to see whether it results from inadequate production of blood cells in the bone marrow, early destruction of blood cells in the blood stream, or loss of blood — bleeding into the gastrointestinal tract or into a hidden part of the body such as the retroperitoneum or hip, or from unusually heavy menses.

Of particular value in distinguishing the possible etiologies is the mean corpuscular volume (MCV), the reticulocyte count, the appearance of the peripheral smear, and the level of iron or ferritin in the blood. Folate and vitamin B_{12} deficiencies also can result in a low blood count.

The main types of anemia are:

Anemia of chronic disease
Aplastic anemia
Hemolytic states, particularly from prosthetic
  heart valves
Iron deficiency anemia
Megaloblastic anemia
Myelofibrosis
Sickling diseases
Sideroblastic anemia
Thalassemia

If the symptoms are severe enough, the patient will require transfusions of packed red blood cells in order to avoid syncope, angina, and increase in congestive heart failure.

Commentary

The foregoing descriptions afford but a handful from the broad spectrum of diseases that constitute the practice of internal medicine, but it is hoped that they provide a picture of the challenges and difficulties of that practice. Ideally, internists must know a great deal more than medicine. They should be well-rounded, broadly educated persons sensitive to the changing panorama of our culture and its shifting values and aware too of the impact of social environment upon the origin and course of disease. Above all, they must somehow contend with the awesome responsibilities of a still inexact science in which perilous probability must be the guide. So too the transcriptionist will often be called upon to resolve doubts and confusions without reliable signs to their correction. The great and vital principle of the profession of each is that its finest realization lies not in impressive facilities or glittering apparatus but in the deep-seated tradition of self-discipline and ongoing education.

Reference Sources

Barker, L. Randol, John R. Burton, and Philip D. Zieve. *Principles of Ambulatory Medicine.* Williams & Wilkins, Baltimore, 1990.

Braunwald, Eugene, et al. *Harrison's Principles of Internal Medicine,* 11th ed., McGraw-Hill Book Company, New York, 1987.

Wyngaarden, James B., Lloyd H. Smith, Jr., and J. Claude Bennett. *Cecil Textbook of Medicine,* 19th ed., W. B. Saunders Company, Philadelphia, 1992.

Paul T. Wertlake, M.D., M.S., M.B.A.

Laboratory Medicine

INTRODUCTION

Clinical laboratories perform in excess of 1000 different assays that detect, diagnose, and monitor disease. Many of the more frequently used tests are briefly described here. It is important to keep in mind that limited information regarding laboratory tests does not permit medical diagnosis.

CHEMISTRY TESTS

These tests may be ordered individually, in a comprehensive profile, or in smaller groups, according to the medical indication. Comprehensive profiles are extensively utilized in health screening.

A/G Ratio ▪ This is a mathematical relationship between the concentrations of albumin and globulin present in the blood. The ratio helps distinguish important protein changes from normal. Ratios of 1 or less should be further evaluated.

Albumin, Globulin, and Total Protein ▪ These tests measure the amount and type of protein in the blood. They are a useful index of overall health and nutrition. The globulin proteins include antibodies important for resisting disease. Protein abnormalities may be further studied by protein electrophoresis, immunoelectrophoresis, isoelectric focusing, as well as measurement of the major immunoproteins: IgG, IgA, and IgM (gamma globulins).

C-Reactive Protein ▪ C-reactive protein (CRP) is an acute-phase reactant and increases with inflammatory processes. It is useful in detecting postsurgical responses and occult infec-tion, including acute appendicitis, and for assessing activity of autoimmune disorders.

Alkaline Phosphatase (ALP) ▪ Alkaline phosphatase is an enzyme that may occur at high levels in the blood as a consequence of disease or physiologic conditions. This occurs with normal, active bone growth of children and teenagers. ALP concentration can be increased up to nine times normal, particularly in young men during a growth spurt. ALP may also be increased in the third trimester of pregnancy, with obstructive jaundice, biliary cirrhosis, tumors within the liver, viral hepatitis and cirrhosis. Bone disorders, primary and secondary, may be the cause of elevated ALP, including metastatic tumor to bone. Elevated ALP with normal gamma glutamyltransferase (GGT) is consistent with bone disease. Elevated ALP with elevated GGT is consistent with hepatic disease.

ALP Isoenzymes ▪ ALP isoenzymes may be helpful in determining the tissue source of increased blood levels of alkaline phosphatase.

Alanine Aminotransferase (ALT [SGPT*]) ▪ ALT is an enzyme, the concentration of which increases in the blood with liver destruction. This occurs with hepatitis, which may be caused by viruses (A, B, C, Epstein-Barr [EBV, mono] and less often herpes, cytomegalovirus, chickenpox, and so forth), alcohol, cancers, drugs of abuse, and chemotherapeutic agents.

Aspartate aminotransferase (AST) and ALT evaluate whether a hepatitis is acute (ALT > AST) or chronic active disease (AST > ALT).

---

*SGPT (serum glutamic–pyruvic transaminase) is no longer in use and has been replaced by ALT (alanine aminotransferase).

Aspartate Aminotransferase (AST [SGOT*]) ▪ AST is an enzyme, the concentration of which increases in the blood with tissue destruction. It may occur in a variety of organs but is more commonly elevated in liver and heart disorders. It is a sensitive indicator of disease but lacks specificity, which means it is not determinative of the site of disease. Clinical correlation and further evaluation are necessary.

Bilirubin ▪ Bilirubin is the primary pigment in bile. High levels of bilirubin in the blood may occur with liver diseases and conditions that obstruct the biliary tract, such as gallstones or cancer. Elevation of bilirubin may also occur with destruction of red blood cells (hemolysis). This occurs with some genetic disorders, acute and severe systemic infections, antibody disorders including autoimmune disease, erythroblastosis fetalis (Rh antibody disease of newborn infants), and incompatible blood transfusion.

BUN and Creatinine ▪ Blood urea nitrogen (BUN) and creatinine are commonly used to screen for kidney disease and to monitor patient management, including hemodialysis. The more common causes of kidney disease are systemic hypertension and diabetes mellitus. BUN represents the major end-product of protein metabolism. Creatinine is the major waste product of creatine (an important muscle metabolite).

In azotemia, BUN, or creatinine, or both are elevated. Prerenal azotemia occurs in conditions such as gastrointestinal hemorrhage, dehydration, and congestive heart failure; the primary problem is not a renal problem. In renal azotemia, the primary problem is a diseased condition of the kidneys. Postrenal azotemia is due to an obstruction of the urinary tract, which might occur as a consequence of malignancy or stone formation.

Creatinine is relatively independent from diet (protein intake), degree of hydration, and protein metabolism and for that reason is a significantly more reliable screening test for compromised renal function.

BUN/Creatinine Ratio ▪ The BUN/creatinine (B/C) ratio is a mathematical expression of the relationship of BUN and creatinine and is

usually in the range of about 10 to 20. A high B/C ratio typically occurs with prerenal azotemia, but it may be seen in postrenal azotemia and in patients with reduced muscle mass. A decreased B/C ratio occurs with renal dialysis and in muscular individuals with renal failure.

Calcium and Phosphate ▪ These tests are indicative of bone function and indirectly of the hormones that influence bone metabolism, in which vitamin D and its metabolites play an active role. Abnormalities can reflect primary bone disease or other disease conditions secondarily affecting bones. The latter include cancers, kidney failure, and parathyroid disorders.

Lipids ▪ Assessment of lipid disorders is best accomplished by performing several analyses, so as to establish a trend.

Triglycerides ▪ Different forms of lipids are measured in the blood. It is preferable that these studies be performed when the patient is well fasted (12 to 15 hours after last eating). Triglycerides, in particular, tend to be transiently elevated following food ingestion.

Moderate elevation of triglycerides only occurs in some individuals, including senior citizens in good health, and does not appear to be a significant risk factor. Elevation of triglycerides associated with other lipid abnormalities is clinically important and is helpful in classification of some types of disorders.

Most lipid disorders are secondary to other conditions, such as diabetes and obesity. The lipid abnormalities often will be alleviated with successful control of diabetes or weight loss. It is recommended that individuals achieve a serum cholesterol level of 200 mg/dL or less.

Cholesterol ▪ Cholesterol is vital to cellular metabolism, and there appears to be a range most compatible with health, perhaps 140 to 200 mg/dL for most individuals. Lower levels may be dangerous. Lower levels are occasionally seen in persons with advanced malignancies.

High-Density Cholesterol ▪ In what might seem paradoxical some individuals with cholesterol levels below 200 mg/dL may be at risk for myocardial infarction and some individuals with cholesterol levels well above 200 mg/dL (e.g., 240 mg/dL) may be at low risk. The latter is sometimes seen in young women in whom the *high-density lipoprotein (HDL) cholesterol* is very high. The former is more likely in men who have very low HDL cholesterol. For this reason it is

*SGOT (serum glutamic–oxaloacetic transaminase) is no longer in use and has been replaced by AST (aspartate aminotransferase).

best to evaluate individuals by measurement of both cholesterol and HDL cholesterol. The relationship between these can be expressed as a ratio of cholesterol to HDL cholesterol. Higher values of this ratio correlate with higher risk for myocardial infarction. Men who measure 4.8 to 5.9 are at moderate risk; less than 3.8 represents the lowest-risk group. For women, 3.7 to 4.6 represents moderate risk, with less than 2.9 the lowest risk.

LOW-DENSITY LIPOPROTEIN CHOLESTEROL ■ *Low-density lipoprotein (LDL) cholesterol* is a calculated value, as determined in clinical practice, and may be expressed as a ratio to HDL cholesterol (LDL/HDL) for assessing risk for myocardial infarction. LDL cholesterol is deposited in tissue, forming atheromata that decrease the elasticity of vessels and obstruct blood flow.

Lipoprotein Electrophoresis ■ Lipid abnormalities may be further investigated by *lipoprotein electrophoresis*, which, combined with the clinical presentation, cholesterol, triglycerides concentration, and presence or absence of chylomicrons, permits categorizing individuals with genetically determined lipid disorders into differing categories with different risks. Patients in different categories require different therapeutic approaches. This is known as the Fredrickson classification of genetically determined dyslipoproteinemias.

Single-gene mutation is relatively rare as a basis for dyslipoproteinemias, with most cases being polygenic or the result of interaction of genetic susceptibility with other conditions such as diabetes, hypothyroidism, nephrotic syndrome, obesity, alcoholism, pancreatitis, obstructive biliary disease, and others. In many patients, these other diseases will prove to be the primary underlying cause of the dyslipoproteinemia, which will improve with successful treatment.

Apolipoprotein ■ *Apolipoprotein A-1* and *apolipoprotein B*, as well as *lipoprotein Lp(a)*, are other tests utilized in assessment of lipid disorders. Lipoprotein Lp(a) structurally resembles plasminogen and may be a lead to the relationship between lipoproteins and the clotting system.

Gamma-Glutamyltransferase (GGT) or Gamma-Glutamyl Transpeptidase (GGTP) ■ Elevations in blood concentration of GGTP occur with liver disorders known as cholestatic conditions, which is obstruction of normal bile flow within the biliary system. The obstruction may be external to the liver or within the liver. GGT is frequently elevated with alcohol abuse. GGT is often used to help evaluate the significance of elevated alkaline phosphatase, which may be elevated in liver disorders as well as in bone disorders. One example is the occurrence of normal concentrations of GGT in pregnant women, although the alkaline phosphatase is elevated owing to the contribution of placental alkaline phosphatase to circulating levels of the total alkaline phosphate. This suggests that the liver of the pregnant woman is normal. Medications may be the cause of increased GGT in the absence of liver disease. These include the antiepileptic agents diphenylhydantoin and phenobarbital.

Glucose ■ The glucose test is a measure of sugar levels in the blood. High values are associated with eating before the test (nonfasted) and with diabetes mellitus. Testing for diabetes may be done by measuring glucose before (fasted) and at different time intervals after ingestion of a standard amount of glucose. This is the *2-hour postprandial glucose test* or the *glucose tolerance test*.

Glucose in the blood binds to blood proteins in proportion to the amount of glucose present. The bound glucose can be measured and indicates the average level of blood sugar over a period of 2 weeks. This is known as *glycated protein* or *protein-bound glucose (PBG)* and is helpful in distinguishing whether a high glucose level is due to diabetes (or a tendency to diabetes) or due to recent eating.

Glucose also attaches to the hemoglobin of red cells in proportion to the amount of glucose in the blood. This test, *glycohemoglobin* or *hemoglobin A1c*, measures glucose binding to hemoglobin over a period of about 60 days. It is used to monitor the adequacy of treatment and the diet compliance of individuals with diabetes. The blood glucose test and the protein-bound glucose test are available as part of automated chemistry profiles.

Human Chorionic Gonadotropin (hCG) ■ Clinical tests for this are often referred to as beta-hCG since assays are directed to one of the two subunits of hCG, alpha and beta. The alpha subunit of hCG is very similar to luteinizing hormone (LH) and follicle-stimulating hormone (FSH).

Pregnancy ▪ Qualitative beta-hCG is tested in the blood or urine for identification of pregnancy. Early detection may be made as soon as 6 to 8 days following conception and implantation. The hCG is secreted by syncytiotrophoblasts.

The hCG has an approximate doubling time of 2 days during the first 10 weeks of a normal pregnancy. Utilization of quantitative measurement of serum levels of hCG, combined with ultrasound, may be very helpful in differentiating ectopic pregnancies from intrauterine pregnancies. When followed by serial measurements, two thirds of patients with ectopic pregnancies will exhibit a fall, a plateau, or an inability to achieve the predicted slope for the increasing hCG production of normal pregnancy. An hCG "discriminatory zone" of approximately 1400 mIU/mL, corresponding to a visualized gestational sac by transvaginal ultrasound, can be achieved for intrauterine pregnancy about 35 days following the last menstrual period. Prior to this time, diagnosis of ectopic pregnancy is a clinical challenge. Following surgical removal of ectopic pregnancies, it is recommended that patients be monitored until nonpregnant levels of beta-hCG (usually 8 to 9 days, with a range of 1 to 31 days) are achieved.

Gestational Trophoblastic Disease (GTD) ▪ This disease, which includes hydatiform mole (HM), chorioadenoma destruens, and choriocarcinoma, is characterized by production of hCG that exceeds that expected for normal pregnancy for similar gestational ages. An enlarged uterus, a variety of possible symptoms, and a characteristic pelvic sonogram help make the diagnosis. The ratio of serum free beta-subunit hCG to total hCG is valuable in prediction of outcome of GTD. Treatment includes use of hCG levels as a measure of response.

Beta-hCG may also be of value as a tumor marker for ovarian germ tumors and testicular tumors. Serial determinations are helpful in monitoring patient response to therapy.

Iron, Total Iron-Binding Capacity (TIBC), Transferrin Saturation, and Ferritin ▪ *Iron (Fe)* in the blood is variable, even from morning to afternoon of the same day, so measurements of iron must be considered together with those of *transferrin*, the blood protein that transports iron. This evaluation includes the total capacity to transport iron (*TIBC*) and the degree to which iron has bound to transferrin (*transferrin saturation*).

Iron deficiency can cause anemia, but it can also be identified before anemia has developed. Iron deficiency can result from blood loss (red cells contain iron) and may be the first indication of an unknown gastrointestinal cancer.

Less well known are the iron overload disorders, including hemochromatosis, a serious, debilitating disease which is difficult to diagnose and afflicts more than one million Americans. Many cases are undiagnosed, which is unfortunate, since hemachromatosis may be successfully treated if diagnosed before irreversible changes occur. Hepatitis can also cause iron overload.

A recent report links high levels of iron and iron storage with increased risk of heart attack. This epidemiologic report was made in Finland. The increased iron was based on increased serum levels of ferritin.

Ferritin, a storage form of iron in the body, is an excellent test to confirm abnormalities detected by the screening tests. Ferritin measures low with iron deficiency and high with iron overload disorders. Ferritin may be increased because of hepatitis or acute inflammatory conditions and is known as an acute-phase reactant.

Lactic Dehydrogenase (LD, LDH) ▪ This enzyme is present in nearly all tissues of the body. Tissue damage of virtually any organ, due to many different causes, may cause LDH to be increased in the blood. It has screening value as an indicator of an existing problem, including problems of the heart, lungs, and liver, as well as hemolysis (destruction) of red blood cells.

LD isoenzymes may be helpful in differentiating heart, liver, and lung diseases.

Magnesium ▪ Magnesium (Mg) is three times more plentiful in red cells than in serum. It may be decreased and is of clinical importance with excessive urinary losses resulting from a variety of problems, such as chronic alcoholism, diuretic therapy, and certain renal problems. Hypomagnesemia occurs from starvation, prolonged intravenous therapy, and decreased intestinal absorption due to malabsorption syndromes such as sprue or massive surgical resection of the small intestine. Prolonged and severe loss of body fluids, as in severe diarrhea, fistulous loss of fluids, prolonged nasogastric suction, and protracted vomiting, also causes significantly decreased magnesium levels.

Increased magnesium levels occur most frequently with renal failure but may occur with pharmacologic doses of magnesium or magnesium-containing compounds, particularly in patients with impaired renal function.

Sodium, Potassium, and Chloride ▪ Measurements of these analytes are known as the blood electrolytes. The functions of many tissues are regulated by electrolyte concentrations. Abnormalities may be associated with a variety of diseases, the hydration of the individual, and effects of therapy. Clinical correlation is necessary.

Thyroxine ▪ Thryoxine (T4) is a hormone produced by the thyroid gland. It is a metabolism indicator. Metabolism can be thought of as how the body uses food. High values may indicate overactivity of the thyroid, and low values may indicate underactivity. Some medications, birth control pills, pregnancy, liver disease, and hormonal therapy can affect values. The T4 may be combined with the *resin T3 uptake* test to provide further information. This combination is also known as T7 or the free thyroxine index (FTI). The T7 or FTI is a calculated value. A variety of tests to further evaluate possible abnormalities are triiodothyronine (T3), thyroid-stimulating hormone (TSH), thyroxine-binding globulin (TBG), thyroid-releasing hormone (TRH), quantitative free thyroxine, and thyroid microsomal antibody.

Uric Acid ▪ This metabolic product is excreted in the urine. High values are associated with gout, kidney problems, certain hematologic disorders, and certain medications, including thiazides. Marked elevations may occur with extensive cellular destruction, as in intensive chemotherapy of leukemic patients with very high cell counts.

HEMATOLOGY TESTS

Complete Blood Count ▪ The complete blood count (CBC) includes red blood cells, white blood cells, and platelets. These components are considered separately.

Red Blood Cells ▪ The principal function of red blood cells is the transport of oxygen. These cells are characterized numerically by three standard indices (MCV, MCH, MCHC) that reflect the average volume of red cells, the hemoglobin content of the average, and the average concentration of hemoglobin in a given volume of packed red cells, respectively.

Automated instruments rank red cells by their volume and produce an RBC histogram (Figure 21–1). If the differing sizes exceed usual parameters, this may be indicative of red cell abnormalities or a second red cell population (transfused cells). The distribution of red cells by volume is referred to as the red cell distribution width (RDW). The red cell volumes are mathematically treated as the coefficient of variation (CV). Marked red cell abnormalities are further evaluated by microscopic examination of stained peripheral smears (Figure 21–2).

The combined data, consisting of the number of red cells, MCV, MCH, MCHC, RDW, and microscopic findings (as required), permit initial characterization of anemic conditions, e.g., iron deficiency, thalassemia trait, anemia of chronic disease, folate or B_{12} deficiencies, and so on. Appropriate confirmation and/or diagnostic tests may be required (e.g., hemoglobin electrophoresis, measurement of folate and vitamin B_{12} blood levels, and so forth).

White Blood Cells ▪ These are characterized by the total number of white cells present, as well as the number and per cent of each type. Normally, the most numerous white cells are neutrophils, followed by lymphocytes and then monocytes. Eosinophils are normally less frequent, and basophils the least. Neutrophils, eosinophils, and basophils are known as granulocytes. The usual distribution of cells may vary remarkably with differing disease conditions and with therapy.

Neutrophils typically increase with acute infections and systemic stress. Neutrophils and other granulocytes are usually increased, moderately to markedly, in various forms of myelocytic leukemia. With some leukemic conditions, the number of cells may be normal or reduced, but they exhibit morphologic immaturity and abnormalities identified by microscopic analysis.

Decreased neutrophils may occur alone or in association with other decreased white cells, red cells, and platelets. Such changes may reflect the effect of therapeutic agents, severe infection, or viral infection. The changes may be mild to severe, be self-limiting, revert to normal, or be life

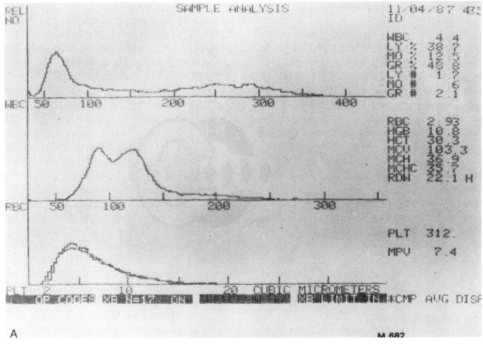

Figure 21–1

A, Macrocytic anemia, Coulter. Coulter S-Plus IV. Macrocytic patient with dimorphic erythrocytes. RBCs are bimodal with macrocytic and normocytic red cell populations and high normal MCHC. The RDW is very elevated as a reflection of increased anisocytosis. WBC and platelet histogram are unremarkable. Manual differential count: 11 n. bands, 47 neutrophils, 21 lymphocytes, 5 atypical lymphocytes, 13 monocytes, 2 eosinophils, 1 basophil.

threatening. Clinical correlation is always required, and further investigation may be necessary.

Lymphocytes may be increased with infectious mononucleosis or other viral infections, as a reaction to medications, and with lymphoproliferative disorders including lymphocytic leukemias and lymphomas.

Decreased lymphocytes may occur in response to severe viral infections, effects of medications, and as a component of generalized bone marrow depression (Figure 21–3).

Eosinophils may be significantly increased owing to allergic phenomena. Basophils are uncommonly increased. This may be seen with chronic ulcerative colitis and autoimmune conditions.

Automated hematology analyzers routinely provide quantitative data regarding the white cells. These data include the absolute count of each cell type and also the relative percentage of occurrence of each cell type of the total white cells present. Absolute cell counts are of particular value for tracking the effects of chemotherapy (Figures 21–4 and 21–5). Microscopic evaluation of white cells by examination of the peripheral smear is very important. This is particularly true for possible leukemic states and for evaluating the response of leukemic patients to therapy (Figures 21–6 and 21–7).

Platelets ▪ Platelets (thrombocytes) are essential for normal coagulation. They are evaluated by determining the number present. Automated hematology analyzers also determine the average volume of platelets.

Platelets are frequently increased (thrombo-

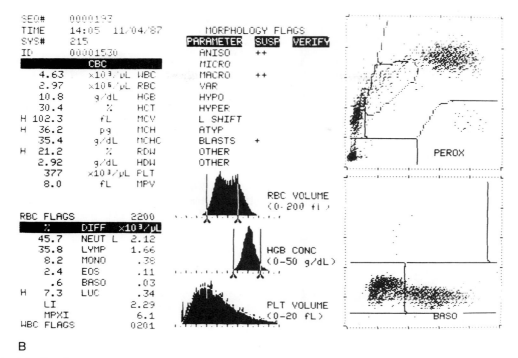

B

Figure 21–1 *Continued*

B, Same specimen as in A, Technicon H-1. The report flags 2+ aniso and macro and shows dimorphic population in the RBC volume histogram. The hemoglobin concentration histogram shows that both RBC populations are normochromic. The false-positive blast flag and true-positive elevated LUCs (large unstained cells) were probably caused by the atypical lymphocytes.

(From Henry, J. B. (ed.): *Clinical Diagnosis and Management by Laboratory Methods.* W. B. Saunders Company, Philadelphia, 1991, p. 572.)

cytosis) as a reactive process to an inflammatory process or infection. However, granulocytic leukemias may cause increases.

Decreased platelets (thrombocytopenia) may occur as a consequence of therapeutic agents, with infections, and with leukemias. A marked decrease of platelets may occur infrequently with no identified cause. This is known as idiopathic thrombocytopenia (ITP).

Automated hematology analyzers perform platelet counts with high accuracy. However, artefactual disturbances of platelet counts (and less frequently white cell counts) can occur due to effects of the anticoagulant EDTA, which is present in the lavender-top tubes used for CBCs. Most frequently this causes platelet counts to be decreased because of the platelets aggregating together — in some instances to levels that are considered medically dangerous (critical values). Less frequently, white blood cells may aggregate.

This condition tends to occur in certain individuals, but delayed mixing can contribute to this phenomenon. For those individuals prone to this condition (no clinical abnormality has been identified), follow-up studies may avoid the problem by use of citrated specimens. Automated instruments usually detect this condition (Figure 21–8). Examination of the stained peripheral smear microscopically permits identification of the platelet aggregates.

An uncommon artefactual condition may arise from improper specimen handling. Markedly elevated platelet counts of 2 million or more may appear, when examined microscopically on stained peripheral smears, as degranulated platelets. The phenomenon has been determined to occur with delayed mixing of the blood, followed by overly vigorous mixing. The white cell count may be increased as well as the platelets.

Unusual findings should be correlated with

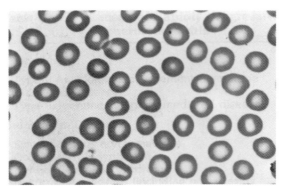

A, Normal blood film (× 875).

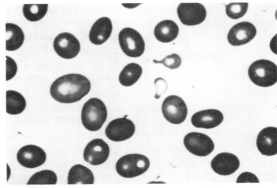

D, Megaloblastic anemia. Macrocytosis. Marked anisocytosis. Note elliptical cells and teardrop-shaped cells (× 875).

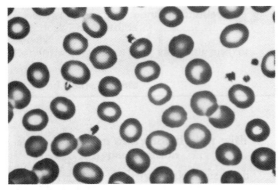

B, This blood film shows a small number of slightly hypochromic red cells; most are normochromic. Cell diameters are normal. MCV and MCHC are normal. The irregular bodies 2 to 3 μm in diameter are normal blood platelets (× 875).

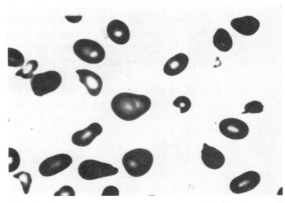

E, Megaloblastic anemia, macrocytosis, marked anisocytosis (× 875).

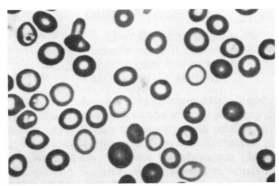

C, Iron deficiency anemia. Most of the cells are hypochromic and microcytic. Note the elliptical cells. Anisocytosis is slight in degree (× 875).

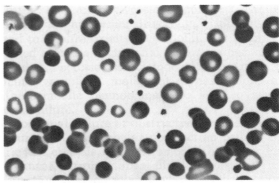

F, Hereditary spherocytosis. The denser cells are more spherocytic. Note that they have minimal and eccentric pallor, moderate anisocytosis. Though the cell diameter is reduced, the MCV is within the normal range (× 875).

Figure 21–2

(From Henry, J. B. (ed.): *Clinical Diagnosis and Management by Laboratory Methods.* W. B. Saunders Company, Philadelphia, 1991, pp. 585–589.)

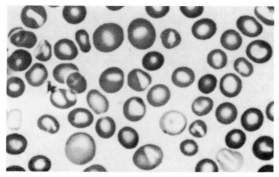

G, Sideroblastic anemia. Dimorphic populations of hypochromic cells and normochromic cells, some of which are macrocytic. Moderate anisocytosis (X 875).

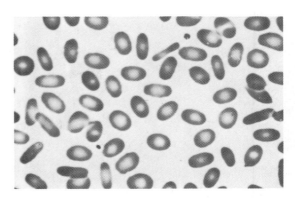

J, Hereditary elliptocytosis. Incidental finding, no anemia (X 875).

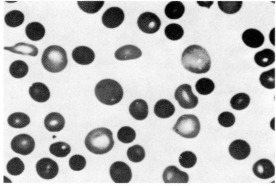

H, Autoimmune hemolytic anemia. The paler, large cells are polychromatic macrocytes (i.e., young reticulocytes). The small, dense cells are spherocytes. Moderate anisocytosis (X 875).

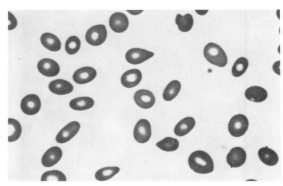

K, Blood film from a patient with myelofibrosis with myeloid metaplasia. Numerous elliptocytes. Teardrop-shaped cells (X 875).

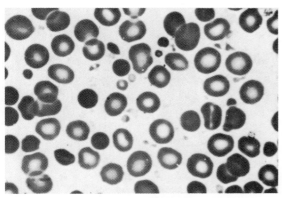

I, Blood film from a patient who has just suffered extensive body burns. Note the many tiny red cell fragments that have budded off the red cells as a result of the heat, leaving spherocytes. Marked anisocytosis (X 875).

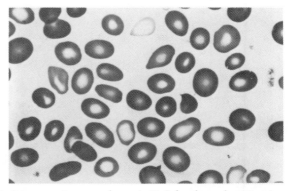

L, Same specimen as shown in K. A few hypochromic microcytic cells are present also (X 875).   *Figure continued*

Figure 21–2 *Continued*

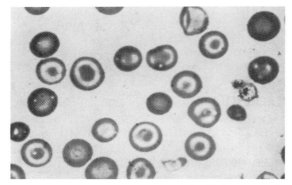

M, Target cells that have an increased cell diameter. Blood film from a patient with obstructive jaundice (× 875).

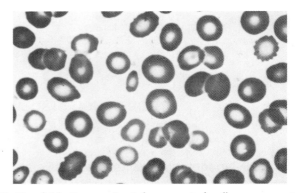

P, Megaloblastic anemia. A few crenated cells are present (× 875).

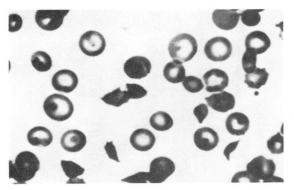

N, Microangiopathic hemolytic anemia; hemolytic-uremic syndrome. Note irregularly contracted cells, schistocytes, a few crenated cells. One nucleated red cell is present (× 875).

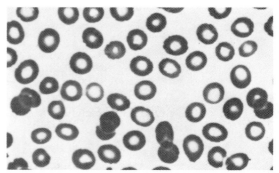

Q, Artifact due to water in the methyl alcohol fixative. If the bubbles are small in size (as here), they cause an indented appearance that may be confused with crenation (× 875).

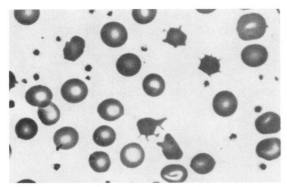

O, Acanthocytes. Note the long spicules that tend to have bulbous ends (× 875).

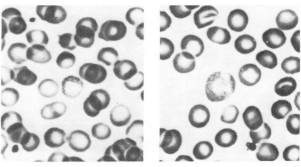

R, Basophilic stippling. One stippled red cell is seen in the center of each field. A, Thalassemia minor; B, lead poisoning (× 875).

Figure 21–2 Continued

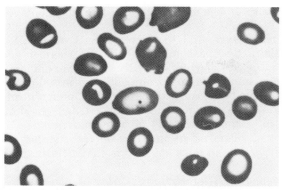

S, Megaloblastic anemia. The central oval macrocyte has four Howell-Jolly bodies; the lower three are touching one another (× 875).

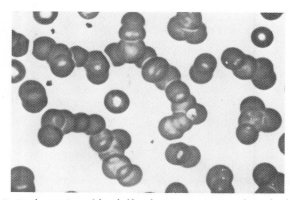

T, Rouleaux in a blood film from a patient with multiple myeloma (× 875).

Figure 21–2 Continued

other information about the CBC and the clinical status of the patient. If a piece of laboratory information does not correlate with the other available information, consideration should be given to possible artefact or other error. The studies should be repeated.

Mean platelet volume (MPV) values may be helpful in assessing likelihood of platelet recovery from thrombocytopenic states. Aplastic anemia, the consequence of total suppression of the bone marrow, causes decreased red cells, white cells, and platelets. It is a critical condition.

The CBC is an important laboratory study for disease detection; it contributes to diagnosis and is important for monitoring treatment of disease. Many ancillary tests are available and necessary for proper diagnosis. *Bone marrow biopsy* and *aspiration* are frequently indicated as the next step in characterizing abnormalities.

Coagulation

Prothrombin Time (PT) ▪ PT is widely used as a screening test for coagulopathies. It is prolonged with coumadin anticoagulation therapy, liver disease, disseminated intravascular coagulation (DIC), and specific coagulation factor deficiencies. The PT is optimally reported using the *International Normalized Ratio (INR),* which permits values reported by laboratories in different parts of the world to be compared.

Activated Partial Prothrombin Time (APTT, or PTT) ▪ The PTT is used as a screening test for coagulopathies and for monitoring heparin therapy. Prolongation of the PTT occurs commonly with vitamin K deficiency, liver disease, disseminated intravascular coagulation (DIC), and deficiencies of coagulation factors. A shortened PTT value may occur with a hypercoagulability state.

Thrombin Time (TT) ▪ The thrombin time evaluates the status of heparin therapy or the presence of heparin substances. It is prolonged with severe hypofibrinogenemia, as may occur with intravascular clotting and fibrinolysis. The thrombin time may be combined with measurement of *protamine sulfate,* which corrects the prolongation due to heparin. This may be helpful in guiding corrective therapy for a patient overheparinized or in the differential diagnosis of other causes of a prolonged PTT.

Thrombolytic therapy (e.g., streptokinase) may be monitored by a combination of tests, including *euglobulin lyis time, thrombin time, PTT, PT* and *fibrin degradation products* (*FDP*). *Fibrinogen, plasminogen, specific factor assays,* and *platelet aggregation studies* are additional coagulation assays that may be necessary to evaluate a wide array of coagulation disorders.

SERODIAGNOSIS OF HEPATITIS A, B, C, D, AND E

Hepatitis A ▪ This disease is caused by a small RNA virus (hepatitis A virus, HAV). Initial testing for HAV detects total antibody (IgG,

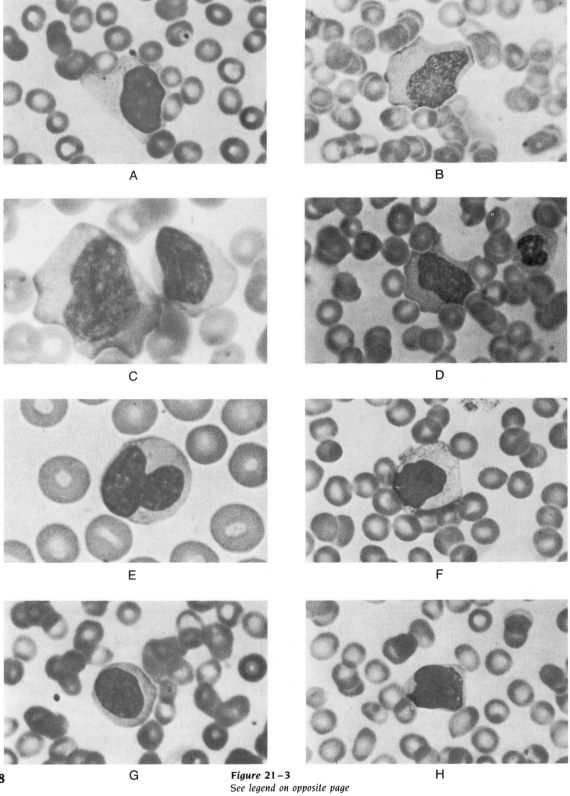

A

B

C

D

E

F

318   G

Figure 21–3
See legend on opposite page

H

IgM, and IgA). If antibody is present, a further assay for IgM HAV is necessary to determine current or recent hepatitis A. IgM antibodies are present with current infection and remain for 3 to 12 months following the acute illness. The IgG antibodies may be detected for years and indicate remote past infection and immunity to reinfection.

Hepatitis B ■ This is caused by a medium-sized DNA virus (HBV). The following serologic tests are used in the diagnosis and monitoring of hepatitis B:

Hepatitis B surface antigen (HBsAg)
Hepatitis B surface antibody (HBsAb)
Hepatitis B core antibodies (HBcAb), IgM
  and IgG
Hepatitis Be antigen (HBeAg)
Hepatitis Be antibody (HBeAb)

HBsAg is present in the blood following exposure and approximately 1 to 7 weeks before illness or elevation of enzymes (AST, ALT) in the blood. With normal resolution of acute hepatitis B, HBsAg may be detectable for 1 to 12 weeks. The presence of HBsAg is indicative of ongoing infection. HBcAb IgM may occur about the same time as enzyme elevations. In some instances, IgM core antibody may be the only marker detected and the patient is referred to as in the "core window." With normal resolution of infection and immunologic response, IgM core antibody will be replaced by IgG core antibody. HBcAb IgM may be present for 3 to 12 months. HBcAb IgG persists for life. Normal resolution is also reflected by disappearance of HBsAg and appearance of HBsAb.

HBeAg is present in the acute phase and may persist with an inadequate immunologic response. The presence of HBeAg is considered to indicate that the person may be infective to others. A normal recovery is characterized by disappearance of HBeAg and the development of HBeAb and HBsAb.

Chronic infection is the consequence of an inadequate immunologic recovery. It is characterized by persistant antigenemia. In addition to persistence of HBsAg and HBeAg, there may be low level persistence of HBcAb IgM. A patient in this status may be infective to others. The patient may develop chronic persistent hepatitis or the more aggressive chronic active hepatitis. Chronic carriers of HBsAg may also have detectable HBsAb. This is not protective antibody, since it is antibody to HBsAg epitopes not shared by the circulating antigen. Long-term sequelae include cirrhosis and the possible development of hepatic carcinoma.

HBsAb may be measured as a determinant of immunity either due to past infection or as a result of vaccination. Vaccination will produce HBsAb only. HBcAb IgG may be tested to differentiate past infection from vaccination.

Hepatitis C ■ Hepatitis C is caused by a RNA virus (HCV) that appears to be responsible for most cases of parenterally transmitted non-A, non-B hepatitis. HCV infection becomes chronic, even if asymptomatic, in about 50 per cent of cases. Long-term sequelae include cirrhosis (up to 25 per cent of cases of chronic infection) and hepatic carcinoma.

Anti-HCV appears approximately 4 to 24 weeks following onset of symptoms. Anti-HCV

Figure 21–3
A, Infectious mononucleosis. All the photographs of the lymphocytes of infectious mononucleosis are from patients with characteristic clinical findings and with positive differential tests. The lymphocyte is larger than any normal so-called large lymphocyte. The cytoplasm is abundant, clear, and moderately basophilic, especially close to the edges of the cell; red azure granules are accumulated along the upper periphery. The cytoplasm is delicate, and the surrounding red cells leave an indentation in the cytoplasm, giving it a scalloped appearance. The nucleus is oval, and the chromatin is delicate and less dense than in normal large lymphocytes. Three nucleoli are seen clearly. The two red cells adjacent on the right made indentations, even in the nucleus, suggesting that it is plastic. There is a light perinuclear zone. The characteristic lymphocytes in infectious mononucleosis are called atypical lymphocytes. B, Atypical lymphocyte, infectious mononucleosis. Notice the sharp separation of nuclear chromatin and parachromatin, and basophilic cytoplasm. C, *Left*, Reticular lymphocyte (nonleukemic lymphoblast); *right*, atypical lymphocyte with greater nuclear maturity. Infectious mononucleosis. D, *Center*, Atypical lymphocyte; *right*, normal lymphocyte. Infectious mononucleosis. E, Atypical lymphocyte with "leukocytoid" nucleus. Infectious mononucleosis. F, Normal monocyte. G, Reticular lymphocyte (nonleukemic lymphoblast); infectious mononucleosis. The nuclear chromatin is uniform and granular (or reticular). Nucleoli are conspicuous. The cytoplasm is deeply basophilic. Note the difference between this cell and the lymphoblast of acute leukemia (H). H, Lymphoblast, acute lymphoblastic leukemia.

(From Henry, J. B. (ed.): *Clinical Diagnosis and Management by Laboratory Methods.* W. B. Saunders Company, Philadelphia, 1991, p. 686.)

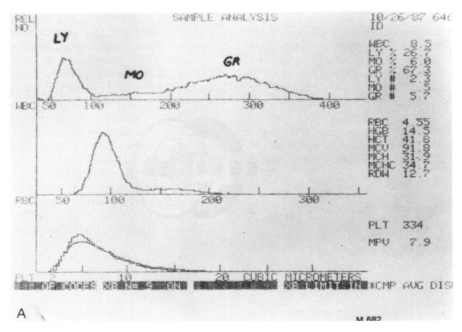

Figure 21-4

A, Normal blood cell histograms (Coulter). In the WBC channel, the altered nuclei larger than 35 fL are counted as WBC. Lymphocytes (LY) are the first peak to the left, about 35 to 90 fL. Mononuclear cells (MO), primarily monocytes, are about 90 to 160 fL. Granulocytes (GR) are mostly neutrophils, about 160 to 450 fL. Absolute counts (#) are calculated from multiplying the percentage of each cell type times the total WBC count. Cells in the RBC channel between 36 and 360 fL are considered erythrocytes; particles in the RBC channel between 2 and 20 fL, extrapolated 0 to 70 fL, are regarded as platelets. Note the typical skewed (log normal) platelet distribution. Manual 100-cell differential count: 64 neutrophils, 33 lymphocytes, 3 monocytes.

may disappear over a period of several years. Persistence of anti-HCV appears to be associated with chronic hepatitis C. At present, we are unable to test for IgG or IgM antibodies. Some patients with chronic hepatitis C (about 20 per cent) do not test positive for anti-HCV. Because anti-HCV arises late, it is advisable to retain a specimen from the acute illness for paired testing of acute- and convalescent-phase samples.

False-positive anti-HCV tests have been associated with the hyperglobulinemia of alcoholic liver disease and autoimmune chronic active hepatitis. Other false-positives have been attributed to storage conditions of specimens. Some false-positives are not explained and have occurred in populations at low risk for disease. A supplemental test is available to confirm positives. The test is a recombinant immunoblot assay (RIBA). A positive anti-HBC RIBA confirms a positive anti-HBC EIA (enzyme immunoassay). The RIBA may be indeterminate. If the RIBA is nonreactive, it favors but cannot be considered proof of a false-positive EIA reaction.

Hepatitis D ■ This is caused by a small, defective RNA virus, the hepatitis delta virus (HDV), that causes hepatitis only in individuals concurrently infected with hepatitis B.

Hepatitis D tends to be a severe disease. There is a high mortality rate in the acute phase, and cirrhosis occurs frequently as a consequence of chronic disease.

HDV may infect a person already infected with HBV, which is known as superinfection. Infection with HDV and HBV may occur simultaneously, which is known as coinfection.

Because anti-HDV arises late in acute delta hepatitis, it is advisable to retain a specimen

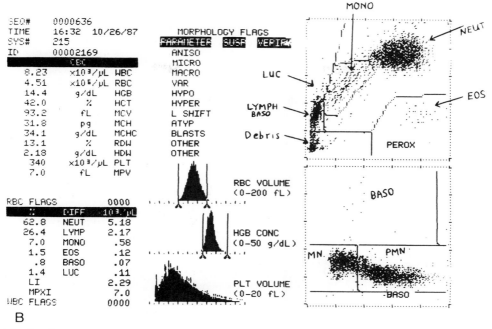

B

Figure 21–4 *Continued*

B, H · I report of same specimen as shown in A. Blood cell counts are essentially identical to those produced by the Coulter. Arrows indicate the cell types in the peroxidase plot. The H · I analyzer computer has segregated the various cells. The basophil/lobularity plot shows the basophils with intact cytoplasm above; below to the left are the mononuclear cells (lymphocytes, monocytes) with granulocytes (bands, eosinophils, and neutrophils) to the right. RBC volume, hemoglobin concentration, and platelet volume histograms are normal, as are the RBC indices and platelet count. Other red cell cytograms of volume versus hemoglobin concentration (not shown) are also available for recall, review, and counting. MONO = monocytes; NEUT = neutrophils; EOS = eosinophils; LUC = large unstained cells; LYMPH = lymphocytes; BASO = basophils; MN = mononuclear cells (lymphocytes, monocytes); PMN = neutrophils.

(From Henry, J. B. (ed.): *Clinical Diagnosis and Management by Laboratory Methods.* W. B. Saunders Company, Philadelphia, 1991, p. 571.)

from the acute illness for paired testing of acute- and convalescent-phase samples (total and IgG). IgM and IgG antibodies may be assayed. A single determination of IgM anti-HDV is considered diagnostic.

Hepatitis D antigen (HDVAg) may also be assayed, and if antigenemia persists, it signals development of chronic HDV infection regardless of whether superinfected or coinfected.

Patients with acute delta coinfection usually clear the HBV and HDV. Less than 5 per cent progress to chronic disease. Patients with acute delta superinfection usually develop chronic delta hepatitis (over 75 per cent).

Hepatitis E ▪ Hepatitis E is caused by a small RNA virus (HEV). The disease may be acute epidemic or enterally transmitted non-A, non-B hepatitis. The disease does not lead to chronic hepatitis or a carrier state. It is associated with fecal-oral transmission of the HEV or with contamination of food or water supplies. The diagnosis is one of exclusion, since serologic tests are under development and not generally available.

TUMOR MARKERS

Many tumor marker assays are available. Most are pending FDA approval and restricted to research or investigational use only. Nonapproved tests are not to be used as diagnostic procedures without confirmation of the diagnosis by other medically established means. The

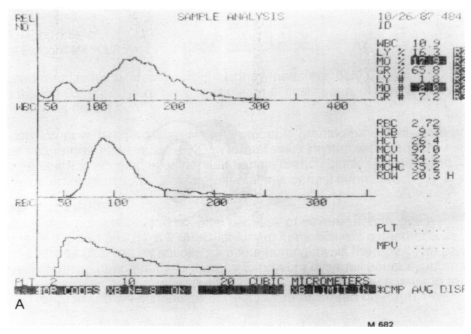

Figure 21–5

A, Acute myeloblastic leukemia with blasts. The WBC histogram shows both R2 (about 90 fL) and R3 flags (about 160 fL). Mononuclear counts above 1500/μL are backlit; here the high mono count and flags are due to the presence of myeloblasts. Chemotherapy has resulted in a macrocytic component to the RBC population and a high RDW (red cell distribution width). The platelet count was 40 × 10⁹/L by phase microscropy. Manual differential count: 50 blasts, 1 myelocyte, 24 neutrophils, 15 lymphocytes, 2 atypical lymphocytes, 1 plasma cell, 7 monocytes, 6 NRBC.

tumor markers discussed here are well known and widely used.

CA 125 ▪ CA 125, a mucin-like molecule detected by radioimmunoassay, is approved for use in the detection of residual ovarian carcinoma in patients who have had first-line therapy and would be considered for diagnostic second-look procedures. It may be elevated in epithelial ovarian carcinoma and in endometrial disorders, including adenocarcinoma and advanced endometriosis.

CA 125 is also useful in monitoring therapy in patients with ovarian or endometrial carcinoma. Rising and falling levels correlate well with progression or regression of disease. It may be elevated in nongynecologic cancers, including pancreatic cancer, lung cancer, gastrointestinal cancer, and adenosquamous cancers of the cervix, and also in advanced liver disease, acute peritonitis, and nonmalignant gynecologic disease.

In association with the menstrual cycle, CA 125 levels may vary from within the reference range to mildly elevated values. These variabilities severely limit the usefulness of this assay as a screening approach to ovarian carcinoma in asymptomatic women. The limited use of CA 125 for early detection of ovarian carcinoma in women who have been determined to be at high risk is being investigated.

Carcinoembryonic Antigen (CEA) ▪ This oncofetal glycoprotein is synthesized by columnar epithelial cells and most frequently measured by immunoenzymatic assay. CEA may be elevated with colorectal cancers (60 to 90 per cent), pancreatic cancers (90 per cent), lung cancers (70 per cent), breast cancers (35 per cent), and ovarian cancers (12 to 14 per cent). It has significant value for monitoring patients with diagnosed malignancies. Persistent elevation following treatment is strongly indicative of residual disease. Declining values generally indicate a favorable response to therapy.

CEA may be elevated in benign liver disease,

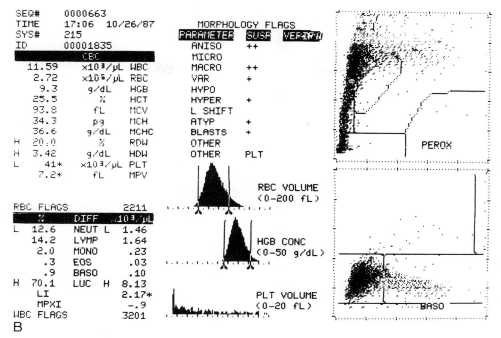

Figure 21–5 *Continued*

B, Same specimen as shown in A. Note the large LUC (70.1 per cent) component above the lymphocyte area in the peroxidase plot and the (correct) blast flag. Also note the predominance of cells (blasts) to the far left in the mononuclear area of the basophil/lobularity plot. The RBC volume histogram shows macrocytosis and anisocytosis (high RDW); the hemoglobin concentraiton histogram indicates a minor hyperchromic RBC population.

(From Henry, J. B. (ed.): *Clinical Diagnosis and Management Laboratory Methods*. W. B. Saunders Company, Philadelphia, 1991, p. 574.)

including cirrhosis, hepatitis, biliary obstruction, and liver abscess. Inflammation, particularly of the gastrointestinal tract, infections, infarction, collagen disease, renal impairment, and smoking may be associated with elevated CEA values. Values obtained by different assays may not be used interchangeably. With change of the assay method, patients being monitored should have sequential testing by the new method to establish a baseline.

Some Investigational Tumor Markers ■ Tumor markers associated with breast carcinoma include CA 15-3, c-erbB-2 (HER-2)/neu, and cathepsin D. CA 19-9 is a tumor marker associated with gastrointestinal and pancreatic adenocarcinomas.

Prostate-Specific Antigen ■ This is a screening test, measuring a glycoprotein produced by the prostate gland. Prostate-specific antigen (PSA) can detect prostate cancers that are non-palpable by digital rectal examination (DRE). Elevations of PSA may be due to conditions other than cancer, such as benign prostatic hyperplasia (BPH), prostatitis, and prostatic infarction. PSA should be combined with digital rectal examination for initial evaluation. Further evaluation of increased PSA, particularly for mild elevations (4.1 to 10.0 ug/L), may be made by transrectal ultrasound (TRUS). Monoclonal PSA values within this range require investigation since serious disease may be present. Nearly half the cancers present in association with moderate increases have extracapsular extension. Definitive diagnosis requires microscopic study of biopsy tissue, usually obtained as cores of prostate tissue by needle biopsy.

Prostatic acid phosphatase (PAP) may be utilized in combination with PSA in the evaluation of prostate disease. PAP is less sensitive and, therefore, less likely to be increased with BPH,

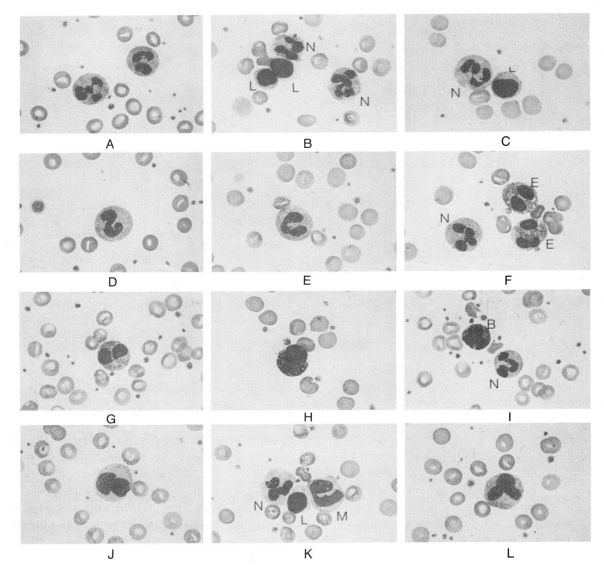

Figure 21–6

These photomicrographs are from buffy coat preparations of blood from a normal individual. Therefore, the number of leukocytes and platelets per field is greater than in blood films made directly. A, Neutrophils. The cell on the right has a few nuclear spicules or extensions. These rather pointed spicules are directed toward the centrosomal region of the cell. Such nuclear extensions may be found in normal individuals but are more frequent in those with chronic illnesses. They should be distinguished from the sex chromatin appendages, which have a drumstick appearance. B, Lymphocytes (L) of slightly different size and chromatin condensation, and neutrophils (N). C, Neutrophil (N) and lymphocyte (L). D and E, Band neutrophils. In E, note the incomplete segmentation. F, Neutrophil (N) and eosinophils (E). Eosinophils have larger granules and, on the average, fewer lobes than do neutrophils. G, Eosinophil. H, Basophil. I, Basophil (B); neutrophil (N). J, Monocyte. K, Neutrophil (N); lymphocyte (L); monocyte (M). The monocyte has more delicately staining chromatin than the other cells; this usually can be appreciated at low magnification. L, Monocyte.

(From Henry, J. B. (ed.): *Clinical Diagnosis and Management by Laboratory Methods.* W. B. Saunders Company, Philadelphia, 1991, Plate 24-1.)

Figure 21–7   *Illustration on opposite page*

A, Acute myeloblastic leukemia (AML), Wright-Giemsa stain. No maturation is evident. This corresponds to the M1 category of the French-American-British (FAB) classification. B, AML, Sudan black B reaction. Same patient as in A. Though granules are not visible with the Wright-Giemsa stain, all the blasts contain sudanophilic material (brown granules). The peroxidase reaction was similarly positive. C, Acute myeloblastic leukemia with partial maturation (M2). Naphthol ASD chloroacetate esterase reaction. All stages of developing neutrophils have a positive reaction. D, Acute myelomonocytic leukemia (AMML),

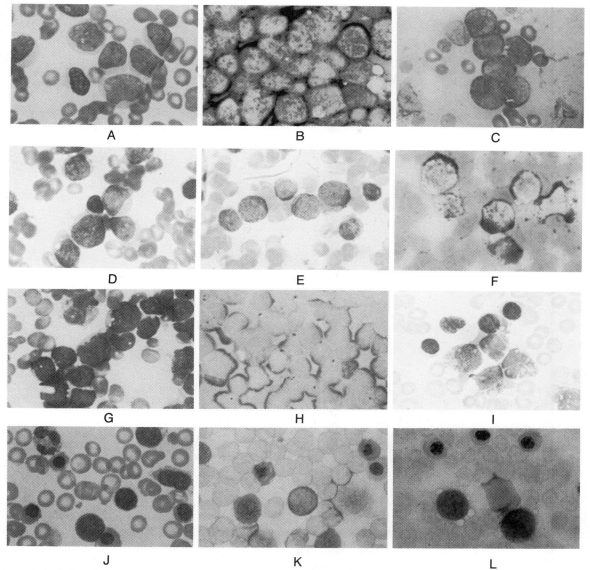

Figure 21-7 *Continued*

Wright-Giemsa stain. No cytoplasmic maturation is evident. This stain alone does not allow a definitive diagnosis. E, AMML, Sudan black B reaction. Same patient as in D. A moderate proportion of the blasts contain sudanophilic material. F, AMML, α-naphthyl acetate esterase reaction. Same patient as in D. Most of the blasts contain nonspecific esterase (which is fluoride sensitive). Cytochemical reactions, therefore, lead to the diagnosis of myelomonocytic leukemia. G, Acute lymphoblastic leukemia (ALL), Wright-Giemsa stain. Most of the blasts are small, and the cytoplasm is scanty. This corresponds to the Ll category of the FAB classification. H, ALL, periodic acid–Schiff (PAS) reaction. Same patient as in G. A moderate proportion of the blasts contains one or more large granules or "blocks" of PAS-positive material. I, Acute promyelocytic leukemia, Wright-Giemsa stain. The majority of cells have abundant azurophil granules, often large. Usually, some cells contain multiple Auer rods, as in the cell at the right. The nuclei are irregularly shaped or indented (Reider forms). This is the hypergranular promyelocytic category M3 of the FAB classification. J, Erythroleukemia, Wright-Giemsa stain. One primitive blast (*lower center*), one abnormal monocyte (*upper right*), one neutrophil, and five nucleated erythroid cells are present. Most of the latter are abnormal. K, Erythroleukemia, PAS reaction. Same patient as in J. Of the six nucleated erythroid cells in this field, five are PAS positive: in the most immature, the reactive material is granular (*lower center*); in the others, it is diffuse. A monocyte and a blast are PAS negative, a neutrophil is PAS positive. L, Erythroleukemia, α-naphthyl butyrate reaction. Same patient as in J. Monocytes are strongly positive for this nonspecific esterase reaction; they were increased in number and morphologically abnormal and part of the leukemic process. Erythroid, granulocytic, and monocytic cell lines are demonstrably involved in this case.

(From Henry, J. B. (ed.): *Clinical Diagnosis and Management by Laboratory Methods.* W. B. Saunders Company, Philadelphia, 1991, Plate 27-3.)

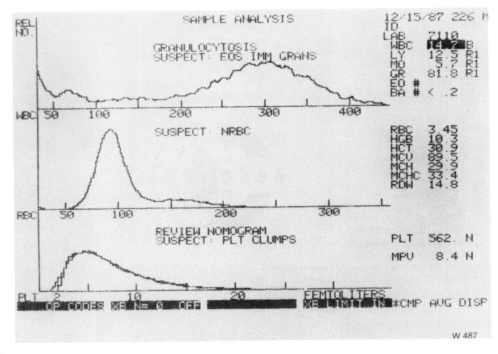

Figure 21–8

Coulter STKR report from a patient with clumped platelets and thrombocytosis. The total WBC count (14.7) is backlit to warn that something is elevating the baseline at about 35 fL, also causing a R1 flag. In this case, clumped platelets are interfering at the left side of the lymphocyte population. This has also resulted in a "SUSPECT: PLT CLUMPS" in the platelet histogram and "SUSPECT: NRBC" in the RBC histogram, since either is a possible cause of the "high take-off" on the WBC histogram. The WBC histogram also gives a true-positive result for granulocytosis (at operator-defined limits) but a false-positive result for eosinophilia (note no EO# printed) and/or immature granulocytes. Although platelet clumps are sometimes seen on the right side of the platelet histogram, they are not seen in this case. Manual leukocyte differential count: 74 neutrophils, 11 n. bands, 9 lymphocytes, 6 monocytes.

(From Henry, J. B. (ed.): *Clinical Diagnosis and Management by Laboratory Methods*. W. B. Saunders Company, Philadelphia, 1991, p. 576.)

but it is also less likely to be elevated with prostatic carcinoma. The combination of PSA and PAP may be useful. PAP may be normal in cases in which the PSA is mildly to moderately elevated and there is a strong probability of BPH. Uncommonly, the PAP may be elevated with some prostatic cancers in which the PSA is normal or moderately increased. These cases should be further investigated. The PAP should not be used as the sole screening test for prostatic carcinoma.

URINALYSIS

A urinalysis (UA) has two major components, the *macroscopic* and the *microscopic*. These findings are illustrated in Table 21–1.

Macroscopic Examination ■ The method for performing the macroscopic examination is as follows:

1. Evaluate specimen according to written guidelines. Record volume of urine received.
2. Pour a standardized volume (10, 12, 15 mL) of urine into an optically clear, labeled centrifuge tube. Make a notation on the report form of volumes less than the standardized volume. Refrigerate remaining urine until examination is completed.
3. Determine color.
4. Determine character (clarity).
5. Report presence of unusual odor and abnormal amounts of or colored foam.
6. Determine specific gravity.
   a. Clean instrument with distilled H_2O before use.

Table 21 – 1 ▪ **Urinalysis Abnormalities Found in Various Urinary System Diseases**

Diseases	Macroscopic Urinalysis	Microscopic Urinalysis
Acute glomerulonephritis	Gross hematuria "Smoky" turbidity Proteinuria	Erythrocyte and blood casts Epithelial casts Hyaline and granular casts Waxy casts Neutrophils Erythrocytes
Chronic glomerulonephritis	Hematuria Proteinuria	Granular and waxy casts Occasional blood casts Erythrocytes Leukocytes Epithelial casts Lipid droplets
Acute pyelonephritis	Turbid Occasional odor Occasional proteinuria	Numerous neutrophils (many in clumps) Few lymphocytes and histiocytes Leukocyte casts Epithelial casts Renal epithelial cells Erythrocytes Granular and waxy casts Bacteria
Chronic pyelonephritis	Occasional proteinuria	Leukocytes Broad, waxy casts Granular and epithelial casts Occasional leukocyte cast Bacteria Erythrocytes
Nephrotic syndrome	Proteinuria Fat droplets	Fatty and waxy casts Cellular and granular casts Oval fat bodies and/or vacuolated renal epithelial cells occurring singly or as cellular clusters
Acute tubular necrosis	Hematuria Occasional proteinuria	Necrotic or degenerated renal epithelial cells Neutrophils and erythrocytes Granular and epithelial casts Broad, waxy casts Epithelial tissue fragments
Cystitis	Hematuria	Numerous leukocytes Erythrocytes Transitional epithelial cells occurring singly or as fragments Histiocytes and giant cells Bacteria Absence of casts
Dysuria-pyuria syndrome	Slightly turbid	Numerous leukocytes, bacteria Erythrocytes No casts
Acute renal allograft rejection (lower nephrosis)	Hematuria Occasional proteinuria	Renal epithelial cells Lymphocytes and plasma cells Neutrophils Renal epithelial casts

Table continued on following page

Table* 21 – 1 ▪ Urinalysis Abnormalities Found in Various Urinary System Diseases *Continued

Diseases	Macroscopic Urinalysis	Microscopic Urinalysis
Urinary tract neoplasia	Hematuria	Renal epithelial fragments Granular, bloody, and waxy casts Atypical mononuclear cells with enlarged, irregular hyperchromatic nuclei and sometimes containing prominent nucleoli that occur singly or as tissue fragments Neutrophils Erythrocytes Transitional epithelial cells
Viral infection	Hematuria Occasional proteinuria	Enlarged mononuclear cells and/or multinucleated cells with prominent intranuclear and/or cytoplasmic inclusions Neutrophils Lymphocytes and plasma cells Erythrocytes

From Henry, J. B. (ed.): *Clinical Diagnosis and Management by Laboratory Methods.* W. B. Saunders Company, Philadelphia, 1991, p. 422.

   b. Check zero calibration with distilled H_2O.

   c. Determine urine specific gravity. Values greater than 1.035 should be diluted 1 : 2 or 1 : 3 with H_2O and rerun. Investigate specific gravities outside the physiologic range (> 1.035).

7. Invert urine to mix and perform reagent strip testing. Use unspun, well-mixed urine equilibrated to room temperature. Follow exact timing. Report results using standardized terminology.

8. Centrifuge capped or sealed urine tubes for 5 minutes at $450 \times g$.

9. Carefully remove supernatant, leaving a fixed sediment volume. The supernatant should be saved for additional testing.

10. Perform confirmatory tests as required. Supernatant is used for:

   a. Sulfosalicylic (SSA) or other confirmatory protein tests.

   b. Ascorbic acid tests.

   c. Ictotest to confirm sugars.

   d. Chromatography to confirm sugars.

   e. Chemical confirmation crystals.

11. Review entire report for inconsistencies/discrepancies. Check patient history when necessary. Make recommendations when appropriate.*

Appearance ▪ The color and clarity are observed and reported. See Tables 21–2 and 21–3.

Specific Gravity ▪ Typical specific gravity results that normally occur are reported. See Table 21–4. Low specific gravity (hyposthenuric) is less than 1.007. This may reflect dilution due to excessive water intake. Renal failure is characterized by a failure to concentrate urine, with specific gravity tending to repeat at about 1.010, that for protein-free glomerular filtrate. A specific gravity above 1.023 indicates an ability of the kidneys to concentrate urine. Dehydration results in high specific gravity, above 1.030.

pH ▪ The urine is normally acid. The kidney normally functions to maintain hydrogen ion concentration in the plasma and extracellular fluid. This function is compromised with renal disease, e.g., renal tubular acidosis results in urine pH greater than 5.3, with acidemia or an

*From Henry, J. B. (ed.): *Clinical Diagnosis and Management by Laboratory Methods.* W. B. Saunders Company. Philadelphia, 1991, p. 398.

Table 21–2 ■ **Appearance and Color of Urine**

Appearance	Cause	Remarks
Colorless	Very dilute urine	Polyuria, diabetes insipidus
Cloudy	Phosphates, carbonates	Soluble in dilute acetic acid
	Urates, uric acid	Dissolve at 60°C. and in alkali
	Leukocytes	Insoluble in dilute acetic acid
	Red cells ("smoky")	Lyse in dilute acetic acid
	Bacteria, yeasts	Insoluble in dilute acetic acid
	Spermatozoa	Insoluble in dilute acetic acid
	Prostatic fluid	
	Mucin, mucous threads	May be flocculent
	Calculi, "gravel"	Phosphates, oxalates
	Clumps, pus, tissue	
	Fecal contamination	Rectovesical fistula
	Radiographic dye	In acid urine
Milky	Many neutrophils (pyuria)	Insoluble in dilute acetic acid
	Fat	
	Lipiduria, opalescent	Nephrosis, crush injury—soluble in ether
	Chyluria, milky	Lymphatic obstruction—soluble in ether
	Emulsified paraffin	Vaginal creams
Yellow	Acriflavine	Green fluorescence
Yellow-orange	Concentrated urine	Dehydration, fever
	Urobilin in excess	No yellow foam
	Bilirubin	Yellow foam if sufficient bilirubin
Yellow-green	Bilirubin-biliverdin	Yellow foam
Yellow-brown	Bilirubin-biliverdin	"Beer" brown, yellow foam
Red	Hemoglobin	Positive ⎫
	Erythrocytes	Positive ⎬ reagent strip for blood
	Myoglobin	Positive ⎭
	Porphyrin	May be colorless
	Fuscin, aniline dye	Foods, candy
	Beets	Yellow alkaline, genetic
	Menstrual contamination	Clots, mucus
Red-purple	Porphyrins	May be colorless
Red-brown	Erythrocytes	
	Hemoglobin on standing	
	Methemoglobin	Acid pH
	Myoglobin	Muscle injury
	Bilifuscin (dipyrrole)	Result of unstable hemoglobin
Brown-black	Methemoglobin	Blood, acid pH
	Homogentisic acid	On standing, alkaline; alcaptonuria
	Melanin	On standing, rare
Blue-green	Indicans	Small intestine infections
	Pseudomonas infections	
	Chlorophyll	Mouth deodorants

From Henry, J. B. (ed.): *Clinical Diagnosis and Management by Laboratory Methods.* W. B. Saunders Company, Philadelphia, 1991, p. 394.

Table 21-3 ▪ **Urine Color Changes with Commonly Used Drugs***

Drug	Color
Alcohol ethyl	Pale, diuresis
Anthraquinone laxatives (senna, cascara)	Reddish, alkaline; yellow-brown, acid
Chlorzoxazone (Paraflex) (muscle relaxant)	Red
Deferoxamine mesylate (Desferal) (chelates iron)	Red
Ethoxazene (Serenium) (urinary analgesic)	Orange, red
Fluorescein sodium (given IV)	Yellow
Furazolidone (Furoxone, Tricofuron) (an antibacterial, antiprotozoal nitrofuran)	Brown
Indigo carmine dye (renal function, cytoscopy)	Blue
Iron sorbitol (Jectofer) (possibly other iron compounds forming iron sulfide in urine)	Brown on standing
Levodopa (L-dopa) (for parkinsonism)	Red then brown, alkaline
Mepacrine (Atabrine) (antimalarial) (intestinal worms, *Giardia*)	Yellow
Methocarbamol (Robaxin) (muscle relaxant)	Green-brown
Methyldopa (Aldomet) (antihypertensive)	Darkening; if oxidizing agents present, red to brown
Methylene blue (used to delineate fistulas)	Blue, blue-green
Metronidazole (Flagyl) (for *Trichomonas* infection, amebiasis, *Giardia*)	Darkening, reddish brown
Nitrofurantoin (Furadantin) (antibacterial)	Brown-yellow
Phenazopyridine (Pyridium) (urinary analgesic), also compounded with sulfonamides (Azo Gantrisin, etc.)	Orange-red, acid pH
Phenindione (Hedulin) (anticoagulant) (important to distinguish from hematuria)	Orange, alkaline; color disappears on acidifying
Phenol poisoning	Brown; oxidized to quinones (green)
Phenolphthalein (purgative)	Red-purple, alkaline pH
Phenolsulfonphthalein (PSP, also BSP)	Pink-red, alkaline pH
Rifampin (Rifadin, Rimactane) (tuberculosis therapy)	Bright orange-red
Riboflavin (multivitamins)	Bright yellow
Sulfasalazine (Azulfidine) (for ulcerative colitis)	Orange-yellow, alkaline pH

*Other commonly used drugs have been noted to produce color change once or occasionally: amitriptyline (Elavil)—blue-green; phenothiazines—red; triamterene (Dyrenium)—pale blue (blue fluorescence in acid urine). An extensive list may be found in Young et al: *Clin. Chem.* 21:379, 1975.

From Henry, J. B. (ed.): *Clinical Diagnosis and Management by Laboratory Methods*. W. B. Saunders Company, Philadelphia, 1991, p. 395.

Table 21–4 ■ Urinary Specific Gravity and Urine Volume Age-Related Reference Values

	Reference Values
Specific Gravity	
Newborn (first few days)	1.012
Infants	1.002–1.006
Adults	1.001–1.035
Adults (normal fluid intake)	1.016–1.022
Volume	
Newborn (1–2 days old)	30–60 mL/24h
Infants	
3–10 days	100–300 mL/24h
10–60 days	250–450 mL/24h
60–365 days	400–500 mL/24h
Children	
1–3 years	500–600 mL/24h
3–5 years	600–700 mL/24h
5–8 years	650–1000 mL/24h
8–14 years	800–1400 mL/24h
Adults	600–1600 mL/24h
Older adults	250–2400 mL/24h

From Henry, J. B. (ed.): *Clinical Diagnosis and Management by Laboratory Methods.* W. B. Saunders Company, Philadelphia, 1991, p. 396.

acute acid challenge. With urine pH 6.1 or more, it can be assumed that bicarbonate is being spilled. In metabolic acidosis, an acid urine is produced. In metabolic alkalosis, an alkaline urine is produced.

In normal individuals, pH can vary from 4 to 8. Meat proteins and some fruits cause a low pH. A diet that is predominantly vegetable will cause an alkaline urine, pH over 6.

Protein ■ Normally, little protein is present in the urine. Strenuous exercise and dehydration can cause protein to increase normally. Proteinuria occurs with:

nephrotic syndrome
nephritis
toxic nephropathies
renal tubular diseases
nephrosclerosis
polycystic kidney disease
pyelonephritis
pre-eclampsia
postural proteinuria
Bence Jones proteinuria

The Dipstik reaction for protein is confirmed by a second test, for sulfosalicylic acid (SSA). The Dipstik test for protein is most sensitive for albumin, compared with globulins. If Bence Jones protein is suspected, immunoelectrophoresis is an excellent test for further evaluation (serum or urine).

Glucose ■ Glucose is not normally present. It may be present in pregnancy because of a lowered renal threshold for glucose. Glucosuria occurs in:

diabetes mellitus
Cushing's syndrome
acromegaly
pheochromocytoma
hyperthyroidism
hemochromatosis
pancreatitis
pancreatic carcinoma
central nervous system disorders
metabolic disturbances
medications: thiazides, corticosteroids, ACTH, birth control pills
renal tubular dysfunction

The Dipstik is specific for glucose. In children, evaluation for reducing substances is done by a copper reduction test.

Ketones ■ The Dipstik measures acetone and acetoacetic acid. Beta-hydroxybutyric acid is not measured. Ketones are elevated in:

uncontrolled diabetes mellitus
nondiabetic ketonuria
  in children:
    acute febrile illnesses
    toxic states with vomiting or diarrhea
alcoholics
rapid weight loss
cachexia

Blood ■ The Dipstik measures hemoglobin and myoglobin. Although intact red cells may be detected, the reagent strip is less sensitive to them. Microscopic examination is more definitive. See Tables 21–5, 21–6, and 21–7.

Bilirubin ■ The bilirubin in urine is bilirubin diglucuronate. Bilirubinuria occurs with liver disease, obstructive biliary tract disease, and congenital hyperbilirubinemias.

Urobilinogen ■ Urobilinogen occurs with hepatitis and liver damage caused by drugs, toxic

Table 21–5 ▪ **Urine and Plasma Findings with Intravascular Erythrocyte Destruction**

Test	Moderate Hemolysis	Marked Hemolysis
Urine		
Bilirubin (conjugated)	Absent	Absent
Urobilinogen	Normal or elevated	Elevated
Hemoglobin	Absent	Present
Hemosiderin	Absent	Present (late)
Plasma		
Bilirubin (unconjugated)	Elevated	Elevated
Haptoglobin	Decreased	Absent
Hemoglobin	Elevated	Elevated (marked)

From Henry, J. B. (ed.): *Clinical Diagnosis and Management by Laboratory Methods*. W. B. Saunders Company, Philadelphia, 1991, p. 410.

substances and congestive failure. It is also seen with hemolytic anemias.

Nitrite ▪ A positive nitrite test indicates the presence of a significant number of bacteria.

Leukocyte Esterase ▪ A positive esterase test gives a good indication of neutrophilic esterases of about 10 or more cells/μL, consistent with pyuria. It is important to note that the specimen must be a clean-catch, midstream specimen, with avoidance of vaginal contamination.

Microscopic Examination ▪ Sediment is examined for red cells, white cells, casts, crystals, microorganisms, and parasites. Normally, 0 to 2 red cells per high-power field are present in men and 3 to 12 in women. The number of white cells normally present is 3 to 5/hpf. Casts are counted per low power field (lpf).

Many artefacts occur in the urine and must be carefully distinguished from legitimate, normal, or abnormal elements of the urine.

Additional findings of importance include renal tubular epithelial cells. These may occur with acute tubular necrosis, ischemic injury, and renal transplant rejection (Figures 21–9 and 21–10).

Red Cells ▪ A very small number of red cells may occur normally in urine, as evaluated microscopically in urine sediment. Increased red cells and aberrant morphology of red cells may occur with glomerular bleeding.

Red cells may be increased in the urine with renal disorders, including glomerulonephritis, lupus nephritis, interstitial nephritis secondary to drug reactions, urinary tract calculi, acute infections, infarction, trauma, and other patho-

Table 21–6 ▪ **Causes of Rhabdomyolysis (Muscle Damage) and Myoglobinuria**

Polymyositis and dermatomyositis (acute, severe)	Toxic substances and drugs
	Acute alcohol overdose, phencyclidine (angel
Trauma and ischemia	dust), other drugs, especially with seizures
Skeletal muscle injuries	Carbon monoxide, ethylene glycol
Crush injury, surgery	Sea snake bite, hornet's venom
Severe exercise	Diuretics causing hypokalemia
Massive muscle ischemia	
Cardiac muscle injury	Hereditary causes
Seizures from any cause	Paroxysmal (Meyer-Betz)
Heat cramps	Anesthesia (halothane), malignant hyperthermia
	Phosphorylase deficiency (McArdle)
Infections	Carnitine palmityl transferase deficiency in children
Influenza, herpes virus	Occasionally in glycogen and lipid storage diseases
Epstein-Barr virus	with myopathies
Legionnaires' disease and other severe bacterial	Occasionally in periodic paralysis
infections	

From Henry, J. B. (ed.): *Clinical Diagnosis and Management by Laboratory Methods*. W. B. Saunders Company, Philadelphia, 1991, p. 411.

***Table* 21–7 ■ Differentiation of Hemoglobinuria, Myoglobinuria, and Hematuria**

Condition	Blood Plasma Findings	Urine Findings
Hemoglobinuria	Color—pink (early) Haptoglobin—low	Color—pink, red, brown Erythrocytes—occasional Pigment casts—occasional Protein—present or absent Hemosiderin—late
Myoglobinuria	Color—normal Haptoglobin—normal CK*—marked increase Aldolase—increased	Color—red, brown Erythrocytes—occasional Dense brown casts—occasional Protein—present or absent

Hematuria	Color—normal	Color—normal, smoky, pink, red, brown
		Erythrocytes—many
		   Renal—red blood cell casts
		      Protein—marked increase
		   Lower urinary tract—no casts
		      Protein—present or absent

*Creatine phosphokinase.
From Henry, J. B. (ed.): *Clinical Diagnosis and Management by Laboratory Methods.* W. B. Saunders Company, Philadelphia, 1991, p. 411.

logic conditions. Red cells also may be present in the urine as a consequence of extrarenal disease. These conditions include acute appendicitis, acute salpingitis, diverticulosis, and various abdominal and pelvic tumors. Toxic reactions to drugs, anticoagulant therapy, and vigorous exercise also may cause increased red cells in the urine.

White Cells ■ The occurrence of 30 or more white cells/hpf is suggestive of an acute infection. White cells may be increased with bacterial or nonbacterial renal disease. White cells may accompany calculi and tumors. Prostatitis in men and the acute urethral syndrome or dysuria-pyuria syndrome in women may cause increased white cells in clean-catch urine specimens.

Casts ■ Casts are initially formed as translucent, colorless gels from proteins in the renal tubules known as Tamm-Horsfall (TH) protein. Normally, few casts are seen in urinary sediment. Vigorous exercise normally can cause an increased number to occur in the urine. Casts are significantly increased in kidney disease. The character of the casts also changes; they become denser and waxy in appearance and entrap red cells, white cells, and tubular epithelial cells according to the renal abnormality. Casts are classified by their appearance and the entrapped elements. See Table 21–8. On occasion, malignant cells may appear in the urine. Viral inclusions may also be observed, e.g., in cytomegaloviral disease.

Crystals ■ A variety of crystals appear in the urine (Figures 21–11 and 21–12). Important ab-

***Table* 21–8 ■ Classification of Casts**

Matrix
   Hyaline—variable size
   Waxy—often broad in use

Inclusions
   Granules—proteins, cell debris
   Fat globules—triglycerides, cholesterol esters
   Hemosiderin granules
   Crystals—uncommon
   Melanin granules—rare

Pigments
   Hemoglobin, myoglobin, bilirubin, drugs

Cells
   Erythrocytes and red cell remnants
   Leukocytes—neutrophils, lymphocytes, monocytes, and histiocytes
   Renal tubular epithelial cells
   Mixed cells—erythrocytes, neutrophils, and renal tubular cells
   Bacteria

From Henry, J. B. (ed.): *Clinical Diagnosis and Management by Laboratory Methods.* W. B. Saunders Company, Philadelphia, 1991, p. 425.

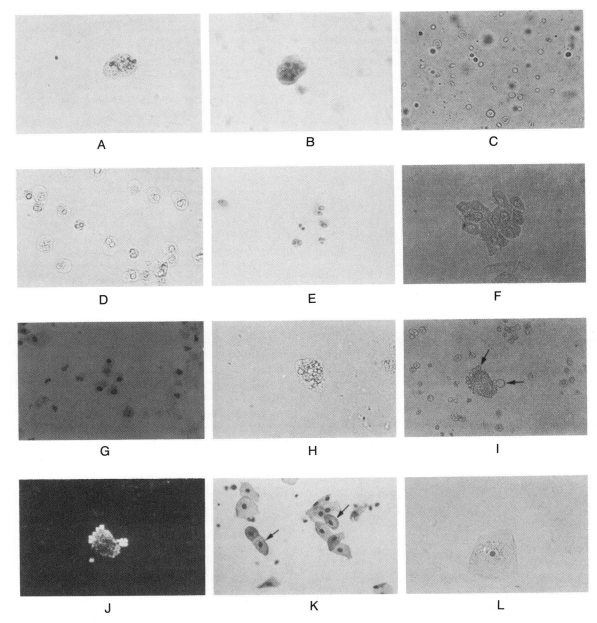

Figure 21–9

A, Renal tubular epithelial cell containing brown pigment; iron, unstained (X 260). B, Renal tubular epithelial cell positive with Prussian blue stain (hemosiderinuria) (X 260). C, Dysmorphic erythrocytes (X 160). D, Neutrophils with dilute acetic acid (X 200). E, Eosinophils (X 500). F, Renal tubular epithelial cells in renal fragment (X 200). G, Renal tubular epithelial cells and neutrophil. Papanicolaou stain (X 430). H, Oval fat body (X 160). I, Oval fat body with attached fat droplets (X 160): brightfield. J, Oval fat body with attached fat droplets (X 160): polarized. K, Transitional epithelial cells. Papanicolaou stain (X 430). L, Squamous epithelial cell. Pyridium-stained (X 200.)

(From Henry, J. B. (ed.): *Clinical Diagnosis and Management by Laboratory Methods.* W. B. Saunders Company, Philadelphia, 1991, Figure 17–1.)

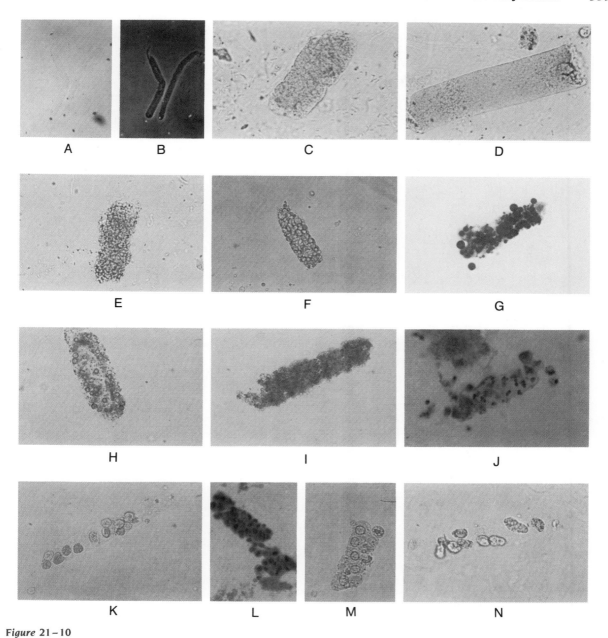

Figure 21–10

Hyaline casts. A, brightfield. B, Phase-contrast microscopy (X 100). C, Finely granular cast becoming waxy (X 200). D, Waxy cast (X 200). E, Granular cast (X 200). F, Fatty cast, nonpolarizing (X 160). G, Fatty cast, nonpolarizing but positive oil red O (X 200). H, Erythrocyte cast (X 200). I, Blood or hemoglobin cast (X 200). J, Leukocyte cast. Papanicolaou stain (X 430). K, Cellular cast (X 200). L, Renal tubular epithelial cast. Papanicolaou stain (X 430). M, Mixed white cell and renal tubular epithelial cast (X 200). N, Cellular cast (X 200).

(From Henry, J. B. (ed.): *Clinical Diagnosis and Management by Laboratory Methods.* W. B. Saunders Company, Philadelphia, 1991, Figure 17–13.)

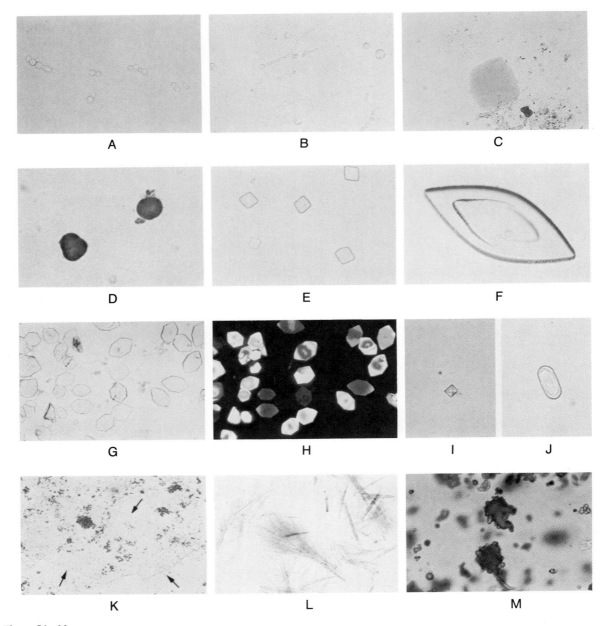

Figure 21–11

A, *Candida*: budding spores (× 200). B, *Candida*: pseudohyphae (× 160, unstained). C, Muscle fiber: patient with rectovesical fistula (× 200). D, Acid urates (× 160). E, Uric acid (× 160). F, Large uric acid plate, laminated (× 160). G, Hexagonal uric acid, unpolarized (× 50). H, Hexagonal uric acid, polarized (× 50). I, Calcium oxalate (× 200). J, Unusual oval form of calcium oxalate (× 200). K, Large, clear plate of calcium phosphate; also amorphous phosphates (× 64). L, Rare, fine sheaves of calcium phosphate (× 160). M, Ammonium biurate (× 160).

(From Henry, J. B. (ed.): *Clinical Diagnosis and Management by Laboratory Methods*. W. B. Saunders Company, Philadelphia, 1991, Figure 17–26.)

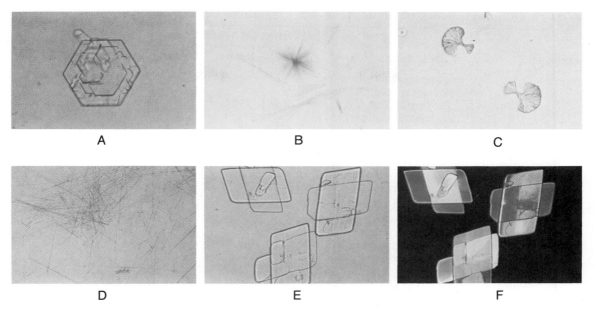

Figure 21–12

A, Hexagonal cystine, laminated (× 200). B, Tyrosine (× 160). C, Sulfadiazine (× 160). D, Ampicillin (× 40). E, Meglumine diatrizoate (Renografin), unpolarized (× 160). F, Renografin, polarized (× 160).

(From Henry, J. B. (ed.): *Clinical Diagnosis and Management by Laboratory Methods.* W. B. Saunders Company, Philadelphia, 1991, Figure 17–38.)

normal crystals include cystine, tyrosine, and leucine. They may be present owing to medication. Commonly, sulfonamide and ampicillin crystals are present. Radiographic media used with intravenous radiographic studies may result in crystalline material. A summary of crystalline material in urine appears in Table 21–9.

Bacteria ▪ In carefully collected specimens, bacterial counts of 100,000/ml suggest bacterial infection. This can be estimated by the observation of bacteria in an oil-immersion field of directly examined, well-mixed urine.

Parasites and Parasitic Ova ▪ These are infrequently observed but may include *Schistosoma haematobium* and *Entamoeba histolytica*. *Enterobius vermicularis* may be seen as a contaminant, particularly in children.

IMMUNOHEMATOLOGY: BLOOD GROUP AND TYPE, ANTIBODY SCREENING AND IDENTIFICATION

ABO Grouping ▪ Blood groups refer to the antigen specificity of red cells. Red cells are also termed *erythrocytes.* These groups are determined by the presence or absence of antigens known as A and B. Individuals whose red cells carry a single antigen, A, are group A, and those carrying the antigen B are group B. Individuals whose red cells carry neither antigen are designated as group O. A lesser number of individuals have red cells carrying both antigens and are designated as group AB. Individuals normally

Table 21–9 ■ **Characteristics of Amorphous and Crystalline Urinary Sediments**

Substance	Description	Acid	Neutral	Alkaline	Solubility Characteristics and Comments
		Urine pH Where Found			
Ampicillin	Uncommon—from high dose; colorless; long prisms that form clusters, sheaves	+	−	−	
Bilirubin	Reddish brown; amorphous needles, rhombic plates, or cubes; may color uric acid crystals	+	−	−	Soluble in alkali, acid, acetone, and chloroform
Cholestereol	Rare; colorless; flat plate with corner notch; accompanies fatty casts and oval fat bodies	+	+	−	Very soluble in chloroform, ether, and hot alcohol
Calcium carbonate	Colorless; small granules in pairs, fours; spheres; rarely needles	−	+	+	Soluble in acetic acid with effervescence
Calcium oxalate	Dihydrate—common; colorless; small refractile octahedron Monohydrate—uncommon; dumbbell and ovoid rectangle	+	+	−	Soluble in dilute HCl
Cystine	Colorless; hexagonal plates, often laminated; rapidly destroyed by bacteria; may be confused with uric acid, but cystine is soluble in dilute hydrochloric acid	+	−	−	Soluble in alkali (especially ammonia) and dilute hydrochloric acid; insoluble in boiling water, acetic acid, alcohol, ether; apply cyanide-nitroprusside reaction
Hematin	Small, biconvex "whetstone" seen with hemoglobinuria	+	−	−	
Hemosiderin	Golden brown; granules in clumps, in cells, casts	+	+	−	Blue with Prussian blue
Hippuric acid	Rare; colorless; needles, rhombic plates and four-sided prisms; distinguish from phosphates	+	+	+	Soluble with hot water and alkali; insoluble in acetic acid
Indigotin	Rare; blue; amorphous or small crystals; colors other crystals	+	+	+	Very soluble in chloroform; soluble in ether; insoluble in acetone

Table 21–9 ▪ **Characteristics of Amorphous and Crystalline Urinary Sediments** *Continued*

Substance	Description	Urine pH Where Found			Solubility Characteristics and Comments
		Acid	*Neutral*	*Alkaline*	
Phosphates					
Amorphous phosphate (magnesium, calcium)	Colorless; fine, granular precipitate	−	+	+	Insoluble with heat; soluble with acetic acid, dilute hydrochloric acid
Calcium hydrogen phosphate	Less common; colorless; star-shaped or long, thin prisms or needles; form rosettes	sl	+	sl	Slightly soluble in dilute acetic acid; soluble in dilute hydrochloric acid
Triple phosophate (ammonium, magnesium)	Common form: colorless; three- to six-sided prisms, "coffin lids" Less often: flat, fern leaf form, sheets, flakes	−	+	+	Soluble in dilute acetic acid
Radiographic media (meglumine diatrizoate)	Intravenous: colorless; thin, rhombic plates, some with notch, resemble cholesterol plates; elongated crystals Retrograde: colorless; long, pointed crystals	+	−	−	Soluble in 10% NaOH: insoluble in ether and chloroform; high specific gravity in urine; polarizes with interference colors
Sulfonamides					
Acetylsulfadiazine	Wheat sheaves with eccentric binding	+	−	−	
Acetylsulfamethoxazole	Brown; dense spheres or irregular divided spheres	+	−	−	
Sulfadiazine	Brown; dense globules	+	−	−	Soluble in acetone
Tyrosine	Rare; colorless or yellow, appears black with focusing; fine silky needles in sheaves or rosettes	+	−	−	Soluble in alkali, dilute mineral acid, relatively heat-soluble; insoluble in alcohol, ether
Urates					
Amorphous (calcium, magnesium, sodium, potassium)	Common; colorless to yellow-brown; amorphous, granular precipitate	+	+	−	Soluble in dilute alkali; soluble at 60 °C or lower; change to uric acid crystal with concentrated HCl or acetic acid
Monosodium urate	Colorless; needles or amorphous precipitate	+	−	−	
Urates (sodium, potassium, ammonium)	Brown; small, spherical; clusters resemble biurates	sl	+	−	Soluble at 60 °C; change to uric acid with glacial acetic acid

Table continued on following page

Table 21–9 ▪ **Characteristics of Amorphous and Crystalline Urinary Sediments** *Continued*

Substance	Description	Urine pH Where Found			Solubility Characteristics and Comments
		Acid	Neutral	Alkaline	
Ammonium biurate	Common in "old" urine; dark yellow or brown; spheres or "thorn apples" (spheres with horns)	−	+	+	Soluble at 60 °C with acetic acid; soluble strong alkali; change to uric acid with concentrated hydrochloric or acetic acid
Uric acid	Common; yellow, red-brown, brown; large variety of shapes—rhombic, four-sided plates, rosettes, "whetstones," lemon shapes; rarely, colorless hexagonals	+	−	−	Soluble in alkali; insoluble in alcohol and acids; polarizes with interference colors
Xanthine	Rare; colorless; small, rhombic plates	+	+	−	Soluble in alkali, soluble with heat; insoluble in acetic acid

sl = Slight.
From Henry, J. B. (ed.): *Clinical Diagnosis and Management by Laboratory Methods.* W. B. Saunders Company, Philadelphia, 1991, pp. 429–430.

do not have antibodies to the antigens present on their red cells. Thus, the person of group AB has no circulating anti-A or anti-B. The person with group O red cells has both anti-A and anti-B. Group A individuals have circulating anti-B. Group B individuals have circulating anti-A. The antibodies to red blood cell antigens are termed alloantibodies and can be naturally occurring, formed because of immunization through transfusion, or induced by exposure to fetal red cells during pregnancy or at the time of birth.

The frequencies of the ABO grouping of red cells in different United States racial populations are shown in Table 21–10.

A few individuals have weaker-reacting A antigen. These are designated as A2, A3, and rare others. Weaker-reacting A may be naturally occurring or may be the consequence of a disease state.

Rh Typing ▪ Red cells may also carry antigens designated as Rh antigens. These antigens are named D, C, E, e, and c, which are also written Rho, rh′, rh″, hr′, and hr″, respectively (Wiener system).

Individuals whose red cells carry the D antigen are spoken of as Rh-positive. These individuals can be transfused with Rh-positive or Rh-negative red cells or carry a baby with Rh-positive blood without danger of developing antibodies against the red cells of the baby. Individuals whose red cells do not carry the D antigen are said to be Rh-negative. These individuals must not be transfused with D-positive red cells, since about two thirds of them will form antibodies (anti-D) against the antigen that is foreign to their system. If carrying a baby that is D-positive, a woman may form anti-D if there is fetal blood loss through the placenta to the maternal circulation.

This is less likely to be a problem in a first pregnancy but can be a problem in any pregnancy. Since some fetal blood enters the maternal circulation with all births, Rho immune globulin (RhIg) is administered to the mother (RhoGAM), which prevents maternal formation

Table 21–10 ▪ Routine ABO Grouping of Erythrocytes

Cells Against Serum with		Serum Against Cells of Group				Frequencies (%) in Major U.S. Population			
Anti-A	Anti-B	A	B	O	Interpretation	Whites	African Americans	Native Americans	Asians
−	−	+	+	−	O	45	49	79	40
+	−	−	+	−	A	40	27	16	28
−	+	+	−	−	B	11	20	4	27
+	+	−	−	−	AB	4	4	< 1	5

Adapted from Henry, J. B. (ed.): *Clinical Diagnosis and Management by Laboratory Methods.* W. B. Saunders Company, Philadelphia, 1991, p. 986.

of anti-D. This safeguards the mother for future pregnancies and possible transfusions. If maternal anti-D forms and acts against the baby's D-positive cells, the red cells of the baby are destroyed (hemolysis). This condition is termed *erythroblastosis fetalis.*

Some individuals have a form of D antigens known as *Du.* Du is detected by testing with an additional procedure known as the antiglobulin test. If Du-positive cells are transfused into a person who is Rh-negative, there is a risk that the person will form anti-D, similar to transfusion of Rh positive blood.

Autoantibodies ▪ Autoantibodies are antibodies that react to antigens that occur in the same subject. They also react with the same antigen found in normal subjects. Antigen-antibody reactions that may occur include hemolytic anemias, leukopenia, and thrombocytopenia, but also there may be no demonstrable clinical symptoms. Tests used to detect autoantibodies include the direct antiglobulin test, which is usually positive, and the indirect antiglobulin test, which may or may not be positive.

Based on the optimal reacting conditions, autoantibodies are classified as warm or cold. Of those autoantibodies causing anemias, warm autoantibodies predominate (85 per cent) and are usually of the IgG class. Cold antibodies (15 per cent) are usually of the IgM class.

Cold Autoantibodies ▪ These include anti-H, anti-I, anti-i and anti-P. Anti-H may be present in low levels in normal persons. Anti-I may occur in normal persons and in cord blood in low titer. It is associated with *Mycoplasma pneumoniae* infections and cold hemagglutinin disease of high titer. Anti-i may occur with in-

fectious mononucleosis, with or without hemolytic anemia. Anti-P occurs with paroxysmal cold hemoglobinuria, a syndrome that occurs with syphilis, mumps, chickenpox, measles, and other viral diseases. It is known as the Donath-Landsteiner (DL) antibody.

Warm Autoantibodies ▪ These are detected by the direct antiglobulin test utilizing anti-IgG serum. They may occur in individuals with anemia or shortened red blood cell survival without anemia. If no other conditions are associated, the condition is designated as primary or idiopathic. If associated with disease conditions, viral infections, or medications, the condition of the autoantibody is designated as secondary.

Drug-Induced Positive Antiglobulin Test ▪ A number of medications are known to induce a positive antiglobulin test. Among them are methyldopa (Aldomet), penicillin (3 per cent of individuals receiving large doses), cephalothin (Keflin), carbromal, chlorpromazine, methadone, cephalothin (Loridine), cephalexin, cefazolin, and other cephalosporins.

Medications may also cause formation of a drug-serum protein complex that adsorbs onto red cells. This condition causes activated C3 and other complement to be fixed to the red cells. This is detected by anti-C3 antiglobulin serum. Medications causing this condition include acetaminophen, aminopyrine (Pyramidon), chloramphenicol, antihistamines, dipyrone, insulin, isoniazid, melphalan, *p*-aminosalicylic acid, phenacetin, quinine, quinidine, rifampin, stibophen (Fuadin), sulfa drugs, sulfonylurea derivatives, methadone, streptomycin, and tetracycline. Insecticides can also cause this condition.

Table 21–11 ▪ Selected Erythrocyte Alloantibodies: Immunoglobulin Class, Optimal Reaction Phase, Clinical Implications, and Chance of Finding a Compatible Donor

Anti-	Immunoglobulin			Optimal Reaction				Hemolysis in			Type	Compatible Donor	
	IgM	IgG	IgA	Sal	Alb	AGT	Enz	Vitro	Recipient	Newborn		White (%)	Black (%)
B	3		1	4				2	4	2	A,O	85	76
A₁	4			4							A₂,O	48	52
A	3	1	1	4				2	4	2	B,O	56	69
A,B	1	3		4				1	4		O	45	49
H*	4			4			3	3	4	0	O$_h$	Very rare	Very rare
I	3	1		3						0	I−	Very rare	Very rare
i	3	2	3	3						0			
P₁	3			3				1	2	0	P₁−	21	6
P	3	2	2								pᵏ	Very rare	Very rare
PP₁Pᵏ (Tjᵃ)	3			3				4	1	1	p	Very rare	
Leᵃ	3	1		3		2	3	2	1	0	Le(a−)	78	77
Leᵇ	4	1		4		3	3	1	1	0	Le(b−)	28	45
Luᵃ	3	1		3				0		1	Lu(a−)	92	96
Luᵇ	3	1	1	3		1		0	1		Lu(b−)	<0.1	<0.1
M	3	1		3		1	0	0	1	0†	M−	22	30
N	3			3			0	0		1	N−	28	26
S	2	2		3		3		0	2	1	S−	45	69
s	1	2				3		0	2	1	s−	11	3
U	1	3				4		0†	2	1	U−	None	1
D	1	3	1	1	3	3	3	0	3	4	D−	15	8
C	1	3		1	3	3	3	0	2	1	C−	30	68
DC	1	3		1	3	3	3	0		1	DC−	13	7
Cᵂ	2	2		1	3	3	3	0	1	1	Cᵂ−	99	100
c	1	3			3	3	3	0	2	2	c−	20	1
E	1	3		1	3	3	3	0	2	2	E−	70	98
e	1	3			3	3	3	0	2	1	e−	2	2
K	1	3		1		3	3	0	2	2	K−	91	97
k	1	4				3	3	0	2	2	k−	0.2	0.1
Kpᵃ	1	4				3	3	0		1	Kp(a−)	98	99.9
Kpᵇ		4				3	3	0		1	Kp(b−)	<0.1	0.1
Jsᵃ		4				3	3	0		1	Js(a−)	>99.9	81
Jsᵇ		4				3	3	0		1	Js(b−)	<0.1	1
Jkᵃ		4				3	3	0		1	Jk(a−)	23	9
Jkᵇ		4				3	3	0		1	Jk(b−)	28	57
Fyᵃ	1	4		1	3	3	1/0	0	1	1	Fy(a−)	34	90
Fyᵇ		4			3	3	1/0	0	1	1	Fy(b−)	17	77
Chᵃ	3					3					Least incompatible		
Sdᵃ	3			3		2		0	1	0	Least incompatible		
Ytᵃ	2	2		3		2		0	1	?	Yt(a−)	<0.1	
Vel	3					3	2	2	0		Vel−	<0.1	
Wrᵃ	3			3		3		0	1	1	Wr(a−)	>99.9	

4 = almost all; 3 = most; 2 = some; 1 = few; 0 = none.
*In Bombay individuals.
†Only one case reported.
Adapted from Henry, J. B. (ed.): Clinical Diagnosis and Management by Laboratory Methods. W. B. Saunders Company, Philadelphia, 1991, p. 982.

342

Other Red Cell Antigens and Antibodies ▪ Over 600 erythrocyte antigens have been reported, organized into 21 blood group systems. Other antigens rarely occur and are referred to as "private" antigens. Antigens that occur on the red cells of almost all individuals are referred to as "public" antigens. Many antigens have no known medical importance. In addition to the ABO and Rh systems, other medically important systems include the Lewis system, I and i antigens, P system, MNS system, Kell system, Duffy system, and Kidd system. Kell antibodies, anti-FYa and anti-FYb (Duffy), and anti-Jka and anti-Jkb (Kidd), and to a lesser degree anti-Lua (Lutheran) are more important in transfusion reactions or hemolytic anemia of the newborn. See Table 21–11 for a summary of erythrocyte alloantibodies.

HIV ▪ The human immunodeficiency virus (HIV-1) is associated with a wide array of clinical presentations. These range from apparently well individuals with serologic evidence of HIV infection to individuals with acquired immune deficiency syndrome (AIDS).

Individuals are additionally classified in AIDS-like syndromes designated as:

AIDS-like disease (illness) (syndrome)
AIDS-related complex (ARC)
AIDS-related conditions
Pre-AIDS
Prodromal AIDS

These designations refer to a variety of symptoms and disorders occurring in individuals with HIV infection, considered to be caused by HIV infection (e.g., abnormal weight loss, anemia, blindness, diarrhea, fever, rash, thrombocytopenia, and many others), and a variety of specific infections (see later section on opportunistic infections). Malignant neoplasms may also occur with HIV infection. These include Burkitt's tumor or lymphoma, immunoblastic sarcoma, Kaposi's sarcoma, lymphoma (histiocytic or large cell), primary lymphoma of the brain, and reticulosarcoma (see first entry in Reference Sources).

HIV infections are characterized by destruction of host *T helper (CD4+) lymphocytes*. Loss of these cells is associated with decreased host cellular defense mechanisms. Higher levels of host *T suppressor (CD8+) lymphocytes* have been reported to be associated with a less virulent clinical course.

HIV-ELISA Test ▪ Laboratory testing is an important part of the diagnosing and monitoring of HIV infection. The HIV screening test is performed as an enzyme-linked immunosorbent assay (ELISA). This is a highly sensitive assay (greater than 99 per cent) that is reactive to HIV, and although highly specific will react to non-HIV specimen immunoglobulins. The latter are false-positive reactions. During 1992, a number of reactive HIV-ELISA assays were attributed to flu infections.

Western Blot Test ▪ Since false-positives may occur, all reactive HIV-ELISA tests must be confirmed by a second confirmatory test, the *Western blot*. The Western blot test develops bands each of which reflects the presence of specimen immunoproteins. These bands include antibodies that have developed to HIV.

The Western blot is nonreactive if no bands are present. This is associated with the status of no infection with HIV, or with recent HIV infection before antibody development.

The Western blot is reported as positive for HIV infection if certain criteria are met. These criteria have been developed by different organizations. See Table 21–12.

Western blot results that do not conform to these criteria but have one or more bands are reported as HIV-Western blot indeterminate. These reports may be further categorized, based on band(s) development, into those reactions that have high probability of HIV infection, those sometimes associated with HIV infection, and those unlikely to be associated with HIV infection (Figures 21–13 through 21–17).

Band development of the Western blot is influenced by the stage of disease. In advanced AIDS, bands may no longer be expressed that were present in earlier Western blot assays. The band intensity may also be related to disease progression, and for that reason it is helpful for bands to be reported with subjective interpretation as to their *strength*. Numerical values are frequently used, ± to 4+, denoting weak to intense bands.

Other HIV-Related Tests ▪ T lymphocyte subsets, T-helper lymphocytes (CD4+) and T-suppressor lymphocytes (CD8+) are measured by *flow cytometry*. The occurrence of significantly decreased CD4+ cells (less than 200 cmm) is considered virtually diagnostic of AIDS.

Other tests useful in monitoring HIV infections are beta-2-microglobulin, which becomes

Table 21–12 ▪ Criteria for Positive Interpretation of Western Blot Tests

Organization	Criteria
Association of State and Territorial Public Health Laboratory Directors *and* Centers for Disease Control	Any two of: o p24 o gp41 o gp120/gp160*
FDA-licensed DuPont test	p24 and p31 *and* gp41 or gp120/gp160*
American Red Cross	≥3 bands: 1 from each gene-product group: o GAG *and* o POL *and* o ENV
Consortium for Retrovirus Serology Standardization	≥2 bands: p24 *or* p31, plus o gp41 *or* o gp120/gp160*

*Distinguishing the gp120 band from the gp160 band is often very difficult. These two glycoproteins can be considered as one reactant for purposes of interpreting western blot test results.

From Centers for Disease Control: Interpretation and use of the western blot assay for serodiagnosis of human immunodeficiency virus type 1 infections. MMWR 38:5–7, 1989.

elevated owing to destruction of lymphocytes and macrophages with exacerbation of disease, and p24 antigen, which may be detectable soon after infection (2 to 6 weeks). The p24 antigen is complexed with antibody following antibody seroconversion and may not be detectable. The antigen-antibody complex may be dissociated by acid treatment, permitting p24 antigen to be detected. Lower levels of antigenemia may test negative due to protein denaturation by the acid treatment. Antibody to p24 is also available.

Human immunodeficiency virus type 2 (HIV-2) also infects humans. This infection is rare in the United States. The American Red Cross (ARC) tests donor blood for HIV-1 and HIV-2.

Opportunistic Infections ▪ Opportunistic infections may occur in immunocompromised individuals, from either therapeutic measures such as intensive chemotherapy or a disease condition such as AIDS. Opportunistic infections include:

candidiasis
cryptosporidiosis
isosporiasis
cryptococcosis
pneumocystosis
toxoplasmosis
coccidioidomycosis
cytomegalic inclusion disease
herpes simplex
herpes zoster
histoplasmosis
microsporidiosis
mycobacteriosis
nocardiosis
salmonella infections
strongyloidiasis
tuberculosis

A variety of laboratory tests are employed to assist identification of these infections. Tests include cultures of blood, tissues (e.g., lymph node, bone marrow), and various body fluids (e.g., cerebrospinal fluid, sputum, bronchial aspirate, urine). Immunoassay of serum antibodies may be employed. Direct examination of specimens for microorganisms may be required, using a variety of staining methods. These include special stains, immunofluorescent techniques, peroxidase-immunoperoxidase procedures, and polymerase chain reaction (PCR).

MEDICAL BACTERIOLOGY

Cultures of virtually all body fluids and tissues are employed in medical diagnosis and care. Common sites and the prevalent, medically important microorganisms are discussed next.

Blood ▪ Indications for culture are manifold: sudden changes in temperature, pulse rate, chills, prostration, hypotension; history of fever associated with a heart murmur; and suspected sepsis. Virtually any microorganism that infects body organs and tissues may be isolated from blood.

Sterile Body Fluids

Cerebrospinal Fluid (CSF) ▪ Meningitis is a medical emergency. *Haemophilus influenzae, Streptococcus pneumoniae* and *Neisseria meningitidis* occur most frequently. In addition to culture, a Gram-stained sediment, from an aliquot of centrifuged specimen, is examined microscop-

Text continued on page 350

LABORATORY REPORT

MYSTERY CLIENT   001.099
*****************   39986
****
***************** , ** 00000

MetWest
Clinical Laboratories
18408 Oxnard Street • Tarzana, CA 91356
(818) 996-7300
Calif. (800) 339-4299

Director and Pathologist
Paul T. Wertlake, M.D.

CLLCT DATE   PANEL(S)
12/06/91

PATIENT	AGE	SEX	PATIENT I.D.	PHYSICIAN	RECEIVED	REPORTED	SPEC. NO.
TEST, TEST					12/06	12/06/91	6000000

REQUESTS	WITHIN RANGE RESULTS	OUT OF RANGE RESULTS	REFERENCE RANGE	UNITS

HIV-1 ANTIBODY RESULTS
    REACTIVE SCREEN TEST(HIV-ELISA)/NEGATIVE CONFIRMATORY TEST(HIV-WB)

REQUESTS	WITHIN RANGE RESULTS	OUT OF RANGE RESULTS	REFERENCE RANGE
HIV ANTIBODY, ELISA		REACTIVE	NON-REACTIVE
HIV-1 AB (W.B.) P24	NONE DETECTED		NONE DETECT.
GP41	NONE DETECTED		NONE DETECT.
P55	NONE DETECTED		NONE DETECT.
GP120	NONE DETECTED		NONE DETECT.
GP160	NONE DETECTED		NONE DETECT.

COMMENTS/RECOMMENDATIONS
IN VIEW OF NEGATIVE WESTERN BLOT STUDY, THE ELISA REACTIVITY IS NOT
RELATED TO HIV ANTIBODIES, BUT REPRESENTS UNIDENTIFIED SERUM ANTIBODIES
TO HLA OR OTHER ANTIGENS.

FURTHER TESTING IS NOT INDICATED IN AN ASYMPTOMATIC PERSON WITHOUT HIV
RISK FACTORS.

HIV INFECTION IS NOT PRECLUDED.

IN PRESENCE OF RISK FACTORS FOR HIV, PERIODIC SURVEILLANCE MAY BE
APPROPRIATE.

REVIEWED BY PATHOLOGIST.

PAGE 1: END OF FINAL   REPORT FOR : TEST, TEST
DATE COLLECTED : 12/06/91 - DATE REPORTED : 12/06/91

FORMS-FREE W/O CHEM 1PT. (NEW) 80219

Figure 21–13
Laboratory report on an HIV-negative confirmatory test.

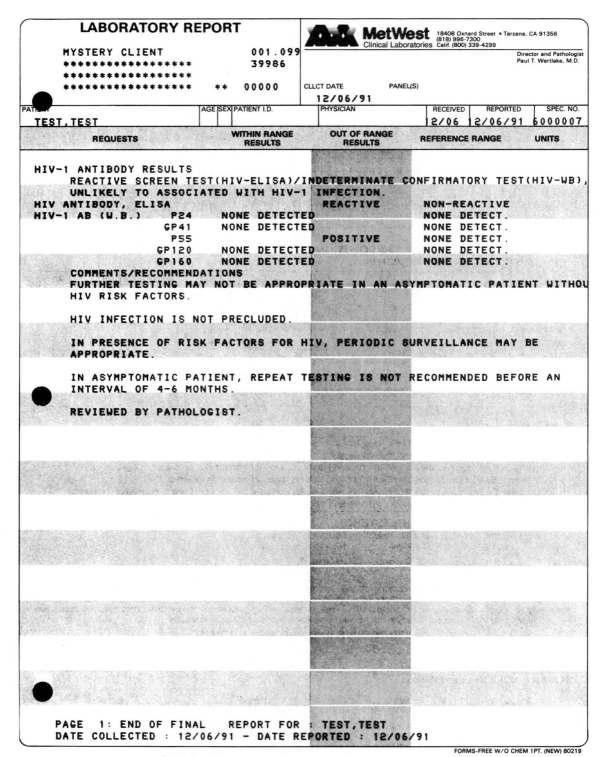

Figure 21–14

Laboratory report on an HIV-indeterminate confirmatory test.

LABORATORY REPORT

MYSTERY CLIENT   001.099

******************   39986

****

***************** , **   00000

MetWest   18408 Oxnard Street • Tarzana, CA 91356
Clinical Laboratories   (818) 996-7300
Calif. (800) 339-4299

Director and Pathologist
Paul T. Wertlake, M.D.

| CLLCT DATE | PANEL(S) |
| 12/06/91 | |

PATIENT	AGE	SEX	PATIENT I.D.	PHYSICIAN	RECEIVED	REPORTED	SPEC. NO.
TEST,TEST					12/06	12/06/91	6000004

REQUESTS	WITHIN RANGE RESULTS	OUT OF RANGE RESULTS	REFERENCE RANGE	UNITS
HIV-1 ANTIBODY RESULTS				

REACTIVE SCREEN TEST(HIV-ELISA)/INDETERMINATE CONFIRMATORY TEST(HIV-WB),
SOMETIMES ASSOCIATED WITH HIV-1 SEROCONVERSION.

REQUESTS	WITHIN RANGE RESULTS	OUT OF RANGE RESULTS	REFERENCE RANGE	UNITS
HIV ANTIBODY, ELISA		REACTIVE	NON-REACTIVE	
HIV-1 AB (W.B.) P24		POSITIVE	NONE DETECT.	
GP41	NONE DETECTED		NONE DETECT.	
P55		POSITIVE	NONE DETECT.	
GP120	NONE DETECTED		NONE DETECT.	
GP160	NONE DETECTED		NONE DETECT.	

COMMENTS/RECOMMENDATIONS
DUE TO POSSIBLE HIV SEROCONVERSION, REPEAT HIV-WB TESTING IS RECOMMENDED
AT 2-4 WEEK INTERVALS, WITH ONSET OF SYMPTOMS, OR WITH PROGRESSION OF
SYMPTOMS, FOR POSSIBLE DEVELOPMENT OF CHARACTERISTIC SEROPOSITIVE PATTER

T CELL SUBSET STUDIES MAY BE INFORMATIVE WITH REGARD TO POSSIBLE IMMUNE
DEFICIENCIES.

REVIEWED BY PATHOLOGIST.

PAGE 1: END OF FINAL   REPORT FOR : TEST,TEST
DATE COLLECTED : 12/06/91 - DATE REPORTED : 12/06/91

FORMS-FREE W/O CHEM 1PT. (NEW) 80219

Figure 21–15
Laboratory report on an HIV-indeterminate confirmatory test.

LABORATORY REPORT

MetWest Clinical Laboratories
18408 Oxnard Street • Tarzana, CA 91356
(818) 996-7300
Calif. (800) 339-4299

Director and Pathologist
Paul T. Wertlake, M.D.

MYSTERY CLIENT   001.099
* * * * * * * * * * * * * * * * *   39986
* * * * * * * * * * * * * * * * *
* * * * * * * * * * * * * * * * *   ** 00000

CLLCT DATE   PANEL(S)
12/06/91

PATIENT	AGE	SEX	PATIENT I.D.	PHYSICIAN	RECEIVED	REPORTED	SPEC. NO.
TEST, TEST					12/06	12/06/91	6000003

REQUESTS	WITHIN RANGE RESULTS	OUT OF RANGE RESULTS	REFERENCE RANGE	UNITS

HIV-1 ANTIBODY RESULTS
    REACTIVE SCREEN TEST(HIV-ELISA)/INDETERMINATE CONFIRMATORY TEST(HIV-WB),
    WITH HIGH PROBABILITY OF HIV-1 INFECTION.

REQUESTS	WITHIN RANGE RESULTS	OUT OF RANGE RESULTS	REFERENCE RANGE	UNITS
HIV ANTIBODY, ELISA		REACTIVE	NON-REACTIVE	
HIV-1 AB (W.B.) P24	NONE DETECTED		NONE DETECT.	
GP41		POSITIVE	NONE DETECT.	
P55	NONE DETECTED		NONE DETECT.	
GP120	NONE DETECTED		NONE DETECT.	
GP160	NONE DETECTED		NONE DETECT.	

COMMENTS/RECOMMENDATIONS
IN A SYMPTOMATIC PERSON, RECOMMEND REPEAT HIV-WB AT 2 WEEK INTERVALS OR
WITH PROGRESSION OF SYMPTOMS, FOR POSSIBLE DEVELOPMENT OF CHARACTERISTIC
SEROPOSITIVE PATTERN.

IN AN ASYMPTOMATIC PERSON, RECOMMEND REPEAT HIV-WB AT 1-2 MONTH INTERVAL
OR WITH DEVELOPMENT OF SYMPTOMS.

T CELL SUBSET STUDIES MAY BE INFORMATIVE WITH REGARD TO POSSIBLE IMMUNE
DEFICIENCIES.

REVIEWED BY PATHOLOGIST.

PAGE 1: END OF FINAL   REPORT FOR : TEST, TEST
DATE COLLECTED : 12/06/91 - DATE REPORTED : 12/06/91

FORMS-FREE W/O CHEM 1PT. (NEW) 80219

Laboratory report on an HIV test with a high probability of infection.

LABORATORY REPORT

MYSTERY CLIENT 001.099
****************** 39986
****
***************** , ** 00000

MetWest
Clinical Laboratories
18408 Oxnard Street • Tarzana, CA 91356
(818) 996-7300
Calif. (800) 339-4299

Director and Pathologist
Paul T. Wertlake, M.D.

CLLCT DATE 12/06/91 PANEL(S)

PATIENT	AGE	SEX	PATIENT I.D.	PHYSICIAN	RECEIVED	REPORTED	SPEC. NO.
TEST,TEST					12/06	12/06/91	6000009

REQUESTS	WITHIN RANGE RESULTS	OUT OF RANGE RESULTS	REFERENCE RANGE	UNITS

HIV-1 ANTIBODY RESULTS
    REACTIVE SCREEN TEST(HIV-ELISA)/POSITIVE CONFIRMATORY TEST(HIV-WB)

    COMMENTS/RECOMMENDATIONS
    THE BANDS PRESENT CONFORM TO CDC CRITERIA FOR AIDS BY HIV-WB TESTING.

    T CELL SUBSET STUDIES MAY BE INFORMATIVE WITH REGARD TO POSSIBLE IMMUNE
    DEFICIENCIES.

REQUESTS	OUT OF RANGE RESULTS	REFERENCE RANGE
HIV ANTIBODY, ELISA	REACTIVE	NON-REACTIVE
HIV-1 AB (W.B.) P24	POSITIVE	NONE DETECT.
GP41	POSITIVE	NONE DETECT.
P55	POSITIVE	NONE DETECT.
GP120	POSITIVE	NONE DETECT.
GP160	POSITIVE	NONE DETECT.

PAGE 1: END OF FINAL   REPORT FOR : TEST,TEST
DATE COLLECTED : 12/06/91 - DATE REPORTED : 12/06/91

FORMS-FREE W/O CHEM 1PT. (NEW) 80219

Figure 21–17
Laboratory report on an HIV-positive confirmatory test.

ically for identification of bacteria. Identification may be confirmed by rapid immunologic tests.

Antigen tests performed by coagglutination and latex agglutination tests may provide rapid evidence of meningitis. False-negative tests may occur, most probably as a result of low concentration of antigen in early infection or prior antimicrobial therapy. Some workers recommend correlation with the Gram stain result.

Other Fluids ■ Pleural fluid, ascitic fluid, and joint fluids are other commonly cultured sterile fluids.

Tissues ■ Surgical tissues are often cultured to distinguish chronic conditions that may be suppurative or granulomatous processes, such as tuberculosis and mycoses. Histopathologic studies not only may identify malignancy, which may be in the differential diagnosis, but also may be helpful in identifying causative microorganisms. Tissues from ulcers, sinus tracts, and abscesses are among the more frequent samples.

Eye ■ Cultures are obtained for the management of bacterial corneal ulcers. Laboratory investigation includes culture and examination of Gram-stained smears.

Respiratory Tract

Ear ■ Acute otitis is most often due to *Streptococcus pneumoniae, S. pyrogenes, Haemophilus influenzae,* or *Branhamella catarrhalis.* In neonates, frequently offending microbes are *Staphylococcus aureus, Escherichia coli,* or *Klebsiella pneumoniae.* Chronic infections are more likely caused by *Staphylococcus aureus* or *Pseudomonas aeruginosa.*

Nasopharynx ■ Pharyngitis is caused by the bacteria *Streptococcus pyogenes* (or a group A), *Neisseria gonorrhoeae, Corynebacterium diphtheriae,* and *Bordetella pertussis.*

Rapid and highly specific tests for detection of streptococcal antigen in throat swab material are available. These tests vary in sensitivity in direct relationship to the number of group A streptococcal antigens present in the specimen. Some workers recommend back-up use of cultures as a prudent practice, particularly in view of a resurgence of acute rheumatic fever in some areas of the United States.

Sputum ■ The usefulness of bacterial cultures is limited by the contamination of the specimen by oral cavity material and bacterial colonization of the oral pharynx in seriously ill patients.

Laboratories employ a system that evaluates the adequacy of the specimen based on the number of squamous cells present (these cells originate from the oral cavity). Mycotic and mycobacterial organisms may also be cultured.

Other specimens may be required; some are collected by specialized techniques: bronchoscopy using a plugged telescoping catheter brush with aspiration or biopsy, transtracheal aspiration, thoracentesis, transthoracic needle biopsy, and open lung biopsy.

Genital ■ The most common infections are due to *Neisseria gonorrhoeae* and *Chlamydia trachomatis.* In symptomatic men, Gram-stained smears are sensitive and specific. Smears are not helpful in cervical or vaginal material.

DNA probe assays are available for identification of *Neisseria gonorrhoeae* and *Chlamydia trachomatis.* These may be assayed from a single specimen and are not dependent on the viability of the microorganisms. These organisms may also be identified by immunoassays.

Haemophilus ducreyi is sexually transmitted and causes a lesion known as a chancroid. This is an uncommon infection.

Bacterial vaginosis is identified by a vaginal pH of 5.0 or greater, a fishy amine odor upon addition of KOH to vaginal secretions, the presence of "clue" cells microscopically, and the character of vaginal secretions. Culture of *Gardnerella vaginalis* is reported as seldom warranted, since this organism is present in up to 40 per cent of normal, asymptomatic women.

Anaerobic organisms are important in female genital tract infections, including pelvic abscesses, septic abortions, tubo-ovarian abscesses, and endometritis. Culdocentesis and laparoscopy may be helpful in obtaining necessary specimens.

Urinary ■ Specimens include clean-voided midstream urine, urine obtained by instrumentation, and suprapubic aspirated urine. The latter is used with infants and small children. Urine should be cultured within 2 hours of collection or refrigerated during storage.

Immediate microscopic examination of the urine has great value in identifying a significant bacteriuria. The presence of at least 2 bacteria per high power field (hpf) correlates well with significant bacteriuria (greater than 90 per cent).

Quantifying cultural growth is important. Colony-forming units (CFU)/mL are determined.

This is dependent on sampling a known quantity of urine. A calibrated loop streak-plate technique is commonly used. The significance of the number of CFU/mL for each culture must be determined by the clinical situation and the sample submitted. In some instances, a small number of CFU/mL are clinically important.

Feces ▪ The important organisms causing diarrheal disease that are successfully identified in the clinical laboratory include those causing salmonellosis, shigellosis, yersiniosis, and campylobacteriosis. The latter may be evaluated by culture (lacks specificity), and latex agglutination for *C. difficile*. The latter is rapid but slightly less sensitive than a tissue culture assay for *C. difficile* cytotoxin.

Invasive *Escherichia coli* is rare in the United States. Enterotoxigenic forms of *E. coli* may cause traveler's diarrhea. Bloody diarrhea may be caused by verotoxinogenic forms of *E. coli* (VTEC).

MEDICAL MYCOBACTERIOLOGY

Infections by mycobacteria occur in two major categories: *Mycobacterium tuberculosis* causing tuberculosis and "atypical" mycobacteria.

M. intracellulare ("Battey bacillus") is closely related to *M. avium*, and differentiation is difficult and may not be important. The *M. avium-intracellulare* complex may cause pulmonary and disseminated infection. This is one of the opportunistic infections affecting individuals with AIDS. *M. kansasii* and *M. haemophilum* also may affect individuals who are immunosuppressed.

A variety of other infections in humans are caused by other mycobacteria.

MEDICAL MYCOLOGY

The importance of mycology has increased because of an increased incidence of disease, particularly with the AIDS epidemic. The clinically important mycosis infections include candidiasis, cryptococcosis, histoplasmosis, coccidioidomycosis, and sporotrichosis. Many of these infections are first manifested as pulmonary infections in individuals with impaired cellular defense. The infections may later become systemic.

Mycoses are recognized in the following groups: superficial, subcutaneous, deep-seated, and opportunistic. Mycoses may be identified by a variety of laboratory studies, including blood cultures (often positive in AIDS patients); culture of drainage, abscess and tissues; and microscopic examination of smears and tissues with use of special stains. Serologic tests also may be helpful in diagnosing offending mycologic agents, particularly when cultural proof is not available.

MEDICAL PARASITOLOGY

Parasitic infections are important, particularly in the immunosuppressed patient (AIDS, transplantation, antineoplastic therapy), in certain populations, and in the international traveler.

Pneumocystis carinii, *Toxoplasma gondii*, and *Cryptosporidium* spp. are causing increased disease in the immunosuppressed. Malaria continues to be an important global pathogen.

Pneumocystis carinii is most frequently identified by microscopic demonstration of the organisms in pulmonary material. Bronchoalveolar lavage (BAL) is widely used. Sputum, bronchial washings, transbronchial biopsy, and open lung biopsy also may be utilized to obtain specimens. The pulmonary material is examined using various stains, including Giemsa, "rapid Giemsa," methenamine silver, toluidine blue, cresyl echt violet, and Papanicolaou. Cultural identification is not clinically available.

Diagnosis of toxoplasmosis may be made by microscopic examination of smears, touch preps, and sections of infected tissues. Giemsa staining is used with smears and touch preps. Hematoxylin and eosin (H & E)-stained tissue sections may be diagnostic. Serologic studies are commonly used in diagnosing toxoplasma infections. Technologies include the indirect immunofluorescence (IIF) and ELISA. IIF may be used to test for IgM, which may be helpful in distinguishing congenital and acute infection.

Isospora and *Cryptosporidium* may cause severe protracted diarrhea in AIDS and other immunosuppressed states. Usually these organisms cause only a self-limited diarrhea in normal individuals. These organisms are usually identified by microscopic examination of stool material.

Microsporidia may cause protracted diarrhea and weight loss in AIDS patients. Examination of stool material is not effective; diagnosis is made by careful light microscopy of intestinal biopsy specimens or by electron microscopy of tissue biopsies. Impression smears stained by Giemsa may permit identification of organisms.

In addition to the parasites discussed above, a wide variety of others cause human disease. More common pathogenic parasites include but are not limited to *Entamoeba histolytica, Giardia lamblia, Balantidium coli, Trichuris trichiura, Ascaris lumbricoides, Enterobius vermicularis* (pinworms), *Ancylostoma duodenale* and *Necator americanus* (hookworms), *Strongyloides stercoralis, Trichostrongylus* sp, *Taenia* spp, *Hymenolepis nana* (small tapeworm), and *Trichinella spiralis*. Other parasites cause medically important disease but are not included here since they occur primarily in other geographic areas of the world.

MEDICAL ENTOMOLOGY

Arthropods are medically important because they transmit a wide variety of infectious agents.

One class, Arachnida, includes mites, scorpions, and spiders. Mites are responsible for a variety of skin disorders, including the common folliculitis (infection of hair follicles), scabies, and allergies to "dust."

Ticks are important as vectors for infectious diseases, including Lyme disease (*Ixodes*) and Rocky Mountain spotted fever (*Dermacentor*). Additionally, ticks may cause an ascending paralysis caused by a toxic substance introduced by the tick. It occurs in occasional patients, especially children. Removal of the tick results in recovery.

Another class of Arthropods, Insecta, includes the medically important lice, fleas, bugs, mosquitoes, flies, bees, and wasps. Bees and wasps may cause severe allergic reactions in sensitive individuals. Lice are named for the region of the body that they usually inhabit. The body louse (*Pediculus humanus corporis*) is the vector for epidemic typhus (trench fever). The head louse (*P. humanus capitis*) and the pubic louse (*Phthirus pubis*) are discovered by a pattern of bites and detection of eggs attached to hairs (nits).

Fleas are bloodsucking, wingless insects. For the majority of people fleas cause little trouble. Some individuals are sensitized and have irritating reaction to flea bites. A human flea (*Pulex irritans*) may infest humans. Humans may also be incidental hosts for the dog flea (*Ctenocephalides canis*) and the cat flea (*C. felis*). The oriental rat flea (*Xenopsylla cheopis*) is the vector for plague.

Bedbugs (*Cimex lectularius*) are bloodsucking insects that may cause wheals of up to 3 cm. in sensitive individuals. The reduviid bugs are vectors of South American trypanosomiasis.

Mosquitoes may transmit infectious agents, most notably for malaria. The plasmodia (*Plasmodium vivax, P. falciparum, P. malariae, P. ovale*) are spread by the female anopheline mosquito.

Bloodsucking flies spread a variety of infectious diseases, including salmonellosis, typhoid fever, shigellosis, and poliomyelitis. Myiases are less frequent problems, caused by invasion of larvae of various flies, which are commonly known as maggots. The eyes, nose, mouth, and gastrointestinal tract may be affected.

MEDICAL VIROLOGY

The infections caused by viruses may be identified by laboratory studies that include cultural isolation from body fluids, scrapings, and tissues. In some instances, typical cytopathic effects (CPE) are evident *in vitro*.

Immunofluorescent or immunoenzyme methods may be effective. Serologic studies are necessary for diagnosis in some instances, including titers, which are increased during the acute infection (a fourfold or greater rise or conversion from seronegative to seropositive). Study of paired (acute and convalescent samples) may be advisable. Additionally, serologic tests may identify IgM antibody indicative of early infection. In mumps, antibodies to "S" (soluble) antigen and modest titer for "V" antigen are considered presumptive evidence of recent mumps infection. In some instances, cytologic or histologic identification may be made.

It is of paramount importance that specimens submitted for laboratory investigation be accompanied by information as to the clinical problem.

Adenoviruses are responsible for up to 5 to 10 per cent of all febrile illnesses in young children and cause sporadic disease in schoolchildren and young adults. The illness often includes conjunctivitis, pharyngitis, and tonsillitis. Illnesses may be severe. Pneumonia may develop and be fatal. Adenoviruses may cause eye infection (follicular conjunctivitis and keratoconjunctivitis), gastroenteritis, urethritis, cervicitis, exanthems, encephalitis, myocarditis, hepatitis, and hemorrhagic cystitis and may be related to childhood mesenteric adenitis, acute appendicitis, and intussusception.

Herpes simplex virus (HSV) is the cause of the cold sore or fever blister (herpes labialis). There are two antigenic types, HSV-1 and HSV-2, which are cross-reacting. HSV-1 occurs primarily in and around the oral cavity and in skin lesions above the waist. HSV-2 usually occurs in the genital tract and in skin lesions below the waist. HSV-2 is the usual cause of neonatal encephalitis, principally due to exposure to an infected birth canal. HSV-1 is the usual cause of adult encephalitis. Not only are antibody reactions of these antigenic types cross-reacting (up to 40 per cent) but also HSV-1 may occur in the genital tract and HSV-2 in the oral cavity.

Cytomegalovirus (CMV) is closely related to herpes simplex and varicella. CMV is probably the most common congenital infection. The effects can vary from mild to severe, including disseminated disease with pneumonitis, chorioretinitis, hemolytic anemia, and growth retardation.

Acquired CMV infections occur with frequency in AIDS, immunosuppressive therapy, postallograft transplantation, and chronic debilitating diseases. Pneumonitis, gastritis, and retinitis may occur, as well as infection in a spectrum of organs and tissues.

Varicella-zoster (V-Z) is associated with chickenpox (varicella) and shingles (zoster). Primary infection results in chickenpox. Upon recovery, the V-Z virus enters a latent phase in neurons of dorsal root ganglia. Reactivation of the virus results in shingles.

Varicella may have serious complications, including pneumonitis, thrombocytopenia with hemorrhage, encephalitis, Reye's syndrome, nephritis, hepatitis, arthritis and myocarditis. Zoster infection may have serious complications, including persistent neuralgia and encephalomyelitis. Acquired neonatal varicella may occur *in utero* or in the perinatal period.

Epstein-Barr virus (EBV) is a herpes-like virus present in many patients with African Burkitt's lymphoma and nasopharyngeal carcinoma. EBV is also associated with infectious mononucleosis (IM). IM is usually a self-limited disease with a 3- to 5-day prodromal period of nonspecific symptoms (fever, asthenia, fatigue, anorexia), commonly followed by pharyngitis, lymphadenitis, and splenomegaly. Mild hepatitis, conjunctivitis, and a rash may occur. Occasionally patients may have severe complications, including severe hepatitis, encephalitis, pneumonitis, thrombocytopenia, splenic rupture, hemolytic anemia, airway obstruction, and transient cutaneous hypersensitivity to penicillin. Patients with immunodeficiency disorders may develop a severe, often lethal lymphoproliferative disorder.

Diagnosis is based on clinical, hematologic, and serologic data. The peripheral blood manifests an absolute lymphocytosis with atypical lymphocytes. The infected cells are B lymphocytes. The atypical cells are uninfected T cells.

The **Mono test** detects heterophile antibody in about 90 per cent of IM cases. Young children are more prone to be negative. False-positives may occur with hepatitis A, hepatitis B, leukemia, lymphoma, and pancreatic carcinoma. About 25 per cent of IM-like illnesses will be heterophile-negative; many of the cases probably represent CMV and *Toxoplasma gondii* infections.

Serologic tests are available for evaluating the status of EBV infections. These include viral capsid antigen (VCA, IgG, and IgM), early antigens (EA), membrane antigens (MA), and Epstein-Barr (virus) nuclear antigens (EBNA). EA antibodies have been subdivided into diffuse (D) and restricted (R) types. Acute infection is usually based on positive IgM-VCA, or seroconversion from negative to positive. Anti-EA is elevated in 80 to 90 per cent of the cases. Fourfold or greater increases in anti-VCA or anti-EBNA may be expected. Table 21–13 presents guidelines for the interpretation of Epstein-Barr viral serologies.

Enteroviruses include poliovirus, coxsackievirus and echovirus species. Some viruses, nonpolio, noncoxsackievirus, have been designated

***Table* 21–13 ■ Guidelines for the Interpretation of Epstein-Barr Viral Serologies**

Clinical Situation	Antibodies			
	IgG-VCA	EBNA	EA	IGM-VCA
No past infection	−	−	−	−
Acute infection	+	−	+	+
Convalescent phase	+	+	+ or −	+ or −
Past infection	+	+	−	−
Chronic or reactivated infection	+	+	+	−

+ = Antibody present; − = antibody absent.
From Henry, J. B. (ed.): *Clinical Diagnosis and Management by Laboratory Methods.* W. B. Saunders Company, Philadelphia, 1991, p. 1235.

as "orphans" and later redesignated as "enteric cytopathogenic human orphans" (ECHO). These viruses are the cause of asymptomatic infections but also illnesses with symptoms, including paralytic disease, aseptic meningitis, encephalitis, pleurodynia, pericarditis, herpangina, and lymphonodular pharyngitis. The most common presentation is with nonspecific fever, malaise, headache, myalgia, and sore throat.

Coxsackie and **echoviruses** cause illnesses with a wide spectrum of clinical symptoms, sometimes following a relapsing course for several weeks. Recurrent infections may occur with Coxsackie B serotypes. Etiologic links have been made to hepatitis, nephritis, acute cerebellar ataxia, and chronic myopathies. Neonates may be affected, and the illness may be severe, occasionally fatal.

Arboviruses are transmitted by hemophagous insects, particularly ticks and mosquitoes. The most important infections in the United States are St. Louis encephalitis, western equine encephalitis, Colorado tick fever, and California (La Crosse) viral infection.

Influenza viruses (A, B, and C) cause periodic local pandemics and major pandemics. Illnesses are usually self-limited, but serious complications may occur, including pneumonia, congestive heart failure with pulmonary edema, disseminated intravascular coagulation, myositis, Reye's syndrome, acute renal failure, encephalopathy, myocarditis, and pericarditis.

Respiratory-syncytial virus (RSV) is the most important respiratory virus affecting infants and young children. Infections may be severe, occasionally fatal, and evidenced as bronchiolitis or pneumonia. Older children and

adults are susceptible, usually with a milder illness, with coryza, cough, and tracheobronchitis. Reinfection is common. RSV has been associated with acute flare-ups of asthmatic bronchitis or chronic bronchitis.

Rhinoviruses are acknowledged as important causes of the common cold.

Coronaviruses are considered to be the cause of mild upper respiratory illness and some acute lower respiratory disease.

Mumps virus causes a parotitis that usually resolves within a week. Complications include epididymo-orchitis in postpubertal men (usually unilateral), pancreatitis, and meningitis. Less common complications may occur: polio-like syndrome, transverse myelitis, cerebellar ataxia, Guillain-Barré syndrome, oophoritis, myocarditis, hepatitis, thrombocytopenic purpura, lower respiratory disease, polyarthritis, and thyroiditis.

Measles virus, or morbillivirus (formerly rubeola), causes an illness characterized by a maculopapular rash, preceded by pathognomonic Koplik's spots on the buccal mucosa. The illness normally resolves in a week. Complications include bronchitis, bronchiolitis, pneumonia, myocarditis, thrombocytopenia, mesenteric lymphadenitis, encephalitis, and more rarely, subacute sclerosing panencephalitis (SSPE, Dawson's or inclusion encephalitis). Infected tissues may contain giant cells (Warthin-Finkeldey cells). SSPE histologically is characterized by intranuclear inclusions of the Cowdry type A (neurons and glial cells of the brain).

Rubella virus is the cause of 3-day, or German, measles. The infection usually results in a benign, mild exanthematous illness. Severe congenital anomalies can result from *in utero* infections occurring in the first trimester of pregnancy. Complications for postnatally acquired infection include postinfectious encephalitis, thrombocytopenia, arthritis, and arthalgias.

Papillomaviruses are the etiologic agents for a variety of cutaneous and mucosal lesions, including warts, and papillomas. They have been associated with cervical cancers and precancerous lesions (known as dysplasias; cervical intraepithelial neoplasia or CIN; or squamous intraepithelial lesion). They also have been associated with anogenital cancers. These lesions are diagnosed by their morphologic characteristics as studied microscopically in cytology preparations or by DNA probes.

Human retroviruses have increased as a worldwide problem and are of paramount medical importance. This group includes HIV-1, human T-cell lymphotrophic virus (HTLV-1), and HTLV-2. HIV-1 is separately discussed. HTLV-2 has been associated with hairy cell leukemia. HTLV-1 is endemic in southwestern Japan, the Caribbean, and areas of Africa. It has been associated with T-cell leukemia/lymphoma. It may also be a cause of myelopathy. This virus has been detected in intravenous drug abusers in the United States.

Other viruses of medical importance include but are not limited to rabies, polio virus, parainfluenza virus, poxviruses, parvovirus B 19, reoviruses, lymphocytic choriomeningitis, arena viruses, and Marburg and Ebola viruses.

Rickettsial infections are characterized by their spread by arthropods and mammals. The human pathogens include the typhus group, spotted fever group, scrub typhus, Q fever, and trench fever. Rocky Mountain spotted fever (wood tick, *Dermacentor andersoni*) and Q fever (*Coxiella burnetii*) are the most common in the United States. Rickettsial infections are usually diagnosed by clinical presentation and by serologic studies.

Chlamydial infections (formerly known as *Bedsonia*) include *Chlamydia trachomatis*, TWAR (*C. pneumoniae*), and *C. psittaci*. *C. psittaci* is associated with psittacosis, a disease of psittacine birds (parrots, parakeets, cockatoos) and other birds including pigeons, chickens, and turkeys. In the latter instances, the term *ornithosis* is preferred. Birds can infect humans via inhalation of fomites. Person-to-person transmission may occur.

TWAR (Taiwan acute respiratory)/*C. pneumoniae* is associated with acute lower respiratory illness.

C. trachomatis is considered the leading cause of pelvic infections in women, including salpingitis and cervicitis. Neonatal conjunctivitis and pneumonitis are linked to passage through an infected birth canal.

Lymphogranuloma venereum (LGV) is caused by chlamydial infection and is characterized by an initial genital vesicle or ulcer that rapidly heals, usually unnoticed, that can be followed by an inguinal adenopathy that may be extensive. The latter may be accompanied by a variety of other symptoms and may occasionally have sequelae of severe proctitis and rectal or urethral strictures.

Spirochetal infections include the three genera of pathogenic organisms, *Treponema*, *Borrelia*, and *Leptospira*.

Treponema pallidum is the etiologic agent of syphilis. The disease occurs with a primary chancre (after an incubation period of 10 days to several months). The chancre is most often on the external genitalia but may occur in the vagina and cervix. A generalized rash occurs 6 to 8 weeks after the chancre appeared and involves mucous membranes as well as the skin (secondary phase). There may be widespread systemic involvement during the secondary phase. The person is infective to others. This phase resolves, and the disease then enters a latent phase, which may be prolonged. About one third of patients with untreated latent syphilis will develop tertiary syphilis (gummas, cardiovascular syphilis, neurosyphilis).

Diagnosis of syphilis is made by clinical findings, demonstration of spirochetes (dark field microscopy) in clinical specimens, or demonstration of antibodies in blood samples or cerebrospinal fluid.

The initial serologic test employed is known as a reagin test, and it may be performed by several different methods: VDRL (Venereal Disease Research Laboratory), RPR (rapid plasma reagin), and a variant, the ART (automated reagin test). These different procedures are equivalent to blood testing. The VDRL should be used with CSF samples for following the response to therapy of proven syphilis. Positive reagin blood tests should be confirmed by specific treponemal antigen tests. The latter include the *Treponema pallidum* immobilization test (TPI) and the fluorescent treponemal antibody absorption test (FTA-ABS). The latter is primarily utilized as the confirmatory test. The TPI is available in only two laboratories in the country. A summary of the commonly used serologic tests for syphilis with respect to the stage of disease appears in Table 21–14.

Biologic-false positives may occur with the reagin tests. The false-positive reaction may be a transient condition related to bacterial or viral infections. Persistent false-positive tests occur in patients with lupus erythematosus and other autoimmune diseases. Other false-positive reactions occur in drug addicts, pregnant women, and individuals over the age of 70 years. Biologic

Table 21–14 ▪ **Commonly Used Serologic Tests for Syphilis**

Test	Primary (%)	Secondary (%)	Late (%)
Nontreponemal (reagin) tests			
Venereal Disease Research Laboratory test (VDRL)	70	99	1*
Rapid plasma reagin card test (RPR); automated reagin test (ART)	80	99	0
Specific treponemal tests			
Treponemal immobilization test (TPI)	50	97	95
Fluorescent treponemal antibody absorption test (FTA-ABS)	85	100	98
T. *pallidum* micro-hemagglutination assay (MHA-TP)	65	100	95

*Treated late syphilis.
Adapted from Henry, J. B. (ed.): *Clinical Diagnosis and Management by Laboratory Methods*, W. B. Saunders Company, Philadelphia, 1991, p. 1095.

false-positives are usually weakly reactive and characterized by a low titer. Borderline reactions may also occur with FTA-ABS. Repeat studies at intervals of 1 or several months are indicated if the clinical history does not suggest infection. Often the borderline reactions will revert to nonreactive.

Other spirochetal infections include yaws and pinta, which are due to *Treponema pertenue* and *T. carateum*, respectively.

Borrelia burgdorferi is the etiologic agent for Lyme disease. The organism is transmitted by *Ixodes dammini* and related ixodid ticks. The disease is prevalent in the northeastern United States and is named for Lyme, Connecticut, where it was first described. Recently a similar but different vector for infection in hillside areas of southern California has been described.

The acute phase of Lyme disease begins with an initial papule at the site of the tick bite, which undergoes annular expansion (erythema chronicum migrans, ECM). The skin lesion is followed by hematogenous dissemination and systemic involvement. The third stage, or chronic infection, develops months after the initial infection and lasts for years. Diagnosis is made by clinical presentation and serologic studies.

Borrelia recurrentis is the etiologic agent for relapsing fever.

Other ▪ Fusospirochetal infections are associated with acute, necrotizing, ulcerative gingivitis (trench mouth, Vincent's angina).

Leptospirosis is an uncommon disease in which serologic tests are helpful in establishing a diagnosis.

Sodoku is a disease in humans that follows infection by *Spirillum minus*, which occurs with a rat or other rodent; the bite could be by a cat or other rodent-eating animal.

SEROLOGIC TESTING FOR AUTOIMMUNE DISORDERS

Autoimmunity and Collagen-Vascular Disorders ▪ These disorders are characterized by multisystem manifestations. Disorders include systemic lupus erythematosus (SLE), rheumatoid arthritis (RA), periarteritis nodosa, progressive systemic sclerosis (SS), Sjögren's syndrome (Sj), mixed connective tissue disease (MCTD), and the combination of calcinosis cutis, Raynaud's phenomenon, esophageal dysfunction, sclerodactyly, and telangiectasia (CREST).

The **antinuclear antibodies (ANA) test** is employed as a screening test utilizing immunofluorescence (also known as FANA, fluorescent antinuclear antibody). It is highly sensitive. It is positive in over 95 per cent of individuals with active, untreated SLE. A persistently negative ANA is strong presumptive evidence against SLE in a symptomatic person who is untreated. The ANA test is not very specific. It may be positive in up to 10 per cent of normal elderly persons (over 70 years), may be positive due to medications (hydralazine, procainamide, others), and may be positive in diseases other than SLE, notably rheumatoid arthritis, Sjögren's syndrome, progressive systemic sclerosis, dermatomyositis/polymyositis, and periarteritis nodosa. Higher titers tend to occur with SLE (more than 1:640).

Anti-dsDNA (double stranded DNA) has a greater specifity than does FANA. Anti-dsDNA is significantly elevated in 65 to 80 per cent of individuals with active, untreated SLE and is infrequently positive in other disorders. Persistently high levels through several months of treatment may be an indication of a subsequent progressive clinical deterioration. This test may be falsely negative during peak disease activity due to full complexing of the antibody by circulating DNA. The test may remain positive after clinical remission of SLE.

Other tests available to evaluate SLE include: **anti-Sm(ith) Ab**, directed against a small nuclear RNA (snRNA). It is present in 30 per cent of SLE patients during active disease, particularly with renal involvement. It is often accompanied by anti-smRNP (**anti-RNP**). The latter may be present in high titer in MCTD in the absence of anti-Sm.

Anti-Ro (SSA) occurs in SLE and Sjögren's syndrome. It is directed against a small, cytoplasmic RNA protein. It is present in about 30 per cent of SLE patients, particularly those with photosensitivity, subacute cutaneous lupus, neonatal lupus, and an lupus-like syndrome with congenital deficiency of C4 and C2. It may also be present in atypical SLE with prominent photosensitivity, serositis, low prevalence of renal and CNS involvement, and negative ANA and anti-DNA tests.

Anti-La (SSB) Ab occurs in SLE and Sjögren's syndrome. The latter usually contains both anti-La and anti-Ro. The presence of both anti-Ro and anti-La tends to be associated with milder forms of SLE.

Additional tests employed in the evaluation of the collagen-vascular disorders include: *anti-Scl-70, anti-PM1, anti-centromere, anti-histone,* and *anti-PCNA.*

Lupus anticoagulant (LA) is present in about 30 per cent of SLE patients; it may occur in other connective tissue disorders and may also be drug-induced. It may be detected by a prolonged aPTT (activated partial thromboplastin time). It may also cause a false-positive reagin for syphilis (e.g., RPR, rapid plasma reagin). It does not cause increased bleeding. SLE patients are at risk for thrombosis. LA also occurs in non-SLE patients, including women with recurrent spontaneous abortions and some young patients with CNS ischemic events.

Rheumatoid factor (RF) is a test utilizing immunoglobulins directed against the Fc fragment of autologous IgG. It is present in over 80 per cent of patients with rheumatoid arthritis (RA). RF may be present at low levels in normal individuals, with increased prevalence in elderly individuals, and may be present in chronic inflammatory conditions or hypergammaglobulinemia. The **latex fixation (LF) test** for RF detects mainly IgM RF and not IgG RF. The LF test in titers of 1:80 or more is considered positive. Very high titers are usually seen in "highly expressed" RA, i.e., patients with subcutaneous nodules, vasculitis, and other findings. Very high levels without evidence of chronic inflammation of joints should raise consideration of a paraproteinemia.

Entities in the differential diagnosis for RF that may present with a negative RF include early RF (first several months), juvenile RA, arthritis associated with systemic disease (Marie-Strümpell ankylosing spondylitis, Reiter's syndrome, colitic arthopathy, and psoriatic arthritis). Additionally, RF may be persistently negative in some cases that are considered definite or classic rheumatoid arthritis.

Cryoglobulins may be classified as monoclonal, mixed polyclonal-monoclonal, and mixed polyclonal-polyclonal. Monoclonal immunoglobulins are paraproteins. IgG commonly occurs in multiple myeloma, IgM in macroglobulinemia and some lymphomas, but IgA and Bence Jones types have been reported. "Benign" monoclonal gammopathy occurs, which may or may not be followed by overt lymphoproliferative malignancy.

Mixed polyclonal-monoclonal cryoglobulins are complexes of IgG "antigen" and monoclonal IgM with anti-IgG (RF activity). They are often associated with IgM lymphoproliferative states.

Mixed polyclonal-polyclonal cryoglobulins are usually IgG-IgM but may be IgG-IgM-IgA. The complement C1q may be present. These cryoglobulins occur with hepatitis B, cytomegalovirus, infectious mononucleosis, and lepromatous leprosy.

A number of assays are used for the immune complexes that may be present in rheumatoid arthritis, childhood nephrotic syndrome, infection, and malignancies. These assays include the *C1q precipitin assay, complement-binding assays,* and the *Raji cell assay.*

ORGAN-DIRECTED AUTOIMMUNE DISORDERS

Thyroid
Immunofluorescence Screening Test ▪ Negative staining of colloid and epithelial cytoplasm is strong evidence against active Hashimoto's thyroiditis or primary myxedema.

Antithyroglobulin Hemagglutinin Test ▪ High titers (more than 1 : 1000) occur in Hashimoto's thyroiditis, Graves' disease and some cases of hypothyroidism.

Antimicrosomal Ab ▪ Positive tests strongly suggest active Hashimoto's thyroiditis or Graves' disease.

Autoimmune Liver Disease ▪ A clinical picture of liver disease in young women with joint, skin, and serosal symptoms, associated with a positive ANA (antinuclear antibodies), has been termed *lupoid hepatitis.*

Idiopathic biliary cirrhosis, which occurs in young to middle-aged women, and primary sclerosing cholangitis, which may be related, are both considered autoimmune disorders.

Autoimmune antibodies may occur in infectious hepatitis, particularly infections with the delta virus.

Tests to evaluate hepatic autoantibodies include:

▪ **Antismooth muscle AB:** Present in up to 90 per cent of individuals with chronic active hepatitis and 25 to 40 per cent of cases of biliary or idiopathic cirrhosis. It may be transiently present in up to 80 per cent of cases of acute hepatitis. It also occurs in up to 80 per cent of patients with infectious mononucleosis who have high-titer heterophil antibodies. Titers of 1 : 100 or more suggest progressive chronic active hepatitis.

▪ **Antimitochondrial Ab:** Present in up to 94 per cent of persons with primary biliary cirrhosis and 25 per cent of cases of chronic active hepatitis.

▪ **Antinuclear ab (ANA):** May be positive in chronic active hepatitis, lupoid hepatitis and idiopathic biliary cirrhosis. The test is usually negative in viral hepatitis or alcoholic cirrhosis.

Multiple Sclerosis (MS) ▪ **CSF immunoglobulin electrophoresis** is highly sensitive for oligoclonal bands in 80 to 95 per cent of patients with MS and positive in 50 to 60 per cent of patients with their first attack. Diagnosis must be made on a combined clinical and laboratory basis. Oligoclonal bands may occur in other conditions, including subacute sclerosing panencephalitis, chronic mycobacterial and fungal meningitis, chronic viral meningitis, neurosyphilis, and optic neuritis.

Other Organ-Related Autoimmune Diseases ▪ Autoimmunity is considered to play a role in diseases of many other organs and systems, although in some instances the evidence is incomplete. These include:

Addison's disease of the adrenal glands
Premature ovarian failure
Infertility (antisperm Ab)
Insulin-dependent diabetes mellitus (IDDM)
Atrophic gastritis and pernicious anemia
Crohn's disease, chronic ulcerative colitis
Skin disorders

    SLE and discoid lupus (DLE)
    Pemphigus vulgaris
    Bullous pemphigoid
    Cicatricial pemphigoid
    Dermatitis herpetiformis

Behçet's syndrome
Vitiligo

Renal diseases

Goodpasture's syndrome
Glomerulonephritis, progressive (some cases)
Glomerular membrane alterations (viral, drug)
SLE
Vasculitides
Infections
Tubulointerstitial nephritis
Membranoproliferative glomerulonephritis

Cardiac disorders

Rheumatic heart disease

Neuromuscular diseases

Multiple sclerosis
Guillain-Barré syndrome
Myasthenia gravis (MG)
Lambert-Eaton mysasthenic syndrome (LEMS)
Dermatomyositis and polymyositis
Paraneoplastic syndromes

THERAPEUTIC DRUG MONITORING (TDM)

Many therapeutic drugs need to be monitored because of possible occurrence of toxic side effects, because the physician needs to determine when the medication has achieved a stable therapeutic effect, and to assess subtherapeutic levels of the drug that may occur with lack of patient compliance.

In general, it will be four half-lives before a medication has achieved the steady state. Prior to the steady state, results may be highly variable. Therapeutic levels may be influenced by hepatic function, particularly if compromised due to liver disease, or possibly if stimulated by other drugs, for example, phenobarbital. Hepatic function is important for the medications that are converted to metabolites in the extramitochondrial, microsomal system of hepatocytes. Therapeutic drugs important to monitor include the following:

Cardiotropics
Digoxin
Digitoxin
Procainamide (Pronestyl)
Quinidine
Lidocaine (Xylocaine)
Propranolol

Anticonvulsants
Phenobarbital
Phenytoin (Dilantin)
Primidone (Mysoline)
Ethosuximide (Zarotin)
Carbamazepine (Tegretol)
Valproic acid (Depakene)

Antiasthmatics
Theophylline

Anti-inflammatory drugs
Acetaminophen (Tylenol)
Acetylsalicylic acid (aspirin)

Immunosuppressives
Cyclosporine

Manic-depressive drugs
Lithium
Tricyclic antidepressants

Neuroleptics, antipsychotic major tranquilizers
Phenazines
Chlorpromazine
Butyrophenones
Haloperidol (Haldol)

Chemotherapeutic agents
Methotrexate

CRITICAL AND ALERT LABORATORY VALUES (Table 21–15)

In the early 1960s, Ernest Cotlove, Ph.D, head of Clinical Chemistry, Clinical Center, National Institutes of Health, Bethesda, Maryland, instituted an **Early Warning System** for abnormal laboratory values that were life threatening. Abnormal results were to be immediately telephoned or personally delivered to the nursing

Text continued on page 368

Table 21-15 ▪ **Critical Values, Alert Values**

Guidelines

Critical Values: Results will be called to the managing physician AT THE TIME OF CONFIRMED RESULTS, regardless of the time of the day or night.

Alert 1: These results are to be called beginning at 7:00 A.M. These results may be given to the authorized office and supportive staff of the managing physician or organization.

Alert 2: These results are to be communicated after completion of all ALERT 1 values. Communication may be in the form of printed results for those clients having point-of-care printers. Results are called to clients not having printers.

Documentation Maintained Shall Include:
- Person making call
- Person taking call
- Date and time called
- Telephone number called
- Test(s) reported

Clinical laboratory areas may use the RED "Critical Values" report form. This is completed and given to Client Services *without delay*. Client services will make the required calls when the department is staffed. Otherwise it is the responsibility of the performing technologist or on-duty manager to call the managing physician.

Critical Values, Alert Values

Acetaminophen, Serum (µg/mL)			≥ 300
Critical		≥ 50	
Alert 1			
Therapeutic Range	10–25		
Albumin, Serum (gm/dL)			
Alert 1	≤ 1.5		
Reference Range	3.5–5.5		
Alcohol, Ethyl, Blood (mg/dL)			
Alert 1		≥ 400	
Reference Range	None detected		
exceptions: 1. All values called as member of Coma Panel.			
2. Industrial drug screens not called unless requested by client.			
ALT (SGPT), Serum (U/L)			
Alert 1		≥ 500	
Reference Range	1–45		
Amikacin, Serum <u>Peak</u> (µg/mL)			
Alert 1		≥ 26	
Therapeutic Range	15–25		
Amikacin, Serum <u>Trough</u> (µg/mL)			
Alert 1		≥ 10	
Therapeutic Range	1–8		
Amitriptyline and Nortriptyline, Serum (ng/mL)			
Alert 1		≥ 500	
Therapeutic Range	120–250		
Amobarbital, Serum (µg/mL)			
Alert 1		≥ 15	
Therapeutic Range	3–12		
Amoxapine, Serum (ng/mL)			
Alert 1		≥ 500	
Therapeutic Range	200–400		

T*able* 21–15 ▪ Critical Values, Alert Values *Continued*

Critical Values, Alert Values

	Critical (low)	Alert (low)	Reference/Therapeutic Range	Alert (high)	Critical (high)
Amylase, Serum (IU/L)					
Alert 1				≥ 200	
Reference Range			16–62		
AST (SGOT), Serum (U/L)					
Alert 1				≥ 500	
Reference Range			1–45		
Bilirubin, Total, Serum Adult (mg/dL)					
Alert 1				≥ 12.0	
Reference Range			0.1–1.5		
Bilirubin, Serum Newborn (mg/dL)					
Critical					≥ 18
Alert 1				≥ 12.0	
Alert 2				≥ 5.0	
Reference Range			0.1–1.5		
Bromide, Serum (µg/mL)					
Alert 1				≥ 1550	
Therapeutic Range			750–1500		
BUN, Serum (mg/dL)					
Alert 1				≥ 60	
Reference Range			6–25		
Butabarbital, Serum (µg/mL)					
Alert 1				≥ 30	
Therapeutic Range			2–14		
Butalbital, Serum (µg/mL)					
Alert 1				≥ 8	
Therapeutic Range			1–7		
Calcium, Total Serum (mg/dL)					
Critical	≤ 6.0				≥ 14.0
Alert 1		≤ 6.5		≥ 12.0	
Alert 2		≤ 7.5			
Reference Range			8.5–10.8		
Calcium, Ionized, Serum (mg/dL)					
Critical	≤ 3.2				≥ 6.4
Alert 1		≤ 4.0		≥ 6.2	
Reference Range			4.5–5.3		
Carbamazepine, Serum (µg/mL)					
Alert 1		≤ 3		≥ 15	
Therapeutic Range			4–12		
Carbon Monoxide, Whole Blood (g %)					
Alert 1				≥ 25	
Reference Range			< 5 Nonsmokers 6–15 Smokers		
Chloramphenicol, Serum (Oral) (µg/mL)					
Alert 1				≥ 15	
Therapeutic Range			3–12 Peak		
Chloramphenicol, Serum (Intravenous) (µg/mL)					
Alert 1				≥ 45	

Table continued on following page

Table 21–15 ▪ Critical Values, Alert Values Continued

Critical Values, Alert Values

	Low Critical	Low Alert	Range	High Alert	High Critical
Therapeutic Range			20–40 Peak 2–10 Trough		
Chlorazepate (as Nordiazepam), Serum (ng/mL)					
Alert 1				≥ 5,000	
Therapeutic Range			400–1500		
Chlordiazepoxide and/or Norchlordiazepoxide, Serum (µg/mL)					
Alert 1				≥ 5.0	
Therapeutic Range			1.0–3.0		
Chloride, Serum (mmol/L)					
Alert 1		≤ 80		≥ 115	
Reference Range			97–107		
Chlorpromazine, Serum (ng/mL)					
Alert 1				≥ 1,000	
Therapeutic Range			50–500		
Clonazepam, Serum (ng/mL)					
Alert 1				≥ 100	
Therapeutic Range			10–80		
CO₂ Content, Serum (mmol/L)					
Critical	≤ 10				≥ 40
Alert 1		≤ 15		≥ 35	
Reference Range			22–34		
CPK, Serum (U/L)					
Alert 1				≥ 1000	
Alert 2				≥ 500	
Reference Range			41–186		
CPK MB, Serum (%)					
Alert 1				≥ 6% Positive band	
Reference Range			0.0–0.0		
Creatinine, Serum (mg/dL)					
Alert 1				≥ 8.0	
Alert 2				≥ 4.0	
Reference Range			0.6–1.4		
Cyanide, Blood (µg/dL)					
Critical					≥ 270
Alert 1				≥ 15	
Reference Range			< 10		
Desipramine, Serum (ng/mL)					
Alert 1				≥ 301	
Thereapeutic Range			50–300		
Diazepam (includes Nordiazepam), Serum (ng/mL)					
Alert 1				≥ 3000	
Therapeutic Range			100–2000		
Digitoxin, Serum (µg/L)					
Alert 1		≤ 9		≥ 26	
Therapeutic Range			9.0–25.0		
Digoxin, Serum (ng/mL)					
Alert 1		≤ 0.4		≥ 2.1	
Therapeutic Range			0.5–2.0		

Table 21–15 ■ Critical Values, Alert Values *Continued*

Critical Values, Alert Values				
Disopyramide, Serum (μg/mL)				
Alert 1		≤ 1		≥ 7
Therapeutic Range			2–5	
Doxepin and N-Desmethyldoxepin, Serum (μg/L)				
Alert 1		≤ 99		≥ 500
Therapeutic Range			100–300	
Ethchlorvynol (Placidyl), Serum (μg/mL)				
Alert 1				≥ 20
Therapeutic Range			2–10	
Ethosuximide, Serum (μg/mL)				
Alert 1				≥ 110
Therapeutic Range			40–100	
Fibrinogen (mg/dL)				
Alert 1		≤ 100		≥ 500
Reference Range			200–400	
Fluorazepam, Serum (ng/mL)				
Alert 1				≥ 500
Therapeutic Range			30–120	
Gentamicin, Serum <u>Peak</u> (μg/mL)				
Alert 1				≥ 12
Therapeutic Range			5–10	
Gentamicin, Serum <u>Trough</u> (μg/mL)				
Alert 1				≥ 2.1
Therapeutic Range			< 2.0	
Glucose, CSF (mg/dL)				
Alert 1		≤ 40		≥ 150
Reference Range			47–80	
Glucose, Serum (mg/dL)				
Critical	≤ 40				≥ 700
Alert 1		≤ 50		≥ 400
Alert 2				≥ 300
Reference Range			65–110	

exceptions: Low glucose with increased potassium due to hemolysis, whole blood specimen with inadequate barrier separation or no barrier.

Glutethimide (Doriden), Serum (μg/mL)				
Alert 1				≥ 10
Therapeutic Range			3–7	
Haloperidol, Serum (ng/mL)				
Alert 1				≥ 20
Therapeutic Range			3–15	
Hematocrit (%)				
Alert 1		≤ 20		≥ 60
Reference Range			37–52	
Hemoglobin (gm/dL)				
Critical	≤ 5			
Alert 1		≤ 8.0		≥ 20
Reference Range			12–18	

Table continued on following page

Table 21–15 ▪ Critical Values, Alert Values *Continued*

Critical Values, Alert Values

exception: Persistence of abnormality prior established, known to client, and part of the medical condition under medical management.

Imipramine and Desiprimine, Serum (ng/mL)		
Alert 1		≥ 500
Therapeutic Range	150–300	
Isopropanol (includes Acetone), Serum (mg/dL)		
Alert 1		≥ 20
Reference Range	None detected	
Ketosis, Urine (Pediatric)		
Alert 1		Trace, 1+ to 4+
Reference Range	Negative	
Lactate (Lactic Acid), Serum (mg/dL)		
Alert 1		≥ 30
Reference Range	9–16	
LDH, Serum (U/L)		
Alert 1		≥ 1000
Reference Range	100–225	
Lead, Blood (Adult) (μg/dL)		
Alert 1		≥ 41
Reference Range	0–40	
Lead, Blood (Pediatric) (μg/dL)		
Critical	≥ 70	
Alert 1		≥ 15
Reference Range	0–10	
Lidocaine, Serum (μg/mL)		
Alert 1		≥ 7
Therapeutic Range	1.5–5.0	
Lipase, Serum (U/L)		
Alert 1		≥ 180
Reference Range	7–60	
Lithium, Serum (mEq/L)		
Alert 1		≥ 1.5
Therapeutic Range	1.0–1.4 Acute therapy 0.5–1.0 Chronic maintenance	
Magnesium, Serum (mEq/L)		
Alert 1	≤ 1.0	≥ 3.0
Reference Range	1.3–2.3	
Malaria, Blood		
Alert 1		Positive
Reference Range	None detected	
Maprotiline (Ludiomil), Serum (ng/mL)		
Alert 1		≥ 1,000
Therapeutic Range	180–450	
Meprobamate, Serum (μg/mL)		
Alert 1		≥ 50
Therapeutic Range	5–30	

Table 21–15 ■ **Critical Values, Alert Values** *Continued*

Critical Values, Alert Values			
Methanol, Serum (mg/dL)			
Alert 1			≥ 10
Reference Range		None detected	
Methotrexate, Serum (uMOL/L)			
Alert 1			≥ 6 24 hr.
			≥ 0.6 48 hr.
			≥ 0.06 72 hr.
Therapeutic Range		≤ 5 24 hr.	
		≤ 0.5 48 hr.	
		≤ 0.05 72 hr.	
Osmolality, Serum (mOsm/kg)			
Alert 1	≤ 240		≥ 320
Reference Range		275–295	
Pentobarbital, Serum (µg/mL)			
Alert 1	≤ 0.9		≥ 6.0
Therapeutic Range		1–5	
Phencyclidine (PCP), Serum (ng/mL)			
Alert 1			≥ 25
Reference Range		None detected	
exception: Industrial or probationary samples not called unless requested by client.			
Phenobarbital, Serum (µg/mL)			
Alert 1	≤ 14		≥ 50
Therapeutic Range		15–40	
Phenytoin (Dilantin), Serum (mcg/mL)			
Alert 1			≥ 25
Therapeutic Range		10–20	
Phosphorus, Serum (mg/dL)			
Alert 1	≤ 1.5		≥ 6.0
Reference Range		2.5–4.5	
exceptions: Associated low glucose and/or low potassium, whole blood specimen with inadequate or no barrier.			
Platelet (× 10^3/cu mm)			
Critical	≤ 30		≥ 1,500
Alert 1	≤ 50		≥ 800
Reference Range		150–400	
exception: Persistence of abnormality prior established, known to client, and part of the medical condition under medical management.			
Potassium, Serum (mEq/L)			
Critical	≤ 2.5		≥ 6.5
Alert 1	≤ 3.0		≥ 6.0
Reference Range		3.5–5.5	
exceptions: Elevated potassium due to hemolysis, whole blood specimen with inadequate or no barrier.			
Primidone, Serum (µg/mL)			
Alert 1			≥ 13
Therapeutic Range		5–12	
Procainamide, Serum (µg/mL)			
Alert 1			> 10
Therapeutic Range		4–10	

Table continued on following page

Table 21–15 ▪ **Critical Values, Alert Values** *Continued*

Critical Values, Alert Values			
Procainamide + NAPA, Serum (μg/mL)			
Alert 1		≥ 35	
Therapeutic Range	5–30		
Protein, Total, Serum (gm/dL)			
Alert 1	≤ 4	≥ 10	
Reference Range	6.0–8.0		
Prothrombin Time (seconds)			
Critical			≥ 40
Alert 1		≥ 25	
Reference Range	10.0–13.0		
Protriptyline, Serum (ng/mL)			
Alert 1		≥ 300	
Therapeutic Range	50–150		
PTT (Partial Thromboplastin Time) (seconds)			
Alert 1		≥ 50.0	
Reference Range	25.0–35.0		
Quinidine, Serum (μg/mL)			
Alert 1		≥ 6	
Therapeutic Range	2.0–5.0		
Salicylate, Serum (mg/dL)			
Critical			≥ 70
Alert 1		≥ 50	
Therapeutic Range	5.0–30.0		
Secobarbital, Serum (μg/mL)			
Alert 1		≥ 6	
Therapeutic Range	1–5		
Sodium, Serum (mEq/L)			
Critical	≤ 120		≥ 160
Alert 1	≤ 125	≥ 155	
Alert 2	≤ 130	≥ 150	
Reference Range	135–148		
Theophylline, Serum (μg/mL)			
Alert 1		≥ 22	
Therapeutic Range	10–20		
Thiothixene, Serum (ng/mL)			
Alert 1		≥ 50	
Therapeutic Range	3–45		
Tobramycin, Serum <u>Peak</u> (μg/mL)			
Critical			> 12
Alert 1		≥ 11	
Therapeutic Range	5–10		
Tobramycin, Serum <u>Trough</u> (mg/L)			
Alert 1		≥ 3	
Therapeutic Range	< 2		
Trazodone, Serum (ng/mL)			
Alert 1		≥ 2000	
Therapeutic Range	750–1600		

Table* 21–15 ▪ Critical Values, Alert Values *Continued

Critical Values, Alert Values			
Uric Acid, Serum (mg/dL)			
Alert 1			≥ 20
Alert 2			≥ 15
Reference Range		3.5–8.0 (Males)	
		2.5–6.0 (Females)	
Valproic Acid, Serum (mg/L)			
Alert 1			≥ 110
Therapeutic Range		50–100	
Vancomycin, Serum <u>Peak</u> (mg/L)			
Critical			> 100
Alert 1			≥ 42
Therapeutic Range		30–40	
Vancomycin, Serum <u>Trough</u> (mg/L)			
Alert 1			≥ 11
Therapeutic Range		5–10	
Vanillylmandelic Acid (VMA), Urine (mg/24 hr)			
Alert 1			≥ 50
Reference Range		1–8	
WBC (× 10^3/cu mm)			
Alert 1	≤ 2.5		≥ 18
Reference Range		4.0–11.0	

Microbiology/Serology Critical Values, Alert Values	
AFB, Culture/Stain	
Alert 2	Any positive
Bacterial Meningitis Antigen	
Critical	Any positive
Beta-Strep Culture	
Alert 2	Any positive
Blood Culture	
Critical	Positive culture, preliminary and final
Bordetella Pertussis	
Critical	Any positive
CSF Culture/Stain	
Critical	Positive culture, preliminary and final
Cryptococcus Culture/Antigen, CSF	
Critical	Any positive
Cryptococcus Culture/Antigen, Other Sources of Clinical Risk	
Alert 1	Any positive
Fungi, CSF	
Critical	Any positive
Fungi (Systemic: Including *Histoplasma*, *Blastomyces*, *Coccidioides*), Other Sources of Clinical Risk	
Alert 1	Any positive
Gram Stain, Sterile Fluids Other Than CSF	
Alert 1	Any positive

Table continued on following page

Table 21–15 ▪ **Critical Values, Alert Values** *Continued*

Critical Values, Alert Values	
Herpes, CSF	
Critical	Any positive
Herpes, Eyes, Other Sources of Clinical Risk	
Alert 1	Any positive
India Ink, Prep, CSF	
Critical	Any positive
India Ink Prep, Other Sources of Clinical Risk	
Alert 1	Any positive
Malaria, Blood	
Alert 1	Any positive
Reference Range	None detected
RSV	
Alert 1	Any positive

Cytology and Tissue Pathology Alert

Alert 1
   Kaposi's Sarcoma
   Malignant Melanoma
   Keratosis with Marked Dysplasia
   Basal Cell Carcinoma
   Squamous Cell Carcinoma
   Dysplasia or CIS or CIN
   All Carcinomas, Adenocarcinomas (Breast, Colon, Prostate, etc.)
   Keratoacanthoma vs. Squamous Cell Carcinoma if SCC favored
   Clinical POC without villi microscopically (or uterine currettings) in suspected ectopic pregnancy
   Bowen's Disease or Bowenoid Features
   Re-Excisions of Previous Malignancies
     ▪ presence or absence of malignancy
     ▪ status of margins as appropriate

From MetWest/Unilab Clinical Laboratories, Tarzana, California.

unit of the patient. The name Early Warning System reflected the geopolitical climate of the world at that time, particularly the nuclear threat posed in Cuba and intensely felt in the Washington, D.C., area. This was perhaps the first such laboratory alert system formally developed and implemented.

The value of the practice has been validated by the implementation of systems in laboratories throughout the world. It is a requirement specified by the Clinical Laboratory Improvement Act of 1988 (CLIA 88). The practice has been updated and extended in scope through the years. It was popularized by George Lundberg,

M.D., editor of the *Journal of the American Medical Association*; he termed the abnormal values "panic" values.

Telephone reporting of selected results is valuable in addition to alerting medical personnel of life-threatening situations. Abnormal values may be an indication for additional tests or changes in patient management. In some laboratories, this type of serious but not life-threatening abnormality is distinguished from the critical values, and the results are reported by telephone at an early opportunity but on a 24-hour basis. Table 21–15 lists Critical and Alert Values for a reference laboratory. Values for assays may be technology- and instrument-dependent and thus may vary for different laboratories.

Reference Sources

Altman, Lawrence K.: High level of iron tied to heart risk. Finnish study backs theory on hardening of arteries. *New York Times*, September 8, 1992.

Clinical Laboratory Improvement Act (42 CFR Part 493, HSQ-176), *Federal Register*, February 28, 1992. U.S. Government Printing Office. ATTN: New Order Desk, P.O. Box 371954, Pittsburgh, PA 15250-7954.

Fariso, K. M., J. W. Buehler, M. E. Chamberland, et al.: Spectrum of disease in persons with human immunodeficiency virus infection in the United States. *Journal of the American Medical Association* 267(13):1798–1805, 1992.

Henry, John Bernard (ed.): *Clinical Diagnosis and Management by Laboratory Methods.* W. B. Saunders Company, Philadelphia, 1991.

Hoofnagle, J. H., and A. M. Di Bisceglie: Serologic diagnosis of acute and chronic viral hepatitis. *Seminars in Liver Disease* 11:(2):73–83, 1991.

Human Immunodeficiency Virus (HIV) Infection Codes and New Codes for Kaposi's Sarcoma. Official Authorized Addenda ICD-9-CM (Revision No. 2). *Morbidity and Mortality Weekly Report (MMWR).* Vol. 40, No. RR-9, July 26, 1991.

Littrup, P. J., F. Lee, and C. Mettlin: Prostate cancer screening: Current trends and future implications. *CA — A Cancer Journal for Clinicians* 42(4):198–211, 1992.

Safai, B., B. Diaz, and J. Schwartz: Malignant neoplasms associated with human immunodeficiency virus infection. *CA – A Cancer Journal for Clinicians* 42(2):74–95, 1992.

For references of specific application to medical transcription, see Appendix 1.

Leslie P. Dornfeld, M.D.

Nephrology

INTRODUCTION

Nephrology, the subspecialty of internal medicine that deals with diseases related to the kidney and its various functions, is a relatively young field of study.

Prior to the 1960s, nephrology was a part of endocrinology or cardiology and was called renology, metabolism, or renophysiology, among other names. With the advent of kidney biopsies, kidney transplantation, and dialysis, the field of nephrology became a separate discipline. The term *nephrology* has been attributed to Dr. Jean Hamberger in Paris, based on study of the nephron, the functioning unit of the kidney (*nephros* is the Greek word for kidney).

Nephrology now encompasses many areas:

- Intrinsic diseases of the kidney
  Glomerulonephritis
  Pyelonephritis
  Renal tubular acidosis
  Congenital abnormalities

- Systemic diseases that affect the kidney
  Diabetes mellitus
  Autoimmune diseases
  Hyperparathyroidism
  Drug reactions

- Hypertension

- Hemodialysis and peritoneal dialysis

- Renal transplantation

- Acid-base disturbances

- Fluid and electrolyte problems

- Metabolic bone problems

Most people do not appreciate that diverse bodily functions, such as the formation and maintenance of bone, the production of red blood cells, blood pressure regulation, and nerve function, depend on normally functioning kidneys.

For these and other reasons, reports, letters, and hospital records coming from the nephrologist contain a much more diverse vocabulary than other subspecialties. However, once it is understood that most of the jargon of the nephrologist derives from either the anatomy of the kidney or physiology, it becomes easy to comprehend.

ANATOMY OF THE KIDNEY

The excretory system, more generally known as the genitourinary tract, normally consists of:

1. Two kidneys
2. Two ureters
3. One bladder
4. One urethra
5. Accessory organs, such as the penis, prostate gland, and testis in the male and the female reproductive organs (uterus, ovaries, cervix, and vagina).

Since the reproductive organs usually fall into the fields of gynecology and urology, this discussion will be confined to the kidneys, ureters, and to a limited degree, the bladder (Figure 22–1).

Kidneys ▪ There are normally two kidneys. Each one weighs approximately 120 to 270 grams and is approximately 11 cm. long by 5 cm. wide by 2.5 cm. deep. The left kidney is slightly

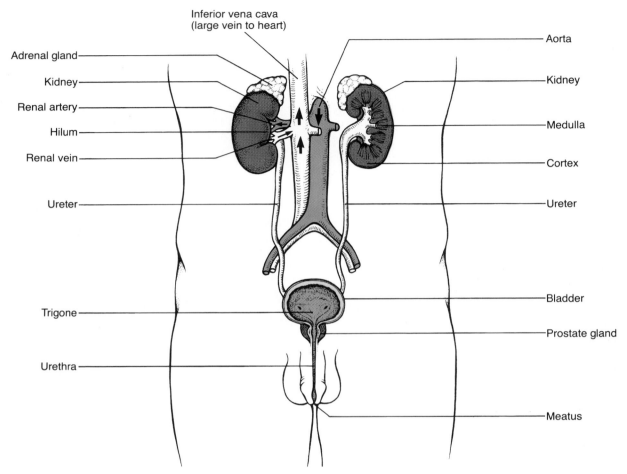

Figure 22–1
The organs of the urinary system.

larger than the right kidney. They usually lie in the retroperitoneal area alongside the vertebral column under the 12th thoracic rib and extend as low as the 3rd lumbar vertebra. There is, however, considerable variability in their location. There may sometimes be only one kidney, or two kidneys may be fused together (horseshoe kidney).

The kidneys are supplied with blood by the renal arteries, which arise directly from the aorta. The kidney is divided into two major parts, the cortex and the medulla. The cortex is the outer rim of the kidney and occupies perhaps the smallest part of the kidney; however, 90 per cent of the functioning part of the kidney, the glomerulus, is located in the cortex. Therefore, any injury to the cortex or glomeruli leads to rapid deterioration of renal function. The medulla, which occupies the largest anatomic space of the kidney, contains mostly tubules and only approximately 10 per cent of the actual filtering system (glomeruli). The diseases of the medulla include interstitial nephritis, pyelonephritis, and various congenital abnormalities.

Within the kidney, the main renal artery divides into lobar arteries, which then divide into lobular arteries, which divide into capillaries and modify to become the glomeruli (Figure 22–

2). The glomeruli are the functioning units of the part of the kidney called the nephron. The other major part of the nephron is the tubule (Figure 22–3).

Blood is filtered at the glomerulus and the plasma is skimmed off. As the fluid proceeds down the tubule, protein, sugar, sodium, potassium, chloride, amino acids, calcium, phosphorus, and other substances are reabsorbed or secreted to prevent loss of these valuable body substances, as well as to prevent an excess accumulation of any one. Excess retention could lead to an abnormal condition; for example, sodium retention could result in swelling (edema) or increased blood pressure (hypertension).

EVALUATION OF RENAL DISEASE

There are many ways to evaluate the function of the kidneys as well as the diseases that occur within the kidney. Diagnostic studies include the following:

Urinalysis

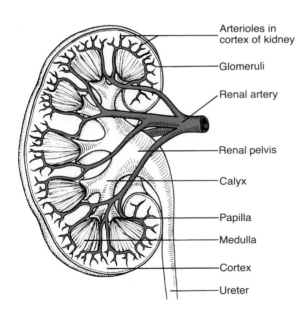

Cutaway illustration of the kidney, showing the renal artery branching to form smaller arteries, arterioles, and glomeruli as well as the medulla and cortex.

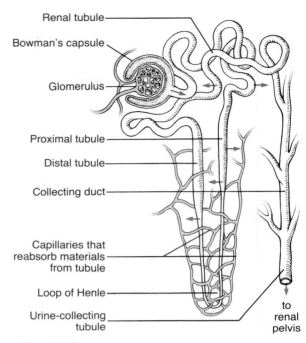

Figure 22–3
Nephron unit showing the renal tubules. Arrows indicate the reabsorption of water, sugar, and salts from the renal tubules into the surrounding capillaries.

- 24-hour collection of urine
- Glomerular filtration rate measurement
- Tubular function testing
- Renal ultrasound
- Excretory urogram (intravenous pyelography [IVP])
- Computed tomographic (CT) scanning
- Magnetic resonance imaging (MRI)
- Renal angiography
- Renal biopsy
- Blood tests

Urinalysis ▪ An examination of a freshly voided urine specimen is the simplest and most convenient way to screen for a kidney disease. Normally, urine is examined for the presence or absence of protein (albumin), sugar, and its pH. Other substances can be evaluated, but these are the most common. Examining the urine under a microscope may reveal the presence or absence of red blood cells, white blood cells, or formed substances that are commonly referred to as casts.

The presence of increased amounts of protein in the urine signifies some disease, usually at the level of the glomerulus. The presence of white blood cells in the urine often signifies infection of the kidney, whereas the presence of red blood cells may mean any disease from glomerular disease to kidney stones. Many other things are seen in the urine, such as crystals and bacteria.

The urine concentration is always analyzed by measuring the specific gravity or osmolality. For further information on urinalysis, see Chapter 21, Laboratory Medicine.

Glomerular Filtration Rate Measurement ■ By determining the ratio of certain substances in the urine in relation to the blood, such as plasma creatinine, the proportion of creatinine that is filtered at the glomerulus and excreted in the urine in relation to how much is in the blood tells the physician the effectiveness of the filtration system—the glomerulus. This is called the glomerulus filtration rate (GFR).

Tubular Function Tests ■ Tubular function can be determined by the pH of the urine or by the concentration (osmolality or specific gravity). An inability to concentrate the urine when it is needed or an inability to excrete extra water when it is ingested is usually the result of a tubular defect. The presence of sugar or amino acids usually means tubular defect.

Ultrasound ■ Ultrasound is another basic test that may determine kidney size, the location of the kidneys, the presence or absence of cystic or solid tumors, or whether there is obstruction to the kidneys.

Excretory Urogram—Intravenous Pyelography (IVP) ■ It was discovered that certain dyes containing iodine, when injected into a vein, were excreted by the kidneys and clearly outlined the kidney on x-ray film as the dye was excreted. Therefore, an IVP is often utilized to determine the size, function, shape, and location of the kidneys (Figure 22–4).

Computed Tomographic Scanning and Magnetic Resonance Imaging ■ These modalities are noninvasive, recently developed techniques that clearly determine the size and shape of the kidney as well as differentiate cysts, tumors, and abscesses. The combination of either of these, plus contrast used in an IVP, makes the studies much more valuable.

Angiography ■ Visualization of the renal artery is infrequently done but is performed to determine lesions of the main renal artery that can lead to hypertension or renal insufficiency. The outline of the venous system is also useful in the diagnosis of renal vein thrombosis. Other diseases, such as polyarteritis nodosa, may be detected by the finding of small microaneurysms in the kidney.

Kidney Biopsy ■ The direct examination of kidney tissue obtained by small needle sampling through the posterior flank or during an open surgical procedure can lead to a definitive diagnosis, especially of glomerular lesions. Renal biopsy is particularly useful in determining the etiology of the nephrotic syndrome, unexplained renal failure, or hematuria of a renal organ. Renal biopsy may be accompanied by complications consisting mostly of gross hematuria (one in ten patients). Occasionally, transfusions are necessary and rarely nephrectomy. For this reason, biopsy is reserved only for those conditions in which a definitive diagnosis would lead to a specific therapy.

Blood Tests ■ By examining the level of certain substances in the blood, one can gauge how effectively the kidney is functioning. The most common tests used in reflecting various aspects of kidney function are

1. Serum creatinine: A simple measure of *glomerulus* filtration rate (GFR).
2. Blood urea nitrogen (BUN): A reflection of the GFR but much cruder.
3. Electrolytes: Sodium (Na^+), potassium (K^+), chloride ($Cl-$), serum bicarbonate (HCO_3^-).
4. Arterial blood gases: The pH of the blood and the arterial PCO_2 are frequent tests used by nephrologists to determine how effectively the kidney is regulating the blood pH.

REPRESENTATIVE DISEASES

Intrinsic Diseases of the Kidney

Glomerular Diseases ■ The glomerulus is the filtering part of the kidney. The glomerulus, when injured, can react in very few ways. There

ABC Radiology Group, Inc.
5400 South C Street
Oxnard, CA 93035-4123

Telephone: 013-430-9877   **Fax: 013-540-8700**

September 29, 1994

Philip S. Brandson, M. D.
3089 Beason Street
Oxnard, CA 93035-4123

Dear Dr. Brandson:

Re: Jennifer L. Chan

Following is the report of the x-ray examination on Mrs. Jennifer L. Chan who was referred to us on September 29, 1994.

INTRAVENOUS UROGRAM:

Preliminary survey films of the abdomen revealed marked bilateral contraction of both kidneys. The right kidney measured 7.8 cm in length as compared to 9.0 cm on the left side. In subsequent films made as the examination progressed, severe bilateral renal parenchymal thinning was noted to be present with a maximum thickness of about 6 mm being present bilaterally. There were no radiopaque urinary tract calculi. Otherwise, the renal and psoas shadows were normal.

Notation is made of a vertically placed liver which extends to the level of the iliac crest. It should be readily palpable.

Following the intravenous administration of 50 cc of Conray 400, films were made with ureteral compression at the five minute and ten minute intervals in the AP and both posterior oblique projections. Because of poor opacification of the collecting systems, an additional 50 cc of Conray 400 was administered and additional films were made with ureteral compression at the ten and fifteen minute intervals in the AP, PA, and both posterior oblique projections. Then, ureteral compression was released, and films were made in the AP and PA projections at twenty minutes and thereafter at twenty-five minutes with the patient upright. The opacified bladder was studied by means of AP, PA, and both oblique projections, followed by an AP view of the bladder region made after micturition.

On this series of films, there was good demonstration of both pyelocalyceal systems, the ureters segmentally, and the bladder shadow.

(continued)

Figure 22–4
Intravenous urogram (IVU) report form, typed in full-block format.

Figure continued

Page 2
Re: Jennifer L. Chan
September 30, 1994

There was moderately severe generalized calycectasis with severe bilateral renal parenchymal thinning. These changes are no doubt the end result of previous infection (pyelonephritis) or pressure atrophy.

Otherwise, both urinary systems were normal.

The opacified bladder was unremarkable; however, on micturition, a small to moderate amount of residual opacified urine remained.

CONCLUSION:

1. Marked atrophy of both kidneys with severe renal parenchymal thinning and moderately severe generalized bilateral calycectasis, findings no doubt the end result of previous infection (pyelonephritis) or pressure atrophy.

2. Diminished renal concentrating ability, moderately severe, secondary to #1.

3. Otherwise normal intravenous urogram except for a small to moderate amount of residua on micturition.

Thank you for referring Mrs. Chan.

Sincerely yours,

Robert M. Gomez, M. D.

mtf

Figure 22–4 *Continued*

can be an increase in the number of cells in the glomerulus, leading to what is called *proliferative glomerulonephritis*.

The filtering surface may become thickened, a condition called *membranous glomerulonephritis*.

The disease may cause both a thickening and an increased number of cells, known as *membranoproliferative glomerulonephritis*.

In addition to injury, the deposition of other substances in the glomerulus may occur in such conditions as diabetes mellitus or amyloidosis. In any event, damage to the glomerulus leads to an increased amount of protein in the urine (proteinuria), which is the hallmark of glomerular disease. Normally, people excrete very little protein in the urine, no more than 150 mg for 24 hours. With glomerular diseases, protein excretion may exceed several grams per day, and it is called a "nephrotic syndrome." The nephrotic syndrome per se is the conglomeration of an increased urinary protein along with a low serum albumin, leading to edema.

The hypoalbuminemia that leads to the edema is not entirely due to losses of protein in the kidney but has to do with the total body catabolism of protein, which is altered in the nephrotic syndrome (Tables 22–1 and 22–2).

A rare type of glomerular disease is called *rapidly progressive glomerulonephritis*. In this disease, the glomerulus is very reactive, and "crescents" are formed between the glomerulus and the tubule. The prognosis of this type of kidney disease is extremely poor (Table 22–3).

Table 22–1 ▪ Causes of Acute Glomerulonephritis

Infectious

Acute poststreptococcal glomerulonephritis
(group A, β-hemolytic streptococcal infection)
Infective endocarditis
Staphylococcal bacteremia
Pneumococcal pneumonia
Meningococcemia
Typhoid fever
Secondary syphilis
Acute viral infection (cytomegalovirus,
Epstein-Barr, hepatitis B, Coxsackie)
Mycoplasma
Trichinosis
Toxoplasmosis
Falciparum malaria

Multisystem Disease

Systemic lupus erythematosus
Mixed connective tissue disease
Rheumatoid arthritis
Henoch-Schönlein purpura
Wegener's granulomatosis
Necrotizing vasculitis
Sjögren's syndrome
Dermatomyositis
Cryoglobulinemia
Amyloidosis (primary and secondary)
Sarcoidosis

Primary Glomerular Disease

IgA nephropathy (Berger's disease)
Mesangial proliferative glomerulonephritis
Membranoproliferative glomerulonephritis

Table 22–2 ▪ Causes of Nephrotic Syndrome

Primary Glomerular Diseases

Minimal change disease (lipoid nephrosis)
Mesangial proliferative glomerulonephritis
Focal and segmental glomerulosclerosis
Membranous glomerulopathy
Membranoproliferative glomerulonephritis
Type I (subendothelial deposits)
Type II (dense deposit disease)
Other types

Multisystem Diseases

Systemic lupus erythematosus
Henoch-Schönlein purpura
Necrotizing vasculitis
Goodpasture's syndrome

Drugs, Toxins, Allergies

Mercury, gold
Penicillamine
Intravenous drugs, e.g., heroin
Probenicid
Captopril

Infectious Diseases

Bacterial
Poststreptococcal glomerulonephritis
Infective endocarditis
"Shunt" nephritis
Syphilis, leprosy, tuberculosis (?)
Viral
Hepatitis B infection
Cytomegalovirus
Epstein-Barr disease
Human immunodeficiency virus
Protozoal
Malaria

Neoplastic

Carcinoma of colon, lung, stomach, breast,
kidney, thyroid, ovary, cervix
Wilms' tumor
Malignant melanoma
Leukemia
Hodgkin's disease
Non-Hodgkin's lymphoma
Multiple myeloma

Miscellaneous

Amyloidosis
Pregnancy-associated (toxemia of pregnancy)
Chronic renal allograft rejection
Malignant nephrosclerosis (essential)

Heredofamilial diseases

Congenital nephrotic syndrome

Systemic Diseases and the Kidney

Diabetes Mellitus ▪ The kidney is involved in many diseases that affect other organs of the body but are not primarily diseases of the kidney. The most common systemic disease affecting the kidney is diabetes mellitus. One of the major complications of diabetes is renal (kidney) failure. Kidney failure occurs in approximately one third of all those with insulin-dependent diabetes and to a lesser extent in the more common type II, or noninsulin-dependent, diabetes. Both of these lead to an increase in proteinuria, resulting in nephrotic syndrome or renal failure. This is probably the most common cause of renal failure in the United States and Western Europe. The five stages of diabetic nephropathy are

Table 22-3 ■ **Causes of Rapidly Progressive Glomerulonephritis**

Idiopathic

Type I: Antiglomerular basement membrane antibody disease
Type II: Immune complex–mediated disease

Multisystem Diseases

Systemic lupus erythematosus
Goodpasture's syndrome
Henoch-Schönlein syndrome
Necrotizing vasculitis (including polyarteritis nodosa and Wegener's granulomatosis)
Cryoimmunoglobulinemia

Infectious Diseases

Poststreptococcal glomerulonephritis
Infectious endocarditis
Sepsis
Hepatitis B infection with vasculitis and/or cryoglobulinemia

Drugs and Toxic Agents

■ Stage I	■ An overworked filter with hyperfiltration
■ Stage II	■ A slightly weak filter with microalbuminuria
■ Stage III	■ A very leaky but still efficient filter with high levels of proteinuria
■ Stage IV	■ An inefficient filter with rise in BUN and creatinine
■ Stage V	■ A filter that has failed with uremia present and excess weight gain due to the accumulation of fluid.

Systemic Lupus Erythematosus Nephritis ■ This disease affects the kidney in many different ways. It can cause an acute proliferative glomerulitis, acute membranoproliferative glomerulonephritis, or pure membranous glomerulonephritis. It can also cause focal sclerosis and various tubular defects. Lupus is most common in women, although it can occur in both sexes and all ages. It is a classic immunologic disease affecting the kidney. In addition, lupus commonly affects joints, skin, heart, and the linings of various organs, such as the lung and the peritoneum. The treatment for lupus glomerulonephritis consists of using corticosteroids in addition to immunosuppressive agents.

The number of systemic diseases that can affect the kidney is extensive; some additional, more common ones include gout, sarcoidosis, amyloidosis, malignancies, and infections.

Acute Renal Failure ■ Acute renal failure is defined as a sudden reduction in renal function due to a severe drop in blood pressure, sepsis or drug-induced injury, or a combination of these. Acute renal failure is usually divided into three groups: prerenal, renal, and postrenal. Prerenal acute renal failure is usually due to losses in the gastrointestinal tract from such causes as vomiting, diarrhea, and severe nasogastric suction. Dehydration, burns, and bleeding also cause prerenal azotemia. Fortunately, most of this does not progress to true acute renal failure (acute tubular necrosis) but is reversible with the restoration of intravascular volume.

True renal failure of the intrinsic renal type can be caused by glomerular diseases, such as rapidly progressive glomerulonephritis, acute postinfectious glomerulonephritis, or that associated with acquired immune deficiency syndrome (AIDS). It can also be due to tubular interstitial disease caused by medications, such as sulfur drugs and some antifungal drugs. Occasionally, it can be due to exposure to certain infections or organic solvents. Acute tubular necrosis is usually associated with severe ischemia, septicemia, or people in a postoperative state. Drugs, like aminoglycosides, contrast agents, and certain antitumor drugs, e.g., cisplatin, can lead to nephrotoxicity. Myoglobin has been reported to cause acute renal failure, as has acute tubular necrosis associated with pregnancy. Acute vasculitis, malignant hypertension, or atheroembolic phenomena also lead to acute renal failure.

Postrenal failure or obstructive uropathy may occur from intratubular obstruction caused by uric acid crystals, obstruction of both ureters due to cancer, retroperitoneal fibrosis, bilateral kidney stones, or papillary necrosis. Obstruction also may be caused by urethral problems, such as benign prostatic hypertrophy or bladder dysfunction that might occur in paraplegics or diabetics. Fortunately, most postrenal or obstructive uropathy is easily reversible by relieving the physical blockage. An example of an inferior vena cavogram (IVC) and renal venogram report is seen in Figure 22–5. A report of a voiding cystogram and cystourethrogram under fluoroscopy is seen in Figure 22–6.

Normal healthy people do not sustain renal injury secondary to nonsteroidal anti-inflammatory agents (NSAIDs). However, when there is heart failure, volume depletion, use of diuretics, hypertension, or diabetes, acute renal failure can

---

St. John's Hospital
2400 Main Street
Anytown, XY 12345-0000

Beatrice K. Hillton
Hosp. No. 543 098759

RADIOLOGICAL CONSULTATION REPORT

2/4/94   INFERIOR VENA CAVOGRAM AND RIGHT RENAL VENOGRAM

After obtaining an informed consent, the right inguinal area was prepped and draped in the usual sterile manner and infiltrated with 1% Xylocaine. Using the Seldinger technique, a red Kifa pigtail catheter was inserted into the inferior vena cava and placed just above the bifurcation into the common iliac veins. Then 40 cc of Reno M76 was injected in two seconds and an inferior vena cavogram obtained. No abnormalities were seen. Contrast material was noted to reflux into the stump of the left renal vein. Following this, the catheter was exchanged for an end-and-side hole, preformed red Kifa catheter and the right renal vein was selectively catheterized and injected with 14 cc in two seconds' time. Again no filling defects or other abnormalities were noted.

Following this, the catheter was removed, and pressure was applied to the right groin until hemostasis was assured. A total of 179 cc of contrast material was used during the exam. The patient was returned to her room in good condition.

IMPRESSION:

1. Negative inferior vena cavogram with evidence of reflux of contrast material into the stump of the left renal vein.

2. Negative right renal venogram with no evidence of thrombus formation.

                                        _____
                                        Clement B. Owens, M. D.
                                        Chief Radiologist

mtf

Figure 22–5
Report form for inferior vena cavogram (IVC) and renal venogram, typed in full-block format.

St. John's Hospital
2400 Main Street
Anytown, XY 12345-0000

Beatrice K. Hillton
Hosp. No. 543 098759

RADIOLOGICAL CONSULTATION REPORT

9/12/94   VOIDING CYSTOGRAM

The preliminary scout film reveals multiple metallic clips overlying the right pelvis. There is a catheter placed within the bladder. The osseous structures and abdominal gas pattern are unremarkable.

Then 300 cc of Cystografin were introduced in a retrograde manner into the bladder. The bladder was shown to be normally distensible. On the micturition film, there was reflux into the left ureter. There is also reflux into the right ileocecal ureter. There was no contrast seen within the right kidney.

CONCLUSION:

1. Reflux of contrast into right ileocecal ureter and left ureter.
2. Marked residual urine.

9/13/94   VOIDING CYSTOURETHROGRAM UNDER FLUOROSCOPY

As compared to previous study of 9/12/94.

Preliminary scout film again reveals multiple metallic clips overlying the right iliac crest. Abdominal gas pattern and osseous structures remain unremarkable.

Then 250 cc of Cystografin were introduced in a retrograde manner into the bladder. Multiple fluoroscopic spot films were taken at various angles of obliquity.

The bladder was normally distensible. There is noted reflux of contrast into the right ileocecal ureter. No contrast was seen within the right kidney.

CONCLUSION:

1. Reflux of contrast into right ileocecal ureter; no contrast seen within right kidney.

_____
Clement B. Owens, M. D.
Chief Radiologist

mtf

Figure 22–6
Report form for voiding cystogram and cystourethrogram under fluoroscopy, typed in full-block format.

develop upon institution of these agents (Table 22–4).

Chronic Renal Failure ▪ This slow, insidious decrease in renal function leads eventually to hemodialysis, peritoneal dialysis, or kidney transplantation. The most common causes of chronic renal failure are those discussed already, such as diabetes mellitus, membranoproliferative glomerulonephritis, systemic lupus erythematosus, severe systemic hypertension, or a congenital hereditary defect such as polycystic kidneys.

Most people with chronic renal failure have some combination of high blood pressure, swelling, nausea, vomiting, anemia, or bone disease. The presence of this combination of symptoms is called uremia (Figure 22–7).

RENAL REPLACEMENT THERAPY

Renal replacement therapy can be accomplished by either kidney transplantation or dialysis. Hemodialysis means using the blood vessel as access to the blood supply: the blood actually leaves the body through a series of tubes, passes through a machine where it is filtered and purified, and returns to the circulation (Figure 22–8). Peritoneal dialysis utilizes fluid introduced into the abdominal cavity: the waste diffuses into the fluid (Figure 22–9). The fluids are removed and new fluids are introduced and recirculated. Both these types of dialyses are effective, have their pros and cons, and are lifesaving procedures. Transplantation of the kidney has been quite successful in the past 40 years and is the preferred means of restoring kidney function, if at all possible. However, there are advantages, disadvantages, and complications with kidney transplantation, just as there are using various dialysis modalities. An example of a discharge summary report of a patient with chronic renal disease with uremia is seen in Figure 22–10. A dialysis review report is given in Figure 22–11.

CONGENITAL ABNORMALITIES OF THE KIDNEY

Many people are born with diseases of the kidney. The most common, agenesis, is the nonformation of one or both of the kidneys. If both

Table 22–4 ▪ Major Causes of Acute Renal Failure

1. Prerenal azotemia due to either hypovolemia (e.g., fluid and electrolyte depletion, hemorrhage) or decreased effective blood volume (heart failure, pericarditis, hypoalbuminuria)

2. Acute tubular necrosis or acute cortical necrosis due to shock

3. Miscellaneous
   Toxins (carbon tetrachloride, toluene, heavy metals, certain antibiotics, anesthetics, and radiographic contrast media)
   Intravascular hemolysis (e.g., mismatched transfusion)
   Myoglobinuria (e.g., crush injuries, prolonged seizures)
   Burns
   Premature separation of the placenta
   Acute glomerulitis and vasculitis (e.g., glomerulonephritis, lupus erythematosus nephritis, periarteritis, Goodpasture's syndrome, RPGN (rapidly progressive glomerulonephritis)
   Acute interstitial nephritis (e.g., severe diffuse pyelonephritis, papillary necrosis, drug-induced nephritis)
   Severe hypercalcemia
   Renal emboli
   Hepatorenal syndrome

kidneys are not formed, the patient dies within a few days of birth. People born with only one normally formed kidney and one nonformed kidney can live all their lives without being aware of the abnormality.

People can also be born with ectopic kidneys that are normal but are in an abnormal location, usually low down in the pelvis.

Horseshoe kidney is a common type of congenital abnormality; both kidneys are fused at the bottom and, therefore, look like a horseshoe. Horseshoe kidneys are compatible with normal life; however, because of the abnormal positioning, sometimes an abnormality of the ureters' draining of the kidney occurs. Because of this, infection or blockages are common.

Hereditary Nephritis ▪ Many diseases of the kidney are inherited, including polycystic kidneys and medullary sponge kidneys. These two conditions may not be obvious at birth but

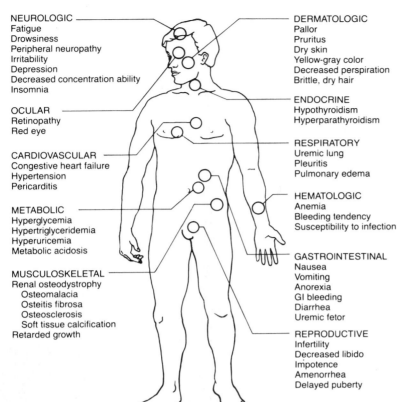

NEUROLOGIC
Fatigue
Drowsiness
Peripheral neuropathy
Irritability
Depression
Decreased concentration ability
Insomnia

OCULAR
Retinopathy
Red eye

CARDIOVASCULAR
Congestive heart failure
Hypertension
Pericarditis

METABOLIC
Hyperglycemia
Hypertriglyceridemia
Hyperuricemia
Metabolic acidosis

MUSCULOSKELETAL
Renal osteodystrophy
   Osteomalacia
   Osteitis fibrosa
   Osteosclerosis
   Soft tissue calcification
Retarded growth

DERMATOLOGIC
Pallor
Pruritus
Dry skin
Yellow-gray color
Decreased perspiration
Brittle, dry hair

ENDOCRINE
Hypothyroidism
Hyperparathyroidism

RESPIRATORY
Uremic lung
Pleuritis
Pulmonary edema

HEMATOLOGIC
Anemia
Bleeding tendency
Susceptibility to infection

GASTROINTESTINAL
Nausea
Vomiting
Anorexia
GI bleeding
Diarrhea
Uremic fetor

REPRODUCTIVE
Infertility
Decreased libido
Impotence
Amenorrhea
Delayed puberty

Figure 22–7
Systemic effects of uremia. (From Miller, Benjamin E., and Claire B. Keane (eds). *Encyclopedia and Dictionary of Medicine, Nursing, and Allied Health,* 5th ed. W. B. Saunders Co., Philadelphia, 1992.)

may develop in later years. Polycystic kidneys is a hereditary form of disease in which multiple cysts form in the kidney and eventually cause problems, such as hypertension or kidney failure. Sometimes these kidneys get so large that they cause massive distention of the abdomen. Transplantation has been very successful in this type of kidney disease. Medullary sponge kidneys is a common disease that is usually quite benign in course and leads only to occasional formation of stones and inability to concentrate the urine. Otherwise, it rarely leads to kidney failure or other serious problems.

Pyelonephritis ▪ Pyelonephritis is an infectious disease of the kidneys most frequently occurring in the presence of some anatomic defect, such as an abnormal ureter, a block in the ureter, or some reason to cause reflux from the bladder back into the kidney. Pyelonephritis is very common. It is most common in women and is usually treatable with antibiotics. Rarely, if ever, does infectious pyelonephritis progress to chronic kidney disease in the absence of obstruction or some other physical anatomic abnormality.

Interstitial Nephritis ▪ This disease of the kidney involves primarily the tubular area of the kidney or the medulla. There are two types of interstitial nephritis, acute and chronic; although some pathologic differences exist between them, the separation is made largely on clinical grounds. The causes of acute and chronic interstitial nephritis are outlined in Table 22–5.

SIGNS AND SYMPTOMS

Patients with renal disease may have no signs or symptoms with chronic and slowly developing diseases, or they may have a sudden onset of

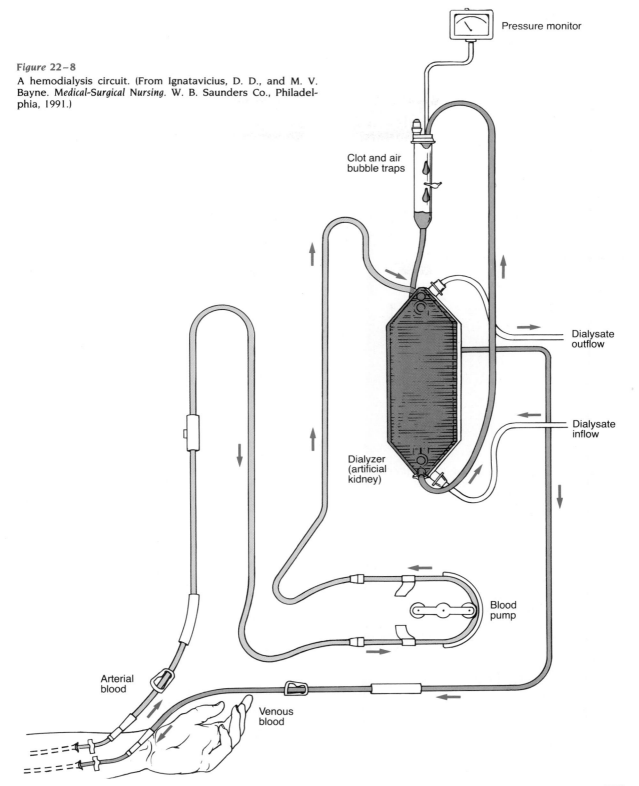

Pressure monitor

Clot and air
bubble traps

Dialysate
outflow

Dialysate
inflow

Dialyzer
(artificial
kidney)

Blood
pump

Arterial
blood

Venous
blood

Figure 22–8
A hemodialysis circuit. (From Ignatavicius, D. D., and M. V.
Bayne. Medical-Surgical Nursing. W. B. Saunders Co., Philadel-
phia, 1991.)

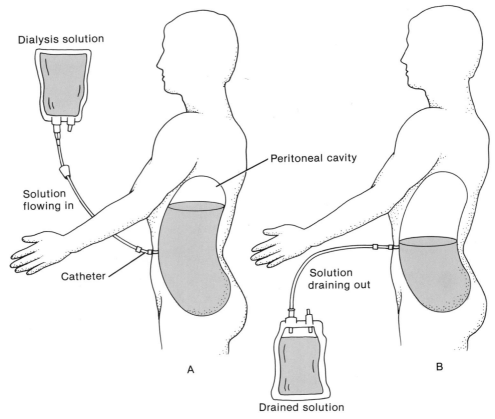

Figure 22-9
Continuous ambulatory peritoneal dialysis (CAPD). A, The dialysis solution (dialysate) flows from a collapsible plastic bag through a catheter into the patient's peritoneal cavity. The empty bag is folded and inserted into undergarments. B, After 4 to 8 hours, the bag is unfolded, and the fluid is allowed to drain into it by gravity. The full bag is discarded, and a new bag of fresh dialysate is attached. (From Chabner, D. E. *Medical Terminology: A Short Course*. W. B. Saunders Co., Philadelphia, 1990.)

inability to urinate, may pass blood in the urine, or may void "cola-colored" urine typical of acute glomerulonephritis. They may present with swelling of the total body or just of the lower extremities. Weakness, nausea, vomiting, fatigue, and getting up at night to urinate are other symptoms. The urine is usually low in volume (oliguria); this occurs more often in children. The type of kidney disease and the stage to which it has progressed determine the symptoms.

Symptoms of nephrotic syndrome may be total body swelling or swelling starting in the legs and progressing to the rest of the body.

Patients with acute pyelonephritis of the infectious type may experience chills, fever, back pain, frequency of urination, and burning upon urination.

Patients with cystitis or a bladder infection may present with urgency (the urge to urinate), frequency (frequent small amounts of urination), pain, or blood upon urination.

Patients with slow, progressive renal disease may have no symptoms until they notice they are getting up more often at night to urinate as the ability of the kidney to concentrate urine diminishes. There may be a change in appetite, with dislike of red meat. The patient may begin to select lighter meats, such as chicken, and finally become a vegetarian. This is because protein in meats contains amino acids, which, when broken down, release other acids, making the

Text continued on page 389

COMMUNITY HOSPITAL
2813 Central Avenue
Philadelphia, PA 19006-0000

DISCHARGE SUMMARY

NAME: Santini, Robert F.
PHYSICIAN: Avery P. Shragg, M. D.

MEDICAL RECORD #450985
DATE OF ADMISSION: 9/20/94
DATE OF DISCHARGE: 9/27/94

HISTORY:
This 77-year-old male was admitted to the hospital because of generalized weakness, fatigue, nausea, and anorexia of several weeks' duration.

For further details, please refer to the admission note and to the cardiology consultation.

PHYSICAL EXAMINATION:
Please refer to the admission note and to the cardiology consultation.

LABORATORY:
Hgb 14.9; hct 44.4; WBC 7.7. Followup on 9/22/94: hgb 13.1; hct 39.4; WBC 8.9; sedimentation rate 8; platelets 105; PT 12.6; PTT 53; repeat 41; bleeding type 3.5.

Urinalysis: WBC more than 200, RBC 10-20, trace protein, specific gravity 1.010. Followup of urinalysis revealed a WBC of only 5-10 and RBCs 50-100, trace protein. Urine eosinophils: None seen. Repeat urinalysis: WBC 5-10; RBC 10-20, negative casts, negative bacteria, specific gravity 1.009.

Serum sodium 130, potassium 4.7, chloride 89, CO_2 15, BUN 276, creatinine 9.1; blood sugar 160; calcium 11; magnesium 2.8; phosphorus 11.8. Followup chem-7 on 9/23/94: glucose 85; sodium 140; potassium 4.7; chloride 98; CO_2 21.9; BUN 107; creatinine 5.7. Repeat calcium 10.8-10.9 with magnesium of 2.5; phosphorus 9.1. CPK was 3971, followup on 9/24/94 2780, and on 9/25/94 was 727. CPK-MB band 245, 203, 81 respectively. B12 level 657; RBC folate 193. Prostate specific antigen 1.6. Hepatitis panel nonreactive. ANA nonreactive.

Serum protein electrophoresis normal. IgA 271; C3 46.4; C4 14.6; total complement 64 (all complement levels were reduced).

Urine for culture unremarkable with no organisms seen and colony count less than 1,000/ml. Albumin 3.6; globulin 2.2; uric acid 4.1; alkaline phosphatase 81; LDH 344; SGOT 128; SGPT 32; total bilirubin 0.9.

Echocardiogram showed cardiomyopathy with severe left ventricular hypokinesis and marked left ventricular enlargement. Renal ultrasound showed dense renal parenchyma bilaterally consistent with chronic renal failure associated with a (continued)

Page 2
Santini, Robert F.
Medical Record #450985

decreased renal sinus bilaterally. Right kidney measures only 6.8 cm in length and on the left 6.5 cm. There were multiple renal cysts seen. There is some mild hydronephrosis on the right.

Chest consistent with atherosclerosis with probable granulomatous disease and bibasilar scarring or atelectasis. EKG: Normal sinus rhythm with frequent premature ventricular complexes and left bundle branch block. Possible old apical myocardial infarction. Old anteroseptal myocardial infarction.

HOSPITAL COURSE:
The patient was admitted to the hospital because of severe uremia with a creatinine of 9.1 and a BUN of 276. Dual-lumen hemodialysis cathether was inserted and was used as an access for acute hemodialysis therapy. The patient was given Mannitol during dialysis therapy to prevent dysequilibrium syndrome and/or seizures. The patient tolerated the dialysis well. Later on a workup for the advanced renal failure was conducted. Results are as stated on Page 1.

During his hospitalization, he was found to have multiple PVCs. Cardiology consultation was obtained. The patient was seen by Dr. Val Brown who felt that the ventricular arrhythmias may not require any treatment as long as it is asymptomatic.

The patient was maintained on the hemodialysis therapy. During the workup, he was found to have bilateral small extremely echogenic kidneys consistent with chronic renal failure and probably end-stage kidney disease. The etiology of his renal failure is not known, but this could be related to nephrosclerosis with or without diabetic nephropathy. It should be noted that in patients with diabetic nephropathy, both kidneys are large; but this is in the early stage of diabetes mellitus. It is possible this patient has a long history of underlying diabetic neuropathy with nephrosclerosis and over the years he has developed more nephrosclerosis with scarring and shrunk kidneys. The low complement may be related to a nutritional factor and under production by the liver. It may not be related to any active glomerulopathy. His sedimentation is normal. Serum protein electrophoresis was normal. A bone scan was done which did not show any specific metastatic lesions. Instead it showed some abnormal increased activities on the anterior rib ends and the mid left thorax probably consistent with old trauma and also increased activity, lateral aspect, mid left rib and increased activity of the left wrist presumably artificial.

General condition of the patient gradually improved. His urinalysis showed gradual resolution of the WBC and RBC. Urine culture was normal. The patient was supported with dialysis therapy during his hospitalization. The BUN this morning was 151 and creatinine of 7.4. He was dialyzed for 3-1/2 hours.
(continued)

Figure 22–10 Continued

Page 3
Santini, Robert F.
Medical Record #450985

DISPOSITION:
He will be discharged home with the dual-lumen hemodialysis in place which will be used as an access for hemodialysis therapy on an outpatient basis. Next week he will be seen by the vascular surgeon, Dr. Hu Ti. An arterial venous Gore-Tex graft will be placed (both the patient and his daughter preferred early discharge to think about the surgery and to be reassessed by the vascular surgeon). The plan at this time is to discharge the patient home and keep the dual-lumen hemodialysis catheter in place. Following the vascular surgery evaluation, he will be admitted as a Same Day Surgery. The dual-lumen hemodialysis catheter will be replaced. A new arterial venous Gore-Tex graft will be placed as per Dr. Hu Ti.

DISCHARGE MEDICATIONS:
Phos-Lo 667 mg po t.i.d.; Reglan 5 mg 1/2 hour prior to meals t.i.d.; Zantac 150 mg po every hs.; multivitamins one tablet po every p.m.; folic acid 1 mg po every a.m.; nitroglycerin 0.4 mg sublingual p.r.n. chest pain; Mexitil 150 mg po b.i.d.

FOLLOWUP:
To be dialyzed on an outpatient basis.

FINAL DIAGNOSIS:
1. Severe advanced chronic renal disease with uremia. The cause of the renal failure is probably secondary to long-standing diabetic nephropathy and nephrosclerosis.
2. Diabetes mellitus, type II.
3. Mild anemia secondary to chronic renal failure.
4. Arteriosclerotic heart disease with cardiac arrhythmias (ischemic cardiomyopathy with left ventricular hypokinesis).
5. History of gout, probable.
6. Severe nausea and recurrent vomiting and some epigastric pains probably related to uremia (resolving).
7. Past history of cholecystectomy.
8. Past history of appendectomy.
9. Past history of transurethral resection of prostate.
10. Status post traumatic injury of left eye, status post artificial eye in place.
11. Probable advanced cataract, right eye.

_____
Avery P. Shragg, M. D.

mtf
D: 9/27/94
T: 9/28/94

Figure 22–10 *Continued*

COMMUNITY HOSPITAL
2813 Central Avenue
Philadelphia, PA 19006-0000

NAME: Helpman, Esme T.
Medical Record #300985

DIALYSIS REVIEW - MONTH OF OCTOBER, 1994

Ms. Esme T. Helpman runs on an EX 29, 2K bath, 3 hours, 3 times a week. Her pre-dialysis weights have increased to 212 with post-dialysis weights of 207. Despite the weight gain, she only shows minimal edema and no evidence of congestive failure. We have discussed the necessity for possibly increasing the length of her runs to insure adequate ultrafiltration. Her pre-dialysis BUN is 56 with a creatinine of 16 and a potassium of 4.6.

Her hematocrit has slipped to 18 and she receives no androgen therapy.

Her pre-dialysis calcium is 8.1 with a phosphorous of 5.5 and an alkaline phosphatase mildly elevated at 197. Her albumin is mildly decreased at 3.2.

She remains antigen positive with her enzymes being normal and her lipids being normal.

This month the patient's weight gains were somewhat excessive because her diarrhea has apparently ceased. She remains on the same Cephulac dose, however. In addition, she has had a marked improvement in her bladder spasms subsequent to the bladder irrigation she is having.

The patient continues on 0.4 mg of Synthroid with a T_4 to be repeated this month. She does not appear to be thyrotoxic on this current dose. Aside from the above-mentioned problems, this has been an uneventful month.

                                        Everett B. Blake, M. D.

mtf
D: 10/16/94
T: 10/16/94

Figure 22–11
Dialysis review report form, typed in full-block format.

Table 22–5 ▪ Causes of Interstitial Nephritis

Acute

Hypersensitivity to drugs (methicillin, penicillin, phenindione, sulfonamides, nonsteroidal anti-inflammatory agents)
Infection (pyelonephritis)
Radiation nephritis

Chronic

Analgesic abuse (phenacetin, usually combined with aspirin)
Metabolic abnormalities (hypercalcemia, hypokalemia, hyperuricemia, oxalate nephropathy)
Immunology (transplant rejection, Sjögren's syndrome)
Obstructive uropathy; vesicoureteric reflux
Nephrolithiasis
Hereditary nephritis
Vascular (arteriolar nephrosclerosis, S-hemoglobinemia)
Neoplastic infiltrates—lymphoma, leukemia, myeloma
Nephrotoxins—lead, cadmium, methoxyflurane
Radiation nephritis
Infection (pyelonephritis)
Idiopathic

blood very acid, thereby causing symptoms and other problems. This trend may progress to total loss of appetite, nausea, vomiting, and even diarrhea, along with swelling, headaches, and fatigue.

Hypertension usually causes no symptoms unless it is of the malignant type, in which case blurry vision and headaches can occur.

People with conditions like diabetes and chronic glomerulonephritis may notice no symptoms until they progress to chronic renal failure or end-stage renal failure and develop a condition called "uremia." This symptom complex consists of nausea, vomiting, diarrhea, weakness, and itching associated with very poor kidney function.

TREATMENT OF RENAL DISEASE

Aside from the treatment of chronic renal failure with dialysis or transplants, many diseases of the kidney can be treated in the early stages with limitation or modification of salt, protein, and potassium intake.

Drugs to control high blood pressure are numerous and fall into many categories. Diuretics control fluid retention. These drug categories and diuretics are shown in Table 22–6.

Infectious complications of renal disease or pyelonephritis may be treated with antibiotics, although often the dose of antibiotics as well as other medications must be modified depending on the degree of renal function. This is true because many drugs are excreted in the urine;

Table 22–6 ▪ Antihypertensive Drugs

Diuretics

Chlorthalidone
Hydrochlorothiazide
Furosemide
Spironolactone
Triamterene
Metolazone

ACE* Inhibitors

Captopril
Enalapril

β-Blockers

Propranolol
Nadolol
Metroprolol
Atenolol
Pindolol
Labetalol

Sympatholytics

Alpha-methyldopa
Reserpine
Clonidine
Prazosin

Calcium Channel Blockers

Nifedipine
Verapamil
Diltiazem

Direct Arteriolar Vasodilators

Hydralazine
Minoxidil

*Angiotensin-converting enzyme.

when the kidneys are not able to excrete the drug, they build up in the system and cause toxicity.

The regulation of the body's sodium content as well as the concentration of sodium in the blood becomes the responsibility of the nephrologist. This is true of most of the body's salts, including potassium, calcium, phosphorus, and magnesium. The terms "hypo-," meaning *under,* and "hyper-," meaning *over,* apply to many minerals or so-called ions.

The conditions of hyponatremia and hypernatremia exist when the serum concentration of sodium is too low or too high. This is usually due to an excess or deficiency of water that dilutes or concentrates the sodium in the blood.

An excess of total body sodium results in edema, and a deficiency of total body sodium leads to dehydration.

Hypokalemia and hyperkalemia refer to a decreased or increased concentration of potassium in the body. Since most potassium is either excreted or retained by the kidney, an elevated serum potassium usually means a disorder of the kidney.

Hypocalcemia and hypercalcemia are conditions that are regulated by the kidney but also include the parathyroid glands and vitamin D metabolism. Hypophosphatemia and hyperphosphatemia are conditions intimately related with calcium and metabolism and are also regulated by the kidney. These are very common conditions encountered in the field of nephrology.

Acid-Base Disturbances ▪ The body carefully regulates the degree of acidity of the blood and the tissues. All enzymes in our body work within a very narrow range of acidity or alkalinity. The ability to regulate the acid condition of our system minute-to-minute, as well as the long-term acid-base milieu, falls to a very complex relationship between the kidneys and the lungs. Acid-base disturbances can be grouped into two major types: acidosis and alkalosis.

In acidosis, too much acid is produced in the body, leading to an acid condition in the blood called acidemia. The causes of this are listed in Table 22–7. When too much acid is lost from the body or too much alkali is added to the body, the condition is known as alkalosis. The causes of metabolic alkalosis are also listed in Table 22–7.

Table 22–7 ▪ Causes of Acid-Base Disturbances

Causes of Acidemia

"Anion GAP" metabolic acidosis
    Ketosis (diabetes mellitus, alcohol, starvation)
    Renal failure
    Drugs: methanol, paraldehyde, ethylene glycol, salicylates
    Lactic acidosis
Hyperchloremic metabolic acidosis
    Diarrhea
    Drugs: acetazolamide
    Urinary diversion
    Renal disease (renal tubular acidosis [RTA])

Causes of Alkalosis

Chloride depletion
    Gastric losses: vomiting, mechanical drainage, bulimia
    Drugs (thiazides, furosemide, ethacrynic acid)
    Diarrheal states
    Posthypercapnic states
Mineralocorticoid excess
    Primary aldosteronism
    Cushing's syndrome
    Secondary aldosteronism
        Adrenal corticosteroid excess
        Renin-secreting tumors
        Renovascular hypertension
    Drugs: licorice, carbenoxolone, hydrocortisone
Excess intake of bicarbonate
Other
    Antibiotics: carbenicillin
    Laxative abuse
    Bartter's syndrome
    Hypercalcemia
    Severe hypoalbuminemia (nephrotic syndrome)

Reference Sources

Brenner, Barry M., and Floyd C. Rector, Jr. *The Kidney.* W. B. Saunders Company, Philadelphia, 1990.

Massry, Shaul, and Richard Glassock. *Textbook of Nephrology.* Williams and Wilkins, Baltimore, Maryland, 1989.

Maxwell, Morton, Charles Kleeman, and Robert Narins. *Clinical Disorders of Fluid and Electrolyte Metabolism.* McGraw-Hill Book Company, New York, 1987.

For references of specific application to medical transcription, see Appendix 1.

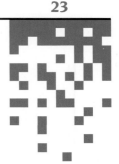

Neurology and Neurosurgery

INTRODUCTION

Neurology and neurosurgery are the medical specialties that diagnose and treat disorders of the central, peripheral, and autonomic nervous systems. The nervous system is responsible for keeping an individual aware of the internal and external environments on a conscious and subconscious level. Further, it integrates all assimilated information and directs the responses to it. The nervous system, after all, is the world's most sophisticated computer.

Adjuncts to the neurologic specialties include a vast armamentarium of diagnostic procedures; the principal ones are outlined in this chapter. Also included are a brief description of common neurologic diseases and therapeutic interventions and sample consultation letters and operative notes.

A glossary of commonly used terms concludes the chapter.

ANATOMY

The nervous system is divided into three principal divisions: central, peripheral, and autonomic. The component parts do not function independently but as a coordinated unit.

Central Nervous System

This includes the brain and spinal cord.

Brain ▪ The brain is compartmentalized into two cerebral hemispheres, the cerebellum, and the brain stem. The hemispheres are demarcated into frontal, parietal, occipital, and temporal lobes (Figure 23–1). The lobe functions are described in a gross overview:

Frontal Lobe ▪ Voluntary muscle movements, elocution, symbolic communication (dominant side), sphincter control, intellect, behavior, and memory. Muscle groups on the left side of the body are controlled by the right side of the brain.

Parietal Lobe ▪ Symbolic communication and calculation (dominant); sensation in all modalities, such as touch, position, pain, and temperature; intellect; memory; and spatial orientation (nondominant).

Occipital Lobe ▪ Vision.

Temporal Lobe ▪ Symbolic communication, hearing, memory, and emotions. The cerebellum, brain stem, and accompanying cranial nerves have many discrete parts.

Thalamus ▪ Sensory information relay station.

Hypothalamus ▪ The endocrine or hormonal control station. Emotional control, memory, and control station for autonomic nervous system.

Midbrain ▪ Origin of the 3rd and 4th cranial nerves. Partially houses the reticular formation, the biologic alarm clock. Portions of all the fundamental sensory and motor (action) nerve pathways are contained herein (Figure 23–2).

Pons ▪ Origin of the 5th cranial nerve. Portions of most of the core sensory and motor nerve pathways. Crucial cardiorespiratory station.

391

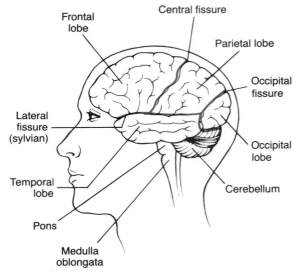

Figure 23–1

Lobes of the cerebral hemispheres. (From A *Primer of Brain Tumors*, 3rd ed. American Brain Tumor Association, formerly Association for Brain Tumor Research, Chicago, 1991.)

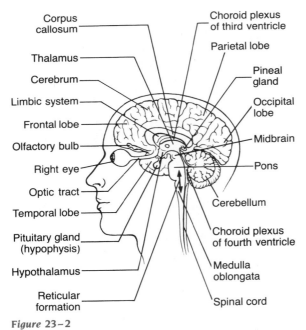

Figure 23–2

Cross-section of the brain. (From A *Primer of Brain Tumors*, 3rd ed. American Brain Tumor Association, formerly Association for Brain Tumor Research, Chicago, 1991.)

Medulla ▪ Origin of the 6th, 7th, 8th, 9th, 10th, 11th, and 12th cranial nerves. Parts of most of the main sensory and motor nerve pathways. Critical cardiorespiratory station locus.

Cerebellum ▪ Principally concerned with balance and coordination.

Cranial nerves ▪

▪ Olfactory (I)	Olfaction, taste
▪ Optic (II)	Vision
▪ Oculomotor (III)	Eye movement
▪ Trochlear (IV)	Eye movement
▪ Trigeminal (V)	Facial sensation, mastication
▪ Abducens (VI)	Eye movement
▪ Facial (VII)	Facial movement, taste
▪ Vestibulocochlear (VIII)	Hearing
▪ Glossopharyngeal (IX)	Gag, taste
▪ Vagus (X)	Heart, intestines
▪ Spinal accessory (XI)	Neck muscles
▪ Hypoglossal (XII)	Tongue movement

Spinal Cord ▪ The spinal cord is divided into cervical, thoracic, lumbar, and sacral segments (Figure 23–3). As a result of differential growth of the spinal cord and spinal column during gestation, the spinal cord does *not* occupy the entire length of the spinal column. The spinal cord terminates in the conus medullaris, usually opposite the 1st lumbar vertebral body. Nerve roots leave the spinal cord from the front (ventral) and enter from the back (dorsal) (Figure 23–4).

The ventral roots are primarily motor (efferent). The dorsal roots are primarily sensory (afferent). The intermediolateral column of the spinal cord is a principal component of the sympathetic nervous system. A major portion of the parasympathetic nervous system is contained within the sacral or lower portion of the spinal cord. The spinal cord functions as the major conduit for information going into and out of the brain. Reflex arcs (e.g., the knee jerk) are also contained within the spinal cord. Portions of most of the primary sensory and motor nervous pathways are found in the spinal cord.

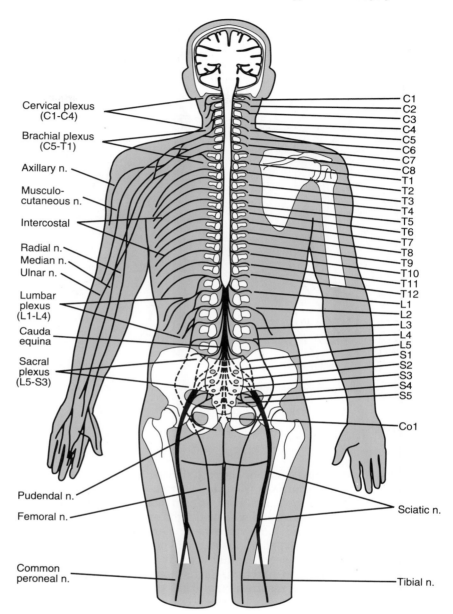

Figure 23–3
The nervous system.

Peripheral Nervous System

This includes all noncranial nerves that supply the body. Peripheral nerves supply sensation and control muscle function throughout the body. The median, ulnar, and radial nerves are examples of peripheral nerves. Peripheral nerves frequently carry components of the autonomic nervous system.

Autonomic Nervous System

This includes the sympathetic and parasympathetic nervous systems. The sympathetic ner-

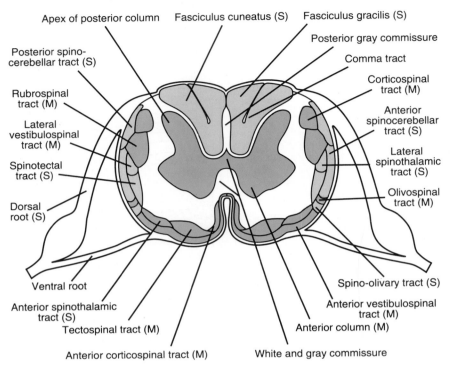

POSTERIOR

Apex of posterior column Fasciculus cuneatus (S) Fasciculus gracilis (S)

Posterior spino-
cerebellar tract (S)

Posterior gray commissure

Comma tract

Corticospinal
tract (M)

Rubrospinal
tract (M)

Anterior
spinocerebellar
tract (S)

Lateral
vestibulospinal
tract (M)

Lateral
spinothalamic
tract (S)

Spinotectal
tract (S)

Olivospinal
tract (M)

Dorsal
root (S)

Ventral root

Spino-olivary tract (S)

Anterior spinothalamic
tract (S)

Anterior vestibulospinal
tract (M)

Tectospinal tract (M)

Anterior column (M)

Anterior corticospinal tract (M)

White and gray commissure

ANTERIOR

S=sensory
M=motor

Figure 23–4
Representative section through
the spinal cord.

vous system originates in the hypothalamus, with significant contributions from the intermediolateral columns of the spinal cord. It controls blood pressure, heart rate, and so-called fight or flight mechanisms. The parasympathetic nervous system has its principal origins in the hypothalamus, medulla, and sacral spinal cord. It is involved in most visceral functions (e.g., intestinal motility, heart rate, respiration, and gastrointestinal secretion).

REPRESENTATIVE DISEASES

Some of the more common neurologic diseases will be briefly described. A more complete rendering of this subject can be found in *Diseases of the Nervous System* by Asbury, McKhann, and McDonald and *Neurosurgery* by Wilkins and Rengachary.

Cerebrovascular Disease

The largest percentage of patients seen by neurologists have cerebrovascular disease. The brain and spinal cord do not store nutrients and are quite sensitive to any interruption in the blood flow that supplies them. Obstruction to the flow of blood to the brain or spinal cord is most commonly due to emboli, which are particulate collections of clotted material, becoming lodged in small blood vessels. This causes neurologic dysfunction of the tissue that depends on the blocked vessel. The type of dysfunction is appropriate to the given area of the nervous system, usually the brain. For example, a clot in the area involved with speech causes difficulty in either understanding or producing speech. This category of symptoms is referred to as aphasia. Symptoms of cerebrovascular disease generally come on suddenly and reach their full extent of severity quickly, within minutes. Sometimes the deficits produced are transient and completely resolve within 24 hours. Such an event is referred to as a *transient ischemic attack*. If the event lasts longer than 24 hours, it is referred to as a stroke. Changes seen on computed tomography (CT) or magnetic resonance imaging (MRI) support the clinical diagnostic impression.

Demyelinating Disease

This class of disease affects the covering surrounding nerve processes, resulting in abnormal electrical conduction. The best-known example of this type of disease is multiple sclerosis. The diagnosis is based on the observation of neurologic deficits separated by site in the central nervous system and time in occurrence. Generally each attack is marked by some recovery although usually not to the premorbid level. Supporting studies include MRI, spinal fluid analysis, and visual evoked responses.

Peripheral Neuropathy

Diseases of the peripheral nerves fall into this category. Although certain diseases affect the peripheral nerves primarily, many systemic diseases affect the peripheral nervous system secondarily. Diabetes mellitus is the leading cause of peripheral neuropathy in the United States, whereas leprosy is one of the more common causes worldwide. Polyneuropathy generally produces symptoms involving the distal aspects (farthest from the body) of the extremities, depriving areas of sensation, motor function, or both. Involvement of the extremities may be symmetric or asymmetric. Electromyography and nerve conduction studies are useful in diagnosing and defining peripheral neuropathies.

Brain Tumors and Spinal Cord Tumors

The most common brain tumors are metastases (representing distant spread from underlying tumors—breast or lung). Of the primary brain tumors, there are benign and malignant brain neoplasms. Within the context of malig-

nant tumors, there are varying degrees of tumor aggressiveness. Tumors may destroy brain tissue or compress it. The symptoms produced will depend on which areas of the brain are affected. The most common malignant tumors are presumably derived from glial cells and are referred to as gliomas, more specifically astrocytomas, oligodendrogliomas, and ependymomas. Glial cells are the so-called supporting cells of the central nervous system. The most frequently occurring benign brain tumor is the meningioma. This type of lesion arises from the meninges or coverings of the brain. Meningiomas are distinctly more common in women and have a tendency to recur after removal. Brain tumors are suspected clinically and confirmed by computed tomography or magnetic resonance imaging.

Spinal cord tumors are distinctly less common than brain tumors in roughly a 1 to 10 proportion; most are benign. The tumor may arise within the spinal cord (e.g., gliomas) or originate in the covering of the spinal cord (e.g., meningiomas). The most common tumors that affect the spinal cord originate in the spinal column and compress the cord. The most common tumor type in this category is a metastasis from an underlying tumor. The common diagnostic tools employed in the diagnosis of spinal cord tumors include computed tomography, magnetic resonance imaging, and myelography.

Vascular Malformations and Aneurysms

Vascular malformations represent abnormal collections of blood vessels. In this category are found arteriovenous malformations, cavernous hemangiomas, telangiectases, and venous angiomas. Of these, arteriovenous malformations and cavernous hemangiomas are the most likely to cause problems, such as intracranial hemorrhage, seizures, and focal or discrete neurologic deficits. Diagnosis is made by magnetic resonance imaging, computed tomography, and arteriography. Surgical therapy may be required once these lesions become apparent. Aneurysms represent a weakening in the wall of a blood vessel, predisposing it to bleeding. Bleeding results in a subarachnoid hemorrhage that may be fatal or manifest only as a headache, with all intermediate points, including a stroke, being possible. Diagnosis of the hemorrhage is made by computed tomography. Arteriography is used to document the presence of an aneurysm and define its vascular anatomy. Surgery is generally required to repair the aneurysm after bleeding has occurred, since there is a strong tendency to rebleed.

Degenerative Disk Disease

This represents one of the most common problems dealt with by neurologists and neurosurgeons. The intervertebral disk separates most of the vertebral bony segments and has a close anatomic relationship with the spinal nerves and spinal cord. Anatomic aberrations (e.g., herniated disk) may produce nerve root compression, causing arm, trunk, or leg pain. Treatment may consist of bed rest, use of nonsteroidal antiinflammatory agents, and/or surgical decompression.

NEUROLOGIC SIGNS AND SYMPTOMS

Neurologic dysfunction may occur primarily or in conjunction with many systemic diseases. Cognitive functions, such as reasoning and memory, may be impaired with dementia of the Alzheimer's type. Involvement of portions of the dominant hemisphere may produce an aphasia or disorder of symbolic communication. This category includes difficulties with calculation. Involvement of the midline cortical structures may produce seizures, which may be quite dramatic in appearance with frothing at the mouth accompanied by rhythmic clonic-tonic movements of the extremities. Other signs and symptoms of brain dysfunction include paralysis of one half of the body, or hemiparesis; and sensory failure of one half of the body, hemisensory loss. These phenomena usually occur on the opposite or contralateral side of the body from the brain involvement.

Involvement of the spinal cord may produce a cord hemisection (Brown-Séquard syndrome), paraparesis (weakness of both legs), or neurogenic bladder. The affected areas may be increased in tone (spastic) or limp (flaccid).

Involvement of the peripheral nerves produces dysfunction in the area served by the individual nerve. Involvement of the median nerve at the carpal tunnel may produce numbness in a portion of the hand. When a peripheral nerve is involved, sensation is generally impaired for all modalities, including touch, pain, and temperature. Involvement of the brain or spinal cord may affect selective modalities while sparing others.

DIAGNOSTIC PROCEDURES AND TESTS

Computed Tomography ■ This study allows evaluation of the skull, brain, and spinal column in a noninvasive manner. With the addition of intravenous contrast, the sensitivity of the technique may be enhanced. Placement of contrast material in the spinal fluid via lumbar puncture substantially improves visualization of the spinal cord and nerve roots.

Magnetic Resonance Imaging (MRI) ■ Unlike computed tomography, no ionizing radiation is involved with this imaging modality. By virtue of perturbations induced in a powerful magnetic field, images of the brain, spinal cord, and other areas of the body may be obtained noninvasively.

Myelography with or Without Adjunctive Computed Tomography (CT) ■ This is accomplished by instilling water-soluble iodinated contrast agents into the spinal fluid by lumbar puncture or spinal tap. A series of x-ray films is then obtained. As the neural elements of the spine are bathed by the spinal fluid, the contrast reveals their outline. With its axial imaging capability, CT improves the imaging resolution of myelography substantially.

Lumbar Puncture ■ This is usually a diagnostic procedure. A small area in the midline of the lower back is infiltrated with local anesthesia. A spinal needle is passed between the bony elements through the dura mater, a covering of the nerve roots, into the subarachnoid space. Fluid is then collected for analysis of cell count. Glucose, protein, and active malignant cells may be encountered.

Electroencephalography ■ This test is accomplished by placing electrical leads or sensors over well-defined areas of the scalp and recording electrical impulses. This reflects the electrical activity of the brain. The test is useful in the diagnosis and management of epilepsy or convulsive disorders. It may also identify areas of focal brain dysfunction.

Evoked Potentials ▪ Tests of this genre apply a fixed and repetitive external stimulus and average the time-locked electrical responses to the stimulus. This allows more discrete analysis of the peripheral and central nervous system function.

Electromyography and Nerve Conduction Studies ▪ These tests are accomplished by placing needle electrodes in various muscles, as well as by applying topical sensors and stimulators over the routes of various nerves. Information about the conduction velocity of the nerves and electrical responses of the muscles is obtained. This testing procedure may separate nervous from muscle diseases. It may further suggest a site of injury if the nervous system is implicated.

Arteriography ▪ This is an invasive test. It involves gaining access to the arterial system at the groin or elbow and inserting a catheter. The catheter is placed in a selected blood vessel and contrast material given. This test allows definition of the vascular anatomy and may demonstrate atherosclerotic lesions, aneurysms, or arteriovenous malformations. It may suggest the presence of a mass lesion but is inferior to CT or MRI for this purpose.

Nerve and Muscle Biopsy ▪ In some cases, a piece of a relatively unimportant peripheral nerve, usually the sural nerve, is removed by a minor surgical procedure under local anesthesia. An analysis of the material may be useful in identifying a disease of the peripheral nervous system or a systemic process. A small portion of the muscle may be sampled for analysis to shed further light on a muscle disease.

SURGICAL PROCEDURES

A few of the more common neurosurgical procedures are outlined here.

Craniotomy ▪ In this procedure an opening in the skull is made to gain access to the brain or supporting structures, and then the bone is re-placed. This differs from a craniectomy, in which the bone removed is not replaced. Once access to the brain has been obtained, a tumor may be resected, an aneurysm clipped, or a cranial nerve decompressed. Depending on the complexity of the procedure, an operating microscope may or may not be used to provide additional illumination and magnification. When a tumor is close to a critical structure, a CO_2 laser may be useful as a precision cutting instrument. Another member of the instrumentation armamentarium is the cavitron ultrasonic aspirator. As the name implies, it breaks up tissue with high-frequency vibrations and aspirates the tissue fragments.

Laminectomy ▪ This procedure involves gaining access to the spinal canal from a posterior approach. The laminae and spinous processes may be removed without compromising stability. In many instances, it is not necessary to remove both laminae. One-sided removal (hemilaminectomy) or partial one-sided removal (hemilaminotomy) may be sufficient to expose a herniated disk or to allow decompression of a nerve root. In the case of spinal cord tumors, the location of the tumor dictates both the approach and the extent of the procedure. Tumors may be outside the dura—extradural; inside the dural tube but outside the spinal canal—intradural, extramedullary; or inside the spinal cord—intradural, intramedullary.

Anterior Approaches to the Spine ▪ These approaches allow access to the spinal canal from the front through the vertebral bodies or the disk spaces separating the vertebral bodies. As column stability may be a concern, a fusion usually accompanies an anterior approach to the spine.

Anterior approaches to the spine may be quite complex. In the neck, the plane between the visceral compartments (trachea, esophagus) and vascular compartments (carotid artery, jugular vein) is entered to expose the front of the cervical spine. The upper 1st and 2nd cervical vertebrae may be approached anteriorly through the mouth. Anterior approaches to the thoracic spine generally necessitate the assistance of a thoracic surgeon to facilitate exposure. Anterior approaches to the lumbar spine are similarly complex.

Peripheral Nerve Surgery ▪ This operation can run from the simple (carpal tunnel release) to the sublime (revamping of the brachial plexus). The bulk of peripheral nerve surgery involves straightforward nerve decompressions. The median nerve, for example, is most commonly compressed at the wrist. Decompression is carried out through a small incision in the palm done under local anesthesia with mild sedation. The ulnar nerve is most frequently compressed at the elbow. Generally, the procedure carried out involves moving the ulnar nerve out of its pocket behind the medial epicondyle of the humerus to an anterior location. This is referred to as a transposition of the ulnar nerve.

Instruments

Various surgical instruments will be referred to repeatedly in operative reports. Table 23–1 categorizes them as to function and is not meant to be either complete or didactic.

GLOSSARY

The following is a glossary of frequently encountered terms used during a neurologic examination.*

abducens: The sixth cranial nerve, which innervates only the lateral rectus muscle of the eye; its action is to deviate the eye laterally.

accommodation: Technically called the *accommodation-convergence synkinesis*, accommodation is elicited by having the patient shift the gaze to some near object after having relaxed the gaze by looking in the distance. Response consists of three parts: thickening of the lens, convergence of the eyes, and pupillary constriction.

adiadokokinesia: The inability to perform rapid alternating movements; usually tested with reciprocal hand or finger movements.

Adson's maneuver: A vascular compression test described by an early neurosurgeon to diagnose the thoracic outlet syndrome; elicited by the following steps: (1) arms hanging down alongside body, with elbows flexed 90° and

*This glossary is adapted from a lecture delivered on March 18, 1989, by Edward A. Smith, M.D., at the annual meeting of the California Association of Medical Transcriptionists (CAMT) in Monterey, California.

Table 23–1 ■ Instruments Used in Neurosurgery

Bone-Cutting Instruments	Forceps
Adson's bone rongeur	Adson's
Hardy's bone rongeur*	bayonet
Horsley's bone rongeur	Cushing's
intervertebral disk rongeur	tissue
Kerrison's rongeur*	**Brain Retractors or Retractor Systems**
Leksell's rongeur	
Schlesinger's rongeur	
Dissectors	brain spatulas
Micropenfield dissectors	Greenberg's retractor system
nerve hook	Layla retractor system
Penfield's numbers 1 through 4	
Rhoton's microdissectors	
Retractors	**Scalp Hemostats**
cerebellar self-retaining retractor	Dandy's hemostats
Markham-Meyerding self-retaining hemilaminectomy retractor	Raney's clips
mastoid retractor	**Scalpel Blades**
Miskimon retractor	Beaver's blade
Scoville's self-retaining retractor	Number 10
Taylor's retractor	Number 11
Weitlaner's self-retaining retractor	Number 15
	Rosen knife
	Scissors
	Iris
	Mayo's
	Metzenbaum's
	microscissors
	Potts'

*This class of rongeurs is sometimes referred to as bone punches.

forearms supinated, (2) neck extended, (3) shoulders retracted, (4) deep inspiration followed by slow expiration. A positive response is diminution of the radial artery pulse. Unfortunately, this test is abnormal in 30 per cent of normal people.

apposition: Placement of two body parts together. Also see *opposition*.

apraxia: The inability to perform skilled movements; assumes that there is no muscular or mechanical impairment to the desired actions.

ataxia: Can be considered to be one form of gait apraxia (there are others) in which equilibrium is disturbed, producing lurches, staggering, collisions, or falls.

Barré's position: For testing postural stability; in a sitting position, the patient elevates both arms overhead and maintains this posture with the eyes closed.

-cephaly: A suffix meaning head. Many prefixes modify this. The adjectival form is cephalic.

> **brachycephaly:** The sagittal diameter of the skull is less than about 1.5 times the transverse (coronal) diameter.

> **dolichocephaly:** The sagittal diameter is more than 1.5 times the transverse diameter.

> **hydrocephaly:** The condition of having increased amounts of cerebrospinal fluid within the cerebral ventricles. There are three types:

>> **communicating:** Ventricular fluid freely communicates with subarachnoid fluid.

>> **ex vacuo:** Enlargement of the ventricular system compensatory to cerebral atrophy.

>> **obstructive:** No communication between intraventricular and subarachnoid fluid.

> **normocephaly:** The sagittal diameter is about 1.5 times the transverse diameter.

choroid: The pigmented middle layer of the three layers of the eyeball; responsible for the reflected glow of light shining in a cat's eyes at night.

Chvostek's sign: A sign said to be characteristic of hypocalcemic tetany; elicited by tapping the facial nerve as it goes around the angle of the jaw from the stylomastoid foramen. Response is ipsilateral contracture of the facial muscles.

conjugate gaze: Both eyes move an equal amount in the same direction; this motion occurs voluntarily and involuntarily.

conjunctiva: The mucous membrane covering the exposed sclera of the eyeball (*bulbar conjunctiva*) and inner aspect of the eyelids (*palpebral conjunctiva*).

convergence: Both eyes deviating medially, as in near vision, such as reading.

cornea: The transparent dome of tissue that lies in front of the pupil. The lateral margin of the cornea is called the limbus.

corneal reflex: Elicited by application of a light touch or puff of air to the cornea; the response is an involuntary blink.

craniostenosis: A skull cavity too small for the usual-sized brain; usually the result of a developmental defect.

craniosynostosis: Premature bony union of skull growth plates, resulting in abnormally shaped skulls and/or craniostenosis.

decerebrate: An adjective describing an abnormal posture in which the arms are adducted at the shoulders, extended alongside the trunk, internally rotated (hyperpronated), and flexed at the wrists; the legs are extended. Muscle tone is rigid. The condition results from brain stem injury at or below the level of the red nucleus.

decorticate: An adjective describing an abnormal posture in which the arms are adducted and internally rotated at the shoulders, with the elbows, wrists, and interphalangeal joints flexed. The legs are usually extended. Body tone is rigid. The usual cause is a stroke.

Ely's test: See FABER test.

-esthesia: A suffix pertaining to the faculty of perception.

> **an:** without.

> **dys:** painful or unpleasant.

> **graph:** perception of writing on skin.

> **hyper:** more than normal, unusually heightened, usually unpleasant.

> **hypo:** less than normal.

> **pall:** vibratory.

> **par:** altered, one sensory modality misperceived as another, often unpleasant.

> **therm:** temperature.

extensor toe signs: A fertile field for neurologists seeking to immortalize their names by discovering a new twist on the elicitation of pathologic great toe dorsiflexion. All have the same meaning: abnormality of voluntary upper motor neuron control of the lower extremities; can be seen in circumstances as diverse as concussion and spinal cord tumors.

> **Babinski's sign:** A sign named for the great Polish-French neurologist who described this premier of all pathologic reflexes. Elicited by stroking the lateral plantar surface of the foot. Elicitation of this sign was initially designed for children, but the response—dorsiflexion of the great toe—applies to any age. In older children and adults, the direction of stroking is from posterior toward the base of the great toe.

Bing's sign: Dorsiflexion of the great toe when the dorsum of that toe is pricked.

Chaddock's sign: A derivation of the Babinski sign for the ticklish; the lateral edge of the foot is stroked toward the little toe in order to elicit great toe dorsiflexion.

Gonda's sign: Depressing, then suddenly releasing, the second or fourth toe elicits dorsiflexion of the great toe.

Gordon's sign: Squeezing the Achilles tendon elicits dorsiflexion of the great toe.

Oppenheim's sign: Stroking the shinbone from knee toward foot elicits dorsiflexion of the great toe.

Schaefer's sign: Squeezing the calf elicits dorsiflexion of the great toe.

Strumpell's sign: Dorsiflexion of the great toe provoked when the patient attempts to perform a straight leg raise against resistance.

FABER test: One of the phantoms of medicine; there is no Dr. Faber. This is an acronym for *f*lexion, *ab*duction, *e*xternal *r*otation of the hip. This is a test to differentiate hip disease from sciatica as it allegedly causes minimal stress on the sciatic nerve. Synonym: Patrick's test.

facial diplegia: The inability to move either side of the face; the cause of the absent motion might be emotional, volitional, or both.

facial spasm: Involuntary exaggerated motion, occurring in response to emotional, volitional, or habitual (e.g., ordinary resting position) stimuli, or any combination of the aforementioned.

femoral stretch test: Elicited by placing the patient prone, then flexing the calf on the thigh; a positive response consists of pain in the anterior thigh, allegedly due to traction on an irritated or compressed femoral nerve.

finger-to-nose test: A coordination test that can be performed in one of two ways: the patient touches the nose with the finger (usually index) or tries to touch the examiner's finger as it is moved (finger-to-finger test).

> **hypometria:** Undershooting the target in the finger-to-finger test, which could reasonably be called "pre-pointing."

> **past-pointing:** An abnormal result in the finger-to-nose or other pointing test in which the patient's finger overshoots the target.

foramen closure test: Usually describing a maneuver to narrow the cervical exit foramina, hence producing compression of entrapped nerve roots, reproducing spontaneous symptoms; elicited by performing vertex compression with the head tilted to one side while turned to the opposite side.

frontal lobe release signs: Any of a large variety of abnormal reflex movements that come about allegedly from loss of inhibitory frontal lobe influences. The abnormalities are usually unilateral and contralateral to the presumably damaged frontal lobe.

> **bulldog sign:** When present, a sign of serious neurologic dysfunction, almost always seen in cases of advanced dementia; elicited by placing a tongue blade between the teeth of the patient, who involuntarily bites down on it.

> **glabellar sign:** A classic sign of Parkinson's disease, occasionally seen in other conditions; elicited by gently tapping on the forehead just above the nasal bridge, resulting in involuntary blinking. The response should be elicited on approximately five consecutive trials since blinks may occur once or twice even in normal individuals.

> **jaw jerk:** Usually representing bilateral frontal lobe dysfunction; elicited by tapping downward on a partially open but relaxed lower jaw, resulting in brisk, involuntary jaw closure.

> **Leri's sign:** Elicited by having the patient flex the elbow and wrist, then applying further passive wrist flexion, resulting in further elbow flexion.

> **palmomental sign:** Elicited by stroking the palm of the hand with a semisharp object, resulting in an ipsilateral retraction of the corner of the mouth and chin.

> **snouting:** Gentle percussion of the philtrum (middle of the upper lip), resulting in puckering.

> **sucking:** By rubbing at the angle of the mouth, a pucker or sucking movement is produced.

Ganslen's test: A sacroiliac joint stress test, by which pain is elicited from a pathologic joint; performed by first flexing both hips and knees of a supine patient, then extending one leg down over the edge of the examination table.

Guillain-Barré syndrome: A syndrome

named for two eminent French neurologists, relating to an inflammatory disease of nerves, both cranial and peripheral, that leads primarily to motor impairment; frequently respiratory embarrassment occurs, which is the usual cause of death. Permanent paralysis results in only a small minority of cases.

heel-shin maneuver: A coordination test performed by first elevating one leg up in the air, then placing the heel onto the knee of the resting leg, and finally sliding the heel down the shin bone to the foot.

hitchhiker sign: A test for compression of the subclavian artery, elicited by externally rotating the shoulder while abducting it 90° with the elbow also bent 90°. A positive response is the reduction of the radial artery pulse.

homonymous: An adjective describing similarity in paired organs but most often referring to similar visual field changes in both eyes.

hyperabduction test: Elevation of the arm above head level, placing the forearm over the head and feeling for reduction of the radial artery pulse.

-kinesia: A suffix meaning (the quality of) movement.
> **a:** without.
> **brady:** slower than normal, as in parkinsonism.
> **dys:** abnormal.
> **hyper:** more than normal, restlessness.
> **hypo:** less than normal.

meningeal (irritation) signs: Produced in the presence of inflammation of the meninges, frequently in the presence of infection or subarachnoid hemorrhage.
> **Brudzinski's sign:** With the patient supine, the neck is passively flexed, resulting in flexion of the patient's hips and knees, to reduce traction on inflamed lumbosacral nerves.
> **Kernig's sign:** The classic meningeal irritation sign; elicited by lifting one or both legs of a supine patient with the hip and knee bent, then extending the knee, resulting in neck flexion.

ophthalmoscopy: Looking at and into the eye with the aid of lenses.

-opia: Suffix relating to the faculty of vision.
> **an:** without vision (blind).
> **hemian:** loss of vision in the right or left half of vision.
> **my:** poor distant vision, i.e., nearsighted.

> **presby:** poor near vision due to age-related loss of ocular accommodation.
> **quadrantanopia:** Loss of vision in one visual quadrant.

opposition: A specific type of apposition in which appendages, usually the thumb and another finger, are placed tip-to-tip. Also see *apposition*.

optic disk: The central retinal depression marking the location of the optic nerve connection to the globe.

paresis: Weakness, from any cause.

Phalen's test: Hyperflexion of the wrist, maintained 30 to 60 seconds, provokes paresthesias in the distribution of the median nerve: thumb, index, middle, and sometimes ring fingers.
> **reverse Phalen's test:** Hyperextension of the wrist to the same purpose.

pinch: Forceful opposition of the thumb and a finger; it requires function of the primary motor cortex.

-plegia: Suffix meaning paralysis, which means total absence of movement, i.e., total paresis.
> **crural:** crossed paralysis, i.e., one arm and opposite leg, or alternatively, paralysis of one leg.
> **di:** paralysis of paired organs, e.g., face or arms (or legs).
> **hemi:** paralysis of ipsilateral arm and leg.
> **mono:** paralysis of one limb.
> **para:** paralysis of both legs, a special case of diplegia.

primary gaze: Position of the eyes looking straight ahead at distance.

ptosis: Drooping of the eyelid(s); technically the lid covers the pupillary margin or limbus.
> **external ophthalmoplegia:** Oculomotor palsy in which the extraocular muscles, including lid movers, are paralyzed. This results in ptosis and mydriasis (pupillary enlargement).
> **Horner's syndrome:** Ptosis, miosis (small pupil), and craniofacial anhidrosis. Due to disease of the carotid sympathetic chain. Anhidrosis usually disappears in a few months whereas the other, ocular abnormalities persist.
> **internal ophthalmoplegia:** A form of oculomotor palsy in which the pupillary and accommodative responses are lost.

-reflexia: A suffix relating to reflex, an involuntary motor response to sensory input, i.e., totally without need for consciousness but which can be consciously altered.

> **a:** without.
>
> **dys:** abnormal, often applied to exaggerated autonomic responses occurring in body segments deprived of spinal cord innervation. Modalities other than contraction of voluntary muscle may be involved, e.g., sweating.
>
> **hyper:** more than normal.
>
> **hypo:** less than normal.

retina: The nerve layer of the eye.

Rinne's test: A hearing test comparing subjective perception of air and bone conduction in one ear with a tuning fork; normally air conduction is more acute.

Romberg's test: A balance test performed in Romberg's position, requiring feet together, head up, hands down to the sides. The test is performed by closing the eyes for 30 seconds and maintaining balance. If the patient cannot assume Romberg's position, the test is invalid.

Schirmer's test: A test of lacrimation (tear formation), performed by placing a strip of filter paper or tissue paper in the inferior fornix of the eye (where the palpebral conjunctiva of the lower eyelid joins the bulbar conjunctiva) and measuring the length of paper moistened by tears after a measured time.

sciatic nerve stretch tests: Designed to elicit pain in cases of irritated lumbosacral nerve roots or of the sciatic nerve itself.

> **Fajersztajn's sign:** The ultimate test of a neurotranscriptionist! This is merely the Lasègue's test to which is added dorsiflexion of the foot to add extra stretch on the sciatic nerve.
>
> **Lasègue's sign:** The straight leg raising test. Performed in the supine position, one leg with a straight knee is elevated above the horizontal and note is made of the angle at which leg or back pain develops and the location of the pain. Probably no test is more confused in the minds of physicians than this.
>
> **reverse:** Prone straight leg raising.
>
> **sitting:** Knee extension of one leg while sitting with hips flexed at 90°; if pain is present, it is always a sign of significant nerve root irritation.

Spurling's sign: Fajersztajn's sign.

sciatica augmentation test: If the physician is not sure that a patient has nerve root irritation due to intraspinal mechanical compression, this test is used. By increasing intracranial pressure through obstruction of cerebral venous drainage, pressure is transmitted through the spinal canal to the lumbar nerve roots. A positive response is reproduction of radicular symptoms.

> **Naffziger's test:** Named after a resourceful San Francisco neurosurgeon who must have had the patient's utmost confidence: both jugular veins are manually compressed until the eyes bulge and the face flushes.
>
> **Viets' test:** As above, with the mechanical refinement of a blood pressure cuff inflated around the neck to provide compression.

sclera: The tough outer layer of the eye.

scotoma: A blind spot; plural is scotomas or scotomata.

> **cecocentral:** in which the scotoma extends from the physiologic blind spot (at the optic disk) to the macular area or fixation point.
>
> **central:** in the center of vision, at the fixation point.
>
> **teichopsia:** a dynamic scotoma, usually peripheral, with flashing lights and multiple colors and patterns.

shoulder depression test: Elicitation of arm pain by pulling down the arm while exerting counterpressure on the patient's axilla indicates nerve root pathology.

Smith's sign: Reproduction of cervical nerve root pain by having the patient reach behind the back, attempting to touch the opposite scapula with the hand.

springing: A maneuver placing ventral stress onto a vertebral spinous process by a sharp thrust, designed to elicit pain from an area of pathology.

stereognosis: The ability to discriminate shapes by touch; requires an intact parietal lobe.

sterno(cleido)mastoid muscle: Attaches from the mastoid bone and inserts on the clavicle and sternum; its action is to rotate the head to the opposite side combined with some forward flexion; innervated by the spinal branch of the spinal accessory nerve (11th cranial nerve). Cleido- is a prefix meaning clavicle.

Sturge-Weber syndrome: A neurocutaneous hereditary malformation arising from the embryonic ectoderm. The full-blown syndrome includes a facial nevus in the distribution of the first division of the trigeminal nerve (forehead, nose) or possibly more extensive. Intracranial involvement consists of a capillary-venous angioma in the gray and white matter of the brain and is manifested by seizures, hemiparesis, mental retardation, intracranial calcification, unilateral exophthalmos, glaucoma, and retinal and choroidal angiomata.

sutures: The adjacent edges of two growth plates of flat bones (enchondral bone). Those composing the cranial vault are:

> **coronal:** the more anterior of the two transverse sutures. The transverse plane also takes its name from this suture.
>
> **lambdoidal:** the more posterior of the two transverse sutures.
>
> **metopic:** an anteroposteriorly directed suture extending anteriorly from the coronal suture.
>
> **sagittal:** the midline anteroposterior suture, which gives its name to the anteroposterior plane.

tandem stance: Standing with the heel of the front foot touching the toes of the rear foot directly behind it. Tandem gait is performed placing each foot in front of the other in such a manner.

Tinel's sign: Named after another neurologist who discovered that percussing a peripheral nerve at the site of local pathology produces a paresthesia in the distribution of that nerve. This test is commonly performed on the median nerve at the wrist in suspected cases of carpal tunnel syndrome.

titubation: Swaying, often in a circular fashion, while in a stationary posture, such as in Romberg's or Barré's tests.

Trendelenburg's sign: Related to a postural abnormality seen in cases of weakness of the gluteus medius muscle. The pelvis on the side opposite the supporting leg during one-legged stance drops. With a normal gluteus medius muscle on the side of the elevated leg, the pelvis rises.

two point discrimination: The ability to perceive the touch of two points separated by variable distances as two discrete points; another test of parietal lobe function.

vertex compression: Pressing downward on the crown of the head to reproduce pain originating in cervical spine disease.

Weber's test: A hearing test performed with a tuning fork placed on the vertex to determine where the vibration is heard (not where it is felt). Normal response is in the middle of the head.

zoopsia: Hallucination in which a patient thinks he or she sees animals.

FORMATS

Letters dictated by a neurologist or a neurosurgeon contain a history, report of a complete neurologic examination, assessment of diagnostic studies, and a plan formulation. Follow-up letters are more limited in scope, detailing the progress of treatment, either surgical or nonsurgical. See Figure 23–5, a consultation letter.

Hospital discharge summaries include:

Name of hospital
Admission and discharge dates
Principal diagnosis
Secondary diagnoses
Procedures
Discharge medications and instructions
History and physical examination
Hospital course, including relevant laboratory data

Figure 23–6 is a sample of a discharge summary.

Operative reports include:

Name of hospital
Date of procedure
Preoperative diagnosis
Postoperative diagnosis
Procedure
Surgeon
Assistants
Anesthesia
Estimated blood loss
Complications
Drains
Operative findings and specimens

Representative operative reports can be seen in Figures 23–7 and 23–8.

Stephen L. Fedder, M.D.
655 Lankenau Medical Building
Philadelphia, PA 19096-0000
215-649-4416

May 4, 1994

David Friedman, M.D.
2365 Logan Street
Philadelphia, PA 19005-0000

RE: Mr. James Wright

Dear Dr. Friedman:

I had the pleasure of seeing Mr. Wright in the office today, May 4, 1994. As you know, he is an otherwise healthy 59-year-old, very active gentleman with a three-week history of right L3 radicular pain. This is accompanied by weakness in the quadriceps area and numbness in the anterior surface of his right thigh. This resulted in his hospitalization at the Hammond Hospital during which time he underwent myelography, CT, and obtained an MRI scan. He has been maintained on Roxicet since then. He indicates that he is having difficulty going on like this although he is usually a stoic person involved in hunting and other very active pursuits.

Past medical history is negative and review of systems is noncontributory.

Neurologic examination shows quadriceps weakness at a level of 4+/5. The deep tendon reflex at the right knee is markedly reduced although present, compared to the left side. Straight leg raising and reverse straight leg raising tests are normal. Posterior tibial pulses are intact and symmetric. There is no tenderness around the hip joints and range of motion of the hips is normal.

MRI, myelogram, and post-myelogram CT are reviewed and all are consistent with a free fragment of disc adjacent to the pedicle at L3 on the right side.

I believe this patient has a clear-cut radicular history associated with appropriate neurologic deficits and supportive radiologic findings. He has failed conservative therapy and, therefore, I feel he is a candidate for microsurgical disc excision. We plan to admit him to the hospital on May 7 for surgery that day.

Thank you very much for your interest and for allowing me to take part in the care of this patient.

Sincerely,

Stephen L. Fedder, M.D.

ssb

Figure 23-5
A consultation letter for a patient with a 3-week history of right L3 radicular pain.

THE LANKENAU HOSPITAL
100 Lancaster Avenue west of City Line
Wynnewood, PA 19096-0000

DISCHARGE SUMMARY

NAME: Dole, Adam
PHYSICIAN: S.L. Fedder, M.D.

MEDICAL RECORD #338964
DATE OF ADMISSION: 8/26/94
DATE OF DISCHARGE: 9/2/94

FINAL DIAGNOSIS:

Colloid cyst of the third ventricle.

PROCEDURES:

1. 8/27/94 - Right frontal twist drill hole for implantation of camino ventricular drain with pressure monitor by Dr. Fedder.

2. 8/29/94 - Right frontal craniotomy and transventricular approach to colloid cyst with excision of colloid cyst by Dr. Fedder.

DISCHARGE MEDICATIONS:

Dilantin, 100 mg. p.o., t.i.d.

HISTORY OF PRESENT ILLNESS: The patient is a 34-year-old white male whose chief complaint has been headaches times three weeks. The patient was feeling fine until he started experiencing sharp pain in the occipital region. The pain was nonradiating and there was no nausea or vomiting at first. The pains persisted and worsened over the past three weeks until they were almost constant. The patient awoke with pain, nausea, and vomiting for the first time on the day of admission. He went to Community Hospital where a CAT scan in the Emergency Room revealed hydrocephalus and a cyst blocking his third ventricle. The patient was referred to Dr. Fedder and admitted.

PHYSICAL EXAMINATION: Physical examination revealed a well--developed, well-nourished 34-year-old white male in only mild distress. Vital signs were stable. Neurological examination revealed an alert and oriented times three person responding appropriately to conversation. Motor strength was 5/5 in both upper and lower extremities and symmetric. Sensation to light touch was

(continued)

Figure 23–6
A discharge summary regarding a patient with a colloid cyst of the third ventricle.

Dole, Adam   Page two
MEDICAL RECORD #338964

intact.   Cerebellar function was normal to alternating fingers and finger-to-nose tests.   Cranial nerves II to XII were intact.

HOSPITAL COURSE: On the day of admission, the camino drain pressure monitor was implanted by Dr. Fedder without complication.   There was immediate relief of major symptoms and the patient was placed in the ICU for close observation overnight.   On 8/28/94, the patient was doing well and Dr. Fedder placed a right subclavian line without difficulty.   Chest x-ray was negative, and the patient was scheduled for surgery for 8/29/94.   On 8/29/94, the patient underwent a right frontal craniotomy and excision of the colloid cyst from the third ventricle.   The operation was carried out without complication.   The patient was awake, alert and oriented in the Recovery Room, and had no drift.   Dressing was dry and intact.

On 8/30/94 the patient remained stable.   All vital signs were stable.   CAT scan revealed no hematoma.   There was no drift.   The patient's dressing was dry and intact and the patient was discharged to a surgical floor.   The patient did well over the next few days, remained alert and oriented times three, with no neurological deficits nor headaches, and was discharged on 9/2/94. Discharge status was good.

_____

STEPHEN L. FEDDER, M.D.

SLF:ssb
D: 9/3/94
T: 9/4/94

Figure 23–6 *Continued*

THE LANKENAU HOSPITAL
100 Lancaster Avenue
Wynnewood, PA 19096-0000

OPERATIVE REPORT

PATIENT: Thomas Clark   DATE: 6/8/94
SURGEON: Stephen L. Fedder, M.D.   RECORD #618256
ASSISTANT: William Green, M.D.

PREOPERATIVE DIAGNOSIS: Colloid cyst, third ventricle.

POSTOPERATIVE DIAGNOSIS: Same.

OPERATION: Right frontal craniotomy and transventricular
                               approach to colloid cyst with excision of colloid cyst.

ANESTHESIA: General endotracheal.

BLOOD LOSS: 150 cc.

COMPLICATIONS: None.

DRAINS: None.

TISSUE TO LABORATORY: Colloid cyst.

PROCEDURE: The risks and complications of the procedure were
                               discussed with the patient and his wife prior to surgery.
They were listed as including, but not limited to: failure to improve, increase in symptoms -
that is headache, stroke, coma; death, infection and bleeding requiring re-operation.

The patient was taken to the operating room and general anesthesia induced and carried on
with precautions for intracranial hypertension. The patient was then placed in a modest
amount of reverse Trendelenburg to facilitate venous drainage. The area over the right frontal
area was shaved and a skin scratch was placed with the midline limb along the superior
sagittal sinus. The previous ventriculostomy incision was in the middle of the field. The area
was prepared as above with surgical drapes applied in the usual manner. A #10 blade was
used to incise the scalp down to the periosteum and Raney clips applied to the scalp edges to
obtain hemostasis. The flap was then reflected over two rolled up sponges to prevent

(continued)

Figure continued

Figure 23-7
An operative report in the style of the Lankenau Hospital.

Thomas Clark
Record #618256   Page two

ischemic necrosis of the flap. Two burr holes were placed along the superior sagittal suture, one just behind the coronal suture and one several centimeters anterior to it. Following this, a cupped curet was used to remove residual bone bits and a #3 Penfield was used to dissect the dura from the overlying calvarium. A bony flap was cut, outer perimeter first and then over the superior sagittal sinus last. The flap was reflected out of the field. Several perimeter holes were placed and #0 Tevdek sutures were placed through them to accommodate the bone flap at the end of the case. Several perimeter holes were also placed in the bone flap. The bone flap was then wrapped in Betadine and placed out of the direct surgical field until needed. Dural tacking sutures were placed to obliterate the epidural space and sewn through the perimeter holes. The dura was opened in a U-shaped manner, hinged on the superior sagittal sinus and retracted out of the field. A bipolar electrocautery was used to coagulate the pia-arachnoid over the proposed site of ventricular tap. A ventricular needle was passed easily into the right frontal ventricular horn, cerebrospinal fluid obtained and obturator replaced. Bipolar electrocautery was then used to coagulate slightly more pia-arachnoid and a #15 blade used to make a pia-arachnoid incision. Suction dissection was then carried down to the level with the ependyma and two Layla retractors were placed to maintain ependymal exposure. The ependyma was opened with a Stecher knife, the ventricle entered and the glistening ependymal surface was noted. The thalamostriate vein was followed back to the level of the foramen of Munro and the choroid plexus identified. At the level of the foramen of Munro, a small amount of choroid plexus was noted to be overlying the colloid cyst. All intraventricular dissecting was done with the operating microscope, using a 300 mm focal length lens.

With the operating microscope in place, the choroid plexus was dissected from over the cyst wall. Some minor adhesions to the fornix were cut with a Stecher knife. Further dissection in the circumference of the foramen of Munro was carried out with a micro Penfield dissector. The colloid cyst was punctured with a Stecher knife and opened more widely with a micro scissors. Gelatinous material was removed and more gelatinous material aspirated. The entire cyst collapsed at this point and was brought out from the third ventricle and passed to the scrub nurse to be sent to pathology. A clear, unobstructed view from the lateral ventricular system into the third ventricle was obtained at this point. A modest amount of bleeding was controlled easily with a small piece of Surgicel. No transgressions of the caudate nucleus or the fornix were noted. The thalamostriate vein and internal cerebral veins were intact at the end of this portion of the procedure. The septum pellucidum was then opened slightly. Retractors were backed out. The area was copiously irrigated with gentamicin-containing saline. A small swatch of Surgicel was placed at the pia-arachnoid incision. Dura was closed with a #4-0 Nurolon running locking suture. The craniotomy flap

Figure 23–7 Continued

Thomas Clark
Record #618256   Page three

was secured with #0 Tevdek sutures. Scalp flap was re-positioned and closed in two layers. The galea and subcutaneous tissue were closed with #2-0 Vicryl in an inverted and interrupted fashion. Skin was closed with #3-0 nylon in a running locking fashion.

_____

STEPHEN L. FEDDER, M.D.

SLF:ssb
D: 6/8/94
T: 6/9/94

Figure 23–7 *Continued*

THE LANKENAU HOSPITAL
100 Lancaster Avenue west of City Line
Wynnewood, PA 19096

OPERATIVE REPORT

PATIENT: Edward Blake   DATE: 5/7/94
SURGEON: Stephen L. Fedder, M.D.   RECORD # 618034
ASSISTANT: William Green, M.D.

PREOPERATIVE DIAGNOSIS:	Herniated free fragment of disc opposite pedicle of L3 on the right side.
POSTOPERATIVE DIAGNOSIS:	Same.
OPERATION:	L3 hemilaminectomy and excision of free fragment of disc.
ANESTHESIA:	General endotracheal.
BLOOD LOSS:	75 cc.
COMPLICATIONS:	None.
DRAINS:	None.
TISSUE TO LABORATORY:	Free fragment of disc in two portions.
PROCEDURE:	Risks and complications were explained to the patient in the presence of his wife.

They were listed as including but not being limited to: failure to improve, increase in pain, paralysis of the legs, bowel and bladder dysfunction requiring catheterization, meningitis, spinal fluid leak and bleeding requiring re-operation. The patient presented voluntarily for surgery. He was brought to the operating room and general anesthesia induced and carried out in the usual manner. He was placed on an Andrews frame. Using anatomic and radiographic landmarks, a skin scratch was placed over the L3 spinous process slightly above and slightly below. The area was prepared with pHisoHex followed by Betadine scrub and solution and surgical drapes were applied in the usual manner. A #10 blade was used to incise the skin down to the dorsal lumbar fascia and a self-retaining retractor placed to maintain incision edge separation and hemostasis. The fascia was carefully defined and depressed just to the right side of the spinous process

(continued)

Figure 23–8

An operative report for an L3 hemilaminectomy and excision of free fragment of disk.

Edward Blake
Record #618034   Page two

with a Cobb periosteal elevator. It was incised with Bovie electrocautery in the coagulation mode. A subperiosteal dissection was then carried out of the L3 spinous process and right sided hemilamina. Sponge packing technique was used to obtain further dissection as well as hemostasis. The cup curette was used to define the inferior hemilamina of the L3 and a Leksell rongeur used to perform a subtotal hemilaminectomy. Following this, a cotton pledget was placed under loupe magnification just beneath the bony surface to prevent dural transgression. The remainder of the L3 hemilamina was removed with an angled Kerrison punch. It was removed laterally to the level of the pedicle at L3 and slightly more laterally below. This having been accomplished, loupe magnification was continued throughout the rest of the case. The thecal sac was gently retracted slightly medially just adjacent to the pedicle revealing a large free fragment of disc as anticipated from the preoperative films. The free fragment was dissected with a #4 Penfield and removed in two bites. A small amount of epidural bleeding was easily controlled with Avitene. The area was then copiously irrigated with gentamicin-containing saline. A Valsalva was delivered by anesthesia and revealed no evidence of spinal fluid leak. The area was copiously irrigated again with gentamicin-containing saline and sponges were removed. Sponge and needle counts were correct. Muscle and fascia were closed with #0 Vicryl in an interrupted fashion. Subcutaneous tissue was closed with #2-0 Vicryl in an inverted interrupted fashion. Skin was closed with #3-0 Vicryl in a running subcuticular fashion.

STEPHEN L. FEDDER, M.D.

SLF:ssb
D: 5/7/94
T: 5/8/94

Figure **23–8** *Continued*

Reference Sources

Asbury, Arthur K., Guy M. McKahnn, and W. Ian McDonald. *Diseases of the Nervous System.* W. B. Saunders Company, Philadelphia, 1986.

Wilkins, R. H., and S. S. Rengachary. *Neurosurgery.* McGraw-Hill, New York, 1985.

For references of specific application to medical transcription, see Appendix 1.

Henry N. Wagner, Jr., M.D.
Julia W. Buchanan

Nuclear Medicine

INTRODUCTION

Nuclear medicine is a medical specialty that uses radioactive materials in diagnosis, prognosis, and treatment. Nuclear medicine studies are often presented in the form of pictures, called nuclear images. These are based on the use of the "tracer principle," invented in 1913 by the Hungarian Georg de Hevesy, for which he was awarded the Nobel prize in 1943. Using the "tracer principle," Hevesy discovered that living organisms, including the human body, are characterized by a continual turnover of the chemical molecules that make up the body. In a healthy person, there is a delicate balance between the rate of formation and rate of breakdown of the chemical constituents of the body. This is called the "dynamic state of body constituents," the examination of which is the basis for the practice of nuclear medicine.

Most physicians who practice nuclear medicine have specialized in other fields, such as internal medicine, radiology, or pathology, prior to their entry into the specialty of nuclear medicine. Patients are referred to nuclear medicine specialists by other physicians who are responsible for the primary care of the patient. Because nuclear medicine is a referral practice, accurate communication between patient and physician, and between multiple physicians and others involved in patient care, is essential.

REQUISITIONS AND REPORTS

Two key vehicles for communication in nuclear medicine are the *requisition* by the refer-

ring physician for the examination(s) to be performed and the *report* of the study by the nuclear physician. Each plays an essential role in the care of the patient, because the referring physician knows more about the specific patient, while the nuclear physician knows more about the technology of nuclear medicine that is being used to care for the patient.

It is essential to have an effective system of communication between physicians who have the primary responsibility for the patient and the nuclear physician who is responsible for the performance and interpretation of the procedures. Requisitions and reports should be problem-oriented, concise, cogent, and complete, not diffuse, superficial, and fragmentary.

The first question is, "What do we want to know about the patient?" The next question is how nuclear medicine tests can help. Complex patient problems should be separated into individual components, and questions formulated that can be addressed by nuclear medicine procedures. After planning the studies, supervising their performance, and recording the results, the nuclear physician must then communicate the results to the referring physician in clear, understandable language.

It is essential that the requisition and report state clearly the patient's problem and the key information available prior to the nuclear medicine procedures. The referring physician should record all the possible diagnoses under consideration, and the probability of each. Initially, the nuclear physician should interpret the results of the nuclear medicine procedure without being aware of the prior information. This is done to achieve independence in the interpretation of the results. After this is done, all the available data are combined with the results of the nuclear medicine study, and a final interpretation is given. Both the unbiased and final diagnoses should be given in the report to the referring physician.

In the report, it is helpful to state clearly a description of the findings, as well as the interpretation of the results, which are expressed in terms of diseases, and the probability of each disease under consideration. A third component of the report is entitled "Comments," and includes any additional information the nuclear physician wants to provide. Qualifying statements about the interpretation are given in this section. Thus, the report to the referring physician is given in three parts:

1. Description. This information consists of both an objective and a subjective description of the findings.

2. Interpretation. This is limited to disease names and probabilities, together with a quantitative assessment of the degree of accuracy of the probability estimate.

3. Comment. This section includes qualifications, suggestions, and any other information that is to be conveyed to the referring physician.

In the interpretation, the first step is to judge the collected data in terms of reproducibility and precision. Then the reliable findings are listed in order of their importance in terms of sensitivity and specificity for different diseases. One or more central findings are selected, and the diseases in which these manifestations occur are listed. The final interpretation is based on selecting the single disease that best explains all the facts, or, if this is not possible, several diseases that account for the findings. Finally, all data are reviewed with the final interpretation in mind.

THE DIAGNOSTIC PROCESS

It is possible to give the results of tests, such as blood chemistry measurements, in absolute units such as millimoles per liter, but interpretation of the results of nuclear medicine procedures includes both quantitative data and subjective interpretations of the results. The latter often express the probability of a specific diagnosis as a percentage of certainty. For example, a report might state that by combining all the available data, there is a 90 per cent probability that the patient has pulmonary embolism.

In the practice of medicine, one must deal constantly with diagnoses that are not 100 per cent certain, and decisions must be made in the absence of complete certainty. The diagnostic process is said to be "probabilistic." The physician often expresses the results as the "most probable" diagnosis. As the diagnostic process proceeds for a given patient, there is a progressive increase in the certainty (probability) that the patient has one or more specific diseases. In the diagnostic process, it is helpful to distinguish between the patient's diagnosis and decisions regarding actions to be taken in the care of the patient.

At times, it will be necessary to get more information about the patient, that is, more tests or more observation of the course of the patient's illness. In other cases, the decision will be that the patient needs surgery or antibiotic or anticoagulant therapy.

A patient may be referred for nuclear medicine studies of the lung when the probability that the patient is suffering from the disease of acute pulmonary embolism is 70 per cent. This is called the "*a priori*" probability—that is, the probability of the diagnosis before the nuclear medicine examination is performed. The results of the lung scanning study may increase the probability of the diagnosis from 70 to 95 per cent (the "*a posteriori*" probability). This is a sufficiently high probability to permit the physician to decide to proceed with anticoagulant drug treatment. Figure 24–1 is an example of a lung study, and Figure 24–2 illustrates a patient undergoing a ventilation study of the lungs.

How certain does the physician have to be before proceeding? The degree of certainty that the physician must have before starting a specific treatment depends on the nature of the different courses of action that are possible. The physician must consider the gains to be made if the diagnosis is correct and the losses incurred if the diagnosis is wrong. For example, the diagnostic certainty would have to be almost 100 per cent before a patient would be operated upon for

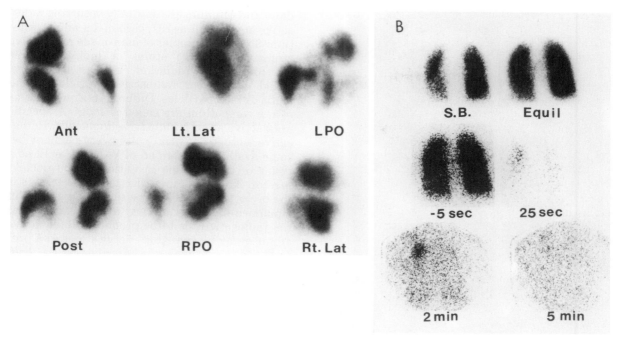

Figure 24–1

The lung study in a 64-year-old woman who had stopped working because she had become so short of breath that she had to stay in bed all day. The perfusion study (A) was performed with technetium (Tc-99m) microspheres and showed multiple large segmental defects in both lungs. The ventilation study (B) was performed by having the patient breathe xenon-133 gas, and it is normal except for a small region of retention of the gas in the left upper lung field. The interpretation of this study was a greater than 90 per cent probability of pulmonary embolism. The patient died two days later and an autopsy revealed large emboli in both lungs.

a brain tumor. On the other hand, the decision to treat the patient for a bacterial respiratory infection might be made when the diagnosis is less certain.

A physician cannot assume that a patient does *not* have a disease, such as pulmonary embolism, when there is still a probability of, say, 20 per cent that the patient has the disease. Before deciding what should be done, the physician must get more information about the patient, in order to lower or increase the likelihood that pulmonary embolism is the correct diagnosis. On the other hand, to wait for absolute certainty before acting may be unacceptable. For example, to wait until one is absolutely certain of the diagnosis of pulmonary embolism without beginning anticoagulant therapy might result in a subsequently fatal embolic episode.

HOW NUCLEAR MEDICINE STUDIES ARE PERFORMED

The patient is injected with a radiopharmaceutical, which is selected to examine a specific biochemical or physiologic process. As the radiopharmaceutical reacts in the chemical process under investigation, the radioactive atom emits gamma rays that are measured with radiation detection instruments. Computers then convert the measurements into "functional" or "biochemical" pictures of processes going on within the patient's body. Table 24–1 lists some radiopharmaceuticals used in nuclear medicine studies.

Radioactive *isotopes* are atoms of a given chemical type that emit gamma, beta, or alpha radiation in the process of *radioactive decay*. Ra-

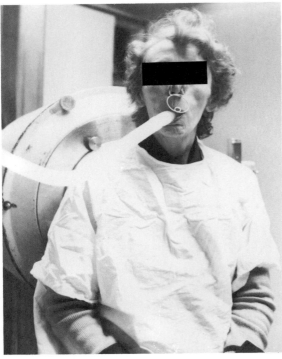

Figure 24-2
A patient undergoing a ventilation study of the lungs. The patient breathes the radioactive gas, xenon-133, and its entry and washout from the lungs are imaged with a gamma camera.

dium and uranium are naturally occurring radioactive atoms; iodine-131, carbon-11, and technetium-99m are examples of man-made radioactive atoms. Radioactive atoms or molecules emit electromagnetic radiation, similar to x-rays, called photons or radioactive particles, called alpha or beta particles. Different chemical forms of the same atom are called *isotopes*. A specific radioactive atom is called a *radionuclide*. Radioactive isotopes of practically every element became available at the end of World War II, as a result of the wartime invention of the nuclear reactor. Another source of radioactive tracers is the cyclotron, which can be turned on and off in a manner similar to an x-ray machine, whenever the radioactivity is to be produced. Radioactive atoms decay by changing energy states in a process, the rate of which is described by the *half-life* of the radionuclide. In the process of radioactive decay, a *parent radionuclide* decays to a *daughter*. Specific parent/daughter systems include the widely used technetium-99m daughter that is obtained from the parent molybdenum-99.

The basic unit of measurement for the dose of radioactivity given to a patient is the curie, named for Marie Curie who, with her husband Pierre, is celebrated as the codiscoverer of radioactivity and of the elements radium and polonium. Usual doses for diagnostic nuclear medicine

Table 24-1 ■ **Commonly Used Radiopharmaceuticals**

Organ System Imaged	Radiopharmaceutical	Abbreviation
Brain		
1. Planar imaging	Technetium-99m diethylenetriamine-pentaacetic acid	^{99m}Tc-DTPA
2. Positron emission tomography	Carbon-11 3-N-methylspiperone	^{11}C-NMSP
	Fluorine-18 2-fluoro-2-deoxyglucose	^{18}FDG
	Carbon-11 L-methionine	^{11}C-MET
	Nitrogen-13 ammonia	^{13}NH$_3$
	Carbon-11 carfentanil	^{11}C-CAR
	Gallium-68 ethylenediamine tetraacetic acid	^{68}Ga-EDTA
3. Single-photon emission	N-isopropyl-(^{123}I)-*p*-iodoamphetamine	^{123}IMP
Cerebral Spinal Fluid	Indium-111-diethylenetriaminepentaacetic acid	^{111}In-DTPA
Heart		
1. Myocardium	Thallium-201	^{201}Tl
2. Cardiac blood pool	Technetium-99m–labeled red blood cells	^{99m}Tc-RBCs
3. Myocardial infarction	1. Technetium-99m pyrophosphate	^{99m}Tc-PYP
	2. Indium-111 antimyosin antibodies	^{111}In-antimyosin Ab

Table 24–1 ▪ **Commonly Used Radiopharmaceuticals (*Continued*)**

Organ System Imaged	Radiopharmaceutical	Abbreviation
Lung		
1. Perfusion	Technetium-99m human serum albumin microspheres	^{99m}Tc-microspheres
2. Ventilation	Xenon-133	^{133}Xe
Thyroid	1. Technetium-99m pertechnetate	^{99m}TcO$_4^-$
	2. Sodium iodide-123	^{123}I
Metastatic survey	Iodine-131	^{131}I
Bone	Technetium-99m methylene diphosphonate	^{99m}Tc-MDP
Liver/Spleen	Technetium-99m sulfur colloid	^{99m}Tc-S-C
Reticuloendothelial System	Technetium-99m sulfur colloid	^{99m}Tc-S-C
Gastrointestinal		
Hepatobiliary	Technetium-99m 2, 6, diisopropylphenyl-carbamoyl-methyl-iminodiacetic acid	^{99m}Tc-disofenin (or diisopropyl IDA)
Gastroesophageal reflux	Technetium-99m sulfur colloid	^{99m}Tc-S-C
Esophageal emptying	1. Technetium-99m diethylenetriamine-pentaacetic acid	^{99m}Tc-DTPA
	2. Technetium-99m sulfur colloid	^{99m}Tc-S-C
Meckel's diverticulum	Technetium-99m pertechnetate	^{99m}TcO$_4^-$
Gastrointestinal bleeding	1. Technetium-99m sulfur colloid	^{99m}Tc-S-C
	2. Technetium-99m–labeled red blood cells	^{99m}Tc-RBCs
Kidney		
1. Function	Technetium-99m diethylenetriamine-pentaacetic acid	^{99m}Tc-DTPA
2. Cortex	Technetium-99m meso 2,3-dimercapto-succinic acid	^{99m}Tc-DMSA
3. Cystography	Technetium-99m pertechnetate	^{99m}TcO$_4^-$
Testes	Technetium-99m pertechnetate	^{99m}TcO$_4^-$
Soft Tissue (abscess or tumor)	Gallium-67	^{67}Ga
Shunts		
1. Le Veen's	Technetium-99m sulfur colloid	^{99m}Tc-S-C
2. Omaya's	Indium-111 diethylenetriamine-pentaacetic acid	^{111}In-DTPA
Salivary Glands	Technetium-99m pertechnetate	^{99n}TcO$_4^-$
Eyes	Technetium-99m pertechnetate	^{99m}TcO$_4^-$
Lymph Glands	Technetium-99m antimony trisulfide colloid	^{99m}Tc-Sb-C
Veins	Technetium-99m human serum albumin microspheres	^{99m}Tc-microspheres
Adrenals	Iodine-131 metaiodobenzylguanidine	^{131}I-MIBG

From Wagner, H. N., Jr., J. W. Buchanan, and D. Espinola-Vassalo. *Diagnostic Nuclear Medicine: Patient Studies.* Year Book Medical Publishers, Chicago, 1986, pp. 415–416.

studies are in millicuries, mCi (1/1000 of a curie) or microcuries, μCi (1/1,000,000 of a curie). The International Unit for expressing radioactivity is the becquerel, defined as one disintegration/second, and it may also be preceded by the milli or micro prefix.

Radiopharmaceuticals can be safely used in medical diagnosis because they disappear rapidly from the body by the process of radioactive decay. Table 24–2 lists the physical half-life of some radionuclides commonly used in nuclear medicine. Many radiopharmaceuticals also have short biologic half-lives, which means they are metabolized and excreted from the body quickly. The combination of the physical and biologic half-life determines the effective half-life of a radiopharmaceutical and the radiation burden to the patient. This is expressed in terms of rads, rems, grays, or sieverts.

DETECTION OF RADIOACTIVITY

The photons emitted from radionuclides are detected by means of simple radiation detectors, often called "probes," or by imaging devices, called cameras or scanners. Nuclear medicine physicians use two types of tests in the diagnosis of disease: *in vitro* (in the test tube) and *in vivo* (in the body) procedures (Figure 24–3). *In vitro* studies in nuclear medicine employ "well-type" radiation counting instruments, into which test tubes are inserted. For example, a radioimmunoassay (RIA) is an *in vitro* procedure that combines the use of radioactive chemicals and antibodies to detect hormones or drugs in a patient's blood.

Most *in vitro* studies in nuclear medicine are based on the use of iodine-125, carbon-14, tri-

Table 24–2 ■ Half-life of Medically Useful Radionuclides

Radionuclide	Half-Life	
^{11}C (carbon)	20.3	min
^{67}Ga (gallium)	78	hr
^{111}In (indium)	2.8	days
^{113m}In	100	min
^{123}I (iodine)	13.3	hr
^{131}I	8.05	days
^{59}Fe (iron)	45	days
^{15}O (oxygen)	124	sec
^{99m}Tc (technetium)	6	hr
^{201}Tl (thallium)	73	hr
^{133}Xe (xenon)	5.3	days

tium, or phosphorus-32. These radionuclides cannot be used for studies of living human beings. The type of radiation they emit—beta emissions—is not able to penetrate the human body and cannot be detected by external imaging devices. Studies with these radionuclides are limited to blood, urine, and feces. Examination of the organs of the living human body requires the use of radiotracers that emit photons that

NUCLEAR MEDICINE TESTS

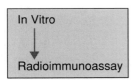

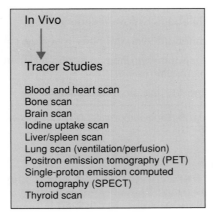

Figure 24–3

Nuclear medicine test: in vitro radioimmunoassay and in vivo trace studies. (From Chabner, Davi-Ellen. *The Language of Medicine,* 4th ed. W. B. Saunders Co., Philadelphia, 1991, p. 732.)

are emitted from radioactive atoms (radionuclides), which can be detected and measured by imaging devices called scanners or scintillation cameras. (The word "scintillation" is used because the radiation produces flashes of light in the process of being detected.)

In vivo tests trace the amount, distribution, and physiologic reactions of radioactive substances within the body. With the technology of nuclear medicine it is possible to examine the chemical reactions occurring within the cells of the body. Radioactive tracers, such as glucose, fatty acids, amino acids, peptides, and nucleic acids, make it possible to examine the growth and development of the organs of the body, their regeneration and repair when injured, and their response to drugs.

SPECT (single photon emission computed tomography) and PET (positron emission tomography) instruments are similar to computed tomography (CT) scanners or magnetic resonance imaging (MRI) devices, but they measure photons coming from decay of a radioactive tracer administered to the patient, rather than from x-rays going through the patient (CT) or radiowaves coming from the patient (MRI). In some cases the imaging detector rotates around the patient. At other times the large radiation detector is kept stationary, which is called planar imaging. Imaging "collimators" are lead devices used to detect only the photons coming from different parts of an organ. In most studies, computers are used to transform the emitted photons into pictures of the chemical reactions going on within the organs being examined. In some patients, large doses of radioactive substances are administered to decrease the rate of a chemical reaction. The classic example is the use of radioactive iodine to treat hyperthyroidism. Radioactive particles or antibodies are used to treat certain types of cancer.

TYPES OF NUCLEAR MEDICINE STUDIES

Among the most common diseases encountered by nuclear physicians are thyroid disease, cancer, and coronary artery disease. The general approach of nuclear medicine is to define normal regional function or biochemistry in normal persons, detect deviations from the normal, and characterize diseases in terms of how the findings differ from normal, using established statistical criteria. This "physiologic" approach is in contrast to the "ontologic" approach, which views disease, such as cancer, as something foreign that has invaded the body.

Modern data processing and analysis make it possible to interpret some of the results of nuclear medicine procedures objectively and express the results as numbers, as well as in the form of images. For example, hyperthyroidism is an increased rate of incorporation of iodine into the thyroid, where it is converted to abnormally increased amounts of the thyroid hormone thyroxine. In hypothyroidism, this reaction is abnormally low, and the patient has a deficiency of thyroxine. See Figure 24–4 for a report on radionuclide thyroid uptake and imaging.

Three types of studies are common: (1) measurement of the blood flow to organs such as the brain and heart; (2) measurement of the accumulation of substances that provide the energy required for all living systems; and (3) molecules involved in intercellular communication. The essence of nuclear medicine is *in vivo* chemistry. Table 24–3 lists studies performed in most nuclear medicine clinics.

Other imaging techniques (Figure 24–5), such as computed tomography (CT) and magnetic resonance imaging (MRI), define disease on the basis of abnormal structure. The anatomic detail obtained from these techniques provides structural detail often surpassing that seen by surgeons at the operating table.

Nuclear medicine techniques can be used to assess the effectiveness of surgical therapy, radiation therapy, and chemotherapy. They can document the extent of disease and the progression or regression in response to different forms of treatment. Such data permit modifications of the treatment plan sooner than can be determined by the clinical response of the patients or changes in the size of the abnormalities. Thus, treatment need no longer be based solely on clinical response, gross morphology of the lesions, and histopathologic examination of biopsy specimens. Biochemical characterization of abnormalities, such as cancer, is becoming a new method for classifying patients and for planning and monitoring their treatment.

DIAGNOSTIC RADIOLOGY GROUP, INC.
2388 Second Street
Baltimore, MD 21207-2178
301/986-4545

REPORT ON NUCLEAR MEDICINE EXAMINATION

Examination Date:	June 23, 1994	Patient:	Cooper, Janice
Date Reported:	June 23, 1994	Age:	43
Physician:	John Relf, M.D.	Hospital #:	80-22-56
		X-ray #:	652096

PROCEDURE: Radionuclide thyroid uptake and imaging.

COMPARISON: None.

TECHNIQUE: Twenty-four hours after the oral administration of 100 µCi of iodine-123, the uptake was calibrated. Following this, scintiphotos were obtained after the intravenous administration of 5 mCi of ^{99m}Tc-pertechnetate.

FINDINGS: The uptake at twenty-four hours is 15.8%. The normal range of uptake is 10-30%.

The scintiphotos demonstrate the thyroid gland to be normal in size, shape, and position, with a uniform distribution of the radionuclide.

CONCLUSION: NORMAL THYROID UPTAKE AND SCAN.

Thank you for referring this patient .

Radiologist_____
                    Evan M. Sanders, M.D.

EMS:ssd
D: 6/23/94
T: 6/23/94

Figure 24–4
A radionuclide thyroid uptake and imaging report.

DIAGNOSTIC RADIOLOGY GROUP, INC.
2388 Second Street
Baltimore, MD 21207-2178
301/986-4545

REPORT ON NUCLEAR MEDICINE EXAMINATION

Examination Date:	May 14, 1994	Patient:	Skinner, Mark
Date Reported:	May 14, 1994	Age:	32
Physician:	John Relf, M.D.	Hospital #:	80-88-23
		X-ray #	642976

PROCEDURE: Radionuclide whole body bone imaging.

COMPARISON: None.

TECHNIQUE: Scintiphotos were obtained after the intravenous administration of 20 mCi of technetium MDP-99m.

FINDINGS: The scintiphotos demonstrate a normal distribution of radionuclide. There were no focal abnormalities.

CONCLUSION: NORMAL RADIONUCLIDE WHOLE BODY BONE IMAGING.

Thank you for referring this patient.

Radiologist_____
                Evan M. Sanders, M.D.

EMS:ssd
D: 5/14/94
T: 5/14/94

Figure 24–5
A radionuclide whole body bone imaging report.

Table 24–3 ▪ Nuclear Medicine Studies

Cardiovascular

Right and left ventricular function
Myocardial perfusion
Myocardial infarction
Myocardial inflammation
Shunt quantification

Central Nervous System

Blood brain barrier integrity
Regional cerebral blood flow
Regional cerebral blood volume
Cisternography
CSF leak
CSF shunt patency
Regional cerebral glucose metabolism
Regional cerebral oxygen metabolism

Endocrine

Thyroid structure and function
Thyroid metastatic survey
Adrenal imaging

Gastrointestinal

Esophageal function
Gastroesophageal reflux
Fat absorption
Gallbladder function (hepatobiliary)
Gastrointestinal bleeding
Gastric emptying
LeVeen shunt patency
Liver and spleen imaging
Meckel's diverticulum

Genitourinary

Renal blood flow and function
Renal function mass

Vesicoureteral reflux
Effective renal plasma flow
Glomerular filtration rate
Testicular blood flow

Hematopoietic System

Bone marrow phagocytic function
In vivo cross-match
Platelet survival and sequestration
Volume — red cell
Volume — plasma
Radioiron kinetics
Splenic sequestration
Vitamin B_{12} absorption

Inflammatory Process and Tumor Imaging

Gallium-67 accumulation
Leukocyte accumulation

Miscellaneous

Lacrimal duct patency
Lymphoscintigraphy
Salivary gland function
Skin ulcer healing
Venography

Respiratory

Perfusion
Ventilation
Aerosol clearance
Pulmonary aspiration

Skeletal

Bone blood flow
Bone metabolic activity

Reference Sources

Freeman, Leonard M. (Ed.). *Freeman and John-son's Clinical Radionuclide Imaging,* Volume 3 update, 3rd edition. Grune & Stratton, New York, 1986.

Maisey, M. H., K. E. Britton, and D. L. Gilday (Eds.). *Clinical Nuclear Medicine,* 2nd edition. J. B. Lippincott, Philadelphia, 1991.

Wagner, H. N., Jr., J. W. Buchanan and D. Espinola-Vassallo. *Diagnostic Nuclear Medicine: Patient Studies.* Year Book Medical Publishers, Chicago, 1986.

For references of specific application to medical transcription, see Appendix 1.

Morgan L. Morgan, M.D.

Obstetrics and Gynecology

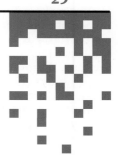

INTRODUCTION

Obstetrics and gynecology (Ob-Gyn) is a combined specialty concerning primarily the general and reproductive health of women. Etymologically speaking, obstetrics originates from the Latin term *obstetrix* for midwife. It is defined as pertaining to the care and treatment of women in childbirth (parturition) and during the period before and after the delivery (*Random House Dictionary of the English Language,* Random House, New York, 1987). *Gyneco* is a Greek root meaning female or denoting relationship to women or to the female reproductive organs. Gynecology is the field of medicine that deals with the health maintenance and diseases of women, especially the reproductive organs.

In the early days of this country, these two disciplines were combined under the purview of the professors of anatomy and surgery. By the beginning of the 19th century, the combined specialties of obstetrics, gynecology, and pediatrics were beginning to be separated from the overall category of surgery. The separation process began with obstetrics, then late in the 1800s gynecology began to stand alone. Pediatrics was defined as a separate entity early in the 20th century.

Residency training programs for the combined disciplines increased in number in the early 1900s, and the establishment of the American Board of Obstetrics and Gynecology in 1930 marked the final merger of obstetrics and gynecology into a major specialty.

The explosion of knowledge, technology, and improving surgical techniques has continued the process of subspecialization. After a 4-year residency in obstetrics and gynecology, specialists may continue and take fellowships in the subspecialties of maternal-fetal health (perinatology, or high-risk obstetrics), reproductive endocrinology, gynecologic oncology (surgery and treatment of cancer of the reproductive organs), and possibly in the future gynecologic urology and pediatric gynecology.

As a result of the rapid changes that are occurring in social and governmental policies concerning the health care field, specialists in obstetrics and gynecology are now being viewed as primary care physicians for the female population — the only medical specialty devoted to one gender.

OBSTETRICS

Obstetrics concerns all aspects of human reproduction from development, sexuality, and fertility to family planning. It is "the branch of medicine that deals with parturition, its antecedents, and its sequels" (*Oxford English Dictionary,* Oxford University Press, 1933). The role of the obstetrician is to promote psychologic, physical, and emotional health within families of childbearing age, to improve quality and help govern quantity of offspring, and to seek to ensure a happy and healthy outcome using the art, current state of knowledge, and technology available.

A thorough understanding of female embryologic development, anatomy, and reproductive physiology is essential to physicians in this specialty. Parts A and B of Figure 25–1 illustrate the basic components of the female reproductive anatomy. Errors of development can lead to anatomic abnormalities and functional disturbances of the sex organs. The onset of puberty signals beginning ovarian function. Breast budding, development of internal and external genitalia, hair growth, and change in the body habitus to that of the adult female, usually with a growth spurt, accompanies the onset of menstruation (menarche). In the United States, this is normally between the ages of 10 and 15 years.

The early years of menstruation are characterized by irregular, heavy (menorrhagia), and frequently infertile (anovulatory) periods. With the onset of ovulation, the menses become regular and may be painful (dysmenorrhea). Conception is possible, and family planning education is helpful in preventing unwanted pregnancies.

Understanding the monthly cycle and the time in the cycle when ovulation is most apt to occur (about 14 days before the next menstrual period [MP]) is essential to knowing when conception can occur. Contraceptive measures, e.g., rhythm, withdrawal, simple barrier techniques (condom, foam, diaphragm), pharmacologic methods (oral

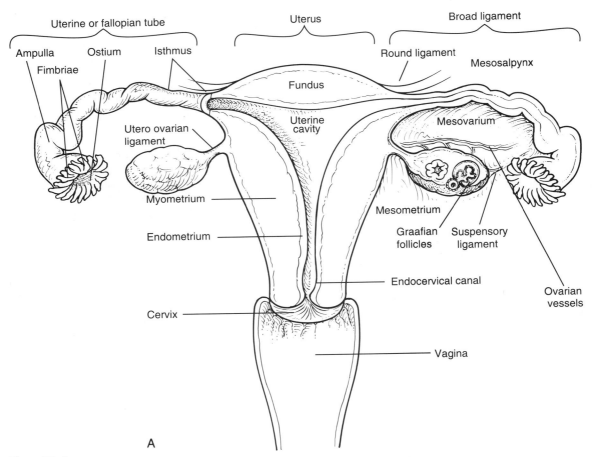

Figure 25–1
A, Anterior view of the female reproductive system. *B,* Lateral view of the organs of the female reproductive system.

contraceptives, Norplant system—subdermal tubes filled with progesterone), and intrauterine devices (IUDs) are covered in this learning process.

When pregnancy is desired, the obstetrician instructs the patient in good health practices and ways to aid and promote the conception process. When a pregnancy is achieved, the obstetrician begins the 9-month education process, training, and care of the gravid woman (Figures 25–2 and 25–3).

The average human gestation lasts about 280 days (40 weeks) from the first day of the last normal menstrual period (LMP). Application of this rule gives the estimated date of confinement (EDC), or due date. Prenatal visits to the physician are usually at 4-week intervals until 32 weeks (Figure 25–4). Then they are every 2 weeks until 36 weeks and then weekly until delivery. Initially, the patient's blood is tested for type and Rh factor as well as for evidence of previous infectious diseases (rubella, syphilis, hepatitis, herpes, AIDS), anemia, and diseases of the fetus. The patient is monitored for weight gain, blood pressure, growth of the uterus, kidney function, and any other problems that might arise. Generally, the fetal heart can be heard by assisted means at the 10- to 12-week stage, and fetal movement can be felt by the mother at 18 to 20 weeks. It is common practice for the patient to have her first ultrasound examination (US, or scan) at between 15 and 20 weeks. During this important examination, a woman will learn whether she is having one or more babies

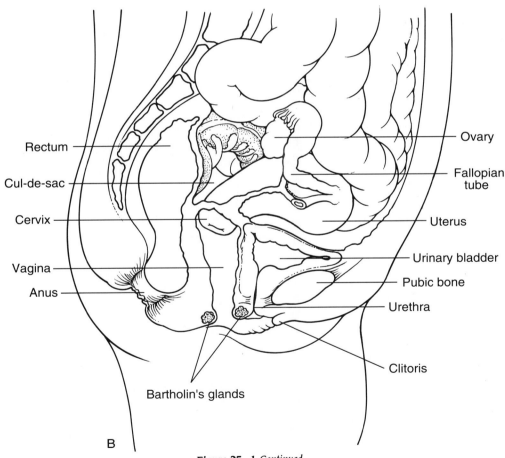

B

Figure 25–1 Continued

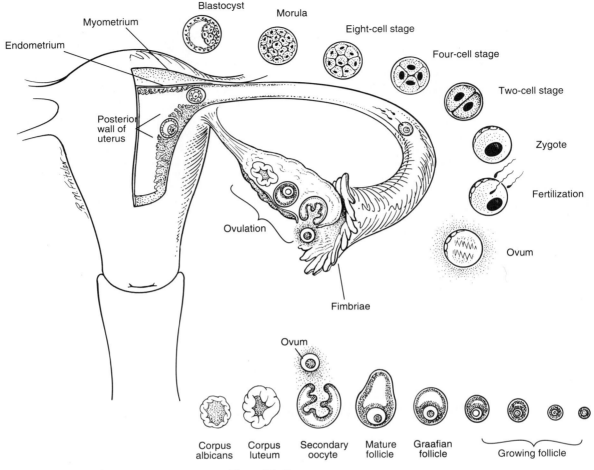

Figure 25–2
Implantation of the embryo.

and the calendar dates will be confirmed with the developmental level of the fetus to further refine the EDC. Anomalies may or may not be apparent at this stage. A second US is frequently done about the 32nd week to determine whether the fetus is developing as expected and whether growth is consistent with the gestational age. Anomalous organs of the fetus are often observable at this time. For information on congenital birth defects, see Chapter 31, Pediatrics.

DISORDERS OF PREGNANCY

During this 40-week pregnancy, the woman is subject to all the familiar health problems that face the nongravid population plus the diseases peculiar to pregnancy. This means that the obstetrician might encounter trauma, infection, system disease, cancer, psychologic dysfunction, problems of abnormal pregnancies, and spontaneous abortion (SAB), as well as unwanted preg-

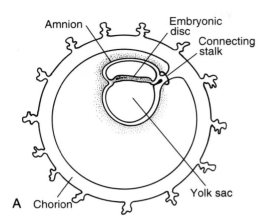

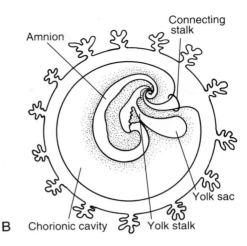

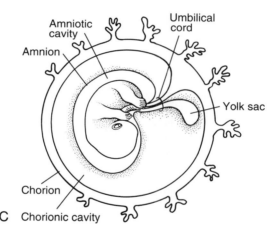

Figure 25–3

Placenta and membranes (chorion and amnion). Development at *A*, three weeks, *B*, four weeks, and *C*, 20 weeks.

nancies. With the advent of antenatal genetic testing, the physician deals with a whole set of potential problems, e.g., amniocentesis and chorionic villi sampling (CVS).

Commonly, the obstetrician encounters simple anemia, respiratory infections, flu, gastroenteritis, cystitis, hyperemesis gravidarum (nausea and vomiting of pregnancy), skin rashes, and allergies. Occasionally, the physician deals with life-threatening illnesses. A relatively common

problem (1:200 pregnancies) is ectopic pregnancy, which implies that the pregnancy is not in its normal location within the uterus but is somewhere else. Often it is found in a fallopian tube (oviduct), which may rupture, causing internal hemorrhage necessitating surgery. About 15 to 20 per cent of all pregnancies are lost in the first trimester by "natural" causes. When a woman begins to bleed in the first weeks of a pregnancy, she is said to be threatening to abort

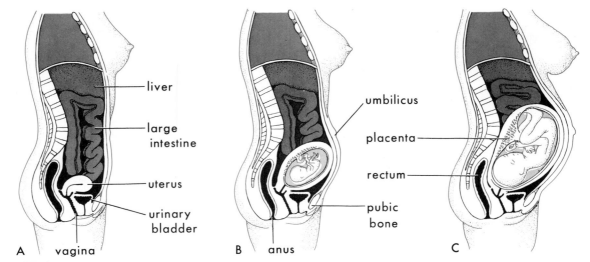

Figure 25-4

Developmental growth of the fetus. *A*, Sagittal sections of a nonpregnant woman; *B*, a woman 20 weeks pregnant; and *C*, a woman 30 weeks pregnant. (From Moore, K. L. *The Developing Human; Clinically Oriented Embryology*, 4th ed. W. B. Saunders Co., Philadelphia, 1988, p. 114.)

(thr. ab.), known to the lay person as a miscarriage. Since 20 to 25 per cent of all women have some vaginal bleeding early in the pregnancy, this is usually cause for great alarm. If the bleeding becomes heavy and there is passage of tissue, it is called an incomplete abortion (inc. ab.). When the entire pregnancy is passed, it then becomes a complete abortion. About 65 per cent of all cases of spontaneous abortion are handled by simple means. One third of aborting patients require a surgical procedure called a dilation and curettage (D & C) to empty the uterine cavity and prevent hemorrhage and infection from developing (Figure 25-5). When a woman chooses to terminate her pregnancy, it is referred to as a therapeutic abortion (TAB).

Other severe problems occurring during pregnancy may involve intra-abdominal surgery (e.g., appendectomy, ovarian cystectomy, myomectomy), cardiac surgery, surgical reduction of fractures, and even brain surgery. In a well-established pregnancy, the fetus is generally very

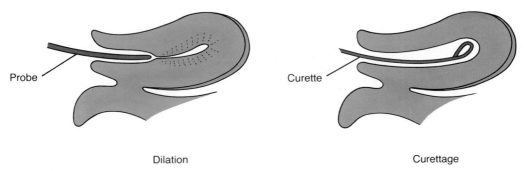

Dilation   Curettage

Figure 25-5

Dilation and curettage. (From Chabner, D. E. *The Language of Medicine*. W. B. Saunders Co., Philadelphia, 1991.)

strong and able to withstand the effects of these disorders and, with proper care, may not abort. When the illness is outside the scope of the obstetrician's expertise, the physician refers the patient to an appropriate specialist or perinatologist or both for consultation and care.

A common medical illness peculiar to pregnancies is gestational diabetes mellitus (GDM), which may result in increased fetal wastage and complications of delivery. Pregnancy-induced hypertension (PIH), known in the past as toxemia or preeclampsia, produces a cluster of signs and symptoms centering on elevated blood pressure, edema (swelling of the tissues), and passage of protein in the urine (proteinuria). If not treated aggressively, this condition may end in loss of the fetus and cause seizures with increased risk of maternal morbidity and mortality. The ultimate treatment is delivery of the fetus.

Obstetric complications include preterm labor (PTL), third-trimester bleeding, and diseases of fetal growth. PTL occurs in about 7 to 10 per cent of all pregnancies and is an enormous cost to the public in both economic and emotional terms. Currently, research is directing attention to the role of intra-amniotic infection and the ability to monitor uterine activity at home. Tocolytic drugs are being employed with increasing frequency to try to quiet the abnormal uterine activity.

Third-trimester bleeding may occur in 2 to 5 per cent of all pregnancies. Because of its potential for serious complications, this bleeding must be accurately diagnosed. The two most urgent problems are placenta previa* and placental abruption. In placenta previa, the placenta partially or totally covers the opening, or internal os, of the uterine cervix (Figure 25–6). The effacement (thinning out) and dilation process may cause the placenta to tear loose and cause severe bleeding. The obstruction of the cervical opening by the placenta may prevent the fetus from passing through.

Abruptio placenta (placental separation, placental abruption) may be of varying degrees from small to total. It may lead to minor complications or to fetal and maternal death. One of the most common complications is severe hem-

---

*Previa means before or in the front of.

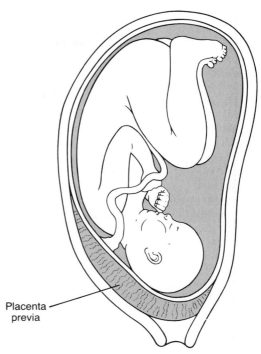

Placenta previa

Figure 25–6
Placenta previa. (From Chabner, D. E. *The Language of Medicine.* W. B. Saunders Co., Philadelphia, 1991.)

orrhage with vascular collapse. Prompt diagnosis is of the utmost importance. Ultrasound has been a vital addition to the diagnosis of both these problems

In the past, the fetus was considered beyond the obstetrician's grasp to treat or influence in any but a general way. Today, fetal diagnosis is commonplace, and fetal treatment is becoming more frequent. With the advent of ultrasound and amniocentesis, the role of the geneticist is established on the clinical team. Fetal blood sampling is now done, and the first steps in surgically treating the fetus in utero have been taken. Ultrasound allows the physician to identify the fetus at risk for intrauterine growth retardation (IUGR), large for gestational age (LGA) fetus, and abnormalities of presentation or position, e.g., breech or occiput posterior.

The electronic fetal monitor (EFM) has brought great change. The obstetrician can test the fetus, in essence ask the fetus how it feels about the intrauterine conditions it finds itself in, by means of nonstress testing (NST) or contraction stress testing (CST). These tests, plus the biophysical profile, may identify the fetus that must be delivered at an early date from those allowed to continue in utero. Continuous fetal monitoring is nearly universal in the labor rooms of the United States. This allows for constant attention to fetal cardiac activity and continuous tracing of the fetal heart rate in relation to uterine contractions.

Normal labor is heralded by the appearance of rhythmic uterine contractions that generally begin far apart and get steadily closer together and stronger in intensity. In the latter weeks of a normal pregnancy, the uterus is frequently irritable and subject to irregular contractions that sometimes can be quite painful. These contractions are called false labor or Braxton-Hicks contractions. At times, it is difficult to differentiate true from false labor patterns.

When the contractions occur at 5- to 10- minute intervals and last 40 to 60 seconds, the patient is admitted to the labor and delivery room for evaluation. Her vital signs are checked and she is placed on a fetal monitor to establish fetal well-being and uterine activity. Her cervix is checked for effacement, dilation, station of the presenting part, and state of the membranes, i.e., ruptured or unruptured. If she is in labor, she will be admitted to the hospital and prepared for labor and ultimate delivery.

First labors normally last 12 to 16 hours, and subsequent labors are usually about 6 to 8 hours in length. Most women are trained in some method of prepared childbirth, e.g., LaMaze, to diminish fear and allow them to control natural reflexes to pain. Epidural block is a popular anesthesia for the labor and delivery process.

Labor is divided into three stages: the first stage is from the onset of labor to full dilation; the second stage is from complete dilation to delivery of the fetus (usually from 1 to 3 hours); the third stage begins after the delivery of the baby and ends with the expulsion of the placenta.

Dystocia (difficult labor) is a relatively common problem encountered by the obstetrician. It may be a result of poor uterine contractions or weak expulsive forces on the part of the mother. It is also associated with a large fetus in a small pelvis, abnormal presentation of the fetus, and contractures of the maternal bony pelvis. Dysto-

cia is one of the most common causes of cesarean* section (C-section) birth, usually described as cephalopelvic disproportion or failure to progress.

When labor contractions weaken or cease, augmentation of labor becomes necessary. This is frequently done by the intravenous administration of oxytocin, a substance that stimulates strong uterine contractions. This method is also used to induce labor in women for medical or obstetric reasons before natural labor begins.

OPERATIVE OBSTETRICS

An episiotomy (surgical incision of the perineum) is frequently done to prevent injury to the maternal pelvic floor and vaginal lacerations. It also hastens the delivery of the fetus. This shortens the time of extreme pressure on the fetal head.

Operative obstetrics is concerned with the use of instruments to facilitate delivery of the fetus. The instruments commonly used are forceps or the vacuum extraction device. Outlet forceps are used to ease the head out from a low position in the birth canal. This occurs often in conjunction with an epidural block when the mother is unable to push effectively. Forceps are employed to overcome dystocias caused by a "tight fit," and specialized forceps are used for rotating the head at a higher station in the pelvis. Sometimes the obstetrician's hand is the instrument of choice when manual rotation of the fetal head is needed to allow descent and delivery of the fetus.

Delivery by cesarean section has become more frequent and accounts for approximately 20 to 25 per cent of all deliveries. The common reasons for cesarean section are fetopelvic disproportion, failure to progress, fetal distress, abnormal presentation (breech), multiple gestation, and maternal infection, e.g., amnionitis or herpes simplex vulvitis (Figure 25–7). Previous cesarean section is no longer an automatic reason to do a repeat section, and vaginal birth after cesarean section (VBAC) is performed successfully in this country in over 60 per cent of cases.

*Optional spellings: caesarean, cesarian, caesarian.

The Puerperium ▪ The puerperium is defined as the 6-week period after delivery. It is a time in which the body literally puts away the baby-making equipment for another day and readjusts itself to the nonpregnant state. Historically, it was a time of danger when the new mother was at risk for postpartum hemorrhage and infection. (Puerperal fever caused the death of many women before Oliver Wendell Holmes and Ignaz Philipp Semmelweis persuaded the profession that precautions of cleanliness could dramatically lower the incidence of this dread disease.) Other problems encountered are breast engorgement, urinary tract infection (pyelonephritis), and postpartum depression. Six weeks after delivery, most women have returned to their normal status. In the nursing mother, the menstrual cycle may not recur until she has stopped breast feeding. However, the majority of women begin their cycle within 3 to 6 months of delivery. Non-nursing mothers usually have their first period within 6 to 12 weeks.

GYNECOLOGY

It is estimated that obstetric and gynecologic problems account for 20 per cent of all female visits to the physician's office. The largest number of these visits are for contraception, pregnancy detection, prenatal care, common genital infections, abnormal menses, sex counseling, and hormonal replacement in the menopausal woman.

History and Physical Examination

The gynecologist begins by obtaining a thorough history, performing a complete physical examination, and doing appropriate laboratory studies, e.g., Papanicolaou smear (Pap smear), urinalysis, and microscopic examination of any unusual discharge. The history begins with the chief complaint that caused her to seek help and is expanded in detail with questions regarding the present illness in terms of pain, fever, nausea/vomiting, abnormal bleeding or discharge, and so forth. The gynecologic history covers menstrual history, sexual activity, sexually transmitted diseases (STDs), and contraceptive use. A pregnancy history is also obtained.

The past history is discussed, including illnesses, surgical history, current medications, allergies to medicines, injuries, and smoking, alcohol, and drug habits. A review of systems is important to define system disease, and a family history is necessary to uncover possible hereditary disorders.

The physical examination begins with vital signs and an overall evaluation of the patient's state of health and is completed by a thorough study of all organ systems. On subsequent visits, the areas of chief concern are examined.

For the gynecologist, the pelvic examination is the main point of interest. It must be done in a calm, professional manner with proper concern for the sensitivities of the patient. At first, the external organs are visually examined for hair distribution, clitoral size, lesions, inflammation, and discharge. A warmed speculum is used to open the vagina and expose the cervix. A Papanicolaou (Pap) smear is obtained from the endocervical canal and portio vaginalis of the cervix. When withdrawing the speculum, the vaginal walls are carefully observed for any abnormalities, and appropriate samples are taken from vaginal secretions for study under the microscope and for culture.

The physician then performs a bimanual examination of the internal genitalia (uterus, tubes, ovaries, ligaments, and cul-de-sac) with a finger in the vagina and the fingers of the other hand on the lower abdomen. The physician should be able to determine the status of pelvic support, size and mobility of the uterus, enlargements (cysts and solid tumors) or fixation (inflammatory reaction or adhesion formation) of the adnexal structures, and the elasticity of the support structures. Determination of the presence or absence of pelvic floor relaxations, i.e., cystocele, rectocele, and enterocele, is also made.

The rectovaginal examination is important to elucidate a mass in the rectum, blood in the stool, and the state of the cul-de-sac. This is the pouch behind the uterus and vagina and anterior to the rectum, where fluids, blood, and pus, for example, will collect.

Normal ovarian function is responsible for orderly progression of female development and a predictable menstrual cycle. Gonadotropin-releasing hormones (GnRH) produced by the hypothalamus in the midportion of the brain stimulate the anterior pituitary to secrete

COMMUNITY HOSPITAL
1234 Main Street
Ventura, CA 93003-1000

OPERATIVE REPORT

Patient: Neema B. Brown
Surgeon: Carlotta F. LaMacchia, M. D.
Assistant Surgeon: Kia Ann Kim
Circulator: Athena K. Onassis, R. N.

Date: 7/18/94
Record # 439078-03

PREOPERATIVE DIAGNOSIS:
1. Intrauterine pregnancy at 41 1/2 weeks, post dates.
2. Fetal macrosomia.
3. Possible early labor.
4. Unengaged fetal head.

POSTOPERATIVE DIAGNOSES:
1. Intrauterine pregnancy at 41 1/2 weeks, post dates.
2. Fetal macrosomia.
3. Possible early labor.
4. Unengaged fetal head.
5. Meconium

OPERATION: Primary low transverse cervical cesarean section.

FINDINGS: The cervix was dilated less than 1 cm, 50 to 60% effaced, with the fetal vertex out of the pelvis. On entry into the abdomen, there was a moderate amount of intraperitoneal straw-colored fluid. Lower uterine segment was markedly thinned out and the bladder flap was normal. The intrauterine examination was normal. There were several scattered small subserosal fibroids on the uterus, none larger than 0.5 cm. The rest of the intra-abdominal exploration was normal.

PROCEDURE: Under satisfactory epidural anesthesia, with the patient prepped and draped in the usual manner, the abdomen was opened through a Pfannenstiel incision and the above findings noted. A bladder flap was developed and reflected inferiorly and a transverse elliptical incision was made in the lower uterine segment. Membranes were ruptured and there was marked meconium staining of the fluid. The fetal head was delivered and the neonatologist was able to perform DeLee suction of the infant prior to delivery.

The baby was then delivered, with stat cry and respiration. He was a male infant weighing 9 pounds, 13 ounces, and he had Apgars of 9 at 1 minute and 9 at 5 minutes. Cord blood was obtained. The placenta was delivered spontaneously

(continued)

Figure 25–7

An operative report of a cesarean section, typed in indented format.

Page 2
Patient: Neema B. Brown
Record # 439078-03

and the uterus was exteriorized. The interior of the uterus was cleansed with a dry sponge and the cervix probed.

The uterine incision was closed in two layers, the first of an #0 chromic interrupted suture, followed by a continuous #0 chromic inverting the first layer. An extra figure-of-eight suture was used at the midpoint of the wound for hemostasis. On completion of these two sutures, the uterine incision was dry to inspection. The bladder flap was closed with a continuous #0 chromic suture and blood and clots were then suctioned from the pelvis. The uterus was returned to its normal position.

The parietal peritoneum was closed with a continuous #0 chromic suture. The fascia was closed with interrupted #0 Vicryl. All bleeders were tied with #000 chromic free-tie and the fat was closed with interrupted #000 chromic sutures. The skin was closed with staples and Steri-Strips. Sponge and needle counts were reported as correct. The patient tolerated the procedure well. The estimated blood loss was approximately 400 to 500 cc. There was no replacement.

Carlotta F. LaMacchia, M. D.

mtf
D: 7-18-94
T: 7-19-94

Figure 25–7 Continued

the gonadotropins: follicle-stimulating hormone (FSH) and luteinizing hormone (LH). These two hormones act on the ovaries, causing ovulation to occur, and force them to produce the sex hormones, estrogen and progesterone. The latter causes the lining tissue of the uterus to respond in a cyclic fashion.

The first 14 days of a 28-day cycle are characterized by estrogen production. This causes growth of the endometrium and is called the proliferative phase. Generally, ovulation occurs on day 14, and the now empty follicle becomes a functioning gland that produces progesterone (pregnancy hormone). Progesterone prepares the endometrium for implantation of a new pregnancy on day 21 and causes endometrial changes that are called the secretory phase. If conception does not occur, the production of es-

trogen and progesterone falls and a menstrual period begins (Figure 25–8).

Gynecologic Disorders ■ Ovarian dysfunction may be characterized by primary or secondary amenorrhea, dysfunctional uterine bleeding (menometrorrhagia), or infrequent menses (oligomenorrhea). Primary ovarian dysfunction may be caused by chromosomal disorders, gonadal dysgenesis, surgical removal, and irradiation effects, and other causes and menses never begin. Secondary ovarian dysfunction may be caused by hormonal abnormalities, infectious diseases, stress, eating disorders (e.g., anorexia nervosa), excessive athletic training, and drugs and may cause a previously functional woman to cease having periods.

The yearly Pap smear has reduced the incidence of cervical cancer enormously. This cancer

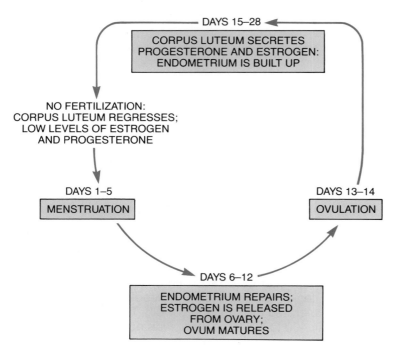

Figure 25–8

The menstrual cycle. (From Chabner, D. E. *The Language of Medicine*. W. B. Saunders Co., Philadelphia, 1991.)

was the most common of female cancers; 2 to 3 per cent of women could be expected to die from it. Today about 20 per cent of the Pap smears collected will be reported as abnormal. The vast majority of these are minimally abnormal and fall into the new classification of abnormal squamous cells of undetermined significance, corresponding to the old Class II smear. Mild infections are frequently the cause of these abnormal smears. Less than 5 per cent are reported as high-grade squamous intraepithelial lesions (SIL). These are studied with the colposcope, a magnifying instrument, and biopsies are frequently taken of the worst-appearing areas. The most commonly reported abnormality today is infection with the human papilloma virus (HPV). Certain types of the HPV virus may be a high-risk factor for developing cancer of the cervix at some future date. Older terms for describing cervical abnormalities are dysplasia, cervical intraepithelial neoplasia (CIN I to III), carcinoma in situ (CIS), and invasive cancer of the cervix. Few women will develop invasive cancer if they have regular smears and have follow-up treatment for irregular smears. When the diagnosis has been determined by colposcopic examination and biopsy, treatment is usually either expectant observation and waiting, cryosurgery (freezing), or conization biopsy of the transformation zone of the cervix (Figure 25–9). The latter procedure is frequently performed in the gynecologist's office with an electrosurgical device called large loop excision of the transformation zone (LLETZ) or loop electrosurgical excision procedure (LEEP). For further information on Pap smear classifications, see Chapter 21, Laboratory Medicine.

Abnormal Bleeding and Pain ▪ One of the most common complaints encountered by the gynecologist is abnormal vaginal bleeding. Causes are lesions of the vulva, vagina, and cervix, endometrial polyps, fibroid tumors of the uterus, hormonal abnormalities, oral contraception breakthrough bleeding, and systemic diseases. An endometrial biopsy or D&C is very important in the diagnosis of the various causes of abnormal uterine bleeding. It may be combined with a procedure called hysteroscopy. A hysteroscope allows the gynecologist to view the interior of the uterus on a video monitor and then biopsy the areas of greatest interest. The D&C is better than 95 per cent effective in diag-

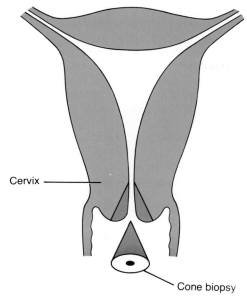

Cervix

Cone biopsy

Figure 25-9

Conization. (From Chabner, D. E. *The Language of Medicine.* W. B. Saunders Co., Philadelphia, 1991.)

nosing the problem and is therapeutic in approximately 60 per cent of the cases of abnormal bleeding.

Pelvic pain is a common complaint; some of the gynecologic conditions commonly associated with pain are described next.

Dysmenorrhea ▪ Dysmenorrhea, or painful periods (cramps), brings many patients to the gynecologist's office. Usually these are "physiologic" in that no pelvic disease is observable. It is thought that the primary cause is the overproduction of a substance of the prostaglandin family that causes the myometrium to contract in a strong and prolonged manner. Painful periods can also be associated with uterine myomas (fibroids) and adenomyosis uteri.

Dyspareunia ▪ Dyspareunia, or painful intercourse, is another commonly encountered problem. No apparent cause may be found, or it may be associated with psychologic disturbances or previously mentioned pelvic disorders.

Premenstrual Tension Syndrome ▪ PMS is a cluster of annoying-to-disabling symptoms associated with the menses in an appreciable number of women. It is characterized by sensations of bloating, cramping, breast tenderness,

difficulty in dealing with stressful events, and emotional irritability and instability. The cause is perplexing, and the condition can be characterized by salt and fluid retention. Treatments aimed at correcting this imbalance are often successful.

Vulvitis and Vaginitis ▪ Vulvitis and vaginitis may be the result of vulvar, vaginal, or urinary infection, allergic reaction, trauma, poor hygiene, and chemical irritations. The patient may experience swelling and inflammation of the tissues and abnormal vaginal discharge. The three most common causes for these disorders are vaginal yeast infections (vaginal candidiasis), trichomoniasis, and nonspecific vaginitis. These infections are easily diagnosed and treated. A dilemma is that familiar symptoms can be experienced by a patient with a serious disease, and she may medicate herself inappropriately and lose valuable time in obtaining the correct treatment. In the menopausal or postmenopausal patient, atrophic changes caused by a lack of estrogen may cause the genital tissues to become weakened in their response to common organisms. The vulvar and vaginal lining will respond nicely to an estrogen creme in most cases.

Cervicitis ▪ Although not usually a source of pelvic pain, cervicitis is indirectly related in that is it often associated with vaginitis.

Acute Salpingitis ▪ Acute salpingitis, or pelvic inflammatory disease (PID), is an infection of the tubes, ovaries, endomyometrium, and supporting structures. Generally, it is caused by an ascending infection by *Chlamydia trachomatis* or *Neisseria gonorrhoeae* contracted through sexual intercourse. It can be mild and easily treated in the ambulatory patient, or it can be severe and may require hospitalization and surgery. In its chronic form, it can be an ongoing source of pain and reinfection and may become life threatening, requiring removal of the pelvic organs.

Endometriosis ▪ Endometriosis and adenomyosis uteri is another commonly encountered, painful disease of the female reproductive organs. In this condition, endometrial tissue is displaced to areas of the body other than the interior of the uterus; in adenomyosis, the aberrant tissue is in the muscular wall of the uterus itself. It behaves like a tissue transplant and continues to respond to the rise and fall of the female hormones wherever it is attached. This tissue will respond on a cyclic basis and bleed once a month. Over a period of time, it will cause the surrounding tissues to react by forming scar tissue or adhesions and possibly solid or cystic tumors of other intra-abdominal organs (Figure 25–10). Examples of a history and physical examination, as well as an operative report for a patient with endometriosis, can be seen in Figures 25–11 and 25–12.

Pain from other organ systems may bring the patient to the gynecologist's office, and these specialists are often the first to diagnose disorders of the urinary and intestinal tracts.

Uterine and Ovarian Tumors ■ Abnormal bleeding, pain, and abdominal enlargement are the common reasons that lead the patient to the physician and the ultimate diagnosis of uterine fibroid tumors called fibromyomata (Figure 25–13), or ovarian tumors (cystic or solid). Fibroid tumors can vary in size from very small to the dimensions of a basketball. They can be single or multiple. They may be symptomatic, causing bleeding disorders, pain, or abnormalities of other organ functions, or totally asymptomatic. About one per thousand has malignant potential. Fibroids are one of the most common indicators for hysterectomy. In women wishing to retain child-bearing function, myomectomy for removing only the tumors is the operation of choice. Usually, these patients are delivered by

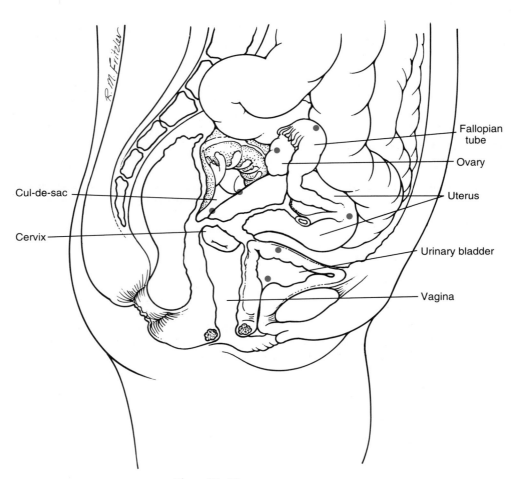

Figure 25–10
Locations of endometrial implants.

COMMUNITY HOSPITAL
1234 Main Street
Ventura, CA 93003-1000

HISTORY AND PHYSICAL

NAME: O'Brien, Brenna M.

MEDICAL RECORD # 9543-587   ADMISSION DATE: 6-20-94

REASON FOR ADMISSION:
This is a 43-year-old Caucasian female whose chief complaint is chronic pelvic
pain and abnormally heavy periods.

HISTORY OF PRESENT ILLNESS:
The patient is gravida 1, para 1, AB 0, whose last normal menstrual period was
approximately the first part of June. She is complaining of severely painful
menstrual periods of 10 years' duration, which have been increasing in severity
over the past six months. The pain with her periods is severe enough for her to
miss work 1 to 2 days per month. She also had pelvic pain like menstrual
cramps when she is not having a period. The patient had an exploratory
laparoscopy done by Dr. Kim in September of 1990 at which time he identified
pelvic endometriosis involving the bladder attachment to the lower uterine
segment and also in the cul-de-sac. She requires Vicodin for relief of the pain,
but lately the Vicodin, even at 1-1/2 tablets at a time, does not relieve the
discomfort. She is now in for definitive treatment of this problem.

PAST HISTORY:
She had the usual childhood diseases and has enjoyed generally good health as
an adult.

REVIEW OF SYSTEMS:
Essentially noncontributory for severe medical illnesses.

ALLERGIES:
She has no known drug allergies.

PAST SURGERY:
She had an appendectomy in approximately 1971. It was unruptured. She had
surgery for a tennis elbow and a dilatation and curettage with laparoscopy in
September of 1987. She has had no fractures or injuries.

SOCIAL HISTORY:
She isnot a smoker. She uses no alcohol and has no history of drug intake.

MEDICATIONS:
The only drug she takes with regularity at this time is Vicodin.

(continued)

Figure 25–11

Report of the history and physical examination of a patient admitted to the hospital with endometriosis, typed in full block
report style.   *Figure continued*

Page 2
NAME: O'Brien, Brenna M.
MEDICAL RECORD # 9543-587

MENSTRUAL HISTORY:
She had menarche at age of 13. Her periods are regular, once a month, lasting five days.

OBSTETRICAL HISTORY:
In 1972 she delivered a male infant weighing approximately 5-1/2 pounds. It was a vaginal delivery at 7-1/2 months with no complications other than prematurity.

FAMILY HISTORY:
Negative for familial diatheses. Mother and father are living and well. She has a sister who is living and well.

PHYSICAL EXAMINATION

VITAL SIGNS:
She is 5' 3" tall and weighs 114 pounds. Her blood pressure is 120/80. Her pulse is 72 and regular.

GENERAL APPEARANCE:
She is a well-developed, well-nourished Caucasian female in no acute distress.

HEENT:
Head, normal. EENT, normal.

NECK:
Supple. There is no adenopathy. Thyroid is not enlarged. Trachea is midline.

LUNGS:
Clear to percussion and auscultation.

HEART:
Regular sinus rhythm, no murmur or enlargement.

BREASTS:
Normal, with minimal fibrocystic change bilaterally.

ABDOMEN:
Soft, flat, with no masses or tenderness. She has a right lower quadrant scar and laparoscopy scars.

PELVIC:
The introitus is marital. The glans are normal. The vagina is healthy with normal secretions. The pubococcygeus muscle is intact. Cervix is smooth. Corpus is in the midline. It is approximately 1-1/2 times normal size and slightly tender to
(continued)

Figure 25–11 *Continued*

Page 3
NAME: O'Brien, Brenna M.
MEDICAL RECORD # 9543-587

palpation. Adnexa: the right ovary is slightly enlarged and there is some bilateral tenderness.

RECTOVAGINAL:
Confirms the aforementioned findings.

EXTREMITIES:
Normal.

NEUROLOGICAL:
Reflexes are normal.

ADMITTING DIAGNOSIS:
Chronic severe pelvic pain with severe dysmenorrhea, probably secondary to pelvic endometriosis.

PLAN:
The patient is to be admitted for total abdominal hysterectomy and bilateral salpingo-oophorectomy. She had a class I Pap smear on May 20, 1994.

_____
Konrad B. Faber, M. D.

mtf
D: 6-20-94
T: 6-21-94

Figure 25-11 Continued

cesarean section as a result of the weakening of the uterine wall from tumor removal. An example of an operative report on a patient with a large fibroid uterus can be see in Figure 25-14.

Tumors of the ovary can be cystic, solid, or a combination of both. They can be simple, arising from a follicle cyst, or complex, arising from germinal tissue (teratomas, dermoid cysts). They can be small to enormous (over 100 pounds), unilateral or bilateral, benign or malignant. About 2 per cent of malignant tumors of the female population are ovarian in origin. They are often silent and discovered on routine examination. Pain, if present, is usually caused by rapid growth and stretching of the tumor capsule, hemorrhage into the tumor, rupture, or twisting of the tumor on its pedicle (torsion).

Ultrasound and magnetic resonance imaging (MRI) are helpful in diagnosing which ovarian tumors are likely to be malignant and in need of specialized patient preparation prior to operation. An example of an operative report on a patient with an ovarian tumor can be seen in Figure 25-15.

Urinary Incontinence ■ Women may seek the gynecologist's advice about problems of urinary incontinence (stress, urgency, overflow, or neurogenic bladder), sexual dysfunction, and pelvic relaxation, i.e., cystocele, rectocele, enterocele, and descensus uteri, or prolapsed uterus. These disorders are associated with injuries incurred during childbirth by descent of the fetal head through the pelvic floor structures and out through the introitus. In the process, the pubo-

COMMUNITY HOSPITAL
1234 Main Street
Ventura, CA 93003-1000

OPERATIVE REPORT

Patient: Annalise T. Rolke   Date: 8/28/94
Surgeon: Casimir Jarek, M. D.   Record # 530078-03
Assistant Surgeon: Kia Ann Kim
Circulator: Athena K. Onassis, R. N.

PREOPERATIVE DIAGNOSIS: Chronic severe pelvic pain secondary to
                                 pelvic endometriosis and dysfunctional
                                 uterine bleeding.

POSTOPERATIVE DIAGNOSIS: Pelvic endometriosis with extensive
                                 adhesion formation.

OPERATION PERFORMED: Exploratory laparotomy, total abdominal
                                 hysterectomy with bilateral salpingo-
oophorectomy, lysis of pelvic adhesions, and coagulation of pelvic endometrial
implants.

FINDINGS: There was an old right lower quadrant
                                 scar. There was evidence of
laparoscopy scars. Upon entry into the abdomen, the uterus was found to be in
an anteverted position and approximately 1-1/2 X normal size. The bladder flap
was advanced onto the fundus with scar formation and adhesions with evidence
of endometrial implants. The right ovary was approximately twice normal size
and bound down posteriorly along the broad ligament. The left ovary was within
the range of normal in terms of size and was moderately adherent to the
posterior leaf of the broad ligament. Endometrial implants were noted in the
posterior left broad ligament and the vesicouterine junction. The appendix was
absent. The upper abdominal exploration was entirely within normal limits.

PROCEDURE: Under satisfactory general anesthesia
                                 with the patient prepped and draped in
the usual manner, the abdomen was opened through a Pfannenstiel incision and
the aforementioned findings were noted. The uterus was elevated with a towel
clip and bowel was packed away. The round ligaments were bilaterally clamped,
cut, and suture ligatured with #0 chromic suture and the bladder flap was
developed with great difficulty because of scarring along the isthmus of the
uterus and the anterior fundus. Nests of bleeders were encountered in the
bladder along this adherent line. These were controlled with free ties of #000
chromic. The bladder was finally dissected by sharp and blunt dissection down
below the level of the cervix and hemostasis was complete. The avascular space
of Graves was then developed on the left side. The left tube and ovary were
elevated and the infundibulopelvic ligament was clamped, cut, and doubly ligated
(continued)

Figure 25–12

Operative report of an exploratory laparotomy of a patient who has endometriosis, typed in indented format.

Page 2
Patient: Annalise T. Rolke
Record # 530078-03

with #0 chromic suture. The same procedure was then carried out on the right.
The peritoneum overlying the posterior uterus was incised and reflected inferiorly.
The uterine vessels were skeletonized and then the left uterine artery was
doubly clamped, cut, and doubly ligated with #0 chromic sutures. The same
procedure was completed with the right uterine artery. Bleeding was further
controlled by this procedure. The endopelvic fascial flaps were then developed
anteriorly and posteriorly and reflected inferiorly below the cervix and the cardinal
ligaments were serially clamped, cut, and suture ligated with #0 chromic sutures.
The uterus was separated from the vaginal cuff by scissor dissection and the cuff
was closed with interrupted #0 chromic sutures. The endopelvic fascial flaps
were then reapproximated incorporating the vaginal cuff with a continuous #0
chromic lock suture. The pelvis was inspected and washed and the surgical area
was dry. Peritonealization was accomplished with a continuous #0 chromic
suture ducking the pedicles. Blood was encountered running into the pelvis. The
pelvis was inspected on several different occasions and no bleeding was seen
from any of the suture lines. It was discovered at this point that a bleeder was
loose in the right fascia. This was clamped and free tied with #000 chromic. The
parietal peritoneum was then closed with a continuous #0 chromic suture. The
fascia was closed with interrupted #0 Vicryl. The subcutaneous fat was
approximated with #000 chromic interrupted suture after coagulating or free-tying
all visible bleeders. The skin was closed with staples and Steri-Strips. The
patient tolerated the procedure well. She lost approximately 350 cc during the
procedure. There was no replacement. She was returned to the postanesthesia
recovery room in good condition. The sponge and needle counts were correct on
three occasions.

Casimir Jarek, M. D.

mtf
D: 8-28-94
T: 8-29-94

Figure 25–12 Continued

coccygeus, or Kegel's muscle is injured and must be restored by a strong program of muscle exercise or surgery. An example of a history and physical examination of a patient with urinary stress incontinence can be seen in Figure 25–16.

Menopause ■ With the "graying of America," the gynecologist will be seeing more women in the postmenopausal years. Treatment of these women consists of hormone replacement therapy to prevent estrogen deficiency–related diseases, such as osteoporosis, coronary heart disease, atrophic vaginitis, and vasomotor and psychologic abnormalities that are the hallmark of this stage of life. It is generally recognized by professionals the world over that women benefit both as to the quality of health and the quantity of years by the administration of hormone replacement therapy (HRT, estrogen and progestin) or estrogen only (ERT) posthysterectomy.

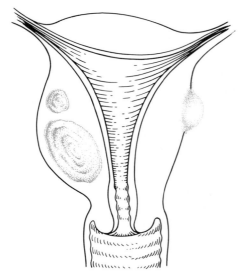

Figure 25–13
Fibroids. (From Chabner, D. E. *The Language of Medicine*. W. B. Saunders Co., Philadelphia, 1991.)

GYNECOLOGIC SURGERY

Some common operations performed by the gynecologist have already been mentioned, e.g., D&C, hysteroscopy, cervical and endometrial biopsy. Opening the abdomen when the diagnosis is unclear is referred to as an exploratory laparotomy. At this time, a total (abdominal) hysterectomy (TAH) may be performed. The lay public misinterprets this as meaning all the pelvic organs. In truth, it means that only the uterus in toto, including the cervix, is removed. If adjacent structures are removed, such as tubes and ovaries, other descriptive phrases are included with total hysterectomy (Figure 25–17). These are salpingectomy and oophorectomy (unilateral [SO] or bilateral [BSO]), meaning the fallopian tubes and ovaries. Often an incidental appendectomy is done at the time of a hysterectomy if there are no complicating factors.

In uterine cancer cases (cervical or uterine), a radical hysterectomy or Wertheim's procedure may be performed in which the uterus and the adnexal structures are removed with wide margins, and extensive pelvic lymph node and periaortic node dissections are performed. For further information on cancer, see Chapter 26, Oncology/Hematology.

Ovarian cysts may be removed alone by shelling the cyst out from the ovarian stroma and repairing the ovary or by including the ovary, ovarian cystectomy, and oophorocystectomy, respectively. In advanced cases of ovarian cancer, debulking of all observable tumor tissue is considered necessary, and sometimes other organs are removed in part or totally, e.g., omentectomy, bowel resection, and removal of the bladder.

In pelvic relaxation cases, operation is often performed through the vagina. This is referred to as a vaginal hysterectomy (VAH). Occasionally adnexal structures can be removed from below, but this is not always possible because of the lack of descent of these organs into the field of view. When a cystorectocele is present, anterior and posterior vaginal repair is almost always done, and this is termed an anterior and posterior colporrhaphy. An example of an operative report is seen in Figure 25–18. This operation brings the tissues together that support the bladder and rectum in the pelvis. In doing so, control of these organs is improved. Another common operation for correction of stress incontinence is the Marshall-Marchetti-Krantz procedure of suspending the urethro-vesicular junction behind the pubic arch. This is done through an abdominal incision.

Laparoscopy or Pelviscopy ■ Gynecologists have pioneered this procedure, and it has been used with increasing frequency in this specialty since the early 1970s. Its beginnings were generally concerned with diagnostic and sterilization procedures (bilateral tubal ligation, [BTL] or coagulation) but in the past 5 years removal of ovarian cysts, myomas, foreign bodies (lost IUDs), appendectomies, ectopic pregnancies, radical lymph node dissections, hernias, and even hysterectomies have been included. Although the operations may take longer to perform, the patient has a shorter hospital stay and leaves with less pain and discomfort.

The laparoscope has been enhanced in its therapeutic range by the advent of improved laser instruments (argon, CO_2, KTP). The laser allows the surgeon to cut and coagulate tissues and to dissect structures for removal. Various methods for the suturing of bleeders and sealing of vessels have been introduced. Miniature and micro video cameras allow the surgeon to view the operation on a large video screen while

Text continued on page 449

COMMUNITY HOSPITAL
1234 Main Street
Ventura, CA 93003-1000

OPERATIVE REPORT

Patient: Adriana F. Bortolussi   Date: 7/8/94
Surgeon: Hyoung Sang Kim, M. D.   Record # 730978-03
Assistant Surgeon: Shirley B. Cassini
Circulator: Athena K. Onassis, R. N.

PREOPERATIVE DIAGNOSIS: Large fibroid uterus, probable
                           endometriosis.

POSTOPERATIVE DIAGNOSIS: Large fibroid uterus, probable
                           endometriosis.

OPERATION: Total abdominal hysterectomy, left
                           salpingo-oophorectomy and incidental
                           appendectomy.

FINDINGS: The uterus was distorted by a single
                           large fibroid measuring approximately
12 to 15 cm in greatest diameter occupying the total volume of the pelvis. The
left adnexa was bound down to the posterior aspect of the broad ligament by
adhesions and what appeared to be endometrial implants. The left ovary and
tube were apparently normal as was the rest of the intra-abdominal exploration.

PROCEDURE: Under satisfactory general anesthesia
                           with the patient prepped and draped in
the usual manner, the abdomen was opened through a Pfannenstiel incision and
the aforementioned findings were noted. The uterus was freed from the pelvis
with a little difficulty and elevated out of the wound with a six tooth tenaculum.
The left adnexal structures, the tube and ovary were bluntly dissected free from
the posterior leaf of the broad ligament and elevated up out of the wound. The
round ligaments were then bilaterally clamped, cut, and suture ligated with #0
chromic sutures. A bladder flap was developed and reflected inferiorly below the
cervix. The avascular space of Graves was developed on the right and the
superior portion of the broad ligament including the tube and utero-ovarian
ligament were doubly clamped, cut, and doubly ligated with #0 chromic sutures.
The avascular space of Graves was then developed on the left and the
infundibulopelvic ligament was doubly clamped, cut, and doubly ligated with #0
chromic sutures. The uterine vessels were skeletonized and the peritoneum over
the posterior isthmus was incised and reflected inferiorly. The uterine arteries
were doubly clamped, cut, and doubly ligated with #0 chromic sutures.
Endopelvic fascial flaps were developed anteriorly and posteriorly and reflected
inferiorly and the cardinal ligaments were serially clamped, cut, and suture ligated
with #0 chromic sutures. The uterus was separated from the vaginal cuff by
(continued)

Figure 25–14
Operative report of a patient with a fibroid uterus, typed in indented report style.   *Figure continued*

Page 2
Patient: Adriana F. Bortolussi
Record # 730978-03

scissor dissection and the cuff was closed with figure-of-eight #0 chromic sutures. The uterus was bivalved open and found to have one large fundal fibroid and probable adenomyosis. Endometrial lining appeared normal. The endopelvic fascial flaps were then sutured closed incorporating the vaginal cuff with a continuous locked stitch of #0 chromic sutures. Bleeding was controlled. Peritonealization was then accomplished with ducking of the pedicles and again the pelvis was inspected and found to be dry.

The cecum was elevated into the wound and the appendix was elevated and a Kelly clamp was inserted through the mesoappendix and a #0 chromic suture was placed around the mesoappendix and tied. The mesoappendix was separated from the appendix and another small clamp was used to clamp the bleeder near the base of the appendix. The appendix was then elevated and a pursestring suture of triple #0 chromic GI was placed around the base of the appendix of the cecum and doubly sutured over the appendiceal artery. The base of the appendix was crushed and then free tied with triple #0 chromic sutures. The appendix was separated from the stump and then the stump was cauterized with a Bovie cautery. The stump was then inverted by means of the pursestring suture. The area was inspected and found to be dry. The cecum was returned to its normal position. Abdominal contents were rearranged in their normal relationships and the parietal peritoneum was closed with continuous #0 chromic sutures. The fascia was closed with interrupted #0 Vicryl and the subcutaneous tissues were reapproximated with triple #0 chromic interrupted sutures after free tying bleeders with triple #0 chromic free ties. The skin was reapproximated with staples and 1/4 inch Steri-Strips cut in half. The patient tolerated the procedure well. She lost approximately 200 cc of blood during the operation and received no replacements. Sponge and needle counts were reported as correct on three different occasions and she was sent to the postanesthesia recovery room in good condition.

Hyoung Sang Kim, M. D.

mtf
D: 7-8-94
T: 7-9-94

Figure 25-14 Continued

COMMUNITY HOSPITAL
1234 Main Street
Ventura, CA 93003-1000

OPERATIVE REPORT

Patient: Sylvia F. Jacobs   Date: 12/8/94
Surgeon: Carrick Morgan, M. D.   Record # 938078-03
Assistant Surgeon: Kia Ann Kim
Circulator: Athena K. Onassis, R. N.

PREOPERATIVE DIAGNOSIS: Large multinodular fibroid uterus, rule out left adnexal mass.

POSTOPERATIVE DIAGNOSES:
1. Large left ovarian fibroma.
2. Benign lesion of the vagina.
3. Multinodular fibroid uterus
4. Cystic cervicitis.

OPERATION:
1. Examination under anesthesia.
2. Dilatation and curettage.
3. Excision biopsy of vaginal lesion with frozen section.
4. Exploratory laparotomy.
5. Left oophorectomy and frozen section.
6. Total abdominal hysterectomy and bilateral salpingo-oophorectomy with cytologic washings of the bilateral pericolic gutters and pelvis.

FINDINGS: The outlet and vagina were normal. The cervix was cystic and slightly inflamed. There was a 1 cm pedunculated papillary lesion of the right fornix which was excised and sent to the laboratory for frozen section. The endometrial cavity sounded to 8 cm and was deviated somewhat to the left. On entry into the abdomen, a large, white smooth wall solid tumor was found occupying the left ovary. There were no excrescences. There was no intraperitoneal fluid. The right adnexa was totally normal. The uterus was distorted by multinodular fibroids. The rest of the intra-abdominal exploration was within normal limits.

PROCEDURE: Under satisfactory general anesthesia, the patient was prepped and draped in the lithotomy position and a weighted speculum was placed in the posterior vagina. The cervix was grasped with a single-toothed tenaculum and the endometrial cavity was sounded. Hegar dilators were used to dilate the endocervical canal to the size of a small curet and sharp curettage was then performed with return of minimal amounts of mucoid material. A 1 cm papillary (continued)

Figure 25–15

Operative report of a patient with an ovarian tumor, typed in indented report style.   *Figure continued*

Page 2
Patient: Sylvia F. Jacobs
Record # 938078-03

lesion was noted in the right fornix, the possibility of metastatic lesion was entertained. This papillary lesion was excised and the base was sutured with #000 suture for hemostasis. The lesion was then sent to the pathologist for frozen section at which point, subsequently, it was reported as benign. This completed the first portion of the surgery.

_____
Carrick Morgan, M. D.

mtf
D: 12-8-94
T: 12-9-94

Figure 25–15 Continued

COMMUNITY HOSPITAL
1234 Main Street
Ventura, CA 93003-1000

HISTORY AND PHYSICAL

NAME: Linter, Teresa F.

DOCTOR: Mary Doe, M. D.

MEDICAL RECORD # 9870-994

ADMISSION DATE: 12-3-94

HISTORY:
This is a 53-year-old Caucasian female who is gravida 5, para 5, AB 0. She has a chief complaint of urinary stress incontinence of approximately 8 years' duration.

PRESENT ILLNESS:
This patient has noticed loss of urine with cough, sneeze, or other exertion over an 8-year period. She has not responded well to exercise in controlling the problem. The patient had a D&C at Community Hospital performed on September 10, 1994 for menometrorrhagia and dysfunctional uterine bleeding. A fractional dilatation and curettage was performed. Findings at the time of surgery were a uterus that sounded to 11 cm and was approximately 3 to 4 times normal size, and symmetrical. The uterine curettings were negative for abnormalities. The patient currently requests surgery for control of stress urinary incontinence.

PAST HISTORY:
She had the usual childhood illnesses and has enjoyed generally good health as an adult.

SYSTEM REVIEW:
Essentially noncontributory.

DRUG ALLERGIES:
She is allergic to Novocain. On one occasion, she was given Novocain in a dentist's chair and is supposed to have had a cardiac arrest.

SURGERY:
In 1975, she had a vein ligation and stripping, and then a fractional dilatation and curettage in 1994.

PAST INJURIES:
She had a skull fracture at the age of 10 and a fractured rib as a child.

MEDICATIONS:
She takes no current medications. She used to take thyroid but has been off of this for years.

(Continued)

Figure 25–16

History and physical examination of a patient admitted to the hospital with stress urinary incontinence.

Figure continued

Page 2
NAME: Linter, Teresa F.
MEDICAL RECORD # 9870-994

HABITS:
She does not smoke. She uses no alcohol.

OBSTETRICAL HISTORY:
She is gravida 5, para 5, AB 0. She had 5 normal term deliveries, and the largest baby weighed 8 pounds, 10 ounces.

FAMILY HISTORY:
Diabetes on her mother's side. Her mother had a mastectomy for breast cancer.

PHYSICAL EXAMINATION

VITAL SIGNS:
Patient is 5' 6" tall and weighs 185 pounds. Blood pressure 148/80. Pulse 72 and regular.

GENERAL:
She is a well-developed, well nourished, Caucasian female in no acute distress.

HEENT:
Normal.

LUNGS:
Clear to auscultation and percussion.

HEART:
Regular sinus rhythm with no murmur.

BREASTS:
Normal with moderate fibrocystic changes bilaterally. There is a soft, indistinct cystic mass in the lateral right breast measuring approximately 1 X 1-1/2 cm and appears to be a moderately dilated duct.

ABDOMEN:
Soft and flat, no scars.

PELVIC EXAMINATION:
The outlet and vagina are normal. The glands are normal. The rectovaginal septum is thin with an attenuated perineal body. The cervix is smooth. The uterus is enlarged 3 to 4 times normal size and is symmetrical. There are no adnexal masses.

(continued)

Figure 25-16 Continued

Page 3
NAME: Linter, Teresa F.
MEDICAL RECORD # 9870-994

RECTAL EXAMINATION:
The finger is able to push the posterior vaginal wall through the introitus without any difficulty. The pubococcygeal contraction is generally good with injuries in the outer one-third bilaterally.

DIAGNOSES:
1. Stress urinary incontinence.
2. Probable adenomyosis uteri.
3. Possible fibroid uterus.

The patient is to be admitted for posterior vaginal repair. She has been advised about the possibility of future hysterectomy for her uterine enlargement and history of abnormal bleeding. She elects not to do that at this time.

_____
Mary Doe, M. D.

mtf
D: 12-3-94
T: 12-4-94

Figure 25-16 Continued

standing upright at the table. This is a great improvement over the early method of peering down the laparoscope while bending over the supine patient.

Open abdominal microsurgery to repair damaged tubes (salpingoplasty) is less frequently employed, and fertility specialists are embracing the laparoscope to perform procedures such as gamete intrafallopian tube transfer (GIFT), zygote intrafallopian tube transfer (ZIFT), and other assisted reproduction methods. In vitro fertilization (IVF) is performed in preference to salpingoplasty.

DISEASES OF THE BREAST

Today breast disease is in a gray area because the gynecologist tends to stay confined to the examination and treatment of diseases of the female reproductive organs. Gynecologists examine more breasts than those in any other specialty but for the most part will not treat breast disease. They will palpate and occasionally drain cysts and order mammograms. If a breast lesion is discovered, the patient is referred to a general surgeon for biopsy and surgical treatment if indicated. Chemotherapy is handled by the oncologist and radiation therapy by the radiologist. In the future, more gynecologists will be trained for definitive breast diagnosis and treatment.

OVERVIEW

The specialty of obstetrics and gynecology continues to find itself at the cutting edge of technology. Techniques and instruments unheard of just a few years ago are transforming the specialty. At the present time, the science and art of obstetrics and gynecology are out in front of current social, ethical, moral, legal, and political thinking regarding reproductive health and population control in this country. The storms of public debate and litigation swirl

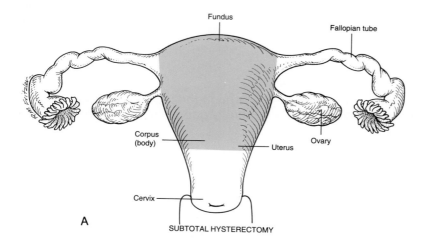

A
SUBTOTAL HYSTERECTOMY

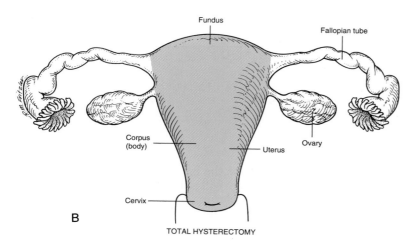

B
TOTAL HYSTERECTOMY

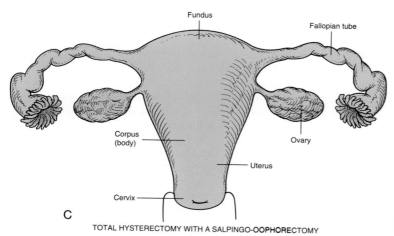

C
TOTAL HYSTERECTOMY WITH A SALPINGO-OOPHORECTOMY

Figure 25–17
Types of hysterectomy.

COMMUNITY HOSPITAL
1234 Main Street
Ventura, CA 93003-1000

OPERATIVE REPORT

Patient: Jane F. Robinson
Surgeon: Carrick Morgan, M. D.
Assistant Surgeon: Kia Ann Kim
Circulator: Athena K. Onassis, R. N.

Date: 12/20/94
Record # 338078-03

PREOPERATIVE DIAGNOSIS: Large rectocele with attenuated perineal body from birth injury.

POSTOPERATIVE DIAGNOSIS: Large rectocele with attenuated perineal body from birth injury.

OPERATION: Extensive posterior vaginal repair and perineorrhaphy.

FINDINGS: The perineum was scarred. The posterior vagina at the introitus was deeply scarred bilaterally. There was marked relaxation of the posterior vaginal wall and almost total absence of the perineal body between the anus, rectum, and vagina. The cervix was smooth. The uterus was approximately 3 to 4 times normal size. As noted previously, there were no adnexal masses.

PROCEDURE: Under satisfactory general anesthesia with the patient prepped and draped in the lithotomy position, an episiotomy was performed and a linear incision was made vertically along the posterior vaginal wall with some difficulty at the introitus due to extensive scar tissue. The mucosa was dissected by sharp and blunt dissection laterally to the lateral pelvic walls bilaterally and for approximately two-thirds the way up the posterior wall of the vagina. With a third glove on the left hand, the operator inserted his index finger in the rectum and then placed interrupted #0 Dexon sutures in the lateral pelvic fascia of the pubococcygeus muscle, bringing the structures together in the midline. This was carried on from the apex of the incision approximately two-thirds of the way up the vagina to the introitus, thus bringing the pubococcygeus together in the midline. The posterior vaginal mucosa was sutured with interrupted #0 Dexon sutures. The perineal body was reconstructed with interrupted #0 Dexon and #0 chromic sutures. Excess vaginal mucosa was trimmed and the procedure was completed with interrupted subcutaneous sutures in the perineum. On completion of the procedure, the bladder was catheterized and the urine was clear. There was a marked improvement in the posterior vaginal support and the perineal body was again intact. The estimated blood loss was approximately 200 cc, no replacement.

mtf
D: 12-20-94
T: 12-21-94

_____
Carrick Morgan, M. D.

Figure 25–18
Operative report of a patient with posterior repair of a rectocele, typed in indented report style.

around us on a daily basis and affect the day-to-day practice of the clinician. It is difficult and trying but exhilarating to be at the center of this intense societal debate.

Reference Sources

Creasy, Robert, and Robert Resnik. *Maternal-Fetal Medicine: Principles and Practice.* W. B. Saunders Company, Philadelphia, 1989.

Cunningham, T. C., P. C. MacDonald, and N. F. Gant. *Williams' Obstetrics,* Appleton and Lange, Norwalk, Connecticut, 1989.

Speert, Harold. *Obstetrics and Gynecology in America: A History.* The American College of Obstetricians and Gynecologists, Chicago, 1980.

Thompson, John D., and John A. Rock. *Te Linde's Operative Gynecology.* J. B. Lippincott, Philadelphia, 1992.

For references of specific application to medical transcription, see Appendix 1.

Thomas G. Gabuzda, M.D.
Carolyn F. Sidor, M.D.

CHAPTER
26

Oncology-Hematology

INTRODUCTION

Medical oncology and hematology are both subspecialties of internal medicine. However, they are often combined because of the close relationships they share. The medical oncologist specializes in the diagnosis, evaluation, and treatment of all kinds of cancers. The hematologist specializes in diseases of the blood cells and the blood-forming organs, many of which are malignancies. Since these specialties overlap, they are commonly practiced by one individual certified in both.

However, the management of cancer is a multidisciplinary effort that involves the coordination of many branches of medicine. Thus, there are surgical oncologists, gynecologic oncologists, radiation oncologists, and pediatric oncologists. Pathology is central to cancer diagnosis. Nursing, social work, and other support components now also have specialization in the field of oncology.

For example, a woman with breast cancer may have the initial lump detected by her gynecologist, family physician, or internist, then she may be referred to a diagnostic radiology center for a mammogram. This is analyzed by a radiologist, and the diagnosis is made by the surgeon from the biopsy tissue that has been interpreted by the pathologist or the cytologist. The tumor will be removed by the surgeon, following which the radiation oncologist may give radiation therapy, and in selected cases the medical oncologist supervises chemotherapy. In the midst of all this the patient needs the support services of technicians specially trained in the skills of mammography, cytology, and radiation therapy, and

nurses specially trained to administer chemotherapy.

THE NATURE OF CANCER

Cancer is a disease in which cell division goes haywire. Cells normally grow through a process of carefully regulated division. When the cell is in a resting, nondividing state, it is in a phase of the cell cycle called G_0. During the next phase of cell division, the cell prepares itself for the major task of doubling the quantity of DNA contained in its chromosomes. This phase is referred to as G_1. During the S phase, DNA synthesis provides this requirement so that each daughter cell receives a full complement of chromosomes. During the subsequent G_2 and M phases, the chromosomes form a spindle and then pull apart into two separate daughter cells identical to the parent cell (Figure 26–1). Normal cell division is very carefully regulated by a series of complex signals mediated by growth factors.

When a cell undergoes malignant transformation, growth occurs in an unregulated fashion, and the cell numbers continue to double. After 20 such doublings, there are a million cells that are still too small to be detected as a discrete tumor, but after 30 doublings a lump forms, which then becomes a 2-pound tumor by the time it goes through 40 doublings (Figure 26–2).

Recent research has shed much light on the reason for malignant transformation. Oncogenes are normally contained in the genes that determine the makeup of the cells. These oncogenes may undergo transformation by a variety of means, leading to an abnormality in the regula-

453

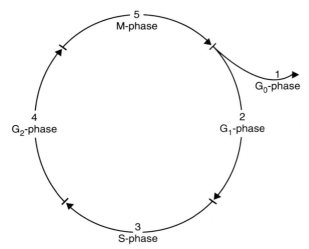

Figure 26–1

The cell cycle. (From Holleb, A. I. *The American Cancer Society Cancer Book*. Doubleday, Garden City, New York, 1986.)

tion of the growth of the cells. Oncogenes are responsible for the production of growth factors, which may have either negative or positive influences on cell growth. Thus the oncogene can do its dirty work either by being absent or by being overly active. In addition to these endogenous factors, exogenous influences also are important in malignant transformation, including tobacco, chemicals, and radiation.

The malignant cancer cell thus has a tendency toward unrestrained growth. It also has a propensity to invade the surrounding structures and to spread to more distant sites in the body, that is, to metastasize. The spread may proceed through the lymphatic system, in which the lymph nodes draining the site of the tumor become involved. Spread also can occur, by means of the blood stream (hematogenous spread), to almost any body organ, such as the liver, bones, lungs, and brain.

The term *benign* may be used to describe a tumor for which the growth is limited, without any propensity either to invade surrounding tissue or to spread. A benign tumor can be the source of a substance like a hormone that could produce significant clinical effects.

Cancers are commonly divided into two major categories, the hematologic tumors and the solid tumors. The latter include all those tumors not involving the blood-forming organs. The hematologic tumors include the lymphomas, the leukemias, and multiple myeloma. The solid tumors include carcinomas and sarcomas. Carcinomas are derived from the epithelial tissues that form surface linings. If they are of glandular origin, they are referred to as adenocarcinomas. If they arise from epithelium of a nonglandular character, like that on the surface of the skin or in the membranes of the mouth or respiratory tract, they are referred to as squamous cell or epidermoid carcinomas. Sarcoma is used to describe cancers arising from the connective tissues, such as muscle, blood vessels, and bone.

For example, the breast may be the site of origin of any of the aforementioned cancers. However, the most common type is an adenocarcinoma, referred to as infiltrating ductal carcinoma. The cytologist and the pathologist are qualified to establish the diagnosis of cancer and to determine what type it is by the appearance of the cells under the microscope. Specimens may be obtained by aspirating material through a fine needle and squirting the material on a slide, which is then stained and examined microscopically by a cytologist, who will determine the diagnosis by the appearance of the individual cells. If a larger piece of tissue is obtained by means of surgical biopsy, the specimen will be fixed in formalin and sliced into very thin sections, which are stained and mounted on slides. The appearance of the intact tissue and its individual cells under the microscope will then be examined by a pathologist, who will in turn determine whether or not it is cancer and what type of cancer it is.

About 90 per cent of cancers are solid tumors, and the remainder are hematologic tumors. Among men, lung cancer is the leading cause of death, followed by colorectal and prostate cancer. Among women, lung cancer has overtaken breast cancer as a cause of death, followed by colorectal cancer (Figure 26–3).

DIAGNOSIS AND EVALUATION OF THE CANCER PATIENT

Cancer Screening: Early Warning Signs ■ When cancer starts as a tiny, undetectable tumor of microscopic size, it will not cause any signs or symptoms. When it grows to the size of

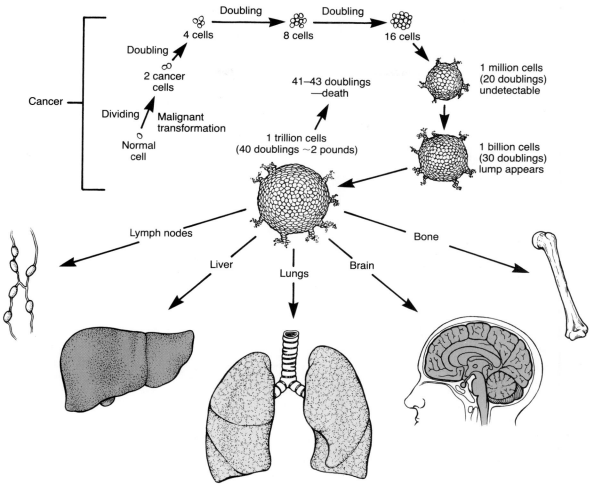

Figure 26–2
Hypothetical model of tumor growth, with cancer metastasis. (From Dollinger, M., E. H. Rosenbaum, and G. Gable. (From *Everyone's Guide to Cancer Therapy*. Andrews and McNeel, Kansas City, Missouri, 1991.)

a small, noticeable lump, it still may not cause any symptoms but it may be in a limited and curable stage of the disease. As it spreads to invade nearby organs and tissues and eventually to the lymph nodes and distant organs, symptoms become progressively more severe and cure less likely. Thus it is crucial to detect cancer in an early and often asymptomatic stage.

The key to early detection is finding the tumor, either through patient self-examination or during the course of the doctor's physical examination. The regular use of certain screening tests also will increase the number of cancers found in an early and curable stage (Table 26–1). For example, early detection of breast cancer by both regular physical examination and mammography has been of proven benefit. Other cancer screening procedures of proven or probable value include periodic pelvic examinations and Pap tests for women; regular digital rectal examinations and checks of the stool for occult blood; and periodic inspection of the lower bowel by sigmoidoscopy. These procedures facilitate early diagnosis of the common cancers affecting

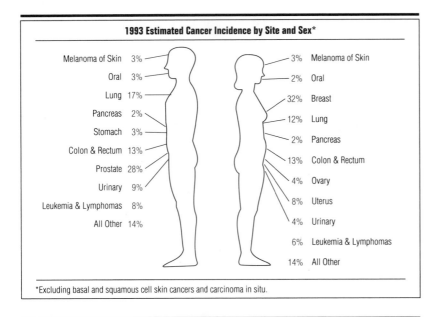

1993 Estimated Cancer Incidence by Site and Sex*

	Male		Female	
Melanoma of Skin	3%	3%	Melanoma of Skin	
Oral	3%	2%	Oral	
Lung	17%	32%	Breast	
Pancreas	2%	12%	Lung	
Stomach	3%	2%	Pancreas	
Colon & Rectum	13%	13%	Colon & Rectum	
Prostate	28%	4%	Ovary	
Urinary	9%	8%	Uterus	
Leukemia & Lymphomas	8%	4%	Urinary	
All Other	14%	6%	Leukemia & Lymphomas	
		14%	All Other	

*Excluding basal and squamous cell skin cancers and carcinoma in situ.

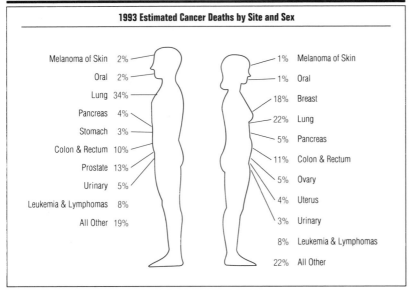

1993 Estimated Cancer Deaths by Site and Sex

	Male		Female	
Melanoma of Skin	2%	1%	Melanoma of Skin	
Oral	2%	1%	Oral	
Lung	34%	18%	Breast	
Pancreas	4%	22%	Lung	
Stomach	3%	5%	Pancreas	
Colon & Rectum	10%	11%	Colon & Rectum	
Prostate	13%	5%	Ovary	
Urinary	5%	4%	Uterus	
Leukemia & Lymphomas	8%	3%	Urinary	
All Other	19%	8%	Leukemia & Lymphomas	
		22%	All Other	

Figure 26–3
Cancer incidence and cancer deaths. (From CA: A Cancer Journal for Clinicians, 73(1):9, 1993.)

the female breast and reproductive organs, prostate cancer in men, and colorectal cancer in both sexes. Screening for lung cancer still has not proved to be of value, probably because of the highly malignant character of most cases.

Asymptomatic patients may see their physicians either for a periodic checkup or because they have had an abnormal screening test that requires further evaluation. Some of the early warning signs and symptoms that may lead to finding cancer are a lump in the breast or elsewhere; a change in bowel or bladder habits; unusual bleeding or discharge from the genital, urinary, or digestive tract; indigestion or difficulty

Table 26-1 ▪ **American Cancer Society Guidelines for Screening**

Test or Procedure	Population		
	Sex	*Age (Years)*	*Frequency*
Sigmoidoscopy	M & F	Over 50	After two negative examinations 1 year apart, perform every 3–5 years
Stool guaiac slide test	M & F	Over 50	Every year
Digital rectal examination	M & F	Over 40	Every year
Pap test	F	20–65; under 20, if sexually active	After two negative examinations 1 year apart, perform at least every 3 years
Pelvic examination	F	20–40 Over 40	Every 3 years Every year
Endometrial tissue sample	F	At menopause, women at high risk*	At menopause
Breast self-examination	F	Over 20	Every month
Breast physical examination	F	20–40 Over 40	Every 3 years Every year
Mammography	F	Between 35–40 40–49 Over 50	Baseline Every 1–2 years Every year
Chest x-ray film			Not recommended
Sputum cytology			Not recommended
Health counseling and cancer checkup†	M & F M & F	Over 20 Over 40	Every 3 years Every year

*History of infertility, obesity, failure to ovulate, abnormal uterine bleeding, or estrogen therapy.
†To include examination for cancers of the thyroid, testicles, prostate, ovaries, lymph nodes, oral region, and skin.
  From CA 35:199, 1985.

in swallowing; persistent cough, especially if productive of bloody sputum, or hoarseness; a sore that does not heal; or an obvious change in a mole or wart. The development of weight loss, loss of appetite, and pain often indicates that the cancer has spread and may be incurable.

Malignant tissues are sometimes capable of synthesizing substances that cause symptoms. Various clinical syndromes produced by these substances are known as paraneoplastic syndromes and often require treatment. One common syndrome is a rise in blood calcium from direct involvement of the bone with metastatic disease or from a circulating hormone produced by the primary tumor. Treatment of this and other paraneoplastic syndromes can alleviate dangerous and disabling symptoms associated with the malignancy.

Although the goal is to detect cancer in an early and asymptomatic stage, some cases defy detection early and remain silent even though they are widespread. Treatment then becomes more difficult or impossible.

Diagnostic Procedures and Tests ▪ Many tests are used to diagnose cancer, but the principal procedure is the biopsy. Biopsies require removal of tissue or cells from a mass or site that is thought to be malignant. Many different types of biopsies exist, including an aspiration biopsy that involves removal of cells with a fine needle attached to a syringe (Figure 26–4), excisional biopsy that requires removal of the entire abnormal area, and incisional biopsy, a removal of a part of a malignant area for the purpose of establishing a diagnosis. The pathologist is then responsible for determining whether the cells are malignant and identifying the primary site of the malignancy (Figure 26–5). Pathologists use several special stains that are specific for cells from various sites in the body to help them identify the origin of the cancer. In addition, substances that serve as tumor markers circulate in the blood in some patients with cancer (Table 26–2). These markers are rarely specific for a type of cancer, but they are often useful in monitoring patients and their response to treatment.

Several special types of x-rays are often used to diagnose cancer. Mammograms are special breast x-ray films used to detect very small lumps and other abnormalities. Ultrasound examinations of breasts and other tissues are used to determine whether abnormalities are solid or fluid-filled cysts. Both these types of imaging procedures are often used to guide needle place-

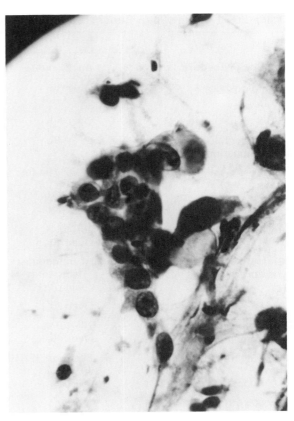

Figure 26–5
Cytologic specimen obtained from brushing the bronchial tree through a bronchoscope. The clump of cells is positive for lung cancer. (Courtesy of Vaidehi Kannan, M.D.)

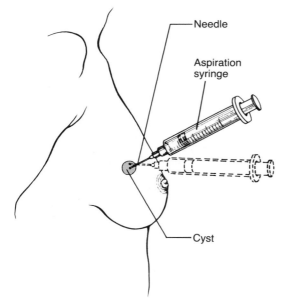

Figure 26–4
Needle aspiration of breast tumor for cytologic examination. (From Holleb, A. I. *The American Cancer Society Cancer Book*. Doubleday, Garden City, New York, 1986.)

ment when a biopsy or cytology specimen is required. Computed tomography (CT) scans, magnetic resonance imaging (MRI) scans, and isotopic scans are frequently used to aid in staging patients and for detecting disease in areas of the body where conventional x-ray studies may be relatively insensitive.

Endoscopes are also being used frequently to aid in the diagnosis of cancer. An endoscope is a flexible instrument that can be inserted into a body orifice to visualize abnormalities and to obtain biopsy specimens and brushings of abnormal areas. A bronchoscope is designed to look into the lungs (Figure 26–6). A colonoscope is used to evaluate the entire colon. Additional instruments visualize the upper gastrointestinal tract as well as the head and neck area. A laparo-

Table 26–2 ▪ Tumor Markers

Type	Abbreviation	Cancer
Carcinoembryonic antigen	CEA	Colon, lung, breast, others
Alpha-fetoprotein	AFP	Liver, germ cell
Human chorionic gonadotropin	hCG	Germ cell
Calcitonin	CT	Thyroid
Prostate-specific antigen	PSA	Prostate
Ovarian carcinoma antigen	CA-125	Ovary
Lactic dehydrogenase	LDH	Germ cell, lymphoma
β_2-microglobulin		Multiple myeloma

scope is used to enter the abdominal cavity without major surgery.

The laboratory is also helpful in diagnosing patients with cancer, as well as patients with benign hematologic diseases. Biochemical profiles obtained on most patients give insight into the function of various organs, particularly the liver and the kidney. Since the liver is often a site of early metastasis, a laboratory abnormality is often the first indication that the cancer has spread to this organ.

Cancer Staging ▪ Once the diagnosis of cancer has been made, it is critical to establish a stage for the disease. Staging helps define future treatment and prognosis. All available information on staging of cancer has been organized into a manual to allow for consistency in describing the extent of various cancers. The TNM system is used to stage most cancers and involves three components:

- T
  - the extent of the primary tumor

- N
  - the absence or presence and extent of regional lymph node metastasis, and

- M
  - the absence or presence of distant metastasis (Figure 26–7)

In addition, numbers added to these letters indicate progressive increase in tumor size or involvement. Thus a cancer patient might have a primary cancer designated T1 through T4, depending upon the size of the primary lesion. In addition, regional lymph nodes designated by N0 through N3 define the extent of lymph node involvement; and M1 indicates distant metastasis to sites other than the primary lesion and its regional lymph node drainage. Once a patient has been adequately staged, decisions are made concerning proper treatment and the goals of such treatment.

For example, the stage of a patient with breast cancer who is found to have a primary tumor less than 2 cm. in size, no involvement of axillary lymph nodes, and no signs of distant metastases is T1N0M0, or Stage I. If the tumor were 3 cm., only 2 of 24 axillary lymph nodes were positive,

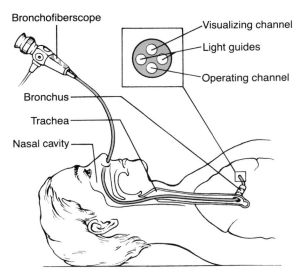

Figure 26–6
Demonstration of flexible bronchoscope for visualizing and taking cell and tissue specimens from the bronchial tree. (From Holleb, A. I. *The American Cancer Society Cancer Book.* Doubleday, Garden City, New York, 1986.)

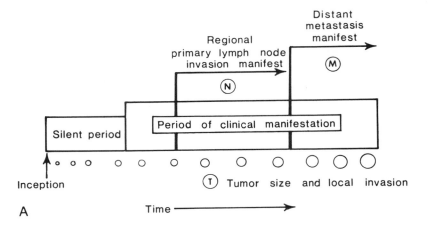

A

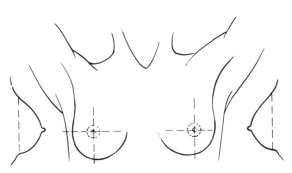

Indicate on diagram primary tumor and regional nodes involved.

Inflammatory
Medullary with lymphocytic infiltrate
Mucinous (colloid)
Papillary
Scirrhous
Tubular
Other
Lobular
  In situ
  Invasive with predominant *in situ* component
  Invasive
Nipple
  Paget's disease, NOS (not otherwise specified)
  Paget's disease with intraductal carcinoma
  Paget's disease with invasive ductal carcinoma
Other

Histopathologic Type

The histologic types are the following:

Cancer, NOS (not otherwise specified)
Ductal
  Intraductal (*in situ*)
  Invasive with predominant intraductal component
  Invasive, NOS (not otherwise specified)
  Comedo

B

Sites of Distant Metastasis

Pulmonary	PUL
Osseous	OSS
Hepatic	HEP
Brain	BRA
Lymph nodes	LYM
Bone marrow	MAR
Pleura	PLE
Peritoneum	PER
Skin	SKI
Other	OTH

Figure 26–7
A, Diagram of the natural history of cancer progression. B, The method of cancer staging. (From Beahrs, O. H., D. E. Henson, R. V. P. Hutter, and M. H. Myers (eds.): *Manual for Staging of Cancer*, 4th edition. Sponsored by the American Joint Committee on Cancer. J. B. Lippincott Company, Philadelphia, 1992, pp. 151–154.)

and there were no distant metastases, the designation is T2N1M0, or Stage II. If the tumor invaded into the structures of the chest wall, it is T4. Even if the lymph nodes were negative and there was no distant spread (T4N0M0), this is Stage III disease (Fig. 26–7B).

Once a patient has started on treatment, it is important to define a response to that treatment. CR, or complete response, is used for those cases in which no further disease can be identified after a course of treatment. PR, or partial response, describes reduction but not

Data Form for Cancer Staging

Patient identification
Name _____
Address _____
Hospital or clinic number _____
Age _____ Sex _____ Race _____

Institution identification
Hospital or clinic _____
Address _____

Oncology Record

Anatomic site of cancer _____
Histologic type _____
Grade (G) _____
Date of classification _____

Chronology of classification
  (use separate form for each time staged)
[ ] Clinical (use all data prior to first treatment)
[ ] Pathologic (if definitively reseted specimen available)

Definitions

Primary Tumor (T)

[ ] TX   Primary tumor cannot be assessed
[ ] T0   No evidence of primary tumor
[ ] Tis Carcinoma *in situ:* Intraductal carcinoma, lobular carcinoma *in situ,* or Paget's disease of the nipple with no tumor.
[ ] T1   Tumor 2 cm or less in greatest dimension
  [ ] T1a 0.5 cm or less in greatest dimension
  [ ] T1b More than 0.5 cm but not more than 1 cm in greatest dimension
  [ ] T1c More than 1 cm but not more than 2 cm in greatest dimension
[ ] T2   Tumor more than 2 cm but not more than 5 cm in greatest dimension
[ ] T3   Tumor more than 5 cm in greatest dimension
[ ] T4   Tumor of any size with direct extension to chest wall or skin.
  [ ] T4a Extension to chest wall
  [ ] T4b Edema (including peau d'orange) or ulceration of the skin of breast or satellite skin nodules confined to same breast
  [ ] T4c Both T4a and T4b
  [ ] T4d Inflammatory carcinoma

Lymph Node (N)

[ ] NX   Regional lymph nodes cannot be assessed
[ ] N0   No regional lymph node metastasis
[ ] N1   Metastasis to movable ipsilateral axillary lymph node(s)
[ ] N2   Metastasis to ipsilateral axillary lymph node(s) fixed to one another or to other structures
[ ] N3   Metastasis to ipsilateral internal mammary lymph node(s)

Pathologic Classification (pN)

[ ] pNX   Regional lymph nodes cannot be assessed
[ ] pN0   No regional lymph node metastasis
[ ] pN1   Metastasis to movable ipsilateral axillary lymph node(s)
  [ ] pN1a Only micrometastasis (none larger than 0.2 cm)
  [ ] pN1b Metastasis to lymph nodes, any larger than 0.2 cm
    [ ] pN1bi   Metastasis in 1 to 3 lymph nodes, any more than 0.2 cm and all less than 2 cm in greatest dimension
    [ ] pN1bii Metastasis to 4 or more lymph nodes, any more than 0.2 cm and all less than 2 cm in greatest dimension

B

[ ] pN1biii Extension of tumor beyond the capsule of a lymph node metastasis less than 2 cm in greatest dimension
[ ] pN1biv Metastasis to a lymph node 2 cm or more in greatest dimension
[ ] pN2   Metastasis to ipsilateral axillary lymph nodes that are fixed to one another or to other structures
[ ] pN3   Metastasis to ipsilateral internal mammary lymph node(s)

Distant Metastasis (M)

[ ] MX   Presence of distant metastasis cannot be assessed
[ ] M0   No distant metastasis
[ ] M1   Distant metastasis (includes metastasis to ipsilateral supraclavicular lymph nodes

Stage Grouping

[ ] 0	Tis	N0	M0
[ ] I	T1	N0	M0
[ ] IIA	T0	N1	M0
	T1	N1*	M0
	T2	N0	M0
[ ] IIB	T2	N1	M0
	T3	N0	M0
[ ] IIIA	T0	N2	M0
	T1	N2	M0
	T2	N2	M0
	T3	N1	M0
	T3	N2	M0
[ ] IIIB	T4	Any N	M0
	Any T	N3	M0
[ ] IV	Any T	Any N	M1

Note: The prognosis of patients with pN1a is similar to that of patients with pN0.

Histopathologic Grade (G)

[ ] GX   Grade cannot be assessed
[ ] G1   Well differentiated
[ ] G2   Moderately well differentiated
[ ] G3   Poorly differentiated
[ ] G4   Undifferentiated

Staged by _____ M.D.
_____ Registrar
Date _____

Figure 26–7B Continued

elimination of tumor following a course of treatment. Some patients will fail to respond at all to treatment.

TREATMENTS

Goals ▪ The primary goal of treatment is to cure the patient. Whether or not a patient may be cured depends on the tumor type and its response to treatment. Curability is determined to a great extent by the degree of spread of the tumor. Therefore after the diagnosis is established, a full staging of the patient for spread of the tumor locally and to other body sites is important. In designing a therapeutic program for cure, surgical therapy, radiation, and medicinal therapy may be used either alone or in various combinations.

Adjuvant therapy refers to the administration of medicinal treatment following the apparent complete removal of local tumor by surgery, radiation, or both. It is based on the premise that certain tumors known to have a propensity to undergo hematogenous spread to various body sites may have done so at a microscopic level undetectable by the usual clinical means of evaluation. The administration of systemic therapy is designed to eliminate such microscopic deposits and to increase the chances for cure or to at least prolong the period of disease-free survival.

When circumstances indicate that cure is impossible, then the treatment goal becomes one of palliation. This is intended to improve the quality and duration of life. This treatment may be used to reduce, although not eliminate, the tumor in order to improve the state of nutrition and overall well being, to alleviate pain, or to relieve obstruction of some vital body site, such as the respiratory tract, the intestinal tract, or the kidneys.

Treatment becomes supportive when it is no longer directed at reducing the amount of tumor but rather only toward the symptomatic treatment of the patient. Supportive treatment includes the use of medications for pain control, antibiotics for infection, transfusions of red blood cells or platelets, and the use of a variety of support services, such as hospice, home care, and physical therapy.

For example, in the case of breast cancer, after the diagnosis is made by either needle aspiration or biopsy of the lump, an evaluation is carried out clinically to exclude signs of spread of the tumor. If such signs are absent, a program is laid out to cure the patient. Tumor is surgically removed either by means of "modified radical mastectomy" (removal of breast and surrounding tissues) or by "lumpectomy" (removal of the tumor and a small amount of surrounding tissue). In either case, the surgeon will also remove lymph nodes from the axilla for pathologic analysis. If the lymph nodes in this site are found to be involved with tumor or if the size of the primary tumor is larger than 2 cm., then the overall prognosis falls significantly. If the surgeon performs a lumpectomy, radiation therapy is necessary to reduce what would otherwise be a rather high rate of recurrence at the site of the orginal tumor. In the case of larger primary tumors or when the lymph nodes are involved, adjuvant hormonal therapy or chemotherapy is often given to increase the chances for cure of the patient and also to delay recurrence in those destined for relapse. Adjuvant therapy is now used even in some patients without exceptionally large primary tumors or involvement of the axillary lymph nodes. If despite these initial efforts to obtain a cure the tumor relapses and spreads to other body sites, such as the lungs, liver, brain, or bones, then treatment can no longer cure and becomes "palliative." Palliative therapy in breast cancer usually consists of radiation therapy, hormonal therapy, or chemotherapy. If even these efforts prove fruitless, then supportive care is carried out to keep the patient as comfortable as possible.

Modality

Surgical Therapy ▪ The surgeon plays a central role in the diagnosis and treatment of many forms of cancer. Surgery of the primary tumor often leads to cure, depending on the accuracy of staging and on the adequacy of the surgical procedure. Surgical cure traditionally has involved removing a great deal more tissue than that of the tumor itself. For example, the operation may involve removal of an entire lobe of the lung, or even the entire lung, a kidney, a large segment of bowel, or the entire female reproductive tract. A recent trend is to design less radical surgery and combine it with other forms of treatment without lessening the chance for cure. The use of lumpectomy in breast cancer, described earlier, is an example.

Surgical reconstruction of the breast after mastectomy is an example of surgery with rehabilitation as its goal.

Occasionally surgery is used for "debulking" the tumor. It is used to remove most of the tumor even though it is impossible to remove it all, but the small amount that remains behind is more readily attacked by radiation therapy and/or chemotherapy.

Occasionally a tumor appears to have spread to a metastatic focus which is isolated in one organ, such as the lung, liver, or brain. If there are no other sites of spread, the surgeon occasionally may remove such a metastatic focus in the hope, usually not fulfilled, that the patient will still be cured.

Surgery is also used significantly for palliation. For example, if an intestinal obstruction occurs, it may be necessary to have the surgeon perform a procedure to bypass this obstruction. The large number of recent developments have often made operation unnecessary for such indications. For example, laser instruments are now used to alleviate obstruction of the esophagus or the bronchus. Endoscopy has been used to insert small catheters, referred to as "stents," into the biliary tree or into the urinary system to relieve obstruction in these sites. These procedures represent major advances in palliative care of the patient.

Radiation ■ In the developed world, radiation therapy is most commonly delivered by means of a large and complex instrument called a linear accelerator, which may have the capacity to treat the patient with either electrons (beta rays) or photons (gamma rays). The linear accelerator has some important advantages, such as a greater depth of penetration into tissues and a more reliable homogeneity of the treatment field, but it also has the disadvantage of being a very complex and expensive instrument requiring much maintenance. The cobalt unit is an older form of radiation therapy still in use in many parts of the world. It is much less expensive, is very durable, and requires very little maintenance but has the disadvantage of a lesser depth of penetration and a somewhat lesser ability to define accurately the radiation field. Both these forms of radiotherapy are "external beam" radiation therapy, which means delivered from some site away from the tumor ("teletherapy"). Brachytherapy means radiation treatment delivered very close to the tumor. This may involve the introduction of radioactive materials within applicators or as needles, wires, or "seeds" into or around the tumor. Brachytherapy is commonly used in the treatment of uterine cancer.

The delivery of radiation therapy into tissues is measured by means of a unit called the gray, which corresponds to 100 rads (1 rad equals 1 centigray).

Radioactive isotopes may also be used to treat malignancies. These are radioactive chemicals that may be delivered into a body cavity or into the circulation, from whence they may treat the entire body, or they may be directed by means of specific antibodies to specific targets in the body. The radioactivity of isotopes is expressed in terms of millicuries. Radioactive iodine is an isotope given into the circulation and taken up by thyroid tissue. It is used in the treatment of thyroid cancer.

Tumors vary in their susceptibility to radiation therapy, some being rather radioresistant and others very radiosensitive. For example, lymphomas are very radiosensitive whereas sarcomas may be very radioresistant. Breast cancer is relatively radiosensitive, and radiation therapy, described earlier, is used both in the primary treatment of the local tumor with curative intent as well as for palliation when the tumor spreads to various body sites and causes symptoms such as bone pain.

Chemotherapy ■ The term *chemotherapy* describes a class of medicinal agents used to treat cancer. These include a wide variety of substances, some of which may be given by mouth, some by injection into the subcutaneous tissues, muscles, or veins, and others only into the circulation. These agents in general have the property of blocking cell growth, thereby leading to reduction in the tumor. However, their action is felt by the normal body cells as well as by the tumor cells.

These therapeutic agents are divided into a number of subclasses, such as alkylating agents, plant alkaloids, antimetabolites, and tumor antibiotics (Table 26–3). They are often used in

Table 26-3 ▪ **Cancer Chemotherapy Agents**

Antimetabolites
Methotrexate
5-Fluorouracil
Cytosine arabinoside (Cytarabine)
6-Mercaptopurine
6-Thioguanine

Alkylators
Nitrogen mustard (Mustargen)
Cyclophosphamide (Cytoxan)
Triethylenethiophosphoramide (Thiotepa)
Ifosfamide
Melphalan (Alkeran)
Chlorambucil (Leukeran)
Busulfan (Myleran)
Nitroso ureas
    BCNU (Carmustine)
    CCNU (Lomustine)
    Methyl CCNU (Semustine)
Cisplatin (Platinol)
Carboplatin

Antitumor Antibiotics
Bleomycin
Anthracyclines
    Doxorubicin (Adriamycin)
    Daunorubicin (Daunomycin)
    Idarubicin
Mitoxantrone
Mitomycin C
Actinomycin D (Dactinomycin)
Mithramycin (Plicomycin)

Plant Alkaloids
Vinblastine (Velban)
Vincristine (Oncovin)
Vindesine
Etoposide (VP-16)
Teniposide (VM-26)

Other Agents
Hydroxyurea
L-Asparaginase
Amsacrine (M-AMSA)
Procarbazine
Dacarbazine (DTIC)
Hexamethylmelamine
Streptozotocin

in long-term palliation in certain lower-grade malignancies and for shorter-term palliation in some of the more aggressive tumors.

Tumors vary a great deal in their sensitivity to chemotherapeutic agents. Leukemia and lymphoma are among the most highly sensitive to chemotherapy, breast cancer and cancer of the ovary somewhat intermediate, while at the other extreme examples of relative resistance to chemotherapy include sarcomas, cancer of the pancreas and bowel, and malignant melanoma.

Since there are a wide variety of chemotherapeutic agents that can be admministered in a variety of dosages and either by mouth or by injection, the side effects will vary a great deal. Some agents must be given directly into the circulation because they would cause significant and sometimes extreme damage if they infiltrated into the surrounding tissues. Most of these agents suppress the bone marrow and therefore cause a lowering of the blood counts, most particularly the white cell count and the platelet count. Many of these agents, but certainly not all of them, cause temporary hair loss of varying degrees. Similarly, the occurrence of nausea, vomiting, and diarrhea is variable and depends a great deal on the particular agent used, the manner in which it is delivered, and the dose selected. Some agents cause temporary damage to the nerves, with weakness and numbness and tingling of the fingers and toes. The oncologist must be thoroughly familiar with the side effects of all these agents and take precautions to avoid serious damage to vital organs, such as the heart, lungs, nervous system, kidneys, or liver. The oncologist must also keep in mind the benefit to be obtained, balancing potential cure against the risk of these side effects (Table 26-4).

These agents are frequently used in combinations referred to by certain abbreviations. One of the most common combinations used in the treatment of breast cancer is CMF, standing for cyclophosphamide, methotrexate, and 5-fluorouracil. Although the details of this regimen may vary, commonly the cyclophosphamide is given in pill form for 2 weeks, and the methotrexate and 5-fluorouracil are given by intravenous injection on the 1st and 8th days of the 14-day cycle. The patient rests for 2 weeks, and then the cycle begins again. When this is used as an adjuvant treatment in breast cancer, the

combinations and are given at various levels of intensity. When the goal is cure or extension of the cancer-free survival of the patient, then the intensity of the treatment tends to be higher. However, many of these agents are also effective

Table 26–4 ▪ **Tumor Response to Chemotherapy**

Cure Possible
Choriocarcinoma
Acute lymphoblastic leukemia
Hodgkin's disease
Large cell lymphoma
Lymphoblastic lymphoma
Testicular cancer
Ovarian cancer
Acute myelogenous leukemia

Responses Often Seen
Small cell lung cancer
Chronic myelogenous leukemia
Chronic lymphocytic leukemia
Multiple myeloma
Follicular lymphoma
Breast cancer
Head and neck cancer

Responses Occasionally or Rarely Seen
Prostate cancer
Bladder cancer
Endometrial cancer
Gastric cancer
Non-small cell lung cancer
Osteogenic sarcoma
Soft tissue sarcoma
Colorectal cancer
Thyroid cancer
Renal cancer
Malignant melanoma

cycles most commonly are administered for 6 months.

Other abbreviations for commonly used chemotherapy regimens are listed in Table 26–5.

Hormones ▪ Among the various hormones that are useful in the treatment of cancer (Table 26–6), the adrenal cortical hormones, such as prednisone, methyl prednisolone, and dexamethasone, have a direct antitumor effect on the lymphomas and lymphocytic leukemias. They may also be used in the palliative sense, for example, to relieve fever, to improve appetite, and to reduce tumor swelling, especially in the brain.

Some of the solid tumors are also controlled by hormones—breast cancer and prostate cancer are two important examples. Tissue taken from the breast cancer biopsy is analyzed for the presence of hormone receptors to estrogen and progesterone. If these are found to be positive, the likelihood of hormonal control of the tumor is much higher.

The hormonal environment may be changed by a variety of ways. For example, in breast cancer the estrogen receptor may be blocked by the use of an agent called tamoxifen, which is effective in many cases of breast cancer. In this case tamoxifen would be considered an antiestrogen. Paradoxically, breast cancer may also respond to large doses of estrogen. Progestational agents are also effective in hormonally responsive cases.

In prostate cancer, the most common traditional means of changing the hormonal environment is orchiectomy, which results in a marked decrease in the levels of the androgenic hormone. Prostate cancer frequently responds to this measure. Estrogens also have been used with great success in prostate cancer. Recently, newer agents have been developed that block the release of the pituitary hormones and also the receptors for androgens at the cell surface. These agents (leuprolide and flutamide) are finding an increasing role in the treatment of prostate cancer and are just as effective as orchiectomy. Progestational agents also are sometimes effective in the treatment of prostate cancer.

The adrenal gland also may be the source of hormones that stimulate breast cancer or prostate cancer; removing this source is yet another, often effective therapeutic maneuver. The adrenal hormones can be blocked by means of an agent called aminoglutethimide. Because of this antihormonal measure, it is generally no longer necessary to remove the adrenal glands, a procedure that once was occasionally done in the treatment of the hormonally responsive tumors.

Biologicals ▪ The field of biologic response modifiers is a rather new one and still, for the most part, an experimental one (Table 26–7). It refers to the use of natural body substances, often now available only through the miracle of recombinant DNA technology, in the treatment of malignant disease. These substances include such factors as interferon, interleukin-2, tumor necrosis factor, and others. Some of the biologicals are very useful as adjunctive treatment for low blood counts, including factors to stimulate the white blood cells and the red blood cells.

The field of immunotherapy is also for the

Table 26–5 ▪ **Abbreviations for Some Commonly Used Chemotherapy Regimens**

ABVD	Adriamycin, bleomycin, vinblastine, dacarbazine
CAF	Cyclophosphamide, Adriamycin, 5-fluorouracil
CAV	Cyclophosphamide, Adriamycin, vincristine
CHOP	Cyclophosphamide, hydroxyldaunorubicin*, Oncovin†, prednisone
CMF	Cyclophosphamide, methotrexate, 5-fluorouracil
CVP	Cyclophosphamide, vincristine, prednisone
FAM	5-Fluorouracil, Adriamycin, mitomycin C
MACOP-B	Methotrexate, Adriamycin, cyclophosphamide, Oncovin†, prednisone, bleomycin
m-BACOD	Methotrexate, bleomycin, Adriamycin, cyclophosphamide, Oncovin†, dexamethasone
MOPP	Mustargen, Oncovin†, procarbazine, prednisone
M-VAC	Methotrexate, vinblastine, Adriamycin, cisplatin
PEB	Platinol, etoposide, bleomycin
ProMACE/CytaBOM	Prednisone, methotrexate, Adriamycin, cytarabine, etoposide, cyclophosphamide, bleomycin, Oncovin†
VAD	Vincristine, Adriamycin, dexamethasone

*Another name for doxorubicin (Adriamycin).
†Another name for vincristine.

most part experimental. A variety of means may be employed to use intact lymphocytes with or without the factors described earlier or specific antibodies to direct the body's immune response to destroy the tumor. This growing field will have an increasing role in the future treatment of cancer.

Clinical Trials ▪ A patient may be asked to participate in a clinical trial. These trials are aimed at answering questions concerning treatment for a specific cancer type. Many times no standard treatment exists for a patient, and various investigational treatments are proposed. These may include new medications in the form of chemotherapy, new surgical techniques, or new combinations of radiation therapy, surgery, and chemotherapy. Patients with similar cancers are randomized to receive one of several treatment modalities, and the information obtained from these trials is used to define how they will be treated in the future. The patients entered into clinical trials are often able to avail themselves of treatment long before it is readily available to others with similar diseases. These trials also serve as a source of information as they are able to accumulate data on large numbers of patients with similar diseases that would

Text continued on page 477

Table 26–6 ▪ **Hormonal Therapy of Cancer**

Adrenal hormones
  prednisone
  methyl prednisolone
  dexamethasone
Estrogens
Tamoxifen
Androgens
Leuprolide
Flutamide
Aminoglutethimide

Table 26–7 ▪ **Biological Response Modifiers Used in Cancer Treatment**

Interferon
Interleukin-2
Tumor necrosis factor
Erythropoietin
G-CSF (filgrastim)
GM-CSF (sargramostim)
Monoclonal antibodies

THE LANKENAU HOSPITAL
101 Lancaster Avenue west of City Line
Wynnewood, PA 19096-0000

DEPARTMENT OF RADIOLOGY

PATIENT'S NAME: Jane Martin   X-Ray No: 6754338
DATE OF BIRTH: 1/17/41

DATE OF STUDY: 12/14/93   PHYSICIAN: James Donald, M.D.
BILATERAL MAMMOGRAM 76984

DIAGNOSIS: Right breast malignancy

COMMENT: Bilateral film screen mammography was performed demonstrating a spiculated mass with microcalcifications located centrally within the upper outer quadrant of the right breast which are highly suspicious for malignancy. No other suspicious areas in the breasts are noted. There are left breast masses again seen as compared to a previous outside mammographic study of 1989. The largest mass within the left breast measures 2 cm. in diameter. These most likely represent cysts of fibroadenomas.

A.   A negative report should not delay biopsy of any clinically significant lesion.
B.   Dense breasts may obscure malignancy.
C.   Ultimate diagnosis of malignancy is histologic.

JOSEPH MILLER, M.D.

JM:rm
D: 12/14/93
T: 12/14/93

Figure 26-8
A radiology report of a bilateral mammogram.

THE LANKENAU HOSPITAL
100 Lancaster Avenue west of City Line
Wynnewood, PA 19096-0000

DEPARTMENT OF PATHOLOGY
SURGICAL PATHOLOGY REPORT

NAME: JANE MARTIN   SEX: FEMALE

MEDICAL RECORD NO.: 6754338   PATHOLOGY NO.: S-93-113013
DATE OF BIRTH: 1/17/41   RACE: WHITE   RM. 207

                                      RECEIVED: 12/28/93
                                      REPORTED: 12/29/93

SURGEON: JAMES DONALD, M.D.

SPECIMEN: A: RIGHT BREAST MASS, NEEDLE LOCALIZATION

GROSS DESCRIPTION:
Labeled right breast mass: Received fresh is a single, roughly ovoid yellow-tan
fibrofatty breast tissue measuring 3.7 x 2.5 x 2.4 cm. The external surface is
inked and sectioning discloses a spherical firm, light tan, gritty mass
measuring 1.5 x 1.5 x 1.5 cm. with attached fibrous streaks centrally. A
section is submitted for receptors and the rest of the specimen is serially
sectioned and entirely submitted.

A1 - A10   Sections of the entire lesion. P.O.T. 11 ALL.
A4 & A5   Two halves of a single section.

H&E: 10

PATHOLOGICAL DIAGNOSIS:
Right breast biopsy: Infiltrating ductal carcinoma, well differentiated,
primarily tubular with foci of infiltrating lobular appearance, histologic Grade
I, nuclear Grade I, measuring 1.5 x 1.5 x 1.5 cm. and focally extending to
inked resection margins. There is a marked desmoplastic stromal reaction.

TP:AW   TIMOTHY PRITCHARD, M.D.
D: 12/29/93
T: 12/30/93

Figure 26–9
A pathology report of breast biopsy.

THE LANKENAU HOSPITAL
100 Lancaster Avenue west of City Line
Wynnewood, PA 19096-0000

OPERATIVE REPORT

PATIENT: Jane Martin　　　　　　DATE: 1/16/94
SURGEON: James Donald, M.D.　　RECORD NO.: 6754338
ASSISTANT: Jonathan Brown, M.D.　ROOM NO.: 207
ANESTHESIA: General
POSITION OF PATIENT: Supine
PREPARATION: Iodine

PREOPERATIVE DIAGNOSIS: Carcinoma of the right breast.

POSTOPERATIVE DIAGNOSIS: Same.

OPERATION: Lumpectomy with axillary dissection.

PROCEDURE: A generous lumpectomy was performed around the site of the previous biopsy and in addition there were numerous cysts encountered in the specimen. An incision was next made in the right axilla and the lower axillary contents were removed. There appeared to be enlarged nodes, but they did not appear to be involved with tumor. A Blake drain was placed and the breast wound was closed with monofilament sutures and the axillary wound was closed with a subcuticular suture and Steri-Strips. Dressing was applied and the patient left the operating room in good condition.

_____
JAMES DONALD, M.D.

JD:bp
D: 1/16/94
T: 1/17/94

Figure 26–10
An operative report of a lumpectomy and axillary dissection.

THE LANKENAU HOSPITAL
100 Lancaster Avenue west of City Line
Wynnewood, PA 19096-0000

DEPARTMENT OF PATHOLOGY
SURGICAL PATHOLOGY REPORT

NAME: JANE MARTIN
MEDICAL RECORD NO.: 6754338
DATE OF BIRTH: 1/17/41

SEX: FEMALE
PATHOLOGY NO.: S-94-54312
RACE: WHITE   RM. 207

RECEIVED: 1/16/94
REPORTED: 1/17/94

SURGEON: JAMES DONALD, M.D.

SPECIMEN: A: RIGHT BREAST LUMPECTOMY, AXILLARY CONTENTS

GROSS DESCRIPTION:
Labeled right breast tissue with axillary contents: The specimen consists of a
7.0 x 4.6 x 2.2 cm. portion of fibrofatty breast tissue with an overlying tan
ellipse of skin measuring 5.6 x 1.2 cm. There is a linear healing scar
measuring 3.7 cm. At the edge of one portion of the specimen is a previously
incised hemorrhagic biopsy cavity, which appears to attach to a second portion
of fibrofatty breast tissue also containing a hemorrhagic biopsy cavity. The
second portion of fibrofatty breast tissue measures 4.5 x 2.8 x 1.5 cm. The
specimen is inked. Sectioning of the larger portion of fibrofatty breast tissue
reveals a 2.2 x 2.0 x 2.0 cm. focally hemorrhagic biopsy cavity displaying areas
of yellow chalkiness, possible fat necrosis. No residual tumor is grossly
identified. Note the biopsy cavity is on the edge of the specimen and thus is
not inked. However, the adjoining portion of fibrofatty breast tissue is inked.
The remainder of the larger portion of fibrofatty breast tissue reveals
predominantly pearly white fibrous breast tissue which is somewhat nodular
and displays several cysts measuring from 0.1 cm. to 0.6 cm. in greatest
dimensions. Also noted is a slightly retracted stellate tan-pink lesion
measuring 0.3 x 0.2 x 0.2 cm. and is located 1.4 cm. from the nearest margin
of resection. Sectioning of the smaller portion of fibrofatty breast tissue, which
abuts the biopsy cavity, reveals focal hemorrhage and yellow chalky areas of
fat necrosis. No gross residual tumor is identified. The specimen is
predominantly yellow lobulated fatty tissue with a moderate amount of pearly
white fibrous breast tissue. Also received is a portion of red-tan to yellow fatty
tissue measuring 6.0 x 4.0 x 1.3 cm. which contains five tan-pink lymph nodes
measuring from 1.5 to 2.5 cm. in greatest dimension.

(continued)

Figure 26–11
A surgical pathology report of a lumpectomy and axillary contents.

JANE MARTIN   Page 2
MEDICAL RECORD NO.: 6754338

Representative sections are submitted:

A1:	One node bisected (2)
A2:	One node bisected (2)
A3:	One node bisected (2)
A4:	One node bisected (2)
A5:	One node bisected (2)
A6-A9:	Representative sections of biopsy cavity from larger portion of fibrofatty breast tissue (4)
A10:	Representative section of small stellate lesion (1)
A11-A12:	Representative sections of fibrous breast tissue (2)
A13-A16:	Representative sections of smaller portion of fibrofatty breast tissue containing a portion of biopsy cavity (4)

PATHOLOGY DIAGNOSIS:

Right breast tissue with axillary contents:
Residual infiltrating ductal carcinoma with tubular features, similar to previous biopsy (S-93-113013), satellite lesions (measuring up to 0.4 cm. in diameter) (A10-12) and metastatic to 4 of 5 axillary lymph nodes. Biopsy site shows primarily granulation tissue with foreign body giant cells.

TIMOTHY PRITCHARD, M.D.

TP:aw
D: 1/17/94
T: 1/18/94

Figure 26–11 Continued

THE LANKENAU HOSPITAL
100 Lancaster Avenue west of City Line
Wynnewood, PA 19096-0000

DISCHARGE SUMMARY

NAME: JANE MARTIN
PHYSICIAN: JAMES DONALD, M.D.

MEDICAL RECORD NO.: 6754338
DATE OF ADMISSION: 1/16/94
DATE OF DISCHARGE: 1/19/94

DIAGNOSIS: CARCINOMA OF THE BREAST

INVASIVE PROCEDURES: Lumpectomy with axillary dissection on 1/16/94.

HISTORY AND PHYSICAL: This is a 52-year-old , white female who had an incisional needle guided biopsy of a lesion found on routine mammogram, revealing a Grade I infiltrating ductal carcinoma. The patient has a history of cystic breast disease and several cysts have been aspirated in the past. She has also had surgical removal of a cyst about 20 years ago. She presents now for lumpectomy with axillary dissection.

PAST MEDICAL HISTORY: As per history of present illness.

PAST SURGICAL HISTORY: As per history of present illness to include dilatation and curettage in 1989 and 1990.

MEDICATIONS: None.

SOCIAL HISTORY: Patient was a smoker up until three years ago.

PHYSICAL EXAMINATION: Is significant for a well-developed, well-nourished, 52-year-old, white female who looks her stated age. No adenopathy appreciated. Right breast with a well healing surgical previous biopsy scar.

(continued)

Figure 26–12
A discharge summary on a patient with carcinoma of the breast.

JANE MARTIN   Page two
MEDICAL RECORD NO.:6754338

HOSPITAL COURSE: The patient was taken to the operating room on 1/16/94 and had a right axillary dissection and lumpectomy. Postoperatively she did well with decreasing drainage in her Blake drain, which was removed prior to discharge. She had been afebrile without erythema, hematoma, or seroma of the incision site.

                                        _____
                                              JAMES DONALD, M.D.

JD:bp
D: 1/19/94
T: 1/20/94

Figure 26–12 Continued

THE LANKENAU HOSPITAL
100 Lancaster Avenue west of City Line
Wynnewood, PA 19096-0000

DEPARTMENT OF RADIOLOGY

NAME: JANE MARTIN   X-RAY NO.: 6754338   SOURCE: OP
DATE OF STUDY: 2/6/94   PHYSICIAN: NANCY DREW, M.D.

BONE SCAN, WHOLE BODY - 87451

(Tc-99m MDP 20 mCi)

FINDINGS:

Imaging was performed in the anterior and posterior positions two hours following radionuclide administration. There are no localized areas of abnormally increased radioactivity to suggest the presence of neoplastic involvement of bone. There is a punctate area of increased radioactivity in the left supraclavicular area. These findings probably represent uptake of radioactive material at an extraskeletal site, possibly in a node.

CONCLUSION:

1. The findings do not suggest the presence of neoplastic involvement of bone.

2. There is a punctate area of extraskeletal uptake of radioactive material in the left supraclavicular region.

_____
STEPHEN BRADLEY, M.D.

SB:rm
D: 2/6/94
T: 2/6/94

Figure 26–13
A report of a whole body bone scan.

THE LANKENAU HOSPITAL
100 Lancaster Avenue west of City Line
Wynnewood, PA 19096-0000

DEPARTMENT OF RADIOLOGY

PATIENT'S NAME: Jane Martin   X-RAY NO.: 6754338
DATE OF BIRTH: 1/17/41
DATE OF STUDY: 2/10/94   PHYSICIAN: Nancy Drew, M.D.

PA AND LATERAL CHEST - 71020

There is again evidence of prior right mastectomy. There are small bibasal discoid atelectases. The heart is normal in size.

IMPRESSION: No active disease seen in the chest.

_____
JOSEPH MILLER, M.D.

JM:rm
D: 2/10/94
T: 2/11/94

Figure 26–14
A PA and lateral chest x-ray film report.

NANCY DREW, M.D.
Lankenau Hospital
100 Lancaster Avenue west of City Line
Wynnewood, PA 19096-0000

February 11, 1994

James Donald, M.D.
1623 Large Street
Philadelphia, PA 19154-0000

RE: Jane Martin

Dear Dr. Donald:

I saw Jane in follow-up for carcinoma of the right breast and to begin adjuvant chemotherapy on February 10, 1994. Piecing together her final pathology report it appears that she has infiltrating ductal carcinoma of the right breast, nuclear grade 1, histological grade 1, with the primary measuring 1.5 x 1.5 x 1.5 cm. In addition, she had a total of 4 out of 5 nodes that were positive for metastatic carcinoma. A bone scan and chest x-ray done prior to her therapy were negative for metastatic disease. Her ER receptors were positive at 18 femtomoles, but the PR receptors were negative.

We will plan six months of adjuvant chemotherapy with Cytoxan, metho-trexate and 5-fluorouracil. Following her chemotherapy she will be placed on tamoxifen and followed. She tolerated day one of her first cycle remarkably well with no adverse effects.

On physical examination the lumpectomy site seems to be well healed with no evidence of any infection or accumulations of fluid. In addition, her right arm shows no edema and her mobility has almost returned to normal at this point. Her only complaint is some soreness and fatigue in that arm.

I will be seeing her again on February 17th, for day eight of therapy and should any changes occur, I will let you know.

Sincerely,

ND:bp

Nancy Drew, M.D.

Figure 26–15
A consultation letter.

be impossible other than through the cooperation of many oncologists, surgeons, and radiation therapists.

FORMATS

Examples are presented here of some of the documentation that characterizes oncology-hematology. These include reports of a mammogram (Figure 26–8) and a pathology report of a breast biopsy (Figure 26–9).

Figure 26–10 is an operative report of a lumpectomy and axillary dissection, and Figure 26–11 is the pathology report on the tissues removed at this operation.

Samples are also provided of a hospital discharge summary (Figure 26–12), a bone scan (Figure 26–13), a chest x-ray study (Figure 26–14), and a consultation letter (Figure 26–15).

Reference Sources

DeVita, V. T., Sr., S. Hellman, and S. A. Rosenberg. *Cancer Principles and Practice of Oncology.* J. B. Lippincott, Philadelphia, 1989.

Dollinger, M., E. H. Rosenbaum, and G. Cable. *Everyone's Guide to Cancer Therapy.* Andrews and McMeel, Kansas City, Missouri, 1991.

Hoffman, R., E. J. Benz, Sr., S. J. Shattil, B. Furie, and H. S. Cohen. *Hematology; Basic Principles and Practices.* Churchill Livingstone, New York, 1991.

Holleb, A. I. *The American Cancer Society Cancer Book.* Doubleday and Company, Garden City, New York, 1986.

Manual for Staging of Cancer, 3rd edition. J. B. Lippincott, Philadelphia, 1988.

For references of specific application to medical transcription, see Appendix 1.

Charles G. Steinmetz, III, M.D.

Ophthalmology

INTRODUCTION

Ophthalmology is an old word derived from the Greek, meaning study of the oculus, or eyeball. Many treatises of the ancient Indians, Greeks, and Arabs discuss ocular problems, surgical therapy, and treatment. Modern ophthalmology began in the late 1700s and early 1800s and rapidly blossomed in Germany, France, and Austria. There were new instruments, such as ophthalmoscopes; new clinical tests, such as bacterial cultures; and new treatments and drugs, such as pilocarpine and atropine. Diseased tissue was studied, and there were new surgical techniques, such as cataract removal. The information was disseminated not only by letters but also by papers, journals, and textbooks. This accelerated tempo of invention, experimentation, discovery, application, and communication is ongoing. It is essential to stay abreast of this expanding world of new disease, new technology, and new words and phrases.

Ophthalmology deals not only with the eyeball but also with vision, eyelids, orbits, and the surrounding face, brain, sinuses, nose, and throat. It is therefore necessary to divide the profession into subspecialties. The assortment of people who work in this field is varied; some are defined here:

- Ophthalmologist. An ophthalmologist has completed 4 years of college, 4 years of medical school, and an internship, and has had specialized training in graduate education at a graduate school or ophthalmic residency and is capable of treating patients and performing surgery.

- Optometrist. An optometrist has completed 4 or more years at a college and has been trained in refraction, diagnosing eye problems, and fitting glasses.

- Optician. An optician has been trained in fitting glasses and understanding the optical principles that produce good, effective, and comfortable glasses.

OPHTHALMOLOGIC SUBSPECIALTIES

Many subspecialties in ophthalmology depend on the anatomic section of the eye that is involved.

A general ophthalmologist treats a variety of ocular conditions and is capable of performing diagnostic procedures as well as surgical procedures.

A retinal specialist is an ophthalmologist who has been highly trained in retinal disease, treatment and surgery and treats only patients with retinal problems.

Corneal specialists limit their practice to treating only conditions of the cornea.

Pediatric and extraocular muscle problems are treated by a specialist in that particular area of care.

A neuro-ophthalmologist deals with problems of the optic nerve, brain, and extraocular muscle deficiencies.

Glaucoma is dealt with by ophthalmologists who are interested in treatment and cure of glaucoma.

479

An ophthalmic pathologist is a physician who specializes in the diagnosis of tissues of the eyes that have been removed because of tumor, infection, or infestation.

An ophthalmic oncologist specializes in diagnosis and treatment of tumors of the eyes and adnexa.

An ophthalmic plastic surgeon is an ophthalmologist whose primary interest is noncosmetic and cosmetic surgery of the eyes, orbits, lids, and adnexa. The major concern is the removal of tumors, correction of congenital deformities, and repair of traumatic insult.

ANATOMY

An ophthalmologist's major anatomic concerns are with the eyeball, lids, and orbits. Each of these areas of the eye are discussed.

The Globe ▪ The eyeball is a globe approximately 24 mm. in length (Figures 27–1 and 27–

2). The anterior one quarter of the globe has a different curvature than the posterior three-quarter section. This anterior one quarter is called the cornea; it is composed of clear tissue permitting light rays to pass through. Because of its shape, it also bends (refracts) these rays. Although a small part of the globe, the cornea is composed of cells divided into five layers that work to keep the tissue transparent.

The posterior three quarters of the globe is formed by a white, opaque tissue known as the sclera. This outer layer of the globe is firm and forms the casing for the vital internal structures.

The internal contents of the globe can be divided into two main areas: the anterior portion —the joining of the cornea with the sclera at the limbus, and the posterior portion, extending from the limbus posterior to the optic nerve. It contains the neuroretinal and vascular elements that are essential to seeing clearly.

The anterior chamber is a space bounded by the cornea anteriorly and the iris posteriorly,

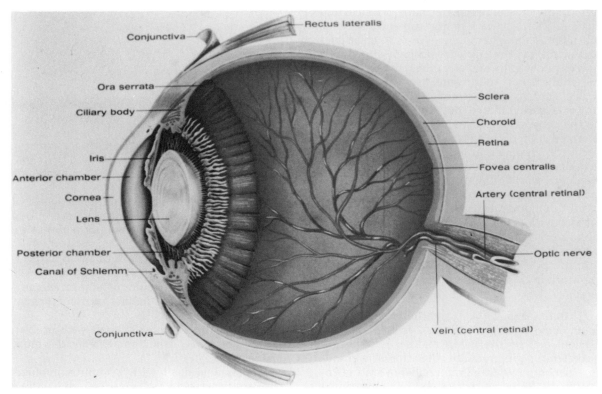

Figure 27–1
Anatomic structure of the eyeball. (Courtesy of Burroughs Wellcome Co., Research Triangle Park, North Carolina.)

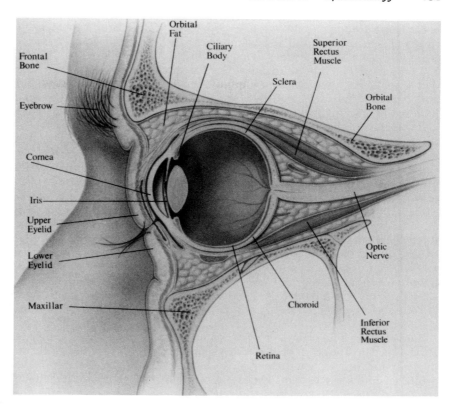

Figure 27–2
Anatomic relationship of the eyeball and adnexa. (Courtesy of Optyl Co., Norwood, New Jersey.)

with the crystalline lens behind the central iris hole, which is known as the pupil. The anterior chamber is filled with a solution known as the aqueous humor. The aqueous humor is constantly changing, being formed in the posterior chamber and flowing between the back surface of the iris through the pupil and into the anterior chamber. It then filters out from the eye through a sievelike structure in the angle where the iris is attached to the cornea and then into collector channels that flow back into the venous drainage from the globe. This sievelike structure is known as the trabecular meshwork.

The posterior portion of the globe begins with a small posterior chamber bounded by the posterior surface of the iris and the anterior surface (hyaloid membrane) of the vitreous humor. In this posterior chamber are the crystalline lens, the lens capsule, and the zonular fibers that hold the lens in place. In younger patients, the lens is capable of becoming round owing to the relaxation of the zonular fibers and thus increasing

the power of the lens for seeing near (accommodation). The aqueous humor is formed in the posterior chamber and flows between the zonular fibers and the posterior and anterior surface of the lens throughout the pupil and into the anterior chamber.

The large posterior globe has three layers: the scleral opaque shell, the choroid that contains blood vessels of varying caliber, and the neuroretina, which contains nine layers of neural and glial cells and whose outer half receives oxygen from blood vessels and capillaries of the choroid. The inner layers receive oxygen from the retinal circulation and retinal artery. The central cavity of the posterior position of the globe is filled with vitreous gel. This gel is transparent and transmits rays of light that have been bent by the curvature of the cornea and crystalline lens to form an image on the retina.

Once the image has been formed on the retina, it is transmitted to the brain via the optic nerve, which exits through the sclera at the scleral optic nerve foramen. The optic nerve is similar to a tract in the brain and, if cut, does not regenerate like peripheral nerves.

The Lids ▪ The lids act like curtains that protect the globe. Constant blinking removes dust and grit from the surface of the cornea and conjunctiva by moving the tear film across the palpebral tissue to the inner corner of the lids and down into the lacrimal punctum, canal, sac, and duct. The quick reflex of the lids protects the globe from approaching objects. The lids also protect the eyes when one sleeps by preventing the cornea from drying. The lids are covered externally by skin, and internally by a soft mucous membrane. The conjunctiva, which joins the loose mucous membrane, covers the globe up to the limbus and the edge of the cornea. The mucous glands secrete mucus that lubricates the membrane and helps entrap dust particles, which roll up into a mucous ball and can usually be found as dried secretion in the inner corner of the palpebral fissure.

The Orbit ▪ The orbit is a long, conical space surrounded by bone in which the eyeball, fat, muscle, and nerves are present. The fat of the orbits cushions the eyeball and permits the extraocular muscles to contract and relax, thereby moving the globe to different directions of gaze. Nerves and blood vessels supply these muscles, and the eyeball passes through the fat in this cone.

REPRESENTATIVE DISEASES

Signs and Symptoms ▪ Most ocular problems are covered by the ensuing classifications and causes:

Red eye: Conjunctivitis, chalazion, subconjunctival hemorrhage, trauma, and glaucoma.

Tearing: Conjunctivitis, chalazion, corneal or conjunctival foreign body, allergy, toxic fumes, sinusitis, and glaucoma.

Headaches: Sinusitis, allergy, refractive error, muscle imbalance, orbital or brain tumors, abscess, and glaucoma.

Blurred vision: Refractive error (astigmatism), double vision, retinal degeneration, orbital and retinal tumors, neurologic problems, retinal diabetes and detachment, cataracts, and glaucoma.

Double vision: Cataracts, macular degeneration, diabetes, muscle imbalance, trauma, and refractive error.

Loss of vision: Retinal vascular accidents, tumors, retinal detachments, trauma, and neurologic catastrophe.

Difficulty with distance vision: Cataracts, macular degeneration, retinal detachment, refractive error (need for corrective glasses), trauma, glaucoma, and neurologic reasons.

Difficulty with near or reading vision: Refractive error (need for bifocal or reading glasses), medication (cycloplegic), cataracts, glaucoma, and retinal problems.

Trauma: Red eye, tearing, blurred vision, loss of vision, expulsion of contents of eyeball, and hemorrhage.

Painful eye: Glaucoma, traumatized eye, referred sinus pain, inflammation of uvea, ciliary spasm, and refractive error.

Congenital conditions: Cataracts, tumors, and malformation of globe and face.

Diagnostic Procedures and Tests ▪ A test of visual acuity is the first procedure performed. This test is carried out with the patient wearing glasses (corrective vision) and not wearing glasses (naked vision), both for near and far. The standard test chart is the Snellen chart, to be read from a distance of 20 feet, and a near vision test chart to be read at 14 inches. The correction can be made with glasses, contact lenses, or telescopic lenses. Whatever the choice, the optical correction must be stated.

Inspection of the eyes must be made to determine the reason for the patient's office visit. Extraocular movements should be checked.

The eye may be refracted for near and far vision to determine the patient's best visual acuity. The pupillary response should be tested and recorded. A slit lamp examination of the anterior portion of the globe should be performed.

Ophthalmoscopic visualization may be made of the posterior segment of the globe, including the optic nerve, macular area, and periphery of the retina. Tonography may be performed to check the pressure of the eyeball. This is the check for glaucoma.

A confrontation field test may be made to determine whether the view of the patient is normally broad or constricted (tunnel vision). Testing of central and peripheral fields may be carried out using computerized analyzers.

Retinal fluorescein photography may be used to determine the viability of retinal tissue and circulation.

Ultrasound may be ordered to measure the length of the globe for determining the power of an intraocular lens implant after cataract surgery, or to see whether hemorrhage is present or retinal detachment has occurred. Electroretinograms may be obtained to determine the function of the retina and optic nerve if no cause for the decrease in vision is found.

Treatment ■ Local medications to the globe and adnexa consist of

1. Local drops — antibiotic, anti-inflammatory, dilating, constricting, pressure-lowering, lubricating, and anesthetic.

2. Local ointments can also be used to accomplish all the aforementioned. They last longer but blur the vision.

3. Injections are used for similar reasons. These injections can be subconjunctival, parabulbar, or retrobulbar. As with any invasive procedure, the risk of hemorrhage is always present and may complicate the treatment.

Systemic medications, such as antibiotics, anti-inflammatories, antiglaucoma drugs, and vitamin therapy may be given in the form of pills or capsules.

Therapeutic glasses may be given: corrective lenses, protective lenses, radiation protection, and cosmetic lenses. Contact lenses can be given for these same uses.

Surgical treatment is used to remove opaque lenses (cataract), correct retinal detachments, replace vitreous, adjust alignment of eyeballs by surgically transplanting extraocular muscles, repair or adjust lids, establish improved drainage of intraocular fluids in glaucoma, and decompress the optic nerve.

SURGICAL PROCEDURES

Surgical procedures may be divided into those for cataract, glaucoma, cornea, retina, trauma, orbit or lid correction, or a combination of all.

Cataract ■ Cataract surgery is for the removal of an opaque or cloudy lens (Figure 27–3). The procedure may be done manually or with phacoemulsification. In manual extraction, the

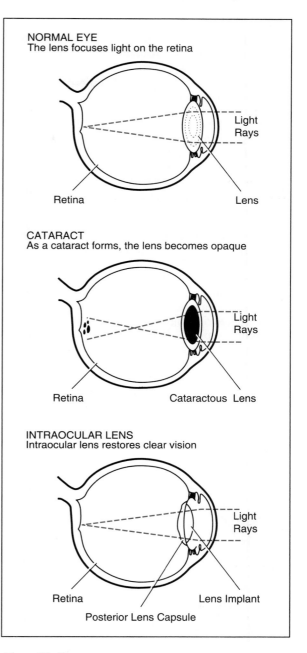

Figure 27–3
The normal eye, the cataractous lens, and an intraocular lens implant.

anterior chamber is entered, the capsule of the lens is incised and the hard nucleus of the lens is slid out, followed by infusion and aspiration of the soft cortex. Material is carried out by suction. An implant lens is then able to slide into the remaining capsular bag or the anterior chamber.

Phacoemulsification uses a small cutting tip that is driven by an ultrasound generator that emulsifies the dense nucleus and sucks the remnant out through an aspiration channel. The advantage of this procedure is that a small entrance into the anterior chamber is made at the limbus (corneoscleral junction), and the eye recovers good vision more quickly. The lens implant can be inserted into the capsular bag after the cortex is removed by aspiration.

An intracapsular cataract extraction may be performed on certain occasions when the cataract is dislocated. This procedure consists of removing the cataract in the capsular bag and necessitates stripping the zonular fibers that hold the lens in place. Following this procedure an anterior chamber lens may be implanted. If vitreous humor is prolapsing, it may be necessary to perform an anterior vitrectomy.

At this time, cataracts *cannot* be removed by lasers. The laser-dissolving technique is a misconception that is perpetrated by false advertising. The bulk of the cataractous lenses is so large and the destruction of the laser rays so small that it would take a great amount of time and energy to destroy both the hard nucleus and cortex.

Glaucoma ▪ The operation for glaucoma is a miniature plumbing procedure to try to direct or reduce the aqueous flow within the eye (Figure 27–4).

Narrow angle glaucoma is caused by the interruption of aqueous flow from the site of its formation in the posterior chamber through the pupil into the anterior chamber and out through the trabecular membrane. The blockage is at the pupil or the iris and is pushed against the trabecular membrane. Therefore, a shunt, or hole, called a peripheral iridectomy (PI), is made in the iris leaf, which permits the aqueous humor to flow directly into the anterior chamber, deepening the anterior chamber and permitting the aqueous to flow from the posterior chamber and out the trabecular meshwork. Lasers are used to make the hole in the iris leaf. If a laser is not available, a surgical peripheral iridectomy can be made by entering the anterior chamber and cut-

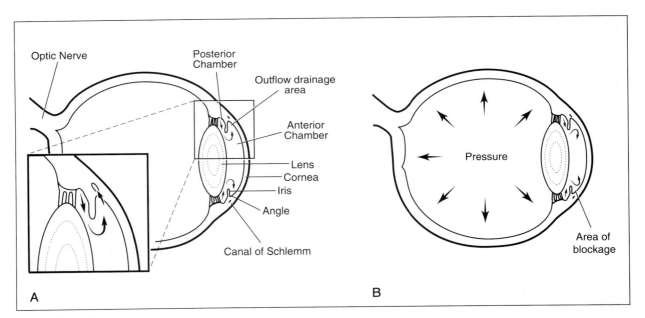

Figure 27–4
A, The normal flow of fluid through the eye; B, reduced flow of fluid with increased pressure, causing glaucoma.

ting a small hole with scissors and suturing the corneoscleral incision to make a watertight closure.

Open angle glaucoma is caused by a nonfunctioning trabecular meshwork. A channel must be formed surgically to drain the aqueous humor from the eye to the subconjunctival tissue, which forms a bleb and lowers the intraocular pressure. The lowering of pressure is carried out by surgically removing a bloc of tissue containing trabeculum and the canal of Schlemm, and then covering the dehiscence with a thin flap of sclera through which the aqueous humor can flow out and under the subconjunctival tissue and form a bleb.

All surgical procedures try to achieve these goals by way of any of the following methods: trabeculectomy, internal goniopuncture, Molteno's implant, or Holman's YAG gonio laser penetration.

Retinal Surgery ■ Replacing a detached retina may be very complicated. The hole or tear must be identified and closed, either by cautery, laser, or cryotherapy. If the detachment is not touching the choroid, the fluid must be drained or the sclera and choroid moved closer by means of an external silicone band or sponge. Silicone oil or gas may be used internally to press the retina into place. Posterior vitrectomy, lifting of the membrane mechanically, and internal laser coagulation may all be used to achieve the desired results.

Repair of Trauma ■ Trauma can occur to the globe by way of contusion, laceration, rupture, or evisceration of global contents. Any such occurrence must be repaired as soon as possible; a trauma team of anterior segment surgeons, retinal surgeons, and plastic surgeons may be used to repair the damaged tissue.

INSTRUMENTS

Ophthalmologists are gadgeteers—more instruments are designed for their use than in all other specialties. Instruments appear in waves and are used for a short period of time until another physician makes a modification, and soon there is a modification of a modification. Since many procedures use a high-power microscope and very fine instruments and sutures,

these modifications are justified. The instruments used today are

- cannula
- cystotome
- disposable knife blades
- fine forceps
- fine hooks
- fine rotators
- fine scissors
- iris retractors
- lid speculum
- microscope
- needle holders
- small caliber needles and thread
- tweezers

Testing instruments include

- camera (tonographic and fundus)
- corneal cell computer
- field tester (computerized)
- keratometer
- ophthalmoscope (direct and indirect)
- slit lamp
- tonometry
- ultrasound imaging devices

Lasers are used in treating glaucoma and retinal problems and for cutting capsular membrane.

FORMATS

Letters ■ With all the methods of communication available today, letters are still the best way to impart the important facts of a case to the referring physician or the physician to whom you are referring a patient.

- Letters inform the physician that the patient was seen. The letter must be current and not sent after a prolonged lapse of time.

- The letter presents the chief complaint or time of accident, initial impression, diagnosis, and plan of treatment. It should close with the expected result and when the patient will be seen before being returned to the physician's care.

- A letter is a courtesy and a thank you to the physician.

- It also advises the referring physician of the treatment the patient received.

CHARLES G. STEINMETZ, III, M.D.
1500 Locust Street
Philadelphia, PA 19102-0000
215/546-0813

January 20, 1994

Daniel Jordan, M.D.
1669 Columbus Street
Philadelphia, PA 19042   RE: Mary Franklin

Dear Dan:

It was my pleasure to see your patient, Mary Franklin, on January 18, 1994. Mrs. Franklin scraped the right cornea with a lash brush that morning. She was in great pain and had severe tearing. After the eye was anesthetized, her visual acuity was obtained and reduced to 20/50. There was corneal lineal abrasion of the central corneal epithelium. The conjunctiva was congested and edema was present.

On slit lamp examination, there was no foreign body seen nor was there a flare or cells in the anterior chamber. The patient was started on Tobrex drops every two hours with patching of the eye between applying the eye drops. An analgesic was ordered to be taken every three hours. I will see Mrs. Franklin tomorrow morning and change her medication as indicated.

I reassured Mrs. Franklin and recommended that she rest at home until the pain and tearing subside.

Diagnosis: Corneal abrasion, right eye (918.10).

Thank you for referring Mrs. Franklin to me. I will inform you of her progress.

Sincerely,

Charles G. Steinmetz, III, M.D.

ssb

Figure 27–5
A letter to a physician from a physician in response to a referral.

WILLS EYE HOSPITAL
9th and Walnut Streets
Philadelphia, PA 19004-0000

OPERATIVE REPORT

PATIENT: Mildred Smithson   DATE: 5/13/94
SURGEON: Charles G. Steinmetz, III,. M.D.   RECORD # 435-023
ASSISTANT: Donald Stern, M.D.

PREOPERATIVE DIAGNOSIS: Cataract, O.D.

POSTOPERATIVE DIAGNOSIS: Same.

OPERATION: Extracapsular cataract extraction with intraocular lens implant in posterior chamber, O.D.

PROCEDURE: After the patient was identified and we spoke with her, a retrobulbar injection of 2.5 cc of Wydase, Carbocaine and Marcaine was given in the superior orbit and a similar injection was given in the inferior orbit.   A block was given over the right facial area using the same amount of medication.

A superior rectus and inferior rectus 4-0 black silk bridle suture was placed. A peritomy ws performed from 12 o'clock to 3 o'clock and 12 o'clock to 9 o'clock and a partial penetrating incison was made into the cornea from 2:30 o'clock to 12 o'clock to 10 o'clock and this was then protected from excessive bleeding by local cautery. The anterior chamber was entered with a superblade at the 9 o'clock position as well as the 12 o 'clock position through the partial penetrating incision. The anterior chamber was filled with Healon and a can-opening type incision made into the capsule with a bent needle. The nucleus was rocked and then the incision was enlarged with scissors making a biplane type of incision. The nucleus was expressed without difficulty, and a large amount of cortex came with it.

Figure 27–6
Operative report for an extracapsular cataract extraction with intraocular lens implant.
Figure continued

Mildred Smithson   Page two
Record # 435-023

Four 8-0 Vicryl sutures were used to close the cornea so that a double cannula could be entered into the anterior and maintain chamber infusion and aspiration. The cortex came out in large chunks and was quickly removed from the eye. The one suture was cut and Healon was instilled into the capsular sac and also into the anterior chamber. A posterior chamber intraocular lens, IOLAB, was introduced into the anterior chamber and easily passed into the capsular space inferiorly and after rotation the haptics were in place and the lens looked good.

The wound was then closed. The Healon was aspirated and myotics were used to bring the pupil down. The corneoscleral wound was then closed using 9-0 nylon and the knots were trimmed and buried. The conjunctival flap was brought down over the suture line and an interrupted suture was used to fashion the conjunctiva over the suture line. The keratoscopy appeared to be round, no prominent sutures were noted. The patient then received gentamicin, steroid, and Ancef and returned to the recovery room in excellent condition.

_____
CHARLES G. STEINMETZ, M.D.

CGS:ssd
D: 5/14/94
T: 5/15/94

Figure 27–6 *Continued*

Letters should contain only important facts and should be brief (Figure 27–5).

Chart notes ■ These may be dictated and typed or written in longhand at the bedside of the patient. Chart notes should contain the date, time of day, the patient's visual acuity, external examination of the patient, ophthalmoscopic examination, and intraocular pressure determination when indicated. The mental status of the patient should be recorded. The diagnosis and prognosis and time when the examiner will see or discharge the patient should be reiterated.

Medical Reports ■ The history and physical examination must include the patient's past ocular history: previous operations, diagnosis, and last ocular examination; the ocular history of the family: glaucoma, cataracts, retinal detachments, diabetes, and congenital visual defects.

The patient's medical history, relating to diabetes, thyroid disease, headaches, and uremia, should be stated, as well as the treatments and medications currently being given: aspirin, Mevacor, beta-blockers, steroids, hormones, birth control pills, diuretics, and the use of alcohol, cigarettes, or other drugs.

Ocular examination includes

- Visual acuity for distance and near, with and without glasses, contact lenses, or telescopic lenses.

- An external examination of lids, conjunctiva, eye movements, convergence, cornea, and pupillary reflexes to light and distance.

- Slit lamp examination of the anterior chamber, cornea, lens, and pupils.

- An ophthalmoscopic examination of the media (which include aqueous, lens, and vitreous), the retina, and optic nerve.

- Measurement of intraocular pressure.

An operative report includes the following information:

Patient's name, hospital number, and date
Which eye was operated on
Name of procedure
Diagnosis
Name of surgeon and assistant
A statement that the patient's identity and mental status were ascertained
A note that the operative permit was reviewed before surgery began

The step-by-step procedure carried out and the instruments used during the operation must be noted, as well as any untoward reactions. The type of closure and antibiotics or steroids injected must also be stated and the patient's condition at the time of return to the room (Figure 27–6).

A consultation report contains

Name of the patient
Date and time the patient was seen
The specific problem
The patient's status as observed by the consultant
Report of the examination that was carried out after the past history was reviewed and findings noted
A diagnosis, including a brief discussion of the mechanisms causing the problem
Recommended treatment, operations, or further follow-up

A discharge summary should state the following:

Name of the patient
Date of admission to hospital or clinic
Diagnosis
Treatment
Operation and complications
Condition on discharge
Disposition of patient
Date and time of discharge

Reference Sources

Boyd-Monk, H., and Steinmetz, III, Charles G. *Nursing Care of the Eye.* Appleton and Lange, Norwalk, Connecticut, 1988.
Obsbaum, S.A. Cataract and intraocular lenses. *Ophthalmol Clin North Am,* June 1991.
Scheie, H. G., and D. M. Albert. *Textbook of Ophthalmology,* 9th edition. W. B. Saunders Company, Philadelphia, 1977.
Tasman, W., and Jaeger, E. *Duane's Clinical Ophthalmology.* Harper and Row, Hagerstown, Maryland, 1991.
Vaughn, D. and T. Asbury. *General Ophthalmology,* 12th edition. Appleton and Lange, Norwalk, Connecticut, 1989.

For references of specific application to medical transcription, see Appendix 1.

John J. Gartland, M.D.

CHAPTER
28

Orthopaedics

INTRODUCTION

Orthopaedics* is the medical specialty relating to the musculoskeletal system and is concerned with disorders and injuries of bones, joints, and muscles and their associated ligaments, tendons, and bursae. Orthopaedics uses both operative and nonoperative treatments to cure diseases and correct deformities affecting the musculoskeletal system.

The word *orthopaedics* derives from the term "orthopaedia" coined in 1741 by Nicholas Andre, dean of the faculty of medicine of the College de France, from the Greek words "orthos" meaning straight and "paidos" meaning child. Andre's premise was that the prevention of deformed adults lies in the development of straight children, and his coined word was eventually adopted as the name of this medical specialty. Modern orthopaedics, however, has expanded from this initial narrow focus and now includes in its scope all the congenital, traumatic, infectious, hereditary, metabolic, neoplastic, and degenerative processes to which the musculoskeletal system is subject.

It is estimated that one of every seven persons in the United States suffers from some form of musculoskeletal impairment. Partially as a consequence of this large volume of patients, some orthopaedic surgeons arbitrarily tend to limit their practices to anatomic areas of special interest to them, such as hip, knee, shoulder, spine, foot, or hand. Of all these anatomic areas, however, only hand surgery requires a special certifying examination.

ORTHOPAEDIC DISORDERS OF CHILDREN

The ability of children's bones to grow in length has particular relevance to orthopaedics. Immature bones, those possessing the ability to grow, are subject to different disorders and responses than adult bone, which is said to be skeletally mature. The officially recognized subspecialty of pediatric orthopaedics deals with the musculoskeletal disorders of childhood that tend to differ in the body's response from orthopaedic problems encountered in adults. Injury or disease affecting children's bones may cause overgrowth, undergrowth, or deformed growth of the involved bone, which may require specialized treatment to correct.

At birth, cartilage masses called epiphyses are found at each end of long bones. An epiphysis consists of a central bony nucleus surrounded by a mass of joint cartilage that enlarges with growth. The part of the cartilage that lies between the epiphysis and adjacent bone is the physis, or growth plate, the cells of which are the source of longitudinal bone growth in children. When bone growth is completed at the time of skeletal maturity, the physis and epiphysis are converted to bone except for a layer of cartilage around the bone ends that persists into adult life as regular joint cartilage. Disorders of bone growth in children, therefore are problems of the physis. It is known that the basic controlling and monitoring mechanism of growth is hormonal.

---

*Some physicians prefer the optional shortened spelling *orthopedics*.

491

However, as an organ system specifically concerned with the single function of longitudinal bone growth, the physis is sensitive not only to local factors, such as injury and disease, but also to the biochemical, physiologic, and pathologic changes that can occur in the body as a whole. Malnutrition, starvation, and severe chronic illnesses, for example, can slow the rate of normal bone growth. Normal bone growth resumes promptly when an adequate diet is provided or normal general health is restored.

ORTHOPAEDIC DISORDERS OF ADULTS

Once bone growth is completed, bone is said to be skeletally mature, or adult, and is no longer subject to the same responses as skeletally immature bone. Adult bones and joints, however, are subject to their own peculiar problems. In addition to skeletal problems associated with infection, trauma, and tumors, adult bones and joints are subject to arthritic and degenerative changes. Arthritis, osteoporosis, fracture nonunion, and bone tumors are among the problems that orthopaedists contend with in the adult skeleton. With the rapidly increasing number of people living beyond the age of 65 years, clinical problems associated with altered bone structure and function, such as arthritis, osteoporosis, and fracture, can be expected to increase markedly.

MUSCULOSKELETAL TRAUMA

Injury involving the musculoskeletal system is a common orthopaedic problem. Each year approximately 25 per cent of the population of the United States report having had to limit their activity or seek medical attention because of a fracture, joint dislocation, sprain or strain, open wound, or contusion involving some part of the body. These injuries occur most commonly at home, at work, as a result of vehicular accidents, or while participating in sports activities. Bone fractures are most frequent in men in the 20- to 40-year age range, with arm and leg bones most often involved. Although forces causing fractures are no respecters of age or sex, certain fractures show characteristic predilections for certain groups of people. Fractures of the clavi-cle (collar bone) and fractures around the elbow are most common in children. Fractures of the shoulder and wrist occur most commonly in middle-aged women. Hip fractures and compression fractures of spinal vertebrae occur mostly in the elderly. Fractures in children, particularly those around joints, carry the added possibility of causing a growth disturbance of the involved bone. Although fracture healing is particularly rapid in very young children, age and the ability and time to heal fractures appear to be virtually unrelated for the rest of the age groups.

Orthodpaedic surgeons are also heavily involved with the care of sports-related injuries and, thus, may be part of a loosely defined subspecialty known as sports medicine. Athletic injuries, particularly to the knee, have always occupied a dominant focus of orthopaedic attention. Athletes differ from nonathletic patients who sustain the same injuries and illnesses only in the higher demand they impose on their cardiovascular, respiratory, and musculoskeletal systems. The primary goals of providing medical care to athletes are to prevent as many injuries and illnesses as possible and to treat injuries and illnesses that do occur with prompt, complete rehabilitation so that athletes have the opportunity to return to their sport.

ANATOMY

The parts of the musculoskeletal system of most concern to orthopaedists are the bones of the neck and spine, upper extremities, pelvis, lower extremities, and the joints associated with these parts; the muscles that pass in front of and behind these joints in order to move them; and the ligaments attached to these joints in order to give them strength and stability. Of all the tissues comprising the musculoskeletal system, the dominant and most interesting one is bone.

Bone ■ A hard, specialized connective tissue with a calcified intercellular substance, bone has an inorganic or mineral portion and an organic portion that is about 95 per cent collagen. Small living cells, the osteocytes, are trapped within this calcified tissue but remain in communication with each other through a network of thin, cellular processes that lie in minute bony canals. Belying its appearance, normal bone is a living tissue in a constant state of physiologic activity.

The sequences of bone formation, bone destruction, and new bone formation are repeated many times in the life cycle of normal bone. Resorption of bone in one region and deposition of bone in other regions are responsible for skeletal growth changes, particularly in bone thickness. Resorption and deposition of bone continues throughout the life of a healthy individual in response to various mechanical and hormonal stimuli.

Bone is also a plastic tissue that responds to stress and is sensitive to changes in its normal mechanical function by adding extra bone where it is needed and by removing bone from where it is not needed. Like other body tissues, bone tissue may react to stimuli in a variety of ways, but these reactions and responses are modified somewhat by its peculiar structure. To heal itself, bone tissue must go through a stage of mineralization and calcification so it can be converted into the hard specialized tissue that is bone.

In addition to serving a mechanical function by forming the skeletal support of the body, bone also protects vital body structures, provides attachment points for muscles and ligaments, and houses the bone mineral for the body. Bone serves as a storehouse for 99 per cent of the body's calcium, 80 to 90 per cent of its phosphate, and 70 per cent of its magnesium. By acting as a storage depot for calcium and phosphorus, bone plays a very significant role in meeting the needs of the body for these vital minerals. Abnormal physiologic demands of the body on bone for these minerals may result in pathologic changes in bone tissue with accompanying weakening of bone structure.

The gross structure of bone is closely related to its function, being strongest in places of greatest stress, such as the legs. Bone is angulated in shape or presents external prominences where such deviations can best serve muscle function or provide for ligament attachment. Bone assumes three general external shapes in the human body:

■ flat bone, such as skull and pelvis

■ cuboidal bone, such as vertebrae and carpal and tarsal bones

■ long bones, such as femur, humerus, and tibia

The ends of long bones are covered with joint cartilage and are broad in shape in order to distribute weight-bearing loads through the joints. Joint cartilage is supported by a bony plate, the subchondral bone, which is the visible margin of a joint as seen on an x-ray film. Grossly, bone occurs in two forms: cancellous (spongy) and cortical (compact). Cancellous bone is a latticework of interconnecting bony trabeculae surrounding bone marrow spaces. Cortical bone is the hard outer surface that gives rigidity and strength to the bone. Almost every bone contains varying proportions of both forms of bone tissue in separate but merging zones. The outer surface of cortical bone is covered with periosteum, a tough, fibrous membrane. The inner surface of cortical bone is lined with a more delicate membrane called endosteum, which also lines the bone marrow spaces.

A long bone can be divided into several anatomic zones by the use of special names (Figure 28–1). The zone at either end of a long bone is called the epiphysis. The metaphysis is that part of the shaft of the bone immediately adjacent to the epiphysis. The diaphysis is the shaft of a long bone and is composed mostly of thick, cortical bone for strength. As the diaphysis merges into the metaphysis, the cortex becomes thinner, with a concomitant increase in the amount of cancellous bone in the marrow area.

Spine and Pelvis ■ The neck, or cervical spine, is a flexible segment of the vertebral column bridging the space between the head and the relatively rigid thorax. The neck consists of seven cervical vertebrae with their joints and intervertebral disks, anterior and posterior spinal ligaments, and anterior and posterior cervical muscles. Cervical vertebrae protect the most vital portions of the spinal cord.

Collectively, the remaining vertebrae, running from the base of the neck to the pelvis, are spoken of as the spine, which is a series of articulated vertebrae assembled to form that part of the vertebral column known as the backbone (Figure 28–2). Its function is to support the weight of the trunk, to transmit the weight of the body to the lower extremities, and to protect the spinal cord and spinal nerve roots from damage. The thoracic segment of the spine (upper back) contains twelve vertebrae and is relatively rigid because of attachments to the ribs. The lumbar segment (low back) is more flexible and contains five vertebrae. The sacral and coccygeal

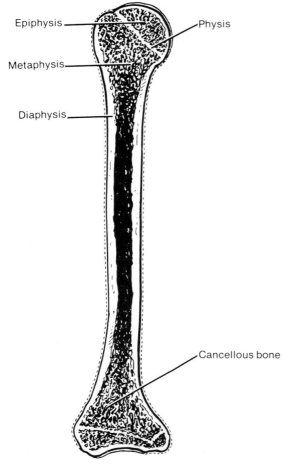

Epiphysis

Physis

Metaphysis

Diaphysis

Cancellous bone

Figure 28–1
Zones and types of bone. (From Gartland, J. J. *Fundamentals of Orthopaedics*. W. B. Saunders Co., Philadelphia, 1987, p. 9.)

vertebrae are fused together in adults and are considered clinically as being two single bones.

Except for the sacrum and coccyx, vertebrae are separated by intervertebral disks, soft tissue cushions acting as shock absorbers for the spine. The spine is further supported by the anterior and posterior longitudinal spinal ligaments and is held erect by the paravertebral spinal muscle masses that arise from the back of the skull, run downward on either side of the vertebral column, and insert on the sacrum and back of the pelvis.

The term *pelvis* is derived from the Latin and means *basin*. The bony pelvis, or pelvic ring, is formed by the right and left ilia, ischia, and pubic bones. These bones join in the front at the symphysis pubis and behind with the first three sacral vertebrae at the sacroiliac joints to form the pelvic ring. The pelvis is attached to the vertebral column through the sacrum and the lumbosacral joint and relates to the lower extremities through the hip joints.

Upper Extremity ■ The term *shoulder* is used clinically to encompass the entire shoulder girdle, which comprises the upper humerus, scapula, clavicle, and sternum, joining through the glenohumeral, acromioclavicular, and sternoclavicular joints (Figure 28–3). Four short muscles, the teres minor, the infraspinatus, the supraspinatus, and the subscapularis, arise closely around the humeral head at the shoulder and function to help lift the arm at the shoulder joint. Their four tendons blend with one another and with the shoulder joint capsule to form the musculotendinous, or rotator, cuff of the shoulder. The long muscles that pass across the shoulder joint are the biceps, coracobrachialis, deltoid, latissimus dorsi, triceps, pectoralis major, and teres major. These are the muscles that move and raise the upper extremity at the shoulder joint. The humerus is the long bone of the arm, and the biceps muscle in front and the triceps muscle behind give shape to the arm.

The elbow is a hinge joint allowing only the motions of flexion, mainly by means of the biceps muscle, and extension, mainly by means of the triceps muscle. The elbow joint is formed by the distal end of the humerus and the proximal ends of the radius and ulna. Because of the anatomic configuration of the elbow joint, the ulnar and median nerves and the brachial artery are susceptible to damage in association with elbow injuries.

The bones of the forearm are the radius and ulna (Figure 28–4). Pronation and supination motions of the forearm, wrist, and hand require a rolling of the radius and ulna on each other along their longitudinal axes, with equal amounts of motion taking place at the superior and inferior radioulnar joints. Pronation is the act of rotating the forearm so the palm is turned backward or downward. Supination is the act of rotating the forearm so the palm is turned forward or upward (Figure 28–5). The muscles that flex the wrist and fingers are bunched together along the volar surface of the forearm and are attached by a common tendon to the medial epi-

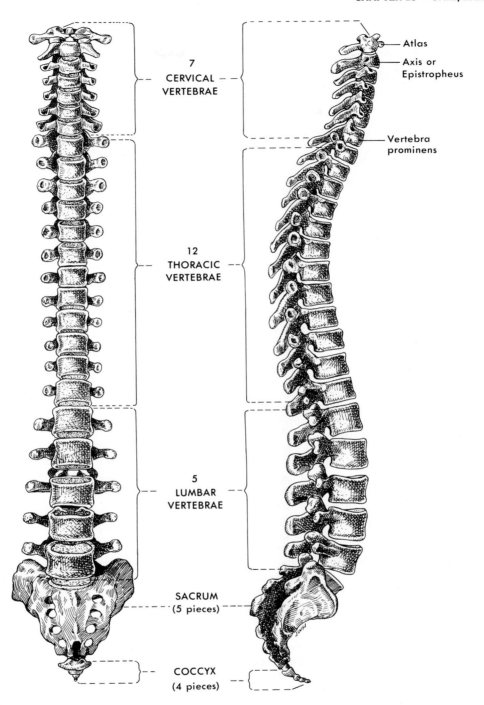

Figure 28-2
Anteroposterior and lateral views of the spine. (From Gartland, J. J. *Fundamentals of Orthopaedics*. W. B. Saunders Co., Philadelphia, 1987, p. 299.)

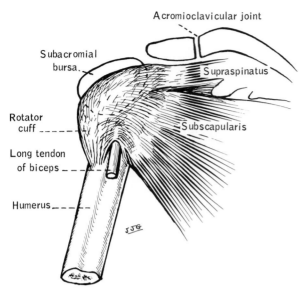

Figure 28–3

Anatomy of the shoulder area. (From Gartland, J. J. *Fundamentals of Orthopaedics*. W. B. Saunders Co., Philadelphia, 1987, p. 231. Redrawn from Marble, H. C. *The Hand*.)

close-fitting, deeply set ball and socket joint between the rounded head of the femur (ball) and the acetabulum (socket) on the side of the pelvic iliac bone and is further supported by a surrounding strong capsule. The principal hip flexor muscle, the iliopsoas, is located in front of the joint. Posteriorly, the gluteus maximus muscle functions as the principal hip extensor. The gluteus maximus and medius muscles abduct the thigh and the adductor muscles (adductor longus, brevis, and magnus, and the gracilis muscles), grouped together along the inner surface of the thigh, adduct the thigh. All muscles moving the femur at the hip joint originate from the pelvis and insert on various prominences of the femur. The shaft of the femur is contained within the thigh. The muscle mass in front of the thigh, the quadriceps muscles (a group of four muscles that function as one muscle), provide extension of the knee and help raise the entire leg. The muscle mass in back of the thigh, the hamstring muscles, provides flexion for the knee and, in association with the quadriceps muscles, helps hold the body in the erect position.

condyle of the humerus. The muscles that extend the wrist and fingers are bunched together along the dorsal surface of the forearm and are attached by a common tendon to the lateral epicondyle of the humerus.

The wrist joint is made up of the distal ends of the radius and ulna plus eight carpal bones arranged in a proximal and distal row of bones. Stability of the wrist is maintained by strong ligaments that lash the carpal bones together. The hand is made up of five metacarpal bones and the phalanges of four fingers and the thumb. Metacarpals and phalanges articulate at the metacarpophalangeal joints (knuckles). The tendons that flex and extend the fingers come from forearm muscles. Tendons that flex the fingers run through fibrous tunnels or sheaths that extend from the distal palm to the fingertips. Short intrinsic muscles to spread the fingers and oppose the thumb arise from the sides of metacarpal bones.

Lower Extremity ■ Because the lower extremities carry the body weight and must provide for locomotion, the joints of this body part are big, tend to be strong and stable, and are served by strong muscles. The hip joint is a

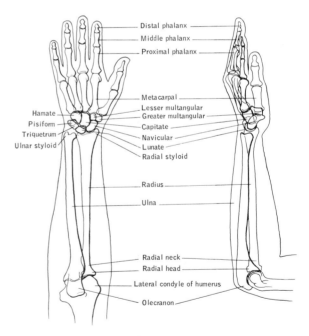

Figure 28–4

Bones of the forearm and hand. (From Gartland, J. J. *Fundamentals of Orthopaedics*. W. B. Saunders Co., Philadelphia, 1987, p. 256.)

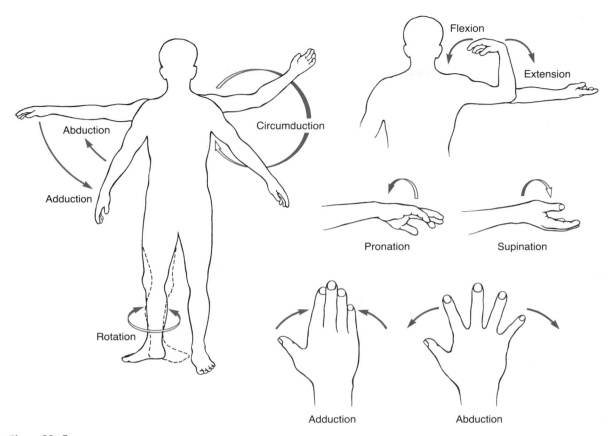

Figure 28–5
Range of motion for upper and lower extremities, including commonly used dictated terms. (From Chabner, M. E. *The Language of Medicine*. W. B. Saunders Co., Philadelphia, 1991.)

The Knee ■ The knee, the largest joint in the body, is a hinge joint between the femur and tibia that permits the motions of flexion and extension (Figure 28–6). In common with other axial joints, the knee joint is lined with a thick, synovial membrane that secretes synovial fluid to lubricate the joint surfaces. With an injury or inflammation of the knee joint, this membrane often produces a large amount of fluid that often causes pain for the individual. Because the knee lacks the inherent bony stability of the hip joint, it must depend on muscles and strong ligaments to bind it together. The knee is braced and stabilized largely by the quadriceps muscles in front in order to support the body weight in the erect position. The quadriceps muscles, inserting on the front of the tibia through the patellar tendon, extend the knee, and the hamstring muscles

in the back of the thigh insert on the posterior surfaces of the tibia and fibula to flex the knee. The knee cartilages (medial and lateral menisci) lie on top of the tibial joint surface and act as seals to promote a closer fit between femur and tibia when the knee is fully extended. The patella (knee cap) is a sesamoid bone lying within the substance of the quadriceps tendon. Its principal function is to act as a fulcrum to increase the mechanical advantage of the quadriceps muscle when it extends the knee and supports the body weight in the erect position.

Medial stability of the knee joint is provided by the joint capsule and the medial collateral ligament, which runs from the medial femoral condyle to the medial tibial condyle. Lateral stability of the knee joint is provided by the joint capsule, the iliotibial band along the outer sur-

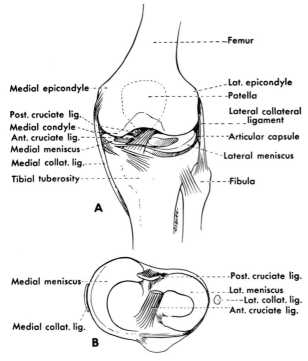

Figure 28–6

Anatomy of the knee joint ligaments. (From Gartland, J. J. *Fundamentals of Orthopaedics.* W. B. Saunders Co., Philadelphia, 1987, p. 365.)

face of the thigh, and the lateral collateral ligament that runs from the lateral femoral condyle to the fibular head. The cruciate ligaments, two binding ligaments lying entirely within the knee joint, are so named because they run in a crisscross fashion from femur to tibia. The anterior cruciate ligament acts to prevent forward displacement of the tibia on the femur while the posterior cruciate ligament acts to prevent backward displacement of the tibia on the femur. The anterior and posterior cruciate ligaments, the medial and lateral collateral ligaments, the two menisci, and the joint capsule all work together to maintain knee joint stability. Twisting injuries, particularly those sustained during athletic and contact sports, may sprain or rupture these structures to produce painful and often disabling conditions of the knee.

The Tibia and Fibula ▪ From knee to ankle, the leg is supported by the tibia and fibula bones and contains the muscles that act on the foot

and ankle. The anterior tibial and toe extensor muscles lie along the front of the leg and act to dorsiflex, or raise, the foot and ankle. The gastrocnemius and soleus muscles lie in the back of the leg, give shape to the calf, and act to plantar flex or bend the ankle and foot downward. These two posterior muscles insert on the back surface of the heel bone (called either calcaneus or os calcis) as the Achilles tendon, or heel cord. Because of its exposed position in the leg, the tibia is the most frequently broken long bone in the body.

The Ankle ▪ The ankle is a hinge joint formed between the lower end of the tibia and the talus, which is one of the tarsal bones (Figure 28–7).

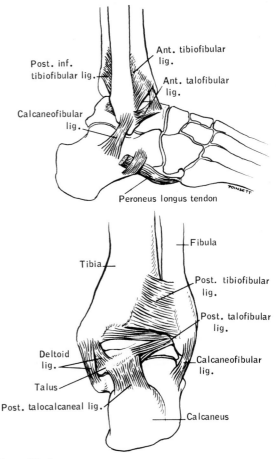

Figure 28–7

Anatomy of the ankle joint ligaments. (From Gartland, J.J. *Fundamentals of Orthopaedics.* W. B. Saunders Co., Philadelphia, 1987, p. 389.)

The distal tibia contributes the medial malleolus to the ankle joint and the distal fibula contributes the lateral malleolus. The two malleoli grasp the sides of the talus to form the ankle joint mortise. As with all hinge joints, the mucles moving the hinge are grouped in front and behind the ankle joint. Six tarsal bones lie between the ankle joint and the foot and are named talus, navicular, cuboid, and three cuneiform bones. The heel bone is called either calcaneus or os calcis. Motions of eversion and inversion of the foot occur through the subtalar complex, which consists of the talocalcaneal, talonavicular, and calcaneocuboid joints. The posterior tibial muscle, acting through these joints, is the chief invertor muscle of the foot while the peroneal muscles, also acting through these joints, function as foot evertors. The subtalar complex also allows most of what rotation of the foot and ankle occurs during walking and running.

The Foot ▪ The foot is the platform that supports the body weight during standing and moves the body during walking, running, and jumping (Figure 28–8). To bear this load most efficiently when the body is in the erect position, the foot is constructed in the form of two resilient arches from the calcaneus, tarsal, and five metatarsal bones lashed together by ligaments. The longitudinal arch of the foot spans the distance between the calcaneus and the metatarsal heads. The anterior or metatarsal arch is formed by the heads of the five metatarsal bones. As noted in the previous paragraph, the muscles moving the foot arise in the leg and are the anterior and posterior tibial muscles, the peroneal muscles, the calf muscles, and the toe flexors and extensors. In addition, short intrinsic foot muscles arise from the sides of the metatarsal shafts to assist in flexing and extending the toes.

REPRESENTATIVE DISEASES AND DISORDERS

Slipped Capital Femoral Epiphysis ▪ This is a fairly common hip joint disorder affecting adolescent children, most frequently overweight boys 10 to 16 years of age. In this condition, the epiphysis of the femoral head (capital femoral epiphysis) gradually displaces outward and backward from the femoral neck, usually in the absence of any specific injury, and for reasons that remain unclear. Slipping of the capital femoral epiphysis occurs through the physis or growth plate on the neck of the femur. If this condition is not recognized early and treated

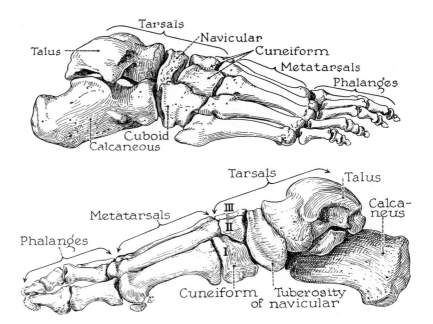

Figure 28–8
Skeletal anatomy of the foot. (From Gartland, J. J. *Fundamentals of Orthopaedics*. W. B. Saunders Co., Philadelphia, 1987, p. 395. Also from Hauser, E. D. W. *Diseases of the Foot*, 2nd ed. W. B. Saunders Co., Philadelphia, 1950.)

rapidly, severe structural deformity of the head and neck of the femur may result in severe disability.

The onset of symptoms is gradual, with the patient often complaining of vague discomfort about the hip with pain that radiates to the groin, medial thigh area, or knee. The child may walk with a painful limp and may complain of a stiff sensation in the involved hip joint.

As the structural deformity of the hip joint progresses, the affected leg tends to shorten a bit and presents an externally rotated appearance. The child's limp may worsen to a lurching type of gait. The telltale physical sign pointing to this diagnosis is the externally rotated position assumed by the patient's thigh and leg as the examining physician flexes the involved hip joint. The examiner also notices that passive internal rotation of the affected hip joint is markedly limited. In an occasional patient, acute and sudden displacement of the capital femoral epiphysis may follow a specific trauma to the hip joint. If this occurs, the physical signs produced by an acute and sudden slipped capital femoral epiphysis are similar to the physical signs produced by a fracture through the neck of the femur in either a child or an adult.

Diagnosis of this condition is made by x-ray examination of both hip joints so the radiologic appearance of the involved hip can be compared with the appearance of the uninvolved hip joint. Slipping of the involved capital femoral epiphysis is most readily identified on the lateral x-ray view of the hip joint and shows downward and backward displacement of the capital femoral epiphysis in relation to the neck of the femur. If the condition progresses before treatment is started, x-ray films may reveal an abnormal rounding of the femoral neck on the affected side.

Occasionally, the presence of this condition about to occur in a child before actual slipping of the capital femoral epiphysis has taken place can be demonstrated on an x-ray film. Called the pre-slip stage, it is characterized by an abnormally widened and irregular physis, or growth plate, associated with x-ray evidence of some bone rarefaction in the metaphysis of the femur but no actual displacement of the capital femoral epiphysis.

Treatment of the slipped capital femoral epiphysis is surgical and is designed to cause premature closure of the growth plate to seal the epiphysis on the femoral neck, thus preventing further slipping of the involved capital femoral epiphysis. Attempts to manipulate the displaced capital femoral epiphysis back to its normal position on the neck of the femur are now known to be unwise, because such attempts are often associated with a high complication rate, particularly avascular necrosis or death of bone tissue. It is considered more appropriate treatment to accept the displaced position of the capital femoral epiphysis and prevent further displacement by surgically closing the involved growth plate and, if needed, by correcting any significant remaining deformity of the hip joint by performing a realignment osteotomy through the intertrochanteric region of the involved femur at a later date.

Premature closure of the involved growth plate is accomplished by surgically introducing finely threaded metallic pins, metallic screws, or bone pegs taken from the patient's femoral neck, across the growth plate. These devices act as forms of internal fixation to hold the capital femoral epiphysis in place until the surgically induced stimulation causes growth plate closure to occur. Metal pins or screws should be removed from the patient's hip joint area once x-ray examination confirms premature closure of the growth plate of the capital femoral epiphysis. Because this condition typically occurs toward the end of the growth cycle in affected children, and because the growth plate of the capital femoral epiphysis contributes less than 30 per cent to the total length of a normal femur, no significant amount of leg shortening follows premature surgical closure of the capital femoral epiphysis growth plate in these children.

Osteoarthritis of the Hip ▪ Osteoarthritis is a degenerative disease process that mostly affects weight-bearing joints. It is a disease mainly of middle and old age and affects women more frequently than men. Involvement of the hip joint by osteoarthritis is a common and usually progressive process, and osteoarthritis of the hip has become the principal indication for performing total hip joint replacement surgery in this country.

When osteoarthritis involves the hip joint as a primary disease process, it causes degeneration and wearing away of joint cartilage, painful joint space narrowing, and bone spurs around the periphery of the joint, which cause loss of joint motion. Osteoarthritis may also develop secondarily in a hip joint in which some mechanical malalignment exists. In this instance, stress of daily wear and tear on a deformed joint gradually erodes the joint cartilage and induces the secondary effects of osteoarthritis, characterized by joint space narrowing and the formation of bone spurs around the periphery of the hip joint.

Regardless of whether osteoarthritis develops in the hip joint as a primary disease process or as a secondary effect of some long-standing mechanical malalignment of the hip joint, the clinical characteristics of the resulting osteoarthritis, the symptoms caused by the osteoarthritis, the x-ray appearance of the hip joint, and the treatment required for the osteoarthritis of the hip are the same.

Osteoarthritis of the hip produces pain, limp, limited joint motion, and deformity of the affected leg. Pain is felt in the area of the groin and may be referred along the anterior surface of the thigh to the knee, along the outer side of the thigh, or posteriorly to the buttock or low back area. Pain is invariably associated with the sensation of the hip joint stiffness. In severe hip joint involvement, the affected leg tends to shorten and turn in the direction of external rotation. The leg is usually flexed and adducted somewhat at the hip joint. Limp may be due to pain, joint stiffness, shortening of the leg, a disturbance in gluteus medius muscle function, or a combination of several of these reasons. The presence of limited hip joint motion is detected by the physician examiner by comparing the range of passive motion allowed by both hip joints. The presence of leg shortening is detected by measuring the length of both legs and comparing the two measurements.

Diagnosis of osteoarthritis of the hip is confirmed by identifying the characteristic features of the disease on anteroposterior and lateral x-ray views. Characteristic joint changes noted on x-ray films include narrowing of the hip joint space, bone spurs around the periphery of the joint, and hypertrophic bone changes around the femoral head and acetabulum that contribute to giving the afflicted hip joint a dense appearance on the x-ray film. In later stages of the disease, the joint space may appear totally obliterated, with grossly deformed and irregular opposing joint surfaces.

In some patients, symptoms of osteoarthritis of the hip may be controlled or relieved by nonoperative measures, such as using a cane in the opposite hand to unload the hip joint in order to relieve weight-bearing pain, or using a shoe or heel lift on the affected side to compensate for the leg shortening caused by the hip disease. Nonsteroidal anti-inflammatory drugs (NSAIDs) by mouth are useful in relieving hip pain temporarily but rarely are effective enough to relieve hip pain on a permanent basis. The majority of patients with symptomatic osteoarthritis of the hip eventually will require some type of surgical treatment for relief. Two surgical procedures, osteotomy of the hip and total hip replacement arthroplasty, are available that seem to have the greatest general usefulness, depending on the severity of the hip joint deformity.

Osteotomy of the Hip ■ This operation works best in patients with minimal hip joint deformity and minimal loss of hip joint motion. The term *osteotomy* means to cut completely through the substance of a bone by using a sharp osteotome and mallet or an electric bone saw. When applied specifically to osteoarthritis of the hip, the bone cutting is through the shaft of the femur at the intertrochanteric line in order to displace the two resulting fragments of bone so as to change the line of weight-bearing thrust on the involved hip joint. The purpose of performing an osteotomy is to change the position of the femoral head so that an area of more normal femoral head cartilage can be brought into contact with the hip socket. Once the desired position is obtained, the two fragments of bone are fixed together in the new position by use of an internal fixation device that remains in place at least until complete bone healing has occurred. The chief patient benefit obtained from an osteotomy of the hip for osteoarthritis is relief of weight-bearing pain. Unfortunately, for most patients, this pain relief is not permanent but lasts, on average, somewhere between 5 and 10 years before hip pain returns.

Total Hip Replacement Arthroplasty ■ This operation is indicated for those patients in whom structural deformity of the hip joint is too advanced for them to be candidates for osteotomy of the hip. The operation of total hip replacement consists of replacing the diseased femoral head and neck with a metallic femoral head prosthesis and resurfacing the diseased hip socket with a plastic cup made of high-density polyethylene. In some total hip operations, both the femoral and acetabular components are fixed to the host bone by bone cement (methylmethacrylate). In other total hip operations, bone cement is not used for bone fixation. Instead the components used in these operations are constructed from porous metals and polymer implants that allow bone to grow into the implants. If successful, this provides for a firm fixation of the components to the host bone.

Total hip replacement has proved to be a very successful operation for patients with disabling osteoarthritis of the hip. Long-term results show about a 90 to 95 per cent success rate, based on relief of pain and ability to regain a useful degree of function. In a small percentage of patients, one or more of the implanted hip components may loosen in time but can usually be successfully replaced in a revision operation.

Herniated Intervertebral Disk ■ Intervertebral disks* in the spine normally function as shock absorbers between vertebral bodies. Each intervertebral disk consists of a soft center mass called the nucleus pulposus and a thick fibrous outer cover known as the annulus fibrosus. Each intervertebral disk is also firmly sealed to the vertebral bodies above and below it, making it impossible for these structures to slip in and out of place in their entirety. In some individuals, for reasons that are not clearly understood, a structural disintegration of the disk occurs that resembles premature aging and results in a cracking and fraying of the thick, fibrous outer cover and conversion of the soft nucleus pulposus into a scarlike tissue. Once begun, degeneration of the intervertebral disk and annulus fibrosus appears to be a progressive and irreversible process that may start as early as the second decade of life in susceptible people.

Abnormal physical stresses placed on a degenerated disk may exceed the mechanical strength of the disk and annulus fibrosus, with resultant tearing of the annulus. Pieces of the nucleus pulposus may herniate through this tear in the annulus fibrosus and extrude into the spinal canal to compress the spinal cord or a lumbar or sacral spinal nerve root as it prepares to exit

---

*Some physicians prefer the optional spelling disc.

from the spinal canal. When herniated nuclear material causes pressure on a spinal nerve root as it passes by the intervertebral disk on its way to exit from the spine, the patient is said to have the clinical condition known as herniated intervertebral disk. This condition occurs most often in patients between 20 and 45 years of age and is more common in men. Because the greatest amounts of motion in the lumbar spine occur at the L4–L5 interspace and at the lumbosacral joint, about 90 per cent of intervertebral disk herniations occur at one or the other of these two spinal interspaces.

A patient with a herniated lumbar intervertebral disk presents with low back pain accompanied by sciatic pain radiating into the posterior buttock area and leg on the side of the disk herniation. Because the lumbar and sacral nerve roots ultimately merge into the sciatic nerve, any pressure on these roots will cause pain to radiate along the sciatic nerve distribution, and such pain is commonly referred to as *sciatica*. The patient may stand with the spine tilted away from the side of the disk herniation. Anything that increases irritation of the affected nerve root, such as bending, lifting, coughing, or sneezing, will cause an increase in sciatic nerve pressure and an increase in the sharpness of the pain. Pressure by deep palpation over the course of the sciatic nerve in the buttock and posterior thigh on the affected side may disclose local tenderness. Straight leg raising and sitting knee extension tests on the affected side are considered positive only if pain over the distribution of the sciatic nerve is reproduced. If back pain only is produced, these tests are considered negative. If pressure on the spinal nerve root is prolonged and severe enough, the Achilles tendon reflex on the side of the nerve root compression may be depressed or absent. Strength of the long toe extensors and anterior tibial muscle may be lessened, even to the point of allowing a complete foot drop. A patient with a herniated lumbar intervertebral disk may complain of a sensation of numbness and tingling in the toes and feet associated with an objective sensory loss in the skin of the associated dermatome.

An intervertebral disk is made up of soft tissue that cannot be visualized on plain x-ray films; only empty spaces between the vertebral bodies are seen. For this reason, plain x-ray examination of the low back is not useful for either confirming or denying the clinical diagnosis of a herniated lumbar intervertebral disk. Localizing the site of a disk herniation for the purpose of confirming the diagnosis is accomplished by the use of specialized tests, such as a myelogram, computed tomography (CT) examination of the suspected spinal level, or a magnetic resonance imaging (MRI) study of the area.

Whether a patient with a herniated lumbar intervertebral disk will need surgical treatment or not depends largely on whether the patient's posterior longitudinal spinal ligament, which lies between the disk material and the spinal nerve roots, is intact or ruptured. If this ligament remains intact, which is the case more often than not, the protruding disk material simply pushes against it and causes the ligament to bulge against the nearest spinal nerve root. On the other hand, if the ligament has ruptured, extruding disk material may push freely into the spinal canal. A high percentage of patients with a clinical diagnosis of herniated lumbar intervertebral disk do retain an intact posterior longitudinal spinal ligament and, consequently, will recover on a well-supervised, nonoperative treatment program that includes a period of absolute bed rest, followed by back-strengthening exercises and instruction in proper back hygiene. Bed rest allows the intradiskal pressure of the intervertebral disk to reduce, which frequently allows the bulging disk to subside and drop away from the posterior longitudinal spinal ligament and the compressed spinal nerve root.

However, if disk material has extruded into the spinal canal through a ruptured posterior longitudinal spinal ligament, most forms of nonoperative treatment usually fail. Generally, these patients require an operation consisting of a hemilaminectomy and excision of the protruding and extruding disk material to decompress adequately the affected spinal nerve root to relieve the patient's back and leg pain.

Carpal Tunnel Syndrome ▪ The carpal bones are bridged by the transverse carpal ligament on the volar aspect of the wrist, thus forming the carpal tunnel, sometimes called the carpal canal. The tendons and tendon sheaths of nine wrist and finger flexor muscles plus the median nerve pass from the forearm into the hand and fingers through this carpal tunnel (Figure 28–9). Anything that causes an abnormal amount of pressure on the median nerve as it passes through this relatively crowded carpal tunnel can give rise to the clinical condition known as carpal tunnel syndrome.

Among the recognized causes of carpal tunnel syndrome are occupational tasks requiring constant and repetitive wrist joint motions. Other causes of abnormal pressure on the median nerve in the carpal tunnel include dislocation of the lunate bone and certain fractures of the navicular bone in the wrist joint, malunited Colles' fractures, arthritic deformities and bone spurs about the wrist, hypertrophy of the transverse carpal ligament, soft tissue masses within the carpal tunnel, such as lipomas and ganglia, and

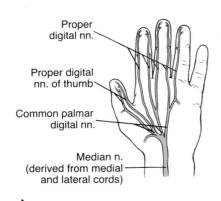
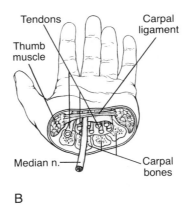
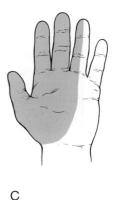

A   B   C

Figure **28–9**
Carpal tunnel syndrome. A, Median nerve supply to the hand. B, Cross-section of the wrist. C, The median nerve's sensory distribution in the thumb, first three fingers, and palm.

thickening of the flexor tendon sheaths secondary to rheumatoid arthritis or chronic tenosynovitis.

Normally, the carpal tunnel becomes tight and narrow when the fingers and wrist are held in a position of forced flexion. If anything in or around the carpal tunnel exerts an abnormal amount of pressure on the median nerve, symptoms characteristic of carpal tunnel syndrome will be produced by wrist motions that tend to constrict the carpal tunnel, such as forced flexion and forced extension of the wrist. Patients with compression of the median nerve in the carpal tunnel complain of pain that radiates along a median nerve distribution pattern in the hand and fingers and may be associated with sensations of numbness and paresthesia. Manual pressure on the carpal tunnel by a physician examiner may accentuate the patient's symptoms of pain and tingling in the hand and fingers. Atrophy of the thenar muscles of the thumb and weakness of thumb opposition motions may develop. Because carpal tunnel syndrome essentially is a soft tissue problem, x-ray examination of the involved wrist is not helpful in making a diagnosis unless the median nerve compression is caused by some type of bone deformity that could be visualized on x-ray films. Diagnosis of carpal tunnel syndrome can usually be confirmed by electromyographic and nerve conduction studies of the median nerve and the muscles the nerve enervates.

Symptoms caused by carpal tunnel syndrome may disappear in some patients following a period of immobilization of the wrist and avoidance of work requiring repetitive flexion of the wrist joint. If this period of enforced rest to the wrist joint is not successful in curing symptoms from median nerve compression at the wrist, the transverse carpal ligament may be surgically divided to unroof the carpal tunnel in order to decompress the constricted median nerve. Refer to Figure 28–10, a history and physical of a case involving carpal tunnel syndrome.

REPRESENTATIVE INJURIES

Supracondylar Fracture of Humerus ▪
The supracondylar area of the humerus is the flared lower end of the bone just above the elbow joint. Falls on the elbow or outstretched arm may cause the humerus to break through the supracondylar area. Fractures through this area of the bone are common in children but not in adults. Supracondylar fractures of the humerus are considered serious and potentially dangerous injuries for children to sustain because of the possibility of associated nerve or artery damage in the area of the elbow joint. The median, ulnar, or radial nerve or the brachial artery may be compressed or lacerated by a fragment of bone or compressed by the extensive swelling that sets in rapidly around the elbow after the occurrence of a supracondylar fracture. The possibility that a child has sustained such a fracture after a fall or injury to the elbow is reinforced by the appearance of a swollen, deformed, and painful elbow. If the brachial artery is compressed by swelling or a fragment of bone, the child's radial pulse on the fracture side will be weak or absent. If compression of the brachial artery is not corrected within a 4- to 8-hour period from the time the fracture was sustained, increased pressure arising within the forearm muscle compartments will lead to a condition known as compartment syndrome. This could result in severe and permanent deformity and crippling of the involved hand and arm.

Diagnosis of a supracondylar fracture of the humerus is made by anteroposterior and lateral x-ray views of the injured elbow. Every child with a suspected elbow fracture should have x-ray films made of both elbows so a comparison of the appearance of both elbows on x-ray films can be made and a possible fracture line distinguished from normally expected growth lines. The normally present epiphyseal or growth lines at the lower end of the humerus sometimes make it difficult to detect a fracture line. If an x-ray film of the uninjured elbow is available for comparison, the detection of a fracture line on the x-ray film of the injured elbow is facilitated. Usually a comparison is not necessary in adults because growth lines are no longer present on x-ray films to cause confusion with a fracture line.

Treatment of supracondylar fractures of the humerus in children should be undertaken as soon as the x-ray films have been reviewed and diagnosis confirmed. Delay in treating this injury is dangerous because of the possibility that increasing swelling about the injured elbow might cause circulatory embarrassment to the arm. Reduction of a displaced supracondylar fracture of the humerus involves restoring the normal forward angulation of the distal end of the humerus, in addition to correcting the rotational spin assumed by the smaller distal fragment of the humerus. If the bone deformity caused by the fracture is not corrected, the child will have a permanently deformed elbow.

The majority of these fractures can be reduced by closed reduction obtained by manipulating the elbow under anesthesia, followed by immobilization of the broken elbow in a plaster (plaster of Paris) cast for 6 weeks. If a supracondylar fracture can be reduced by a closed reduction but proves to be unstable after reduction, fixation of the bone fragments in the reduced position can be achieved by introducing metal pins percutaneously into the medial and lateral humeral epicondyles and advancing them across the fracture line under x-ray control. Patients with severe displacement of the fracture with severe swelling of the elbow or with multiple fracture fragments may have to be treated in the hospital in skin or skeletal traction. The prognosis for the return of normal elbow function is excellent in children whose supracondylar fracture is well reduced and heals without complication.

Hip Fracture ▪ Fracture of the hip refers specifically to fractures occurring through the neck of the femur or through the intertrochanteric region of the femur (Figure 28–11). Women experience 70 to 80 per cent of hip fractures, and the incidence of the two types is approximately equal. This is a common injury in older adults, with a doubling of the fracture rate for each decade of life after age 50 years. Management of a hip fracture is complicated by the fact that at least one third or more of the injured patients have an associated medical disorder of some significance, such as diabetes or heart disease, or are of advanced age. This is a serious injury for older patients, and mortality rates of 20 per cent within 6 months of breaking a hip are reported. Hip fracture may follow a twisting injury to the leg or a fall directly on the hip, or just may occur in the seeming absence of specific injury in patients with osteoporosis. Patients with hip fractures may experience severe pain in the area and inability to move or bear weight on the injured leg. Following hip fracture, the affected leg tends to assume a characteristic position of shortening, adduction, and external rotation. It is not

possible to distinguish between a fracture through the neck of the femur and a fracture through the intertrochanteric region of the femur solely on clinical signs. Anteroposterior and lateral x-ray views of the affected hip joint are required to confirm the diagnosis and to identify the type of fracture sustained.

Except in unusual circumstances, the treatment of hip fractures is surgical. Treatment for fractures through the neck of the femur consists of accurate reduction of the two fracture fragments by either closed or open methods, followed by operative insertion of some metallic internal fixation device, such as a compression screw or multiple threaded pins to fasten the two broken bone fragments together until bone healing occurs. The use of an x-ray image intensifier in the operating room greatly aids in the accurate placement of the metallic internal fixation device. Effective and secure internal fixation allows the patient to be out of bed early in the postoperative period, but full weight bearing on the operated leg is prohibited until subsequent x-ray examination shows complete healing of the fracture, a process that may take as long as 6 months.

Fractures occurring through the neck of the femur are difficult to treat and slower to heal than fractures occurring through the intertrochanteric region of the femur. This is because in femoral neck fractures, the proximal fragment (femoral head) is small, contains a high proportion of hard, dense cortical bone, and has a relatively poor blood supply. Even under the best of circumstances, about 25 per cent of patients with fractures through the neck of the femur will develop nonunion of the fracture site following treatment. In selected frail, aged, or senile patients, the femoral head can be excised and replaced with a metallic femoral head prosthesis anchored to the remaining femoral neck by bone cement.

Fractures through the intertrochanteric region of the femur are treated by closed reduction of the fracture carried out on a fracture table with the aid of an x-ray image intensifier and a C-arm. Once adequate closed reduction has been achieved, a metallic nail-plate device, with or without a compression telescoping element, is inserted through a lateral incision for the purpose of internal fixation of the reduced intertrochanteric fracture. If satisfactory closed reduc-

Telephone: 805/956-8009   **JOHN SMITH, M. D.**   Fax: 805/982-0900
4500 College Avenue
Oxnard, CA 93035-4123

January 28, 1994

St. Paul Insurance
20800 Swenson Drive, Suite 300
Waukesha, WI 53186-0980

ATTENTION: Mr. Aaron Sterling, Claims Adjuster

Dear Mr. Sterling:

RE: Jason Owen
EMPLOYER: ABC Tool and Die Company
DATE OF INJURY: October 6, 1993

Mr. Jason Owen is seen with your authorization for evaluation of a problem with
his right hand.

HISTORY:
The patient is currently 39 years of age. In October of 1993, he states he was
unloading a box load of freight from a truck when he lifted a 40-50 pound box. It
twisted his hand, and he states he developed numbness and tingling in his
fingers. He believes he was given a diagnosis of acute carpal tunnel syndrome.
He believes neurologic studies were obtained before his surgery. It was
recommended by his surgeon, Dr. Doe, that he undergo a carpal tunnel release.
A faxed copy of the operative report from College Hospital, dated November 8,
199X, reveals that he had a preoperative diagnosis of acute right carpal tunnel
syndrome, and he underwent right carpal tunnel release with epineurolysis of the
median nerve. Findings of surgery indicated acute carpal tunnel syndrome;
however, he was found to have thickened tenosynovium secondary to overuse
syndrome. The patient states that prior to being released to return to work, he
relocated to the Tulsa area. He has not worked since his injury. The patient
states that he underwent physical therapy for approximately one month after his
surgery. He states he has been released to return to work; however, jobs are
currently unavailable.

CURRENT SYMPTOMS:
The patient states he has numbness in the thumb, index, and long finger of his
right hand which persists subsequent to the surgery. He states he has weakness
of the right hand compared to the left. Currently, he has no other symptoms.

EXAMINATION:
Physical examination reveals a healed incision which is 4 1/2 cm in length in the
proximal portion of the palm of the hand along the thenar crease. The incision

Figure 28-10
History and physical examination report of a patient with carpal tunnel syndrome.

Page 2
Jason Owen
January 28, 1994

itself is nontender. There is no evidence of hypertrophic scar formation. He has full range of motion of all digits and of the wrist in dorsiflexion, palmar flexion, and radial and ulnar deviation. Tinel's sign over the base of the palm causes a tingling which he feels in the palm. Two point discrimination was tested and is 4 mm on the radial and ulnar halves of all digits, including the thumb, index, long, ring, and little fingers. Allen's test performed at the wrist reveals normal feel from the radial and ulnar arteries within four seconds. Grip strength was tested with the Jamar dynamometer and was listed as follows:
Right/left: 25/80; 50/70; 35/80. Pinch strength: (right/left) two finger pinch 7/9; three finger pinch 17/18; lateral pinch 26/20. Motor examination reveals normal motor strength of abductor pollicis brevis, opponens pollicis, first dorsal interosseous, and abductor digiti quinti.

IMPRESSION:
The patient has symptoms of numbness in the thumb, index, and long fingers of his right hand subsequent to carpal tunnel release. The symptoms of numbness are not confirmed by sensory examination, and, in fact, two point discrimination is found to be normal. Motor evaluation fails to reveal any evidence of weakness or atrophy. However, the patient has a weakness of grip strength which seems to be inconsistent with the physical examination, in that he does not grossly appear to have any disuse, weakness, or atrophy of the hand which would coincide with his weak grip.

RECOMMENDATIONS:
It is my opinion that the patient had carpal tunnel release for what was likely chronic carpal tunnel syndrome. It would be important to review the nerve conduction velocities which were performed at that time. However, in order to settle his case and confirm the objective nature of his median nerve function at this time, I would recommend carpal tunnel studies repeated in order to assess the nerve conduction velocities of the median and ulnar nerves of the right hand. There is an inconsistency in the patient's current symptoms and the physical findings, namely relating to sensation. I am concerned that the patient may not be motivated to maximize the results of his grip strength testing when performed with the Jamar dynamometer. I recommend that the nerve conduction velocities that were performed prior to his surgery be forwarded for review and comparison to current studies. Current studies are necessary in order to formulate his permanent and stationary evaluation. Upon their receipt, an addendum report will be necessary in order to complete this review.

If any further information is required in the interim, please do not hesitate to contact this office.

Sincerely,

John Smith, M. D.

mtf

Figure **28–10** *Continued*

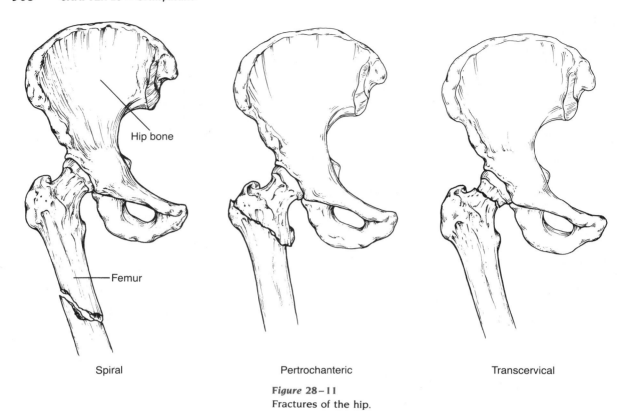

Spiral   Pertrochanteric   Transcervical

Figure 28–11
Fractures of the hip.

tion cannot be achieved, the fracture can be reduced by open reduction, followed by insertion of the nail-plate device. Effective and secure internal fixation of intertrochanteric fractures of the femur allows early ambulation for patients, but full weight bearing on the operated leg is discouraged until subsequent x-ray examination shows complete healing of the fracture, a process that occurs within a 3- to 4-month period postoperatively. Generally, patients sustaining fractures through the intertrochanteric region of the femur are older than those patients sustaining fractures through the neck of the femur. However, healing of the fracture is more favorable at the intertrochanteric region, because this anatomic area of the bone contains a high proportion of vascular cancellous bone tissue.

Colles' Fracture ■ The most frequent bone injury produced by a fall on the outstretched hand in the adult is a wrist fracture called a Colles' fracture. This injury is a fracture through the distal end of the radius, with or without an

associated fracture of the ulnar styloid. This common fracture was first described, before the discovery of x-rays, by an Irish surgeon named Abraham Colles.

The wrist of a patient with a Colles' fracture appears puffy and deformed. The distal radial fragment is displaced upward and tilted backward, giving rise to a characteristic hump on the back of the wrist, the so-called "silver fork" deformity, best seen when the injured wrist is viewed from the side. Backward tilting of the distal radial fragment causes shortening of the radius and an alteration in the normal position of the radial styloid in relation to the position of the ulnar styloid. The normal volar concavity of the radius is lost, and the area feels distended when palpated. The median nerve may be compressed in the carpal tunnel as a consequence of a Colles' fracture. Usually there are no accompanying circulatory complications with this fracture. Because this fracture is sustained by a fall on the outstretched hand, an occasional patient may suffer an associated fracture of the elbow or shoulder.

Although the presence of a Colles' fracture can be suspected in an adult patient on the basis of a history of a fall on the outstretched hand and the appearance of a swollen, painful, and deformed wrist, the diagnosis can be confirmed only by anteroposterior and lateral x-ray views of the injured wrist. Examination of the x-ray films is needed to identify the position and number of fracture fragments in the injured wrist.

Most patients with a Colles' fracture can be treated satisfactorily by closed manipulative reduction under local or general anesthesia, with immobilization of the fracture in a plaster cast for 6 to 8 weeks. Because the forearm and hand motions of supination and pronation can cause the fracture fragments to move at the wrist and because supination and pronation motions of the forearm arise from the elbow joint, the immobilization cast generally extends above the patient's elbow, at least for the first 4 to 6 weeks. In some patients, a Colles' fracture may be so comminuted and unstable it cannot be immobilized satisfactorily in a plaster cast. External fixation devices, using pins drilled into bone above and below the fracture area, are quite satisfactory for holding such fractures in the reduced position until healing occurs.

Ankle Fractures ■ Although frequent in occurrence, these are often quite complicated injuries that pose difficult treatment problems. Many complex mechanisms of injury may be applied to the ankle joint by forces arising from vehicular, pedestrian, or athletic trauma to produce a variety of fracture combinations. Ankle fractures include fractures of the lateral malleolus, medial malleolus, both malleoli (Pott's fracture), and, if a vertical compression force is part of the mechanism of injury, of the posterior lip of the tibia (trimalleolar fracture). These fractures may occur singly or in various combinations, depending on the mechanism of injury and how it is applied to the ankle joint. In addition to the bone injury at the ankle, one or more of the supporting ligaments of the ankle, including the tibiofibular syndesmosis, which holds the tibia and fibula together at their distal ends, may be ruptured (see Figure 28–7). Rupture of a medial or lateral supporting ligament may allow the talus to shift either medially or laterally in the ankle joint mortise. Rupture of the tibiofibular

syndesmosis may cause an associated diastasis or widening of the ankle joint mortise.

The mechanism of injury by which an ankle fracture is produced is important to know because the principle underlying successful reduction of ankle fractures is based on reversing the injuring forces. For example, fractures produced by external rotation and abduction forces on the ankle will be easily reduced by internal rotation and adduction forces applied to the injured ankle by the treating physician.

Most ankle fractures occur when the force applied to the foot and ankle is transmitted through the talus, displacing it beyond the normal elasticity of the ankle ligaments. The mechanism of injury can be delivered to an ankle joint in the directions of external rotation, abduction, adduction, vertical compression, or in various combinations of these force directions. For example, slipping on ice or a wet floor produces a combination of external rotation and abduction forces on the ankle and is the most common mechanism by which ankle fractures are produced. In addition, a fracture produced by an injuring mechanism is further modified by the position of the patient's foot at the time of injury. For example, internal rotation forces applied with the foot supinated injure the lateral side of the ankle first, but the same forces applied with the foot pronated injure the medial structures of the ankle first.

Ankle fractures produce pain, swelling, disability, and varying degrees of deformity of the ankle area. Most patients who sustain an ankle fracture cannot bear weight on the injured part. Associated vascular or nerve damage is rarely encountered. Specific details regarding the type and severity of the ankle fracture are identified by reviewing anteroposterior, lateral, and mortise x-ray views of the injured ankle. Details regarding the bone injury can be identified on these x-ray films but not details about any possible associated ligament damage at the ankle joint. The latter can be assessed by stress x-ray films of the ankle joint, an MRI study of the ankle, and, possibly, an arthrogram of the ankle joint.

The most satisfactory long-term results following treatment of displaced ankle fractures are obtained by anatomic restoration of the contours of the ankle joint. For some fractures, this condition may be obtained by closed reduction of the fracture followed by several months in a long leg cast. However, for most ankle fractures, exact reduction of the fracture fragments can be achieved and maintained more predictably by open reduction of the fracture and internal fixation of the fracture fragments with metallic plates, screws, or wires. The goals of treatment for displaced ankle fractures include anatomic positioning of the talus in the ankle mortise, a joint line that is parallel to the ground, and a smooth joint surface. Careful review of long-term results of ankle fracture treatment clearly demonstrates that acceptance of lesser goals frequently results in patients with poor clinical outcomes and chronically painful ankle joints.

GLOSSARY OF SURGICAL TERMS

amputation: The removal of part or all of a limb by cutting through the bone.

arthrodesis: The operation by which fusion is obtained between the bony parts of a joint. This term can be used interchangeably with the word "fusion."

arthroplasty: A reconstructive operation performed on a joint previously damaged by trauma or disease. The operation is designed to restore the integrity and functional power of the joint, usually by insertion of metallic or plastic implants.

arthroscopy: The technique of looking inside a joint through an arthroscope for diagnostic or therapeutic purposes.

arthrotomy: The operation of cutting into a joint.

aspiration: The act of withdrawing fluid material from a joint through a needle inserted through the skin.

bone grafting: The operation by which bone tissue is transplanted from one site in the body to another place in order to give added strength to the recipient bone or to induce healing in an area of fracture nonunion. Bone that comes from the same person who is to receive it is called an autogenous bone graft. Bone that comes from a different person is called an allograft.

capsulectomy: The surgical act of excising or resecting the capsule of a joint.

capsulotomy: The surgical act of cutting into a joint capsule.

closed reduction: A nonoperative method of treating fractures or joint dislocations by manually restoring normal alignment to the broken bone or dislocated joint.

curettage: The surgical scraping of bone tissue with a sharp, cup-shaped instrument called a curette.

debridement: The surgical cleansing of a wound to remove dead, devitalized, infected, or soiled tissue.

disarticulation: The removal of a limb by cutting through a joint.

displacement osteotomy: The operation of cutting through a bone and shifting the position of the bone fragments to change the alignment of the bone or to alter the weight-bearing stresses applied to the associated joint.

epiphysiodesis: The operation of creating permanent premature closure of a growth plate (physis) by passing finely threaded metallic pins, metallic screws, or bone pegs across the growth plate.

excision: The surgical act of cutting out and removing soft tissue or bone. This term and the word *resection* can be used interchangeably.

fusion: The operation by which joint cartilage is removed from bones of a joint and the bone ends opened so new bone will join the bone ends together, thus obliterating the joint as a functioning unit. This term has the same orthopaedic significance as the word *arthrodesis*.

hemilaminectomy: The operation of removing a portion of the vertebral lamina to gain exposure to an underlying spinal nerve root or intervertebral disk.

internal fixation: The surgical act of introducing metallic pins, wires, screws, nails, plates, or rods into bone for the purpose of holding two or more bones fragments securely in apposition and alignment until bone healing occurs.

laminectomy: The operation of removing a vertebral lamina to gain exposure to an underlying spinal nerve root or intervertebral disk or to decompress a compressed spinal cord and spinal nerve roots occurring in patients with spinal stenosis.

lavage: The surgical cleansing of a joint or an area of exposed bone by washing with copious amounts of fluid, frequently delivered to the part under mechanical pressure.

neurectomy: The surgical excision of a part of a nerve.

neurolysis: The surgical freeing of a nerve from surrounding scar tissue.

open reduction: A surgical method of treating fractures or joint dislocations by restoring normal bone alignment or joint integrity under direct vision through a surgical incision.

ostectomy: The surgical act of excising or resecting bone tissue.

osteotomy: The surgical act of cutting completely through a bone, usually by employing an osteotome and mallet or an electric bone saw.

prosthetic replacement: The surgical act of inserting a prosthetic implant, usually metal or plastic, as a replacement for a part of a bone or joint that is diseased, damaged, or deficient. The term *prosthetic replacement* is also correctly used when applied to an artificial limb.

resection: The surgical act of cutting out and removing soft tissue or bone. This term has the same meaning as the word *excision*.

revision: In its most frequently applied orthopaedic usage, revision refers to the surgical procedure of correcting or revising some mechanical difficulty encountered in a previously performed total joint replacement arthroplasty. Revisions of previously performed total joint replacement arthroplasties are performed because of mechanical malalignment of the inserted components, because of mechanical loosening of previously inserted prosthetic joint components, or because of other factors that prevent the prosthetic device from functioning as it was designed to function.

spinal fusion: The operation of fusing together two or more vertebral segments to eliminate motion between them.

synovectomy: The operation of excising or resecting the synovial membrane of a joint.

tendon graft: The operation by which tendon tissue is transplanted from one tendon in the body to another tendon in order to replace diseased or damaged tendon tissue or to fill a gap in the host tendon. If the tendon graft comes from the same person who is to receive the tendon graft, it is called an autogenous graft. If the tendon graft comes from a different person, it is called an allograft.

tendon lengthening: The operation of lengthening a tightened or contracted tendon.

tendon repair, flexor: The term "no man's land" may be dictated by some physicians when describing a flexor tendon repair of the hand. This phrase is an accepted anatomic term for one of the six designated zones of the hand and is used to reference visually the underlying tendons.

tendon transfer: The surgical relocation of the tendon of a normal muscle to another nearby site in the body to take over the function of a muscle permanently inactivated by trauma or disease.

tenotomy: The surgical cutting of a tendon.

total joint replacement: A special type of arthroplasty in which both sides of a diseased or damaged joint are replaced by metal and plastic implants. The implants may be made of a specialized porous metal or plastic that allows bone to grow into the implants in order to anchor them firmly to the host bone. Other implants may be anchored to the host bone by bone cement (methylmethacrylate).

SURGICAL INSTRUMENTS

Orthopaedic surgeons use some surgical instruments that are common to most surgical procedures and other instruments especially designed to be used with bone. Many of these especially designed bone instruments have proper names attached to them, such as Kerrison's bone punch.

General Instruments

forceps: These come in various types and styles. Forceps used frequently in surgical procedures include the following: Allis' tissue forceps, bayonet forceps, sponge-holding forceps, towel forceps (also called towel clips), and coagulation forceps (bipolar) used with electrical equipment to coagulate bleeding vessels to obtain hemostasis.

hemostat: A clamp used to grasp a bleeding vessel so it can be tied off or coagulated.

Kocher's clamp: Resembles a large hemostat but is a heavier instrument with toothed blades; it is generally used for holding or putting traction on various tissues.

needle: These come in various sizes and curvatures and are used for sewing tissue together.

needle holder: A surgical clamp used to hold the needle when engaged in sewing tissue together.

retractor: These come in various types and sizes and frequently have proper names attached to them. They are used to hold noninvolved tissue away from the surgical field.

scalpel: Usually an individual knife handle to which knife blades of various sizes and shapes are attached.

scissors: A straight or curved instrument used to cut soft tissue and suture material. A popular surgical dissecting scissor is called a Metzenbaum's scissor.

Special Instruments

Some specialized instruments used in orthopaedic surgery, such as bone saws, bone drills, and screwdrivers, can be manually operated or electrically driven. Special use instruments include:

bone biter: This instrument is used to bite off small pieces of bone. The instrument may be straight or angled.

bone chisel: A flat, sharp bone-cutting tool that may be straight or curved in shape.

bone drill: An electrically operated device to which drill bits of varying sizes can be attached for the purpose of drilling holes in bone.

bone forceps: A tool used to pick up pieces of bone.

bone fragment clamp: Generally, this is used to hold two bone fragments together until they can be stabilized by an internal fixation device.

bone-holding clamp: This tool has essentially the same purpose as a bone fragment clamp.

bone punch: An instrument to remove small pieces of bone.

bone rasp (raspatory): A bone file.

bone rongeur: This tool is used to remove larger pieces of bone and may be straight or angled in shape.

bone saw: This device may be operated manually or electrically.

cast equipment

    cast cutter: An electrically driven saw used to cut casts open.

    cast spreader: An instrument used to spread or force cut edges apart after cast has been cut through.

curette: A sharp, cup-shaped instrument of various sizes used to scrape bone and hardened soft tissue.

internal fixation device: A device used to hold two broken or cut fragments of bone together until healing occurs. It is made from special metals or metal alloys that are nonreactive in body tissues. Among the internal fixation devices in common use are nails, pins, plates, rods, screws, and Kirschner's wires. These devices come in various sizes, and many have attached proper names.

intramedullary fixation device: These internal fixation devices can be either metallic rods or thick metal pins introduced into the marrow cavity of long bones, i.e., Kuntscher's rods, Lottes' nails, and Rush's pins.

mallet: A surgical hammer.

microsurgery instruments.: Specialized instruments and equipment used for microsurgery.

nerve root and spinal cord retractor.: A device used to protect the nerve root and spinal cord structures during intervertebral disk surgery.

nerve root elevator: A device used to mobilize or free a spinal nerve root from adhesions during intervertebral disk surgery.

osteotome: A broad, sharp, flat, straight, or curved instrument of various sizes that is used to cut bone when tapped with a mallet.

periosteal elevator: A flat instrument that resembles a paddle, used to raise the periosteal membrane from bone before the bone is cut or drilled.

plaster of Paris bandages: Rolls of crinoline-like bandage of varying sizes, impregnated with anhydrous calcium sulfate. When dipped in lukewarm water and wrapped around a body part, these bandages harden to become a plaster cast.

prosthesis: An artificial replacement for part of the body that is diseased, damaged, or deficient. It can be made from special metals, metal alloys, or high-density polyethylene plastic, all of which are nonreactive to human body tissues.

    total hip prosthesis: This device has a metal or metal alloy femoral component and a plastic acetabular component.

    total knee prosthesis: This device has a metal or metal alloy femoral component and a plastic tibial component.

reamers: These heavy drill bits of varying sizes are used to ream out the marrow cavity of a long bone preparatory to introducing an intramedullary nail into the cavity. Drill bits used for reaming are attached to electrically operated drills.

retractor: This tool comes in various sizes and shapes and is used to hold uninvolved tissue away from the surgical field. Some surgical retractors are self-retaining.

screwdriver: This instrument may be operated manually or electrically.

sheet wadding: A soft, cotton-like material wrapped around a body part before applying plaster of Paris bandages in the construction of a plaster cast. The function of sheet wadding is to protect the skin from being rubbed by a hardened plaster cast.

stockinette: A woven, stocking-like material pulled over a body part before applying sheet wadding and a plaster cast. Stockinette is folded back over plaster cast edges to lessen skin irritation and rubbing.

tendon retriever: A tool used to probe for and locate a tendon end that has retracted after being cut.

tendon stripper: An instrument used to strip the sheath away from a tendon.

wire instruments: Generally, tools used in conjunction with inserting or extracting Kirschner's wires from bone. These include wire cutters, wire drills, wire extractor pliers, and wire tighteners.

FORMATS

Letters ▪ Letters written to referring physicians by orthopaedic surgeons should be factual and objective, with built-in, logically derived sequences in a narrative writing style.

1. State how the patient described the problem for which assistance is sought.

2. List the symptoms and signs found as a result of the history, physical examination, and ancillary tests performed or reviewed on behalf of the patient.

3. State what the findings mean and what the patient's problem is.

4. Give recommendations of what should be done to correct or alleviate the problem.

5. Mention what the patient was advised to do and, if appropriate, the arrangements made for the patient to receive treatment.

6. End the letter by thanking the referring physician for the opportunity of assisting in the management of the patient's care and, if appropriate, advise the referring physician that he or she will be kept informed of the patient's progress and response to orthopaedic treatment.

Progress Notes
Hospital Charts ▪ The purpose of progress notes in a patient's hospital medical chart is to record the progress or lack of progress of the physician's treatment plan in solving or ameliorating the medical problem for which the patient was admitted to the hospital. Progress notes should be pertinent, relevant, and material, recorded in a narrative writing style using clear and understandable language, and signed or initialed by the progress note writer. Entries should be made in a timely fashion, in chronologic order, with date and time when the progress note is written.

Usually written daily, progress notes record any change in the patient's complaints or physical findings and evaluate radiologic and laboratory studies as the results relate to the patient's diagnosis, treatment, or response to treatment. Physicians comment on findings recorded by consultants, on any unexpected laboratory or radiologic results, and on any untoward clinical events sustained by the patient. They respond to any contradictory observations by nurses or other health care professionals. Any change in the physician's thinking in regard to diagnostic impression, diagnostic efforts, or patient management must be explained in a progress note.

Office Medical Record ▪ Information about a patient gathered by a physician in the history taking and physical examination part of the diagnostic interview in the office should be recorded in a style and format with which the physician is comfortable. Once a comfortable and satisfactory writing style and format for office medical records has been adopted, the physician should stick to it so other readers can follow a patient's course with a minimum of difficulty. Notes made in office medical records must be written in clear, easily understood, and uncomplicated words that are made into sentences that flow in a continuous and sensible fashion. Generally, progress notes made in office medical records are short and concise and tend to emphasize critical and important points about a patient's diagnosis, treatment, and progress or lack of progress toward recovery. Office medical records should specify tests, radiologic examinations, or consultations that have been ordered, the reasons for ordering them, and the results when the information becomes available.

Medical Reports
History and Physical Examination

1. Chief complaint

2. History of present illness

3. Past medical history

4. Family history

5. Personal history, habits, occupation, and environmental factors

6. Review of systems

7. Summary and working diagnosis

8. Signature of physician writing the medical record

9. A physical examination recorded in the chart of a patient with an orthopaedic complaint or problem is confined to the musculoskeletal system and, specifically, to the body part involved in the complaint or problem.

In a general orthopaedic examination, the patient's general posture and body alignment, as viewed from both front and back, are observed and recorded. Any physical abnormalities associated with walking, standing, sitting, or lying down are noted and recorded. In a local orthopaedic examination, the examiner notes and records contour, appearance, color, or deformity of a part and its general relationship to the body as a whole. The examiner detects by palpation tenderness, swelling, muscle spasm, local temperature changes, or gross alterations in the shape of a body part.

RANGE OF MOTION ■ Each joint has characteristic motions that can be measured manually by the examiner while the patient is lying relaxed in bed or on an examining table (Figure 28–5).

Joint motion is measured and recorded in degrees of a circle. Active joint motion represents the degree to which a patient can move the particular joint by virtue of his or her own muscle power without assistance from the examiner. Passive joint motion is measured manually by the examiner while the patient lies relaxed. The examiner tests the range of motion the joint is normally capable of achieving and compares these degrees with those obtained in the opposite joint. When the patient's complaint involves an arm or leg, the physical examination always includes measuring and recording the range of motion found in the comparable joint in the opposite arm or leg.

MEASUREMENT ■ Atrophy or hypertrophy of a part may be determined by comparing circumferential tape measurements made at the same points on opposite sides of the body. Limb lengths are measured, recorded, and compared in order to assess any inequality in length that may be present.

NEUROLOGIC EXAMINATION ■ The strength of muscle power should be assessed and recorded whenever the presence of muscular weakness is suspected in a body part. The quality of the superficial and deep tendon reflexes and the integrity of cutaneous sensation should be determined and recorded when indicated.

Figure 28–10 is an example of a history and physical examination in letter style.

Operative Reports ■ Language used in operative reports should be crisp and clearly understandable, so readers are provided with a lucid picture of what took place during the operative procedure. A dictated operative report contains the following bits of factual information:

Patient's name, medical record number, date of hospital admission, and date of operation
Names of surgeon and assistants
Name of surgical procedure performed
Type of anesthetic agent used
Name of anesthetist
Preoperative diagnosis (spelled out with no abbreviations)
Postoperative diagnosis (spelled out with no abbreviations)
Indication for operation
Position of patient on the operating table and type of skin preparation carried out
Type of skin incision used

UNIVERSITY HOSPITAL
1234 Main Street
Oxnard, CA 93030-0000

OPERATIVE REPORT

PATIENT: Matthew Bowles   ANES: Robert Doe, M.D.
SURGEON: John Smith, M. D.   RECORD #   540809-01
ASST SURGEON: None.

PREOPERATIVE DIAGNOSIS: Tear of the medial meniscus right knee.

POSTOPERATIVE DIAGNOSIS: Tear of the posterior horn of the medial
                                                          meniscus right knee, peripheral, and
chondromalacia of the right medial tibial and fibular condyles.

MATERIAL FORWARDED TO LAB: None.

OPERATIVE PROCEDURE: After the patient was under adequate
                                                  mask anesthesia, the left leg was placed
in a stirrup, and the right leg was placed in a leg holder and a tourniquet. The
tourniquet was elevated to 400 mm of Mercury, and the leg was prepped and
draped in a sterile fashion. The procedure was done in the bent knee position.
Standard mediolateral and superolateral portals were made after injecting the
skin sites with quarter percent Marcaine with epinephrine. The suprapatellar
pouch did not reveal any pathology, and the undersurface of the patella appeared
normal. The medial compartment had a significant posterior horn tear of the
medial meniscus which pulled into the joint. With great difficulty, the posterior
horn of the medial meniscus was removed, utilizing the suction basket, Shutt
basket forceps, and the turbo meniscal trimmer. The hook knife had to be used
to get the most lateral portion of the posterior horn loose, and then attention was
directed to the medial tibial and femoral condyles. They were trimmed, utilizing
the suction basket and the whisker trimmer. I would grade the chondromalacic
changes there at Grade II to III where the meniscus had been moving in and out
of the joint. After the medial compartment was completely cleaned with the
whisker trimmer, the scope was then taken into the notch where the anterior
cruciate ligament was intact and tightened appropriately with drawer testing. The
lateral compartment appeared entirely normal as did the lateral gutter. The
patient seemed to tolerate the procedure well. The tourniquet time was a total of
2 hours and 35 minutes, with the first tourniquet time being 1 hour and 15
minutes. That tourniquet failed, and so after five minutes, the tourniquet was re-
inflated, and it lasted for another hour and twenty minutes. The knee had 20 cc
of 0.25% Marcaine and epinephrine instilled prior to bandaging the wounds. The
wounds were closed with 3.0 Dexon S subcuticular sutures and Steri-strips.

(continued)

Figure 28–12
A, An operative report of an arthroscopy, typed in indented format. B, The arthroscopy procedure.

Figure continued

Page 2
Matthew Bowles
Record # 540809

A sterile pressure dressing was applied. Patient seemed to tolerate the procedure well and was in good condition when taken to the recovery room.

John Smith, M. D.

mtf
D: 7-26-94
T: 7-27-94

A

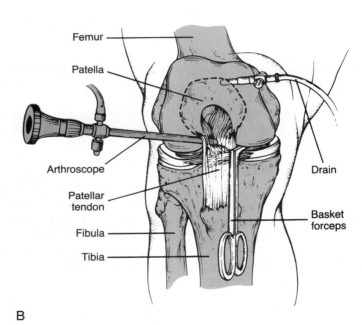

B

Figure 28–12 *Continued*

Telephone: 805/956-8009   **JOHN SMITH, M. D.**   Fax: 805/982-0900
4500 College Avenue
Oxnard, CA 93035-4123

February 18, 1994

Kevin North, M. D.
4000 Main Street
Woodland Hills, XY 12345-0000

Dear Dr. Smith:

Re: Harry Garcia

Thank you for your kind referral of Harry Garcia who was seen in my office today.

Mr. Garcia is a 23-year-old male injured at work on November 11, 1993. The patient has been off work since the injury. He describes the injury as follows. He was carrying a piece of drywall, weighing approximately 100 pounds. He slipped on some electrical conduit and fell backwards onto his buttocks, back, and head. He states that part of the electrical conduit, which was round, was impacted into his lumbar spine as well. He denies any loss of consciousness. He states he noted immediate onset of low back pain which has been present ever since. He has been to see Dr. David Ross who is a chiropractor. He did manipulations and other therapies with adjustments. He states he had mild relief but has been unable to return to work because of his discomfort. The pain is nonradiating and localized to his lumbar spine. It is present most of the time. It does not wake him up at night. He denies any bowel or bladder symptoms. He denies any previous episodes of low back pain prior to this. He states he is otherwise healthy. Other treatments which have been tried include a corset which gave him no relief and bed rest which gave him only light relief. Presently, he takes Tylenol for discomfort.

Physical examination reveals a 23-year-old male, looking his stated age. His gait is normal. He can heel and toe walk without difficulty. Lower extremity muscle strength is 5/5 throughout. Sensory examination is normal to light touch. Straight leg raising is 90° bilaterally with reproduction of low back symptoms at 90°. His reflexes are symmetric, and both toes are down going.

Lumbar spine x-rays done at your office reveal a spondylolysis bilateral at L5-S1 with a minor slip, less than Grade I. Flexion/extension views done today show no motion at the L5-S1 junction.

It is my impression that the patient sustained a lumbosacral strain following work injury with incidental findings of a spondylolysis and Grade I spondylolisthesis.

Figure 28–13
A consultation report in letter style, typed in full block format.   *Figure continued*

Page 2
Harry Garcia
February 18, 1994

Although a fusion may be of benefit, the source of his pain cannot be completely attributed to the spondylolysis. This is an unknown at this time. Preferably, I would continue to treat him nonoperatively. I do not consider chiropractic manipulations adequate nonoperative treatment. I believe he should be tried on a course of anti-inflammatories and have supplied him with Naprosyn, 500 mg, p.o., b.i.d. with full disclosure discussed. In addition, I believe Med-X program for lumbar evaluation and strengthening would be of great benefit. This would avoid possible surgery to his spine. Should he require surgery or should his symptoms not resolve and he continues to have severe pain, then diagnostic tests to try to identify the source, such as local blocks into the lytic areas and possibly discograms would be indicated. I have made him aware of this, and he is quite satisfied to proceed with Med-X and anti-inflammatories. He will require clearance from his workers' compensation carrier prior to this.

Again thank you for referring this patient to me. I will keep you informed of his progress.

Sincerely,

John Smith, M. D.

mtf

cc: Workers' Compensation and Indemnity

Figure 28–13 Continued

Findings at operation
Surgical procedure performed
Technical points of operation, such as type of suture material and drains used
Type of wound closure performed
Description of tissue removed and its disposition
Volume of fluids lost by patient
Amount of fluids or units of blood administered to patient
Condition of patient on conclusion of operative procedure
Signature of the surgeon. Residents may dictate operative reports as part of the learning process, but the surgeon retains the obligation of signing the report

Figure 28–12 shows an orthopaedic operative report.

Consultation Reports ■ The following format can be used for consultation reports in hospital medical records:

1. A statement of the patient's description of the problem for which the consultation was requested.

2. The symptoms and signs found as a result of the examination and after reviewing the medical history, recorded physical examination, and ancillary tests performed on behalf of the patient.

3. The findings and what the medical problem is.

4. Recommendation to correct or alleviate the problem for which the consultation was requested.

5. Thanks to the attending physician for being asked to assist in the management of the patient's care.

Figure 28–13 is an example of a consultation report.

Discharge Summary ■ The discharge or narrative summary is an account of the patient's medical experiences while hospitalized and is written in past tense using a narrative writing style. Chapters 12 through 38 feature illustrations of discharge summaries for various medical specialties. For further detailed information on discharge summaries, refer to the end of Chapters 16, 17, 23, 27, 29, 31, 34, 36, 37, and 38.

Reference Sources

Edmonson, A., and A. H. Crenshaw (Eds.). *Campbell's Operative Orthopaedics,* 7th edition. C. V. Mosby Company, St. Louis, 1987.
Gartland, J. J.. *Fundamentals of Orthopaedics,* 4th edition. W. B. Saunders Company, Philadelphia, 1987.
Lovell, W., and R. B. Winter. *Pediatric Orthopaedics,* 2nd edition. J. B. Lippincott Company, Philadelphia, 1986.

For references of specific application to medical transcription, see Appendix 1.

Otorhinolaryngology

INTRODUCTION

An otorhinolaryngologist is a doctor of medicine who subspecializes in the medical and surgical management of diseases of the ear, nose, throat, and related areas of the head and neck.

Otorhinolaryngology derives its name from the Latin roots of the word. *Oto* is the Latin root for the word ear, *rhino* is the Latin root for nose, and finally *laryn* is the Latin root for throat.

Many years of advanced training are necessary for otorhinolaryngologists, since many medical specialties overlap otorhinolaryngology, such as general surgery, general plastic surgery, oral surgery, dermatology, maxillofacial surgery, ophthalmology, neurosurgery, allergy, and thoracic surgery. Although training programs differ somewhat in their emphasis of subspecialty areas, all areas are covered in most residency programs. When otorhinolaryngologists begin their practices, they may subspecialize in a smaller area of the specialty.

Otorhinolaryngologists are trained to perform a great variety of surgical procedures in the treatment of head and neck diseases. These procedures range from microsurgery, through which operation on the stapes bone in the middle ear can restore hearing, to extensive cancer surgery in the head and neck area. Because of the extensive training that otorhinolaryngologists receive in head and neck anatomy and physiology, many perform facial plastic and reconstructive surgery.

ANATOMY

Ears ▪ The anatomy of the ear is divided into three parts: the external ear, which is the visible portion on the outside of the head; the middle ear, which contains the small bones, or ossicles, that transmit sound waves; and the inner ear, which contains sensory organs for both hearing and balance. The middle ear and inner ear are located within the temporal bone of the skull. (AD [auris dextra] refers to the right ear; AS [auris sinistra] refers to the left ear.)

External Ear ▪ The external ear is made up of the auricle and the external auditory canal. The visible auricle on the side of the head is made up of elastic cartilage with skin attached very closely in most areas (Figure 29–1). The external auditory canal extends from the external acoustic meatus to the tympanic membrane. The superior wall is slightly shorter than the inferior wall, causing the tympanic membrane to be positioned obliquely. The outer half of the ear canal is composed of cartilage, the inner half is surrounded by bone. The skin that lines the bony portion of the ear canal is very thin and contains no hair or cerumen glands. The outer cartilaginous portion is lined by thicker skin in which both cerumen glands and hair follicles may be found (Figure 29–2).

Middle Ear ▪ The middle ear is a cavity in the temporal bone of the skull that is bounded by the tympanic membrane laterally, by the floor of the middle cranial fossa superiorly, and medially by the structures contained within the inner ear. Inferiorly and anteriorly the eustachian tube connects the middle ear to the nasopharynx and is important in providing adequate ventilation to the middle ear space (see Figure 29–2). Three small bones, or ossicles, in the middle ear space transmit sound to the inner ear. The malleus is attached to the tympanic membrane and articulates with the incus, which in turn articulates with the stapes, forming an intricate ossicular

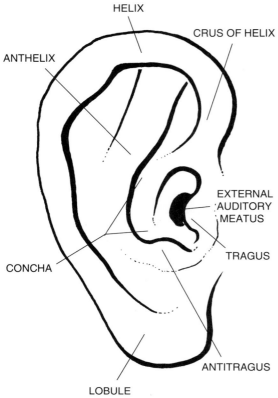

Figure 29–1
The auricle and external meatus of the ear.

chain that utilizes principles of mechanical advantage to amplify sound (Figure 29–3).

Two muscles attach to the ossicular chain. The tensor tympani muscle attaches to the neck of the malleus. The action of this muscle is to make the tympanic membrane tense by pulling the malleus inward. The stapedius muscle is the smallest muscle in the body and attaches a small process in the posterior wall of the middle ear to the neck of the stapes. This muscle contracts during loud sound to prevent excessive noise vibrations from being transmitted to the sensitive inner ear. Posteriorly, there is an extension of the middle ear space through the area of the aditus into mastoid cells within the temporal bone (Figure 29–4). This honeycomb mass of air cells is lined with the same thin mucous membrane layer that covers the middle ear. Inflammation and infection present in the middle ear can therefore extend into the mastoid.

Inner Ear ■ The inner ear contains the sen-

sory organs for both hearing and balance. Both these structures are found deep within the petrous portion of the temporal bone (see Figure 29–2). The cochlea is the sensory organ of hearing that resembles a snail shell. Within the cochlea are three compartments. The *central compartment* contains the organ of Corti, which is the sensory organ of hearing (Figure 29–5). The *labyrinth* contains the sensory receptors for equilibrium. The *vestibular portion* of the inner ear is made up of the three semicircular canals and the utricle. The ends of the semicircular canals open into the utricle, connecting to the endolymphatic duct and saccule, which has a membranous extension through the cochlear duct to the cochlea (Figure 29–6). The three semicircular canals are important in maintaining equilibrium. The eighth cranial nerve divides; the cochlear portion carries impulses from the cochlea and functions as the nerve of hearing; and the vestibular portion travels to the vestibule to provide a pathway for the labyrinth to send nerve impulses to the brain regarding equilibrium (see Figure 29–2).

Nose ■ The external portion of the nose consists of the dorsum, that portion of the nose lying between the nasal tip and the root of the nose. The base of the nose includes the nares, or nostrils, and laterally contains the nasal ala (Figure 29–7). Two paired nasal bones make up the upper third of the external nose. The lower two thirds of the nose is composed of both upper and lower lateral cartilages. The nasal dome is the portion of the cartilage that makes up the nasal tip along the lowermost portion of the nasal dorsum (Figure 29–8). The nasal septum is the partition in the center of the nose that divides it into two chambers. The anterior portion of the nasal septum is composed of cartilage; posteriorly, both superiorly and inferiorly the septum is made of bone (Figure 29–9).

Laterally along the walls of the nose are structures called turbinates. Although the inferior turbinate is a separate bone, other turbinates are portions of the ethmoid bone. The recess beneath a turbinate is called a meatus (plural: meatus). The various sinuses drain into the meatus (Figure 29–10). There are four paired sinuses: the maxillary, ethmoid, frontal, and sphenoid sinuses. These are air-filled spaces lined by mucous membranes. The sinus cavities all drain into the nose along the lateral wall. Ethmoid sinuses are composed of a honeycomb

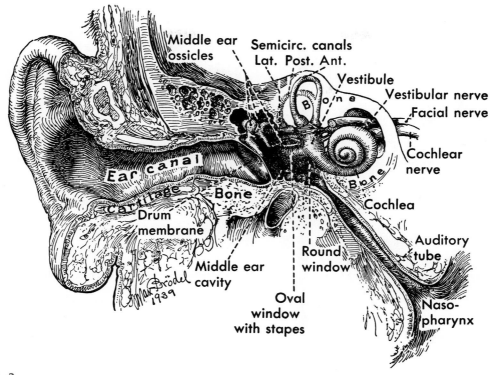

Figure 29–2

A diagram of the external, middle, and internal ears. (From Brödel, Max. *Three Unpublished Drawings of the Anatomy of the Human Ear.* W. B. Saunders Co., Philadelphia, 1946.)

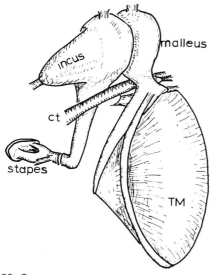

Figure 29–3

Sound conduction mechanism of the middle ear. (From Ballenger, John. *Diseases of the Nose, Throat, and Ear,* 11th ed. Lea & Febiger, Philadelphia, 1969.)

of small cells that lies beneath the bony portion of the external nose and surrounds the medial portion of the orbit. Mucous membrane lines the nose and the paranasal sinuses and extends through the eustachian tube into the middle ear and mastoid. This same lining also extends into the pharynx and lower respiratory areas.

The roof of the nasal vault contains the sensory cells of smell, or olfaction. These delicate nerve fibers extend from the upper recesses in the nose to the olfactory portion of the frontal lobe of the brain.

Throat ▪ The oral cavity extends from the opening of the mouth posteriorly to the tonsils. The tongue lies along the floor of the oral cavity and contains muscles in three planes as well as a very rich blood supply. The tongue contains both motor and sensory nerves and is the organ of taste. Motion of the tongue is also important in moving food during both chewing and initiation of the swallowing process. Beneath the tongue are two small ducts that allow saliva made in the

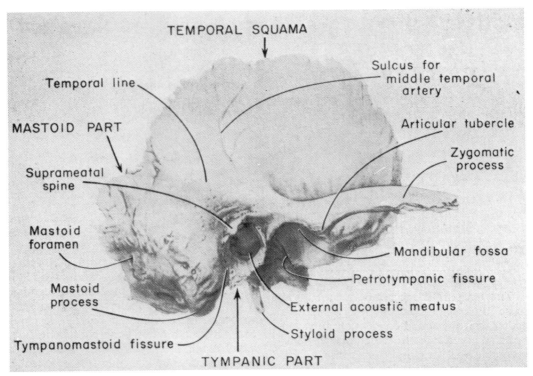

Figure 29-4
Right temporal bone, lateral view. (From Ballenger, John. *Diseases of the Nose, Throat, and Ear,* 11th ed. Lea & Febiger, Philadelphia, 1969.)

submaxillary glands to enter the mouth and aid in digestion. The roof of the oral cavity is formed by the hard and soft palate. The hard palate is the anterior portion that is formed by bone. The soft posterior portion of the palate is a fibrous area that attaches posteriorly to the pharynx (Figure 29-11). The lateral walls of the oral cavity are formed by the lips and buccal mucosa. An opening in the posterior portion of the buccal mucosa allows saliva from the parotid glands to enter the oral cavity.

The pharynx is commonly divided into three parts: the nasopharynx, the portion of the pharynx that is present behind the posterior choanae of the nose; the oropharynx, the portion of the pharynx beneath the nasopharynx that opens into the oral cavity; and the laryngopharynx, or hypopharynx, the lower portion of the pharynx that leads to the larynx and to the opening of the esophagus (Figure 29-12).

The parotid gland is the largest of the salivary glands and extends from an area just anterior to the external canal of the ear to the midface. The facial nerve, which provides animation to the muscles of the face, separates this gland into a superficial and a deep lobe. The parotid duct enters the oral cavity through a small opening just above the second upper molar tooth (Figure 29-13). The submandibular and the submaxillary glands are found beneath the anterior portion of the mandible. The submandibular duct, or Wharton's duct, enters the mouth through small openings near the lingual frenulum. The sublingual glands are found beneath the anterior portion of the floor of the mouth, and very short ducts allow saliva secreted in these minor salivary glands to enter the mouth directly.

The larynx, or voice box, is formed by the thyroid cartilage above and the cricoid cartilage below. These structures lie in the midline of the neck, and the U-shaped hyoid bone, which is found directly above the thyroid cartilage, provides attachment for both tendons and muscles from the tongue and mandible to connect to the

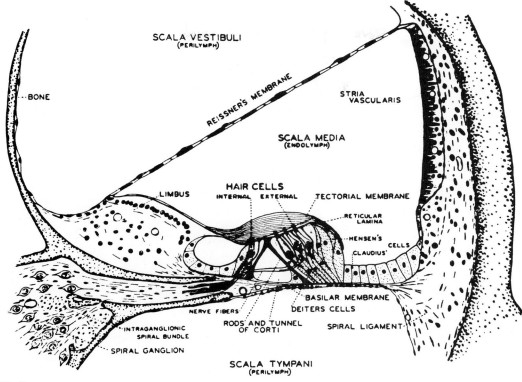

Figure 29–5
Cross-section of the cochlear partition in the guinea pig. (From Best, C. H., and N. B. Taylor. *The Physiological Basis of Medical Practice.* Williams & Wilkins, Baltimore, 1953.)

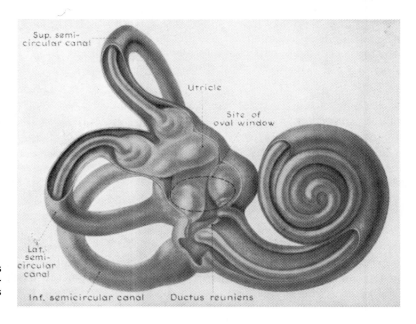

Figure 29–6
The osseous and membranous labyrinths of the ear. (From Boies, L. R., Jr. *Fundamentals of Otolaryngology*, 5th ed. W. B. Saunders Co., Philadelphia, 1978.)

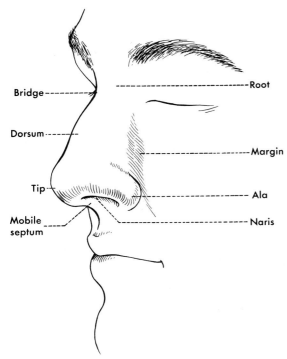

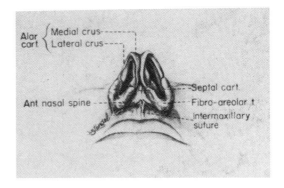

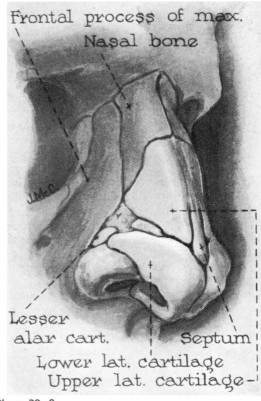

Figure 29–7

Parts of the external nose. (From Hollinshead, W. Henry. *Anatomy for Surgeons*; Vol. 1/*The Head and Neck*, 2nd ed. J. B. Lippincott, Philadelphia, 1968.)

Figure 29–8

The external framework of the nose. (From Ballenger, John. *Diseases of the Nose, Throat, and Ear*, 11th ed. Lea & Febiger, Philadelphia, 1969.)

larynx and elevate it during the swallowing process (Figure 29–14). The thyroid cartilage, or "Adam's apple," looks like a shield; the smaller cricoid cartilage is shaped like a signet ring. The epiglottis is a flap of cartilage that functions in a protective way to divert food from the airway. The valleculae are two small recesses just anterior to the base of the epiglottis, separating it from the base of the tongue. The larynx contains the true vocal cords, which are innervated by the recurrent laryngeal nerve (Figure 29–15). Motion of the vocal cords and trapping of air beneath the cords when they are fully abducted allow for speech. The piriform sinuses are two recessions along the lateral posterior portion of the larynx that empty into the esophageal inlet.

REPRESENTATIVE DISEASES

Diseases of the External Ear
Preauricular Fistula and Cysts ▪ A preauricular fistula occurs as a result of a devel-

opmental defect of the first branchial arch and appears as a small, pinpoint depression, usually just in front of the helix of the ear. Frequently a fistula is bilateral, and on occasion it may become infected. An acute infection is treated with

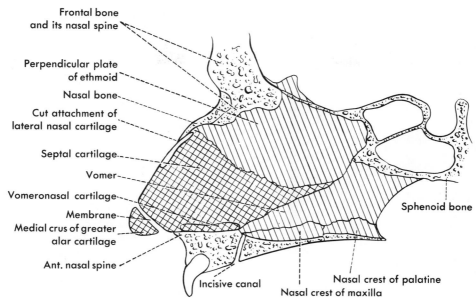

Figure 29-9
Composition of the nasal septum. (From Hollinshead, W. Henry. *Anatomy for Surgeons*; Vol. 1/*The Head and Neck*, 2nd ed. J. B. Lippincott, Philadelphia, 1968.)

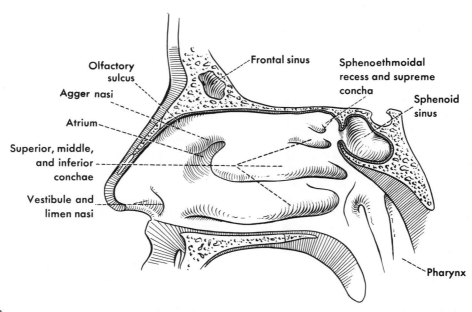

Figure 29-10
The lateral nasal wall. (From Hollinshead, W. Henry. *Anatomy for Surgeons*; Vol. 1/*The Head and Neck*, 2nd ed. J. B. Lippincott, Philadelphia, 1968.)

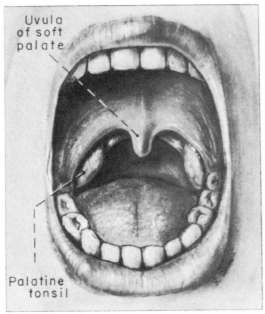

Figure 29–11

Oral cavity, soft palate, and palatine tonsils. (From Hollinshead, W. Henry. *Anatomy for Surgeons; Vol. 1/The Head and Neck*, 2nd ed. J. B. Lippincott, Philadelphia, 1968.)

antibiotics, but with recurrent infection, excision of the fistulous tract may be necessary. Frequently the developmental defect will not terminate in a fistula's opening to the outside skin, but rather a cyst will be present just beneath the surface. As with a fistula, a cyst may become infected, and antibiotic therapy may be necessary. Repeated infections of the cyst also require surgical excision.

Congenital Aural Malformation ▪ Congenital aural atresia and malformation of the auricle are also seen as a result of a developmental defect. The malformation may range from complete absence of the external ear to a deformed auricle. This also may be associated with malformation of the external canal and, if bilateral, may require surgery or a prosthesis for cosmetic effect as well as surgery or the use of a hearing aid to correct a hearing loss.

Keloid of the External Ear ▪ Injuries of the external ear may result in keloid formation after trauma to the skin. Following trauma, excessive collagen in certain predisposed individuals may form a hypertrophic scar. This hypertrophic

scar, or keloid, is usually treated with injections of steroids, but surgical excision followed by steroid injection therapy is frequently done.

Auricular Hematoma ▪ Trauma to the external ear may result in bleeding and formation of a hematoma between the cartilage and the perichondrium. Treatment of the hematoma consists of aspiration or surgical drainage, followed with application of a pressure dressing. If the hematoma is not treated and subsequently organizes into fibrous tissue, a "cauliflower ear" may result, with surgical correction necessary for cosmetic reasons.

Perichondritis ▪ This is an inflammation that involves the perichondrium, or lining of the cartilage of the external ear. It may follow a surgical procedure or trauma, or extension of infection from the external canal. Treatment consists of antibiotic therapy and drainage of any areas of accumulated purulent secretions.

Allergic Eczema ▪ Allergic eczema is frequently seen at the opening of the external canal and presents as a dry, scaly rash with associated itching. Steroid creams are frequently useful to treat this condition. Avoidance of the offending allergen is also necessary to prevent recurrence.

Diseases of the External Auditory Canal ▪ The external auditory canal is lined with skin or squamous epithelium and is therefore subject to many forms of dermatitis, as well as self-inflicted problems due to the tendency of some individuals to pick at the ears with fingers or sharp objects. Water may also enter the ear canal and increase the risk of infection. Cerumen may be present in the external canal. Water frequently becomes trapped in this canal, and efforts to remove the cerumen and trapped water may result in infection.

Impacted Cerumen ▪ The most common cause of obstruction of the external canal is cerumen impaction. Cerumen glands are located in the cartilaginous ear canal, providing it with a protective surface that tends to have antibacterial activity. Formation of cerumen is extremely variable among individuals, and some people may need to have the canals cleaned periodically. Removal of the cerumen is performed with either irrigation or blunt instruments.

Foreign Bodies ▪ Many foreign bodies have been found in ear canals. The tendency of a small child to place a foreign body in the ear canal is well known. The major problem with a

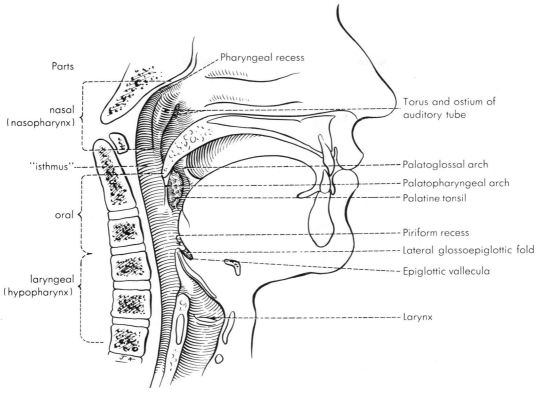

Parts

nasal
(nasopharynx)

"isthmus"

oral

laryngeal
(hypopharynx)

Pharyngeal recess

Torus and ostium of
auditory tube

Palatoglossal arch

Palatopharyngeal arch

Palatine tonsil

Piriform recess

Lateral glossoepiglottic fold

Epiglottic vallecula

Larynx

Figure 29–12

The pharynx and larynx. (From Hollinshead, W. Henry. *Anatomy for Surgeons*; Vol. 1/*The Head and Neck*, 2nd ed. J. B. Lippincott, Philadelphia, 1968.)

foreign body is its removal from the narrowed area of the isthmus, which is the constricted area at the junction of the bony and cartilaginous canal.

External Otitis ▪ All inflammatory processes in the external auditory canal are generally referred to as external otitis and may be either acute or chronic. They may be further classified as infectious, eczematous, or seborrheic. The symptoms are usually itching, which progresses to pain as edema in the canal causes pressure. Increasing edema will result in hearing loss because of obstruction of the canal. Acute external otitis, or swimmer's ear, is usually caused by *Pseudomonas aeruginosa* and responds to cleaning of the ear canal and acidification or the use of antibiotic ear drops. Fungal ear infections, especially *Aspergillus niger,* may also be found, with a wet, grayish exudate frequently seen in

the external canal. Cleaning of the ear canal, acidification, and topical antifungal agents are effective treatment.

Traumatic Perforation of the Tympanic Membrane ▪ This can occur secondary to blows to the ear, diving, water skiing, or a foreign object that has been pushed into the external canal. Rarely, perforation can be caused by a loud explosion or forceful irrigation of the ear. Hot metal-welding sparks have also been known to cause perforations because the edges of the perforation are cauterized by the welding spark. This type of perforation will frequently not heal, resulting in a persistent perforation. Traumatic perforations usually heal spontaneously in a few weeks; if they do not, stimulation of the edges of the perforation by cautery or with a sharp instrument and placement of a small patch of paper or Gelfoam may result in healing. If the

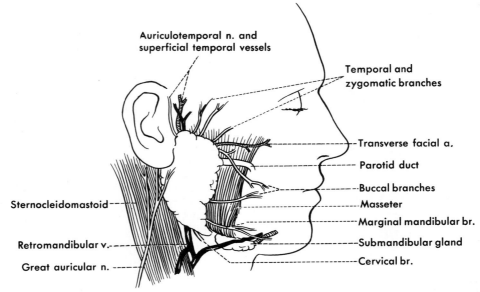

Figure 29–13
Superficial relations of the parotid gland. (From Hollinshead, W. Henry. *Anatomy for Surgeons*; Vol. 1/*The Head and Neck*, 2nd ed. J. B. Lippincott, Philadelphia, 1968.)

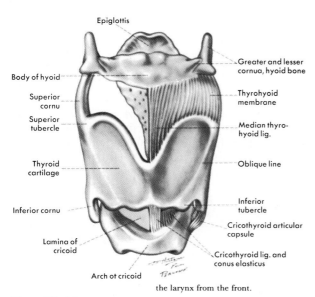

the larynx from the front.

Figure 29–14
Cartilages and ligaments of the larynx from the front. (From Hollinshead, W. Henry. *Anatomy for Surgeons*; Vol. 1/*The Head and Neck*, 2nd ed. J. B. Lippincott, Philadelphia, 1968.)

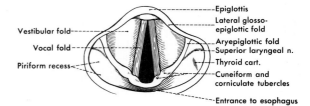

Figure 29–15
Piriform recesses, pharynx, and larynx from above. (From Hollinshead, W. Henry. *Anatomy for Surgeons*; Vol. 1/*The Head and Neck*, 2nd ed. J. B. Lippincott, Philadelphia, 1968.)

perforation is persistent, tympanoplasty, usually with a graft of temporalis fascia, may be performed with a high success rate of closure.

Tumors ■ Both benign and malignant tumors may be found in the external canal. Osteoma is a common bony growth found in the bony portion of the external canal. These rounded growths occur in individuals with a history of cold-water swimming. They cause symptoms only when they trap cerumen or become large enough to block the external canal.

Adenomas are small, benign growths arising from the cerumen or sebaceous glands of the external canal. When symptomatic, they may require surgical excision.

Malignant tumors include squamous cell carcinoma, adenocarcinoma, and basal cell carcinoma. Treatment is surgical excision, radiation therapy, or both.

Diseases of the Tympanic Membrane and Middle Ear

Infection ▪ Inflammatory conditions of the middle ear space are all reflected in the tympanic membrane. Generally five types of diseases are characterized as causing middle ear infection:

▪ Acute suppurative otitis media

▪ Acute necrotic otitis media

▪ Acute viral otitis media and bullous myringitis

▪ Tuberculous chronic otitis media

▪ Nontuberculous chronic otitis media

ACUTE SUPPURATIVE OTITIS MEDIA ▪ This bacterial inflammation of the middle ear space is characterized by pain and inflammation of the tympanic membrane. Infected fluid increases in the middle ear space, and with pressure spontaneous rupture of the tympanic membrane may result. This condition is treated with antibiotic therapy; however, when the tympanic membrane is bulging, myringotomy or drainage of the middle ear space may be necessary to relieve the pressure and speed resolution of the disease process.

ACUTE NECROTIC OTITIS MEDIA ▪ This infection is frequently seen in young children and has a more rapid course than the acute suppurative variety. Necrosis of the ossicular structures in the middle ear as well as the tympanic membrane may result. Beta-hemolytic *Streptococcus* is commonly the organism responsible for this condition. Treatment consists of antibiotic therapy and myringotomy if the tympanic membrane is bulging.

ACUTE VIRAL OTITIS MEDIA (BULLOUS MYRINGITIS) ▪ Bullous myringitis is a type of viral involvement of the tympanic membrane that causes extreme pain and is frequently seen in younger children. Multiple blebs are present on the surface of the tympanic membrane that are noted on otoscopy to be extremely erythematous. This is a self-limiting condition, and treatment consists of pain medication. Antibiotics may be used to prevent secondary bacterial infection.

TUBERCULOUS CHRONIC OTITIS MEDIA ▪ This condition is extremely rare now that pulmonary tuberculosis has been controlled with medical therapy. A patient who has continuing perforations while on antibiotic therapy should cause the clinician to suspect a tuberculous etiology, and frequently multiple perforations may be found in the early stages. Culture of the organism will confirm the diagnosis, and therapy consists of antituberculous medication.

NONTUBERCULOUS CHRONIC OTITIS MEDIA ▪ Various chronic causes of otitis media must be considered when other etiologies have been excluded. Collagen vascular diseases such as systemic lupus erythematosus and Wegener's granulomatosis must be considered.

Tympanosclerosis ▪ This benign condition results from inflammatory conditions in the tympanic membrane that cause calcification to build up in mucous membranes of the middle ear and mastoid as well as the fibrous layer of the tympanic membrane. Tympanosclerotic plaques may then cause problems with conduction of sound through the tympanic membrane and the ossicular chain.

Keratitis Obturans ▪ In this condition, epithelium forms a mass in the ear canal, and with repeated desquamation a cystic structure may obliterate the external canal. Treatment consists of removal of the accumulated desquamated debris.

Cholesteatoma ▪ A cholesteatoma is a sac consisting of an ingrowth of squamous epithelium that enlarges and through pressure necrosis can destroy bony structures of the middle ear and mastoid, as well as being a source of chronic infection. Cholesteatoma may be either congenital, formed from a remnant of squamous epithelium present at birth, or acquired, the most common variety. Acquired cholesteatomas may be found in either the middle ear, the area of the attic, or in the mastoid. Erosion of the ossicular chain or destruction of the air cells in the mastoid may result in persistent infection that may spread to contiguous structures in the ear, including the labyrinth, to the facial nerve, or to the brain. Treatment consists of removal of the cholesteatoma through a surgical procedure.

Otosclerosis ▪ Otosclerosis is a condition of the middle ear in which a vascular type of abnormal bone may invade the stapes, causing fixation of the ossicular chain with resultant hearing loss. This condition usually develops in young adults and frequently has a familial association. Exacerbation of otosclerosis can occur following pregnancy. The diagnosis is made with tuning forks and hearing tests, which indicate a conductive hearing loss, and by finding fixation of the stapes bone at time of surgery. Hearing may be restored either by use of a hearing aid or by stapedectomy (Figure 29–16).

Granulomas of the Ear and Temporal Bone ▪ A granuloma is a tumor-like mass of granulation tissue due to a chronic inflammatory process. Several specific types of granuloma have been identified in the ear and temporal bone. Granulation tissue secondary to infection is the most frequent cause of granulomas seen in the ear; however, eosinophilic and tuberculous granulomas may also be encountered. Following diagnosis, treatment varies depending on the etiology of the granuloma.

Glomus Jugulare ▪ This benign vascular tumor arises from the jugular bulb in the inferior portion of the middle ear cavity. Although the tumor is benign, its location near the cranial nerves may cause progressive neurologic symptoms, and profuse bleeding also may be present. Diagnosis is made by computed tomography (CT) scan and angiography (dye injection into the blood vessels that feed the tumor). Treatment is surgical resection.

Malignant Tumors of the Middle Ear and Mastoid ▪ Squamous cell carcinoma is the most common malignant tumor of the middle ear and mastoid. Pain and bleeding are frequently the only symptoms of this disorder, and treatment requires radical resection of the tumor with or without radiation therapy. The cure rate, however, is extremely low.

Disorders of the Eustachian Tube ▪ An abnormally patent eustachian tube may be found in individuals who have lost a significant amount of weight over a short period. The patients will have a sensation of fullness in the ear and their own voice will sound abnormally loud to them. Weight gain usually relieves the symptoms.

OBSTRUCTION ▪ Eustachian tube obstruction can occur secondary to a variety of problems, such as allergies, with resultant swelling of the mucous membrane of the eustachian tube, and inflammatory illnesses and tumors. Treatment consists of therapy to the underlying cause.

AEROTITIS ▪ Aerotitis, also known as "middle ear squeeze," is an inflammatory condition in the middle ear in which the middle ear pressure is less than that of the surrounding atmosphere. This happens when the eustachian tube fails to open. The condition may be experienced during descent on an airplane or during ascent on diving. Treatment consists of re-establishing a normal middle ear pressure. The symptoms may be relieved by chewing gum, drinking liquids, or decongestant therapy. A persistently blocked eustachian tube may require a myringotomy and placement of a ventilation tube.

SEROUS OTITIS MEDIA ▪ Serous otitis media is a very common otologic problem in young children. In patients under the age of 6 years, re-

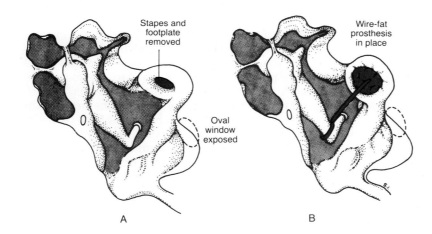

Figure 29–16
Stapedectomy for hearing loss caused by otosclerosis. (From Miller, B. F., and Claire B. Keane. *Encyclopedia and Dictionary of Medicine, Nursing, and Allied Health.* W. B. Saunders Co., Philadelphia, 1992.)

peated upper respiratory infections, eustachian tube obstruction, and the anatomically small, horizontally positioned eustachian tube may result in persistent middle ear effusions that may not clear with medical management. Treatment consists of antibiotic therapy. If middle ear effusions persist and are not cleared with medical management, myringotomy and placement of a ventilation tube may be necessary to decrease the incidence of infection as well as to restore hearing.

Facial Nerve Paralysis ▪ The facial nerve (the seventh cranial nerve) runs a course through the brain, entering the inner ear via the cerebellopontine angle, where it courses the internal auditory canal before terminating extracranially as branches to the face, which result in facial movement. The facial nerve has a significant tympanomastoid course in which innervation is given to the stapedius muscle and chorda tympani, which provides taste sensation. Branches are also given off to the sublingual, submaxillary, and submandibular glands for salivation. The tympanomastoid portion of the facial nerve may be involved in various disease processes. Inflammatory diseases of the middle ear and mastoid may cause a paralysis of the facial nerve. Tumor and cholesteatoma in the middle ear and mastoid similarly can place pressure on the facial nerve and cause a facial paralysis. Depending upon the location of the injury to the nerve, decreased salivation and taste can also be noted.

BELL'S PALSY ▪ This idiopathic condition is manifest in a peripheral facial nerve paralysis. Studies suggest a viral etiology for the condition, and more than half the patients have complete remission of the paralysis. Treatment generally consists of medication to reduce the swelling in the nerve.

TRAUMA ▪ Another common cause of facial nerve paralysis is trauma. Fractures across the petrous bone of the skull may cause injury to the facial nerve. Facial nerve paralysis also may occur from injury to the skull at birth.

Diseases of the Inner Ear

Sensorineural Hearing Loss ▪ This is caused by pathology within the cochlea or along the central connections from the cochlea to the auditory nucleus in the brain. Congenital sensorineural loss can be due to genetic factors as well as injury to the fetus during pregnancy, such as

drug injury, rubella infection, and RH incompatibility problems. At the time of delivery, convulsions and lack of oxygen to the baby may also cause sensorineural loss.

PRESBYCUSIS ▪ Presbycusis is a gradual, symmetric sensorineural loss that develops with aging and is caused by damage to the sensory cells and the organ of Corti. Acoustic trauma also may cause sensorineural loss. Noisy machinery and gunfire at a frequency higher than 4000 hertz usually cause hearing loss.

Tumors in the area of the cerebellopontine angle may affect the auditory as well as the vestibular nerve. This type of tumor frequently results in markedly decreased auditory discrimination.

OTOSCLEROSIS ▪ Otosclerosis may involve the labyrinthine capsule as well as the middle ear. Coexisting stapedial otosclerosis may also be found. CT scan of the cochlea will frequently make the diagnosis. Treatment consists of fluoride in an attempt to control the active vascular new bone formation. Hearing aids also may be helpful. Infections, both viral and bacterial, that may be associated with elevated temperatures can cause sensorineural loss. Measles, mumps, and acute febrile illnesses may result in sensorineural hearing loss in both children and adults.

MÉNIÈRE'S DISEASE ▪ This fluctuating, usually low-frequency sensorineural hearing loss is associated with tinnitus, or ringing in the ears, as well as recurrent vertigo. Endolymphatic hydrops or dilation of the endolymphatic space within the cochlea is seen pathologically. This condition is thought to be related to a defect in the potassium-sodium active transport mechanism in the inner ear. Sodium restriction and administration of diuretics are usually helpful in treating this disorder.

Tinnitus ▪ Tinnitus, or ringing in the ear, can be caused by many disorders. Objective tinnitus can be heard by both the patient and the examiner. It may be caused by arteriovenous malformation or aneurysm of the arteries in the area of the ear. Treatment of objective tinnitus requires treatment of the underlying cause. In subjective tinnitus, the patient hears noises that cannot be heard by the examiner. It has many causes. It may be noted secondary to impacted cerumen in the external canal and frequently is seen after drug toxicity. No specific drug therapy is useful in treatment. Various medications, including vitamins and vasodilators, have been used in the past. Tinnitus is usually treated by masking. One masking technique is playing a radio at night to mask out the annoying sounds that the patient hears. Tinnitus maskers are devices that resemble a hearing aid; biofeedback techniques are also used.

Dizziness and Vertigo ▪ Dizziness is a sensation of unsteadiness with a feeling of movement within the head. Orientation of the body in space is controlled by a number of body systems that include the inner ear (labyrinth), the muscle-tendon-joint system, and the visual system. In addition to these three distinct systems, disorders of the central auditory pathways in the brain stem and their connections to the nuclei in the brain may also produce a sensation of disorientation.

It is important to distinguish between true vertigo, which is a turning sensation, and dizziness. True turning vertigo is produced by disorders of the semicircular canals, the utricle, and the vestibular nuclei and their connections within the brain. Nystagmus, or rapid movement of the eye, is the most important physical sign noted with true vertigo. Vertical nystagmus is said to be diagnostic of central nervous system disease, whereas horizontal nystagmus is frequently seen with peripheral vestibular disturbance.

True vertigo has many causes: foreign bodies of the ear canals, trauma to the middle ear, and infection. A fistula in the footplate of the stapes may also cause vertigo and may be associated with a positive fistula test. In this test, positive ear pressure is placed against an intact tympanic membrane, resulting in vertigo. An audiogram is also an important test, even though no complaint may be made of hearing loss. Severe loss of auditory discrimination may suggest an acoustic neuroma or a tumor in the area of the cerebellopontine angle. Electronystagmography is a method of evaluating the function of the inner ear. Alternate warm and cold air or water is placed in the external canals, and the labyrinth is stimulated. Recordings of nystagmus are made from electrodes placed lateral to and above the eyes and may indicate unilateral weakness of the labyrinth. Tumors in the brain stem and especially in the cerebellum may produce a turning type of vertigo. Vascular occlusions to the arteries that supply the vestibular system may also give rise to a sensation of turning vertigo.

Diseases of the Nose and Paranasal Sinuses

Congenital Defects of the Nose ▪ Dermoid cysts and medial nasal fistulas are congenital defects secondary to rests of epidermal elements that occur during the growth of the nasal bones in the embryo. Fistulas and connecting cysts are usually found along the midline of the dorsum of the nose and extend to the ethmoid sinuses or occasionally to the frontal sinus area. The cysts frequently become infected, and the acute infection is treated with antibiotics. Only a complete surgical excision of the cyst will result in a cure.

Congenital Tumors of the Nose ▪ Congenital tumors of the nose arise from neural elements, which include neurofibromas and encephaloceles. Neurofibromas are a group of tumors derived from neural elements that may be localized or occasionally part of a more generalized von Recklinghausen's neurofibromatosis. Multiple neurofibromas and the presence of coffee-colored spots, café-au-lait spots, will also help make the diagnosis. Congenital encephaloceles may be found both inside and outside the nose and represent a cystlike structure that is filled with cerebrospinal fluid communicating directly with the ventricles of the brain. On straining, the size of an encephalocele will usually increase; transmitted pulsations can be helpful in making the diagnosis. Following careful radiographic studies, surgical resection is necessary for cure.

Other congenital tumors may contain mesodermal elements. These include cavernous hemangiomas, which are blood vessel tumors in the nose, and plasmacytomas, which may be a localized tumor or part of a systemic disease. Systemic disease may be associated with punched-out lesions in bone noted on skeletal bone radiographs.

Diseases of the External Nose ▪ Many bacterial and viral infections may affect the external nose. Impetigo is a staphylococcal infection that presents as inflammation and a pustular infection of the external nose. It is extremely contagious. Treatment consists of topical antibiotic ointments and systemic antibiotic therapy. A furuncle is an acute infection in the base of a hair follicle, usually just inside the vestibule of the nose, frequently caused by *Staphylococcus aureus*. Pain and swelling just inside the vestibule of the nose, as well as occasional swelling on the tip of the nose, are frequent signs. Treatment consists of antibiotic ointment in the nasal vestibule and appropriate antistaphylococcal antibiotics. If an abscess develops, incision and drainage are frequently necessary. Herpetic ulcerations may be seen around the nose, usually as part of a more generalized herpes simplex infection. This virus causes ulcerations that may appear when an individual is under stress. The disease is self-limited, and local anesthetics and analgesics are used to provide pain relief. Rhinophyma is an unsightly enlargement of the nose caused by hypertrophy of the skin and engorgement of the underlying sebaceous glands. Treatment is usually surgical and usually results in a much improved cosmetic state.

Nasal Tumors ■ The most common malignant tumors of the skin of the nose are basal cell and squamous cell carcinomas. Both types of tumor may be caused by prolonged exposure to harmful ultraviolet rays of the sun over many years. Although basal cell carcinomas do not metastasize, they can become locally aggressive and can destroy significant parts of the nose if untreated. Squamous cell carcinomas may metastasize to local lymph nodes as well as to systemic areas. Treatment of these malignant tumors consists of surgical resection.

Nasal Fractures ■ The most common injury to the nose is nasal fracture. The paired nasal bones may be broken secondary to trauma to the face, and the midline nasal septum frequently is displaced. The type of fracture seen depends on the intensity and direction of the force injuring the nose. Because the nasal lacrimal system, as well as the cribriform plate, is closely connected to the nasal bone, injuries to the lacrimal system and cerebrospinal leak may be seen in significant nasal injuries. Nondisplaced fractures require no treatment; however, displaced fractures require surgical reduction. The reduction may be closed: simple manipulation of the nasal bones back to the midline position and proper splinting, or if an injury is severe, open surgical reduction and splinting may be necessary. Severely comminuted nasal fractures may require open reduction with surgical splinting until stabilization has occurred.

Epistaxis ■ Probably the most common emergency involving the nose is epistaxis. Epistaxis can be secondary to local effects, such as trauma to the lining of the inside of the nose, to bleeding tumors located within the nose or adjacent paranasal sinuses, or to acute inflammation of the lining of the nose. Epistaxis can also be a sign of systemic disease, such as blood dyscrasias, coagulation defects, or hypertension. Most nose bleeds seen in children occur along the anterior portion of the nasal septum in an area known as Kiesselbach's plexus. This bleeding is usually successfully treated with local cautery or occasionally with anterior packing.

More significant bleeding can occur from the posterior portion of the nose, which may be secondary to bleeding from branches of the internal maxillary artery or the anterior ethmoidal artery. Frequently a posterior nasal pack is necessary to control this vigorous bleeding. This may be made by preparing a rolled-up piece of gauze to which three silk sutures are attached. After a rubber tube is passed through the nostril into the pharynx, two of the sutures may be tied to the catheter, which is pulled back through the nose, leaving the third silk suture remaining in the pharynx for later retrieval of the pack. An anterior pack is then placed in the nose, and the two silk sutures are tied over a gauze pack in the front of the nostril. The anterior opening of the nose, as well as the posterior choanae, is therefore firmly occluded with packing, which almost always controls the bleeding. Specially designed epistaxis balloons may also be used to control posterior bleeding. Balloon catheters usually contain both an anterior and a posterior balloon, which will occlude both the anterior and posterior openings of the nose after the balloons are filled with saline solution. Care should be taken to be certain that pressure caused by the balloons is not excessive, as tissue necrosis and later scarring may result.

Rarely, surgical intervention may be necessary upon failure of a posterior pack. Ligation of branches of the external carotid artery, either in the neck or through the posterior wall of the maxillary sinus, may be necessary. Bleeding from the anterior ethmoid artery may be controlled after direct visualization of the artery is made through a small incision over the lateral portion of the nose.

Recurrent epistaxis can also occur in hereditary disorders. Hereditary hemorrhagic telangiectasia, also known as Rendu-Osler-Weber disease, is an inherited disorder in which multiple abnormal small blood vessels may be found in the body where the wall of the vessel lacks elastic and muscular tissue. These thin-walled vessels frequently bleed and can be the site of recurrent, persistent epistaxis of significant severity. Among the multiple treatments is septal dermoplasty, in which a graft of dermis from a donor site is used to cover a portion of the nasal septum after the diseased mucosa has been removed. Other techniques, such as nasal cautery and ablation by laser, have also been successful.

Foreign Bodies of the Nose ■ These are common in children, less frequent in adults. The usual symptom is unilateral nasal obstruction that may be associated with foul-smelling discharge. Treatment consists of topical vasoconstrictors to shrink the mucosal lining of the nose and physical removal of the foreign body with nasal forceps.

Rhinitis ■ Rhinitis, or inflammation of the nasal mucosa, is commonly seen secondary to a viral upper respiratory infection. Symptoms include sneezing and a watery nasal discharge, and the nasal mucosa is noted on examination to be swollen and inflamed. Treatment consists of decongestants and analgesics. Bacterial rhinitis is treated with antibiotic therapy, with the choice of antibiotic guided by culture and sensitivity testing of the nasal discharge. Allergic rhinitis represents a hypersensitivity of the lining of the nasal mucosa secondary to an antigenic stimulus. The presence of eosinophils in nasal secretions may help make the diagnosis. Allergy testing is helpful in identifying the offending allergens, and desensitization therapy may be very helpful. Treatment with antihistamines and decongestants frequently provides symptomatic relief. Topical nasal steroid sprays can also be quite effective.

Nasal Septal Deformities ■ A deviated or obstructing nasal septum is a frequent cause of nasal obstruction. The nasal deformity may be secondary to congenital factors, birth injury, or acquired traumatic deformity. The most common symptom is frequently unilateral nasal obstruction. Direct inspection of the nasal septum confirms the diagnosis. Treatment requires septoplasty in which the obstructing portion of the nasal septum is replaced into the midline.

Septal Hematomas and Abscesses ■ Septal hematoma is a collection of blood along the septal cartilage. Drainage is necessary. Frequently septal hematomas will become infected and develop into an abscess, for which incision and drainage are necessary to prevent necrosis of the septal cartilage, which may result in saddle deformity of the nose.

Sinusitis ■ This infection of the paranasal sinuses may spread from the nasal cavity into the paranasal sinuses or may be caused by obstruction of the ostium, or drainage site, of the sinus. Anatomic deformities or mucosal inflammation and swelling frequently cause obstruction, which may lead to secondary infection. Typically a patient presents with nasal congestion and dull pain and pressure over the involved paranasal sinus. Maxillary sinusitis frequently presents as a feeling of pressure over the midface, with pain occasionally noted in the upper teeth. Infection of the ethmoid sinus presents with discomfort across the bridge of the nose, with pain occasionally radiating toward the orbit. Frontal sinusitis presents as pain or pressure across the forehead area. Sphenoidal sinusitis may cause a sensation of pressure or pain in the occipital area of the head. A low-grade fever is typically present, and purulent drainage may be noted in the area of the involved sinus ostium. Frontal sinusitis may cause purulent drainage, noted under the anterior portion of the middle turbinate. The maxillary sinus ostium is located in the midportion of the middle meatus, and frequently purulent secretions will be found in this area. The ethmoid sinus drains into the middle meatus from the anterior cells, and the posterior cells may drain into the superior meatus. The sphenoid sinus drains into the sphenoid ethmoidal recess.

Diagnosis of the sinusitis is made after a careful history and physical examination. Tenderness is usually present over the involved sinus, and the diagnosis can be confirmed by radiographic studies. Medical treatment consists of antibiotics and decongestants. Nasal humidification is also helpful. Symptomatic fluid levels within the maxillary sinus may require antral lavage for both diagnostic and therapeutic reasons. A sample of the fluid is useful for culture and sensitivity testing. Persistent fluid level in the frontal sinus may require a frontal sinus drainage procedure.

Chronic sinusitis may require surgical intervention. External sinus surgery, such as the Caldwell Luc operation; external ethmoidectomy; and frontal sinus obliteration procedures traditionally have been used to treat chronic sinus disease. Functional endoscopic sinus surgery is assuming an increasing role in re-establishing drainage to the paranasal sinuses through the areas of their natural ostium without need for external incisions. Intranasal endoscopy for diagnostic purposes as well as intranasal sinus surgery has become an increasingly valuable surgical method of evaluating and treating sinus disease that is refractory to medical management.

Tumors of the Paranasal Sinuses ▪ Benign tumors of the paranasal sinuses may include papillomas, mixed tumors, and a multitude of connective tissue tumors including fibromas, hemangiomas, and neurilemomas. Bone tumors such as osteomas, giant cell tumors, and bony cysts may also be present. Tumor-like lesions such as mucoceles, pyoceles, and polyps frequently present in the paranasal sinuses. These conditions are all usually treated with surgical intervention if they are symptomatic.

Malignant Tumors of the Paranasal Sinuses ▪ Although malignancies of the paranasal sinuses are rare, frequently they are large when first diagnosed. Typically the tumor within a sinus breaks through a bony wall before symptoms are present. A patient may present with nasal obstruction, numbness, and swelling over the sinus; bloody or purulent drainage; and occasionally pain. The maxillary sinus is most frequently involved, and the most common tissue type is squamous cell carcinoma. CT scan of the paranasal sinuses is helpful to evaluate the tumor and to ascertain the degree of bone involvement. Biopsy of the tumor is necessary prior to planning definitive treatment. The prognosis for carcinoma of the maxillary sinus is poor, and radical resection combined with radiation and chemotherapy is often the mode of treatment.

Diseases of the Throat

Diseases of the Oral Cavity and Pharynx ▪ Congenital cleft lip and cleft palate cause functional as well as cosmetic problems. Cleft lips are commonly paramedian and extend through the lip to the floor of the nostril. Congenital clefts of the palate are variable in extent and are caused by failure of fusion in the embryo of the palatal processes. Cleft lip, cleft palate, or both are seen in approximately 1 in every 700 births. Clefts are more common on the left side. Treatment for both cleft lip and cleft palate is surgical correction.

Ankyloglossia ▪ Ankyloglossia is a congenital condition resulting in a very tight lingual frenulum that fixes the tip of the tongue. This causes problems with both speech and eating. Treatment consists of surgical incision of the frenulum.

Macroglossia ▪ Macroglossia is frequently seen in mongolism and can also be idiopathic or due to lymphangioma or hemangioma. This condition, in which the tongue is too large for the mouth, may rarely require surgical intervention with reduction in the size of the tongue.

Median Rhomboid Glossitis ▪ This is neither a glossitis nor an inflammation of the tongue. This condition represents faulty development, in which the tuberculum impar of the tongue lies in front of the foramen cecum. Because of a lack of papillae on the tongue, the tongue appears to be red. No treatment is necessary.

Gingivitis ▪ Gingivitis, or inflammation of the gums, can be either acute or chronic. It can result from a number of factors, including infection and leukemia. It may also be seen in certain drug therapies, most notably with the use of Dilantin.

Necrotizing Gingivitis ▪ Necrotizing gingivitis is inflammation of the gums caused by Vincent's organisms. Spirochete and fusiform bacteria cause painful, bleeding gums, occasionally covered by a gray pseudomembrane. Treatment consists of careful cleaning of the oral cavity and antibiotic therapy.

Hairy Tongue ▪ This condition is frequently seen following antibiotic therapy. It results from hypertrophy of the filiform pili of the tongue and discoloration secondary to the growth of fungi following oral antibiotic therapy. Treatment consists of local cleaning of the tongue. Once antibiotic therapy is discontinued and the normal oral bacteria return, the condition almost always clears.

Geographic Tongue ▪ This refers to deep fissures and ill-defined discoloration of the dorsum of the tongue, which requires no specific treatment and is usually self-limiting. The cause of this condition has not been established with certainty.

Ranula ▪ A ranula is a fluid-filled cyst found on the undersurface of the tongue, usually displaced to one side or the other, that requires surgical removal.

Papilloma ▪ A papilloma is a benign tumor commonly found in the oral cavity. It may be caused by viral infection; treatment is by surgical removal.

Leukoplakia ▪ Leukoplakia is a white patch

in the oral cavity that may be seen with a variety of conditions, including local irritation and tobacco and alcohol use. Treatment consists of eliminating any local irritating factors; excision is necessary to rule out the possibility of malignant disease.

Squamous Cell Carcinoma ▪ This is the most common malignant tumor of the oral cavity. This tumor can be found on the lips and on any part of the oral cavity. It frequently presents as a hard mass that may be friable and ulcerated. Tobacco and alcohol use have been associated with oral carcinoma. The treatment is surgical resection, radiation therapy, or both. Spread of the cancer from the oral cavity usually results in local involvement of the lymph nodes of the neck. This local metastatic disease can be treated with either surgery or radiation therapy. Widespread metastatic disease can also occur.

Pemphigus ▪ Pemphigus is a disease of the oral cavity, resulting in thin-walled bullae that rupture, causing painful oral lesions. Treatment consists of steroid therapy.

Lichen Planus ▪ Lichen planus is a disorder of the mucous membranes of the oral cavity, resulting in a lacelike white pattern seen in the oral mucosa. Frequently this condition is asymptomatic; however, if it is extensive and symptomatic, medical therapy may be necessary.

Diseases of the Salivary Glands

Mumps ▪ Mumps, or epidemic parotitis, is an acute viral disease of the salivary glands that may involve systemic organs. Although usually seen in children, it can occur in adults, in whom the disease process may be more virulent. The disease starts with chills, fevers, and swelling of the major salivary glands. Treatment is symptomatic, as there is no specific cure for this viral disorder. Complete recovery usually occurs; however, sensorineural hearing loss or sterility secondary to involvement of the gonads may occur. A vaccine is available for small children who have not had the disease.

Acute Suppurative Sialadenitis ▪ This acute infection of the salivary glands presents with inflammation and tenderness of the salivary glands. The process may be initiated by an impacted stone in the salivary gland duct, resulting in secondary bacterial infection. Treatment consists of stone removal, heat applied to the gland, adequate hydration, and appropriate antibiotic therapy. Should an abscess develop within the gland, surgical drainage may be necessary if response to antibiotic therapy is poor.

Benign Lymphoepithelial Sialoadenopathy ▪ This disorder has been referred to in the past as "Mikulicz's disease." It is seen most commonly in middle-aged women. It presents with recurrent swelling of the salivary glands with no systemic signs of sepsis. The ducts within the gland display delayed emptying. The exact cause is not known, and treatment consists of increasing the salivary flow and preventing blockage of the ducts with mucous plugs. Treatment is almost always conservative medical management.

Benign Mixed Tumor ▪ The most common tumor of the parotid gland is the benign mixed tumor. This tumor, generally slowly growing, is a mass usually presenting in the superficial portion of the parotid gland. The mass may extend into the deep lobe and may pass through the stylomandibular ligament, entering the parapharyngeal space. Because the entrance into the space is narrow, the tumor frequently assumes a dumbbell appearance; it is therefore called a "dumbbell tumor." Benign mixed tumors can also occur in the other salivary glands, although the frequency of this tumor in the parotid gland is much higher. Treatment consists of surgical resection. Since branches of the facial nerve pass through the parotid gland, extreme care in identifying the nerve and preserving all branches of the nerve is necessary during parotid surgery.

Warthin's Tumor ▪ Warthin's tumor, also called papillary cystoadenoma lymphomatosum, is a benign tumor usually found in the parotid salivary gland. It usually presents as a soft mass in the tail of the gland and may be confused with benign mixed tumor. Treatment is surgical removal.

Oncocytoma ▪ Also called acidophilic cell adenoma, this is a benign, slowly growing tumor of the salivary glands. Treatment consists of surgical removal, with preservation of the facial nerve during the operative procedure.

Squamous Cell Carcinoma ▪ Squamous cell carcinoma is a firm, poorly defined, malignant mass that may be found in the salivary gland. It is more commonly found in the parotid gland, and, because of its infiltration into the gland, involvement of the facial nerve with paralysis of the face may occur. Metastatic spread to the local cervical lymph nodes is common, and the tumor may extend posteriorly into the ear canal. Treatment is surgical excision of the tumor, with neck dissection when lymphatic metastatasis has occurred. Radiation therapy is also frequently used in combination with surgical treatment.

Adenocystic Carcinoma ■ Adenocystic carcinoma is also called cylindroma; it is a malignant tumor that may be found in the salivary glands. Although the tumor grows slowly, pain is a common presenting symptom, and early involvement of the facial nerve with facial paralysis may be seen. Local metastatic spread to the adjacent lymph nodes and distant metastases to the liver, lungs, brain, and bone may be seen. A combination of surgical therapy and radiation is the usual treatment choice.

Acinic Cell Adenocarcinoma ■ This aggressive tumor of the salivary glands occurs most often in the parotid gland. The lesion has a characteristic appearance on light microscopy and presents as a solitary mass within the salivary gland. Local metastatases to the neck and systemic metastatases may occur; treatment consists of surgical resection.

Mucoepidermal Tumor ■ Mucoepidermal tumor may be either high grade or low grade with variable aggressiveness. The behavior of the tumor may not be predicted by it pathologic appearance. Treatment consists of surgical removal. Local metastatic disease to the neck is also removed at operation.

Diseases of the Pharynx

Acute Pharyngitis ■ This acute inflammation of the lining of the mucous membrane of the pharynx may be caused by either a virus or a bacteria. This condition usually presents with a sore throat and frequently is associated with swallowing problems. An elevated temperature and generalized weakness may also occur. Examination of the pharynx reveals diffuse redness, and occasionally a white exudate may be seen over the mucosal surface. Viral pharyngitis is treated symptomatically with pain medication and increased fluid intake. Topical anesthetics are also frequently used. Bacterial pharyngitis is treated with appropriate antibiotic therapy that can be guided with culture and sensitivity testing.

Acute Tonsillitis ■ This inflammation of the tonsils shows diffusely swollen tonsils frequently covered with a white exudate. It may be viral or bacterial. Viral tonsillitis is treated symptomatically, and bacterial tonsillitis is treated with antibiotic therapy guided by the results of culture and sensitivity testing. Beta-hemolytic streptococcal infections are frequently seen, and adequate antibiotic therapy is necessary, since a prolonged infection may result in rheumatic fever and kidney disease.

Chronic Recurrent Tonsillitis ■ Chronic recurrent tonsillitis, or hypertrophic tonsils that symptomatically obstruct the oral airway, may require tonsillectomy, or surgical removal of the tonsils.

The adenoids are lymphoid tissue found in the nasopharynx directly behind the posterior choanae of the nose. When this tissue becomes hypertrophic, nasal obstruction may ensue. Excessive adenoid tissue may also obstruct the opening of the eustachian tube and serve as a source of infection or cause physical obstruction of the tube in children with chronic otitis media. Treatment is adenoidectomy. Tonsillectomy and adenoidectomy are frequently performed simultaneously, as the indications for both procedures are frequently present.

Moniliasis ■ Moniliasis, or thrush, is a fungal infection of the oral cavity and pharynx caused by *Candida albicans*. This condition is frequently seen after antibiotic therapy. Examination of the oral cavity and pharynx reveals a whitish friable plaque over inflamed mucous membranes. Treatment consists of oral suspensions of nystatin. Improvement also occurs after antibiotic therapy is discontinued and the normal bacterial flora is allowed to repopulate the area.

Chronic Pharyngitis ■ This chronic inflammatory disease of the mucous membranes of the pharynx may be due to repeated attacks of viral or bacterial infection; irritation from tobacco smoke, alcohol, or other irritants; or chronic drainage secondary to allergy. Although pain may be less severe than that seen in acute pharyngitis, it generally is of a long-standing nature and may be intermittent. Occasionally, the symptoms are accompanied by noticeable posterior nasal drainage. Treatment consists of eliminating the factorial cause. Antibiotics following appropriate culture and sensitivity testing are used when indicated, irritants that may cause irritation of the walls of the pharynx are avoided, and allergic workup and management may be necessary to control irritation caused by chronic allergic drainage.

Infectious Mononucleosis ▪ This systemic viral disease caused by the Epstein-Barr virus presents with low-grade fever, fatigue, and frequently acute pharyngitis and tonsillitis. The diagnosis is confirmed by heterophil antibody testing, and treatment is symptomatic. Antibiotics are used only for secondary bacterial infections in the pharynx. Significant cervical lymphadenopathy is a common presenting finding in this disorder.

Thornwaldt's Cyst ▪ This cyst, found in the posterior midline of the nasopharynx, may become infected and symptomatic. When infected, it may cause persistent purulent drainage and occipital headaches. Examination of the nasopharynx will confirm the diagnosis, and treatment consists of surgical excision or wide marsupialization.

Nasopharyngeal Angiofibromas ▪ These are rare vascular neoplasms in the nasopharynx that may present with severe epistaxis and nasal obstruction. The angiofibroma may extend into adjacent bone and cause paralysis of cranial nerves. Radiographic studies, including CT scan, magnetic resonance imaging (MRI), and arteriograms to delineate the vessels that feed the angiofibroma, are necessary prior to surgical removal, since operative blood loss can be considerable. Frequently feeding vessels are embolized during arteriography in an effort to reduce the operative blood loss.

Thyroglossal Duct Cyst ▪ This congenital cyst is usually found in the midline of the neck near the hyoid bone. It can become infected and may present as an inflamed mass in the midline of the neck near the hyoid bone. A fistulous tract may extend near or through the hyoid bone and can extent to the base of tongue. The treatment is surgical excision with removal of the midportion of the hyoid as well as excision of the tract if present beyond the hyoid.

Zenker's Diverticulum ▪ Zenker's diverticulum is a pulsion diverticulum of the hypopharynx that may be due to a congenital muscular weakness in the wall of the lower pharynx. It affects men more often than women and is usually seen in people over the age of 40 years. Symptoms include dysphagia with choking sensations and regurgitation of undigested food. Surgical treatment may be necessary if the diverticulum is symptomatic, and frequently cricopharyngeal myotomy or an incision through the cricopharyngeus muscle is a helpful adjunct in restoring normal swallowing function.

Acute Epiglottitis ▪ Acute epiglottitis is an inflammation of the epiglottis, seen more commonly in children. The patient can present in acute respiratory distress, and physical examination reveals a swollen red epiglottis obstructing the airway. The progression of the disease may be rapid, so treatment must be initiated promptly. Most cases of epiglottitis respond to medical management, including antibiotic therapy, steroids, and respiratory care. Endotracheal intubation and occasionally tracheostomy may be necessary to ensure an adequate airway.

Laryngitis ▪ Laryngitis is an inflammation of the larynx due to infection of the laryngeal mucosa. It may be viral or bacterial. Patients present with hoarseness and occasionally may have a low-grade fever and cough. Examination of the vocal cords reveals edema and erythema. Treatment consists of voice rest, analgesics, increased hydration, and antibiotic therapy when the etiology is bacterial.

Chronic Laryngitis ▪ Chronic laryngitis is an inflammatory disorder of the lining of the vocal cords, which may be secondary to excessive smoking or other irritants as well as vocal abuse. Hoarseness is usually the presenting symptom. Treatment consists of eliminating the irritants that have caused the problem and voice rest. Chronic laryngitis may result in polyp formation if the irritating factors are not controlled.

Croup ▪ Croup, or acute laryngotracheobronchitis, is inflammation of the lining of the larynx and tracheobronchial tree, usually caused by a viral infection. The initial symptoms are similar to those seen in a cold or upper respiratory infection. A very typical "croupy" cough may result secondary to edema at the subglottic level. Treatment consists of placement of the patient in a high-humidity tent, administration of steroids if necessary to decrease the edema, and antibiotic therapy for those cases caused by bacteria or for secondary bacterial infections.

Leukoplakia ▪ Leukoplakia is a premalignant, thickened white epithelial layer that may be seen in the larynx secondary to chronic irritation. Patients may present with hoarseness. Treatment consists of removal of the leukoplakic lesions during direct laryngoscopy.

Vocal Cord Nodules ■ Vocal cord nodules are an inflammatory reaction usually occurring at the junction of the anterior and middle one third of the vocal cords. This condition is usually caused by excessive voice use, and hoarseness is the usual presenting symptom. Examination of the vocal cords reveals a small nodule that is usually bilateral. Treatment consists of adequate voice rest; with appropriate rest, the nodules almost always clear. Rarely, direct laryngoscopy with surgical removal of the nodules is necessary.

Vocal Cord Polyps ■ A vocal cord polyp is the most common benign tumor of the vocal cord. Polyps are usually secondary to prolonged vocal abuse or irritation of the cords. Smoking is a common cause. Hoarseness is the most common presenting symptom, and surgical removal with the aid of an operative microscope is the treatment of choice.

Vocal Cord Paralysis ■ Vocal cord paralysis can be unilateral or bilateral. Paralysis may be due to a local infiltrating tumor, a central etiology, or stretching of the recurrent laryngeal nerve. Patients present with hoarseness and occasionally will aspirate as the posterior commissure does not completely close. Many cases of vocal cord paralysis are idiopathic, and spontaneous recovery will usually occur within 6 months. Persistent vocal cord paralysis associated with significant hoarseness may be treated surgically by injection of the paretic vocal cord with various materials to approximate a more midline position.

Laryngeal Cysts ■ Laryngeal cysts, or laryngoceles, are cysts in the area of the ventricle that may interfere with the airway and cause voice abnormalities. The diagnosis is made with direct visualization of the larynx. Surgical removal may be necessary if the cyst is symptomatic.

Laryngeal Papillomas ■ Laryngeal papillomas may be seen in both adults and children, but the juvenile variety may be quite extensive and interfere with the airway. Papillomas are thought to have a viral etiology. Surgical removal of the lesion, especially in children, should be conservative, as multiple surgical procedures are usually necessary. The use of laser surgery on vocal cords for papillomas has proved to be of benefit.

Carcinoma of the Larynx ■ The most common laryngeal carcinoma is squamous cell carcinoma, although other types of malignancies may be seen. The most common presenting symptom is hoarseness, although patients may present with referred ear pain, difficulty in swallowing, and bloody sputum. Evaluation consists of direct laryngoscopy and biopsy as well as radiographic studies, including CT scan. Treatment depends upon the extent of the tumor. Early tumors confined to the vocal cords are usually treated with radiation therapy. More extensive tumors with local neck metastases are usually treated with surgery and radiation therapy.

SURGICAL PROCEDURES

A large variety of surgical procedures are performed in the field of otorhinolaryngology:

- Procedures performed in the head and neck
- Common otologic procedures
- Plastic and reconstructive procedures
- Endoscopic procedures
- A general category

Head and Neck

Salivary Glands

Superficial Parotidectomy—surgical removal of the superficial lobe of the parotid gland or that portion of the gland that lies superficial to the branches of the facial nerve.

Total Parotidectomy, Seventh Nerve Preserved—removal of the entire parotid gland with preservation of the seventh nerve. This requires removal of parotid tissue both above and below the facial nerve.

Parotidectomy with Nerve Graft—removal of the parotid gland and a portion of the facial nerve with a nerve graft interposed between the resected ends of the facial nerve.

Submandibular Gland Excision—surgical removal of the submandibular gland. This is usually performed for tumor, chronic infection, or stones in the hilum of the gland.

Parapharyngeal Space tumor—resection

of a tumor in the parapharyngeal space, which is a deep space in the neck.

Sialolithotomy—removal of a stone impacted in the drainage system of a salivary gland.

Nose and Maxilla

Rhinectomy—surgical removal of the nose.

Lateral Rhinotomy—exposure to the nose and maxilla through a surgical incision coursing along the lateral portion of the nose.

Maxillectomy—surgical removal of the maxillary sinus, usually for malignant disease.

Maxillectomy with Orbital Exenteration—removal of the orbit as well as the sinus, usually for extensive malignant disease that has invaded the orbit.

Excision Angiofibroma—surgical removal of a highly vascular angiofibroma usually found in the area of the nasopharynx.

Lips

Lip Shave—resection of the vermilion surface of the lip.

Wedge Resection, Primary Cause—wedge resection of a portion of a lip with direct closure, usually performed for malignant lesions.

Excision with Flap Reconstruction—excision of a portion of the lip, usually for malignant disease, with reconstruction of the resected portion utilizing adjacent tissue surgically positioned to fill the operative defect.

Local Resection for Carcinoma of the Mouth—removal, usually by wide excision, of a malignant tumor in the oral cavity.

Hemiglossectomy—surgical removal of one half of the tongue, which may be performed with or without reconstruction.

Composite Resection of Primary Tumor in Floor of Mouth, Alveolus, Tongue, Buccal Region, Tonsil, or Any Combination—surgical removal of a carcinoma in the oral cavity, which may be combined with radical neck dissection for involved local neck metastases.

Mandibular Resection—removal of a part of the mandible, for benign or malignant disease.

Ear

Excision of Pinna—surgical removal of the outer ear.

Temporal Bone Resection—surgical removal of the temporal bone. This is an extensive procedure, and it is usually done for malignant disease.

Neck

I & D, Neck Abscess—incision and drainage of an abscess cavity in the neck.

Radical (Complete) Neck Dissection Without a Primary—radical neck dissection that includes the removal of lymph nodes in the neck, the sternocleidomastoid muscle, and the internal jugular vein as it courses through the neck.

Radical (Complete) Neck Dissection with a Primary—a radical neck dissection that also includes removal of the head and neck primary tumor.

Modified Neck Dissection Without a Primary—a modified neck dissection in which the internal jugular vein and sternocleidomastoid muscle may be spared, with removal of the lymph nodes of the neck.

Modified Neck Dissection with a Primary—a modified neck dissection that also includes removal of the primary head and neck tumor.

Transsternal Mediastinal Dissection—removal of the lymph nodes in the mediastinum with surgical access through the sternum.

Cervical Node Biopsy—biopsy of a neck node.

Scalene Node Biopsy—biopsy of a scalene node or a node in the lower part of the neck just above the clavicle, or collar bone.

Larynx

Thyrotomy (Laryngofissure)—surgical splitting of the larynx for access to remove a tumor or growth.

Vertical Hemilaryngectomy—removal of one half of the larynx, usually for malignant disease.

Supraglottic Laryngectomy—removal of

that portion of the larynx above the vocal cords that includes the epiglottis, usually for malignant disease.

Total Laryngectomy—removal of the entire vocal box.

Laryngopharyngectomy—removal of the voice box and pharynx, most commonly done for malignant disease.

Surgical Speech Fistula—creation of a small opening or fistula in the cervical esophagus for implantation of a device to restore speech following laryngectomy.

Repair of Laryngeal Fracture—surgical repair of fractures in the cartilaginous portion of the larynx following injury.

Section of Recurrent Laryngeal Nerve—surgical interruption of the recurrent laryngeal nerve, which is the nerve that innervates the vocal cord.

Arytenoidectomy / Arytenoidpexy—removal or surgical fixation of the arytenoid, which is the cartilage adjacent to the posterior portion of the vocal cords.

Thyroid Lobectomy—surgical removal of a lobe of a thyroid gland.

Subtotal Thyroidectomy—incomplete removal of the thyroid gland.

Total Thyroidectomy—complete removal of the thyroid gland.

Parathyroidectomy—removal of the parathyroids, which are glands located on the posterior surface of the thyroid gland.

Pharyngoesophagectomy—surgical removal of the pharynx and esophagus to the extent required to resect malignant disease.

Cervical Esophagostomy for Feeding—an opening made into the cervical esophagus to allow for feeding when oral feeding cannot be initiated.

Pharyngeal Diverticulectomy—removal of a diverticulum, or pouch, in the pharynx.

Tracheotomy—opening into the trachea to allow for a secure airway.

Tracheal Resection with Repair—removal of a portion of the trachea with subsequent repair of the resected area.

Congenital Cysts

Branchial Cleft Cyst—removal of a congenital cyst in the head and neck area secondary to a persistent congenital remnant. The location of the cyst is dependent upon the location of the congenital defect.

Thyroglossal Duct Cyst—removal of a persistent congenital rest of thyroid tissue usually found in the midline of the neck near the hyoid bone. Frequently the cyst penetrates the hyoid bone and may extend toward the base of the tongue.

Common Otologic Procedures

Myringotomy and Tube—surgical incision in the tympanic membrane with placement of a ventilation tube.

Tympanoplasty I, or Myringoplasty—surgical repair of a perforation of the tympanic membrane, usually performed with a graft of temporalis fascia.

Tympanoplasty II–IV Without Mastoidectomy—in a Type I tympanoplasty, the graft will generally rest on the malleus. In Type II, the graft rests on the incus. In Type III, the graft attaches to the head of the stapes bone. In Type IV, the graft attaches to the footplate of the stapes.

Tympanoplasty with Mastoidectomy—repair of the tympanic membrane, associated with surgical resection of the mastoid.

Simple Mastoidectomy—surgical opening into the mastoid cavity without removal of the bony wall separating the middle ear and mastoid.

Modified Radical Mastoidectomy—opening of the mastoid air cells, usually for removal of a cholesteatoma, with lowering of the facial ridge or that portion of bone above the facial nerve that separates the mastoid and middle ear space. The tympanomeatal flap, or flap of tissue containing the reflected eardrum and a portion of the canal wall skin, can be rotated over the area of excised bone, as in Bondy's modified radical mastoidectomy.

Radical Mastoidectomy—usually performed for patients with chronic middle ear and mastoid disease that is suppurative, but on occasion neoplastic. No effort is made to restore hearing or to obliterate the mastoid cavity; radical removal of the mastoid cortex, tympanic membrane, and ossicular chain are all components of this procedure.

Ossiculoplasty—surgical repair through one of many methods to re-establish the ossicular chain.

Stapedectomy—surgical opening in the footplate of the stapes with placement of a prosthesis, usually performed for otosclerosis with fixation of the stapedial footplate.

Facial Nerve Decompression—opening of the bony canal that the facial nerve passes through to relieve pressure caused by swelling of the nerve.

Facial Nerve Graft, Repair, or Substitution—surgical grafting or repair of a damaged facial nerve.

Repair of Fistula (Oval Window or Round Window)—surgical repair of an opening in the oval or round window, usually accomplished by placing a fat graft.

Labyrinthectomy—surgical destruction of the labyrinth, or inner ear, performed for cases of intractable vertigo.

Endolymphatic Sac Operation—procedure to decompress the endolymphatic sac, performed for the intractable vertigo seen in Ménière's disease.

Resection of Cerebellopontine Angle Tumor—surgical removal of a tumor, usually an acoustic neuroma or less often a meningioma, found at the entrance of the internal auditory canal as the eighth cranial nerve courses toward the inner ear.

Eighth Nerve Section (Translabyrinthine, Retrolabyrinthine, Midfossa)—surgical resection or cutting of the eighth cranial nerve through one of three surgical approaches.

Reconstruction of Congenital Aural Atresia—surgical reconstruction of a deformed external ear, usually performed in stages.

Plastic and Reconstructive Procedures

Otoplasty—cosmetic surgical reconstruction of the outer ear.

Rhinoplasty—surgical and usually cosmetic reconstruction of the outer portion of the nose.

Mentoplasty—surgical and frequently cosmetic reconstruction of the area of the chin.

Rhytidectomy—face-lift procedure.

Blepharoplasty—surgical correction of eyelid deformities.

Reduction Facial Fractures

Frontal—surgical repair of a fracture through the frontal bone and/or frontal sinus.

Nasal—reduction of a displaced nasal fracture.

Maxilla–Le Fort I—separation of the hard palate, lower portions of the pterygoid processes, and nasal septum from the rest of the facial and cranial skeleton. Also referred to as Guerin's fracture.

Le Fort II—separation of the mid-portion of the facial skeleton from the cranial skeleton with the zygomatic compound attached to the cranial skeleton bilaterally.

Le Fort III—separation of the entire facial skeleton from the cranial skeleton.

Malar (Zygomatic)—fracture of the zygomatic arch or cheek bone.

Orbital Blowout—fracture through the floor of the orbit with displacement of fat and orbital contents into the maxillary sinus below.

Mandibular (Closed)—fracture of the mandible that is repaired through manipulation, without surgical exposure.

Mandibular (Open)—fracture of the mandible that requires repair through an open incision.

Laryngoplasty—surgical reconstruction of the larynx, usually following trauma or cancer surgery.

Tracheoplasty—surgical reconstruction of the trachea following trauma or repair following removal of malignant disease.

Pedicle Flap Procedures

Local—reorientation of local tissue to fill a surgical defect where the tissue is adjacent to the defect.

Regional—reorientation of tissue in the region of the surgical defect that is rotated to fill the surgical defect.

Myocutaneous—a pedicle flap of tissue that includes muscle with overlying skin on a dominant vascular pedicle to fill surgical defects.

Grafts

Split-Thickness Skin Graft—removal of less than the entire thickness of skin for purposes of reconstruction.

Full-Thickness Skin Graft—removal of a full thickness of skin to be used as donor tissue for skin loss.

Microsurgical Free Flap—a free flap of tissue transposed to another area with an anastomosis of the vessels of the free flap and recipient area through microsurgical techniques.

Fascial Sling Procedures—use of a segment of fascia to support a structure.

Oroantral Fistula Repair—repair of an opening between the oral cavity and the maxillary antrum, which can be seen following dental extractions.

Choanal Atresia Repair—surgical opening of blockage of the posterior portion of the nose.

Cleft Lip Repair—cosmetic surgical repair of a cleft lip.

Cleft Palate Repair—surgical repair of a cleft palate, which may or may not be associated with cleft lip.

Pharyngeal Flap—surgical correction of a short palate, accomplished by attaching a flap from the pharynx to the posterior palate.

Endoscopic Procedures

Direct Laryngoscopy, Diagnostic—direct inspection of the larynx with a laryngoscope for diagnostic purposes.

Laryngoscopy with Excision—direct laryngoscopy with surgical removal of a lesion contained within the larynx.

Laser Laryngoscopy—laryngoscopy performed with a laser used for the surgical procedure.

Vocal Cord Injection—injection of the vocal cord with one of a number of materials to allow a paralyzed vocal cord to assume a more midline position and improve voice quality.

Esophagoscopy, Diagnostic—direct inspection of the esophagus with an esophagoscope for diagnostic purposes.

Esophagoscopy with Foreign Body Removal—direct inspection of the esophagus with removal of a retained foreign body.

Esophagoscopy with Stricture Dilation—direct inspection of the esophagus with serial dilation, or stretching, of a narrowed area of stricture.

Bronchoscopy, Diagnostic—direct inspection of the tracheobronchial tree with either a fiberoptic or a rigid bronchoscope for diagnostic purposes.

Bronchoscopy with Foreign Body Removal—direct inspection of the tracheobronchial tree with removal of a foreign body.

Bronchoscopy with Stricture Dilation—direct inspection of the tracheobronchial tree with dilation for an area of stricture.

Panendoscopy (Multiple Concurrent Endoscopic Procedures)—usually includes bronchoscopy, esophagoscopy, and direct laryngoscopy. Frequently performed for diagnostic purposes in patients with head/neck malignant disease.

Mediastinoscopy—surgical inspection of the mediastinum, performed by passing a mediastinoscope through an incision in the midline of the lower part of the neck.

General Procedures

Adenoidectomy—surgical removal of the adenoid tissue or the lymphoid tissue found in the nasopharynx directly behind the posterior portion of the nose.

Tonsillectomy—surgical removal of the palatine tonsils.

T & A—tonsillectomy and adenoidectomy.

Nasal Polypectomy—surgical removal of nasal polyps.

Submucous Resection of the Septum—resection of the cartilaginous and/or bony septum through an incision made on the inside of the nose through the mucoperichondrium.

Nasal Septoplasty—surgical correction of a deformed nasal septum, using plastic surgical techniques with minimal removal of cartilage.

Turbinectomy—surgical removal of the nasal turbinates or structures on the lateral portion of the nose, usually to increase the nasal airway.

Intranasal Antrotomy—a surgical opening created in the nose, connecting the maxillary sinuses for the purpose of drainage.

Caldwell-Luc Operation—surgical exposure of the maxillary sinus, performed through an incision made in the canine fossa.

Transantral Ligation of Vessels—ligation of blood vessels, usually branches of the internal maxillary artery, for epistaxis through a Caldwell-Luc procedure and removal of the posterior wall of the sinus.

Intranasal Ethmoidectomy—intranasal removal of disease in the ethmoid sinus.

External Ethmoidectomy—removal of diseased ethmoid sinus cells through an external incision.

Frontoethmoidectomy—surgical exposure and removal of diseased tissue through an external incision through the brow line and lateral portion of the nose, providing exposure to both the frontal and the ethmoid sinuses.

Frontal Sinus Trephine—an opening made into the floor of the frontal sinus for drainage purposes.

Osteoplastic Frontal Sinusectomy—procedure performed on a frontal sinus in which a bone flap, usually inferiorly based, is replaced following the procedure on the sinus.

Frontal Sinus Ablation—ablation of the frontal sinus, usually with fat, after all the diseased mucosa has been removed, usually seen as part of an osteoplastic frontal procedure.

Sphenoidotomy—surgical opening into the sphenoid sinus.

Hypophysectomy, Transnasal Approach—approach to the pituitary gland through the nasal septum and sphenoid sinus.

Nasal Endoscopy—visualization of the anatomy of the nose through fiberoptic endoscopes.

Functional Endoscopic Sinus Surgery—surgery on the paranasal sinuses performed with fiberoptic nasal endoscopes.

INSTRUMENTS

The most commonly used instruments for examination are listed under three categories: ears, nose, and throat.

Ears

Otoscope—device used to examine the ear canal and tympanic membrane.

Ear Curettes—used for cleaning out debris from the ear canal.

Suction Tubes—tubes that are used to suction out fluid from the ear.

Tuning Forks (256 Hz and 512 Hz)—devices that when struck at the forked end vibrate; used in testing hearing.

Ear Forceps—instrument used in removing foreign bodies from the ear canal.

Nose

Nasal Speculum—instrument used to examine the nose internally.

Nasal Forceps—instrument used to place nasal packing or to remove foreign bodies from the nose.

Throat

Laryngeal Mirror—a mirrored instrument used to examine the larynx.

Tongue Depressor—instrument used to depress the tongue and facilitate examination of the oropharynx.

FORMATS

Letters ■ Letters are written to the patient's referring physician after examination has taken place. These letters contain the patient's history of the problem, finding of the examination, diagnosis, and treatment. An example of a letter is shown in Figure 29–17.

Physical Examination—Otolaryngology ■ An otolaryngologic physical examination form includes those areas of the head and neck routinely examined and also provides anatomic diagrams for chart notations. A sample is shown in Figure 29–18.

Reports

Consultation Report ■ Reports are written to the physician who requested a consultation on a patient. Such a report, giving the opinion of a consultant, is shown in Figure 29–19.

Operative Report ■ Figure 29–20 provides an example of a typical operative report on a patient with chronic otitis media on whom a myringotomy with insertion of ventilation tubes was performed.

Discharge Summary ■ This must give the patient's full name, medical record number, admission and discharge dates, discharge diagnoses, procedures performed, history of present illness, physical examination, impression, laboratory and surgical procedures performed, condition at the time of discharge, and medications

Text continued on page 553

WILLIAM J. LEWIS, M.D.
33 Lankenau Medical Building West
100 Lancaster Avenue west of City Line
Wynnewood, PA 19096-0000
215/896-6800

February 12, 1994

John R. Green, M.D.
111 Baker Street
Philadelphia, PA 19109

RE: Eliot Stenton

Dear Dr. Green:

It was my pleasure to see your patient, Eliot Stenton. Mr. Stenton came to see me for evaluation of bothersome postnasal drainage and intermittent nasal congestion. My examination revealed the following:

EARS: The external auditory canals and tympanic membranes were normal appearing. There was no evidence of otologic pathology. Rinne test with a 512 Hertz tuning fork was positive in both ears.

NOSE: The nasal mucous membranes were allergic appearing and congested, but otherwise unremarkable. Nasal polyps were not present and posterior rhinoscopy was
unrevealing.

THROAT: Examination of the oral cavity revealed a scant amount of clear drainage along the lateral pharyngeal walls. Indirect examination of the larynx was unremarkable. There was no evidence of vocal cord pathology.

It was my impression that Mr. Stenton has allergic rhinitis with intermittent postnasal drainage as the cause of his symptoms. He was given a prescription for a mild antihistamine to be taken at bedtime. I suggested that he call me in a few weeks and report his progress to me. I expect he will do quite well.

Cordially,

William J. Lewis, M.D.

ssb

Figure 29–17
A referral letter.

OTOLARYNGOLOGY — **HISTORY & PHYSICAL** — DATE — **Formedic**

NAME — S M W D — DATE OF BIRTH

ADDRESS — PHONE (H) — (O)

OCCUPATION / EMPLOYER

REFERRED BY — PHONE — INS.

HISTORY C.C.

EAR – NOSE – THROAT   [N] – NORM / N.A. — **PAST MEDICAL / SURGICAL HISTORY**

EARS– ☐ HEARING LOSS
☐ PAIN ☐ PRESSURE ☐ RINGING
☐ VERTIGO ☐ NOISE EXPOSURE
☐ FREQ. INF. ☐ DISCHARGE
☐
NOSE– ☐ TRAUMA ☐ SURGERY
☐ OBST. ☐ DISCHARGE
☐ EPISTAXIS ☐ PND
☐ SNORING ☐ SMELL
☐
THROAT– ☐ SORENESS
☐ FREQ. INF. ☐ ODYNOPHAGIA
☐ DYSPHAGIA ☐
LARYNX– ☐ SORENESS
☐ VOICE CHANGE
☐ SINUS INF. ☐
HEADACHE–

ALLERGIES
☐ HAYFEVER
☐ ASTHMA
☐ DESENSITIZATION
☐
Rx ALLERGIES

FAMILY HISTORY
☐ ALLERGIES ☐ BLEEDING
☐ ASTHMA ☐ CANCER
☐ HEARING LOSS ☐ DIABETES
☐ HEART DIS. ☐ HYPERTENSION

CURRENT Rx

SOCIAL HISTORY — CIG / DAY — ALCOHOL OZ / DAY — COFFEE CUPS / DAY

SUMMARY

Formedic — FREE PATIENT RECORD FORMS PARTNERS WITH PHYSICIANS SINCE 1982 — *Your Supplier of Free Patient Record Forms*

12-D WORLDS FAIR DRIVE • SOMERSET, N.J. 08873

CHART # PAGE # 12D WORLD'S FAIR DRIVE, SOMERSET NJ 08873 PRINTED IN CANADA FORMEDIC © 1988 OTHPLE

Figure 29–18

An example of a history and physical examination form. (Reprinted with permission from Formedic, Ltd., Somerset, New Jersey.)

548

THE LANKENAU HOSPITAL
100 Lancaster Avenue west of City Line
Wynnewood, PA 19096-0000

CONSULTATION REQUEST

PATIENT: Jonathan Stevens   DATE: 1/11/94
DESIRE FOR CONSULTATION WITH: William J. Lewis, M.D.
REASON FOR CONSULTATION: Epistaxis
REQUESTED BY: Henry Seaforth, M.D.

REPORT AND OPINION OF CONSULTANT

HISTORY: The patient is a 56-year-old white male who was admitted to the hospital for acute respiratory failure. The patient has had a history of nasal airway obstruction in the past said to be secondary to a deviated nasal septum. At the present time, he is receiving oxygen (O_2) by a nasal cannula. The patient is a two pack-per-day smoker with a history of emphysema.

EXAMINATION
EARS: Both external canals and tympanic membranes were unremarkable. The tympanic membranes were translucent and there was no evidence of middle ear effusion. Rinne test with a 512 Hertz tuning fork was positive in both ears.

NOSE: The nasal septum was noted to be deviated toward the right side with moderate nasal airway obstruction on that side. The nasal mucosa was noted to be dry and a bleeding vessel was noted along the anterior portion of the right side of the nasal septum. Epistaxis was controlled with silver nitrate cautery.

THROAT: The examination of the oral cavity including indirect laryngoscopy was unremarkable. There was no evidence of endolaryngeal pathology.

IMPRESSION: Epistaxis controlled with nasal cautery.

SUGGEST: Humidification with oxygen to prevent mucosal dryness.

Thank you for the opportunity to evaluate this patient.

_____
WILLIAM J. LEWIS, M.D.

WJL:bp
D: 1/1/94
T: 1/3/94

Figure 29-19
A form for a consultant's report and opinion.

549

THE LANKENAU HOSPITAL
100 Lancaster Avenue west of City Line
Wynnewood, PA 19096-0000

OPERATIVE REPORT

PATIENT: James Drummond   MEDICAL RECORD NO. 434 441
STATUS: ASU
DATE OF PROCEDURE: 1/2/94

PREOPERATIVE DIAGNOSIS: Chronic otitis media

POSTOPERATIVE DIAGNOSIS: Chronic otitis media

OPERATION: Bilateral myringotomy and insertion
                                    of Paparella ventilation tubes.

SURGEON: William J. Lewis, M.D.
ASSISTANT: Timothy Trent, M.D.
ANESTHESIA: General

COMPLICATIONS: None
TISSUE FOR LAB: None
BLOOD LOSS: None

PROCEDURE: Under satisfactory general
anesthesia with the patient in the supine position, the tympanic membranes
were directly inspected with the Zeiss operative microscope after the patient
had been draped in routine manner for myringotomy. The drums were noted
to be dull and retracted and there appeared to be mucoid purulent material in
both middle ear spaces. Myringotomy incisions were made in the anterior and
inferior quadrant and mucopurulent material was aspirated from both middle
ear spaces. The middle ear mucosa appeared to be hyperplastic. Paparella
ventilation tubes were placed without incident. The patient tolerated the
procedure well and left the operating room in satisfactory condition.

_____
WILLIAM J. LEWIS, M.D.

WJL:bp
D: 1/2/94
T: 1/3/94

Figure 29-20
An operative report for a bilateral myringotomy and insertion of Paparella ventilation tubes.

THE LANKENAU HOSPITAL
100 Lancaster Avenue west of City Line
Wynnewood, PA 19096-0000
DISCHARGE SUMMARY

PATIENT: JANICE LANE

UNIT HISTORY NO: 758-905

ADMITTED: 1/2/94

DISCHARGE DATE: 1/3/94

PHYSICIAN: William J. Lewis, M.D.

DISCHARGE DIAGNOSES:
1. Bilateral Otosclerosis
2. History of Cholecystectomy

PRINCIPAL PROCEDURE: Right Stapedectomy, 1/2/94

CONSULTATION: None

HISTORY OF PRESENT ILLNESS: The patient is a 40-year-old female who was admitted 1/2/94 with a history of progressive conductive hearing loss. The patient had noted decreased hearing loss over the past 15 years which has become increasingly symptomatic over the past five years. There is a history of familial hearing loss and one brother and two sisters have undergone stapedectomy procedures for otosclerosis. The patient had noticed increased hearing loss with pregnancies. The past medical history was essentially unremarkable. The patient had a history of chickenpox at age six. There was no history of measles or mumps. The patient has no known drug allergies. She had undergone cholecystectomy eight years ago under general anesthesia with no anesthetic or surgical complications. The family history is significant in that there is a history of otosclerosis. The patient is a nonsmoker and nondrinker. Review of systems is unremarkable.

PHYSICAL EXAMINATION: The patient appeared to be a well-developed and well-nourished female in no acute distress. The examination of the head, eyes, ears, nose, and throat revealed the patient to be normocephalic. The pupils were equal, round, reacted to light, and accommodation. The extra-ocular muscles were intact. Rinne test with a 512 Hertz tuning fork was negative in both ears and Rinne test lateralized toward the right ear. No significant nasal septal deformity was present. The nasal mucosa was unremarkable and nasal polyps were not present. The examination of the oral cavity was unrevealing. The neck was supple without thyromegaly or lymphadenopathy. The lungs were clear to percussion and auscultation. The heart rate was 72 and regular without murmurs, rales or gallops. The abdomen was soft without organomegaly or tenderness. The extremities were unremarkable. Neurologic examination was grossly intact.
(continued)

Figure 29–21

A discharge summary for a patient with bilateral otosclerosis.

Figure continued

JANICE LANE   Page two
UNIT HISTORY NO. 758-905

The impression at the time of admission was bilateral conductive hearing loss, right greater than left, secondary to otosclerosis.

Preoperative laboratory studies were obtained. A CBC and urinalysis were within normal limits. A chest x-ray was clear with no evidence of pulmonary pathology. An electrocardiogram was unremarkable. Normal sinus rhythm was present. A preoperative audiogram revealed bilateral conductive hearing loss with a more significant loss noted on the right side. A 30dB air/bone gap was present on the left and a 45dB air/bone gap was present on the right. Speech reception threshold was 45 dB on the left side and 65 dB on the right. Auditory discrimination was 92% bilaterally. Impedance tympanometry was unremarkable.

The patient was taken to the operating room on 1/2/94 and underwent a right stapedectomy with placement of a 4.0 mm. Shea Teflon cup prosthesis. The patient's postoperative course was unremarkable and she ambulated on the first postoperative day without difficulty. Postoperatively, she had no nystagmus or vertigo. She was discharged the following morning, 1/3/94, on no medications with instructions to return to see her attending physician in one week for follow-up postoperative care.

_____
WILLIAM J. LEWIS, M.D.

WJL:bp
D: 1/3/94
T: 1/4/94

Figure 29–21 Continued

given with instructions for follow-up care. An example is shown in Figure 29–21.

Reference Sources

Ballenger, John J. *Diseases of the Nose, Throat, Ear, Head and Neck,* 14th edition. Lea and Febiger, Philadelphia, 1991.

Cummings, Charles W., et al. (Eds.) *Otolaryngology–Head and Neck Surgery.* C. V. Mosby, St. Louis, 1986.

DeWeese, David D., et al. (Eds.) *Otolaryngology–Head and Neck Surgery,* 7th edition. C. V. Mosby, St. Louis, 1988.

Glasscock, Michael E., and George E. Shambaugh, Jr. *Surgery of the Ear,* 4th edition. W. B. Saunders Company, Philadelphia, 1990.

Stammberger, Heins. *Functional Endoscopic Sinus Surgery.* B. C. Decker, Philadelphia, 1991.

For references of specific application in medical transcription, see Appendix 1.

Paul T. Wertlake, M.D.

Anatomic Pathology

WORK FLOW FOR INFORMATION GENERATION AND REPORTING

The work flow outlined in this chapter occurs in a well-organized laboratory. Users of the laboratory appreciate the ready availability of written information involving collection and processing procedures, contact persons, proper containers and fixatives, and pertinent requisition forms. The provision of support materials is a responsibility of the anatomic pathology laboratory.

The anatomic pathology department and the individual tasks executed within it interlock into the overall function of the medical facility. This can be appreciated by viewing the entire spectrum of what occurs with a single report, for example, a breast biopsy report. The chronology of events begins with the patient, starting when the physician determines that a biopsy is indicated, including any further testing or procedures. The patient is scheduled and admitted to a medical facility. This is followed by performance of the surgical procedure, immediate postoperative care, discharge, billing, follow-up management and counseling, and peer review and quality assurance activities of the medical facility.

Anatomic pathology functions should integrate with and support all aspects of the full chain of service. This is essential to the success of continuing quality improvement.

A typical flow chart of major steps is shown in Figure 30–1. In practice, many details are determined by procedures of the medical facility.

PATIENT CARE REPORTS

The conformation, style, and specific language of these reports is quite variable. Nevertheless, certain elements are uniformly included as a standard of practice.

Patient care forms for anatomic pathology serve two differing functions: the REQUEST for service and the REPORT of results, and often occur as separate forms for each. The two functions may be combined in a single turnaround document. The following discussion deals with these two major functions as separate forms.

Tissue Request Forms ▪ Surgical pathology request forms should be received with the following information:

1. Demographic information, including the patient's name, age, sex, primary and secondary patient identifiers, ordering physician, and other physicians.
2. Billing information.
3. Date of procedure.
4. Tissue specimen identification.
5. Procedure performed.
6. Relevant clinical information.
7. Request for pathology examination to be performed, including any special requests.
8. Operating room consultations, with or without frozen section, including diagnoses rendered, procedures performed, and additional studies initiated.

Cytology Request Forms
Nongynecologic Specimens ▪ Cytology request forms for nongynecologic sources, for example, fine needle aspirations, bronchial brush-

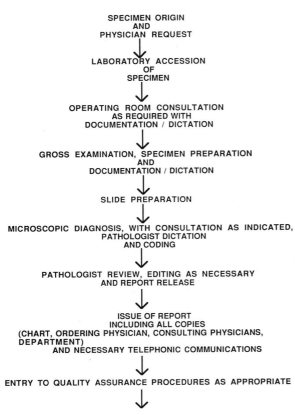

SPECIMEN ORIGIN
AND
PHYSICIAN REQUEST

↓

LABORATORY ACCESSION
OF
SPECIMEN

↓

OPERATING ROOM CONSULTATION
AS REQUIRED WITH
DOCUMENTATION / DICTATION

↓

GROSS EXAMINATION, SPECIMEN PREPARATION
AND
DOCUMENTATION / DICTATION

↓

SLIDE PREPARATION

↓

MICROSCOPIC DIAGNOSIS, WITH CONSULTATION AS INDICATED,
PATHOLOGIST DICTATION
AND CODING

↓

PATHOLOGIST REVIEW, EDITING AS NECESSARY
AND REPORT RELEASE

↓

ISSUE OF REPORT
INCLUDING ALL COPIES
(CHART, ORDERING PHYSICIAN, CONSULTING PHYSICIANS,
DEPARTMENT)
AND NECESSARY TELEPHONIC COMMUNICATIONS

↓

ENTRY TO QUALITY ASSURANCE PROCEDURES AS APPROPRIATE

↓

EXECUTION OF BILLING FUNCTIONS

Figure 30–1
Typical flow chart of major steps of specimen origin to billing.

ings, and urinary bladder washings, are similar in many respects to the content of tissue study requests (Figure 30–2). The following information should be included:

1. Demographic information, including the patient's name, age, sex, primary and secondary patient identifiers, ordering physician, and other physicians.
2. Billing information.
3. Date of procedure.
4. Specimen identification.
5. Procedure performed.
6. Relevant clinical information.
7. Request for cytology examination to be performed, including any special requests, e.g., silver stain for *Pneumocystis carinii*.

Gynecologic Papanicolaou (Pap) Smear Request Forms

■ The following information is important for inclusion within the Pap smear request form (Figure 30–3):

1. Demographic information, including the patient's name, age, sex, primary and secondary patient identifiers, ordering physician, and other physicians.
2. Billing information.
3. Date of procedure.
4. Specimen identification: cervical and/or endocervical and/or vaginal, endometrial sampling.
5. Sampling performed: endocervical brush or swab; specify other type of sampling.
6. Date or estimate, last menstrual period (LMP).
7. Pregnant: yes, estimated date of confinement (EDC); or no.
8. Postpartum: Yes or no.
9. Postmenopausal: Yes or no.
10. Abnormal bleeding: Yes, specify; or no.
11. Hysterectomy: Yes, total or partial (supracervical); or no.
12. Intra-uterine device (IUD): yes or no.
13. Oral contraception (OC): Yes, specify; no.
14. Previous abnormal Pap smear: Yes, this laboratory, previous cytology number; other laboratory; or no.
15. Previous biopsy: Yes, this laboratory, previous biopsy number; other laboratory; or no.
16. Relevant history: Squamous intraepithelial lesion (SIL), low grade, high grade.
17. Cancer: specify type.
18. HPV* infection: Yes, specify HPV DNA studies, date, types detected: 6, 11 _____, 16, 18 _____, 31, 33, 35 _____, other _____ .
19. Treatment: Laser therapy: Yes, give date; or no.
    Cryotherapy: Yes, give date; or no.
    LEEP:† Yes, give date; or no.
    Hormonal: Yes, specify type, give date; or no.
    Other: Yes, specify type, give date; or no.
20. Other risk factors: Yes, specify; or no.

---

*Human papillomavirus.
†Loop electrocautery excision procedure.

Design of Test Request Forms ■ Good design of requisition forms is essential. Providing complete information may prove vital to optimal processing of specimens or diagnostic considerations in case study. In some instances, lack of the proper information may lead to loss of opportunity for certain specialized studies to be performed, e.g., estrogen and progesterone receptor sites, cultures, or certain genetic studies. In some instances, additional procedures may still be performed, but the turnaround time (TAT) of the final report may be delayed.

The desired elements, such as those enumerated under the Pap smear request form, should be carefully considered in the composition of request forms. Forms are most successful when they are designed by someone actively involved in many aspects of the laboratory. Considerations include ease of reading, space for write-in information, the number of copies necessary, modifying some for functions such as billing, and time/date stamping for receipt of specimens.

Tissue Reports

Gross Description ■ These reports include a description of materials received in the laboratory. This is commonly referred to as the gross description and includes whether a tissue was received fresh or in a container of formalin or other fixative, the number of tissues received, the size by weight or volume, description of the specimen (surfaces, texture, color, visible abnormalities — tumors, ulcerations). Sizes of abnormalities are noted as well as relationships to specific structures and margins of excision or resection.

Prior removal of tissue for frozen section or other studies is noted, with specification of the site. Frozen-section diagnoses rendered are included in the report, as well as identification of the performing pathologist.

Microscopic Description ■ Dissection of the specimen by the examining pathologist is described. Tissues selected for microscopic examination are specified.

Photographs, radiologic examinations, and tissue selected for other specialized studies are stated. The latter include estrogen and progesterone receptor assays, other tumor marker studies by immunocytochemistry procedures, electron microscopy, and enzymatic studies.

Tissues selected for routine microscopic examination are identified by code letters or numbers stated in the report, which correspond to the paraffin blocks and slides prepared. It is good practice to identify the number of cassettes utilized for processing tissue from a given case. This may be done as a summary of tissues at the conclusion of the specimen description, or it may be incorporated into the description.

The microscopic diagnosis also includes the tissue, the site, and the procedure. Some reports will have only a gross description and gross diagnosis. However, some reports, especially those consisting of multiple parts, may have both microscopic and gross diagnoses.

Reports of cases examined intraoperatively include specific diagnoses for all tissues examined by frozen sections, touch preparations, or smears, together with identification of pathologists making the diagnoses.

Many reports give only microscopic diagnoses, not microscopic descriptions, when the information in both is essentially the same. If additional and significant information is conveyed by a microscopic description, it is appropriate to include this as a separate section of the report.

Microscopic diagnoses that include complete reporting of important information offer significant advantages:

■ Telephone requests from individuals other than pathologists can very likely be fulfilled by reading the microscopic diagnoses to the person.

■ Accessibility to on-line information within computer systems is significantly extended by long-term retention of microscopic diagnoses, together with comments, addenda, revisions, and corrections. The deletion of gross and microscopic descriptions is space conserving. Full reports may be permanently retained off-line. Access to off-line reports is generally delayed compared with on-line information, which is immediately available.

Facilities may determine the length of time that full reports should be available on-line, perhaps 4 months, before being formatted to long-term storage. It may be desirable, therefore, to include in the microscopic diagnosis the following elements:

■ Lesion as clinically identified.

■ Anatomic site.

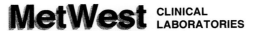

MetWest CLINICAL LABORATORIES

18408 Oxnard Street • Tarzana, CA 91356
(818) 996-7300   (800) 382-3322
Medical Director: Paul T. Wertlake, M.D.
Co-Medical Directors: Alex W. Ngo, M.D.   Donald R. Simpson, M.D.

PHYSICIAN NAME

PATIENT NAME _____
    LAST   FIRST   M

ADDRESS _____

CITY _____ STATE _____ ZIP _____

AGE ____   SEX ____

BILLING INFORMATION

☐ BILL DOCTOR   ☐ BILL PATIENT (Address Required)   ☐ INSURANCE
☐ BILL MEDI-(CAL/CAID) (Copy of ID Card or POE Sticker required)
☐ BILL MEDI-CARE (Address and Medicare No. req)   NO: _____

CYTOPATHOLOGY CONSULTATION, NON-GYNECOLOGIC SOURCES

SPECIMEN TYPE

ASPIRATE _____; BRUSHINGS _____; FNA: PASS 1_____, PASS 2 _____, PASS 3 _____
FLUID _____; SCRAPING _____; SMEAR _____; TOUCH PREP _____; WASHINGS _____

SPECIMEN SOURCE

BLADDER: CYSTOSCOPY URINE _____; CYTOSCOPY FLUID _____

BREAST: CYST _____; MASS _____; NIPPLE _____; RIGHT _____; LEFT _____;
        LOCATION: UOQ _____; UIQ _____; LOQ _____; LIQ _____; CENTER _____

BRONCHUS: Specify: (1) _____;(2) _____; (3) _____; (4) _____; (5) _____; (6) _____

COLON: MASS _____; POLYP _____; ULCER _____; OTHER _____
        ANORECTAL _____; LOCATION in cm. (1) _____ (2) _____ (3) _____ (4) _____

DISCHARGE: _____ SPECIFY _____

ESOPHAGUS: MASS _____; **ULCER** _____; **OTHER** _____
        LOCATION in cm. (1) _____ **(2)** _____ **(3)** _____ **(4)** _____

EYE: LESION _____; RIGHT _____; LEFT _____

FLUIDS: CSF _____; CUL de SAC _____; CYST: _____ SPECIFY _____
        DRAINAGE _____ SPECIFY _____
        GASTRIC _____; PERICARDIAL _____; PERITONEAL _____;
        PLEURAL: RIGHT _____ LEFT _____

LUNG: MASS: _____ INFILTRATE: _____ PLEURAL _____ OTHER _____

LYMPH NODE: SPECIFY _____

ORAL CAVITY: SPECIFY _____

PROSTATE: SPECIFY _____

SKIN: LESION _____; LOCATION: _____

SOFT TISSUE MASS: SUPERFICIAL _____; DEEP _____

SPUTUM: EARLY AM _____; INDUCED _____; SACCOMANNO _____

THYROID: RIGHT LOBE _____; LEFT LOBE _____; OTHER SPECIFY _____

URINE: RANDOM URINE _____; EARLY AM URINE _____; CLEAN CATCH URINE _____

OTHER SITES, SOURCES: SPECIFY _____

CONCURRENT BIOPSY: _____ **PREVIOUS BIOPSY:** _____ **THIS LAB:** _____

PREVIOUS CYTOLOGY: _____ **THIS LAB:** _____

RELEVANT HISTORY: _____

PLEASE COMPLETE FOCUSED HISTORIES ON REVERSE SIDE

80001

Figure 30-2
Example of cytology request form for nongynecologic specimens. (Reprinted with permission of MetWest Clinical Laboratories, Tarzana, California.)

PLEASE COMPLETE FOCUSED HISTORIES

RESPIRATORY LESIONS

PRESENT SMOKER: _____ PAST SMOKER: _____ PACKS PER DAY: _____

YEAR STARTED: _____ YEAR STOPPED: _____ PIPE ONLY _____

INDUSTRIAL EXPOSURE TO CARCINOGENS: _____

BREAST LESIONS, WOMEN

HISTORY OF BREAST CARCINOMA: MOTHER _____; SISTER(S) _____

CONCURRENT MAMMOGRAM: MASS _____ CALCIFICATIONS _____ LOCATION _____

THYROID LESIONS

CYST _____; SINGLE NODULE _____; MULTIPLE NODULES _____

HOT NODULE _____, COLD NODULE _____; ENLARGED GLAND _____

TREATMENT: SPECIFY _____

PROSTATE LESIONS

SINGLE NODULE: _____ MULTINODULAR: _____ INDURATION: _____ RIGHT: _____ LEFT: _____

PROSTATIC ACID PROSPHATASE: NORMAL _____; ELEVATED _____

PROSTATIC SPECIFIC ANTIGEN: NORMAL _____; ELEVATED _____

GENITO-URINARY LESIONS

URINE RETENTION: _____ CYSTITIS: _____ BPH: _____ PELVIC RELAXATION: _____ HEMATURIA: _____

CONCURRENT CALCULI: _____ PRIOR CALCULI: _____ DEMONSTRATED LESION: _____

PRIOR UROTHELIAL CARCINOMA: _____ PRIOR UROTHELIAL DYSPLASIA: _____

Figure 30–2 *Continued*

■ Procedure performed.

■ Preparations examined.

Examples of such a microscopic diagnosis may appear as:

■ Pigmented lesion, right cheek, excisional biopsy:
  Intradermal nevus.

■ Polyp, colon at 50 cm., polypectomy:
  Tubulovillous adenoma.

Often a Comment section is given following the microscopic diagnoses for discussing problematic aspects of a case, risks that the patient may be subject to, follow-up actions that may be required, and the like. The Comment section may state that case material has been provided for expert consultation or that certain follow-up procedures, such as immunocytochemical assays or special stains, are in progress, as well as a statement that there will be a subsequent report. Special stains or other specialized procedures that have been utilized in study of the case should be identified.

Generally, reports consist of multiple parts. An original report is provided for the patient's chart; copies go to the requesting physician, who usually performs the surgical procedure, other physicians concerned with medical management of the patient, and the department. In addition, the report will usually include a billing copy.

Preliminary Reports ■ In some instances, it may be important to issue a preliminary report indicating the status of the case and the actions in progress. Certain bone tumors require an extended decalcification time before microscopic sections and slides can be prepared. It is helpful to the managing physicians to have a timely preliminary report identifying this situation. In other instances, unusual lesions may require expert consultative opinion before a final diagnosis is reported. A preliminary diagnosis may be helpful or, if it is necessary to defer diagnosis, it is important for that to be reported in a timely manner. Such preliminary reports should include identification of expert consultants to whom the case has been referred.

Tissue cases related to prior or concurrent cytologic studies should include a correlation

MetWest
UNILAB
18408 Oxnard Street
Tarzana, CA 91356
(818) 996-7300
Southern California
(800) 339-4299

Medical Director:
Paul T. Wertlake, M.D.

Co-Medical Directors:
Alex W. Ngo, M.D.
Norman M. Williams, M.D.
Kenneth H. Francus, M.D.
John H. Yoell, M.D.
Prospero B. Pilar, M.D.

ACKNOWLEDGEMENT OF SPECULOSCOPY CHARGES

I UNDERSTAND THAT METWEST WILL BE BILLING ME OR MY INSURANCE COMPANY DIRECTLY FOR THE PAP SMEAR PROCEDURE (INCLUDING SPECULOSCOPY MATERIALS) PERFORMED DURING MY VISIT TODAY. I AGREE TO PAY ALL AMOUNTS NOT PAID BY MY PRIVATE INSURANCE COMPANY OR HMO. NOT APPLICABLE FOR PATIENTS WITH MEDICARE, MEDI-CAL, OR CHAMPUS INSURANCE.

PHYSICIAN NAME

SIGNATURE:

PATIENT'S LAST NAME   FIRST   M.I.   PATIENT ID / SS #

ADDRESS

CITY   STATE   ZIP   D.O.B.   AGE   DATE COLLECTED

COMPLETE FOR ALL BILLING TYPES
PLEASE PRINT CLEARLY
ALL INFORMATION MUST BE PROVIDED OR ACCOUNT WILL BE BILLED
COMPLETE FOR ALL THIRD PARTY BILLING

BILL TO: ☐ OUR ACCOUNT ☐ PATIENT ☐ INSURANCE ☐ IPA / HMO ☐ MEDICARE ☐ MEDI-CAL / CAID (Please attach card of P.O.E. Sticker)

AUTHORIZATION
BY SIGNING THIS AUTHORIZATION, I UNDERSTAND THAT I AM RESPONSIBLE FOR PAYMENT OF CHARGES FOR LABORATORY WORK REQUESTED BY MY PHYSICIAN. IF INSURANCE COVERAGE IS INDICATED ABOVE, I ALSO AUTHORIZE THE RELEASE OF ANY INFORMATION NECESSARY FOR THIS CLAIM. I ACCEPT AND UNDERSTAND THAT I AM RESPONSIBLE FOR ANY CO-INSURANCE AND/OR DEDUCTIBLE AMOUNTS NOT PAID IN FULL. BE ADVISED THAT CURRENT CHANGES IN PAYMENT POLICY HAVE EXCLUDED CERTAIN TESTS AS BENEFITS UNDER MEDICARE

INSURANCE COMPANY / IPA / HMO   DOB

ADDRESS

PT./RESPONSIBLE PARTY SIGNATURE

CITY / STATE / ZIP CODE

RESPONSIBLE PARTY

CERTIFICATE NO.   GROUP NO.

PHONE NO.   ICD-9 CODE (DX)   MEDICAID / MEDICARE NO.   STATE

STATE LAW 1050(g) (2A) REQUIRES PATIENT NAME, COMPLETE PATIENT HISTORY AND SLIDES PROPERLY LABELED WITH PATIENT IDENTIFICATION. UNLABELED SLIDES WILL BE RETURNED UNPROCESSED

GYN CYTOLOGY REQUEST

TEST ☐ PAP ☐ PAP PLUS SPECULOSCOPY

SOURCE   LMP
HORMONAL ESTIMATE REQUIRES
VAGINAL WALL SAMPLE

☐ VAGINAL (SPATULA)
☐ CERVIX (SPATULA)
☐ ENDOCERVIX   ☐ SWAB   ☐ BRUSH
☐ COMBINED CERVIX, ENDOCERVIX SAMPLE
☐ OTHER
PATHOLOGIST RECOMMENDATION (for patient follow- up): ☐ YES ☐ NO

CLINICAL HISTORY

☐ ROUTINE CHECK-UP
☐ CURRENT DIAGNOSTIC PROBLEM (PROVIDE ICD-9 ABOVE)
☐ PREGNANT   EDC
☐ POST PARTUM
☐ TOTAL HYSTERECTOMY
☐ SUB-TOTAL HYST (CERVIX IN PLACE)
☐ POST MENOPAUSAL
☐ ABNORMAL BLEEDING
☐ CERVICITIS / VAGINITIS

☐ DES EXPOSURE
☐ ORAL CONTRACEPTIVES
☐ HORMONAL REPLACEMENT
☐ POST-ESTROGEN TRIAL
☐ CRYOTHERAPY
☐ LASER TREATMENT
☐ STD
DATES OF THERAPY

☐ LEEP
☐ RADIATION THERAPY
☐ CHEMO/HORMONAL THERAPY
☐ HPV
☐ L SIL
☐ H SIL
☐ MALIGNANT

NON - GYN CYTOLOGY REQUEST

SOURCE   LEFT RIGHT   COLLECTION METHOD
☐ BREAST   ☐   ☐   ☐ FNA
☐ NIPPLE   ☐   ☐   SITE
☐ BRONCHUS   ☐   ☐   ☐ BRUSHING
☐ PLEURAL FLUID ☐   ☐   ☐ WASHING
☐ THYROID   ☐   ☐   ☐ VOIDED   # OF SPECIMENS
☐ URINE   ☐ CATHETERIZED
☐ SPUTUM   ☐ SMEAR
☐ PERITONEAL FLUID   ☐ SCRAPING
☐ CSF   ☐ OTHER SPECIFY
☐ OTHER, SPECIFY

CLINICAL INFORMATION CYTOLOGY / BIOPSY

PREVIOUS: CYTOLOGY/BIOPSY SPEC #

DATE: THIS LAB: ☐ YES ☐ NO ☐ ABNORMAL
DIAGNOSIS:
OTHER:

BIOPSY REQUEST

BIOPSY SITE (S)

OF SPECIMENS:

SPECULOSCOPY
RESULTS: ☐ POSITIVE ☐ NEGATIVE
CERVIX   VAGINA
PLEASE INDICATE AREAS OF ACETO - WHITENING

COLPOSCOPY
RESULTS: ☐ POSITIVE ☐ NEGATIVE
CERVIX   VAGINA
PLEASE INDICATE AREAS OF ABNORMAL CHANGES

☐ SATISFACTORY
☐ UNSATISFACTORY
☐ WHITE EPITHELIUM
☐ PUNCTATION
☐ MOSAIC PATTERN
OTHER

MetWest Pap Plus System Form 80022 (REV 3/93)

LAB COPY

Figure 30–3
Example of cytology request form for gynecologic specimens. (Reprinted with permission of MetWest Clinical Laboratories, Tarzana, California.)

560

CYTOTECH_____ RESCREENING CYTOTECH _____ PATHOLOGIST_____

DATE _____ DATE _____ DATE _____

PRIOR SMEARS/PRIOR BIOPSIES / REVIEW DX   GROSS DESCRIPTION / PRELIMINARY DX / COMMENTS

\# _____

\# _____

\# _____

SAMPLE ADEQUACY

1001	☐ SAT	1020	☐	ENDOCX CELLS PRS
1002	☐ SAT/LIMIT ➡	1021	☐	NO EC PRESENT
1003	☐ UNSAT ➡	1022	☐	NO EC IN PMENO
1004	☐ SCANT CELLS	1015	☐	DRY EFFECT
1005	☐ INSUF CELLS	1016	☐	THICK SM
1006	☐ POOR FIX/PRES	1017	☐	OBS INFL/BLD
1007	☐ OBSC INFL	1018	☐	THK OBS BLD OR INFL
1008	☐ OBSC BLD	1019	☐	OBSC BACT
1009	☐ MENS SM	1023	☐	SCANT SQ CELLS
1010	☐ FOREIGN MAT	1024	☐	EXCESSIVE CYTOLYSIS
1011	☐ NO ENDOCX 1030 ☐ NO LMP	1025	☐	BROKEN AREA/ EST ____
1012	☐ NOT REP SITE 1031 ☐ NO AGE	1026	☐	SUG EC, ? HYST
1013	☐ BROKEN SL 1032 ☐ NO SOURC	1027	☐	SUG EC, ? VAG SAMPLE
1014	☐ INSUF PT HX ➡ 1033 ☐ NO DOC	1028	☐	DEGEN GLAND VS PSEU

CLASSIFICATION

2001 ☐ WITHIN NORMAL LIMITS
2002 ☐ W.N.L./ REACTIVE/REPARATIVE/SEE DESC DX
2003 ☐ ABNORMAL/SEE DESC DX/RECOMMENDATIONS

MICRO-ORGANISMS   REACTIVE REPARATIVE

4000	☐ BACT FLORA POLYMORPHIC	5000	☐	ENDOCX CHG R/R> DYSPL?
4001	☐ MIXED BACTERIA	5001	☐	META CELLS
4002	☐ COCCOID	5002	☐	REACT ENDOCX
4003	☐ BACILLARY	5005	☐	ENDOCERVICITIS/REACT EC
4005	☐ ACTINO	5006	☐	FOLLICULAR CXITIS
4006	☐ LEPTO	5011	☐	POST PARTUM
4008	☐ FUNGUS NS	5012	☐	REPAIR
4009	☐ SPORES ONLY	5013	☐	INFL CHG
4010	☐ CANDIDA	5014	☐	INFL CHG/TRICH
4011	☐ SUSP TRICH	5015	☐	INFL CHG/CANDIDA
4012	☐ TRICH	5021	☐ MILD	
4013	☐ HERPES	5022	☐ MOD	
4018	☐ BACT FLORA HEAVY	5023	☐ SEV	
4020	☐ FEW RBC	5017	☐	ANUCL SQUAMES? LESION
4021	☐ MOD RBC	5018	☐	CELLULAR CHG/HERPES
4022	☐ MANY RBC	5019	☐	CELLULAR CHG/CHLAMYDIA
4050	☐ NO POLYS	5020	☐	REACT SQUAMES
4051	☐ OCC POLYS	5025	☐	ATROPHIC MILD
4052	☐ MOD POLYS	5026	☐	ATROPHIC MOD
4053	☐ NUM POLYS	5027	☐	ANUCL SQ W/BACT COLONIZ
4060	☐ BACT VAGINOSIS/4000	5028	☐	ANUCL SQ W/ATROPHY
		5029	☐	REACT META

HORMONAL EVALUATION

6000	☐ MIXED E.E.	6026	☐	COMPAT W.POST PARTUM
6001	☐ MATURATION: HIGH	6028	☐	NO H.E./POOR PRESERV
6002	☐ MATURATION: MODERATE	6029	☐	NO H.E./CANDIDA
6003	☐ MATURATION: LOW	6030	☐	NO H.E./VAG SAMPLE REQ
6007	☐ ATROPHIC	6031	☐	NO H.E./INFLAMMATION
6004	☐ MI: P ___ I ___ S ___	6032	☐	NO H.E./EXCESS BLOOD
6005	☐ COMP W/AGE/HX	6033	☐	NO H.E./NUM ANUCL SQUAMES
6006	☐ INCOMP W/AGE/HX	6034	☐	NO H.E./HEAVY BACT FLORA
6008	☐ ATROPHIC W/AUTOLYTIC PAT	6035	☐	NO H.E./AUTOLYSIS
6009	☐ EQUIVOCAL ATROPHIC PATTERN	6036	☐	NO H.E./ENDOCX POPULATION
6010	☐ MIXED EE/PERIMENO	6037	☐	NO H.E./INSUFF PT HISTORY
6011	☐ MIXED EE/PMENO/HORM RX	6038	☐	NO H.E./TRICHOMONAS
6012	☐ MIXED EE/PMENO/?HORM RX	6039	☐	NO H.E./SMALL SQUAMOUS POP
6013	☐ ELV EE/PMENO/HORM RX	6040	☐	NO H.E./HPV
6019	☐ ELV EE FOR AGE/HX	6041	☐	NO H.E./ ABNORMAL CELLS
6020	☐ LOW EE FOR AGE/HX	6042	☐	NO H.E./METAPLASTIC CELLS
6021	☐ ELV EE FOR AGE/?HORM RX	6045	☐	MIXED EE/NO HORM HX.

CR ☐,☐   U ☐,☐   O ☐,☐   MO ☐,☐   MDX ☐,☐

EPITHELIAL ABNORMALITIES
SQUAMOUS CELLS

3001	☐	ASCUS. MIN
3002	☐	ASCUS. MILD
3003	☐	ASCUS, MOD/DYS?
3004	☐	NUM META SQ CELL
3005	☐	ATYP META SQ CELL/DYS?
3006	☐	PARAK CELLS
3007	☐	ATYP PARAK CELL
3010	☐	ATROPHIC NEOPL VS R/R
3012	☐	LO SIL W/HPV
3013	☐	LO SIL/CIN 1 HPV
3014	☐	LO SIL CIN 1
3015	☐	LO SIL CIN 1 RAD
3016	☐	HI SIL CIN 2 W/HPV
3017	☐	HI SIL CIN 2
3018	☐	HI SIL CIN 2 RAD
3019	☐	HI SIL CIN 3 W/HPV
3020	☐	HI SIL CIN 3
3021	☐	HI SIL CIN 3/CIS W/HPV
3022	☐	HI SIL CIN 3/CIS
3023	☐	C/W SQUAMOUS CA
3024	☐	DYS META TYPE
3045	☐	DYS KERAT TYPE

GLANDULAR CELLS

3025	☐	ENDOM OUT PHASE
3026	☐	ENDOM/PMENO
3027	☐	ENDOM/PMENO/EXOG HORM
3028	☐	SUG ENDOM HYPERPL
3029	☐	SUG ATYP ENDOM HYPERPL
3030	☐	SUG ENDOM ADCA
3031	☐	C/W ENDOM ADCA
3032	☐	SUG ENDOCERV DYSPL
3033	☐	SUG ENDOCX ADCA
3034	☐	C/W ENDOCX ADCA
3037	☐	SUG XTRAUTERINE ADCA
3038	☐	ENDOCERV VS ENDOMET
3039	☐	ATYP GLND EC VS ENDOMET
3043	☐	ENDOM STROMAL HIST
3044	☐	ATYP ENDOM STROM HIST
3046	☐	POSS GLND, INVOLV
3047	☐	DYSPL/CA NOT PRECLUD
3070	☐	ATYP ENDOCX CELLS

SPECULOSCOPY FINDINGS

3080	☐	SPECULOSCOPY NEG
3081	☐	SPECULOSCOPY POS ➡
3082	☐	ACETO WHITE 12-3
3083	☐	ACETO WHITE 3-6
3084	☐	ACETO WHITE 6-9
3085	☐	ACETO WHITE 9-12
3086	☐	ACETO WHITE OS
3087	☐	ACETO WHITE 12
3088	☐	ACETO WHITE 3
3089	☐	ACETO WHITE 6
3078	☐	ACETO WHITE 9

COLPOSCOPY FINDINGS

3090	☐	COLP NEG
3091	☐	COLP POS ➡
3092	☐	ABNORM 12
3093	☐	ABNORM 3
3094	☐	ABNORM 6
3095	☐	ABNORM 9
3096	☐	ABNORM OS

RECOMMENDATIONS/COMMENTS

7000	☐	REPEAT
7003	☐	REPEAT 12 MONTHS
7004	☐	REPEAT MID-CYCLE
7005	☐	REPEAT 6 WKS-3 MONTHS
7006	☐	REPEAT 6 MONTHS
7007	☐	REP/POST RX/INFL
7008	☐	REP/POST RX W/EXTROGEN
7009	☐	REP POST PARTUM 6 WKS
7010	☐	REC BRUSH SAMPLING
7011	☐	REC VAG WALL SAMPLING
7012	☐	REC SM/COLP/BX
7013	☐	REC BX
7014	☐	REC COLP/BX
7050	☐	PERSISTENT ATYPIA/COLP
7051	☐	REC COLP/FRACT CURRET
7052	☐	REC COLP EVAL
7015	☐	REC CERV CONE
7016	☐	REC ENDOMET SAMPLING
7017	☐	REC ENDOM EVAL
7018	☐	REC F/U
7023	☐	EVAL FOR ENDOG/EXOG EST
7024	☐	CRYOSURGERY EFFECT
7025	☐	ELECTROCAUTERY EFFECT
7026	☐	EVAL DES HX
7027	☐	DES VAG SAMPLING
7028	☐	CLIN. EVAL REQ
7029	☐	ENDOM CELLS IN PHASE
7030	☐	REC SAMPLE LEUPLAKIA
7031	☐	CONFIRM LMP/ENDOM PETUR
7032	☐	REC F/U BACT VAGINOSIS
7034	☐	HX NOTED.
7039	☐	REC COLP/ ESTROG TRIAL
7040	☐	DNA PROBE/CHLAMYDIA
7045	☐	REACT CHANGE W/OUT ATYP
7046	☐	MILD/ MOD INFL CHANGE
7047	☐	DEGEN CHANGE
7055	☐	ENDOMET ? LMP
7035	☐	ENDOM CELLS NOS
		PREVIOUS REV. _____
7019	☐	CHANGES SIM TO PREV SMEAR
7020	☐	ATYP < PREV SMEAR
7021	☐	PREV ATYP NOT EVIDENT
7022	☐	SAMPLE VARIANCE /LOSS ATYP
7070	☐	PS/REC COLP/BX.PAP NOR
7071	☐	PS/REC COLP/BX.PAP
7072	☐	REC COLP/BX.PAP INDET
7073	☐	PS/REC COLP/BX PAP LSIL
7074	☐	PS/REC COLP/BX PAP HSIL
7075	☐	PS/REC COLP/BX.PAP GLND
7076	☐	PS/REC COLP/BX.PAP LMT
7077	☐	PS/REC COLP/BX.PAP UNSAT
7078	☐	COLP/BX.HPV/DNA POS
7079	☐	HPV 6, 11
7080	☐	HPV 16, 18
7081	☐	HPV 31, 33, 35
7082	☐	HPV, SPECIFY
7086	☐	SPECULOSCOPY INDET
7087	☐	SPECULOSCOPY NC

_____
_____
_____
_____
_____
_____

Figure 30–3 *Continued*

561

statement. This should occur for nongynecologic and gynecologic studies. The correlation should state whether the cytology and tissue studies were concordant or discordant. If concordant, no further comment is necessary. If discordant, a number of considerations must be made and reported. These considerations include whether the variance was due to:

1. Lack of abnormal cellular elements in the cytologic preparation, which might be a consequence of
   a. Cytologic sampling.
   b. Obtaining of the cytologic material preceding the manifestation of the lesion.
2. Presence of abnormal cells in the cytologic material, confirmed by a quality assurance review with no corresponding lesion in the tissues examined. The report should reflect whether the abnormal cells are from a low-grade lesion, particularly if a Pap smear with features of HPV that may have regressed.
   a. The abnormal cells, any grade, may have originated from an area not sampled in the tissue studies, and there is indication for further evaluation and tissue studies.
   b. Identification of abnormal cells, not previously reported, in the cytologic material upon quality assurance review. Comment should identify limiting factors, such as few cells, poor preservation, obscuring inflammation, and the like.

Tissue reports may include diagnostic and procedure codes.

Addenda Reports ▪ Addenda reports are not unusual and reflect additional information from special studies, consultants, and the like. The additional information is specific with regard to procedures, consultants, diagnoses, or important differential diagnoses for the patient.

Occasionally revised or corrected reports are required. Such reports must be clearly identified and state that prior reports should be superseded. It may be necessary to revise a diagnosis because of follow-up information obtained by a specialized study or as a consequence of expert consultation. Care must be taken that the distribution of the corrected report is made to all the physicians receiving the original report.

Surgical Pathology Reports

Biopsies ▪ Usually, these reports are short (Figure 30–4). They often consist of a brief gross description and microscopic diagnoses. The turnaround time for these reports is short. Often the microscopic diagnoses for biopsies are needed to determine and schedule further diagnostic studies or therapeutic measures for the patient. For this reason, it is common for physicians to seek the results of these studies the morning of the day following acquisition of the tissue for study. Biopsy results are telephoned to physicians in order to convey this important information promptly.

If possible, the diagnoses made from biopsied material should be correlated with the findings of subsequent surgical specimens.

Excisional biopsies are intended to remove lesions. The report will state whether the lesion is present in the margins of the tissue or whether the entire lesion appears removed. This is particularly important with small malignancies or lesions that may be precancerous.

Resections ▪ These are larger specimens and may be complex, multiple-part specimens. These cases often require a substantial gross description, including a key of tissues submitted for microscopic examination, the initiation and identification of special stains and other specialized studies, inclusion of frozen-section results, identification of photographs taken, and identification of retained tissues for possible further study.

In many of these cases, there may be preceding biopsy reports, the results of which should be correlated with the gross and microscopic findings of the resection specimen.

Adequacy of resection is of paramount importance. This is true for resection of a malignancy or with regard to viability of tissue at margins in the event of infarcted tissue. Reports must clearly state whether the margins are adequate.

Cytologic Reports

Nongynecologic ▪ These reports resemble tissue biopsy reports (Figure 30–4). They include a description of the material received. The material may consist of fluid or semisolid material, small fragments of apparent tissue, or previously prepared slides with smeared cellular material. The description is reported as a gross description. The comments should identify processing of material, such as centrifugation, preparation of smears, and filters. The number of preparations should be identified.

Such reports include a microscopic diagnosis.

```
                                    HOSPITAL                        PAGE 1
RUN ON




     PROFESSIONAL BILLING      <PTW
        88331
        88307

     GROSS DESCRIPTION     <PTW
        Right breast tissue received on ice, unfixed, for frozen section. The
        specimen consists of a single tissue. The tissue measures 2.0 x 2.8 x 5.5
        cm. The surfaces of the specimen consist of approximately 70% fat tissue
        and the remainder moderately firm pale tan to white tissue. Blue dye is
        applied to the periphery of the specimen. The specimen is sectioned. The
        tissue is 60% fat and 10% white stromal tissue and the remainder a firm to
        brawny pale tan tissue which is not well demarcated from adjacent breast
        tissue. Representative tissue is examined by frozen section. Carcinomatous
        tissue is prepared for estrogen and progesterone receptors, DNA ploidy and
        DNA synthesis phase fraction assays. The frozen section control tissue is
        submitted. 1 cassette. Representative tissue additionally submitted.   3
        cassettes.
        Frozen section diagnosis:
        -intraductal carcinoma, extensive, with areas of possible invasion. Focal
        areas of intraductal necrosis present. To be further evaluated by
        permanent sections.
        -margins of excision, gross evaluation: tumor present
        -(PTW)
           Dictated By: Paul T. Wertlake,M.D.

     MICROSCOPIC DIAGNOSIS    <PTW
        Breast, right, excisional biopsy:
        -Comedocarcinoma, with focal invasion of stroma
        -Extensive atypical lobular and ductal hyperplasia
        -Margins of excision: Carcinoma present
        -Breast carcinoma predicative assays: pending
           Dictated By: Paul T. Wertlake,M.D.

     SPECIMEN DESCRIPTION    <PTW
        Right breast lesion

     PATH PROCEDURES    <LAB/RD
        BREAST CA PROG  (1,1)
        HIST SEND OUT (1,1)
        SURGICAL BLOCK (4,4)
        SURG PATH CLERI (1,1)
```

Figure 30–4
Sample form for a pathology report on a biopsy specimen.

In certain instances, a microscopic description or comment section or both may be shown, stating unusual findings, limiting factors, and recommendations for further actions.

If special stains or other specialized procedures have been utilized in study of the case, they are identified. These reports may include diagnostic and procedure codes.

Gynecologic Studies

Papanicolaou (Pap) Smears ▪ In 1988, a National Cancer Institute–sponsored workshop developed a standardized system for reporting Pap smears.[1] This system replaces what was commonly known as the Pap class system, which is no longer recommended. The new system is based on narrative reporting of descriptive diagnoses and resembles the reporting of tissue studies. The common usage of pathologic terminology in tissue and Pap reports permits effective correlation studies. The standardized reporting of Pap smears by this method, known as The Bethesda System (TBS), makes possible more effective communication of clinically relevant cytologic findings (Table 30–1). A second workshop was held in 1991 to assess the use of TBS in actual practice, and several modifications were introduced. In addition, areas for continued investigation and development were identified.[2] The style and formatting of Pap smear reports utilizing The Bethesda System vary widely.

Bone Marrow Reports ▪ Generally, bone marrow request and report forms follow a format similar to that of tissue biopsy studies. A specialized request form for bone marrow studies is helpful and may include specific items of history, the presenting clinical problems, and certain requests for stains and chromosomal studies.

Bone marrow reports optimally segregate and describe microscopic observations with regard to sections of core biopsies, sections of clotted bone marrow aspirate, smears prepared from particulate material of bone marrow aspirates, special stains of sectioned material, and smears as well as analysis of a concurrent complete blood count (CBC) study, including a peripheral blood smear. These findings are integrated and correlated with the relevant clinical status of the patient. Based on this body of information, diagnoses are made and reported.

The report identifies special stains and other specialized studies that may have been performed.

These reports may include diagnostic and procedure codes.

Autopsy Reports ▪ Autopsy reports may vary considerably in style and will reflect the extent of the postmortem study, which may be limited by authorization to a single organ, such as the heart. In a forensic study, the autopsy may be very extensive in scope and documentation. In addition to tissue studies, a variety of studies may be made, such as cultures or analysis of fluids for toxic agents and drugs.

A death certificate signed by the managing physician should be available in a medical autopsy.

Many special circumstances apply to forensic autopsies. Reference should be made to forensic pathology literature for relevant information.

The autopsy report includes as a minimum the following elements:

- A statement as to authorization for the procedure that includes the person/agency granting legal authorization and the extent of examination authorized.

- The date of examination.

- The person(s) performing the examination.

- The managing and consulting physicians' names.

- A concise statement as to the relevant clinical status of the deceased and any circumstances known to be contributory to death.

- An accurate gross description of the body and all organs and cavities examined.

- A preliminary report upon completion of the gross examination.

- A list of all photographs taken and other studies conducted.

- A list of tissues examined microscopically, together with the number of tissue blocks prepared for each organ/tissue. It is advisable to include special stains performed.

- Diagnoses based on gross, microscopic, and other studies, as correlated with the clinical status.

- Optional: Microscopic description and comments.

Table 30–1 ▪ **The 1991 Bethesda System**

Adequacy of the Specimen
  Satisfactory for evaluation
  Satisfactory for evaluation but limited by . . . (specify reason)
  Unsatisfactory for evaluation . . . (specify reason)
General Categorization (Optional)
  Within normal limits
  Benign cellular changes: see descriptive diagnosis
  Epithelial cell abnormality: see descriptive diagnosis
Descriptive Diagnoses
  Benign cellular changes
    Infection
      Trichomonas vaginalis
      Fungal organisms morphologically consistent with *Candida* sp.
      Predominance of coccobacilli consistent with shift in vaginal flora
      Bacteria morphologically consistent with *Actinomyces* sp.
      Cellular changes associated with herpes simplex virus
      Other
    Reactive changes
    Reactive cellular changes associated with:
      Inflammation (includes typical repair)
      Atrophy with inflammation ("atrophic vaginitis")
      Radiation
      Intrauterine contraceptive device (IUD)
      Other
  Epithelial cell abnormalities
    Squamous cell
      Atypical squamous cells of undetermined significance: qualify*
      Low-grade squamous intraepithelial lesion encompassing HPV† mild dysplasia/CIN 1
      High-grade squamous intraepithelial lesion encompassing moderate and severe dysplasia, CIS/CIN 2, and CIN 3
      Squamous cell carcinoma
    Glandular cell
      Endometrial cells, cytologically benign, in a postmenopausal woman
      Atypical glandular cells of undetermined significance: qualify*
      Endocervical adenocarcinoma
      Endometrial adenocarcinoma
      Extrauterine adenocarcinoma
      Adenocarcinoma, not otherwise specified
  Other malignant neoplasms: specify
  Hormonal evaluation (applies to vaginal smears only)
    Hormonal pattern compatible with age and history
    Hormonal pattern incompatible with age and history: specify
    Hormonal evaluation not possible due to . . . (specify)

*Atypical squamous or glandular cells of undetermined significance should be further qualified as to whether a reactive or a premalignant/malignant process is favored.
†Cellular changes of human papillomavirus (HPV) (previously termed "koilocytosis," "koilocytotic atypia," or "condylomatous atypia") are included in the category of low-grade squamous intraepithelial lesion.
From Luff, R.D. The Bethesda System for reporting cervical/vaginal cytologic diagnoses: Report of the 1991 Bethesda Workshop. *Human Pathology* 23(7):719–721, 1992.

- Clinical-pathologic correlation.

- Signature of the pathologist(s) performing and making the final autopsy report.

Report Signatures ▪ All reports must be signed by the pathologist taking final responsibility for the case. Reports may be issued with electronic signature. This requires compliance with federal and state regulations as well as the policies of the hospital. The reports must be reviewed and released by the pathologist.

It is good practice to include identification of pathologists who provide consultative opinions for the case, whether internal or external to the department.

Codes in Reports ▪ Optionally, reports may include Systematized Nomenclature of Medicine (SNOMED) codes for pathologic diagnoses and Current Procedural Terminology (CPT) for billing codes.

The SNOMED optional coding is effective in retrieval and subsequent analysis of diagnostic material. This system is favored by pathologists, and reference material is available from the College of American Pathologists, 325 Waukegan Road, Northfield, Illinois 60093-2750.

Another coding system used for clinical diagnoses is the *International Classification of Diseases, Adapted, 9th edition, Clinical Modification* (ICD-9-CM), Volumes I, II, and III.[2] These codes are required for billing Medicare, Medicaid, CHAMPUS, and private insurance carriers. ICD-10-CM has been developed, and this may be implemented beginning in the year 2000. A color-coded edition is also available from St. Anthony's Hospital Publications.[3]

A procedural coding system developed by the American Medical Association for hospital outpatient and physician billing is found in a book entitled *Current Procedural Terminology* (CPT). Another publication produced quarterly is the *CPT Assistant*.[4] CPT codes are required for billing Medicare, Medicaid, CHAMPUS, and private insurance carriers. A summary of CPT pathology codes was published by the College of American Pathologists.[5]

Unique Physician Identifier Number ▪ Medicare assigns each physician a Unique Physician Identifier Number (UPIN). The ordering physician's UPIN must be included on the billing report submitted.

WORD PROCESSING AND COMPUTERIZED REPORTING

Proper application of word processing and computer-assisted reporting needs to be made according to the workload and financial and space resources of each medical facility. Affordable and effective computerized word processing is widely available and can be expected to provide significant benefits. Most software programs offer good flexibility and are rather easily learned. Through their wide use, many employees and prospective employees have word-processing skills.

With transcribed dictation, the use of word processing makes corrections a quick and easy task. The ability to make multiple printings is a distinct advantage. The ability to store short or long-term material electronically provides increased flexibility and assurance.

Many applications can be used. Some are as simple as pre-formatting repetitive material so it can be recalled with a few key strokes. In some instances, the majority of a report may be recalled and modified. More complex applications may be effected with more word-processing skills, such as formatting for completion of pre-printed forms (Figure 30–5).

Text-processing systems that are available on large computer systems are usually less flexible and more difficult to use. Nevertheless, effective reporting can be achieved with reasonable effort. These systems permit substantial pre-formatting of narrative material for recall by a few keystrokes. In addition, these systems permit substantial report retention (Figure 30–6).

For medical facilities with very large volumes, particularly of reports with the same formatting and high recurrence of certain findings, computerized reporting is essential to cost-effective and accurate documentation.

The ability to pre-format narrative comment offers three valuable advantages in pathology transcription:

1. Extensive comments that may include highly technical language and data in formats that are difficult and time-consuming to type, as well as material that is prone to error and difficult to proofread, e.g., tables and literature references.

DNA INDEX AND CELL CYCLE ANALYSIS REPORT

METHODOLOGY: Computerized image analysis of tissue sections.

STUDY MATERIALS: Results represent analysis of tissue
sections prepared from:
        Case identification No.:
        Tissue block identification:

RESULTS:

DNA INDEX (DI)	1.0
PROLIFERATION INDEX	23.5%
DEGREE OF HYPERPLOIDY	0.0%

INTERPRETATIVE COMMENT:

These results indicate that the tumor cell population
analyzed in this tissue section is diploid with a high
proliferation index and no hyperploidy peaks.

                         _____M.D.
                         Pathologist

The DNA Index (DI) is the ratio of the average amount of DNA
in a given cell population to DNA content in normal diploid
cells. A DNA Index of 1.0 ± 0.1 indicates a diploid
population. Aneuploidy is indicated by a DNA Index which is
either < 0.9 or greater than > 1.1. A tetraploid population
is indicated by a DNA Index of 2.0 ± 0.1 and corresponds to
a normal population in mitosis (G2M).

REFERENCES:
1. Wied GL et al: Image Analysis in Quantitative
     Cytopathology and histopathology. Human Pathol 1989,
     20: 549-571.

2. Merkel DE, McGuire WL: Ploidy, Proliferative Activity and
     Prognosis. DNA Flow Cytometry of Solid Tumors. Cancer
     1990, 65: 1194-1205.

The results of this test are for research / investigational
use only and should be evaluated in conjunction with
information available from other medically established
procedures.

Histograms: forwarded under separate cover.

Figure 30–5

Example of a pathology report using a complex computer software application to format completion of a preprinted form.

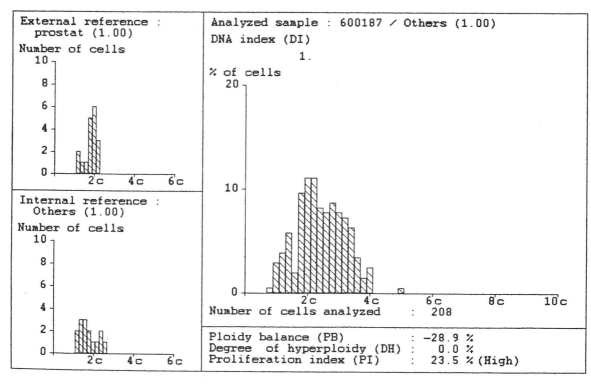

MetWest Tarzana
Att: Pathology Dept.
18488 Oxnard Street
Tarzana, CA 91356

ACCESSION NOS: 92-PLO-129
                       600187

                    PLOIDY ANALYSIS

Date   : 08/04/92
Slide reference   : 600187
Sample received on : 08/03/92
Organ   : prostate
Preparation   : fine needle biopsy
Stain   : feulgen

External reference :
  prostat (1.00)
Number of cells
10
8
6
4
2
0
      2c   4c   6c

Internal reference :
  Others (1.00)
Number of cells
10
8
6
4
2
0
      2c   4c   6c

Analyzed sample : 600187 / Others (1.00)
DNA index (DI)
                1.
% of cells
20

10

0
          2c   4c   6c   8c   10c
Number of cells analyzed   : 208

Ploidy balance (PB)   : -28.9 %
Degree of hyperploidy (DH) :   0.0 %
Proliferation index (PI)   : 23.5 % (High)

Comments

These results indicate that the tumor cell population analyzed is diploid DI=1
with a high proliferation index PI=23.5 (PI correlates with S-phase of the cell
cycle) and no hyperploid peaks.

Figure 30-6
A ploidy analysis showing the computer printout of substantial preformatted material recalled by a few keystrokes. (Reprinted with permission of MetWest Clinical Laboratories, Tarzana, California.)

2. Standardization of language as used by multiple persons, making reports uniform in content, thus less likely to be misunderstood by physicians receiving reports.

3. Coded and pre-formatted narrative may be electronically stored and available for incorporation into quality assurance systems without recourse to redundant data entry.

QUALITY ASSURANCE REPORTS

Correlations, Cytology and Tissue Reports ▪ Content of cytology and tissue correlations was described previously on page 556. In preparing quality assurance reports, the data are systematically analyzed for the laboratory as a whole and by individual cytotechnologists and pathologists, deficiencies and trends are identified, and corrections made. Ongoing monitoring is required with documentation.

Correlations, Frozen Sections and Final Reports ▪ Reports include final microscopic diagnoses as well as frozen-section diagnoses. Ongoing monitoring of these correlations is required. Each case must be categorized as concordant or discordant. Discordant results must be further categorized as to whether the frozen section was not representative of the lesion due to a sampling variance, or whether the permanent sections did not represent the lesion although it was present in the frozen section and confirmed by a quality assurance review. This may occur because a lesion is small, the tissue obtained represented only a small part of the lesion, lesional tissue was submitted for studies other than paraffin section, and so forth. Misinterpretation of the frozen or paraffin section material must be considered. The systematic review must be formally documented.

Correlations, Biopsy and Resection Reports ▪ These correlations are similar to those described in the two aforementioned correlations. Discordant results must be analyzed to determine the basis for variance. The review process must be ongoing and documented.

Correlations, Primary Report and Consultative Reports ▪ The original reports must be correlated with the diagnostic findings and recommendations of consultant reports (Figure 30–7). Analysis for significant disparities must be made. Review of materials and other corrective actions may be required. This must be ongoing and documented.

Problems and Corrective Action Logs ▪ Problems may be identified in many different ways. Some can be identified and responded to through the previously described quality assurance programs. Problems may be identified by physicians or other staff members, including members of the nursing staff. These problems and the corrective action measures must be documented.

Periodic review of problems and corrective actions must be effected. This is done to assess the adequacy of corrective actions and identify trends. Reviews must be documented.

ADMINISTRATIVE REPORTS AND RECORDS

Administrative functions and record keeping for the anatomic pathology department are as essential as the generation of patient reports. In fact, these elements as well as quality assurance activities are integral to a department's ability to serve its physician-clients and patients properly. Achieving quality work requires effectiveness in all these areas.

This includes the general work of the department, such as file maintenance of patient reports, accurate maintenance of various logs (e.g., cases requested for review by others, cases referred for consultation, cases out of the file for quality assurance reviews), management of slides, maintenance of telephone records reporting diagnoses, logging and sequestering medicolegal sensitive case materials, preparing and maintaining minutes of all departmental meetings (administrative, quality assurance, safety), communication and coordination with the facility's Quality Assurance/Continuing Quality Improvement program.

The accomplishment of these very substantial tasks requires excellent organization and support combined with close collaboration of the secretarial staff and pathologists.

```
LABORATORY REPORT                              MetWest         18408 Oxnard Street • Tarzana, CA 91356
METWEST-TARZANA-MAIN          001.099          Clinical        (818) 996-7300
18408 OXNARD STREET           09581            Laboratories    Calif. (800) 339-4299
TARZANA, CA  91356                                                          Director and Pathologist
                                                                            Paul T. Wertlake, M.D.


                                        DATE COLLECTED      PANEL(S)
                                          02/19/93

PATIENT                    AGE SEX  PATIENT I.D.    PHYSICIAN         RECEIVED   REPORTED   SPEC. NO.
SAMPLER,SUSIE               31  F  ANY ID          ANY DOCTOR        02/19    02/19/93   K888884
                              WITHIN RANGE        OUT OF RANGE
         REQUESTS              RESULTS              RESULTS       REFERENCE RANGE      UNITS
```

                    C Y T O P A T H O L O G Y   R E P O R T
****

GENERAL CATEGORIZATION
                                          ABNORMAL

     EPITHELIAL CELL ABNORMALITY.
     CLINICAL CORRELATION REQUIRED.
     SEE DESCRIPTIVE DIAGNOSIS BELOW.

****

SPECIMEN ADEQUACY
     SPECIMEN IS SATISFACTORY FOR INTERPRETATION
     ENDOCERVICAL COMPONENT PRESENT

DESCRIPTIVE DIAGNOSIS
     LOW-GRADE SIL (SQUAMOUS INTRAEPITHELIAL LESION) WITH
     HPV CYTOPATHIC CHANGES

MICRO-ORGANISMS/INFECTION
     BACTERIAL FLORA: MIXED COCCOID AND BACILLARY
     MODERATE ERYTHROCYTES PRESENT
     MODERATE NUMBER OF POLYS PRESENT

HORMONAL EVALUATION
     MODERATE MATURATION
     HORMONAL PATTERN IS COMPATIBLE WITH AGE AND HISTORY

SPECULOSCOPY
     SPECULOSCOPY FINDINGS: POSITIVE
          ACETO-WHITENING PRESENT: CIRCUMFERENTIAL ABOUT CERVICAL OS

RECOMMENDATIONS/COMMENTS
     RECOMMEND COLPOSCOPIC GUIDED TISSUE EVALUATION INCLUDING ENDOCERVICAL
     CURRETTING

PATIENT HISTORY
     SPECIMEN: 1 SLIDE
     SOURCE: VAGINA,CERVIX,ENDOCX
     LMP   :   2/18/93   PREGNANT: NO
     PREVIOUS ABNORMAL: K777777

                                              PAUL T. WERTLAKE, M.D.
EMELYN BENNETT, CT(ASCP)   SIGNATURE ON FILE

     PAGE 1: END OF REPORT FOR : K888884

                                              FORMS-FREE W/O CHEM (REV 11/92) 80219

Figure 30–7
A sample of cytopathology consultative report. (Reprinted with permission from MetWest Clinical Laboratories, Tarzana, California.)

570

POSITION DESCRIPTION OF A PATHOLOGY SECRETARY

The following is an example of what some of the job duties might encompass for a person working as a pathology secretary.

Qualifications

1. Must have effective basic comprehension regarding medical conditions. Must have effective pathology knowledge, such as anatomic pathology, relevant clinical diagnoses, symptoms and abnormalities, particularly as applicable to anatomic pathology. These skills must be sufficient to permit telephone communication with physicians and other medical care workers.

2. Must have good communication skills. These skills must extend to effectiveness in stressed communications with external and internal clients. Must communicate effectively with persons concerned with laboratory inspections and licensing and legal interests, vendors, and financial persons regarding budget planning and management. Must effectively network with internal staff members of the facility regarding the conduct of interrelated functions, issues resolution, and future planning.

3. Must have ability to maintain organization of files, both for a conventional filing system as well as within a computer system.

4. Must have good organizational skills in maintaining a department calendar that includes key personnel, key activities, training and education, and vacation. This includes monitoring of follow-through actions for responsible personnel.

5. Must have good typing (keyboarding), transcribing, and composing skills in order to communicate messages and announcements, prepare letters and bulletins, and produce reports.

6. Must be able to take and transcribe minutes of meetings.

7. Must have basic skills in use of a personal computer. This includes knowledge of word processing and spread sheet software computer programs. Must have attentiveness and commitment to perform accurate data entry of medically important information.

8. Desirable to have knowledge and experience in quality assurance and total quality management, particularly with regard to an organizational system with ongoing monitoring, setting of standards, resolution of variances, and education of personnel to system use.

9. Desirable to have business orientation to assist budget monitoring, determination of unit costs, measurement of productivity, and analysis of variances.

10. Desirable to have ability to conceptualize and effect measures and displays of key indicators for departmental performance, e.g., turnaround time for reporting, error rates, and the like.

11. Must have ability to train personnel and monitor ongoing performance for compliance with performance standards.

12. Must be able to supervise effectively reporting staff personnel, including work performance, assignment of work, development of personnel skills, counseling as required, and formal periodic evaluations.

Duties and Responsibilities ■ The pathology secretary reports to the chief pathologist of the department or pathology facility and is in liaison with the following:

Administration and management staff of medical facility
Pathologists
Supervisory staff, all departments
Laboratory personnel, all departments
Purchasing staff
Warehouse staff
Quality Control/Assurance/Safety manager
Billing/accounting personnel
Off-site personnel, satellite facilities, affiliated facilities
Security personnel
External persons as required

The pathology secretary supports the chief pathologist in the following:

A. Maintains calendar, communications, files, and records and monitors activities and programs, including continuous quality improvement.

B. Performs data entry functions for quality assurance programs of the department.

C. Accepts calls from physicians or their supporting staff, particularly if the chief pathologist is not immediately available. Directs calls for immediate response if possible or, if necessary, obtains pertinent information to facilitate follow-up response by obtaining the following information:

- Physician's name or contact person
- Patient's name
- Specimen number and client number
- Specific interest or question

Routes calls to the appropriate person for prompt response, including supportive information that is available.

D. Makes entries of quality/service issues to Quality Assurance Log system

E. Maintains legal, literature, and correspondence files.

F. Maintains licenses and inspection records.

G. Maintains coordinated calendar for pathologists' vacations and educational absences.

H. Prepares measure and display graphics.

I. Monitors monthly supervisor reports for timely completion.

J. Monitors quality assurance activities, including documentation of timely corrective actions.

K. Monitors department budget(s) and assists in preparation of new department budgets.

L. Recommends system enhancements, including equipment, software, and procedural changes.

M. Prepares clinical bulletins, letters, memos, announcements.

N. Schedules meetings, with provision of notification, and prepares and distributes meeting agendas.

O. Takes, transcribes, and distributes minutes.

P. Other duties as required.

Additional Job Information

Salary ▪ Position is an exempt (salaried) position. Salary is commensurate with professional qualifications and experience.

Hours ▪ Usually Monday through Friday, 9:00 A.M. to 6:00 P.M. Special projects or situations can be anticipated to require attendance at other times, more often later than 6 P.M. On occasion, some weekend duty may be required. Duties may require attendance and support at meetings or functions of importance to the department and/or the medical facility, on- or off-site. Attendant expenses will be paid by the medical facility.

Continuing Education ▪ Approved training and continuing education will be provided, with attendance expenses paid by the medical facility.

Benefits ▪ Those that are standard for the medical facility.

Reference Sources

1. Luff, R. D. The Bethesda system for reporting cervical/vaginal cytologic diagnoses: Report of the 1991 Bethesda Workshop. *Human Pathology* 23(7):719–721, 1992.
2. *International Classification of Diseases, Adapted, 9th edition, Clinical Modification* (ICD-9-CM), P. O. Box 991, Ann Arbor, Michigan 48106-0991.
3. St. Anthony's Hospital Publications, P. O. Box 14212, Washington, D. C. 20044.
4. American Medical Association, 515 North State Street, 11th Floor, Chicago, Illinois 60610-4377.
5. *Relative Value Schedule (RVS) Final Rule.* The College of American Pathologists, 325 Waukegan Road, Northfield, Illinois 60093-2750, November 1991.

For references of specific application to medical transcription, see Appendix 1.

Pediatrics

INTRODUCTION

Pediatrics is the medical discipline concerned with the growth, development, adaptation and function of infants, children, adolescents, and youth from birth through 21 years of age. Pediatricians have a major interest in disease prevention and health promotion, as well as in the diagnosis and management of biomedical and psychosocial disease and illness. Each of the principal pediatric age groups — newborn, infancy, early childhood, middle childhood and adolescence — is characterized by differences in anatomy, cognition, physiology, biochemistry, immunology, and emotional and social development.

NEONATOLOGY

Neonatology is the subspecialty concerned with the care of newborn infants, especially those who are premature, small for gestational age, or sick. The disorders discussed in this section exemplify the symptoms and disease states frequently encountered by the neonatologist.

Respiratory Distress ▪ Asphyxiation of the neonate should be evaluated at birth by the Apgar score (Table 31–1), measured at 1 and 5 minutes. A score of 0 to 3 implies severe distress and is an indication for immediate resuscitation. Apgar scores of 4 to 7 indicate moderate distress. With a score of 7 to 10, continued observation is all that is required.

The signs of respiratory distress in the newborn infant include rapid respiratory rate, cyanosis, grunting, retractions, and nasal flaring. Tachypnea, or rapid respiration, in the neonate is defined as a respiratory rate of over 60 breaths per minute.

Common nonsurgical causes of neonatal respiratory distress include hyaline membrane disease, meconium aspiration, transient tachypnea of the newborn, pneumonia, and persistent pulmonary hypertension.

Idiopathic respiratory distress syndrome, or hyaline membrane disease, occurs in premature infants because of the surfactant deficiency associated with lung immaturity. In this disorder, signs of respiratory distress occur within minutes or hours after birth. Findings include expiratory grunting, nasal flaring, retractions in the intercostal and subcostal spaces, and cyanosis. The chest x-ray film demonstrates a characteristic fine, reticular granular pattern diffusely present in both lungs. Determination of arterial blood gases shows hypoxemia, accompanied at times by acidemia.

Treatment of the respiratory distress syndrome includes provision of adequate oxygenation. This may require mechanical ventilation. A neutral thermal environment and intravenous glucose administration are other supportive therapeutic measures employed. The advent of exogenous surfactant treatment, which causes an immediate improvement in lung function, has resulted in lower mortality in this disorder.

Transient tachypnea of the newborn is caused by a delay in the resorption of normal lung fluid. Symptoms, which begin within hours after birth, include rapid respiratory rate, grunting, nasal flaring, and soft tissue retractions. The chest roentgenogram is diagnostically helpful but not specific. Symptoms last for 24 to 48 hours. Supplemental oxygen and other supportive measures are indicated.

Table 31–1 ▪ **APGAR Score**

Sign	0	1	2
Heart rate	Absent	Slow (below 100)	Over 100
Respiratory effort	Absent	Slow, irregular	Good, crying
Muscle tone	Flaccid	Some flexion of extremities	Active motion
Reflex irritability	No response	Grimace	Vigorous cry
Color	Blue, pale	Body pink, extremities blue	Completely pink

The *meconium aspiration syndrome* may occur as a complication of meconium staining of the amniotic fluid. The respiratory rate is rapid, and hypoxia may be marked. Prevention of meconium aspiration by immediate suctioning of the nose, mouth, and oropharynx before delivery of the chest is an important intervention.

Persistent pulmonary hypertension, or persistent fetal circulation, and neonatal pneumonia, perhaps accompanied by sepsis, are other causes of respiratory distress in the newborn infant.

Bronchopulmonary dysplasia is a poorly understood, chronic pulmonary disorder that has its onset in the first month of life, especially in infants exposed to such lung injury factors as oxygen therapy, positive pressure ventilation, and respiratory infections. Clinical manifestations include a rapid respiratory rate, respiratory distress, abnormal gas exchange, and a characteristic chest x-ray film. Therapy includes the use of bronchodilator agents, corticosteroid therapy, and nutritional support.

Neonatal Sepsis ▪ The clinical indicators of sepsis in the newborn are often subtle and nonspecific. They include poor feeding, jaundice, apnea, respiratory distress, abdominal distention, lethargy, seizures, fever, hypothermia, and petechiae. Laboratory evaluation of an infant suspected to have sepsis includes blood cultures, analysis of cerebrospinal fluid, urine culture, complete blood count, and chest x-ray film.

The pathogens that cause neonatal sepsis include group B beta-streptococcus, *Escherichia coli*, *Listeria monocytogenes*, and group D streptococcus, among others. Treatment involves the use of the appropriate antibiotic.

Congenital Heart Disease ▪ Cyanotic heart disease in the newborn infant may be caused by several congenital anomalies. Transposition of the great vessels is the most frequent cause. Severe cyanosis is usually present within 2 to 3 days after birth.

Hypoplastic left heart syndrome causes cyanosis and congestive failure in the first 24 to 48 hours of life.

Persistent pulmonary hypertension of the newborn (persistent fetal circulation syndrome), owing to continuing postnatal pulmonary hypertension, is characterized by abnormal right-to-left shunting through a patent foramen ovale or patent ductus arteriosus. The infant, usually term or near-term, may appear normal at birth but then develops cyanosis accompanied by tachypnea and acidemia in the first 24 hours of life.

Tetralogy of Fallot consists of pulmonary stenosis or atresia, a ventricular septal defect, a dextroposed aorta that overrides the septal defect, and right ventricular hypertrophy. Although cyanosis is present at birth in about one third of these patients, in most instances it does not appear or become persistent until the child begins to walk or run.

Ventricular septal defect is the most common acyanotic congenital health malformation in children. Small defects are usually detected in infancy on auscultation of the chest whereas larger defects may present with symptoms of congestive heart failure. Atrial septal defects, either isolated or accompanied by other anomalies, are another of the more common congenital heart defects. Patent ductus arteriosus is most commonly noted on physical examination when a continuous murmur is heard. Coarctation of the aorta may be asymptomatic except for causing hypertension or may be a cause of cardiac failure in infants. Pulmonary stenosis is another relatively frequent cardiac anomaly (Figure 31–1).

Diagnostic measures useful in the evaluation of acyanotic congenital cardiac defects include electrocardiography, echocardiography, and cardiac catheterization (Figure 31–2).

Surgical Disorders in Neonates ▪ *Pneumothorax* is a frequent cause for respiratory distress in the newborn infant, occurring in 0.5 to 2 per

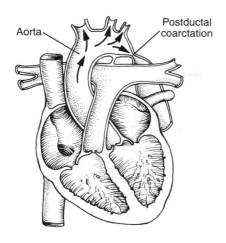

COARCTATION OF THE AORTA

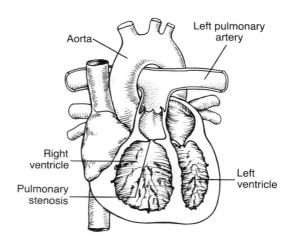

PULMONARY STENOSIS

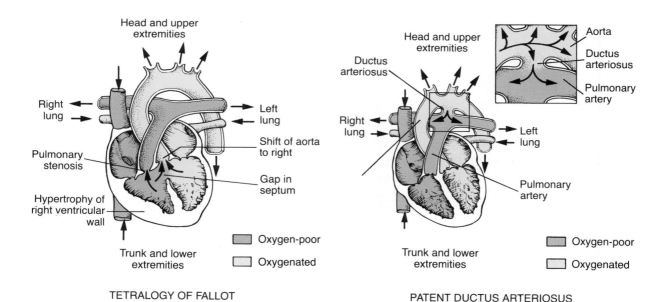

TETRALOGY OF FALLOT

PATENT DUCTUS ARTERIOSUS

Figure 31–1
Congenital heart defects.

cent. The diagnosis may be suggested by transillumination and established by a chest roentgenogram. Treatment includes oxygen administration for mild distress, needle aspiration of the pneumothorax, or chest tube placement.

Esophageal atresia and tracheoesophageal fistula may be suspected because of excessive drooling and salivation in the newborn infant and confirmed by the physician's inability to pass an orogastric tube. The management is surgical.

Necrotizing enterocolitis is characterized by abdominal distention, poor feeding, bilious vomiting, respiratory distress, jaundice, diarrhea, apnea, lethargy, hypothermia, and blood in the stools. The infant appears septic and in shock.

THE WILSON HOSPITAL
843 Barnaby Road
Indianapolis, IN 46202-5225

CARDIAC CATHETERIZATION PROCEDURE NOTE

RE: FORMAN, Janice
DOB: 2-1-94
MR #: 6490876
CATH #: 47932
CATH DATE: 2-4-94
WEIGHT: 2.7 kg.

OPERATORS: James Jackson, M.D.
                     Charles Kroger, M.D.

PROCEDURE: Right and left cardiac catheterization.

PRECATH DIAGNOSIS:
1.   Moderate left ventricular and mitral valve hypoplasia.
2.   Ventricular septal defects.
3.   Patent ductus arteriosus on PGE1.
4.   Coarctation of the aorta.
5.   Moderate right atrial enlargement.
6.   Moderate right ventricular hypertrophy and dilatation.
7.   Intact atrial septum.

POSTCATH DIAGNOSIS: As above plus good sized aortic annulus and ascending aorta; very hypoplastic aortic arch from the origin of the right innominate artery to the isthmus; coarctation (1.5-2.9 mm in diameter). Ventricular septal defects, at least one muscular and one membranous, both moderate-sized. Aortic saturation 89 to 95% on 80 to 100% FIO2.

CATH MEDICATIONS: PGE1 I.V. drip, heparin 200 cc. I.V.
SEDATION: Morphine sulfate.
CONTRAST: 24.5 cc.
ESTIMATED BLOOD LOSS: 14 cc.; no transfusion
COMPLICATIONS: None. Transient supraventricular tachycardia resolved with catheter manipulation.

(continued)

Figure 31–2
A cardiac catheterization procedure note on a 3-day-old infant.

INTRODUCTION:

Janice Forman is a 3-day-old white female who was born by normal spontaneous vaginal delivery at 37 weeks' gestational age. Mother had three ultrasound examinations during pregnancy, one at 22 weeks' gestational age which was reported as normal; a second one a week prior to delivery with a diagnosis of oligohydramnios and a third one a day prior to delivery. No cardiac lesion was suspected. The infant was born with poor tone and required bag and mask ventilation. Apgars were 5 at one minute and 8 at five minutes. The patient was taken to the special care nursery for observation. A cardiology consult was obtained at 12 hours of age when the first arterial blood gases from the left radial artery showed a pH of 7.32, pCO_2 47, and pO_2 43 on 24% FIO2. A repeat ABG on 100% FIO2 showed pO_2 of 64. On 30% O_2 via hood, saturation was 98%.

On examination, she had some dysmorphic features. There were bilateral neck folds, bilateral dislocated hips and bilateral dislocated knees. Chest examination revealed a quiet precordium, normal S1 and S2. There was a grade 1-2/6 high-pitched systolic murmur heard best at the left lower sternal border. There was symmetrical chest movement. No gallop or click was heard. Lungs were clear to auscultation. Abdomen was soft with no hepatosplenomegaly. There were palpable femoral pulses. The blood pressure in four extremities showed systolic blood pressure 30-40 mm Hg higher in the upper extremities than the lower extremities. Chest x-ray showed pulmonary vascular congestion. Heart size was normal. An echocardiogram was performed which showed a large right ventricle and large atrium with a relatively small left ventricle, at least one muscular and one membranous ventricular septal defect, bidirectional patent ductus arteriosus, coarctation of the aorta from the origin of the right innominate artery ending in a coarctation. At this point, the patient was started on prostaglandin E1 and after half an hour, because the CO_2 was climbing up, the patient was intubated. The catheterization was performed to delineate her anatomy and hemodynamics in preparation for surgery.

DESCRIPTION OF PROCEDURE:

The baby was taken to the cardiac catheterization laboratory on full respiratory support. The areas over the right and left groins were prepped and draped in the usual sterile manner. Local anesthesia was accomplished with 1% xylocaine in the right groin. The left femoral vein was accessed percutaneously and a #5F sheath was placed into the vessel. Through this sheath, a #5F Berman catheter was advanced to the inferior vena cava, right atrium, superior vena cava, and back to the right atrium and right ventricle where pressures and saturations were recorded. At this time, the first angiogram was performed in the right ventricle. Then, the catheter was maneuvered from the right ventricle to the main pulmonary artery and passed through the ductus arteriosus to the descending aorta where the second angiogram was

(continued)

Figure 31–2 Continued   *Figure continued*

FORMAN, Janice   Page three
MR #: 6490876

performed in the descending aorta with balloon occlusion. The umbilical artery catheter was
exchanged for a #5F sheath and then a #4F high flow pigtail catheter was advanced
retrograde from the descending aorta toward the isthmus but could not pass beyond the
isthmus. A third angiogram was performed at the level of the isthmus. During the
procedure, the baby had transient supraventricular tachycardia and it resolved by pulling back
the catheter with catheter manipulation. The saturations were 89 to 95% on 80 to 100%
FIO2.

FINDINGS:
1. BLOOD GAS DATA: ABG on 100% FIO2: pH 7.35, pCO$_2$ 36, pO$_2$ 72, when sitting,
PIP 22, PEEP 3, IMV 15.
2. SATURATIONS (in %): SVC 74, RA 76, RV 86-89, descending aorta 95.
3. PRESSURES: (in mmHg): Right atrium A=9, V=7, Mean=6. Right ventricle 78/7.
Ascending aorta 78/42, mean 55. Descending aorta 78/42, mean 55.
4. ANGIOGRAPHY: Three angiograms were performed, one in the right ventricle, the
second one in the descending aorta with balloon occlusion and the third angiogram was
performed via retrograde arterial catheter at the level of the isthmus. The findings were a
dilated right ventricle, right atrium, large patent ductus arteriosus, no atrial septal defect,
moderate left ventricle and mitral valve hypoplasia, good sized aortic annulus and ascending
aorta, very hypoplastic aortic arch from the origin of the right innominate artery to the
isthmus which measured 1.5-2.0 mm in diameter.

IMPRESSION:
1. Moderate left ventricle and mitral valve hypoplasia.
2. Good sized aortic annulus and ascending aorta; very hypoplastic aortic arch from the
origin of the right innominate artery to the isthmus.
3. Ventricular septal defects, at least one muscular and one membranous, both moderate-
sized.
4. Dilated right atrium, right ventricle, large patent ductus on PGE1, no atrial septal defect.
5. Aortic saturation 89 to 95% on 80 to 100% FIO2.

---------------------------------   ---------------------------------
          James Jackson, M.D.   Charles Kroger, M.D.

JJ:ssb
D: 2/04/94
R: 2/11/94 - 2/24/94
T: 2/12/94 - 2/25/94

Figure 31–2 Continued

X-ray studies reveal free peritoneal air, pneumatosis intestinalis, or hepatic portal venous gas. Necrotizing enterocolitis occurs most frequently in premature infants on the third to fifth day of life, especially in those who have experienced perinatal stress, but it may also occur in the term infant. Signs of peritonitis — resistance to palpation, induration, discoloration and edema of the abdominal wall — may be present.

Gastrointestinal Obstruction ▪ The signs of gastrointestinal obstruction in the newborn infant include bile-stained vomitus, abdominal distention, failure to pass meconium, and maternal polyhydramnios. Obstruction may be complete due to atresia or partial caused by intestinal stenosis. Volvulus associated with malrotation of the intestine is a surgical emergency. Colonic obstruction may be caused by the meconium plug syndrome, Hirschsprung's disease, and imperforate anus.

Abdominal Wall Defects ▪ *Omphalocele*, a defect of the umbilical ring usually more than 4 cm. in circumference, is covered by both peritoneum and amnion and contains eviscerated organs, such as the liver and the intestines.

Gastroschisis is a paraumbilical, full-thickness abdominal wall defect, usually a few centimeters in diameter, to the right of the umbilicus and between the rectus muscles, with evisceration of the bowel through the defect. The stomach, urinary bladder, uterus, and adnexa may also be extruded as an adherent, dark purple mass covered by a thick, gelatinous or fibrinous material.

REPRESENTATIVE DISEASES

The following discussions are synopses of selected medical and surgical pediatric disorders, with notes on their signs and symptoms, diagnosis, and treatment.

Jaundice ▪ Jaundice, or icterus, refers to a yellowish discoloration of the sclera, mucous membranes, and skin owing to an excess of bilirubin in the blood. Jaundice is evident in most newborn infants with a serum bilirubin concentration of 5 to 7 mg./dL. In older children, jaundice appears when the serum bilirubin level reaches about 2 mg./dL.

The appearance of jaundice in the first 24 to 48 hours of life or intense icterus at any time in the neonatal period raises the possibility of hemolytic disease of the newborn owing to maternal/infant blood group incompatibility. Such incompatibilities include those due to A, B, O, Rh, and other blood groups.

Physiologic jaundice of the newborn appears commonly in newborn infants between the second and fifth days of life. Jaundice in the first 24 hours in the term infant or the first 48 hours in the premature baby is not physiologic and requires investigation. The serum bilirubin level in full-term infants with physiologic jaundice generally is less than 7 mg./dL. and rarely exceeds 10 mg./dL. Physiologic jaundice usually disappears by the fifth to eighth day, except in the premature, in whom it may persist into the second week of life.

Neonatal jaundice associated with breast-feeding may appear between the sixth and eighth days of life.

Viral *hepatitis* or hepatitis A in older children may demonstrate such prodromal symptoms as anorexia, fatigue, headache, nausea, vomiting, fever, enlargement of the liver, and right upper quadrant pain. Depending upon the level of severity, jaundice may or may not be present. Hepatitis B is transmitted through the infusion of blood contaminated with the virus. Newborn infants may become infected from their mothers.

Atresia of the extrahepatic bile ducts is one of the causes of obstructive jaundice in the newborn infant. The diagnosis usually is not suspected until the infant is about 3 weeks of age.

Neonatal hepatitis and neonatal jaundice with giant cell transformation of the hepatic parenchyma are terms applied to a clinical and histologic pattern associated with obstructive jaundice in the newborn. Jaundice begins in the early weeks of life and, along with dark urine and acholic or white stools, may persist for months.

Hemorrhage and Purpura ▪ Hemorrhage may have local causes, such as Meckel's diverticulum, or be caused by systemic disorders, such as thrombocytopenic purpura. In most instances, the cause can be identified readily through the history, the physical examination, and selected laboratory procedures. The two chief processes involved in the pathogenesis of hemorrhagic disorders are an increase in capillary fragility (vascular factors) and a defect in the blood-clotting mechanism (intravascular factors).

Purpura refers to hemorrhage into the skin or

mucous membranes. Pinpoint- or pinhead-sized, scarlet or bluish purple extravasations of blood are referred to as petechiae. Larger areas are usually termed ecchymoses.

Hemorrhage and purpura may be caused by either vascular or intravascular factors. Allergic, anaphylactoid or Henoch-Schönlein purpura may be characterized by a distinctive rash with purpura; severe, cramping abdominal pain; painful, hot, swollen joints; localized edema; and, possibly, melena, epistaxis, hematemesis, or hematuria.

Intravascular factors or defects in the blood-clotting mechanism include a quantitative deficiency of platelets (thrombocytopenia) or qualitative platelet disorders, inherited deficiencies of coagulation factors, and acquired clotting factor deficiencies.

Thrombocytopenia may be idiopathic, a diagnosis made by exclusion of other specific etiologies, or secondary to infections, leukemia, and multiple other disorders.

The inherited deficiencies of coagulation factors include a deficiency of antihemophilic globulin (factor VIII), the cause of hemophilia A, and deficiency of factor IX, the cause of hemophilia B, or Christmas disease.

Acquired clotting factor deficiencies include disseminated intravascular coagulation, or consumptive coagulopathy, characterized by the intravascular consumption of factors I, II, V, VIII, and platelets; deposition of fibrin thrombi within the vascular system; and a generalized hemorrhagic state.

Hemorrhage or purpura in the newborn infant may have several causes. Hemorrhagic disease of the newborn occurs on the second or third day of life owing to transient deficiencies of vitamin K–dependent clotting factors or congenital deficiency of clotting factors. Neonatal thrombocytopenic purpura may be immune-mediated and associated with fetal-maternal platelet antigen incompatibility or maternal idiopathic thrombocytopenia. Intrauterine infections and sepsis are other causes of neonatal thrombocytopenia.

Laboratory tests that may be used in the diagnosis of hemorrhagic states include the clotting time, the bleeding time, white and red blood cell counts, hemoglobin, hematocrit, platelet count, peripheral smear, prothrombin time, partial thromboplastin time, and fibrinogen level. In some cases, examination of the bone marrow may be indicated.

Cystic Fibrosis ▪ Cystic fibrosis is a genetically transmitted disease that affects many body systems, especially the gastrointestinal and respiratory tracts. The diagnosis is made usually by the first year of age. The gastrointestinal symptomatology includes meconium ileus, a cause of intestinal obstruction in the newborn infant, malabsorption with resultant failure to thrive, and steatorrhea. The diagnosis is also suggested by a persistent cough and recurrent pneumonia, most frequently caused by *Staphylococcus aureus*, *Haemophilus influenzae*, and *Pseudomonas aeruginosa*.

In patients with a history of chronic lung disease or pancreatic insufficiency, the diagnosis is established by the finding of a sweat chloride level greater than 60 mEq./L.

Therapeutic management includes nutritional supplements. The formula prescribed for infants with steatorrhea contains partially hydrolyzed protein and medium-chain triglycerides. In addition to multivitamins, the diet is supplemented with a pancreatic enzyme preparation to obtain more normal stools.

Pulmonary therapy includes chest percussion and postural drainage. Bronchodilators and aerosolized antibiotics may be used selectively. The lung complications of bronchitis and pneumonia are aggressively treated with appropriate antibiotics. Continuity of care with regular evaluations is essential.

Asthma ▪ Asthma, or reactive airway disease, is characterized by recurrent episodes of wheezing, cough, and dyspnea, and an increase in sputum production. The pathophysiology consists of bronchoconstriction, hypersecretion of thick mucus, and mucosal edema. In addition to the history, the physical examination, principally auscultation, and a chest roentgenogram, pulmonary function testing in children old enough to cooperate is an important part of the initial diagnosis and continuing assessment. The chest x-ray film may show air trapping, atelectasis, and increased perihilar bronchovascular markings. During episodes of asthma, arterial blood gas measurement is useful in evaluation of the patient's status.

Since asthma is a chronic disease, a long-term management plan is essential. Allergens known or suspected of triggering episodes of asthma, including cigarette smoking by adults in the household, should be avoided whenever possible. Drug therapy includes the use of beta-agonists such as albuterol by aerosol inhalation, cromolyn, theophylline, and steroids. Children with asthma are encouraged to live normal lives, including participation in sports.

Apnea ▪ Apnea, or transient cessation of respiration, occurs commonly in normal preterm and full-term infants. However, older infants may experience apneic episodes that constitute an apparent life-threatening event (ALTE). These spells are characterized by cessation of breathing, cyanosis or other skin color change, limpness, and choking or gagging.

Because of the possibility of sudden infant death, infants with a history of ALTE should be evaluated in the hospital with monitoring of the cardiorespiratory status. Such evaluation may include a complete blood count, serum electrolytes, chest radiograph, electroencephalogram, electrocardiogram, and pneumocardiogram with air flow and oximetry. In selected infants, additional evaluations, such as an upper gastrointestinal contrast study, may be indicated.

For infants in whom a treatable cause cannot be found, home apnea monitoring may be prescribed if there is a significant risk of sudden death or intense parental anxiety. Some patients with abnormal respiratory patterns may be treated with drugs, such as theophylline or caffeine.

Respiratory Tract Infections ▪ The most common pediatric infectious disorders are those of the respiratory tract. These are usually viral in etiology.

Acute otitis media, which accounts for most sick visits to the physician, is characterized by otalgia, fever, irritability, and purulent fluid in the middle ear. Nonsuppurative or serous otitis media is characterized by a nonsuppurative effusion in the middle ear. The diagnosis of this disorder is made by visualization of the tympanic membrane. Tympanometry has also been helpful in differentiating a normal middle ear from one with effusion.

Streptococcus pneumoniae is the most frequent cause of suppurative acute otitis media. *Haemophilus influenzae* is a frequent etiologic agent in children under 4 years of age. Other possible causes include *Branhamella catarrhalis*, group A streptococcus, *Mycoplasma*, and viruses.

Therapy may include such antimicrobial agents as ampicillin, erythromycin in combination with sulfisoxazole, cefaclor, cefuroxime, and clavulanate. Serous otitis media is also treated with antibiotics. If the effusion persists more than 3 months, myringotomy and placement of tympanotomy tubes may be indicated.

Pneumonia ▪ Pneumonia refers to an inflammation of the pulmonary tissue beyond the terminal bronchioles. The etiology of pneumonia varies with the age of the patient. In the newborn period, bacterial pneumonia is usually accompanied by bacteremia, with group B streptococcus, *Escherichia coli*, and *Listeria monocytogenes* among the more common pathogens. In young infants over 1 month but less than 3 months of age, pneumonia characterized by rapid respiration and a staccato cough may be caused by *Chlamydia trachomatis*.

After 3 months of age, most pneumonias in children are attributable to viruses or *Mycoplasma*. Respiratory syncytial virus, which occurs in seasonal outbreaks in the winter and early spring, is the most common viral etiologic agent. Symptoms of viral pneumonia may include coryza, cough, fever, and wheezing.

Bacterial pneumonias are accompanied by high fever, lethargy, cough, headache, and abdominal pain. Diagnostic studies include a chest roentgenogram, a white blood cell count, and, possibly, a blood culture. Bacterial causes of pneumonia include *Pneumococcus*, *Haemophilus influenzae*, *Staphylococcus aureus* and group A streptococcus. Intravenous antibiotics are indicated in the treatment of seriously ill patients.

Bacterial Meningitis ▪ In infants and children, this is most commonly caused by *Haemophilus influenzae* type b, *Streptococcus pneumoniae*, and *Neisseria meningitidis*.

Young infants with meningitis may not demonstrate the nuchal rigidity, opisthotonos, and positive Kernig's and Brudzinski's signs seen in older children. A tense or bulging fontanel is an important finding in this age period. The baby may be unusually irritable or drowsy. Fever, vomiting, diarrhea, jaundice, or a convulsion may occur. The older child with meningitis may present with headache, nausea, vomiting, confusion, coma, a stiff neck, and back pain.

The diagnosis is established by examination of the cerebrospinal fluid, including a leukocyte count, differential, protein, glucose, and culture. Antibiotic treatment should be initiated before the result of the culture is known. Steroids may be used as an adjunct to antibiotic therapy.

Diarrhea ▪ Diarrhea refers to the passage of frequent, abnormally liquid stools. The infectious agents that cause diarrhea may be viral, e.g., rotavirus, or bacterial, e.g., *Escherichia coli*, *Shigella*, and *Salmonella*, among other agents. Diarrhea may also be caused by parasites, e.g., *Giardia lamblia*, by noninfectious causes such as a side effect of antibiotics, and food intolerance. Diagnostic measures in the case of acute diarrhea may include stool cultures and examination for ova and parasites.

The chief concern in patients with acute diarrhea is the patient's state of hydration. In most cases, oral rehydration is successful. When dehydration is severe, intravenous hydration may be necessary. Most acute infectious diarrheas have a self-limited course.

Failure to Thrive ▪ Weight gain during early infancy is relatively rapid, amounting to 5 or 6 and sometimes up to 10 ounces a week. In the latter half of the first year, the weight gain is slower, amounting to from 3 to 5 ounces a week. During the first year of life, failure of infants to demonstrate a steady weight gain calls for prompt investigation.

Some babies experience poor weight gain (Figure 31–3) because of inadequate caloric intake. This may be attributable to feeding difficulties associated with physical factors such as a cleft palate. Breast-fed babies may fail to gain because of an inadequate breast milk supply.

Maternal/infant transactional difficulties and lack of mutuality are the most frequent cause for failure to thrive. The malnutrition in these infants is attributable to an inadequate caloric intake, either because they are not offered sufficient calories or because they do not eat or drink adequate amounts of what is offered.

Other causes of failure to thrive include inadequate digestion. For example, failure to gain in spite of hunger and a large food intake is an early symptom of cystic fibrosis. The cause may also be inadequate absorption as in celiac syndrome or loss of food intake because of regurgitation, vomiting, or diarrhea.

Failure of utilization or increased metabolism is illustrated by such disorders as repeated or chronic infections, cardiac disease in infants, chronic pulmonary disease, renal disease, and inborn errors of metabolism such as galactosemia. Some infants with cerebral damage, mental retardation, or cerebral palsy also may not thrive.

Anemia ▪ Anemia is characterized by a diminution in the hemoglobin concentration, or oxygen-carrying capacity, of the blood. For general purposes, a hemoglobin level below 10 gm./dL. of blood or a red blood cell count below 4 million indicates the presence of anemia. Symptoms of anemia may include paleness, irritability, lethargy, and lightheadedness.

Classification of anemia may be based on red cell size or on the underlying mechanism for the anemia. The cell size classification of anemia includes those that are microcytic, e.g., iron deficiency anemia; macrocytic, e.g., megaloblastic anemia; or normocytic, e.g., those caused by production defect, hemolysis with shortened red cell life span, or blood loss. Classification based on mechanism includes decreased red cell production, shortened life-span of the cells, or blood loss through hemorrhage. Anemias may also be categorized as acute or chronic.

Iron deficiency anemia, which occurs principally in infants between the ages of 6 months and 2 years, is caused by insufficient intake of iron-containing foods. The principal chronic anemias of childhood are sickle cell disease, thalassemia, or Cooley's anemia, and hereditary spherocytosis.

Laboratory tests may include determination of the hemoglobin, hematocrit, a blood smear, a reticulocyte count, osmotic fragility, hemoglobin electrophoresis, serum iron, iron-binding capacity, and serum ferritin. Management depends on the specific etiology.

Acute Leukemia ▪ Leukemia is the most common malignancy in childhood. Acute lymphoblastic leukemia (ALL) is the predominant form of leukemia in children, with acute nonlymphocytic leukemia (ANLL) accounting for most of the other cases.

Presenting symptoms include pallor, fever, petechiae, bruising, skeletal pain, anorexia, and fatigue. Lymphadenopathy and hepatosplenomegaly also may be noted on the physical examination.

Laboratory findings include anemia, thrombocytopenia, and abnormal white cell counts. Bone marrow examination establishes the diagnosis.

Treatment consists primarily of combination chemotherapy. Bone marrow transplantation may be indicated in the presence of persistent bone marrow relapse.

Urinary Tract Infections ▪ After the early infancy period, urinary tract infections occur more commonly in girls than in boys. The symptoms associated with these infections differ in

BOYS FROM BIRTH TO 36 MONTHS

WEIGHT FOR AGE

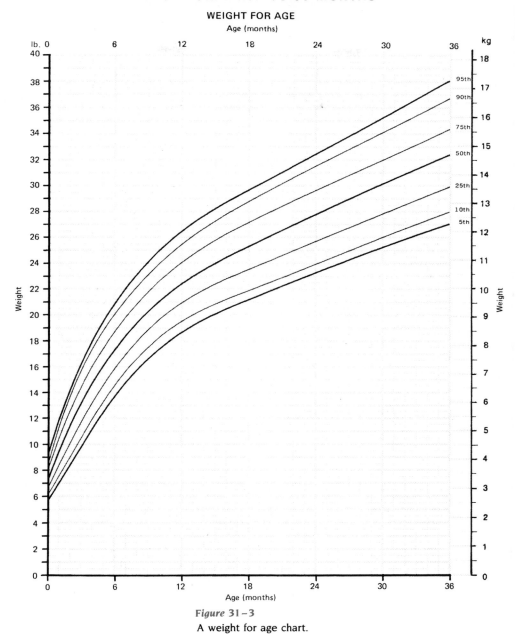

Figure 31–3
A weight for age chart.

infants and young children from those in adults. In the newborn period, urinary tract infections may be accompanied by vomiting, diarrhea, jaundice, or sepsis. The symptoms in older infants and toddlers with urinary tract infections may include fever, abdominal pain, irritability, and diarrhea. Older children may present with abdominal pain, urgency, and enuresis.

A urinalysis may suggest the presence of infection by the finding of pyuria—that is, white cells and bacteria in the sediment. The urine culture is the best laboratory examination for establishment of the diagnosis. When a urinary tract infection is suspected, urine for culture may be obtained by a clean-catch midstream urine specimen in the older child or by either catheterization or suprapubic aspiration in the infant or young child. Radiographic studies utilized in the diagnosis and management of urinary tract infections may include an intravenous pyelogram and a voiding cystourethrogram.

The most frequent pathogenic organism is *Escherichia coli.* Other bacteria that may be cultured in urinary tract infection include *Klebsiella, Enterobacter, Proteus,* and enterococcus. Antimicrobial agents commonly prescribed include sulfisoxazole, nitrofurantoin, cephalexin, trimethoprim and sulfamethoxazole, and ampicillin.

Juvenile Rheumatoid Arthritis ▪ This is the most common cause of chronic arthritis in children. Characteristics needed to establish the diagnosis include persistent swelling, pain, and morning stiffness that continues for 6 weeks in one or more joints.

Juvenile rheumatoid arthritis has three major subtypes. The systemic type, which usually starts before the age of 6 years, is characterized by daily or twice-daily temperature spikes of 39.5° C (103° F) or higher, a salmon-colored macular or maculopapular rash, and symmetric involvement of multiple large and small joints and the cervical spine.

The polyarticular-onset subtype is characterized by the involvement of more than five joints but without systemic effects. About 40 per cent of patients demonstrate a pauciarticular onset with involvement of four or fewer joints; these patients are at special risk of developing chronic iridocyclitis.

Treatment of juvenile rheumatoid arthritis includes the use of nonsteroidal anti-inflammatory drugs (NSAIDs), occupational therapy, and physical therapy.

Cerebral Palsy ▪ This neuromotor disorder is often accompanied by other handicaps such as epilepsy, mental retardation, strabismus, hearing impairment, and speech problems. An etiologic or pathologic classification is not feasible, so clinical designations are usually employed, e.g., spastic (hemiparesis, diplegia), athetoid, rigid, atonic, ataxic, or mixed forms.

Once the diagnosis is recognized, referral to an early intervention or multidisciplinary cerebral palsy center for an integrated rehabilitation program is indicated. This may include occupational and physical therapy, speech therapy, developmental assessment, orthopedic evaluation, and parental counseling.

Mental Retardation ▪ Mental retardation has been defined by the American Association on Mental Deficiency as "significantly subaverage general intellectual functioning existing concurrently with deficits in adaptive behavior, and manifested during the developmental period." Significant subaverage performance is defined as an I.Q. of 70 or below. Levels of mental handicap are defined as mild (I.Q. 50 to 55 to approximately 70), moderate (35 to 40 to 50 to 55), severe (20 to 25 to 35 to 40), and profound (below 20 or 25).

About 25 per cent of children with mental retardation have a syndrome recognizable at birth or early in infancy or childhood; however, most are not identified until school entrance.

The list of possible etiologies for mental retardation is a lengthy one, including chromosomal abnormalities such as Down's syndrome or the fragile X syndrome, biochemical abnormalities such as phenylketonuria, metabolic abnormalities such as Williams' syndrome, infections, toxic agents, cerebral malformations, trauma, autism, and cultural-familial factors.

Evaluation includes a determination of intellectual function and the performance of appropriate diagnostic tests in an attempt to identify a specific etiology. Although the latter are unlikely to identify a treatable cause, a specific diagnosis is useful in determining prognosis and in genetic counseling. The principal approach to management is an educational one, including infant development stimulation programs, preschool experiences, and special education classes.

Epilepsy ▪ Convulsive seizures affect between 3 and 5 per cent of children. Most of these episodes are febrile convulsions, but others are afebrile epileptic seizures.

Convulsive seizures accompanying acute febrile illnesses in children occur more commonly in boys under the age of 3 years, and especially in the first 2 years of life. The febrile seizure usually follows a rapid rise of temperature. Most children who have one or two febrile convulsions never experience another; however, about one third have a subsequent febrile seizure, and 2 to 3 per cent have recurrent afebrile convulsions.

Epileptic seizures may be generalized or partial. Generalized seizures are characterized by bilateral involvement and loss of consciousness. The patient with generalized tonic-clonic or grand mal seizure may suddenly cry out and fall to the floor. Stiffening of the body may then occur with rolling of the eyes, tongue-biting, cyanosis, drooling, and, perhaps, involuntary urination and defecation. The clonic phase that follows is characterized by violent jerking movements of the trunk and extremities.

Absence or petit mal seizures, which are most common between 4 and 8 years of age, are characterized by transient lapses of consciousness. Myoclonic seizures represent another type of generalized seizure. Infantile spasms, one type of myoclonic epilepsy in infants, are characterized by brief episodes in which sudden jerks of the extremities and head dropping occur.

Partial seizures may be simple or complex. The former, which do not alter consciousness, may be motor, sensory, or a mixture of both psychic or autonomic. Complex partial seizures (psychomotor) are characterized by some alterations of consciousness.

The diagnosis of epilepsy is established by the history, the physical examination, and the electroencephalogram. In selected patients, additional diagnostic measures such as imaging studies and laboratory tests for metabolic and other disorders may be obtained.

Treatment includes the appropriate selection of anticonvulsant drugs and attention to the healthy adaptation of the child and family to this long-term disorder.

Hyperactivity; Attention Deficit ▪ Hyperactivity is a common presenting complaint in children. It may be merely the manifestation of a constitutionally high level of motor activity or may be associated with anxiety, depression, or other psychosocial factors. Neurologic impairment, autism, the fragile X syndrome, and learning disorders are other considerations in the differential diagnosis.

Attention deficit, hyperactivity disorder (ADHD) is the diagnostic term applied to a group of behavioral symptoms having onset before 7 years of age and persisting for at least 6 months. Symptoms include inattention, impulsiveness, and motor hyperactivity. These children are unable to sit still for long periods of time and are always moving about. They have a short attention span and are easily distracted. School problems may be secondary to the child's short attention span and distractibility or may be attributable to a concomitant learning disorder.

The diagnosis is based on clinical judgment, since no specific tests are available. However, a variety of parent and teacher rating scales are useful in the evaluation of the child's attention span and social adjustment.

Treatment includes several approaches. Pharmacologic treatment is stimulant medication with the choice being made between methylphenidate (Ritalin), dextroamphetamine (Dexedrine), and pemoline (Cylert). Behavioral therapy, an appropriate academic environment, and support of the child's self-esteem are additional therapeutic measures.

Headaches ▪ These are frequent complaints in children. Muscle contraction or tension is the most common cause of recurrent or chronic headaches in this age group. A persistent headache is almost always psychogenic, owing to anxiety or depression. Both migraine and muscle contraction headaches may be precipitated by stressors.

Common or classic migraine headaches have an incidence of 2 to 4.5 per cent in children and adolescents. Classically, the migraine headache is periodic, unilateral, and retro-orbital, and frontal or temporal in location. Complicated migraine includes ophthalmoplegic migraine, hemiplegic migraine, and basilar artery migraine.

Other causes of headache include intracranial tumors, brain abscesses, pseudotumor cerebri, head trauma, ocular disorders, sinusitis, and temporomandibular dysfunction.

The interview is the most helpful tool in understanding the cause of headaches. Careful funduscopy, testing of visual fields, and screening of visual acuity are important aspects of the physical examination. Computed tomography or magnetic resonance imaging is indicated if the symptoms suggest a brain tumor.

Diabetes Mellitus ▪ Type I or insulin-dependent diabetes affects 1 in 500 school age children. This disorder is an autoimmune disease precipitated in genetically susceptible children by such environmental factors as viruses or certain chemicals.

In children, the onset of diabetes is generally sudden, with such symptoms as frequent urination, thirst, nausea, vomiting, abdominal pain, lethargy, and in some cases coma.

The diagnosis is established by the finding of a random blood glucose level of 200 mg./dL. or greater. Occasionally, an oral glucose tolerance test may be indicated.

The goal of treatment in diabetes mellitus is restoration of near-normal carbohydrate metabolism through insulin administration, glucose monitoring, diet, and activity or exercise. Recombinant or biosynthetic human insulin is available. Generally, patients are begun with two or more insulin injections a day with a mixture of insulins, generally rapid-acting regular insulin and the intermediate NPH or lente form.

Self-blood glucose monitoring four to five times a day is necessary to determine insulin dosages. Determination of glycosylated hemoglobin levels helps assess the level of glucose control over a period of weeks. Acute complications of diabetes include hypoglycemia and ketoacidosis. Testing of urine for ketones is indicated when the child is ill or has blood glucose levels over 240 mg./dL. Dietary consultation is required to develop an appropriate diet plan. Regular exercise and social activities are important for physical fitness and good self-esteem.

Understature ▪ Understature is a common normal variant. Children with normal variant, familial, or constitutional short stature tend to be short at birth and follow the normal growth pattern but remain below the fifth percentile on growth charts. The bone age is normal, and puberty is not delayed. Usually the parents and other close family members are short, with a height of 5 feet or less.

Children with normal variant constitutional delay are of normal length at birth but shift to at or below the third percentile channel between 3 and 36 months of age. The rate of growth is then normal for their age and parallels the standard growth pattern. Over 90 per cent of these patients are boys. The onset of puberty and the adolescent growth spurt are delayed. Bone age is moderately retarded. Normal adult height is eventually attained.

Skeletal disorders, chronic malnutrition, chronic renal and other systemic diseases, inflammatory bowel disease, and chromosomal abnormalities are other causes of short stature (Figure 31–4). Hypopituitarism may be caused by developmental, genetic, or acquired defects in the production or action of growth hormone. Retardation of growth attributable to isolated growth hormone deficiency may be noted in the first year of life or during early childhood. After this onset, the velocity of growth is slow—less than 4 to 5 cm. annually.

The diagnosis of hypopituitarism requires a minimum of two definitive stimulation tests of plasma growth hormone. A low somatomedin C or plasma IGF-I level suggests the possibility of growth hormone deficiency in the absence of inflammatory bowel disease, hypothyroidism, or other disorders.

Growth arrest or marked slowing may be the chief or only clinical manifestation of hypothyroidism acquired after age 2 years.

The most useful clinical assessment in the evaluation of possible short stature is a record of serial heights and weights. At 4 years of age, the third percentile of height velocity is 5 cm. per year. The velocity at age 7 years is 4 cm. per year.

A roentgenogram of the left hand for determination of bone age is useful in determining whether the understature is attributable to normal variant short stature or to constitutional delay. A lateral skull x-ray film may also be indicated. A karyotype determination is indicated in dysmorphic children who are understatured and in girls with unexplained short stature, to rule out Turner's syndrome.

Other laboratory studies may include a complete blood count, sedimentation rate, serum electrolytes, thyroxine, thyroid-stimulating hormone, calcium, phosphorus, creatinine, and blood urea nitrogen.

Treatment is determined by the specific cause of the understature. Human growth hormone produced by using recombinant DNA technology is used for the treatment of growth hormone deficiency.

Surgical Disorders ▪ A list of pediatric surgical procedures is provided in Table 31–2.

Intussusception ▪ This is an important diagnostic consideration in infants with abdominal pain. Immediate diagnosis and treatment are imperative. The history of abdominal pain, sudden in onset, lasting several seconds and recurring

GIRLS FROM 2 TO 18 YEARS

STATURE FOR AGE

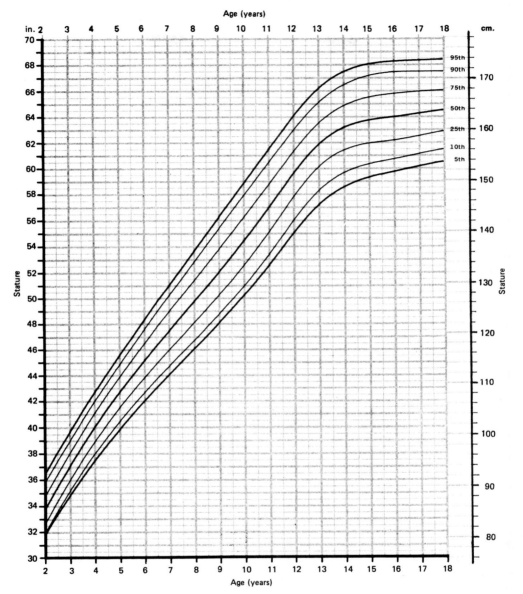

Figure 31–4

A stature for age chart.

Table 31–2 ▪ **Common Pediatric Procedures**

Abdominal paracentesis	Esophagogastroduo-
Angiography	denoscopy
Arterial line placement	Exchange transfusion
Arthrocentesis	Kidney biopsy
Audiometry	Laryngoscopy
Bladder tap	Liver biopsy
Bone marrow aspiration	Lumbar puncture
Bone marrow	Myringotomy
transplantation	Peripheral artery
Bone marrow biopsy	puncture
Brain stem evoked	Peritoneal dialysis
potential	Proctoscopy
Bronchoscopy	Psychometric testing
Cardiac catheterization	Respiratory function
Central venous catheter	tests
Chest tube insertion	Skin biopsy
Colonoscopy	Subdural tap
Echocardiography	Thoracentesis
ECMO (extracorporeal	Umbilical vein
membrane	catheterization
oxygenation)	Umbilical artery
Endotracheal intubation	catheterization
	Ventilatory care

challenging. The classic history begins with abdominal pain followed by nausea, vomiting, and fever. Initially the pain may be periumbilical or epigastric. After a time, perhaps a few hours, it may become localized in the right lower quadrant or in the region of the umbilicus. The pain is rarely severe and is usually constant, but it may be colicky or intermittent. If the appendix ruptures, the child may complain less of pain for an hour or two. The symptoms associated with abdominal pain and appendicitis in infants and very young children are irritability, restlessness, unexplained crying, refusal of feedings, and vomiting.

Vomiting with or without nausea, almost a constant feature in children with appendicitis, may occur once, twice, or repeatedly. Fever is usually low grade.

The physical findings are of great importance in deciding whether or not a "surgical" abdomen is present. If these findings have not developed when the child is first seen, repeated examinations are indicated over a period of a few hours.

every 5 to 15 minutes always means intussusception until ruled out. In some instances, pain is not a prominent feature, or it is persistent rather than intermittent. Between the paroxysms of pain, the child may appear completely normal. Vomiting occurs early in many of these patients. Blood in the stools is usually a relatively late finding. At times, infants with intussusception present with limpness, lethargy, listlessness, obtundation, or stupor. A sausage-shaped tumor or an unusual fullness may be palpated in the upper abdominal quadrants in some infants and children with intussusception (Figure 31–5). Although the diagnosis usually can be made readily on the basis of the history and physical examination, a barium enema is diagnostic and usually therapeutic.

Pyloric Stenosis ▪ In infants with pyloric stenosis, regurgitation in the first week of life is frequently the initial symptom. Usually, vomiting begins gradually in the second and third weeks. Vigorous gastric peristalsis is commonly visible. The presence of a palpable pyloric tumor is diagnostically helpful.

Appendicitis ▪ The diagnosis of appendicitis is often not difficult, but it may at times be most

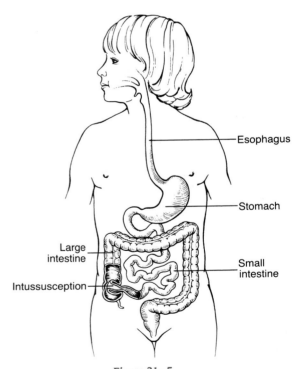

Figure 31–5
Intussusception.

SAMUEL J. MILLER, M.D.
1314 Grant Road
Indianapolis, IN 46209-0000
317/578-9043

Joseph Smithson, M.D.
7098 White River Parkway
Indianapolis, IN 46208-0000

RE: Donavan, Arthur
MRN: 0067438X

Dear Dr. Smithson:

Your patient, an 11-week-old infant, has just been seen in the Pediatric Clinic for evaluation of possible premature fusion of his cranial sutures.

He is the product of a 36-week gestation with a spontaneous vaginal delivery and a birth weight of six pounds, three ounces. Initially, he exhibited some respiratory expiratory grunting, but this cleared spontaneously with observation in a special care nursery. A cranial ridge was noted by the parents shortly after his delivery. Since that time, the parents have noticed that he has developed fullness in the right anterior portion of his face and frontal bone with some posterior narrowing of the skull.

Development is notable with a social smile and recognition of his mother. His head control is developmentally normal. His head circumference is 40.7 cms. There is a ridge along the sagittal suture. The right nares appears slightly larger than the left. The remainder of the physical examination is normal. A skull x-ray demonstrated premature fusion of the sagittal suture.

The baby was then seen by our pediatric neurosurgical consultant, Dr. John Johnson, who concurred with the diagnosis of premature closure of the sagittal suture. The baby has been scheduled for sagittal craniotomy. You will receive a report following that admission.

Thank you for your kind referral of this patient.

Sincerely,

Samuel J. Miller, M.D.

cc: Dr. John Johnson
SB:ssb

Figure 31–6
Consultation letter on an 11-week-old infant seen in the pediatric clinic for evaluation of possible premature fusion of his cranial sutures.

THE WILSON HOSPITAL
843 Barnaby Road
Indianapolis, IN 46202-5225

DISCHARGE SUMMARY

PHYSICIAN:	MORTON GREGG, M.D.
PATIENT'S NAME:	MARCIE JOHNSON
HOSPITAL NUMBER:	2-782538
ADMISSION DATE:	10/15/94
DISCHARGE DATE:	10/18/94
DISCHARGE DIAGNOSIS:	SOMATIZATION DISORDER

This 15-year-old girl was admitted with a history of dizzy spells. These were said to begin three months before admission. Initially, they were intermittent and occasionally associated with occipital headaches. During the last three months, the episodes gradually increased to the point where the patient was continuously feeling dizzy and had constant occipital headaches. At times this symptomatology was worse, particularly when the patient would lie flat in bed. The child is also said to have blacked out during a chemistry examination. Most of her severe episodes have been relieved by lying down.

The physical and neurological examinations were within normal limits. The child was begun on a detailed schedule consisting of activities which kept her active most of the day. These included school, child life activities, physical therapy, occupational therapy, library activities, and social/recreational room activities. The patient improved steadily over time and reported that she felt much better now than she had in the past three years. During the hospitalization, the child was able to study once again, although she had not been able to do so for some time. In addition, she began to play the clarinet up to an hour a day.

The child reported a number of stressors including those at school. They were algebra, Spanish, and activity with her fellow students. She feels that the students do not allow her to enter their clique. She often feels left out. In spite of this, she reported that "nothing bothers me." I think the child tends to be somewhat angry and self isolated in these contacts. In terms of activities

(continued)

Figure 31–7
A discharge summary for a 15-year-old girl with a somatization disorder.

MARCIE JOHNSON   Page two
HOSPITAL NUMBER: 2-782538

outside the school and family, she would like to have a part-time job, learn to
drive and increase physical activities such as swimming, biking, running and
basketball. We talked to her about her need to develop a means to express her
anger, how she might make more friends and the importance of continuing her
activities. I also advised her and her parents of the advisability of mental
health counseling in her community. They are to advise me as to how things
go.

_____

MORTON GREGG, M.D.

CC: Joseph Smith, M.D.

MG:ssb
D: 10/18/94
T: 10/19/94

Figure 31–7 *Continued*

A white blood cell count, urinalysis, and chest roentgenogram are indicated in the workup.

Abdominal tenderness, especially localized or point tenderness, is the finding of greatest diagnostic significance in children with acute appendicitis and is almost always present. Abdominal rigidity, usually in the right lower quadrant, indicates that extension of the inflammatory process to the peritoneum has occurred.

Mesenteric lymphadenopathy may cause abdominal pain that closely resembles that of acute appendicitis.

FORMATS

Consultation Letters ■ An example of a pediatric consultation letter is seen in Figure 31–6.

Discharge Summary ■ A pediatric discharge summary should contain the following information:

- Physician's name (spell it) and service.
- Patient's name (spell it).
- Chart number.
- Date admitted and date discharged or expired.
- Discharge diagnoses—list in order of descending importance.
- Procedures.
- Consultations.
- History—state concisely the relevant background history, the present illness, and the reason for hospitalization.
- Physical examination—include only the pertinent findings on admission.
- Laboratory data—include only pertinent laboratory, x-ray, or electrocardiographic findings at admission.

SOUTHEAST MEMORIAL HOSPITAL
1726 Columbia Road
Indianapolis, IN 46208-0000

OPERATIVE REPORT

NAME OF PATIENT: CRANE, ROBERT
HOSPITAL NUMBER: 008728X
DATE OF OPERATION: 4/7/94
DATE OF DICTATION: 4/7/94

SURGEON: RONALD HELLER, M.D.

PREOPERATIVE DIAGNOSIS: Sagittal synostosis
POSTOPERATIVE DIAGNOSIS: Same
NAME OF PROCEDURE: Sagittal and occipital craniectomy

PROCEDURE: The operation was done under general
                          anesthesia with the patient in the prone
position. The head was prepared and draped in the usual manner. The skin was infiltrated
with .24% Xylocaine with Adrenalin 1:200,000. An incision was made in the midline from a
point approximately at the apex of the occipital projection anteriorly to the posterior edge of
the anterior fontanel. The incision was carried down to the periosteum. The scalp was
reflected laterally. The periosteum was then incised just anterior to the lambdoid suture, just
posterior to the coronal suture and 3 cm. lateral to the midline. The periosteum was stripped
in the corner and midway anterior posterior. Bur holes were then made in each of these
areas. The dura was freed, and an osteotomy was then carried out just anterior to the
lambdoid suture using a Ruskin rongeur. Similarly, the osteotomy was carried out just
posterior to the coronal suture, again using a Ruskin rongeur. The bur holes were
interconnected laterally using the craniotome after freeing dura with a saw guide. The sagittal
section of bone was then freed and removed, and sent for pathologic examination.
Hemostasis was obtained with bipolar cautery and thrombin spray. The periosteum was then
incised posteriorly from a point approximately 1 cm. lateral to the sagittal craniectomy
extending posteriorly to the summit of the occipital projection. The dura was then freed
along the edge of the lambdoid suture. The occipital bone superiorly was then removed with
the aid of a Fulton rongeur. The dura was then freed in the posterior fossa. Radial cuts were
then made in the remaining occipital bone just posterior to the lambdoid suture

(continued)

Figure 31-8

An operative report for a patient with sagittal synostosis, typed in indented format.

CRANE, ROBERT   Page two
HOSPITAL NUMBER: 008728X

bilaterally, and two radial cuts midway anterior posteriorly. The dura was then freed lateral to the sagittal craniotomy. Here again, radial cuts were made laterally using the Tessier scissors with cuts being made just anterior to the lambdoid suture, just posterior to the coronal suture with two cuts between. This was carried out bilaterally and hemostasis was obtained with the aid of bone wax and Gelfoam powder soaked in thrombin. The wound was then thoroughly irrigated using bacitracin solution. Hemostasis was again obtained using bipolar cautery, Gelfoam powder soaked in thrombin, bone wax and thrombin spray. The wound was then closed in the usual manner using interrupted 4-0 Dexon for galea, 5-0 nylon for skin. The patient tolerated the procedure satisfactorily.

STAFF SURGEON AND DICTATED BY: RONALD HELLER, M.D.

cc: John Smith, M.D.

Figure 31−8 *Continued*

- Hospital course — concisely review diagnostic procedures and findings, the treatment plan, and the patient's response.

- Discharge plan — state the patient's condition on discharge and specific instructions given to the patient and family, including prescriptions for physical activity, medications, diet, and follow-up care.

- Copy distribution — include full name of attending physicians, referring physician(s), and major consultant physician(s).

This list is intended to be only a guide. Inclusion of material varies, depending on the dictating physician as well as the particular case history (Figure 31−7).

Operative Report ■ An operative report includes the physician's name, the patient's name and hospital number, the date of operation, the preoperative and postoperative diagnosis, and the name of the procedure. Figure 31−8 is an example of a pediatric operative report.

Reference Sources

Behrman, R. E. (Ed.). *Nelson Textbook of Pediatrics,* 14th edition. W. B. Saunders Company, Philadelphia, 1992.

Green, M. *Pediatric Diagnosis; Interpretation of Symptoms and Signs in Infants, Children and Adolescents,* 5th edition. W. B. Saunders Company, Philadelphia, 1992.

Oski, F. A. (Ed.). *Principles and Practice of Pediatrics.* J. B. Lippincott, Philadelphia, 1990.

Rudolph, A. M. (Ed.). *Rudolph's Pediatrics,* 19th edition. Appleton & Lange, Norwalk, Connecticut, 1991.

For references of specific application to medical transcription, see Appendix 1.

Plastic Surgery

INTRODUCTION

The field of plastic and reconstructive surgery has evolved since ancient times, largely as a result of attempted correction of facial and other soft tissue injuries resulting from burns, trauma, disease, and congenital deformities. The important principles of the specialty have gradually become established and accepted since the mid-18th century. Many of the developments in the field of reconstructive surgery came about in an effort to treat injuries sustained in wars, especially after World War I. The American Board of Plastic Surgery was established in 1937.

The areas of training now include the care and treatment of the following:

Burns
Skin malignancies, including melanoma
Reconstruction of various facial deformities, including congenital abnormalities, such as cleft lip and palate
Head and neck cancer surgery and reconstruction
Maxillofacial trauma
Hand surgery
Microsurgery, including replantation of amputated body parts, as well as the free transfer of soft and hard tissue in reconstruction
Reconstruction of the trunk, including breast reconstruction following mastectomy
The care and treatment of pressure sores
Surgery of the genitourinary system, including hypospadias and reconstruction of the external genitalia
Cosmetic surgery

Plastic surgery is often confused with cosmetic surgery. Cosmetic surgery is only one area within the broader area of the specialty of plastic surgery. Even though various synthetic materials are often used in both cosmetic and reconstructive surgery, the word plastic is actually derived from the Greek words *plastos* and *plastikos,* which mean forming or molding, especially in a sculpturing or creative sense.

Although some plastic surgeons specialize in only one area within the field, such as hand surgery or cosmetic surgery, the majority of the practicing physicians are involved in both cosmetic and reconstructive surgery.

GENERAL PRINCIPLES OF RECONSTRUCTION

A number of factors must be taken into consideration in any reconstructive procedure. Important among these are the age and sex of the patient, the skin type and quality, and the general health of the patient. There are usually several possible choices for reconstruction of a particular defect. It is essential that the patient be involved in the decision-making process. For example, a person who is the primary source of income for a family may be less interested in a multistaged reconstruction, even if it gives a somewhat better cosmetic result, than in a single-staged reconstruction, because of the economic hardship of losing time from work.

As a general rule, the restoration of function is given more weight in the decision-making than the cosmetic appearance. Of course, all efforts

595

are made to restore both form and function as optimally as possible. Wherever possible, reconstruction is accomplished in a single stage to save recovery time and costs.

A principle of reconstruction is to "replace like tissue with like tissue." While this is not always feasible, the surgeon will strive to satisfy this principle for aesthetic* as well as functional concerns. For example, the extremely specialized skin that occurs on the plantar aspect of the foot and palmar surfaces of the hand is not found anywhere else on the body. This skin is the most durable coverage for these areas, and whenever possible the rule of "replace like tissue with like tissue" should be adhered to. This is especially true on the soles of the feet, where coverage with lesser quality skin could lead to pressure problems such as ulcers, chronic skin breakdown, and infections. Appearance in these situations is secondary to achieving satisfactory functional coverage. Another example is coverage of the upper eyelid, such as needed following a deep burn. When the scar tissue is excised, the defect is best grafted with skin borrowed from the excess skin from the opposite upper eyelid. Here again the tissue is extremely specialized and is not found in this precise texture, quality, and appearance at any other location on the body. It is exceedingly thin, mobile, and elastic, to serve the functional needs of the defective eyelid. It is also the perfect color match and identical quality.

In eyelid reconstruction, an older patient may have already developed extremely heavy, redundant upper lid skin folds, which would be the most suitable donor site for grafting. The donor site would benefit as well. Removal of all the excess skin would enhance the appearance of the donor eyelid, as well as correcting possible functional problems, such as lash ptosis and partial visual field obstruction due to hooding.

On the other hand, in a younger patient the same procedure could foreshorten the upper lid, resulting in permanent lid lag, leading to chronic corneal exposure and dry eye syndrome. Secondary donor site areas must then be given consideration and would vary depending on the skills, experience, and comfort level of the surgeon. Some other sites that could be selected for cover-

age of an upper eyelid are free skin grafts from behind or in front of the ear, the upper inner arm or thigh, the supraclavicular area, and the groin. Sometimes local or distant skin flaps might be used, such as the lower eyelid (if there is sufficient redundancy of tissue), the temple region, or the area just above the eyebrow.

The donor site in reconstruction must also be given careful consideration because of the different long- or short-term effects it might have on a male or female patient. For example, a nasolabial flap that includes some cheek skin could be an excellent choice for covering a nasal defect in a young girl. However, in a young male that same tissue would prove unsatisfactory after the onset of puberty, when eruption of the beard cilia would prove unmanageable and cosmetically unacceptable.

A certain amount of what might be referred to as the "luck of healing" must also be taken into account when a donor site is selected. Some surgeons have chosen the instep of the plantar aspect of the foot to resurface large defects of the palmar aspect of the hand and fingers. However, on occasion these donor areas have developed thick, painful, or pruritic hypertrophic scars that have seriously hindered the wearing of certain footwear or even impeded ambulation. As a general rule, the favored donor sites are those that heal rapidly and predictably and are hidden in natural folds or creases or by hair. Furthermore, tissues that will not affect function of the donor site will be preferred over those that might affect function.

Other principles of reconstruction include the idea that autogenous tissues are generally chosen over heterologous, xenographic, or synthetic materials (see the section on Implant Materials that follows). Operative procedures that will entail less blood loss, anesthesia, and operative time are favored. The economics of medicine also apply in determining which procedures can be done on an outpatient basis or with the least amount of hospitalization required.

In every reconstructive situation, the surgeon must anticipate the possible failure of the first choice for reconstruction. This usually means loss of a graft or flap, and the surgeon should be prepared with secondary and tertiary possibilities for effective salvage of a failure or a poor result from the initial reconstructive effort.

---

*Also spelled esthetic.

IMPLANT MATERIALS

A patient's skin and tissues, as well as tissues and materials other than the patient's own, have long been used in reconstruction. Autogenous tissues are those from the patient. A skin graft is referred to as an autograft. Heterologous tissues are tissues that come from another individual, such as blood, corneal grafts, heart, lung, and liver for transplantation purposes, and irradiated cartilage. In identical twins, tissues can be transplanted freely, but the rejection phenomenon makes this difficult in many other situations. A graft from another individual is called an allograft. Xenografts are tissues from a species other than a human being. Examples are pigskin grafts used for temporary coverage of burns, and pig heart valves used in cardiac surgery. Again, the limitations most frequently encountered have to do with the phenomenon of rejection.

Alloplastic materials are synthetic materials that are used in human reconstruction (or in some cases, cosmetic surgery). No material has been found to be ideal, but the search continues, and a variety of substances have been tried with varying degrees of success. In the past, ivory, silver, gold, paraffin, amber, and various inorganic rubbers were used, but for the most part they have been abandoned. Another example of an outdated substance is Ivalon, a polyvinyl alcohol-formaldehyde sponge that was used in breast augmentation surgery many years ago.

Materials currently being used include metals such as vitallium (an alloy of chromium, cobalt, molybdenum, nickel, and tungsten) and stainless steel. Textiles include Teflon, in a cloth form often used in vascular prostheses, and Dacron, a polyester fiber with little reactivity. The solid form is called Mylar. Plastics include methylmethacrylate, which is used extensively in orthopedic surgery as a cement but is also useful in filling cranial defects; Teflon in solid form; polyurethane in solid or foam form; and polyethylene in a surgical-grade material known as Marlex, which is often used to reinforce the abdominal wall, chest, or other areas.

Rubbery materials known as elastomers are usually derived from the silicones, which can take on many forms, from watery and oily to gel-like, adhesive, rubbery, or very hard. These materials are used in many different types of prosthetic implants, including finger-joint prostheses, cardiac pacemakers, and breast, chin, cheek, ear, and nose implants. The nature of the material depends upon the vulcanizing process used. A silicone rubber termed Silastic is often used, and this usage is often found in transcription: "A Silastic chin implant was inserted."

GRAFTS

A graft of human tissue is tissue that has been removed from one area of the body and transplanted into another area. Almost any type of body tissue from the simplest to the most complex may be involved. Synthetic materials, as seen in a vascular bypass "graft," should probably best be termed implants or prostheses.

A graft may be skin, but nerve grafts, vascular grafts, cartilage or bone grafts, fat grafts, and hair replacement grafts are also used. All these are removed from their blood supply and so are not vascularized at the time of surgery. Some grafts, such as skin grafts, will survive for a day or two until capillary circulation has been restored from the donor site. Thinner skin grafts, which are referred to as split-thickness grafts, have a better chance of survival than do thick ones, which are referred to as full-thickness skin grafts (Thiersch graft for split grafts and Wolfe graft for full-thickness grafts). If circulation is not quickly established these grafts will die and eventually slough away. Other types of grafts, such as bone grafts, are not capable of picking up a blood supply and, therefore, will never become viable. In fact, they may, in some cases, be slowly broken down and reabsorbed. However, before this happens, they serve as a scaffolding to allow adjacent bone tissue to grow over and through to fill a gap or allow healing to take place. This type of graft may be used to achieve a bony fusion of a nonunited fracture or to close the separation in a cleft palate.

The term *compound graft* refers to a more complex type of graft consisting of more than one tissue type. An example is the skin-cartilage graft that is taken from the rim of the ear to replace a defect in the alar rim of the nose. There is a limit to the size of the defect that can be filled. If the graft size exceeds the ability of the body's capacity to revascularize the graft, then it will be lost. Therefore, when large or complex types of tissue are needed, flaps are used instead of grafts.

FLAPS

Most of the major reconstructive work carried out today is accomplished through the use of various types of flaps. Unfortunately, there is no simplified or universally accepted terminology for flaps. Flaps may be classified in a number of ways. Most commonly this is done anatomically, using a description of the tissues involved. Some particular flaps have been in use so long that they have evolved a commonly accepted name that is based on historical usage. For example, the Indian forehead flap is used for nasal reconstruction. This term has been used for centuries, although it may simply be referred to as a forehead flap (Figure 32–1).

Another long-established flap, still occasionally used for nasal reconstruction, is the so-called Italian flap or Italian method of reconstruction. The specific name often given to this

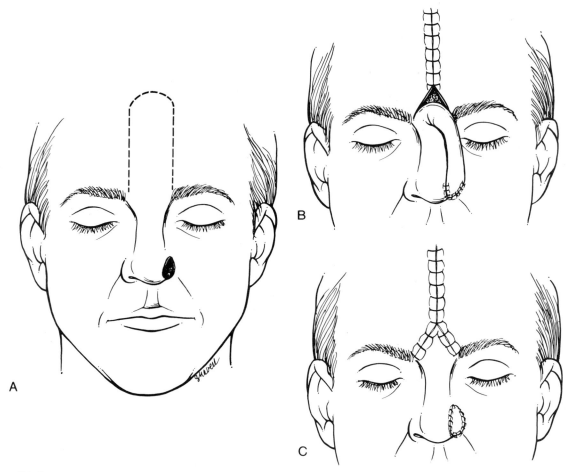

Figure 32–1
Midline forehead flap, or Indian flap. A, Outline of midline forehead flap, showing the blood supply from the supratrochlear vessels. B, Flap rotated into position, with the midline defect of the forehead closed by a direct advancement flap. The flap is being used to cover a defect of the left side of the nose and alar rim. C, Appearance following division and inset of flap to lower nose and alar region, with return of unused portion to the glabellar area.

particular flap is the Tagliacozzi flap, named after the innovator, Gaspar Tagliacozzi, who popularized its use. A skin flap from the upper arm is attached to the nasal area requiring soft tissue. After an appropriate waiting period, during which the hand is strapped to the head to immobilize the extremity, the flap is detached, and the tissue left at the site of reconstruction is reshaped to fit the needed contours. The donor site is easily closed, since the upper inner arm skin is quite mobile. The scar is fairly well hidden. The disadvantage of this method is that the patient's arm is immobilized in a rather uncomfortable position for 1 to 2 weeks.

A third flap used in nasal reconstruction is the scalping flap, in which the skin from one side of the forehead is used to reconstruct the entire nose, or at least a very large portion of it. To transfer this highly satisfactory tissue safely to the nasal area, the major portion of the scalp is raised, along with the forehead skin. The scalp portion serves as the blood supply to the forehead skin, which is reshaped to reconstruct the nose in its new position. After an appropriate delay period, the forehead tissue is detached from the scalp and the scalp is placed back into its normal anatomic position. The donor area in the forehead is usually covered with a full-thickness skin graft.

Most commonly, flaps are described according to tissues utilized, such as skin flap or skin-muscle flap. Though not stated, it is understood that the skin flap contains the underlying subcutaneous fat, which is the majority of the blood supply to the skin. The skin flap is commonly given the name of the anatomic areas involved. For years the deltopectoral flap has been the workhorse of head and neck reconstruction (Figure 32–2). This skin flap is still often referred to as Bakamjian's flap for the physician who popularized its use.

The terms musculocutaneous flap or myocutaneous flap are often used interchangeably with skin-muscle flap (Figure 32–3). Carrying this phrasing one step further, an osteomyocutaneous flap would contain bone as well as skin and muscle.

To further clarify the particular flap being chosen, the anatomic site completes the terminology of a particular flap. For example, the fat of the lower abdomen is now commonly transferred to the upper chest area for reconstruction, particularly for breast reconstruction. The blood supply used to transfer this large portion of the lower abdominal skin and fat to its new location is the rectus abdominis muscle. This type of flap is thus a rectus abdominis myocutaneous flap, but it is commonly referred to as a transverse rectus abdominis myocutaneous (TRAM) flap because the skin portion is usually taken in a

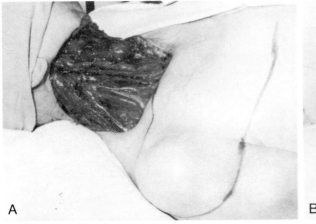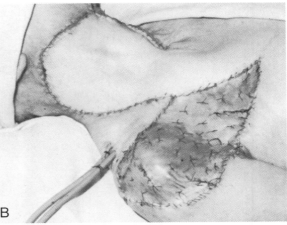

Figure 32–2
Deltopectoral flap in open transposition for a total resurfacing of one side of the neck. A, The defect from a radical neck dissection, with sacrifice of involved skin with cancer in the neck. B, The repair with the deltopectoral flap on the neck and skin graft on its donor bed. (From Grabb, William C., and M. Bert Myers. *Skin Flaps.* Little, Brown and Company, Boston, 1975, p. 231.)

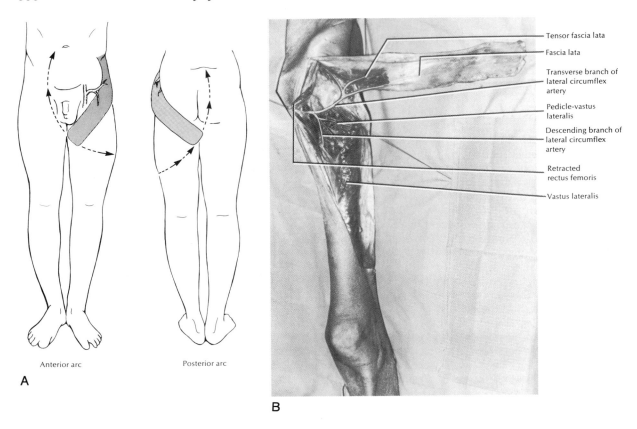

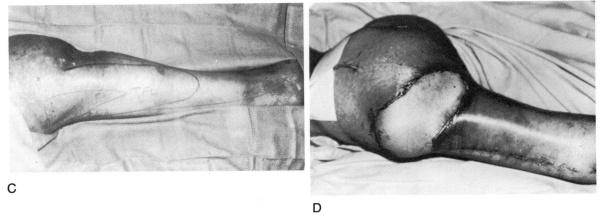

Figure 32–3
A, Arcs of rotation of anterior and posterior skin flaps for the tensor fascia lata muscle. B, The anatomy of the tensor fascia lata muscle from the anterior thigh in preparation of a skin flap. C, Tensor fascia lata musculocutaneous flap design for a patient with a trochanteric pressure ulcer. D, The trochanteric defect is closed with a tensor fascia lata island musculocutaneous flap (posterior arc). The secondary defect is closed directly. (From Mathes, Stephen J., and Foad Nahai. *Clinical Atlas of Muscle and Musculocutaneous Flaps*. C. V. Mosby, St. Louis, 1979, pp. 66–68.)

horizontal or transverse direction (see Figure 32–10). Another flap used for breast reconstruction is the latissimus dorsi myocutaneous flap.

The fasciocutaneous flap is essentially a skin flap that derives its blood supply from the vessels that come from the underlying fascial tissues, usually between the muscles as on an extremity. Another generalized term for a flap based on a particular blood supply is the island flap. This describes the flap that has had its blood supply reduced, usually to a single artery and vein, which are the pivot point from which the tissue needed can be rotated from one position to another. Use of this method is common in the hand, where often a nerve is included with the artery and vein so that sensation can be restored along with the skin that is being used for coverage (Figure 32–4).

In flap terminology, the word *pedicle* is often used. The pedicle contains the blood supply. When a particular flap is being elevated to rotate into its new position, the pedicle is that part of the flap that is still attached. In the TRAM flap, the pedicle is the upper end of the rectus abdominis muscle; in the deltopectoral flap, it is the medial portion of the flap near the sternum and chest junction; in the island flap, it is the artery, vein, and nerve at their point of attachment, usually in the midpalmar area; and in the fasciocutaneous flap, it is in the filmy fascial tissues between the muscular planes.

In breast reduction surgery, the nipple must usually be transferred to a new, higher position. It may be left attached to some portion of the dermis, fat, or sometimes the breast tissue itself. This blood supply to the nipple is referred to as the pedicle, and it is usually described by its point of attachment: bilateral breast reduction using an inferior pedicle or a superomedial pedicle or a central pedicle, and so forth.

With the advent and refinement of microsurgery, it immediately became possible to transfer almost any type or quantity of tissue from one area of the body to any other. This sophisticated and demanding technique requires that the tissue to be transferred has a known and predictable blood supply (artery and vein), and that these vessels are large enough to work with so that they can be plugged into a new blood supply at the recipient site. The tissues so transferred are referred to as free flaps, and the vessels, as in the island flap, are the pedicle. Such flaps are known as free flaps because they have been removed completely free from the body before reattaching at the recipient site. Flaps that have been previously used for reconstruction may now be detached at their blood supply and moved to any location where the tissue is needed. Thus, one can have a free TRAM flap or a free fasciocutaneous flap, and so forth.

Types of Flaps

A number of flaps are now in common usage and the terminology of them is frequently utilized in operative reports, consultations, and admitting history and physical examinations. Flaps are described here according to their anatomic location.

Head and Neck Flaps

Abbé's Flap ■ This useful flap usually involves two stages and is used for reconstruction of the lips or eyelids. In the first stage, the needed amount is borrowed from the donor area and turned on a pedicle 180 degrees to be fitted into the recipient site. After an appropriate delay period, the pedicle is divided and the remaining portion is inset into the defect. Usually about 20 to 40 per cent of the donor site can be used without loss of function and with reasonable cosmetic appearance, depending on the age and tissue characteristics of the patient (Figure 32–5).

Estlander's Flap ■ This is similar to Abbé's flap but usually involves the corner of the mouth. A portion of the donor lip is cut at the commissure and rotated around to the recipient site. The angle usually is blunted, and often a second stage is performed to improve the appearance of the corner of the mouth. This procedure is usually referred to as a commissuroplasty, and this term also applies to correction of congenital or acquired macrostomia or microstomia. Some other names associated with local flaps to reconstruct the lip areas include Kazanjian's, Bernard's, Karapandzic's, Webster's and Von Brun's.

Scalp Flaps ■ Larger scalping flaps have various names attached according to size and direction; three examples of these are Converse's, Gillies', and Millard's. Some scalp flaps are used for hair replacement in male pattern baldness, such as Juri's flap. Others, such as Orticochea's

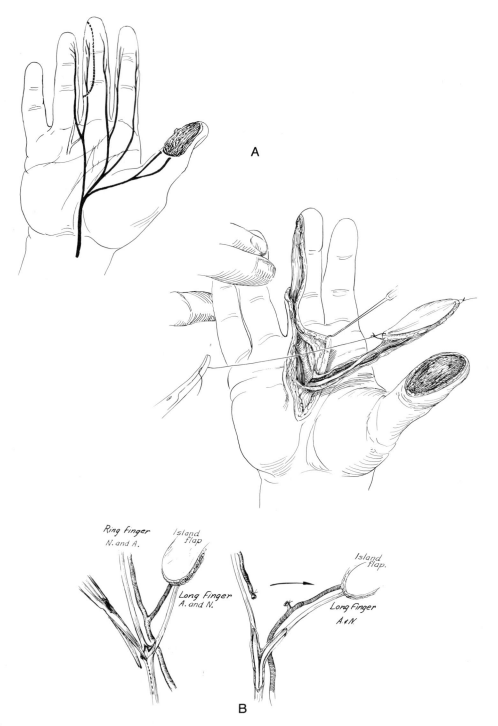

Figure 32–4

Island flap. A, Loss of tissue along with sensation to the right thumb. The donor island flap is outlined from the ulnar side of the right long finger and the nerve supply to this region. B, The island flap from the long finger, showing the dissection of the artery and nerve in the transposition of the island from the long finger to the thumb. Not depicted but included in this type of flap are the venae comitantes.

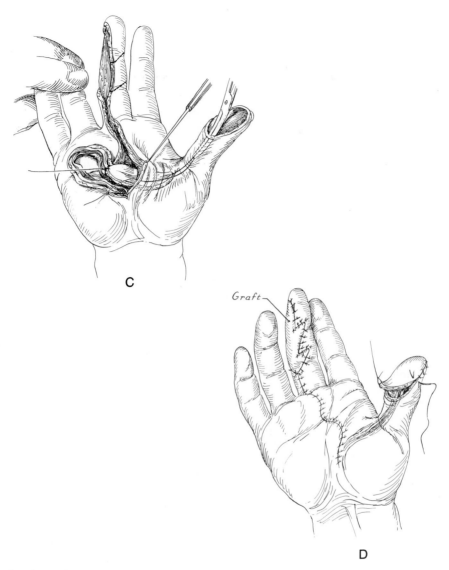

C

D

Figure 32–4 Continued
C, The island flap is being brought through a subcutaneous tunnel from its donor site of the long finger to the recipient thumb touch pad. D, Completion of the procedure, showing inset of the island pedicle flap to the thumb and closure of the defect on the ulnar side of the long finger with a skin graft. (From Chase, Robert A. *Atlas of Hand Surgery*. W. B. Saunders Co., Philadelphia, 1973, pp. 79–80.)

flaps, consist of multiple hair-bearing scalp flaps to reconstruct more massive scalp defects.

Washio Flap ■ This flap is based on the posterior branch of the superficial temporal artery and its anastomosis with the retroauricular artery. It allows the nonhair-bearing skin of the posterior auricular region to be transferred to the midfacial region and is, therefore, quite useful in nasal reconstruction.

Forehead Flap ■ The entire forehead from hairline to brows is occasionally used in a single- or multistaged procedure based on the temporal artery and vein. It may be used to line the inner oral cavity in place of mucosa for head and neck

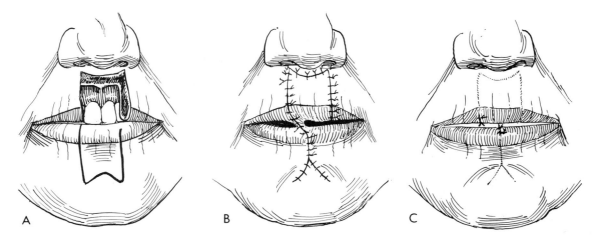

Figure 32–5

The modified Abbé operation. A, A large, prong-shaped Abbé flap is prepared to repair a defect of the upper lip. B, The flap after transposition. Note that the blood supply is at the small pedicle at the midline of the lower lip. C, Completion of the operative procedure and division of the pedicle in a second stage. (From Converse, John M. *Reconstructive Plastic Surgery*, Vol. 4. W. B. Saunders Co., Philadelphia, 1977, p. 1551.)

cancer reconstruction or to replace skin and subcutaneous tissue for the nose and cheeks.

Temporalis Muscle Flap ▪ Used for soft tissue fill in the cheek area.

Cervical Visor Flap ▪ This flap can slide up to the chin or lip area from the neck because it is based on two lateral pedicles for its blood supply.

Platysma Myocutaneous Flap ▪ This flap allows thin, pliable skin to be used in the cheek area or as an intraoral lining in women.

Sternocleidomastoid Myocutaneous Flap ▪ The arc of rotation of this flap allows coverage of the anterior neck, face, and forehead as well as the posterior neck, skull, and posterior mastoid regions.

Nasolabial Flaps ▪ These skin flaps are used often for reconstruction about the nose, especially the ala nasi, upper lip, and cheek. They can also be used intraorally.

Deltopectoral Flap (Bakamjian Flap) ▪ As previously noted, this classic skin flap is based on the perforating vessels of the internal mammary artery. This pedicle is over the upper medial half of the chest at the sternal junction, and the flap can be extended to reach the upper neck and facial regions as well as to serve as lining for closure of large defects of the oropharyngeal area. The reliability of this flap is based on the fact that the perforating vessels run parallel along the flap toward the deltoid region, giving what is referred to as an "axial pattern blood supply" over most of the length of the flap. Flaps that do not have this type of pattern have instead a "random pattern blood supply," and these types of flaps are much more limited in the range of length to which they can be raised.

Pectoralis Major Myocutaneous Flap ▪ There are several versions of this flap; a portion of the flap and its blood supply may be utilized, or the entire muscle unit and its overlying skin can be transferred. For head and neck reconstruction, most commonly a skin-muscle island flap is utilized, based on the pectoral branch of the thoracoacromial vessels.

Latissimus Dorsi Myocutaneous Flap ▪ This flap is supplied by the thoracodorsal artery and vein. It has a reliable blood supply, with a long useful pedicle, and good range of mobility to service many areas of the head and neck, as well as the trunk and upper extremities. It has also proved quite useful for free microvascular flap transfers. As with the pectoralis major myocutaneous flap, the muscle alone can be used, or a large island of skin can be included with the flap.

Trapezius Myocutaneous Flap ▪ The posterior arc of this muscle will cover defects in the skull and posterior neck, while the cervical humeral flap that extends down the dorsolateral arm and is based on the trapezius muscle medially has an extensive range and can resurface anterior neck and facial defects.

Shoulder Flap ■ This is a skin flap that is based over the nape of the neck and runs toward the shoulder between the clavicle and the scapula. It is quite useful for coverage in the anterior neck, especially after release of severe contractures as seen in burn victims. This flap has a number of variations, and the names of Zovickian, Kazanjian, Converse, and Bakamjian, among others, have been associated with its use.

Free Flaps ■ It is now commonplace to reconstruct head and neck defects with various free flap tissue transfers. Especially useful flaps include the radial forearm flap (sometimes referred to as the Chinese flap), the subscapular flap, and free omental flap transfers. Segmental microvascular transfers of jejunum or portions of the stomach can reconstruct portions of the pharynx and upper esophagus.

Trunk Flaps

Pectoralis Major Flap ■ This flap is especially useful for the anterior trunk and can be advanced medially to cover sternal defects, such as sternotomy dehiscences after cardiac surgery.

Serratus Anterior Flap ■ This flap is supplied by the long thoracic artery as well as the thoracodorsal artery. It can be used as a muscle flap, a musculocutaneous flap, or a composite flap, including a segment of rib. Facial reanimation can be obtained using slips of muscle that have the nerve branches preserved in the flap. Disadvantages of this flap are the diminished arm movements and winged scapula deformities that can result from its use.

Rectus Abdominis Flap ■ The two major pedicles supplying the rectus abdominis flap come from the superior epigastric artery above and the inferior epigastric artery below, which anastomose and run on the deep surface of the muscle. This is an extremely versatile flap and can rather reliably transport large amounts of skin from the lower abdominal region to the upper chest. It has had its greatest use in postmastectomy reconstruction, and in some cases both muscles are used to increase the vascular supply to the overlying tissues. It is being used commonly as a free flap.

Latissimus Dorsi Flap ■ This flap is still very useful in breast reconstruction cases, and the narrow, mobile pedicle allows for a great range of application to the anterior as well as the posterior and lateral trunk. This is in addition to its usefulness in head and neck reconstruction and free flap transfers, as previously noted.

Groin Flap ■ This was one of the first flaps used for microvascular free flap transfer. Its use as a free flap has diminished with the establishment of other flaps that have more reliable vascular pedicles. It is still useful as a pedicle flap, since the donor site is reasonably well hidden and the nonhair-bearing, elastic, and pliable nature of the skin represent real advantages, as does the size of the flap that can be raised and the arc of rotation afforded by the pedicle. It can reach the upper thigh as well as the upper and contralateral abdomen (Figure 32–6).

Extremity Flaps

Deltoid Flap ■ The deltoid upper arm flap is a fasciocutaneous flap based on the posterior circumflex humeral artery. The donor defect requires a skin graft for closure that is cosmetically deforming.

Medial Arm Flap ■ The blood supply to this flap is less reliable than that of the deltoid flap, but the donor defect can be closed primarily in most cases, and the skin quality of the upper inner arm has advantages in neck and facial free flap situations.

Lateral Arm Flap ■ This flap is based on the profunda brachii artery. It can be based on a long vascular pedicle, and a neurosensory flap can be used in free flap transfer situations owing to a reliable neurovascular pedicle. The donor site often can be closed directly.

Radial Forearm Flap ■ Provided there is adequate blood supply to the donor extremity from the ulnar artery, the radial forearm, or Chinese flap, has great reliability and usefulness, particularly as a free flap. The radial artery itself is the vascular supply, along with large venous tributaries that make microanastomosis easier than with other free flaps. Segments of distal radius can be included, with overlying skin making up a fascio-osteocutaneous flap. The drawbacks of this flap are the need for skin grafts with larger defects to cover the donor site and the cosmetic deformity resulting from its use.

Biceps Brachii Flap ■ This flap is used only if alternatives fail, as this muscle is not expendable. It can be used to cover defects in the axilla and upper arm.

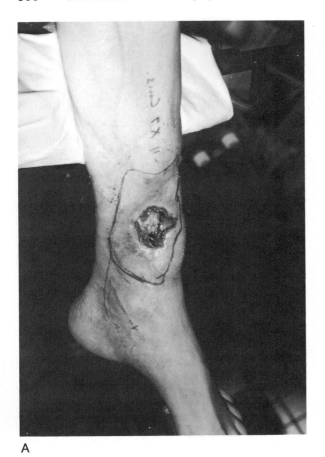

A

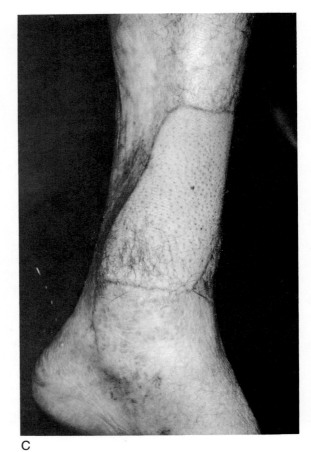

C

Outline of groin flap

Femoral artery

Femoral vein

Superficial circumflex artery and vein

B

Figure 32–6

Free microvascular groin flap to the right lower leg. A, Chronic ulceration of the right lower leg with osteomyelitis. The recipient artery and veins are labeled near the instep. B, Diagram of the groin flap, showing the superficial circumflex artery and vein as they come off the femoral artery and vein in the medial groin. This area can supply a large soft tissue cover, and the skin laxity often allows for a primary closure of the wound without need for a skin graft. C, The completed groin flap in place at 5 months postoperatively shows complete healing of bone with good soft tissue coverage.

Brachioradialis Flap ▪ This flap is suitable to cover defects in the upper forearm, lower arm, and antecubital fossa. Unlike the biceps brachii muscle, this flexor of the forearm is relatively expendable.

Flexor Carpi Ulnaris Flap ▪ Coverage of the antecubital fossa, arm, and forearm are the applications of this flap as a muscular flap or a myocutaneous flap.

Hand Flap ▪ Several hand muscles can serve for coverage of critical structures or to restore function, but their usage is rare. Among these units are the first dorsal interosseous, the abductor digit minimi, and the abductor pollicis brevis.

Lower Extremity Flaps

Cross-Leg Flap ▪ For years the most challenging problems in reconstruction in plastic surgery dealt with defects in the lower extremity. The dependent nature of the lower extremity and the relatively poor blood supply contributed to these problems. The vascular supply to the skin territories as well as the functional muscle units was not adequately understood. Serious fractures of the anterior tibial region requiring open reduction often led to skin necrosis, exposure of hardware, and osteomyelitis. The cross-leg flap was the major method for reconstruction, including coverage of defects of the forefoot and heel areas. This was a two-stage method in which a random skin flap was elevated from the good leg, according to comfort and position, and the flap was then sutured over the defect on the injured leg. After a delay of about 2 weeks, during which time the patient remained at complete bed rest, the flap could be safely divided, and the donor area was usually covered with a skin graft. This method still has its advocates but has been largely supplanted by various muscle flaps or skin-muscle units or free flaps.

Gracilis Flap ▪ This flap has a good arc of rotation and a proximal vascular pedicle that allows excellent coverage in the perineal area, groin, lower abdominal wall, and ischium. It has been used for vaginal reconstruction as well as coverage of pressure ulcers. This is an expendable muscle unit.

Sartorius Flap ▪ This muscle flap is another expendable unit. It has applicability for coverage of the groin, femoral area, and knee.

Rectus Femoris Flap ▪ This can serve as a muscle flap, myocutaneous flap, or free flap and can cover the abdominal wall, groin, perineum, trochanter, and ischium. The latter two areas are the sites of pressure ulcers, and this muscle is expendable in that situation.

Vastus Lateralis Flap ▪ This flap has use in pressure ulcers, especially the trochanteric and ischial types.

Tensor Fascia Lata Flap ▪ This flap has had extensive use and has one of the widest applications of lower extremity flaps. It can be used with the overlying skin safely and also as a free flap. Its arc of rotation can reach the upper abdomen and medial and posterior thigh and buttock region, and it can comfortably be used as staged reconstruction for the forearm and hand (see Figure 32–3A)

Gluteus Maximus Flap ▪ This flap, along with the posterior thigh muscles, the biceps femoris, the semitendinosus, and the semimembranosus, finds great usage in the coverage of pressure ulcers of the sacrum, ischium, perineum, buttocks, and trochanteric areas.

Gastrocnemius Flap ▪ This versatile flap may be used as a muscle, myocutaneous, or free flap. Its coverage range includes the knee and the upper one third of the lower leg. It can be used as a skin-muscle cross-leg flap in a two-stage procedure that is similar to the previously mentioned cross-leg flaps. However, it is safer because there is a more reliable blood supply, and a longer pedicle can improve the position and, therefore, patient comfort during the delay period. Either the medial or lateral head of the gastrocnemius muscle can be used, allowing for coverage to either side of the extremity.

Soleus Flap ▪ This flat, fish-shaped (sole) muscle flap serves for coverage of the middle third of the leg.

Tibialis Anterior (Anticus) Flap ▪ This flap can serve as a muscle or skin-muscle flap for coverage of the middle third of the leg.

Extensor Digitorum Longus Flap ▪ This muscle flap, along with the extensor hallucis longus muscle flap, can cover defects of the lower third of the leg.

Peroneus Longus and Peroneus Brevis Flaps ▪ These are utilized for smaller defects of the middle third or lower third of the lateral or medial leg.

Abductor Hallucis Flap ▪ The muscles in the foot, including the flexor digitorum brevis, the abductor digiti minimi, and the extensor digitorum brevis, have all found purpose in the coverage of small to moderate-sized areas in the heel, medial ankle, and lateral ankle. Free functional muscle transfer, as for facial reanimation, has also been described.

Fibula Flap ■ The fibula is an excellent donor site for vascularized bone, and an osteocutaneous flap can be taken if skin is also needed.

Dorsalis Pedis Flap ■ This is a skin flap and has usage for local coverage in the medial and lateral foot and ankle, as well as a free flap. The donor area requires a skin graft, and this can be a troublesome area postoperatively with regard to footwear comfort.

Toe-to-Thumb Flap ■ This free tissue flap transfer is used to reconstruct a missing thumb. The great toe or second toe is commonly used, and the nerves as well as the vessels are anastomosed to restore sensation to the new thumb. This is referred to as a pollicization procedure.

RECONSTRUCTION OF CONGENITAL DEFORMITIES

Cleft Lip and Palate ■ The most common serious congenital deformity of the head and neck is cleft lip and palate. Either can occur as an isolated condition but more commonly they occur together. There is a definite hereditary tendency, and it is seen in about 1 in 700 to 1000 births, although some racial groups have an occurrence rate almost twice that. The term *harelip,* a reference to the cleft in the midline of a rabbit's upper lip, is antiquated and demeaning and should not be used.

A cleft lip may be partial or complete, depending on whether or not it goes completely through the nostril. Furthermore, it may be unilateral or bilateral. Simonart's band is that bridge of tissue in an incomplete cleft that holds the medial and lateral nostril together.

Clefts of the palate also may be described as complete or incomplete. The palate is divided into the primary palate, that portion anterior to the incisive foramen, and the secondary palate, that portion behind the foramen. About one third is anterior to the foramen and two thirds posterior.

A number of names are associated with repairs of the cleft lip. Commonly performed procedures bear the names of Randall-Tennison, Rose-

Thompson, Lemesurier, Millard, Skoog, and Manchester. Secondary repairs as the child grows are common and often have as much to do with residual nasal deformities as they do with lip deformities. Some of the names used in various secondary repairs are Schjelderup, Wilkie, Dibbell, and Cronin. In severely deficient clefts, an Abbé flap from the lower to upper lip is used to add length (see Figures 32–5 and 32–7).

Cleft lip repairs are performed when the child is about 3 months of age, whereas palatal repairs are generally performed at closer to 1 year of age. In the hard palate, the function of the jaws and dentition are important, but in the soft palate the primary function is speech. Cleft palate speech is characterized by escape of air through the nose, which is referred to as nasal emission. The soft palate, or velum, may not close properly to the posterior pharyngeal wall in a cleft patient, which leads to the speech abnormality. This abnormality is described as velopharyngeal incompetence, or VPI*. Operative procedures to close the hard and soft palate are concerned with avoiding or minimizing VPI. Common procedures are Von Langenbeck's procedure, Wardill-Killner repair, and more recently the double-opposing Z-plasty technique described by Furlough. Peristent VPI not corrected by speech therapy may require additional operations using an inferiorly or superiorly based pharyngeal flap to the velum to direct airflow from the nose to the mouth. A technique known as pharyngoplasty, particularly one described by Orticochea, has produced good speech in secondary cases.

Other Congenital Abnormalities ■ Less common anomalies of the head and neck are seen in plastic surgery, such as the first and second branchial arch syndrome, also known as hemifacial microsomia. Children with this condition have varying degrees of microtia (underdevelopment of the external ear), hypoplasia of the middle ear, often with hearing loss, and underdevelopment of the facial bones and muscles.

Treacher Collins syndrome is associated with hypoplasia of the facial bones and external and middle ears, macrostomia (enlarged mouth), a

---

*Two words that transcriptionists sometimes have difficulty in understanding when transcribing dictation are the words "velopharyngeal" and "alveolopalatal." *Velopharyngeal* means pertaining to the soft palate and pharynx; *alveolopalatal* means pertaining to the alveolar process and palate.

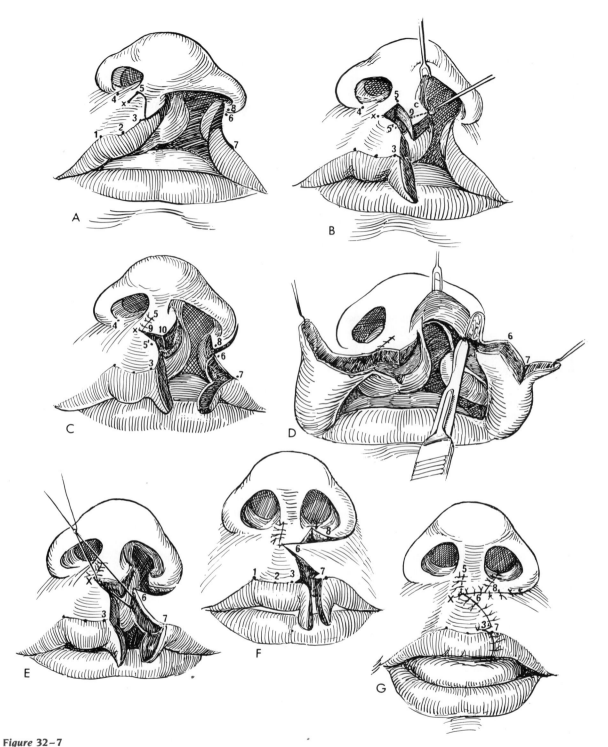

Figure 32–7

The Millard II rotation-advancement repair. A, Design of flap. B, C, and D, Incisions made and tissues mobilized. E and F, Layered closure of tissues. G, Final appearance at completion of repair. (From Converse, John M. *Reconstructive Plastic Surgery*, Vol. 4. W. B. Saunders Co., Philadelphia, 1977, p. 2044.)

high-arched palate with abnormal dentition, an abnormal slant to the eyes with notching (colobomas) of the lower eyelids, and other facial abnormalities.

Crouzon's syndrome has similar abnormalities, including a high prominent forehead with exophthalmos and hypertelorism. In Apert's syndrome (the "t" in Apert is silent), the deformities are much like those in Crouzon's but there also are hand anomalies such as syndactyly, polydactyly, and clinodactyly.

An acquired deformity, hemifacial atrophy (Romberg's disease), bears mention as it is common and can occur in younger individuals. The cause is unknown but it involves progressive atrophy of the soft tissues of one side of the face. The characteristic depressions along the forehead, medial cheek, and chin produce a sabre-like indentation referred to as the "coup de sabre." Free flap transfers are now frequently used to correct the soft tissue deficits.

BURN RECONSTRUCTION

Burns are among the most severe injuries a person can sustain. They can be from chemicals, scalds, electricity, and heat. Classification utilizes the first, second, and third degrees as the burn type, with the first degree being the most superficial (sunburn) and the third degree being deepest (loss of skin down to the subcutaneous level). Prior to grafting, burned areas are dressed with topical antimicrobial agents, such as silver nitrate, mafenide acetate cream (Sulfamylon), or silver sulfadiazine cream (Silvadene). Most of the surgical effort is directed toward obtaining healing by skin grafting. Debridement of the nonviable tissue (referred to as eschar, meaning "scab" in Greek) is often done by tangential excision using a freehand guarded blade. Most often split-thickness skin grafts are harvested, but certain critical areas, especially the face, require full-thickness grafts for mobility as well as appearance.

The late surgical treatment of burns may be for functional or aesthetic reasons. Burns cause severe restrictive contracture, particularly in flexor areas such as the anterior neck, axilla, and antecubital fossa. Multiple Z-plasties and other tissue rearrangements are performed to eliminate the scar and break up the contractures.

Local flaps, including skin and myocutaneous flaps, may be used in late reconstruction as may free flaps. Eyelid, perioral, nasal, and auricular burn deformities and contractures often present the most challenging areas of reconstruction.

BREAST SURGERY

Breast cancer has been increasing in incidence in the past few decades, and despite the increase in earlier detection and nonsurgical treatment, such as lumpectomy and radiation, a great number of mastectomies are performed each year. In addition, many women who are at high risk owing to strong family histories for the disease or a particular type of mastopathy (i.e., intraductal papillomatosis or atypical hyperplasia) undergo prophylactic total or subcutaneous mastectomy. Methods of reconstruction have become increasingly more sophisticated, and the results are gradually improving. In some communities, immediate reconstruction following mastectomy is becoming more commonplace.

Reconstruction of the female breast can be undertaken with an internal prosthesis, or implant, by the use of autogenous tissue, such as skin-muscle flaps, or with both. The trend has been toward less radical soft tissue resection in ablative breast surgery, and in some cases the use of a specialized mammary implant can serve as a simple and effective method to reconstruct the breast mound. Implants are filled with saline or silicone gel, or sometimes they are compartmentalized and have both saline and gel. Becker's implant can be inflated in situ with saline and left in position until the desired size has been achieved. Some physicians have stacked implants of differing sizes to achieve a more natural shape and projection. When skin coverage is tight, the use of soft tissue expanders has become quite common. They are gradually inflated and often overinflated for several weeks or months. After the skin has sufficiently relaxed, they can be replaced with a permanent implant. The position of an implant or an expander may be under the subcutaneous fat or under the muscle, depending upon the thickness of the subcutaneous fat and the preference of the surgeon. The technique of subpectoral-subserratus muscle implantation following subcutaneous mastectomy has been refined by Jarrett.

Mammary implants were traditionally smooth surfaced. One type of implant had a textured polyurethane covering on the surface that allowed tissue ingrowth. This seemed to diminish the incidence of contracture of the scar tissue that would normally build up around the implant. When the scar tissue would contract, referred to as a capsular or spherical contracture, the implant and, therefore, the breast would feel hard or firm. Other manufacturers have textured the surfaces of their implants in order to decrease the incidence of capsular contracture, but that problem still represents the most common complication of breast implant surgery. A contracture severe enough to be uncomfortable or disfiguring usually requires surgical management (Figure 32–8).

More recent advances in breast reconstruction involve the use of specialized flaps that can be used alone to reconstruct the breast mound or in some instances used with an implant. Examples of such flaps include the transverse rectus abdominis myocutaneous flap (TRAM flap); the latissimus dorsi myocutaneous flap; and more recently free flaps, including the free TRAM flap, the superior gluteal flap, the inferior gluteal flap, and the lateral thigh flap (Figures 32–9 and 32–10).

The art of nipple reconstruction has evolved over the decades. Autogenous tissues included grafts harvested from the labia majora and labia minora, the earlobe, the tip of the toe, and the opposite nipple. The areola has been reconstructed using skin grafts from various areas; techniques of sharing skin from the opposite areola, if it is large enough, have been successful. Tattooing has also been successfully used to create an areola. Most recently the use of local flaps, such as the skate flap, the S-flap, and the Maltese cross–patterned flap, has become popular.

Reduction Mammaplasty ■ Macromastia, hypermastia, mammary hyperplasia, gigantomastia, mammary hypertrophy, and juvenile mammary hyperplasia are all terms used to describe enlargement of the female breast. Having breasts that are proportionately larger than a woman's frame can be both embarrassing as well as debilitating. Breast reduction surgery is quite reliable, and satisfying results can be expected in most cases. In many cases, it is not possible to preserve normal nipple sensation or lactational function, so the alternatives must be carefully weighed by the patient (Figure 32–11.)

Surgeons have a number of methods from which to choose. These differ primarily in the means by which the nipple is transferred to its new location. In extremely large breasts, the nipple-areolar complex may be removed as a full-thickness graft and then replaced over a deepithelialized circular area in the appropriate position, after the breast has been reduced. It is more common, however, to leave the nipple-areola complex attached to a vascular pedicle

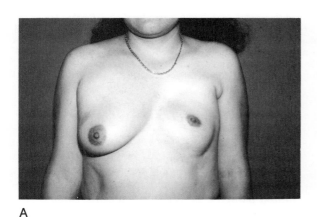

A

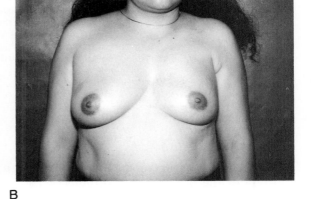

B

Figure 32–8

Reconstruction of the breast from a congenital deformity. A, The congenital deformity of a 22-year-old woman with absence of the left pectoralis major muscle and hypoplasia of the left breast (Poland's syndrome). B, Postoperative result after correction of the deformity, using a polyurethane breast implant along with creation of the left mammary fold.

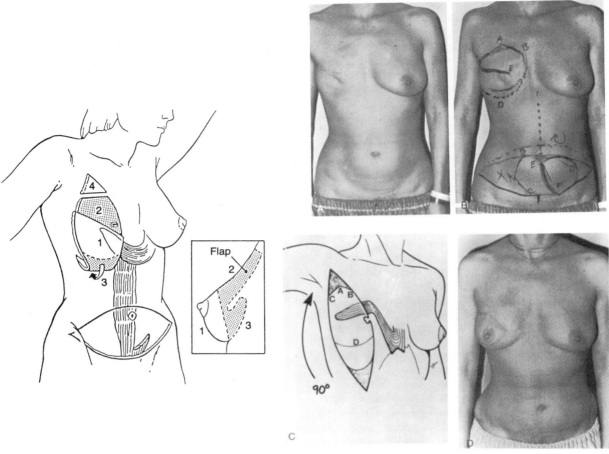

Figure 32–9

Technique of vertical inset in breast reconstruction with the transverse rectus abdominis myocutaneous (TRAM) flap. (After Hartrampf, C. R., Jr. *Transverse Abdominal Island Flap Technique for Breast Reconstruction After Mastectomy.* University Park Press, Baltimore, 1984, p. 106.) A and B, Preoperatively, showing the mastectomy defect and markings. The flap will be elevated on a contralateral muscle pedicle. C, The flap is rotated clockwise along an 80- to 90-degree arc for transfer to the chest wall. Shaded areas will be discarded. D, Postoperatively, after nipple reconstruction and areolar tattooing. (From Hartrampf, C. R., Jr. The transverse abdominal island flap for breast reconstruction. A 7-year experience. *Clinics in Plastic Surgery* 15(4):703, 1988.)

consisting of dermis, subcutaneous fat, and a portion of the breast tissue. Strombeck used a horizontal bipedicle dermal flap to transpose the nipple, whereas McKissock used a vertical bipedicle flap. Superior, lateral, and medial pedicles have been championed by some and central breast tissue pedicles by others. Recently, a method using an inferior pedicle has been promoted as being better in preserving innervation to the nipple-areola complex while maintaining a reliable blood supply. The majority of these techniques use the pattern first described by Wise to help resect the excess skin and underlying breast tissue.

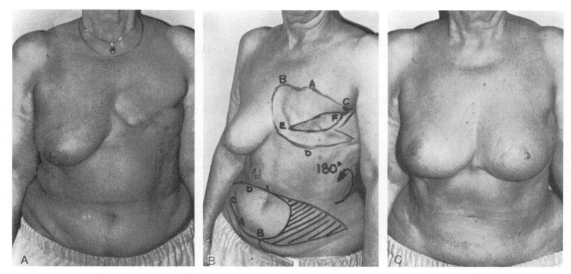

Figure 32–10
Breast reconstruction with the lower TRAM flap. A, The mastectomy defect is wide and extends into the lateral chest. B, To avoid the atypical appendectomy scar, the flap is designed higher on the abdomen. The transfer involves 180-degree counterclockwise rotation of the flap on a contralateral rectus pedicle. C, One year after reconstruction and simultaneous reduction of the opposite breast. (From Hartrampf, C. R., Jr. The transverse abdominal island flap for breast reconstruction. A 7-year experience. *Clinics in Plastic Surgery* 15(4):703, 1988.)

Mastopexy ■ Breast ptosis is usually categorized as first, second, or third degree, depending upon the laxity and droop of the breast tissues. *Mastopexy* is the term used to describe the uplift procedure that involves removal of the excess skin, tightening of the internal breast tissue, and transposing the nipple-areola complex into a new and higher position. Wise's pattern is still popularly used, but some have sought to use patterns that would diminish the length and number of scars. The "donut"* mastopexy is carried

_____

*Also spelled doughnut.

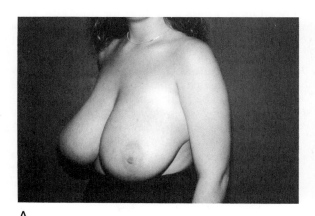

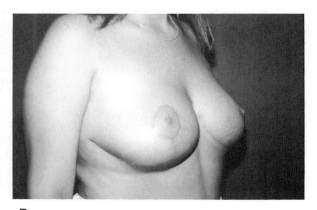

A   B

Figure 32–11
Breast reduction. A, Oblique view of a 20-year-old woman with marked juvenile mammary hyperplasia. B, Postoperative result of a reduction mammaplasty using the inferior pedicle technique to transfer the nipples to a new position.

out through the areola, and some prefer this for minor degrees of correction. In some ptotic breasts, an implant may be placed at the time of mastopexy or in the second stage.

One unusual developmental deformity worthy of note is Poland's syndrome. This syndrome consists of absence of the pectoralis major muscle and a severely underdeveloped breast on the affected side. The latissimus dorsi, as a muscle flap, can be rotated into the chest to provide coverage under the chest wall skin as well as an anterior axillary fold. A mammary implant may then be placed beneath the muscle to create the breast mound.

Another variation in development is the tuberous breast, often referred to as the "Snoopy" breast after the cartoon character. The subareolar area is greatly expanded in this condition, giving a "double-bubble" effect. The areola itself is often greatly enlarged, and that area may be larger than the breast itself. Correction consists of a reduction in the size of the areola and a telescoping inward of the areolar breast tissue. If the breast is quite small, an implant can be employed in the correction.

Figure 32–12 is an example of an operative report on a reduction mammaplasty.

Augmentation Mammaplasty ■ Breast enlargement usually involves placement of a mammary implant beneath either the breast or the pectoralis major muscle. Surgical approaches include transaxillary, periareolar inframammary, and, more recently, an umbilical approach involving laparoscopy, which has shown promise.

COSMETIC SURGERY

The past quarter of a century has seen the refinement and gradual acceptance of cosmetic surgery. Results are becoming more natural and predictable, and most of the procedures can be performed safely and comfortably in an outpatient setting. Many physicians have developed private and accredited ambulatory surgical centers that appeal more to the public than the traditional hospital setting. Anesthetic techniques have now been geared to the outpatient setting, and newer agents afford a quicker recovery and lower incidence of side effects, such as nausea and vomiting, than was seen in the past.

Otoplasty ■ Otoplasty is the term used for correction of prominent ears. The technique involves weakening of the cartilage to allow the ears to fold back into a more natural position. The usual cause of the deformity is the lack of a fold in the superior crus of the antihelix. A cartilage morselizer, which is an instrument that can weaken cartilage much like a tenderizer, is often used along the area in which the fold is desired. Horizontal mattress sutures, described by Mustardé, will hold the position of correction until scar tissue secures it. In some cases, the concha of the ear must be recessed also.

Rhinoplasty ■ The technique of rhinoplasty has evolved greatly in the past few years. The trend has been to a more natural and less surgical look, and this has led to greater use of cartilage shaping and cartilage grafting and a more conservative approach to the bony aspect of the procedure. Fewer osteotomies are performed, thus avoiding the overly narrowed or collapsed look over the nasal dorsum. The open rhinoplasty approach has become increasingly popular for difficult and secondary rhinoplasty because it affords a direct look at the structures involved and allows grafts to be accurately placed and fixed. Some use this method almost exclusively, arguing that the midcolumellar scar is inconsequential compared with the benefits of this approach. Septal cartilage, vomer, and outer table cranial bone grafts have been used in contouring the nasal dorsum. When insufficient cartilage is available, ear cartilage and occasionally rib cartilage have been used successfully as dorsal onlay grafts as well as for tip grafts. Septoplasty and inferior turbinate resection can be performed at the same time as rhinoplasty if functional improvement in airway is needed.

Chin Augmentation ■ This is commonly performed with rhinoplasty if the chin profile is weak. This sets a balance to the facial configuration and often further enhances the result of the rhinoplasty. A Silastic or other synthetic conforming implant is placed from either the intraoral or submental approach. Occasionally, a sliding genioplasty is performed to increase or decrease chin prominence through the intraoral route, using wire fixation of the sliding segment.

Facelift Procedures ■ These have become much more sophisticated in the past few decades. This procedure, often termed *rhytidectomy* or *meloplasty,* involves pre- and postauricular incisions extending into the temple and occipital areas. Wide undermining of the neck and facial skin allows access to underlying structures, including the platysma muscle and the superficial musculoaponeurotic system (referred to as the SMAS layer). Submental incisions are also used to allow access to the platysmal muscle bands and the submental fatpad. Liposuction or direct defatting is common in the neck and submental region and occasionally along the margin of the mandible and the cheek. The SMAS system and platysma muscles may be folded upon themselves (plication) or undermined and overlapped (imbrication) to tighten the deeper layers. A deep-plane rhytidectomy at or beneath the layers of the facial muscles is now being performed by some as well as a deeper subperiosteal approach, although the latter is more commonly performed with forehead lifts (Figures 32–13 and 32–14).

Forehead and brow lifts have become increasingly more common in conjunction with facelifts and are occasionally performed alone. The incisions may be in the forehead itself, usually at the hairline (the pretrichial incision) and less commonly just above the brows (supraciliary) or even the midforehead. If the forehead is not high, the approach most often used is about 6 cm. behind the hairline of the frontal scalp. This incision, usually called a coronal forehead or browlift approach, can conveniently connect with the standard facelift incisions in the temple regions. The undermining is carried deep to the glabellar and brow regions, and care is taken to preserve the supraorbital and supratrochlear nerves. The muscles in the area, including the frontalis, the procerus, and the corrugator, may be incised, removed, or cauterized to weaken their activity. Skin staples are often used to close the defect in the hair-bearing portion of the incision.

Lid Procedures ▪ Upper and lower lid corrective surgery is termed *blepharoplasty* and may be performed along with other corrective facial procedures, such as rhytidectomy and coronal brow lift. Deep to the muscle is the orbital septum, which may be approached transconjunctivally or through an infraciliary (also called a subciliary) incision. Behind this thin layer are the orbital fat compartments that contribute to excessive fullness and, especially in the lower lids, the "baggy eyes" look. In the lower lids,

removal of the excessive fat will smooth out the appearance, and usually only a small amount of skin and/or muscle is also resected. Excessive resection, weak lid tone, and other factors may lead to ectropion or an increased scleral show. In the upper eyelids, the primary objective is to remove the excessive skin (and occasionally excessive orbicularis oculi muscle) that creates a heavy or tired appearance to the eyes. In some individuals, the redundant skin folds can rest on or over the lashes, causing functional problems such as lash ptosis or even visual field obstruction.

Skin Peels ▪ Chemical peels and dermabrasion have had long-standing popularity as methods of improving the texture and appearance of the skin. Peels, in general, have been used for aging and sun-damaged skin, whereas dermabrasion has been used for acne and other facial scarring. The phenol peel has had several decades of usage; the trichloroacetic acid, or TCA, peel has become widely used more recently. Some physicians will use dermabrasion after a phenol peel as a combined procedure.

Body Contouring and Liposuction ▪ Body contouring is the shaping of specific areas of the body into more aesthetically pleasing outlines. Traditionally, this was done by direct surgical excision alone, but now additional refinements can be made with the use of liposuction (also referred to as suction-assisted lipolysis or SAL, suction lipectomy, and fat suction) and fat reinjection.

Liposuction has become an accepted procedure in the United States since its introduction from Europe in 1981. The uses and limitations have become more familiar to the plastic surgeon, and it is among the safest procedures performed. The most common complication is surface irregularity in the treated areas. This may be very minor or extreme. The use of smaller cannulas allows for a more controlled evacuation, which can minimize unsightly depressions. Some advocate the use of the syringe technique to avoid the higher pressures and what they believe to be greater soft tissue injury with the suction pumps. The Illouz blunt-tipped cannulas are primarily used. There is a great variation in size, length, number of holes, position of the openings, and shape of the tip. Some tips are flattened somewhat and are given descriptive names, such as cobra tip or spatula tip. Cannulas

UNIVERSITY HOSPITAL
1234 Main Street
Oxnard, CA 93030-0000

Patient: Jane Doe   Time started: 7:00 A.M.
Surgeon: David Smith, M. D.   Time finished: 9:30 A.M.
Assistant Surgeon: Ray Jonson, M. D.   Record # 39090-03
Circulator: Beth Evans, R. N.

OPERATIVE REPORT

PREOPERATIVE DIAGNOSIS: Macromastia.

POSTOPERATIVE DIAGNOSIS: Same.

OPERATION: Bilateral reduction mammaplasty.

ANESTHESIA: General endotracheal.

FINDINGS: The patient is a 34-year-old transcriptionist
                               with double D-cup sized breasts with
symptoms of upper back, neck, and shoulder problems. She had approximately
750 grams resected from each side. An inferior pedicle was used to transfer the
nipple areolar complex into its new position. Mild fibrocystic disease was noted
on both sides and the specimens were submitted fresh for evaluation. There was
no evidence of malignancy and permanent histology is pending.

PROCEDURE: Following infiltration of 1% Xylocaine   with
                               epinephrine along the incision lines
preoperative markings were followed using the Wise pattern and the inferior
pedicle was developed by de-epithelializing the overlying skin. Remaining
incisions were then made and the lateral and medial portions of breast tissue to
be resected were then removed using the cautery. The central breast tissue
was also removed as was a portion superiorly.

After careful control of bleeding, the breast was reshaped using interrupted #4-0
Vicryl sutures to join the lateral and medial flaps with the mid-inferior suture line.
The vertical incision was closed in layers of #4-0 Vicryl interrupted and a running
subcuticular #5-0 Prolene. The inframammary incision was closed with
interrupted #4-0 Vicryl and running subcuticular #4-0 Prolene. The nipple-
areolar complex was positioned and closed in layers with #5-0 Vicryl interrupted
at the dermal layer and a running horizontal mattress #6-0 Prolene for the skin.
Suction drains were brought out through separate stab wounds and a bulky

(continued)

Figure 32–12
An operative report of a bilateral reduction mammaplasty, using the indented format.

Page 2
Name: Jane Doe
Record # 39090-03

dressing was applied. Blood loss estimated at 150 cc. Nipple color was good at the end of the procedure. The patient was discharged to the recovery room in satisfactory condition.

_____
                    David Smith, M. D.

mtf
D: 11/21/94
T: 11/21/94

Figure 32–12 Continued

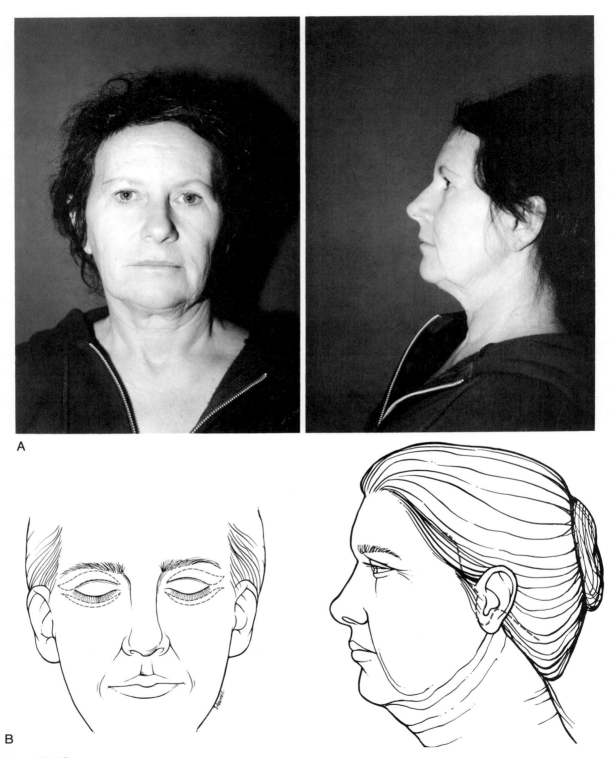

A

B

Figure 32–13

Cosmetic surgery. A, Front and side view photographs of the patient before the operative procedure. B, Diagrams for cosmetic surgery, showing the incisions made on either side of the face from inside the hairline at the temples, around the earlobe, to the lower scalp. The incisions follow natural contour lines in the upper and lower lids to provide access to skin and fatty tissue.

618

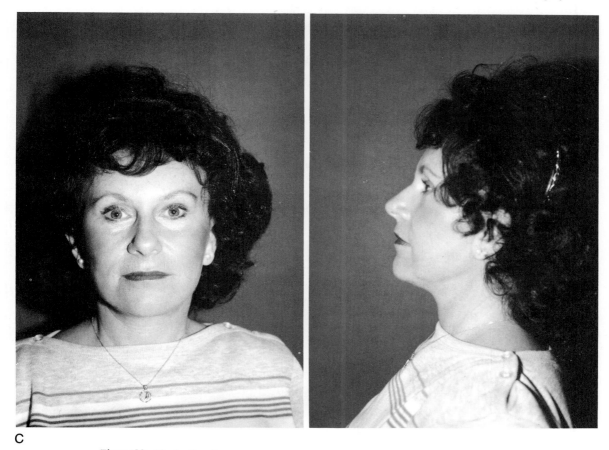

C

Figure 32–13 *Continued*
C, Front and side view photographs of the patient after the operative procedure.

with three holes around the tip are called the Mercedes tip. Fluid replacement is critical, particularly when large volumes of fat are aspirated (2000 to 3000 cc. or more). Some physicians are using freshly aspirated fat to reinject as filler for various contour deformities.

Abdominoplasty ▪ Abdominoplasty (also referred to as abdominal dermolipectomy and tummy tuck) is probably one of the most commonly performed of the body-contouring procedures. Tightening of the abdominal wall fascia is usually performed along with the resection of a good portion of the lax abdominal skin and subcutaneous fat. Many skin incisions have been used, but most popular is the lower incision that lies just above the pubic area and within the bikini bathing suit area. The French-cut bathing suit has required some modification: it has re-

quired that the lateral portions of the incision be brought outward in a higher position. In patients with massive abdominal aprons, the incisions may extend almost circumferentially about the patient. Liposuction may be performed with abdominoplasty to remove fullness in the resulting lateral folds, also referred to as "dog ears."

Thigh Lift ▪ Medial and lateral thigh lift has been refined more recently by Lockwood, who advocates anchoring the flaps in the medial lift to Colles' fascia and combining liposuction where necessary.

Brachioplasty ▪ This is the term describing the procedure for correction of flaccid, hanging arm skin, often termed the "batwing deformity." Variations abound, but the most common incisions are along the inner aspect of the arm from the axilla to the elbow. Liposuction may enhance

UNIVERSITY HOSPITAL
1234 Main Street
Oxnard, CA 93030-0000

Patient: Jane Jones
Surgeon: David Smith, M. D.
Assistant Surgeon: Ray Jonson, M. D.
Circulator: Beth Evans, R. N.

Time started: 7:00 A.M.
Time finished: 8:30 A.M.
Record # 28090-03

OPERATIVE REPORT

Preoperative Diagnosis:
Facial cutaneous laxity with bilateral upper lid blepharochalasis and lower lid fat compartment fullness.

Postoperative Diagnosis:
Facial cutaneous laxity with bilateral upper lid blepharochalasis and lower lid fat compartment fullness.

Operation:
Rhytidectomy with bilateral upper and   lower lid blepharoplasty.

Anesthesia:
IV sedation with Versed, Nubaine, and Ketamine; 0.5% Xylocaine and 0.25% Marcaine with epinephrine 1:200,000 local infiltration.

Findings:
The patient is a 47-year-old female with excessive skin redundancy of the upper lids and fullness of the lower lids due to excessive medial and mid-compartment fat excess. She had moderate jowl formation and fullness in the submental region as well as prominent platysmal bands in the mid-anterior neck.

Procedure:
Following infiltration of local, skin-muscle flaps were developed through an infraciliary lower lid incision. The orbital septum was divided and with gentle pressure on the globe the prominent fat was displayed. The mid and medial fat compartment excess was removed by clamping across the base, resecting the excess and treating the pedicle with bipolar. No bleeding was encountered upon release of the pedicle and the premarked redundant skin and muscle was removed. The wound was closed with running horizontal mattress 7-0 Prolene.

Next, a generous ellipse of upper lid skin was removed following preop markings. Bleeding was controlled with bipolar and the medial compartment fullness was dissected free and removed as in the lower lids. The wound was closed with a running subcuticular 7-0 Prolene reinforced with Steri-strips.
(continued)

Figure 32–14
An operative report of a rhytidectomy and blepharoplasty, prepared in full-block format.

Page 2
Hosp. No. 28090-03
Patient's Name: Jane Jones

A submental incision was made next and wide undermining carried out just superficial to the platysma muscles. The medial borders were plicated from the mentum toward the cervical crease with 4-0 Vicryl interrupted. A Z-plasty was then designed in the muscle edges, and then cut with the elements rotated into their new positions using 4-0 Vicryl. Direct defatting in the submental region was carried out next. The wound was closed with running subcuticular 5-0 Prolene and Steri-strips.

Standard facelift incisions were then made from the temple hairline, along the inner aspect of the tragus and then at the postauricular crease into the occipital hairline. Extensive undermining was carried out at the subcutaneous level connecting to the midline area previously undermined. Some direct defatting was done beneath the margin of the mandible. The SMAS layer in the mid-facial level was incised laterally and undermined for several centimeters medially. The platysma at the level of the mastoid muscle medially was incised and undermined to the midline. The SMAS was then sutured to the surrounding preauricular tissues with 4-0 Vicryl figure-of-eight sutures and the platysma was sutured in a similar fashion to the mastoid fascia. The skin flaps were then rotated into their new position and held in place with key sutures of 5-0 Prolene. The redundant pre- and postauricular skin was then resected and these wounds were closed with a few interrupted 5-0 Prolene sutures and the rest with running subcuticular 5-0 Prolene. The temple and occipital skin excess was then removed and closed in the temple with interrupted 5-0 Prolene and in the occipital area with interrupted 4-0 Vicryl in the dermis and running subcuticular 4-0 Prolene in the skin. Light bulky dressings were then applied along with cool saline compresses to the eyes. EBL - negligible; no drains. Patient tolerated the procedure well and was discharged to the recovery room in good condition.

David Smith, M. D.

mtf
D: 11-20-94
T: 11-20-94

Figure 32–14 Continued

the result, but the primary drawback of this procedure is the resulting scars that are often quite prominent.

INSTRUMENTS USED IN PLASTIC SURGERY

Many physicians do not necessarily dictate the eponymic names of instruments. However, for reference, some of the common instruments used in plastic surgery, including their eponymic names, are listed here.

- Adson forceps
- Aufricht nasal retractor
- Ballenger swivel knife
- bayonet forceps
- Blair cleft palate elevator
- Castroviejo needle holder and forceps
- Cottle septum elevator
- Dingman mouth gag
- Fomon rasp
- Freer elevator
- Gorney facelift scissors
- iris scissors
- Killian septum forceps
- Maltz rasp
- Parkes rasp
- pituitary rongeurs
- Rubin cartilage morselizer
- Senn retractor
- strabismus scissors
- tenotomy scissors
- Webster needle holder

Reference Sources

Baylor University. *Selected Readings in Plastic Surgery.* Baylor University Medical Center, Dallas, Texas, 1986–1991.

Furlow, L. T., Jr. Cleft palate repair by double opposing Z-plasty. *Plastic and Reconstructive Surgery* 78: 724, 1986.

Jarrett, J. R., R. G. Cutler, and D. T. Teal. Subcutaneous mastectomy in small, large, or ptotic breasts with immediate submuscular placement of implants. *Plastic and Reconstructive Surgery* 62: 702-704, 1978.

Juri, J. Use of parieto-occipital flaps in the surgical treatment of baldness. *Plastic and Reconstructive Surgery* 55: 456, 1975.

Lockwood, T. E. Fascial anchoring technique in medial thigh lifts. *Plastic and Reconstructive Surgery* 82: 299, 1988.

Mustarde, J. C. The treatment of prominent ears by buried mattress sutures; a ten-year survey. *Plastic and Reconstructive Surgery* 39: 382, 1967.

Orticochea, M. Construction of a dynamic muscle sphincter in cleft palates. *Plastic and Reconstructive Surgery* 41: 323, 1968.

Wise, R. J. A preliminary report on a method of planning a mammaplasty. *Plastic and Reconstructive Surgery* 17: 367, 1956.

For references of specific application to medical transcription, see Appendix 1.

Michael A. DiGiacomo, D.P.M.

Podiatry

INTRODUCTION

Podiatric medicine is that branch of the healing arts concerned with the diagnosis and treatment of conditions affecting the human foot and ankle, including the local manifestations of systemic conditions, by all appropriate systems and means. The modern podiatrist has undergone the minimum requirements of a baccalaureate degree, successful completion of a medical college admissions test (M.C.A.T.), and four years of podiatric medical education. These four years include 4000 didactic hours, the same as for a medical doctor. In addition, the podiatrist, unlike the dentist, must sit for a residency in foot and ankle surgery in many states for a minimum of 1 year before taking the licensure examination. Podiatric residencies range from 1 to 4 years.

The history of foot care dates back to the earliest records of human history. In 2500 B.C., a picture in a tomb of an Egyptian pharaoh showed foot care being rendered.

The subsequent centuries have seen depictions and descriptions of foot care remedies and treatments. For instance, in 1500 B.C. a discourse on the treatment of the common corn appears in a text entitled *The Evers Papyrus*. This treatise outlined the use of olive oil and cow fat for the treatment of the common corn. Leonardo da Vinci said that "the feet are a mirror of the human body."

In 1686, Fuchs wrote a book, *De Clavo Pedis*, devoted entirely to the condition of the digital corn. President Abraham Lincoln had a foot care provider named Issachar Zacharie for his often-mentioned painful feet. Many podiatry offices display a plaque with a copy of the testimonial Lincoln wrote about the treatments of Dr. Zacharie.

The initial field of foot care in the United States was known as chiropody. This term was coined by an Englishman, Dr. David Lowe, in 1784 and was derived from the French words *chirurgien* (surgeon) and *pied* (foot). In the 1830s and 1840s, many itinerant doctors of the foot were making the rounds throughout the larger cities of the United States, and in 1843, Dr. John Littlefield opened an office in New York.

An organized field of chiropody practice began in the late 1890s when the Pedic Society of New York was organized and developed its own board of examiners. From 1895 to 1912, this board issued certificates to practice after successful completion of an examination. In 1905, New York state created the first legislation authorizing licensure for chiropodists.

The national association changed its name in 1958 to the American Podiatry Association, dropping the word chiropody in favor of podiatry. In 1984, this association became known as the American Podiatric Medical Association.

During the Korean War, podiatrists were given commissioned officer status, and in the late 1960s, foot services provided by podiatrists were covered under the Federal Medicare Act. Medicare recognizes the doctor of podiatric medicine (D.P.M.) as a physician. At present there are approximately 12,000 podiatrists in the United States, contrasted to the 615,000 medical doctors. Approximately 50 per cent of all hospitals in America have podiatrists with staff privileges.

Podiatric residency programs can be found in 181 institutions in 34 states and the District of Columbia. The seven colleges of podiatric medicine maintain affiliations with one or more teaching hospitals accredited by the Joint Commission of Accreditation of Health Care Organizations.

The future needs for podiatrists are ever increasing as our population ages, and the projection is that the more than 50 million patient visits to podiatrists in 1990 will be exceeded greatly by the year 2000.

Podiatrists may be certified by one of three certifying boards recognized by the American Podiatric Medical Association: the American Board of Podiatric Orthopedics, the American Board of Podiatric Public Health, and the American Board of Podiatric Surgery. The typical podiatrist is a solo practitioner; however, podiatrists are integrated with other specialties in many group settings. A study conducted by Johns Hopkins University in 1987, utilizing Medicare Part B data, indicated that podiatric physicians were the physicians of choice for the following procedures: 82 per cent of all hammer-toe operations, 71 per cent of all metatarsal operations, 68 per cent of all bunionectomies; 56 per cent of all rear foot operations, and 77 per cent of all foot care.

ANATOMY

The human foot consists of 26 bones, 33 joints, 11 muscles, and a myriad of nerves, arteries, veins, and lymphatic channels. The foot bones (Figure 33–1) are:

talus (ankle bone)
calcaneus or os calcis (heel bone)
cuboid
cuneiform bones (three in number)
navicular
metatarsals (five in number)
phalanges (two for the hallux, or great toe; three for each of the other digits)

Other bones include two sesamoid bones beneath the first metatarsophalangeal joint (a me-

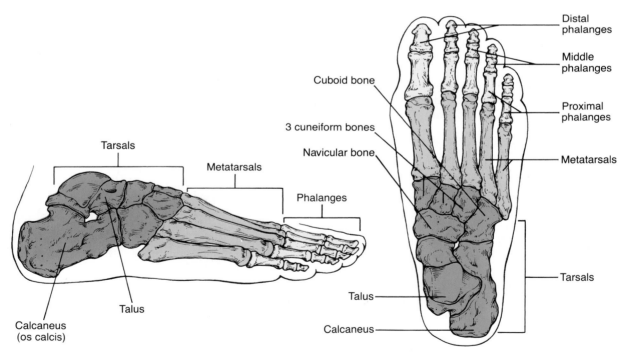

Figure 33–1

Bones of the foot. A, Lateral view. B, View of the dorsal aspect of the right foot (from above).

dial and lateral sesamoid bone, also known as a tibial or fibular sesamoid bone). Additional bones infrequently seen in the human foot are the os navicularis (an extra bone medial to the navicular bone), the os trigonum (behind the talus), and the os peroneus (lateral to the cuboid bone).

Collectively, bones in the toes are known as phalanges, and bones proximal to this are known as metatarsals. Bones in the mid-foot to the rear foot are known as tarsal bones. The talus, or ankle bone, articulates with the two lower leg bones — on the lateral side or outer side as the fibula and the inner border as the tibia. The distal ends of these bones where they articulate with the ankle bone are known as the lateral malleolus for the fibula and medial malleolus for the tibia.

The top of the foot contains only one intrinsic muscle, known as the extensor digitorum brevis muscle. It sends tendons to the great toe, or hallux, and to the next three toes. This muscle is known as brevis because it inserts at the more proximal aspect of the toes in its job of extending or bringing up the toes. Extrinsic muscles that arise outside the foot end as tendons and insert into the distal phalanges. They have the same function of extension and are known as longus tendons. These are the tendons sent forth from the extensor digitorum longus muscle, which arises in the front of the lower leg.

The bottom of the foot consists of four complete layers of muscles. The first layer on the bottom of the foot contains the abductor hallucis, abductor digiti quinti, and flexor digitorum brevis muscles. The second layer consists of the quadratus plantae and lumbricalis muscles. The third layer consists of the flexor hallucis brevis, adductor hallucis, and flexor digiti quinti brevis muscles. The fourth layer consists of the dorsal and plantar interossei muscles. The other important structure on the plantar aspect of the foot is the plantar fascia, which arises from the bottom of the calcaneus, or heel bone, and extends distally into the base of the digits. It is frequently seen in pathologic conditions known as fasciitis or plantar fasciitis and is associated with the formation of a heel spur and the heel spur syndrome.

The primary blood vessels involved with the foot and ankle are the medial and lateral plantar arteries on the bottom of the foot, which extend distally into the toes, there being called the plantar metatarsal and digital arteries. These are an extension of the posterior tibial artery. On the top of the foot, the main supply is by the dorsalis pedis artery, which is an extension of the anterior tibial artery. It bifurcates distally at the toes, extending into the proper digital arteries.

The venous structures important to the foot and ankle are veins on the top of the foot that form the dorsal venous arch, which extends proximally into the saphenous veins. The short saphenous vein begins on the lateral or outer side of the foot and courses proximally, ending in the popliteal vein. The long saphenous vein begins on the medial or inner side of the foot and passes proximately to end in the femoral vein.

REPRESENTATIVE DISEASES

The feet, which on an average take 8,000 to 10,000 steps every day and travel 115,000 miles in a lifetime, can suffer from more than 300 ailments. Four organ systems are represented in the feet — integumentary, neurologic, musculoskeletal, and peripheral vascular. It is convenient to classify ailments or diseases as they afflict the feet into these organ systems.

Integumentary Problems ▪ Integumentary problems deal with all the appendages to the skin as well as the skin itself, that is, the epidermis, nails, and hair. The most common digital deformity associated with the skin is corns (Figure 33–2). Corns on top of the toes are compacted epidermal tissue, usually in an inverted cone shape, with the point being deepest within the foot. These are known as hard corns when on top of the toes and soft corns when between the toes. The most frequent site for a soft corn is between the small and fourth toes. Technical terms for corns are *heloma durum* (hard corn) and *heloma molle* (soft corn).

Calluses are compacted tissue lesions on the bottom of the foot beneath the metatarsal bones; they are referred to as intractable plantar keratomas (IPKs). Porokeratomas are deep plugs of hard epidermal tissue extending into the dermal-epidermal junction of the foot. These are usually thought to be a manifestation of an aberrant sweat duct that becomes keratinized.

Warts are a viral infection of the skin, often

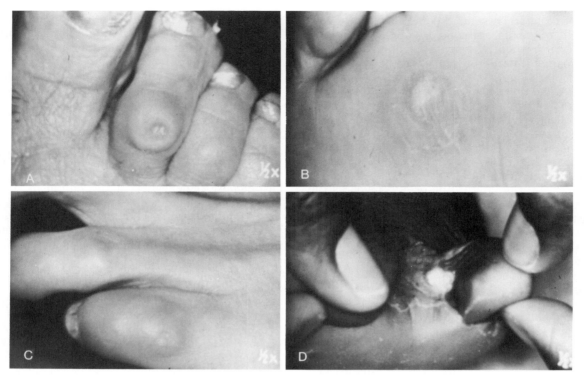

Figure 33–2
Foot corns. A, Heloma durum (hard corn) on top of second toe. B, Corn on the plantar aspect of the foot. C, Heloma durum (hard corn) on top of fifth toe. D, Interdigital heloma molle (soft corn). (Reprinted with permission from The Podiatry Institute, Tucker, Georgia.)

cauliflower in shape (Figure 33–3). If they are on top of the foot, they are known as verruca vulgaris (common warts). Another name is gym warts, as in something that could be picked up in gym class. Warts on the bottom of the foot do not extend outward but are embedded within the foot (verruca plantaris). The bottom of the foot is known as the plantar surface; therefore, a wart on the bottom of the foot is called a plantar wart. A plantar wart is more difficult to treat than a verruca vulgaris, because it is embedded. Treatment with conservative measures is prolonged. Deep enucleation or laser ablation, if needed, is done surgically.

Infrequently, hair follicles on the feet can become infected; this manifestation of an integumentary disease is known as folliculitis. Nails are commonly associated with pathology, most commonly onychomycosis, a fungal infection of the toenail (Figure 33–4). The ingrowing toenail

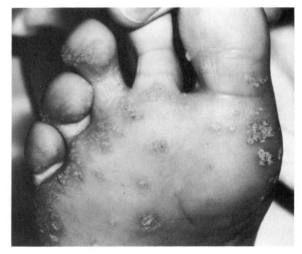

Figure 33–3
Verruca plantaris (plantar foot warts). (Reprinted with permission from The Podiatry Institute, Tucker, Georgia.)

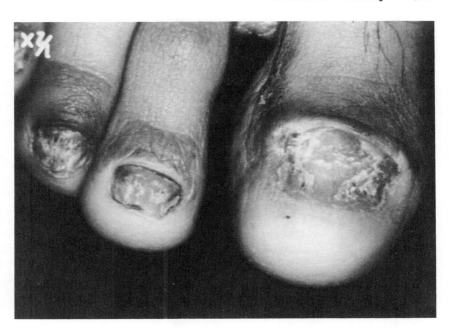

Figure 33–4
Onychomycosis (fungal infection) of the right foot. (Reprinted with permission from The Podiatry Institute, Tucker, Georgia.)

is called onychocryptotic, and the offending border is usually denoted as a medial or lateral border or a tibial or fibular border of the respective toe. Psoriasis is a systemic skin disease that can be manifested in the foot, and nails can become involved with the psoriatic process. These often mimic an onychomycotic toenail in appearance. They are usually differentiated by taking a fungal culture of a suspect toenail; if positive for mycoses, the toenail is known as onychomycotic. An ingrown toenail is called a paronychia; less frequently, a felon (Figure 33–5). Simple thickening of a toenail without evidence of infection or disease is known as onychauxis. A toenail loosened from the nail bed is onycholytic, and the process of the nail separating from the nail bed is onycholysis. Fungal infection involving the skin of the feet is known as tinea pedis. This is sometimes associated with secondary bacterial infection, which can lead to an inflammation of the soft tissues known as cellulitis.

Peripheral Vascular Problems ▪ The peripheral vascular system involving the foot also exhibits numerous pathologic conditions and diseases, the most common of which are associated with diabetes mellitus. Of the 2.1 million people aged 65 and over who have diabetes, more than 63,000 have diabetic foot diseases, and 20 per cent of all people with diabetes who enter a hospital are admitted for foot problems. Diabetes is an insidious disease that involves thickening of the basement membrane of the capillary, the very smallest of the blood vessels. It is at this blood vessel level that red blood cells squeeze between the cells into tissues to bring nourishment and oxygenation. The subtle thickening of the basement membrane that occurs with diabetes ultimately involves malnourishment of peripheral nerves, leading to a progressive and inevitable diminished sensation in the extremities known as diabetic neuropathy. Diabetic patients are prone to arteriosclerotic plaque formation within the arteries and arterioles. It is often noted on radiograph examination that arteries in the ankle and foot can be seen because of the extensive calcification usually associated with diabetes. This is known as arteriosclerosis obliterans (ASO).

Lymphatic problems in the foot are manifested by edema, or fluid collection in the soft tissues (Figure 33–6). This is more pronounced in the afternoon. When a thumb is pushed into the swollen area, a deep impression is made, leaving a pit, which is known as pitting edema. Pitting edema is differentiated from brawny

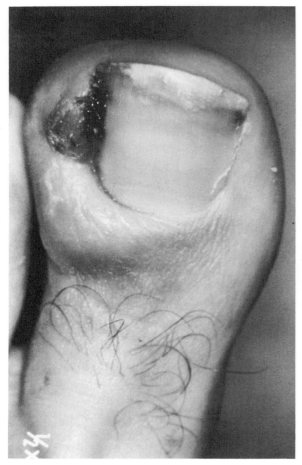

Figure 33–5
Paronychia (ingrown toe nail) of the first toe. (Reprinted with permission from The Podiatry Institute, Tucker, Georgia.)

edema, a more woody or fibrous type of edema in which pressure does not leave any indentation in the soft tissues.

The veins are blood vessels that direct blood back to the heart and have very delicate one-way valves. When these valves become compromised, they allow leakage of fluid backward, creating more back pressure on the veins farthest from the heart. This is manifested as varicosities, or varicose veins, and is associated with a darkening of the skin about the malleoli. It is also associated with deposition of hemoglobin from red blood cells that have leaked out into the soft tissues. When hemoglobin breaks down, it turns into a brown substance known as hemosiderin.

Associated with both arterial and venous problems are various types of compromises in the skin known as ulcerations. These ulcerations, if associated with the veins, are around the ankle, and if they are associated with the arterial supply or with diabetes due to neuropathy, they are on the plantar aspect of the foot. The bed of an ulcer consists of tissue that is devitalized, or lacking a proper blood supply, and is described as necrotic. If an ulcer is in a healing phase and is filled with good, richly endowed tissue with new growth of capillaries, it is known as granulation tissue.

Commonly performed tests for circulatory problems are those of palpation of the pulses. The pulses can be felt in two areas of the foot, one on the top of the foot over the midtarsal joint for palpation of the dorsalis pedis artery, and the other behind the medial malleous, for the posterior tibial artery. Both arteries are graded as 4/4, the strongest, to 0/4, nonpalpable (Figure 33–7). The next test of circulation is that of the capillary filling time (CFT); it is noted as subpapillary venous refill time. In this test, the end of the toe is compressed with digital pressure for a few seconds until all the blood is squeezed out and the area blanches. Then it is noted how fast the color returns to the area. Capillary filling time is usually considered to be normal if it is 3 seconds or less. In a person with arteriosclerosis or diabetes, the capillary refill is delayed.

Neurologic Problems ▪ The neurologic system as manifested in the foot consists of sensory and motor nerves. The sensory nerves are seen in pathologic conditions as having diminished ability to create appropriate sensation signals that are sent to the brain. The motor nerves can also be afflicted with the effects of diabetes and other diseases that affect the peripheral nerves, manifested as muscle wasting and atrophy. The diminished ability of peripheral sensory nerves is also associated with lack of proprioception, or the sense of where a joint is in space. This lack is especially important in such diseases as diabetes and the alcoholic neuropathies, as well as Hansen's disease (leprosy). If the nerves of the peripheral joints do not provide a spatial sense, the patient tends to stand with the foot in one position too long, ultimately breaking down the soft

VASCULAR EVALUATION

Patient's Name_____ Age _____

Date_____

( )   Preoperative vascular evaluation re: healing potential

( )   Investigation of objective finding/subjective complaint suggestive of vascular pathology.

OBJECTIVE FINDINGS

	Right	Left

A. Pulses: Popliteal   _____

Posterior tibial   _____

Dorsalis pedis   _____

B. Subpapillary venous plexus filling time_____

C. ( ) Varicosities present, location_____

D. ( ) Ulceration(s) present, location_____

E. ( ) Trophic changes

    1. ( ) Hair growth absent

    2. ( ) Integument ( ) pale ( ) dry ( ) thin ( ) inelastic

                     ( ) dystrophic nails ( ) cool with gradient

F. ( ) Edema: ( ) pitting   ( ) nonpitting

G. ( ) Color abnormalitiy: ( ) erythema/hyperemia ( ) cyanosis

               ( ) temperature related: ( ) cold ( ) heat

PAST HISTORY

A. ( ) Cold injuries ( ) frostbite ( ) trench foot

B. ( ) Repeated cellulitis/ulcerations in lower extremities

C. ( ) Thrombophlebitis ( ) deep   ( ) superficial

D. ( ) Systemic disease traditionally associated with vascular disease:

    ( ) diabetes ( ) hypertension ( ) rheumatoid arthritis

    ( ) other_____

HABITS

A. ( ) Smoking (quantity_____duration_____)

B. ( ) Alcoholic beverages (quantity_____duration_____)

PRESENT HISTORY

A. ( ) Intermittent claudication (claudication distance_____)

B. ( ) Ischemic neuropathy_____

C. ( ) Ischemic-type pain at site of lesion

D. ( ) Nocturnal cramping

Blood pressure:_____ Pulse:_____ Room Temperature:_____

Figure 33–6

A vascular evaluation form.

Jose L. Alvarez, D. P. M.
A Professional Corporation
1234 Main Street
Anytown, XY 12345-0000
Diplomate, American Board of Podiatric Surgery
Fellow, American College of Foot Surgeons

DOPPLER ULTRASOUND ARTERIAL EVALUATION

ANKLE SYSTOLIC PRESSURE: Right_____   Left_____

ANKLE PERFUSION INDEX   Ankle systolic pressure

Right_____   Left_____

RIGHT FOOT   LEFT FOOT

CONCLUSIONS:_____
_____
_____
_____
_____
_____
_____
_____

Figure 33–7
A Doppler ultrasound arterial evaluation report.

tissues, causing ulcerations, and creating the breakdown of bones and joints.

Examination of the peripheral nerves is done by testing the ankle and knee jerk reflexes, which can indicate loss of lower motor neuron function. Usually the response to the knee or ankle jerk is rated at a gradation of anywhere from 0/4 to 4/4, the latter being the most brisk. Babinski's response is a test done by stroking the plantar aspect of the foot with a sharp object from the heel toward the toes and from the outer side of the foot to the medial side. A downward response of the foot is normal. An abnormal or positive Babinski's sign is when the digits fan apart and extend dorsally. This indicates an upper motor neuron lesion (Figure 33–8). Proprioceptive sensation is tested by moving a digit independently up and down or side to side with the patient's eyes closed. The subject is then asked to state the last position of the digit. In addition, the peripheral nervous system is tested for ability to discriminate between light touch and deep pressure. When the foot is touched with a sharp object with the patient's eyes closed, the test is to determine whether the subject withdraws in response to the stimulus. Another commonly performed test of peripheral sensation is ability to distinguish hot from cold.

Tarsal tunnel syndrome is an entrapment neuropathy in which the posterior tibial nerve is entrapped in the canal behind the medial malleolus. Generally, the history reveals a complaint of burning pain in the toes and sole of the foot. Tapping the tarsal canal creates either a Valleix phenomenon (pain radiating proximally and distally) or Tinsel's sign (distal radiation only.)

Musculoskeletal Problems ▪ The musculoskeletal system is the fourth organ system examined in a podiatric evaluation. If a patient has presented with trauma, perhaps a serious athletic injury or an industrial accident and the mechanism of the injury is questioned, then the musculoskeletal examination is very specific, very detailed, and much more in depth than for the average patient. The mechanism of the injury is a very important part of the initial history. This is because the position of the foot or ankle during a traumatic event will predict type and severity of injury regardless of what physical signs or symptoms show. In a sports or industrial injury the circumference of the calf muscle on the affected side is measured versus the unaffected side to see whether atrophy or wasting due to antalgic or painful gait has occurred. In addition, range of motion of all peripheral joints is

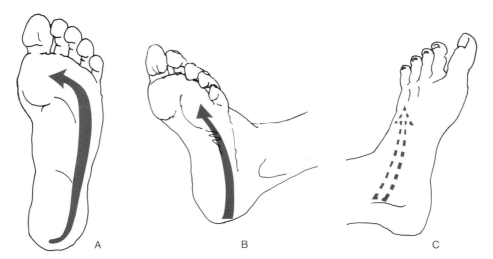

Figure 33–8
Normal and Babinski reflexes. A, Line of stimulation: Outer sole, heel to little toe. B, Plantar (normal) reflex. Toes curl inward. C, Positive Babinski reflex (always abnormal). Great toe bends upward; smaller toes fan outward. (From O'Toole, Marie (Ed.). Miller-Keane Encyclopedia and Dictionary of Medicine, Nursing, and Allied Health, 5th edition. W. B. Saunders company, Philadelphia, 1992.)

examined in detail and compared with the normal range of the contralateral side.

If an ankle injury is the presenting chief complaint, the specific lateral ankle ligaments are examined. On the outer side of the ankle are the anterior talofibular, calcaneofibular, and posterior tibiofibular ligaments. In a simple ankle sprain, the anterior talofibular ligament is usually injured to some degree (Figure 33–9). In a more complex sprain, the injury involves the ligaments as they go from front to back: the calcaneofibular and posterior talofibular ligaments. This can be seen in an inversion-type injury in which the foot turns inward, with the sole of the foot pointing toward the other foot. The subject is examined by palpation of the ligaments for point tenderness, and then the foot is gently but forcibly inverted to see whether the ankle or talus will come out of its relationship with the tibia and fibula. This is also examined in relation to the contralateral or uninjured side.

Injury to the inner side of the ankle involves the deltoid ligament, which holds the tibia to the talus and calcaneus on that side. This broad, dense ligament consists of two layers and usually is not injured, but if it is, it is a more serious injury. The anterior aspect of the ankle joint's integrity is tested by letting the back of the leg rest on the examiner's hand: the foot is forcibly pushed forward to see whether the talus will come out of the ankle socket anteriorly. If it does, this is called a positive drawer sign, which indicates a lateral collateral ankle rupture, or loss of integrity of the anterior aspect of the ankle joint.

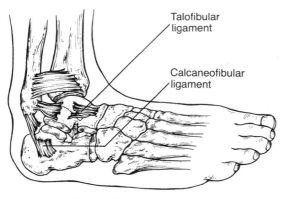

Talofibular ligament

Calcaneofibular ligament

Figure 33–9
A severely sprained ankle.

Gait analysis is a typical part of any biomechanical or musculoskeletal examination. A common problem encountered in gait analysis is equinus deformity, manifested by the patient's having an early heel-off or bouncing type of gait. This indicates that the Achilles tendon is shortened and means that the heel is on the ground for less time than normal. This unseats the talus or ankle bone from the calcaneus and allows the foot to go into a pronated, pes planus, or flattened position. A patient who has had an upper motor neuron lesion or a cerebrovascular accident often loses the ability to dorsiflex the foot or bring the foot up on the leg. This is manifested as weakness in the anterior tibial muscle, the main dorsiflexor muscle on the front of the leg. This is evidenced by a slap foot or drop foot gait and is noted in the gait analysis.

If noted in the gait analysis, these conditions are further studied with the patient in a seated position and testing of muscle strength in all four quadrants of motion: dorsiflexion, plantar flexion, inversion, and eversion. Dorsiflexion means bringing the foot up on the leg, and plantar flexion means pulling the foot down and away from the leg. Inversion is tested by having the subject draw the foot inward; eversion, by having the patient use the peroneal muscle group and pulling the foot outward (Figure 33–10).

Examination of stance and gait evaluates the patient's foot posture. A foot rolled over or flattened in the arch exhibits pes planus, or pronation. A foot that is high-arched, slightly everted, or turned outward exhibits pes cavus (Figure 33–11). Radiographic studies will show that the pes planus foot has a calcaneus or heel bone with an upward inclination of less than 15 degrees, so that the calcaneus parallels the ground rather than being upwardly inclined. This is associated with equinus, or shortness of the Achilles' tendon, and leads to the talus being unseated off the calcaneus. This chain of events allows the front part of the foot to be loose. The first metatarsal can drift medially or inward toward the other foot, ultimately creating a metatarsus primus adductus deformity usually associated with a bunion.

In the pes cavus foot, a lateral x-ray finding of the calcaneus is an exaggerated pitch upward in excess of 25 degrees. In this type of foot, weight is borne mostly on the heel and ball of the foot,

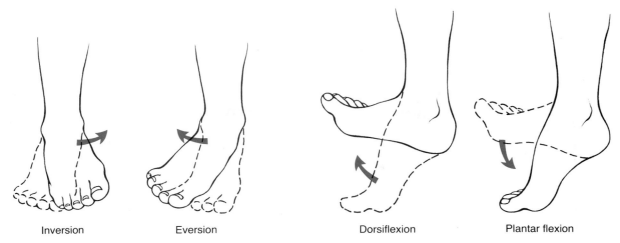

| Inversion | Eversion | Dorsiflexion | Plantar flexion |

Figure 33–10
Range of motion of the foot.

which is known as a poor shock absorber. It is associated with plantar callus formations under the first and fifth metatarsal bones.

A bunion is the prominence on the inner border of the foot at the first metatarsal head. The lateral drifting of the big toe or hallux often associated with this is known as hallux valgus. In dictating reports, doctors will often refer to one or all of these as the same thing, i.e., a bunion might have hallux valgus associated with it, a hallux valgus might or might not be associated with a bunion, and a metatarsus primus adductus is associated with both.

After examination of the gait and stance, the foot is examined for the presence of digital deformities aside from hallux valgus (Figure 33–12). A common digital deformity is hammertoe, which is a contracture of the proximal interphalangeal (PIP) joint, leaving the first bone or proximal phalanx dorsiflexed onto the metatarsal bone behind it, with the middle and distal phalanges being plantar flexed. This is associated with formation of a hard corn (heloma durum) at the dorsal aspect of the proximal interphalangeal joint. Another digital deformity is a mallet toe, a contracture of the end joint or distal interphalangeal joint (DIPJ), which is the end bone being plantar flexed toward the ground. This is associated with formation of a hard corn on the dorsal aspect of the DIP joint.

In the biomechanical and musculoskeletal ex-amination, one frequently encounters either suspected or occult fractures. A stress fracture can be suspected by history when the patient has acute, persistent pain at the distal aspect of one of the metatarsal shafts. This may or may not be associated with x-ray findings indicative of a fracture on earlier examination. This kind of fracture is known as an occult or hairline fracture and is not seen on radiographic examination until 2 to 4 weeks after initial insult or injury. In many instances, there is no history of initial insult or injury but an insidious pain that began with activity. The typical gross fracture encountered is Jones' fracture, a fracture of the fifth metatarsal base, which is avulsed or pulled away from the rest of the metatarsal bone. In Pott's fracture, both the medial and lateral malleoli are fractured (Figure 33–13).

Fractures are identified in one of the following seven ways:

- simple fracture, in which two fragments are created, one proximal and one distal;
- comminuted fracture, when there are more than two fragments;
- compound fracture, in which there is a break of skin by the fractured bony pieces;
- compression fracture, which is a compressing or crushing type of fracture;

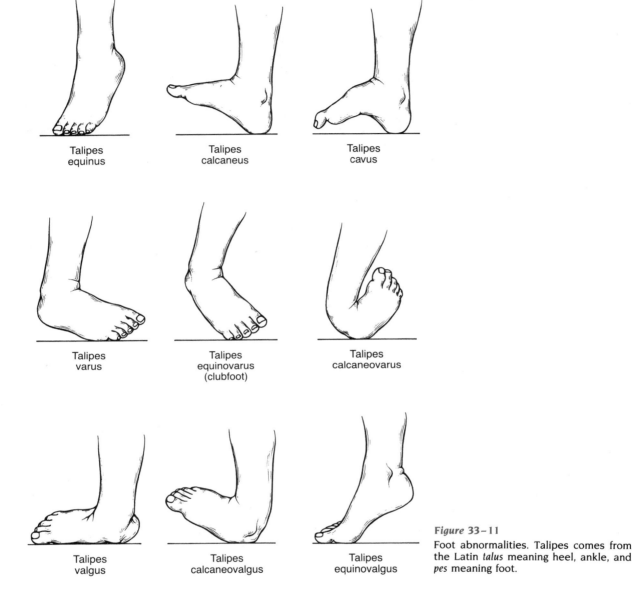

Talipes
equinus

Talipes
calcaneus

Talipes
cavus

Talipes
varus

Talipes
equinovarus
(clubfoot)

Talipes
calcaneovarus

Talipes
valgus

Talipes
calcaneovalgus

Talipes
equinovalgus

Figure 33–11
Foot abnormalities. Talipes comes from the Latin *talus* meaning heel, ankle, and *pes* meaning foot.

- stress fracture;

- avulsion or chip fracture, when a tendon or ligament pulls a piece of bone away from larger bone;

- greenstick fracture, seen in children when one cortex is broken and the other bows but does not give.

In the musculoskeletal examination, one needs to differentiate etiologies of pain in and around the metatarsophalangeal joints. Inflammation in a metatarsophalangeal joint is called capsulitis, or inflammation of the capsule. This can be affiliated with a periarticular bursitis or bursa formation and is sometimes associated with or found to be a cause of neuritis, an in-

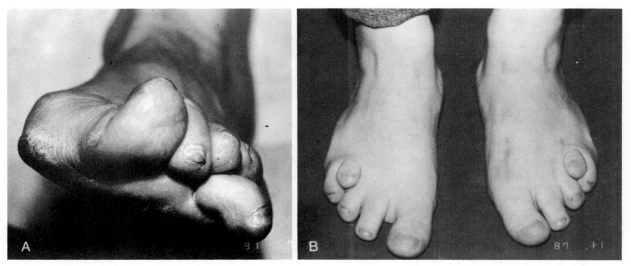

Figure 33–12
A, Digital abnormality. B, Brachymetatarsia. (Reprinted with permission from The Podiatry Institute, Tucker, Georgia.)

flammation of the nerve that runs between the metatarsophalangeal joints. If a neuritis between the metatarsophalangeal joints is chronic in nature, it develops into a rather firm, fibrous adhesion within the nerve substance called a neuroma (Figure 33–14). The most common is Morton's neuroma, found between the third and fourth metatarsal heads. This is examined by pushing the metatarsal heads together while a thumb is placed between the metatarsal heads. If sharp pain is elicited, the patient is found to have a positive Mulders sign. A patient with

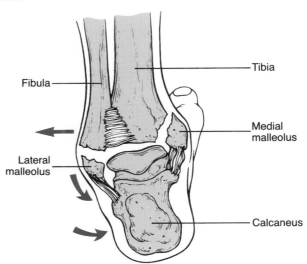

Pott's fracture

Figure 33–13
Pott's fracture. The lower part of the fibula is illustrated, with serious injury of the lower tibial articulation, usually a chipping off of a portion of the inner malleolus or rupture of the internal lateral ligament.

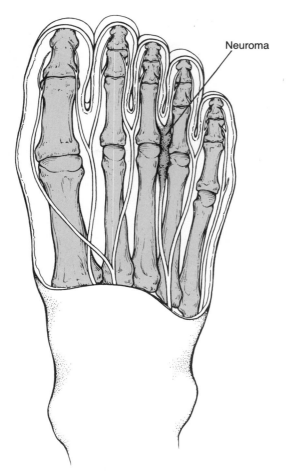

Neuroma

Figure 33–14
Digital neuroma (nerve irritation and enlargement).

Morton's neuroma experiences pain or numbness between the third or fourth toes or cramping in this region. This is caused by wearing close-toed shoes and is relieved by rest and removing the shoe.

Another common pathology in the musculoskeletal system is pain at the plantar aspect of the heel with stiffness or inability to walk early in the morning. This gradually gets better and goes away with activity. It is associated with the radiographic finding of a heel spur or a projection from the bottom of the heel bone pointing forward. This calcification originates from the plantar fascia and is accompanied with or diagnosed as a plantar fasciitis. The heel pain can be present with or without evidence of a heel spur on radiograph examination. Patients are examined by deep palpation to the plantar medial aspect of the calcaneus. This is done with the foot in an extreme dorsiflexed position and the digits in a forcibly dorsiflexed position, which tightens the plantar fascia. This exacerbates symptoms.

TREATMENT

Nonsurgical Procedures ▪ Common nonsurgical treatment for some of the aforementioned pathology includes digital pads for treatment of a heloma durum and felt padding or a lamb's wool pad applied to or around the toe to alleviate pressure from the contracted joint. This is done after the corn is trimmed. A soft corn, or heloma molle, is treated with packing of the interspace with lamb's wool to separate the proximal phalanges of the two digits involved. The treatment of intractable plantar keratosis (IPK) is trimming the lesion, putting a pad around it, or fabrication of an orthotic device. Orthotics are custom-molded inserts taken from a cast of the patient's foot; if the orthotic alleviates pressure or is for cushioning or comfort, it is known as an accommodative orthotic (Figure 33–15C). Orthotic devices used for biomechanical purposes—attempts to change the mechanics of the foot—are known as rigid, biomechanical, or functional orthotics (Figure 33–15D).

For treatment of insensitive feet with associated chronic ulcerations, as in patients with diabetic neuropathy, accommodative orthotics are utilized, and the area of bone creating the ulceration is accommodated or floated by elevating it with soft elevations built into the orthotic. Another way of treating this problem is to put a bar across the front of the shoe so that as the patient walks, the ball of the foot does not bear weight but rocks over this area. This is known as an anterior heel, rocker bar, or metatarsal bar.

For treatment of venous stasis and ulcerations of the malleoli, it is common to use a dressing of gauze impregnated with zinc oxide paste, known as an Unna boot, medicopaste bandage, or soft cast. These are sequentially applied from the base of the toes proximally to help gently com-

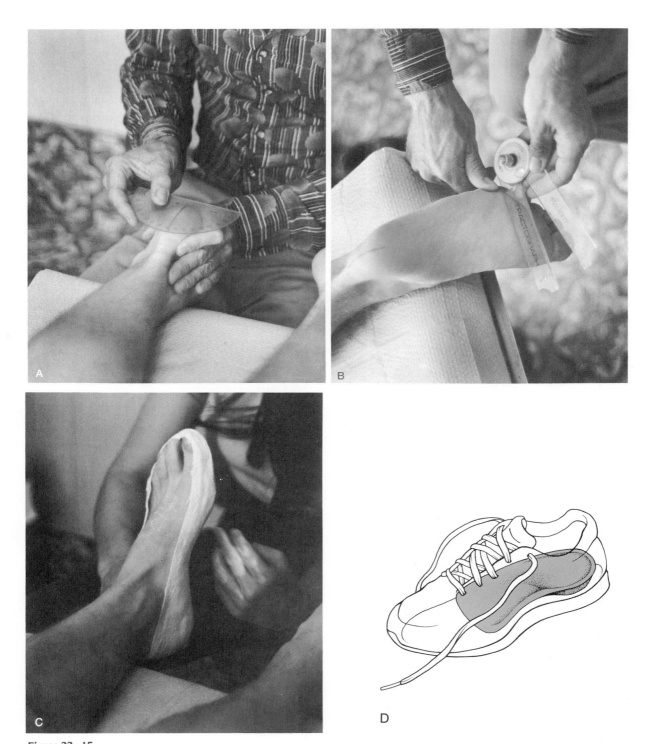

Figure 33-15

Orthotic devices. A, Measuring the heel for an orthotic device. B, Measuring across the metatarsal for an orthotic device. C, Making a plaster foot impression. (A, B, and C courtesy of John W. Pagliano, B.P.M., and California Orthopaedic Laboratory, Inc., Lakewood, California.) D, A flexible orthotic device to be worn inside a shoe.

press the veins, alleviate edema, and help the wound granulate.

Treatment of fungal toenails involves grinding down the toenail with a motor driven bur attached to a vacuum. Simple treatment for an ingrowing toenail, or onychocryptosis, is manual avulsion, which means the offending side of the nail is removed with or without local anesthetic.

If the patient has an equinus type of gait, a stretching exercise program is used to alleviate the equinus. If the patient has a drop foot type of gait, a drop foot brace is made from polypropylene molded plastic that goes from the back of the calf down underneath the foot, holding the foot at a right angle. There are also spring-loaded T-strap braces, in which the foot is sprung dorsally by a spring mechanism as the heel strikes the ground. Some children have in-toeing deformities, with soft tissue contractures or muscle imbalances. These are sometimes treated with cables that are spring-loaded and begin at the waist with a belt and end at the shoe. These are known as twister cables. Children who have simple intoeing or out-toeing problems are treated with a Denis Browne (D-B) bar or night splint. These are fixed to a pair of shoes with angles set to create a passive stretch on the muscles as the child sleeps.

In nonsurgical treatment of hallux valgus, or bunion deformity, a molded shoe known as a space shoe, custom-made by a shoemaker, is prescribed and fitted. This is done from a plaster casting made of the foot. Other nonsurgical treatment might include use of a foam sleeve that pulls over the big toe and helps support or protect the bunion from shoe pressure. An additional nonsurgical treatment is to use a latex molded shield that incorporates a foam padding around the bunion, made from a casting of that part of the foot.

Nonsurgical treatment of neuritis or Morton's neuroma is injection of a cortisteroid and local anesthetic into the affected interspace. Combined with this is use of a metatarsal pad, a teardrop-shaped pad placed in the shoe behind the offending metatarsal bones. This has the tendency, as the foot bears weight, to separate the metatarsal bones, alleviating pressure on the interdigital nerve.

Bunions are often detected at an early stage (Figure 33–16). A bunion is due to a biomechanical fault in the foot and, thus, treatment is use of a functional orthotic device in an attempt to control or alter the function of the foot. A bunion deformity of the foot is evaluated with the patient lying on the stomach with the foot in a relaxed attitude and the rear foot to lower leg in the neutral position. If the foot is inverted, the inversion can cause a bunion deformity, because as the foot hits the ground, it goes through an abnormal amount of pronation-type motion. The remainder of the examination concerns the relationship of the forepart of the foot. The examiner looks from the heel to the toes: if the forepart of the foot is elevated on the inner border, this is forefoot varus. The opposite is forefoot valgus when the first metatarsal bone is plantarly deflected or sticking down. Patients with forefoot or rearfoot varus may be prone to a bunion deformity. Patients can have a combined deformity. These deformities are treated with a functional orthotic in which a post or addition to the bottom of the device is placed to bring the ground up to the elevated bony part. This keeps the bony part from undergoing a compensatory motion that leads to an unbuckling of the first metatarsophalangeal joint and the inevitable bunion formation.

Surgical Procedures ■ Surgical procedures can be categorized under four organ systems: integumentary, neurologic, peripheral vascular, and musculoskeletal.

Integumentary Procedures ■ The most typical type of podiatric surgery performed is for ingrown toenails. Removal of the offending border, if only one border is involved, is called simple partial nail avulsion. If avulsion is permanent, then the underlying nail matrix is excised or obliterated. This is known as a partial matricectomy if one edge is involved. If both sides of a nail are involved, then both borders of the nail, defined as the medial and lateral borders, may be treated (keep in mind that the hallux, or big toe, is called the first toe). A complete nail removal is

Figure 33–16
A, Tailor's bunion of the fifth toe. B, Hallux valgus (bunion deformity). (A and B reprinted with permission from The Podiatry Institute, Tucker, Georgia.) C, Skeletal anatomy of hallux valgus (bunion deformity). D, Appearance of foot bones after bunionectomy.

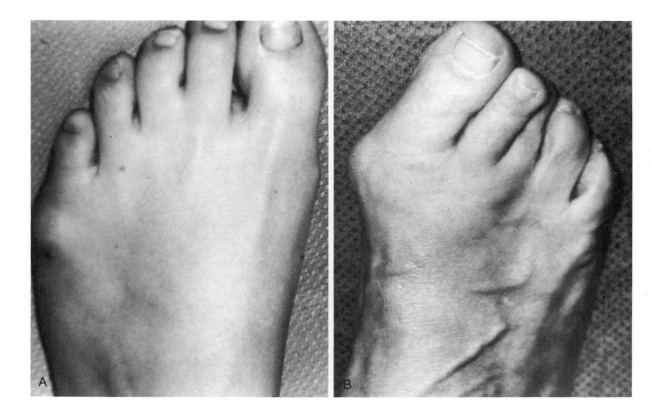

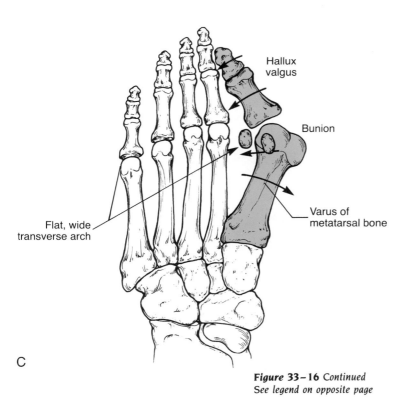

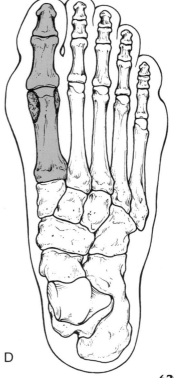

Hallux
valgus

Bunion

Varus of
metatarsal bone

Flat, wide
transverse arch

C

D

Figure 33–16 Continued
See legend on opposite page

known as total nail avulsion. If this is associated with an obliteration of the nail root, it is called total matricectomy. The word matricectomy means obliteration of the matrix; it is done by sharp dissection and excision, closed with Steri-Strips or sutures. It requires a surgical scrub.

Another way to obliterate a nail root is with chemical matricectomy, in which the nail is manually avulsed and the nail root obliterated with use of a chemical, phenol (89 per cent carbolic acid). Phenol is applied to the nail matrix for approximately 1.5 minutes after the nail has been avulsed and then washed with alcohol. This is called a P & A procedure. Another form of treatment for nail deformities is a laser matricectomy. The matrix of the nail is manually avulsed and obliterated with a carbon dioxide laser. This is a nonsterile procedure.

A new procedure for treatment of onychomycosis is waffling or perforation of the nail with a carbon dioxide laser. The nail is treated with a liquid antifungal medication that permeates through the perforations created in the infected nail matrix. This is known as a simple laser treatment, although it is defined as a surgical procedure.

For treatment of plantar warts, or verruca vulgaris, that are encountered on the dorsal aspect of the foot, there are many procedures. The tissue infected with the wart virus must be destroyed. This can be done by surgical excision and suturing if the lesion is very large. Or the wart can be destroyed with liquid nitrogen, which creates a vesicle-type formation, and the tissue is eventually sloughed off. Other forms of treatment for a verruca are the carbon dioxide laser beam; use of a hyfrecator, in which an electrical spark is generated, creating desiccation and destruction as it is absorbed into the verrucous tissue; and chemical cautery, a simple application of salicylic acid over a period of time.

Plantar keratoses of the plugged sweat duct variety are treated with simple excision or eradication by the same method used for treatment of a plantar wart.

Treatment of hard and soft corns is related to bone surgery discussed in the section on musculoskeletal surgery. Dermal lesions suspicious in origin are treated with biopsy. The biopsy can be excisional, removing the entire lesion, incisional, removing only part of the lesion, or a punch biopsy, in which a special surgical punch is inserted to remove a small cylindric piece of soft tissue. This is then submitted for pathologic examination.

Neurologic Procedures ■ The most frequently encountered neurologic problem in the foot is Morton's neuroma. If this does not respond to conservative treatment, surgical excision is performed (Figure 33–17). This is done with sharp dissection starting over the dorsal aspect of the affected interspace, exploration for either bursa or neuroma formation, and finally excision of the affected tissue. In Great Britain and in some areas of the United States, the incision for Morton's neuroma is on the plantar aspect of the foot, between the metatarsal bones to avoid weight bearing on the scar. In either instance, the deep transverse intermetatarsal ligament is incised as the exploration and excision is performed, because this is the ligament going from side to side that impinges on the neuroma.

Tarsal tunnel syndrome, if not effectively treated by conservative measures, requires operation in which a large, J-shaped incision is made posterior to the medial malleolus. The laciniate ligament that overlies the tarsal canal is incised. The contents of the tarsal canal are examined, and also the posterior tibial artery, the two posterior tibial veins, any associated communicating veins, and the posterior tibial nerve. The nerve is examined proximal to the medial mal-

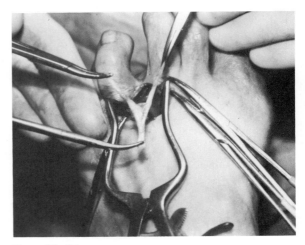

Figure 33–17
Excision of a digital neuroma. (Reprinted with permission from The Podiatry Institute, Tucker, Georgia.)

leolus and then distally into the area where the nerve trifurcates into the medial calcaneal, plantar, and medial branches.

Neurotrophic ulcers are sharply excised to get rid of necrotic tissue and allow granulation tissue to form. In some instances, there is a prominent metatarsal bone or other bony prominence, and this is sharply excised through the chronic ulceration site. If the bony part is partially excised, this is called saucerization of the affected bone. If the ulcer is partly excised, this is known as saucerization of the ulcer or ulcer bed.

Peripheral Vascular Procedures ▪ In the realm of peripheral vascular problems, sometimes dilated, varicose, or tortuous veins need to be excised. This is not done by a podiatrist because these veins communicate with the femoral vein. Such problems require more proximal operation by a peripheral vascular surgeon.

Musculoskeletal Procedures ▪ Musculoskeletal surgery is the most common podiatric surgery performed. The most common procedures, ranging from digital to more proximal, are described here.

HAMMERTOE ▪ When hammertoe is associated with hard corns, treatment is excision of the hard corn via two semielliptical incisions and resection of the head of the proximal phalanx after the extensor tendon has been tenotomized, or cut through. This is known as Post's procedure. If a patient has a more distal hard corn and a mallet toe deformity, the procedure is excision of the distally placed hard corn — a tenotomy of the extensor tendon at the level of the distal interphalangeal joint and a total or partial excision of the head of the middle phalanx, with simple interrupted suture closure.

KERATOMA ▪ For an intractable plantar keratoma associated with either a hammertoe or an independent plantarly deflected metatarsal bone, an osteotomy or cutting through of the metatarsal bone is performed. An incision is made directly over the metatarsal at its neck and carefully carried by layers down to the periosteum. This is reflected medially and laterally, and an osteotomy or cut through the bone is performed. This cut can be in many different shapes. A typical one is a V-shaped osteotomy from dorsal to plantar through all cortices of bone, and the site is closed simply. As the patient walks on the foot, this metatarsal head will translocate dorsally to approximate the other

metatarsals on the bottom of the foot. This alleviates the pressure that causes the intractable plantar keratoma.

Another form of osteotomy is a straight-through cut from medial to lateral at the metatarsal neck from side to side without having the shape of a V. This cut is either allowed to float freely or can be fixated with the use of a K-wire driven across the osteotomy site. Another is done at the more proximal end of the metatarsal, known as the base of the metatarsal. In this case, a bony wedge is taken out, with the base, or wider part, at the top, or dorsal, aspect of the bone and the apex, or point, at the plantar aspect. As the intervening wedge of bone is removed, the distal or end part of the metatarsal elevates and is fixated with a K-wire driven across the osteotomy site. This is a smooth, straight wire that projects from the foot and is removed later when sutures are extracted. It can be fixated by using a screw or stainless steel wire passed through a pair of drill holes, one on either side of the osteotomy site. It is cinched up to elevate the metatarsal bone, with the residual part of the wire placed into a third hole made on the base of the metatarsal bone.

SOFT CORN ▪ Part of the bone on either or both of the phalanges of the affected toes is removed. This can be performed with an excision of the intervening wedge of soft tissue between the bones and joining together soft tissue of the two affected bones, known as a webbing procedure, or syndactilization.

BUNION ▪ Treatment of hallux valgus or bunion deformity has many alternatives. Entire textbooks have been written on this subject. The typical bunion deformity is evaluated for its extent and severity by studying the foot, x-ray studies, and patient's history. If a bunion deformity is associated with a high intermetatarsal angle or metatarsus primus adductus (or the first metatarsal has drifted medially toward the other foot away from the other metatarsals), an osteotomy is performed to bring the metatarsal back into correct alignment. Extra bone growth that created the prominence at the end of the first metatarsal is removed. To bring the first metatarsal back into alignment, the osteotomy can be placed at the base of the first metatarsal bone; it is then an osteotomy performed by the removal of a wedge of bone, the base being on the lateral side and the apex being on the medial side.

When this wedge of bone is excised and the osteotomy is closed, the first metatarsal is closer to the second metatarsal at a high intermetatarsal angle.

An alternative is the modified crescent osteotomy at the base of the metatarsal, where bone distal to the cut is shifted into a corrected position and a fixation device (screw, K-wire, or pin) is placed across the osteotomy to hold it. Regardless of the type of osteotomy performed, usually a partial resection of the first metatarsal head is performed. The most distal osteotomies are described as a chevron or Austin's procedure. The apex of these osteotomies is distal and the osteotomy goes from medial to lateral across the foot in the shape of a V. In this procedure, the bone is cut entirely through, and the entire metatarsal head is shifted laterally to get closer to the second metatarsal bone for correct alignment. The bone in this type of osteotomy is compacted or pushed together manually, allowing for fixation. If the compaction does not allow for good fixation, pins, screws, or wires can be used.

If there is a bunion deformity, but the intermetatarsal angle is not very high or the first metatarsal is not spread very far from the second metatarsal bone, a procedure known as McBride's bunionectomy is performed (see Figure 33–16C & D). This consists of removal of bone on the medial aspect of the first metatarsal head and tightening the medial capsule or loosening the lateral capsule with or without excision of fibular or lateral sesamoid bone. If it is a dorsal bunion, exostosis of extra bone growth on the first metatarsal top, a simple excision of bone across the top of the first metatarsal, is performed. This is known as a cheilectomy.

For grossly arthritic first metatarsophalangeal joints with long-standing bunions, the entire base of the first proximal phalanx is removed in Keller's procedure. If it is grossly arthritic, sometimes the first metatarsal head is partially resected (Mayo's procedure).

In the last 20 years, there has been a proliferation of artificial joints by various manufacturers for replacement of the first metatarsophalangeal joint. Treatment for an arthritic first metatarsophalangeal joint is Keller's procedure with insertion of a hemi-implant or Silastic implant that fits into the residual of the base of the proximal phalanx of the great toe. This interfaces with the first metatarsal head. Hinged, double-stemmed implants also are available that place a hinge where the first metatarsophalangeal joint used to be and stems into both the proximal phalanx and the first metatarsal bone. This is a combined Keller-Mayo procedure in which bone is removed from the bones on either side of the joint. Some surgeons prefer to fuse the joint rather than implant it.

A deformity associated with a bunion that is known as hallux valgus interphalangeus means there is a curvature of the first bone or proximal phalanx in the great toe laterally. This structural deformity can be corrected by an osteotomy. In this case, the wedge of bone is spaced on the medial side, with the apex on the lateral side, and when the intervening wedge of bone is removed, the distalmost part of the toe is brought medially into a corrected alignment. The osteotomy can be left unfixated and treated with splinting or bandaging, or fixated with any of the aforementioned measures. This procedure is known as Akin's procedure.

CYSTS AND SPURS ▪ Other musculoskeletal procedures frequently performed involve the excision of ganglions or fluid-filled cysts, often encountered on the dorsal aspect of the foot. These are treated with simple excision. Heel spurs infrequently require surgical treatment; however, heel spur resection is associated with a plantar fasciotomy or cutting through of the plantar fascia. This is performed by an incision on the medial plantar aspect of the heel. Dissection is directed toward the inferior aspect of the calcaneus, and the forward-pointing calcaneal spur is resected with a hammer and chisel, known as an osteotome and a mallet. This procedure is a cutting away of the plantar fascia from the spur, called a fasciotomy. Many podiatric surgeons now perform the fascia release through an endoscope with instruments used in endoscopic carpal tunnel procedures in the hand.

HEEL PROBLEMS ▪ The heel can have an angular deformity where it does not sit in a straight line with the lower leg. The heel can be in an attitude of varus (far inwardly rotated) or valgus (far externally rotated). If these are significant pathologic conditions creating other abnormalities, they can be treated with various forms of osteotomies or cutting through of the heel bone. They can be either sliding-type osteotomies where a simple cut is made completely through the body of the bone and the two segments are rotated into correct alignment and fixated, or an osteotomy where a wedge of bone is taken out on the lateral or medial side for a varus or valgus attitude of the heel. An osteotomy of the calcaneus for angular correction is known as the Dwyer osteotomy.

ANKLE PROBLEMS ▪ The subtalar joint, or the joint between the ankle or talus and the calcaneus or heel bone, is often associated with arthritic changes. This joint is composed of three separate articulations between the ankle bone and the heel bone. If the arthritis is significant and untreatable by nonsurgical methods, the joint is fused. In this fusion, one or all of the articulations are resected and fused in a procedure known as a subtalar arthrodesis. Arthritis encountered in this area is arthritis of the joint between the calcaneus and the cuboid and the talus and the navicular. All these joints are fused in advanced arthritis or if there is severe angular deformity not correctable in any other fashion. This is called a triple arthrodesis procedure. If the ankle joint is involved and is significantly arthritic or has an angulation deformity, it and the other joints are often fused, which is known as a pantalar fusion. The ankle can be independently fused without surgery on the more distal joints.

For treatment of fractures within the ankle joint, known as talar dome fractures, or for the treatment of certain arthritic conditions of the ankle joint, arthroscopy is the usual procedure. The arthroscopist uses various approaches in treating known anatomic deformities, depending on their location.

For the treatment of gait abnormalities known as equinus, in which the heel is not on the ground as long as it should be during the gait cycle or is not amenable to soft tissue passive and active stretching activities, lengthening of the Achilles tendon can be performed. This procedure is known as a tendon Achilles lengthening (TAL) and is often associated with a capsulotomy of the posterior aspect of the ankle joint. The following exercises for stretching the Achilles tendon can be done twice a day, once in the morning and once in the evening, ten times on each foot. They are done barefoot at a very slow pace.

1. Stand facing the wall and place both hands against the wall.

2. Step back an arm's length from the wall and bring the right foot forward one step toward the wall.

3. Bend the right knee and raise the heel.

4. The left foot should remain flat on the floor, and the left leg should remain straight.

5. Press up against the wall, lean forward.

6. Change feet and repeat this exercise.

When the collateral ankle ligaments are injured, avulsed, or ruptured, and if surgical treatment is elected, they are repaired by primary suturing. If the collateral ligaments are injured beyond surgical repair, the tendon of the peroneus brevis is rerouted on the backside of the ankle joint through the fibula, back onto itself in a circumferential fashion. Procedures done utilizing this tendon, and variations thereof, are known as Elmslie's or the Watson-Jones procedure for lateral ankle stabilization.

IMBALANCES ▪ When severe neuromuscular imbalances leave the foot in a badly balanced position, osteotomies or stabilizations are performed. In addition to this, major tendons from the leg that insert into the foot are rerouted to create more balanced function. For instance, the anterior tibial tendon courses down from the outer side of the lower leg to the inner side of the foot and inserts into the first metatarsal base–navicular area. It can be rerouted to the lateral or outer side of the foot when the peroneal muscles are found to be malfunctional due to neuromuscular disease.

Various wedges and osteotomies are performed that involve the entire forefoot. In a foot with a local cavus deformity in which the forepart of the foot is entirely plantar flexed on the rear part of the foot, a wedge-type osteotomy is performed. This is done through all the bones of the midpart of the foot so that the foot from midfoot distally can be elevated onto the rearfoot to make the entire foot approach the ground in a balanced fashion. Japas' procedure is an osteotomy done for this deformity.

INSTRUMENTS

A reusable surgical handle on which a disposable blade for surgical incision is attached is the Bard-Parker handle. The No. 15 blade is the smallest, No. 10 is medium sized, and No. 20 is the largest.

To grasp the soft tissues once they have been incised, the podiatrist uses a tissue forceps. The most popular is a Brown-Adson forceps, which looks like a long tweezers.

Retractors used in podiatry are simple skin hooks—very fine-pointed, single-edged hook-type instruments with a handle to hold just the skin or superficial tissues.

Another type is Senn's retractor, which has a rake-like, three-pronged edge on one side, a handle in the center, and an L-shaped blunt solid end. Senn retractors have sharp or dull ends on the rake end and are held by an assistant surgeon. If there is not an assistant surgeon, a self-retaining retractor is used; the most common variety is Weitlaner's retractor.

To grip large fibrous or bony tissues held for surgical dissection and excision, Kocher's hemostat is sometimes used. This long hemostat has a toothed end that locks. Smaller hemostats used for clamping vessels are a mosquito (the smallest) or Kelly's (medium-sized). These can be straight or curved.

An instrument used to hold sterile surgical drapes in place is a Backhaus towel clamp. It is also used to hold large fibrous or bony parts while they are being surgically dissected.

Heavy Mayo's scissors, curved or straight, are used in foot and ankle surgery. Smaller scissors are used for dissection around the sesamoid bones during a sesamoidectomy for bunion surgery. They are curved collar and crown scissors. A smaller scissors for dissection of the finer tissues or for suture removal is the iris scissors.

Forceps are instruments used for cutting bone. A typical bone-cutting forceps is Liston's. An instrument that looks like a bone-cutting forceps and is used to gouge or sculpt bone is known as a bone rongeur. Both the bone-cutting forceps and the rongeur are available in various sizes. To scoop and help sculpt bone, there are bone curettes that have a small, cuplike end and a large, broad handle. These come in various sizes from a 60 to a 6 and are used for removing or saucerizing bone. Once bone is removed, it is smoothed with a file or rasp. A file has straight serrated edges from one side to the other, whereas a rasp has crosshatch-type endings. A typical podiatry rasp is Joseph's nasal rasp.

To elevate the periosteum, various forms of instruments pry up the skinlike covering of the bone. They are called periosteal elevators; a popular one is Sayre's elevator.

The bone can be sculpted with a chisel or an osteotome. A chisel is an instrument with a sharp edge on one side and a straight edge apposing it, whereas an osteotome bevels to a point, with the bevel on either side. Osteotomes and chisels are available in various widths and lengths. A typical osteotome used in podiatric surgery is Lambotte's osteotome.

Mallets are shaped like a small hammer. They may have heads of solid steel or replaceable fiber, or have plastic inserts on the face.

Biopsies are performed with a small instrument that makes a cylindric excision known as a punch biopsy.

Foot and ankle surgery requires the use of power instrumentation; the most popular type is that of gas-powered or electrically driven saws. The three most commonly used saws are the power oscillating saw, in which the saw blade is at a right angle to the handle and goes from side to side; the sagittal saw, which reciprocates in and out of the handle in a straightforward fashion as the operator uses it in a straight downward manner; and the reciprocating saw, utilized for a crescentic-type osteotomy in the base of the first metatarsal, for reduction of a high intermetatarsal angle.

Surgical drills are rotary-driven instruments used to drive in K-wires or make holes for screws. Three popular drills and saws are Hall's, Stryker's, and Ritter's. These are driven by nitrogen gas or by electricity.

Podiatrists use needles of from 0.5 to 2 inches in length in gauges varying from 18 to 30. The higher the gauge, the thinner the needle.

For closure, a needle holder is used. It can be a simple needle holder that holds the needle, or it can be a combination needle holder and scissors used by a surgeon operating alone.

Since the mid-1980s, podiatrists have been performing soft tissue surgery with the use of a carbon dioxide–generated laser. It is used for a wide variety of surgery, including excision of Morton's neuroma, dissection of ganglia and other soft tissue foreign bodies, removal of warts, eradication of ingrown toenails, and treatment of fungus-infected toenails.

Podiatrists most often use local anesthetic and anesthetic blocks for their procedures, rather than general anesthesia. A popular local anesthetic is bupivacaine, known by the brand name Marcaine. Other local anesthetics are Xylocaine and Carbocaine. All these can be used with or without epinephrine, which is a vasoconstrictive agent useful to control bleeding. Podiatrists often inject proximal to the operative site after surgery with a corticosteroid. Commonly used is Decadron, a short-acting corticosteroid that controls swelling and inflammation and helps diminish need for postoperative pain medications. Most podiatric surgery is done with a localized tourniquet in place. This can be inflated with a pneumatic carbon dioxide canister known as a kiddie cuff, or it can be a simple wrapping with a 3- to 4-inch-wide rubber Esmarch bandage. This can be used to milk the foot, as with the use of a kiddie bandage, or it can milk the foot and then be maintained about the level of the ankle to create hemostasis during operation.

After operation on bone, it is common to take postoperative radiographs in the weight-bearing position, for standardization and to make the bones appear as they really are during function. Most standard radiographic examinations are taken in the anteroposterior (AP) position: the patient stands on a small platform, and the head of the x-ray machine projects downward from front to back with the beam centering on the center of the talus. When patients are examined in this fashion, the view is called the angle and base of gait. The angle of gait means the amount of external rotation the patient ordinarily has, and the base of the gait means the separation of one foot from the other, seen when the patient is ambulatory.

Study of the plantar aspect of the foot, specifically the sesamoids, is done with the rear part of the foot raised on a plastic block as the tube head of the x-ray machine shoots from the back of the foot toward the toes. In the axial sesamoidal view, the plantar aspect of the metatarsal heads as well as the sesamoids under the first metatarsophalangeal joint can be visualized. A Harris-Beath view is taken at various angles to get one picture that will show all the facets of the subtalar joint.

As an adjunct to surgery, the foot is dressed in soft gauze squares 2 or 4 inches square known as 2x2s or 4x4s. A roll gauze known as Kling and the product known as Coban are then applied for soft tissue dressings. Coban adheres to itself without stickum. It affords mild compression and protects the inner dressings against disruption. Osteotomy or other bone work is stabilized with a cast. Casts can be made of fiberglass or plaster of Paris. Cast configurations can be either a slipper cast or below the malleoli, a B-K cast for below the knee to the toes with the foot held at a right angle, or an A-K cast that goes from the toes to above the knee, with the knee flexed and the foot at a right angle to the leg. This type of cast is used in an ankle fusion, Achilles tendon lengthening, or subtalar arthrodesis.

FORMATS

Chart Notes ■ The typical podiatry chart is organized in the SOAP (subjective, objective, assessment, and plan) format (Figure 33–18). The initial office visit of a podiatry patient includes a complete medical history of the patient's present illness, current medications, allergies, past medical history, systems review, traumatic history, surgical history, social history, family history, vital signs, and a complete physical examination. Each subsequent visit is arranged in the SOAP manner, i.e., the patient enters with a subjective complaint and an objective finding is made by the examiner. Then an assessment is made that indicates what the probable diagnoses are, and a treatment plan is formulated and enacted.

Of note to transcriptionists are systems for automated charting, dictation on a daily basis, and storing of the record in the computer, known as a paperless charting system. In addition, there are charting systems in which a wand is drawn across the patient's chart to note the patient's inventory control number. This wand is drawn over a series of statements that help reflect the correct SOAP charting for that day's visit. This is immediately entered into a computer software program and can be retained or printed for entry into the chart.

Disability Reports ■ If the podiatric medical report reflects an injury, a subsequent report to an industrial carrier documenting the nature

Bradshaw, Tiffany P.   AGE: 83

04-18-94

SUBJECTIVE: An 83 y.o. female complains of pain @ end of 3rd digit left foot X
               1 month with drainage noted in the shoe. Has history of poorly
controlled insulin dependent diabetes.

OBJECTIVE: Exam reveals a poorly nourished female who is alert as to place
               and time.
               P.V. exam reveals +1/4 D.P. pulses trace to 0 P.T. pulses. CFT
is +4 sec Ⓑ. Has varicose veins Ⓑ c̄ stasis dermatitis.
               Integumentary exam reveals skin that is tense, shiny, and
devoid of hair. Skin turgor is diminished. Nails are thickened, discolored. There
is a 1.5 cm ulcer on distal aspect of 3rd digit left c purulent exudate. The distal
phalanx is exposed.
               Neuro exam: downgoing plantar responses. Light touch and
sense of hot-cold are diminished. Protective response to sharp stimulus is
absent. DTRs are +1/4 Ⓑ.
               M.S. exam: Has Ⓑ pes planus with multiple hammer toes. 3rd
left is rigidly hammered.

ASSESSMENT: Insulin dependent DM. PVD: micro as well as large vessel
               disease; hammer toes; pes planus; ulcer 3rd digit left; diabetic
neuropathy; rule out osteomyelitis.

PLAN: To x ray; to lab: CBC/ Sed rate/ glucose/ gram stain & C & S.
               Debrided & dressed ulcer site. Rx'd Dicloxacillin 500 #28 1
q.i.d.; wet to dry dressing orders; retn 48 hrs.

_____
Hoon Wu, D.P.M.

mtf

Figure 33–18
Sample chart entry using the subjective, objective, assessment, plan (SOAP) method.

Jose L. Alvarez, D.P.M.
1234 Main Street
Anytown, XY 12345-0000
Telephone: 013-320-8977 Fax: 013-329-6755

OPERATIVE REPORT

NAME OF PATIENT: John Doe

PLACE OF SURGERY: 1234 Main Street
Anytown, XY 12345-0000

DATE AND TIME: June 30, 1993 10:00 a.m.

SURGEON: Jose L. Alvarez, D.P.M.

ASSISTANT SURGEON: None.

PREOPERATIVE DIAGNOSIS: Possible Morton's neuroma, 2nd interspace, right foot.

POSTOPERATIVE DIAGNOSIS: Possible Morton's neuroma, 2nd interspace, right foot.

SURGICAL PROCEDURE: Exploration and removal of Morton's neuroma, 2nd interspace, right foot.

HEMOSTASIS: An ankle tourniquet was placed at the level of the ankle at 250 mmHg.

DESCRIPTION OF OPERATION: The patient was brought into the operating room and placed on the table in a supine position. The operative site was prepped and draped in the usual sterile manner. The site was anesthesized with approximately 2 cc of 0.5% Marcaine plain with 4 cc of Lidocaine.

PROCEDURE NUMBER 1: Exploration and removal of neuroma, 2nd interspace, right foot.

A longitudinal incision was made from the intermetatarsal space proximally. The incision was carefully carried by layers down to the intermetatarsal space. The deep transverse intermetatarsal ligament was incised and then, with pressure from below, I noted that there was a large white fibrous mass in the intermetatarsal space. This consisted of a central nerve body with extension into the toes and extending proximally between the metatarsal necks. It was dissected proximally as far as the metatarsal necks and distally as far as the digits and these margins were then transected using the CO2 laser set at 15

(continued)

***Figure* 33–19**
Operative report of a Morton's neuroma, or a Post procedure.

Figure continued

John Doe
Page 2
June 30, 1993

watts of continuous power. The neuroma was then removed from the surgical site in toto. The subcutaneous layer was then closed with simple interrupted sutures of 5-0 nylon.

When the surgery was complete a dry sterile, slightly compressive bandage was applied to the surgical site. The tourniquet was released and the vascular status of the foot examined and found to be intact. The patient tolerated surgery and anesthesia well and was escorted to the waiting room ambulatory with vital signs normal. The patient was given an appointment for followup and a prescription for analgesics. Postoperative instructions were expressed verbally and given in printed form.

Jose L. Alvarez, D.P.M.

mtf

Figure 33–19 *Continued*

and extent of the injury is made, along with an apportionment of disability with an indication of whether it is temporary, permanent, or stationary. The report outlines a plan of treatment and a prognostication of the length of the treatment plan.

Surgical Reports ■ Reports of operations and procedures outline the date, time, and place of surgery, names of the patient, surgeon and assistant surgeon, anesthesia, type of hemostasis used, preoperative diagnosis, postoperative diagnosis, length of surgery, and findings (Figure 33–19). This is usually summed up with a description of the dressings applied, the condition of the patient, and neurovascular status of all the digits.

Reference Sources

Ballow, Edward B. *Laser Surgery of the Foot.* International Society of Podiatric Laser Surgery, Doylestown, Pennsylvania, 1988.

Donick, Irvin I. *Podiatry for the Assistant,* 2nd edition. Baltimore, Williams and Wilkins, 1988.

Scher, Richard K., and C. Ralph Daniel, III. *Nails: Therapy, Diagnosis, Surgery.* W. B. Saunders Company, Philadelphia, 1990.

Yale, Irving. *Podiatric Medicine.* Williams and Wilkins Company, Baltimore, 1980.

For references of specific application to medical transcription, see Appendix 1.

Zigmond M. Lebensohn, M.D.

Psychiatry

INTRODUCTION

Psychiatry, more than any other medical specialty, depends heavily on precise, evocative prose to describe the many subtleties of the mental and emotional states with which it deals. For this reason, the skills of the transcriptionist play an important role in the preparation of accurate and useful reports.

The term *psychiatry* is of relatively recent origin. First used by the German physician Reil in the early 19th century, it is derived from the Greek *iatreia*, meaning medical treatment, and *psyche*, meaning the mind or soul. Therefore, a psychiatrist by definition is a doctor of medicine who specializes in the study and treatment of disorders of the mind, usually referred to as mental and/or emotional disorders or more simply psychiatric disorders.

The field of psychiatry itself, just as any other field of medicine, is further divided into numerous subspecialties. A few of the best known subspecialties are listed below:

- Administrative psychiatry
- Adolescent psychiatry
- Biologic psychiatry
- Child psychiatry
- Geriatric psychiatry
- Group therapy
- Psychoanalysis
- Substance abuse (subspecialty dealing with addictions)

The field of mental health professionals has exploded in recent years. At present, psychotherapy (the so-called talking cure) is conducted by clinical psychologists, social workers, nurse practitioners, pastoral counselors, sexual and marital therapists, and other health professionals. These therapists usually have a master's degree (M.S.) or a doctorate (Ph.D.) in their chosen area and are most often licensed by their specialty licensing board. However, they do not have a medical degree and therefore are not permitted to write prescriptions for psychopharmacologic agents, although this restriction is currently being challenged by clinical psychologists in some quarters, particularly in the military.

"Psychoanalysis" when used without a modifier (such as Jungian or Adlerian), means Freudian psychoanalysis. This is a system of psychologic theory, investigation, and treatment elaborated in the early 1900s by the Viennese psychiatrist Sigmund Freud and his followers. It depends on frequent sessions (three to five times weekly), free association, interpretation of dreams, development of a very special relationship between analyst and patient called transference, and considerable emphasis on early childhood memories. Most psychoanalysts in the United States have an M.D., but there are many lay analysts here and abroad who have made significant contributions to the field. Erich Fromm, author of such well-known books as *Escape from Freedom* and *Psychoanalysis and Religion*, is a well-known example. A practicing psychiatrist may use the services of a clinical psychologist for conducting various personality and intelligence tests to obtain more data about a particular patient or refer a patient to a psychoanalyst or other mental health professional for treatment if it is considered appropriate.

REPRESENTATIVE DISEASES

The vast number of psychiatric disorders are listed and described in the *Diagnostic and Statistical Manual III, Revised* (DSM-III-R), published by the American Psychiatric Association. This reference book should be in the library of every practicing psychiatrist. Its terminology will be used here. The disorders are divided into the following broad groups:

1. Developmental Disorders. These include many forms of mental retardation and autistic behavior, among others.
2. Behavior Disorders of Children.
3. Organic Mental Disorders. These include all disorders in which the direct cause is a demonstrable circulatory, toxic, atrophic, infectious, or traumatic lesion of the brain. Examples include Alzheimer's disease and senile dementia, as well as alcohol-, drug-, or chemical-induced organic brain disorder.
4. Substance Abuse. This group includes dependency on or addiction to alcohol, cocaine, narcotics, or similar substances (Table 34–1).
5. Schizophrenia. This major disorder accounts for approximately 50 per cent of all patients residing in state hospitals. The precise cause of this condition is still unknown, but the symptoms may include paranoid delusions (false beliefs of being persecuted), auditory or visual hallucinations (hearing voices or seeing things that are not there), and pervasive disorders of thinking.
6. Mood Disorders. These are the manic depressive (or bipolar) disorders and the various types of depression. Extremes of elevated mood (mania) or depressed mood (suicidal depression) often warrant hospitalization. Milder forms of these disorders may be treated by the psychiatrist in the office on an outpatient basis.
7. Anxiety Disorders. This large group (formerly known as the psychoneuroses) includes panic disorders, obsessive-compulsive disorders (such as obsessional handwashing), social phobias, and PTSD (posttraumatic stress disorder).
8. Somatoform Disorders. This group includes disorders with physical symptoms, such as paralysis, weakness, anesthesia, or inability to speak, which are caused by deep, unre-

solved emotional conflict in the absence of any demonstrable physical cause.
9. Dissociative Disorders include multiple personality disorder, cases of amnesia, and depersonalization.
10. Sexual Disorders include exhibitionism, pedophilia (abnormal sexual involvement with children), voyeurism (peeping Toms), sexual sadism, and masochism.
11. Sleeping Disorders include the various forms of insomnia, hypersomnia (excessive need for sleep), and narcolepsy (attacks of falling asleep).
12. Factitious Disorders. In these disorders, the patient consciously and deliberately makes up physical or psychiatric complaints for specific purposes.
13. Impulse Control Disorders. These include kleptomania (shoplifting), compulsive gambling, pyromania (firesetting), and trichotillomania (compulsive pulling out of one's hair).
14. Adjustment Disorders include episodes of anxiety, depression, and/or altered conduct, which result from difficulty in adapting to a new or stressful life situation.
15. Personality Disorders. These are long-standing disorders, often present since childhood or early adulthood, which result in serious difficulty with relating to others. Patients with personality disorders rarely seek help until their behavior creates such problems that they are urged or ordered to seek help.

A word about format in using diagnostic terms; the usual format for writing out a diagnosis is as follows: "The patient is suffering from Generalized Anxiety Disorder, 300.02 (DSM-III-R)."

Many psychiatrists preparing formal reports will summarize their results in the form of a multiaxial evaluation that is carefully explained on page 21 of DSM-III-R. Axis I lists the primary psychiatric disorder or disorders. Axis II gives the diagnosis of any underlying personality disorder. Axis III lists any significant concurrent medical disease. Axis IV describes the nature of any stressors present, together with an estimate of the severity of these stressors (mild, moderate, or extreme.) Axis V describes Global Assessment of Functioning (GAF). Here, an assessment is made of the current level of functioning and the highest assessment attained during the

Table 34–1 ▪ **Commonly Abused Drugs**

Drug	Street Name	How Used	Symptoms and Signs
Marijuana Hashish	Pot, grass, reefer, weed, hash, sinsemilla, joint	Smoked Ingested	Loss of interest Recent memory loss Dry mouth and throat Mood changes Increased appetite
Alcohol	Booze, brew, hooch	Ingested	Impaired coordination Impaired judgment
Nicotine	Smoke, butt, coffin nail	Smoked Chewed	Tobacco smell Stained teeth
Amphetamines	Speed, uppers, pep pills, bennies, dexies, black beauties, meth, crystal	Ingested Injected Sniffed	Dilated pupils Increased energy Irritability Nervousness Needle marks
Cocaine	Coke, crack, snow, white lady, toot	Snorted Injected Ingested Smoked	Dilated pupils Increased energy Restlessness Intense anxiety Paranoid behavior Needle marks
Barbiturates	Downers, barbs, yellow jackets, red devils, blue devils, double trouble	Injected Ingested	Constricted pupils Confusion Impaired judgment Drowsiness Slurring of speech Needle marks
Methaqualone	Ludes, sopors, Quaaludes	Ingested	Slurring of speech Drowsiness Impaired judgment Euphoria Seizures
Heroin Morphine	Junk, scag, dope, horse, smack, dreamer	Injected Smoked Sniffed Skin popped	Constricted pupils Needle marks Drowsiness Mental clouding
Codeine	School boy	Ingested Sniffed	Constricted pupils Drowsiness
Demerol Methadone Percodan Pentazocine		Ingested Injected	Constricted pupils Drowsiness Mental clouding Needle marks
PCP (phencyclidine)	Angel dust, hog, killer weed, supergrass	Smoked Snorted Injected Ingested	Dilated pupils Slurring of speech Hallucinations Blurring of vision Uncoordination Agitation Confusion Aggressive behavior

Table continued on following page

Table 34–1 ▪ **Commonly Abused Drugs (***Continued***)**

Drug	Street Name	How Used	Symptoms and Signs
LSD (lysergic acid diethylamide)	Acid, cubes, purple haze	Ingested Injected	Dilated pupils Hallucinations Mood swings Increased alertness Acute panic reactions
Mescaline	Mesc, cactus	Ingested	Dilated pupils Hallucinations Mood swings
Psilocybin	Magic mushrooms	Ingested	Dilated pupils Hallucinations Mood swings
Airplane glue*		Inhaled	Poor motor coordination
Paint thinner*		Sniffed	Impaired vision Violent behavior
Nitrous oxide	Laughing gas, whippets	Inhaled Sniffed	Hilarity Euphoria Lightheadedness
Amyl nitrite	Poppers, rush, locker room, snappers, amies	Inhaled Sniffed	Hilarity Dizziness Headache Impaired thought

*The active agent in airplane glue and paint thinner is toluene. Naphtha, methyl ethyl ketone, and gasoline may produce similar symptoms.
From the Department of Transportation Emergency Medical Technician National Standard Curriculum, 1985.

past year, to indicate whether the patient has shown any functional change. The scale (which is found on page 12 of DSM-III-R) runs from 1 to 90, with 90 representing absent or minimal symptoms.

An example of the format for recording the results of a complete multiaxial evaluation is this:

Axis I: 296.23 Major Depression, Single Episode, Severe, Without Psychotic Features
303.90 Alcohol Dependence
Axis II: 301.60 Dependent Personality Disorder (Provisional, rule out Borderline Personality Disorder)
Axis III: Alcoholic cirrhosis of liver
Axis IV: Psychosocial stressors: anticipated retirement and change in residence with loss of contact with friends

Severity: 4 — moderate (predominantly enduring circumstances)
Axis V: Current GAF: 44
Highest GAF past year: 55*

DIAGNOSTIC PROCEDURES AND TESTS

Signs and Symptoms ▪ The kinds of psychiatric disorders seen by a psychiatrist will depend largely on the type of practice and subspecialty. For example, the state hospital psychiatrist will see the sickest patients, including those suffering from severe, chronic schizophrenia, major

---

*Reprinted by permission of the American Psychiatric Association.

suicidal depressions, and gross dementia with organic brain disorders. On the other hand, the psychoanalyst in solo practice will see patients suffering from the various psychoneuroses, milder depressions, and disorders of living that may interfere with the patient's ability to adjust but do not require hospitalization.

Some of the signs and symptoms of the most commonly encountered disorders are listed here. The list is by no means complete and is presented primarily to give examples of the major categories.

1. *Schizophrenia.* Symptoms may include flatness of affect, thought disorder, verbal blocking, mutism, catatonic stupor, waxy flexibility, paranoid delusions, auditory hallucinations, lack of insight, impaired judgment.

2. *Bipolar Disorder (Manic Phase).* Symptoms may include psychomotor overactivity, motor restlessness, lack of impulse control, euphoric mood, rapid speech, clang association, impaired insight and judgment, buying sprees, denial of need for sleep or rest.

3. *Bipolar Disorder (Depressed Phase).* Symptoms may include psychomotor retardation, depressed mood, suicidal thoughts or attempts, slow or retarded speech, thought blocking, feelings of hopelessness and despair, delusions of guilt or self blame.

4. *Generalized Anxiety Disorder.* Symptoms may include severe anxiety about almost everything (pananxiety) or about specific items that produce phobias, such as mysophobia (fear of dirt) or claustrophobia (fear of closed spaces).

5. *Organic Brain Disorder.* Symptoms may include disorientation for time, place or person, varying degrees of memory impairment (especially for recent events), impaired retention, impaired ability to do simple calculations, slurred speech.

Psychiatric Evaluation

The extended psychiatric evaluation based on a sufficient number of sessions conducted by a well-trained psychiatrist is still the method of choice and the most frequently used diagnostic procedure. Occasionally, a patient may need medical, neurologic, or psychologic testing, and these tests will be noted later.

A complete physical examination together with appropriate laboratory tests may reveal a physical disorder that influences mental functioning, such as uncontrolled diabetes or hypertension.

Radiographic Studies

X-ray films, computed tomography (CT), magnetic resonance imaging (MRI) of the head and positron emission tomography (PET), a complex procedure used primarily in brain research centers.

Psychologic Testing

These tests are performed by a trained clinical psychologist. A battery of these tests may include any one or several of the following:

- Beck Depression Inventory
- Bender-Gestalt test (BGT)
- Draw-A-Person drawing
- Halstead-Reitan tests (for evidence of organic brain disease)
- House-tree-person inkblot test
- Minnesota Multiphasic Personality Inventory (MMPI)
- Rey-Osterreith Complex Figure test
- Rorschach Inkblot test
- Rotter Sentence Completion test (RSCT)
- Stanford Achievement Test (SAT)
- Thematic Apperception Test (TAT)
- Wechsler Adult Intelligence Scale (WAIS)

TREATMENTS

A large number of treatment modalities are available in the field of psychiatry. The task of the psychiatrist is to decide which of the various treatment methods is most effective for a given patient. Some of the more commonly used treatments are listed here. This list should by no means be considered complete.

Psychologic Treatments

Psychotherapy
Psychoanalysis
Cognitive therapy
Supportive therapy
Group therapy
Desensitization therapy
Behavior therapy

Psychopharmacologic Treatments

Minor tranquilizers, including benzodiazepines such as diazepam, alprazolam, or lorazepam, for severe anxiety or panic.

Mood stabilizers such as lithium carbonate (used primarily for the manic phase of bipolar disorder).

Neuroleptic and antipsychotic agents such as chlorpromazine, thioridazine, or haloperidol.

Antidepressants. There are several classes of antidepressants, including tricyclic antidepressants (TCAs), monoamine oxidase inhibitors (MAOIs), and agents such as fluoxetine hydrochloride.

Cortical stimulants. Methylphenidate is often used in the treatment of attention deficit disorder (ADD) in hyperkinetic children and also as a stimulant for adults.

Somatic Therapies

ECT (electroconvulsive therapy) may be used successfully in cases of severe suicidal or delusional depressions. Certain other somatic therapies such as insulin shock therapy and psychosurgery, which were used during the 1930s and 1940s, are no longer or rarely used.

FORMATS

Reports ▪ Reports of psychiatric evaluations are often six to ten pages in length. These reports contain exceedingly confidential material and are subject to strict medicolegal regulations. For this reason, no psychiatrist should send any report, even to the referring physician, without the patient's written consent. Because of the potential for harm, many jurisdictions provide special forms for the release of mental health information. Many psychiatrists refuse to send complete reports unless the legal requirements are meticulously followed. In some instances, the psychiatrist may show a report to the patient prior to sending it to the authorized party or parties concerned.

Letters ▪ One of the most important formats used in psychiatric practice is the letter written by the psychiatrist to the referring physician. This letter serves several purposes:

1. It tells the referring physician that the patient has, in fact, consulted the psychiatrist.

2. It gives the referring physician the diagnosis or initial impression and a proposed plan of treatment.

3. It acknowledges the referral as a courtesy to the referring physician.

Chart Notes (or Progress Notes) ▪ Many psychiatrists write their progress notes in longhand and prefer this method for reasons of confidentiality. In hospitals and institutions, chart notes are often dictated and transcribed periodically. The note is always dated and contains the doctor's assessment of the patient's condition at the time the patient was seen. The note should indicate whether it was a long, intermediate, or brief interview. In some instances the doctor indicates the number of minutes spent with the patient. In addition to the description of the patient's appearance, behavior, and speech, any changes in medication are noted. Figure 34–1 is an example of a chart note.

Medical Reports

Psychiatric History ▪ The psychiatric history differs from the history of most other medical specialties in that it is much more detailed and covers every aspect of the patient's life that could possibly explain the present condition. The following outline, followed in full or in part depending on the circumstances, represents the format used in most treatment centers.

MAIN FACTS ▪ This section consists of a brief paragraph giving the age, occupation, and the circumstances that led to the patient's coming for help.

PRESENT ILLNESS ▪ This section describes in greater detail the events that led to the patient seeking treatment.

CHART NOTE

Flanaghan, Donna S.   Age : 32

January 15, 1994
Patient was seen on the unit for approximately 20 minutes. Chart reviewed.
She is eating and sleeping well. States that her spirits are up. Thinks she
"turned the corner" sometime during the night. Tolerating doxepine HC1 very
well. No adverse reactions other than dry mouth which is subsiding. Will
continue doxepine HC1 100 mg. for a few more days but will taper off night
time sedation and consider extension of hospital privileges if she continues to
hold her gains.

                                        _____
                                        Zigmond M. Lebensohn, M.D.

Figure 34–1
A chart note following a hospital visit by the attending physician.

FAMILY HISTORY ▪ Parents and siblings are listed and briefly described in terms of age, state of health, occupation, and special relationship to the patient.

PERSONAL HISTORY

Birth and Early Development ▪ Date and place of birth, and any unusual complications attending birth and early development, such as delays in walking, talking, or sphincter control.

Educational History ▪ A list of all schools attended in chronologic order, including dates, academic standing, learning problems, honors, and academic degrees, if any.

Military History (If Applicable) ▪ Branch of service, enlisted or drafted, length and type of service, highest rate or rank attained, disciplinary record, if any, and date and type of discharge.

Occupational History ▪ A chronologic list of all jobs held, together with details regarding salary, type of occupational adjustment, problems with superiors, colleagues, or subordinates, and the reasons for leaving or changing jobs.

Psychosexual Development ▪ Here are recorded the appropriate details of the patient's basic sexual history and present sexual orientation and sexual problems, if any.

Marital History (When Applicable) ▪ Date of marriage, length of acquaintance prior to marriage, age of patient and spouse at time of marriage, number of children listed by name, age, and state of health. Description of the quality of marriage (satisfying or unsatisfying), specific problems.

Past Medical History ▪ Here all illnesses, surgical procedures, and serious accidents are listed in chronologic order. A history of previous psychiatric illness and treatment is also included. Women are asked to give a menstrual history together with a history of all pregnancies and children, if any. If there has been a series of marriages and divorces, this section can become quite complicated.

Habits ▪ Use of tobacco, alcohol, and drugs is described in detail.

Social Adaptability ▪ Member of clubs, organizations; leader or follower, socially active or inactive.

ZIGMOND M. LEBENSOHN, MD.
2015 R. Street, N.W.
Washington, DC 20009-0000

July 21, 1994

Dr. Jonathan Jones
2589 Suffix Lane
Baltimore, MD 20085

RE: Jane Rose

Dear Dr. Jones:

I should like to report to you on your patient, Mrs. Jane Rose, who consulted me on January 16, 1994, at your kind suggestion.

I shall not repeat the lengthy history with which you are thoroughly familiar by virtue of having been her attending physician for the past ten years. Suffice it to say, we are dealing here with a 45-year-old single librarian who has experienced numerous anxiety attacks since her early thirties. Most of her anxieties are concentrated on her gastrointestinal tract, and symptoms include nausea, gagging on food, and vague discomfort in the epigastrium. She fears she may have an undetected cancer growing in her abdomen. However, studies of the upper and lower gastrointestinal (GI) tract carried out under your supervision have all been within normal limits.

I have made a tentative diagnosis of Somatization Disorder 300.70 (DSM-III-R), with marked anxiety features. A course of supportive psychotherapy accompanied by judicious use of a mild benzodiazepine was recommended. She states that she would like to discuss the situation with you before making a decision, and I have encouraged her to do so.

With many thanks for asking me to see Mrs. Rose, I am,

Sincerely,

Zigmond M. Lebensohn, M.D.

ZML:rm

Figure 34–2

A consultation report to a physician regarding a patient with a long-standing history of anxiety attacks.

DEPARTMENT OF PSYCHIATRY
Sibley Memorial Hospital
5255 Loughboro Road, N. W.
Washington, DC 20016-0000
202/537-4000

DISCHARGE SUMMARY

NAME OF PATIENT: Davis, Richard   DOB: 1/10/30

ADDRESS: 135 Orchard Street,
Washington, DC 20854

MEDICAL RECORD NO: 56-61-10

ADMITTED: 1/16/94   DISCHARGED: 2/7/94

To: √1. Home
      2. Other Hospital
      3. Nursing Home

DIAGNOSIS: (Multiaxial evaluation)

Axis I 296.2x   Major Depression, Single Episode, Severe with
Psychotic Delusional Features.

Axis II 301.40 Obsessive Compulsive Personality Disorder.

Axis III Atrial Fibrillation, Chronic, Controlled by Medication.

Axis IV Psychosocial Stressors: Threatened dissolution of his
business enterprise.

CONSULTANTS: T. H. Jones, M.D. (Cardiology)

REASON FOR ADMISSION: Mr. Davis is a 62 year-old business man who was admitted to the psychiatric unit as an emergency following a serious suicidal attempt by cutting both wrists. A perfectionist all his life, he was successful in business until recently when key personnel left his organization in substantial numbers. He had never seen a psychiatrist before but began consulting a psychiatrist for depression about two months prior to admission. He was treated by outpatient psychotherapy and antidepressant medication. In spite

(continued)

Figure 34–3
Discharge summary for a 62-year-old man who was admitted to a psychiatric unit following a suicide attempt.

Figure continued

Richard Davis
Medical Record No. 56-61-10   Page two

of therapy his condition worsened and following his suicidal attempt he was
referred to my service on the psychiatric unit for observation and possible
electric convulsive therapy (ECT).

SUMMARY OF FINDINGS ON ADMISSION: Patient was still grossly depressed
on admission. The lacerations of his wrists had been sutured and dressed in
the emergency room prior to arrival on the unit. At times he felt hopeless and
expressed regret about not having been successful in his suicidal attempt. At
other times he appeared ashamed of what he had done.

PHYSICAL EXAMINATION: Physical examination revealed recent lacerations of
both wrists (tendons intact) and atrial fibrillation which the patient has had for
at least 12 years. Blood pressure 130/90. He is taking Lanoxin 0.125 mg.
b.i.d. and Inderal 20 mg. t.i.d. Dr. Johns, his cardiologist, was notified and
saw the patient in consultation for medical clearance for ECT. All laboratory
findings except the electrocardiogram (EKG), which confirmed the diagnosis of
atrial fibrillation, were within normal limits. Frequent checks by nursing staff
were ordered until his condition improved.

COURSE IN HOSPITAL: Patient received medical clearance for ECT from Dr.
Jones on 1/18/94. He then received a course of six ECT's, each treatment
preceded by IV Brevital anesthesia and succinylcholine as a muscle relaxant.
Patient tolerated the treatments well with no complications. His mood began
to lift after the fourth treatment. Memory impairment following the sixth
treatment was mild and confined to recent events.

CONDITION ON DISCHARGE: Patient was considered greatly improved at time
of discharge. His last treatment was on 2/1/94. He was mildly euphoric and
did not appear concerned about the fuzziness of memory which, he was
assured, would clear up in a matter of weeks.

INSTRUCTION TO PATIENT: Patient was told he could have a normal diet with
no restrictions. He was told to continue his cardiac medication and keep in
touch with Dr. Jones, his cardiologist. He was also advised to avoid all
alcoholic beverages and told not to drive a motor vehicle until considered ready

(continued)

Figure 34–3 *Continued*

Richard Davis
Medical Record NO. 56-61-10   Page three

by his attending psychiatrist. He will be seen in my office at weekly or
biweekly intervals together with his wife who has been very supportive.

PROGNOSIS: Good.

ZML:ssb   Zigmond M. Lebensohn, M.D.
D: 2/7/94
T: 2/8/94

Figure 34–3 Continued

Antisocial Trends ▪ Conflicts with authority, arrests, prison terms, charges and disposition.
Avocational Interests ▪ Hobbies, sports, reading matter, cultural interests.
Religious Background ▪ Observant or nonobservant; religious conflicts; how important is religion in the patient's life?
MENTAL STATUS EXAMINATION
General Appearance ▪ Dress, demeanor, cooperative or uncooperative, mannerisms, tics.
Stream of Speech ▪ Clear? Relevant? Coherent? Slurred? Echolalia? Word salad? Flight of ideas?
Affect and Mood ▪ Elated? Depressed? Euthymic? Anxious?
Abnormal Mental Trends ▪ Delusions? Hallucinations? Obsessive-compulsive ruminations?
Mental Grasp and Capacity

▪ Orientation: Time, place, and person.

▪ Memory: Remote events, recent events, retention.

▪ Ability to perform simple calculations.

▪ General fund of knowledge: Compatible or incompatible with patient's educational background?

▪ Insight and judgment.

Dreams ▪ Recurrent? Subject matter? Affect? Nightmares?
Consultation Report ▪ As noted in the section under Letters, such a report is of great importance to the psychiatrist and to the referring physician. A sample of such a consultation appears in Figure 34–2.
Discharge Summary ▪ This should be no longer than one or two pages at the most and should include the following data:

Name of institution, address, and telephone number
Full name of patient, address, and date of birth
Dates of admission and discharge
Final diagnosis in form of multiaxial evaluation
Consultants, if any
Reason for admission
Summary of findings of physical and psychiatric examination on admission, plus any significant laboratory findings
Course in hospital, including special procedures
Condition on discharge
Instructions to patient

See Figure 34–3 for an example.

Reference Sources

Diagnostic and Statistical Manual III, revised. American Psychiatric Association, Washington, D.C., 1987.

Freedman, A. *Comprehensive Textbook of Psychiatry,* 3 volumes. Williams & Wilkins, Baltimore, 1989.

Gay, Peter. *Freud; A Life for our Times.* Norton, New York, 1988.

Grinspoon, L. (Ed.). *Psychiatry Update,* Volumes I, II, and III. American Psychiatric Press, Washington, D.C., 1982, 1983, and 1984.

Karasu, T. B. *The Psychiatric Therapies.* American Psychiatric Press, Washington, D.C., 1984.

Kolb, L., and A. Noyes. *Modern Clinical Psychiatry,* 8th edition. W. B. Saunders Company, Philadelphia, 1982.

McKinnon, R. A., and R. Michels. *The Psychiatric Interview in Clinical Practice.* W. B. Saunders Company, Philadelphia, 1991.

Menninger, K. A. *The Human Mind,* 3rd edition. Alfred A. Knopf, New York, 1946.

For references of specific application to medical transcription, see Appendix 1.

Raymond L. Del Fava, M.D.
Frank L. Hussey, Jr., M.D.
Kerano J. Sperry

Radiology

INTRODUCTION

The first part of this chapter will deal with diagnostic radiology and the last part will discuss radiation oncology.

DIAGNOSTIC RADIOLOGY

The first x-ray examination was done in 1895 by a physics professor who stumbled upon the power of the unknown or "x" ray. Wilhelm Conrad Roentgen was experimenting with light when he discovered the mysterious ray that was to advance the practice of medicine. Within three months of Roentgen's discovery, x-ray images were being used to detect "bullets, bones, and gallstones."

Diagnostic radiology is medicine's eye into the human body. Diagnostic radiologists help the referring physician detect disease using a variety of techniques. They act as consultants in the care of patients. The education of a radiologist begins with a four-year college degree. Four years of medical school follows that to earn the doctoral degree. Then a transitional year may be required. The next step is a four-year radiology residency. Following residency, most radiologists go into practice as physicians specializing in the use of roentgen rays and other forms of energy in the diagnosis and treatment of diseases.

The diagnostic radiologist has a variety of techniques to choose from — plain film x-rays, mammography, computed tomography, magnetic resonance imaging, ultrasound, and nuclear medicine — to provide the best look inside the human body.

Plain Film X-ray Studies ▪ Film x-ray studies are the most common radiologic procedures. The image on an x-ray film is produced when a very small amount of ionizing radiation passes through the patient's body to expose film on the other side. Dense tissue, such as bone, does not let much radiation pass through the body — bone absorbs or blocks a greater amount of radiation so it appears white on the x-ray film. On the other hand, fatty tissue and air-containing structures, such as the lungs, are not very dense so they allow nearly all the x-rays through. These structures appear darker on the x-ray film.

Some structures, such as the liver, heart, and kidneys, have about the same density. They are difficult to distinguish from one another. This problem can be solved by introducing a contrast medium into the organ. Contrast media (sometimes called contrast agents, contrast material, or dyes) block or partially block the passage of x-rays so the radiologist can distinguish certain anatomic structures from surrounding tissues of similar density.

Barium compounds and iodine-containing solutions are the most common groups of contrast agents. Barium compounds can be swallowed to highlight the esophagus, stomach, and intestine. Iodine compounds may be injected into the bloodstream to accentuate blood vessels or kidneys. Rarely patients may have a reaction to the iodine-based contrast. Research continues, and recently some new contrast agents have been developed that seem to be even better tolerated by these patients.

The most common type of film x-ray examination is the chest x-ray view to examine the heart and lungs. This examination has left its mark in social history by helping control tuberculosis, pneumonia, and coal miner's "black lung" disease (see Figure 35–1 on pages 664 and 665).

Another common type of x-ray film examination is mammography, which is an x-ray examination of the breasts. Mammography is the most effective means for detecting breast cancer at an earlier and more curable stage. Major national medical organizations, including the American Cancer Society and the American College of Radiology, recommend that women begin having regular screening mammography by the time they are 40 years of age (see Figure 35–2 on pages 666 and 667).

Many of these x-ray films are "snapshots" of internal organs or tissues. They do not show any movement, such as the heart beating or diaphragm moving.

The radiologist can do fluoroscopy to create "motion pictures." These studies also use x-rays to create images. The radiologist can watch these "motion pictures" on a video screen while the examination is being performed. These pictures can be taped so they can be reviewed after the examination. The gastrointestinal series and the barium enema are the most common fluoroscopic studies. These studies are done to diagnose ulcers, tumors, and other abnormalities in the stomach and intestine (see Figure 35–3 on pages 668 and 669).

Computed Tomography (CT) ■ This is the computerized version of the film x-ray (see Figures 35–4, 35–5, 35–6, and 35–7 on pages 670 to 675). This technique also uses x-rays to create images. To produce the images (also called CT scans), a patient is put on a narrow table, which then slides into the CT scanner. An x-ray beam inside the scanner rotates around the part of the patient being examined. X-rays passing through the body are detected by sensors that also are inside the scanner. Information from the sensors is processed by an attached computer, which then displays the CT scan on a video screen. Film copies also may be made so the radiologist can review the scans after the examination is completed.

Standard computed tomography creates two-dimensional image slices. It allows radiologists to separate overlapping structures precisely. Sometimes oral or intravenous contrast medium is given to the patient to further enhance the CT image.

CT is useful in examination of virtually any part of the body.

Special computer software can create three-dimensional CT images. These images are especially useful in planning reconstructive surgery.

Magnetic Resonance Imaging (MRI) ■ This procedure is like computed tomography in that it produces images that show slices of the human anatomy (see Figure 35–8 on pages 676 and 677). However, MRI does not use any ionizing radiation to create its images. Instead it uses magnetic fields and radio frequencies. During the MRI examination, a patient is placed on a narrow table, which is then placed inside the MRI scanner. The patient is surrounded by a magnetic field up to 30,000 times stronger than that of the earth.

The human body is made of tiny particles called atoms. At the center of the atoms are spinning particles called nuclei. Normally, nuclei spin at many different angles. The magnetic field of the MRI scanner makes the nuclei spin at the same angle. The scanner then subjects the nuclei to a radio signal, temporarily knocking them out of alignment. When the signal stops, the nuclei return to the aligned position, releasing their own faint radio frequencies. The scanner receives these frequencies; a computer attached to the scanner turns the information into very detailed images of the human anatomy.

MRI produces remarkable images of the brain and spine. It is also being used to evaluate joints, bone, and soft tissue abnormalities, as well as abnormalities of the chest and abdomen.

Three-dimensional MRI images are also possible.

Ultrasound ■ Ultrasound imaging does not use x-rays to create images (see Figure 35–9 on pages 678 and 679). It uses high-frequency sound humans cannot hear. In most ultrasound examinations, a transducer, a lightweight device that produces sound waves, is placed on the patient's skin. There are also special transducers that can be placed into the vagina (transvaginal ultrasound) or rectum (transrectal ultrasound) to image these areas of the body. The transducer produces sound waves that penetrate the skin to reach tissues and organs. Echoes are produced in tissues and organs in varying degrees of intensity, depending on the density of the material. They are sent back to the transducer, which electronically converts the echoes into an image displayed on a video screen. These images on the video screen show motion. The images can also be recorded on film.

Ultrasound imaging is commonly used to view a growing fetus and to check for position and approximate age of the fetus. Ultrasound imaging can show whether multiple fetuses are present and whether there are any developmental abnormalities in the fetus. Such studies are also used to further detect breast cancer and are often used after abnormal mammograms.

Ultrasound images can show the shape, texture, and composition of tumors and cysts. This technique provides a new way to examine the musculoskeletal system. Such studies also are used to diagnose disease in children and to examine the gallbladder and kidneys.

Doppler ultrasound shows the flow of blood through veins and arteries, so it can be used to detect clogged blood vessels.

Cardiac ultrasound uses sound waves to determine how well the heart is working.

Nuclear Medicine ▪ Nuclear medicine studies use radioactive chemicals called radiopharmaceuticals to show whether certain organs are working properly. They are also used for therapeutic purposes (see Figure 35–10 on pages 680 and 681). Nuclear medicine studies are different from most other radiology studies because they document organ function rather than particular anatomy.

Organs such as the heart, kidneys, brain, thyroid gland, and lungs may be studied. The patient's bones also may be examined.

In a typical nuclear imaging procedure, a small amount of a radioactive substance is given to a patient. Usually, it is injected into the patient's vein. It may be swallowed or inhaled. Special substances that have been tagged with radioactive compounds emit gamma rays (a type of ionizing radiation). These compounds are formulated to collect, for a very short time, in the parts of the patient's body to be studied. Images of the patient may be taken immediately or they may be taken several hours or even days later.

In most studies, a patient lies comfortably on a table. A large instrument called a scintillation or gamma camera is put over the organ to be imaged. The camera can be moved around a patient if necessary. The camera detects the radiation being emitted from the radioactive compound and creates a picture on a display screen or on film (called a scan or scintigram).

Heart and bone studies are two common nuclear medicine examinations.

Heart studies are done to evaluate blood flow to the heart muscle and also to evaluate cardiac function. A single photon emission computed tomography (SPECT) study also may be done to evaluate the heart. During this study, the patient exercises to get the heart pumping faster. A radioactive compound is injected into the patient and then one or two sets of images are taken. A special computer turns these images into two- or three-dimensional displays showing how well the heart is working.

Bone studies are accurate methods for evaluating the skeleton. Before the examination, a radioactive compound is given to the patient. The bones absorb the compound and then images are taken. The bone scan may show whether cancer, infection, or trauma is present.

Positron emission tomography (PET) studies are being done in some radiologic facilities to study the metabolic activity inside an organ. PET has been shown to be useful in the study of brain-related disorders such as epilepsy and dementia. For further information on nuclear medicine as well as examples of reports, see the section entitled Nuclear Medicine.

Interventional Radiology ▪ A relatively recent extension of radiology is into the area of interventional radiology. In this field, the radiologist is no longer just an observer of the patient's imaging findings but assumes a more active role in the diagnosis and treatment. Balloon angioplasty is a common interventional procedure that is done to open blocked arteries. The interventional radiologist threads a balloon-tipped catheter to the part of an artery which is blocked by plaque. The balloon is inflated, then removed, so normal blood flow resumes. Interventional radiologists also use catheters to drain pus or pockets of blood and to remove kidney stones from the urinary tract and gallstones from the bile duct. Refer to the report of the CT biopsy of the pancreas and liver in Figure 35–7 on page 674. Note the use of proprietary names for instruments used in this invasive procedure and the concluding statement regarding a clinical assessment of the patient following the procedure.

Radiation Safety

Radiologists and the others who work in the radiology department are specially trained in radiation safety. The workers within the department wear a radiation badge that is tested regularly to ensure that the level of radiation exposure each worker receives is well within safe limits. Examinations are done to produce the best images using the least amount of radiation possible. There has never been convincing proof that this very small amount of radiation poses any health risk. Some examinations, such as ultrasound and magnetic resonance imaging, do not use any radiation at all. Ultrasound examinations rather than x-ray examinations are frequently done on children and fetuses because children and fetuses are growing rapidly so they may be more susceptible to x-ray radiation. In almost all x-ray examinations, the radiation beam is limited to only the part of the body being imaged. In addition, lead shielding, which blocks radiation, may be placed around the area being x-rayed to protect surrounding organs or tissues.

RADIOLOGY REPORTS

The written radiology report is the most important communication between the radiologist and the referring physician. The radiology report must contain the appropriate identification of the patient (name, birthdate, date of examination, x-ray number, address or hospital bed, and the referring physician or physicians). Such documents also must indicate the type of examination, the modality used, and the views obtained (i.e., PA and lateral), as well as the areas included in the imaging examination. The words chosen for the headings of the reports vary a great deal from office to hospital to clinic.

The importance of a strong knowledge of anatomy in radiology transcription cannot be overstressed. It also helps to have some knowledge of physiology, biology, and chemistry. A transcriptionist who is unaware of the various anatomic landmarks cannot be aware of any "slips of the brain or tongue" the radiologist might make. Three examples spring to mind: (a) The greater and lesser tuberosities are on the humerus; the greater and lesser trochanters are on the femur; (b) the metacarpals are in the hand; the metatarsals are in the foot; (c) mammography reports frequently include references to a clock face and/or a specific quadrant. For example, "In the right upper outer quadrant, in the 10 o'clock position . . ." The transcriptionist needs to be aware that the quadrants and time references will not be the same for both breasts: the 10 o'clock position on the left breast is in the upper inner quadrant. All these exam-

ples can lead to confusing reports if the radiologist misstates the location and the transcriptionist does not perceive the error and question the dictator (or leave a blank and flag it, depending on the standard policy of handling such instances in a particular institution).

The following documents illustrate examples of a few of the imaging studies and the reports that might be made. There are certainly a wide variety of reporting styles, depending upon the reporting radiologist, but a common method is to begin the report with a description of the findings and to complete it with a conclusion or impression of the findings that have been described.

With the introduction of the newer modalities, many new words are being used in radiology reports. A few examples of these words and phrases are pointed out here.

Chest X-ray Film ▪ This report includes pertinent negative findings (i.e., the heart size and contour are normal and the costophrenic angles are clear), as well as the positive pathologic descriptions (Figure 35–1). If any earlier radio-

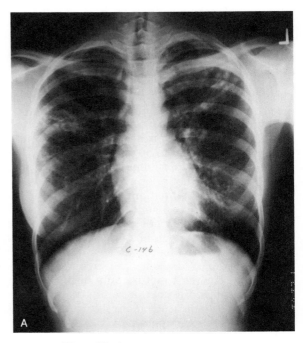

Figure 35–1

A, Posteroanterior (PA) chest x-ray.

University Radiological Medical Group, Inc.
1234 Main Street
Los Angeles, CA 90012-0000

NAME: Jane Doe   B/D: 03/17/15   RM/BD: 513301   EDP# 75033   ORD#00034

REFERRING PHYSICIAN: John Smith, M. D.   PERFORMED BY CMK

DATE: 04/16/94   TIME: 1735

MJ DATE: 04/17/94   TIME: 1012

RADIOLOGIST: James Jones, M. D.

DATE AND TIME OF FINAL REPORT: 04/18/94 1036

X-RAY #000097959

EXAMINATION: CHEST PA & LATERAL

The heart size and contour are normal. There is streaky infiltration in the left infraclavicular region extending back down toward the left hilar area. There is somewhat similar interstitial infiltration in the projection of the 2nd right anterior interspace. There are several smooth, rounded areas of radiolucency within the infiltrate.

There are also interstitial infiltrations in the right mid and left paracardiac regions.

The costophrenic angles are clear.

Impression: BILATERAL UPPER LOBE INFILTRATIONS WITH PROBABLE CAVITY FORMATION WITH BRONCHOGENIC SPREAD TO THE RIGHT MID AND LEFT LOWER LUNG FIELDS.

THE FINDINGS ARE MOST LIKELY ON THE BASIS OF TUBERCULOSIS, BUT THE EXACT ETIOLOGY AND ACTIVITY MUST BE ESTABLISHED CLINICALLY.

James Jones, M. D.
RADIOLOGIST ELECTRONIC SIGNATURE

JJ/alb
D: 04/18/94
T: 04/18/94

B

Figure 35–1 *Continued*
B, A final chest x-ray report.

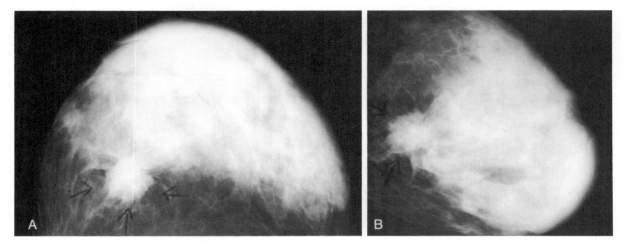

Figure 35–2
Screening mammography, showing a spiculated density that must be considered malignant until proved otherwise. A, Craniocaudad view. B, Oblique-lateral view.

graphic studies of the chest had been available, some comment would have to be made about a comparison. Notice that the radiologist sometimes indicates what other imaging studies might be done and, at times, what other appropriate clinical data might be helpful.

Mammography ▪ An example of a screening mammography may be seen in Figure 35–2. The report illustrates a type of case in which the radiologist might recommend further testing, using ultrasound of the dense area of the left breast.

Barium Enema ▪ A report of a barium enema should include the date and time of the examination and transcription, along with the signature of the radiologist. The radiologist must sign the report after proofreading. He or she may sign directly, use a rubber stamp (the rubber stamp must be under strict control of only the radiologist), or imprint an electronic signature if computer reporting is utilized (Figure 35–3).

Computed tomography (CT) Scan ▪ These studies utilize words and phrases not commonly found in plain film studies, such as "hypodense" and "with and without infusion" (Figures 35–4 and 35–5.)

In Figures 35–6 and 35–7, note the use of proprietary names for instruments used in this invasive procedure and the concluding statement regarding a clinical assessment of the patient after the procedure was concluded.

Magnetic Resonance Imaging (MRI) ▪ In Figure 35–8, note that MRI has introduced terms such as "T1 and T2," "ring enhancement," and "flow-void."

Ultrasound Imaging ▪ Figure 35–9A illustrates an ultrasound image of the gallbladder. Note that ultrasound also has added words to the radiology jargon, examples in Figure 35–9B being "echogenic" and "acoustical shadowing."

Single Photon Emission Computed Tomography (SPECT) ▪ When evaluating the heart, some practices get two dictations, one from the cardiologist describing the treadmill stress test and a second from a radiologist describing the results of the imaging procedure (Figure 35–10). In regard to terminology, the field of nuclear medicine has made additions to the jargon, such as "millicuries," "SPECT," and "planar images."

Text continued on page 682

University Radiological Medical Group, Inc.
1234 Main Street
Los Angeles, CA 90012-0000

NAME: Jane Doe   B/D: 03/17/15 RM/BD: 513301 EDP# 75033 ORD# 00034

REFERRING PHYSICIAN: John Smith, M. D.   PERFORMED BY CMK

DATE: 04/16/94   TIME: 1735

MJ DATE: 04/17/94   TIME: 1012

RADIOLOGIST: James Jones, M. D.

DATE AND TIME OF FINAL REPORT: 04/18/94 1036

X-RAY # 000097960

CRANIOCAUDAD, OBLIQUE-LATERAL, FILM SCREEN.

EXAMINATION: MAMMOGRAPHY
The breasts show a large amount of fibroglandular density (Wolfe's classification DY).

There is a spiculated mass density measuring approximately 2.0 cm x 2.5 cm x 2.5 cm in the deep portion of the left breast just medial and very slightly below the line of the nipple. There are a few small, smooth calcifications, both within the mass density itself and in the adjacent area.

The remaining portions of the left breast and the right breast are within normal limits.

Impression: SPICULATED DENSITY IN THE LEFT BREAST WHICH MUST BE CONSIDERED MALIGNANT UNTIL PROVEN OTHERWISE.

IF THE LESION IS NOT PALPABLE, BIOPSY SHOULD BE DONE AFTER RADIOGRAPHIC LOCALIZATION.

JJ/alb
D: 04/18/94
T: 04/18/94

C

_____
James Jones, M. D.
RADIOLOGIST ELECTRONIC SIGNATURE

Figure 35–2 *Continued*
C, The mammography report of the films shown in A and B.

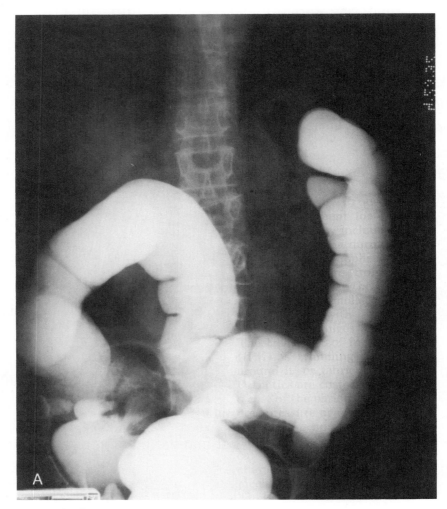

Figure 35–3
A, Barium enema with no demonstrable disease of the colon or terminal ileum.

University Radiological Medical Group, Inc.
1234 Main Street
Los Angeles, CA 90012-0000

NAME: Jane Doe   B/D: 03/17/15 RM/BD: 513301 EDP# 75033 ORD#000343
REFERRING PHYSICIAN: John Smith, M. D. PERFORMED BY CMK
DATE: 04/16/94   TIME: 1735
MJ DATE: 04/17/94   TIME: 1012
RADIOLOGIST: James Jones, M. D.
DATE AND TIME OF FINAL REPORT: 04/18/94   1036
X-RAY #000097959

EXAMINATION: BARIUM ENEMA

The colon filled quite readily and did not show evidence of stenosis, ulceration, neoplastic filling defect, diverticula, or abnormal irritability.

The cecum showed a minor malrotation with the ileocecal valve being located laterally. A short segment of the terminal ileum filled and appeared normal.

IMPRESSION: NO DEMONSTRABLE DISEASE OF THE COLON OR TERMINAL ILEUM.

NO CLINICAL SIGNIFICANCE IS ATTACHED TO THE MINOR MALROTATION OF THE CECUM MENTIONED ABOVE.

_____
James Jones, M. D.
RADIOLOGIST ELECTRONIC SIGNATURE

JJ/alb
D: 04/18/94
T: 04/18/94

B

Figure 35–3 *Continued*
B, Barium enema x-ray report.

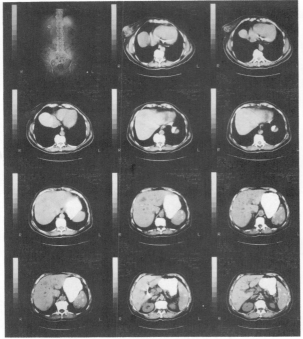

A

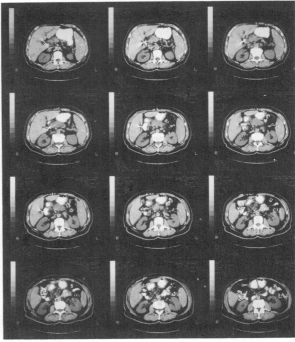

B

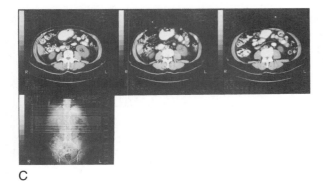

C

Figure 35–4

A–G, Computed tomography (CT) scans of the abdomen and pelvis with and without the use of intravenous contrast.

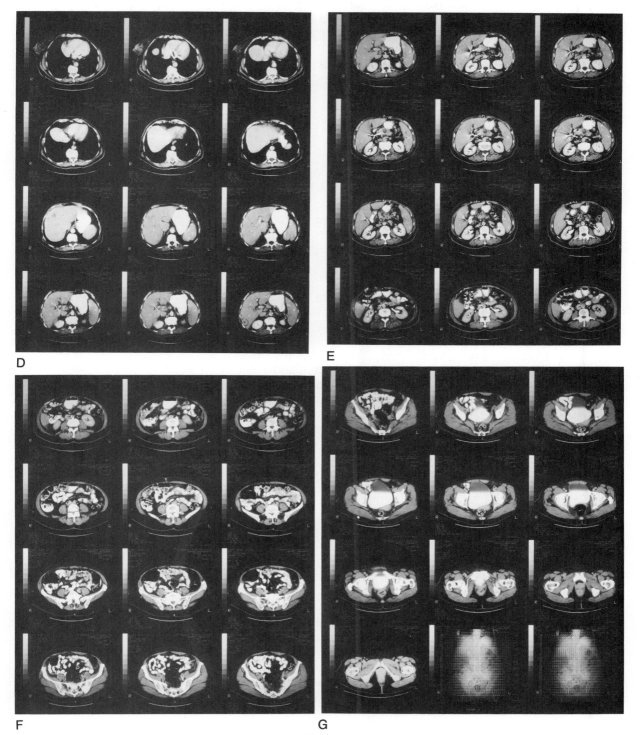

D

E

F

G

Figure 35–4 Continued

University Radiological Medical Group, Inc.
1234 Main Street
Los Angeles, CA 90012-0000

NAME: Jane Doe   B/D: 03/17/15 RM/BD: 513301 EDP# 75033 ORD#000343
REFERRING PHYSICIAN: John Smith, M. D. PERFORMED BY CMK
DATE: 04/16/94   TIME: 1735
MJ DATE: 04/17/94   TIME: 1012
RADIOLOGIST: James Jones, M. D.
DATE AND TIME OF FINAL REPORT: 04/18/94 1036
EXAMINATION: CT ABDOMEN W & WO IV CONTRAST   X-RAY #000097959

CT OF THE ABDOMEN AND PELVIS WITH AND WITHOUT USE OF IV
CONTRAST.

The patient is post left mastectomy.

There are multiple hypodense lesions throughout the right and left lobes of the
liver. The largest lesion is 3 cm and is located in the anterior segment of the right
lobe of the liver.

Multiple calcifications, many of which have a ringed contour, are identified in the
spleen. Several hypodensities are identified in proximity to these calcifications.
This appearance would be atypical for granulomatous disease and suggests
calcified and necrotic metastatic lesions to the spleen.

Surgical clips are seen in the gallbladder fossa consistent with the history of
cholecystectomy.

At the junction of the head and body of pancreas, there is a 5 cm inhomogeneous
mass which is encasing the superior mesenteric vein. The pancreatic head and
tail are relatively atrophic.

There are multiple small lymph nodes identified in the peripancreatic and
periaortic regions.

There is a small amount of peritoneal fluid identified in the left paracolic gutter
and cul-de-sac.

The kidneys excrete contrast in a normal fashion and no mass lesions are
identified. The left adrenal gland size is within the upper limits of normal but
maintains a relatively normal contour. The right adrenal gland appears normal.

There is a 2.5 cm right adnexal hypodensity which most likely represents a cyst.
(continued)

Figure 35-5
Computed tomography (CT) report of the abdomen and pelvis with and without use of intravenous contrast, typed in full block
format.

Page 2
Re: Jane Doe
Xray # 000097959

CONCLUSION:
1. PANCREATIC MASS, AS DESCRIBED, WITH EVIDENCE OF REGIONAL LYMPH NODE INVOLVEMENT AND ENCASEMENT OF THE SUPERIOR MESENTERIC VEIN.

2. METASTATIC LESIONS WITHIN THE LIVER AND SPLEEN. DIFFERENTIATION BETWEEN METASTASES FROM THE BREAST VERSUS THE PANCREAS CANNOT BE MADE.

Biopsies of the liver and pancreatic lesions are recommended for further investigation.

                                            James Jones, M. D.
                                            RADIOLOGIST ELECTRONIC SIGNATURE

JJ/alb
D: 04/18/94
T: 04/18/94

Figure 35–5 Continued

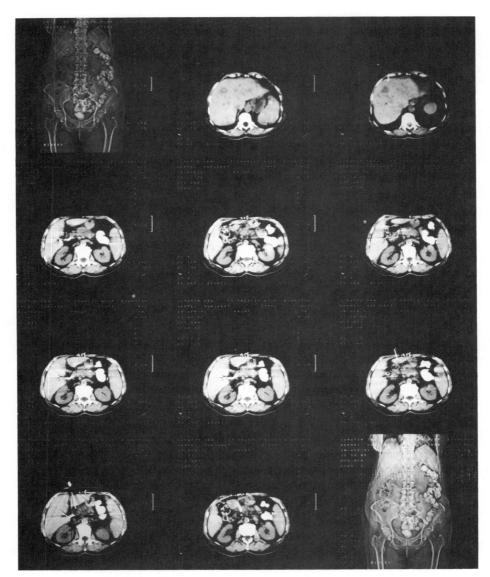

Figure 35–6
CT-guided biopsy of the pancreas and liver.

University Radiological Medical Group, Inc.
1234 Main Street
Los Angeles, CA 90012-0000

NAME: Jane Doe   B/D: 03/17/15 RM/BD: 513301   EDP# 75033 ORD#000343

REFERRING PHYSICIAN: John Smith, M. D. PERFORMED BY CMK

DATE: 04/16/94   TIME: 1735

MJ DATE: 04/17/94   TIME: 1012

RADIOLOGIST: James Jones, M. D.

DATE AND TIME OF FINAL REPORT: 04/18/94   1036

EXAMINATION: CT BIOPSY   X-RAY #000097959

CT - GUIDED BIOPSY OF THE PANCREAS AND LIVER:

The right anterior abdomen was prepped and anesthetized in the usual manner. Using CT guidance, the previously noted pancreatic and liver masses were biopsied.

Using a BioP-T needle, two specimens were obtained from the largest hypodensity in the right lobe of the liver.

Using a Menghini 21-gauge needle, the pancreatic mass was biopsied.

The specimens were sent to pathology.

The patient tolerated the procedure and left the department in good condition.

_____
James Jones, M. D.
RADIOLOGIST ELECTRONIC SIGNATURE

JJ/alb
D: 04/18/94
T: 04/18/94

Figure 35–7
Computed tomography (CT) report of a biopsy of a pancreas and liver, typed in full block format.

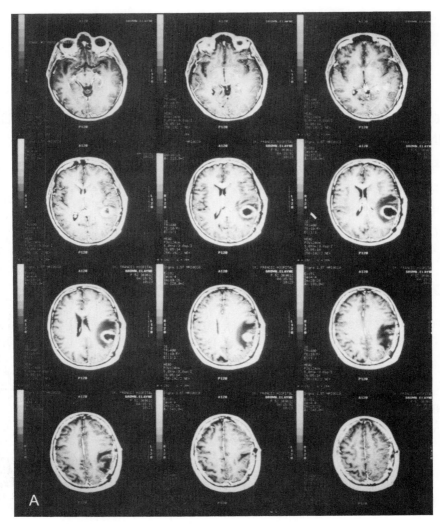

Figure 35–8
A, Magnetic resonance imaging (MRI) of the brain with and without contrast, showing a 4-cm. mass in the left parietal lobe.

University Radiological Medical Group, Inc.
1234 Main Street
Los Angeles, CA 90012-0000

NAME: Jane Doe   B/D: 03/17/15 RM/BD: 513301   EDP# 75033 ORD#000343

REFERRING PHYSICIAN: John Smith, M. D. PERFORMED BY CMK

DATE: 04/16/94   TIME: 1735

MJ DATE: 04/17/94   TIME: 1012

RADIOLOGIST: James Jones, M. D.

DATE AND TIME OF FINAL REPORT: 04/18/94   1036

EXAMINATION: MRI BRAIN W & WO CONTRAST   X-RAY #000097959

MRI EXAMINATION OF THE BRAIN WITH AND WITHOUT CONTRAST
SHOWS AS FOLLOWS:

There is noted a 4 cm mass in the left parietal lobe with ring enhancement after
contrast, surrounded by well-defined edema. Both a necrotic tumor or an
abscess could give this appearance; however, the ring enhancement is
somewhat irregular and nodular in portions. There are also a few flow-voids
seen in the spin echo images which suggest feeding vascularity. These findings
favor a neoplastic process over an inflammatory abscess.

IMPRESSION: THERE IS A 4 CM MASS IN THE LEFT PARIETAL LOBE WITH
MARKED T1 PROLONGATION AND SLIGHT T2 SHORTENING WITH RING
ENHANCEMENT AFTER CONTRAST SURROUNDED BY EDEMA. I FAVOR A
NEOPLASTIC PROCESS OVER AN INFLAMMATORY ABSCESS.

_____
James Jones, M. D.
RADIOLOGIST ELECTRONIC SIGNATURE

JJ/alb
D: 04/18/94
T: 04/18/94

B

Figure 35–8 *Continued*
B, The report of this MRI study of the brain.

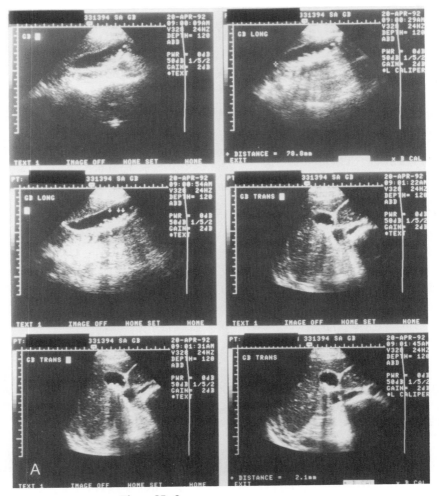

Figure 35–9
A, Ultrasound image of the gallbladder.

University Radiological Medical Group, Inc.
1234 Main Street
Los Angeles, CA 90012-0000

NAME: Jane Doe   B/D: 03/17/15 RM/BD: 513301 EDP# 75033 ORD#000343
REFERRING PHYSICIAN: John Smith, M. D. PERFORMED BY CMK
DATE: 04/16/94   TIME: 1735
MJ DATE: 04/17/94   TIME: 1012
RADIOLOGIST: James Jones, M. D.
DATE AND TIME OF FINAL REPORT: 04/18/94   1036
EXAMINATION: ECHO GALLBLADDER   X-RAY #000097959

ECHO GALLBLADDER

The gallbladder, which is not enlarged, contains numerous gravity dependent echogenic densities which produce acoustical shadowing and would be indicative of cholelithiasis.

NO BILIARY DUCTAL DILATATION IS SEEN.

_____
James Jones, M. D.
RADIOLOGIST ELECTRONIC SIGNATURE

JJ/alb
D: 04/18/94
T: 04/18/94

B

Figure 35-9 *Continued*
B, The report of the study.

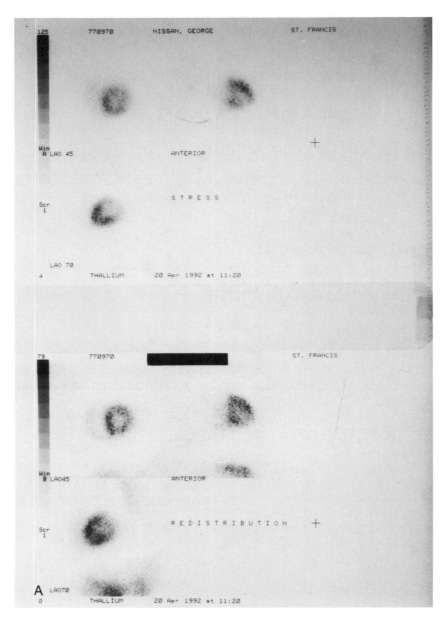

Figure 35–10
A, Thallium S/R single photon emission computed tomography (SPECT) evaluation of the heart.

University Radiological Medical Group, Inc.
1234 Main Street
Los Angeles, CA 90012-0000

NAME: Jane Doe   B/D: 03/17/15 RM/BD: 513301 EDP# 75033 ORD#000343

REFERRING PHYSICIAN: John Smith, M. D. PERFORMED BY CMK

DATE: 04/16/94   TIME: 1735

MJ DATE: 04/17/94   TIME: 1012

RADIOLOGIST: James Jones, M. D.

DATE AND TIME OF FINAL REPORT: 04/18/94   1036

EXAMINATION: THALLIUM S/R SPECT - HEART   X-RAY #000097959

EXAMINATION: RADIONUCLIDE THALLIUM MYOCARDIAL PERFUSION
IMAGING

The patient was brought to stress under the direction of the cardiologist at which time 3.5 millicuries of thallium 201 were injected intravenously and the patient allowed to stress for an additional minute. Immediately thereafter planar images were obtained in the anterior, 45 and 70 degree LAO projections. SPECT tomograms were also made. The patient returned at three hours and the images repeated as above.

The patient exercised for 10 minutes. The target heart rate was achieved. There are no areas of reversible ischemia demonstrated on the planar or tomographic images. A small area of thinning is seen at the apex which can be seen normally.

IMPRESSION: NO EVIDENCE OF REVERSIBLE ISCHEMIA.

_____
James Jones, M. D.
RADIOLOGIST ELECTRONIC SIGNATURE

JJ/alb
D: 04/18/94
T: 04/18/94

B

Figure 35–10 *Continued*
B, Report of this evaluation.

RADIATION ONCOLOGY

Cancer is a group of diseases that affects millions of people each year. In fact, the American Cancer Society estimates that one person in every three will develop cancer sometime during his or her lifetime. Cancer is characterized by the unusual growth and spread of abnormal cells. If the spread of these cells is not stopped, death can occur.

On the other hand, if the cancer is found early, before the abnormal cells have spread, the cancer patient usually survives and lives a normal life.

There are hundreds of different types of cancer. They are identified by the type of body tissue involved or by the body part involved. The major classifications are:

- Carcinoma: a malignant tumor found in the outermost covering or lining of body surfaces. These solid tumors are commonly found on the skin, in the mouth and throat, or in organs like the breast and prostate.

- Sarcoma: a malignant tumor found in connective tissues, such as bone, muscle, and cartilage.

- Leukemia: malignant disease found in bone marrow and other blood-forming organs.

- Glioma: cancer in the brain, spinal cord, or nerves.

- Lymphoma: a malignant tumor of the lymph glands or other lymphatic tissues.

Cancer patients can be treated in a number of ways. The three most common approaches are surgery, radiation therapy, and chemotherapy. Today, many patients are being treated with a combination of these three methods.

For example, a breast cancer patient may undergo a lumpectomy—removal of the cancerous lump—and then undergo radiation therapy. The radiation helps destroy any cancer cells that were not removed during the surgery. This cooperative effort provides the patient with the best care.

Only cancer specialists, such as radiation oncologists, who have carefully reviewed a patient's medical records, can determine which treatment or treatments are best for any patient. Sometimes there is a choice, such as when two or more of the treatments get the same result.

Some patients with larynx cancer can choose between surgery and radiation therapy, for example. The survival rate for these patients would be about the same if they chose either treatment. The advantage of radiation therapy is that patients can keep their voice box. With surgery, they might well need a mechanical device to help them speak.

About half of all cancer patients are treated with radiation at some time during their disease. Radiation can be used to cure the disease. It also

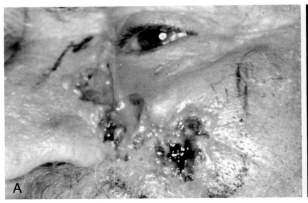 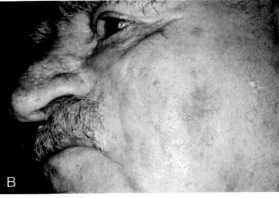

Figure 35–11

A, A malignant skin lesion of the cheek. B, The same patient after radiation therapy.

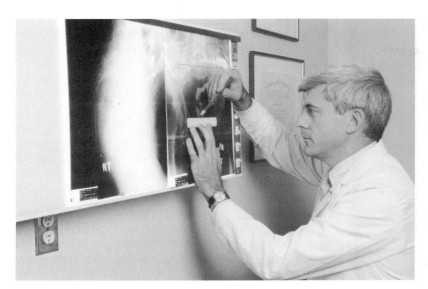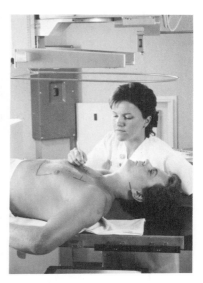

Figure 35–12
A, A radiation oncologist studies the x-ray image to determine where and how to direct the radiation. B, A radiation technologist marks the tumor site on the patient.

can be used to relieve pain. For example, radiation can shrink a tumor in the hip, decreasing pain, thereby making it easier for a patient to walk.

Radiation therapy has been practiced for almost 100 years. It involves the careful use of high-energy radiation (usually x-ray radiation) to treat cancer. Radiation therapy is effective in treating a wide variety of cancers, including skin (Figure 35–11), prostate, and breast cancer.

Most patients undergo external beam radiation treatment. Before actual treatment can begin, a patient first undergoes simulation. During simulation, a radiation therapy technologist takes a series of x-ray images of the patient. The radiation oncologist (the physician) studies these images to determine where and how to direct the radiation (Figure 35–12A). Frequently, the technologist marks the tumor site on the patient. These markings later will help the technologist aim the radiation at the area being treated (Figure 35–12B).

Most radiation therapy patients receive external beam therapy four or five times a week, for a

few minutes each day. Some patients are treated twice a day; others are treated only once or twice a week. Each treatment is painless (Figure 35–13). The entire course of treatment can last from one to nine weeks, depending on what type of cancer the patient has and whether the physician is trying to cure the disease or relieve the patient's pain. Most patients can go home after each treatment and continue with their normal daily activities.

During treatment, the patient lies on a treatment table. The radiation oncologist uses linear accelerators and cobalt machines — machines that produce ionizing radiation, such as x-rays, gamma rays, and electron beams — to destroy tumors at different sites within the body. The radiation is directed to the tumor and surrounding area. The linear accelerator treatment machine may rotate 360 degrees around the patient so the radiation can hit the tumor from all angles.

Some radiation therapy patients undergo brachytherapy, in which the radiation source is placed as close to the tumor site as possible. This

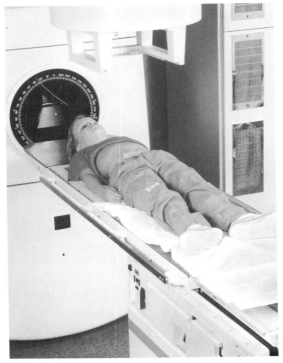

Figure 35-13
A patient is positioned on a linear accelerator for treatment.

big area surrounding the tumor. Brachytherapy then delivers a higher dose of radiation to help destroy the main mass of tumor cells.

RADIATION ONCOLOGY TEAM

Radiation oncologists are the physicians who specialize in the use of radiation to treat cancer patients. Radiation oncologists have completed four years of college, four years of medical school, one year of general medical training, then three to four years of residency training in radiation oncology. They must pass a special examination to be certified by the American Board of Radiology. Radiation oncologists are in charge of the patient's treatment. They decide what type of radiation is best, plan the treatment, and then carefully monitor patients during treatment.

A whole team of medical professionals work with radiation oncologists to provide patients with quality care. Each team of experts may also include physicists, radiation therapy technologists, dosimetrists, nurses, social workers, and dietitians.

Medical physicists help plan each patient's treatment. In addition, they are responsible for developing and directing quality control programs for equipment and procedures. They over-

technique is very effective in treating cancers of the eye, cervix, uterus, vagina, rectum, head, and neck (Figure 35-14).

In intracavitary brachytherapy, containers, such as metal rods or wires that hold radioactive sources, are put in or near the tumor.

In interstitial brachytherapy, the radioactive sources alone are put into the tumor.

The radioactive sources may be left in the patient for only a few days or they may remain permanently. While the radioactive sources are inside the patient, the patient may have to stay in the hospital. Newer devices allow the radiation oncologist to put the radioactive source in the patient and then remove it on the same day, or soon thereafter. The patient usually goes home shortly after the procedure.

Brachytherapy can be done alone or in conjunction with external beam therapy. The external beam radiation destroys cancerous cells in a

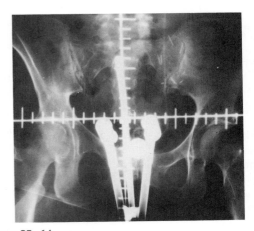

Figure 35-14
In brachytherapy, radioactive sources are placed in or near the tumor. In this case, cancer of the cervix, the metal rod and round containers hold the radioactive sources.

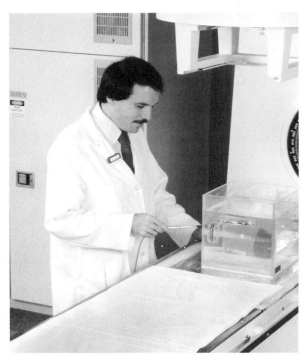

Figure 35–15
The medical physicist regularly checks treatment machines to make sure they work properly.

see the daily checkups of the treatment equipment and are responsible for making sure the equipment works properly (Figure 35–15).

Medical physicists have doctorates or master's degrees. Qualified physicists have gone through four years of college, two to four years of graduate school, and, typically, one to two years of clinical physics training. They are certified by the American Board of Radiology or the American Board of Medical Physics.

Radiation therapy technologists also help plan a patient's treatment. Under the radiation oncologist's prescription and supervision, a radiation therapy technologist carefully and accurately treats each patient. Radiation therapy technologists work closely with each patient. They make sure the radiation therapy service is efficient and of high quality.

Radiation therapy technologists go through a two- to four-year educational program following high school. They take a special examination and can be certified by the American Registry of Radiologic Technologists (A.R.R.T.). Some states also require that radiation therapy technologists be licensed.

Dosimetrists perform calculations to insure that each patient's tumor is getting the dose prescribed by the physician. They also work with other members of the treatment team to determine how the radiation will be given to best destroy the tumor but spare the normal tissues nearby.

Many dosimetrists start as technologists, then, with on-the-job training, become dosimetrists. One- to two-year dosimetry programs also are available following high school. Most dosimetrists are certified by the Medical Dosimetrist Certification Board (Figure 35–16).

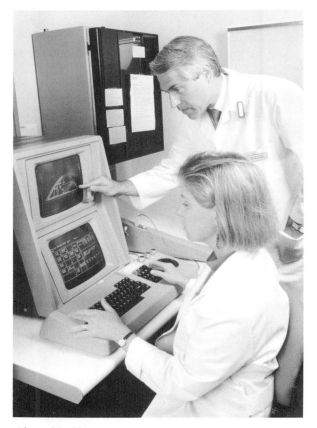

Figure 35–16
The medical physicist and the dosimetrist work with a computer to help design a treatment plan.

Radiation therapy nurses are registered nurses. They help educate the patient and family about radiation treatment and also provide them with emotional support. Radiation therapy nurses do general nursing duties as specifically related to patients undergoing radiation therapy (Figure 35–17).

Social workers also may be available to provide emotional support to each patient and their family. Social workers may be licensed. Licensed social workers must have a master's degree with two years' experience. They also must pass an examination.

Dietitians help each patient eat properly during treatment. They attend four years of college, then usually take part in a one-year internship. Dietitians who pass a professional examination

are registered by the American Dietetic Association.

FUTURE THERAPIES

Radiation oncologists and other medical professionals are researching new and better ways to treat cancer patients using radiation and radioactive sources. The practice of radiation oncology, like all of medicine, continues to grow and change.

Stereotactic radiation therapy is now being used to treat brain tumors and other types of cancer. It allows the radiation oncologist to focus the radiation beams precisely on the tumor volume so more normal brain cells are spared than is possible with conventional external beam radiation.

Intraoperative radiotherapy also is being studied. Here, the radiation treatment is given in the operating room. A surgeon temporarily moves the normal organs out of the way so radiation can be used directly on the tumor.

Heat (hyperthermia) and radiosensitizers (certain drugs) are being reviewed as possible means to make cancer cells more sensitive to radiation.

Other drugs, called radiation protectors, may help protect normal tissue during radiation treatment.

Research is underway using radiolabeled antibodies. Antibodies are made radioactive and then they are injected into the patient. These antibodies search out and destroy tumor cells. This technique is called radioimmunotherapy.

The field of radiation oncology has seen enormous changes in its first 100 years. It will continue to grow and change as researchers learn more about cancer. Radiation oncologists and others who are part of the radiation oncology team are committed to providing cancer patients with quality treatment.

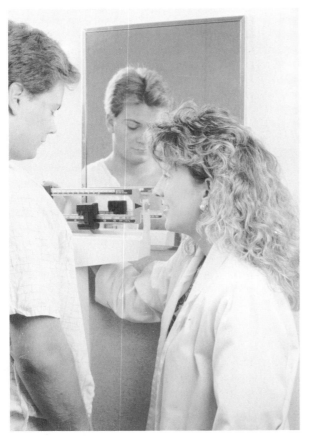

Figure 35–17
A radiation therapy nurse helps collect information on the patient.

Reference Sources

For further information on radiology or for copies of or information on the ACR Standard of Communications mentioned in this chapter, contact the American College of Radiology (ACR), Attention: Public Relations, 1891 Preston White Drive, Reston, VA 22091.

Brecher, Ruth, and Edward Brecher. *The Rays.* Williams and Wilkins, Baltimore, 1977.

Grigg, E. R. N. *The Trail of the Invisible Light.* Charles C Thomas Publisher, Springfield, Illinois, 1965.

Hagen-Ansert, Sandra L. *Textbook on Diagnostic Ultrasound,* 3rd edition. Mosby/Year Book, St. Louis, 1989.

Lee, Sevngho H., and Krishna C. Rao. *Cranial Computed Tomography and MRI,* 2nd edition. McGraw-Hill, New York, 1987.

Lee, Joseph K., et al., *Computed Body Tomography with MRI Correlation,* 2nd edition. Raven Press, New York, 1989.

For references of specific application to medical transcription, see Appendix 1.

William G. Figueroa, M.D.
Ethel L. Wise, B.S., R.R.T., R.P.F.T.

Respiratory and Pulmonary Medicine

INTRODUCTION

The respiratory system performs many vital functions 24 hours a day, the most important of which is the exchange of the gases carbon dioxide and oxygen. Other functions include filtering the air breathed, filtering the blood from the systemic circulation, and production and breakdown of substances that affect the blood's conducting system.[1]

Throughout a lifetime of breathing, the respiratory system is exposed to a variety of substances, such as gaseous pollutants, and particulate matter from the environment, including bacteria, viruses, fungi, mold, and other irritants like cigarette, cigar, and pipe smoke, dust particles, and toxic chemicals.

The constant exposure to substances foreign to the respiratory system and particularly the lungs often causes respiratory disease(s). This chapter provides an overview of representative diseases: asthma, chronic bronchitis, emphysema, carcinoma, and sleep disorders. The diagnostic and surgical instruments and procedures utilized in respiratory medicine to identify the type of respiratory disorder and to quantify the amount of respiratory impairment are described. Sample letters, chart notes, and medical reports are presented here as guidelines.

ANATOMY

The gas conduction portion of the respiratory system is composed of a tracheobronchial tree, or airways, a sequential series of approximately 22 to 25 branching tubes. Their main function is to conduct gases into and out of the lungs. The airways also provide defense mechanisms that protect the airway surfaces, or mucosa, and the gas exchange portions of the lung from noxious agents in the environment.

The trachea, or windpipe, and the main stem bronchi lie in the center of the chest (mediastinum) outside the lungs, while the remaining branches of the tracheobronchial tree lie within the lung and are referred to as intrapulmonary structures. The conducting airways and the lungs lie within the chest wall, or bony thorax, which consists of the spine, ribs, and sternum. These structures are connected by ligaments and cartilage that are responsible for the movement of the ribs during inspiration and expiration. The chest wall and mediastinum are lined by a membrane called the parietal pleura, which contains many pain fibers. These fibers sometimes get irritated, then pain is experienced as a result of the motion of the chest wall. This pain is referred to as *pleuritic chest wall pain*.

The respiratory muscles are skeletal muscles that are essential for life. Normally, the active work of inspiration is provided by the diaphragm and external intercostal muscles. The accessory muscles (the scalene and sternocleidomastoid) come into play during disease and severe respiratory distress.

As the respiratory muscles contract, the chest wall and lungs expand, pressure contained in the lungs drops, and gas moves into the lungs until the pressure inside the lungs equals the pressure in the atmosphere. As the respiratory muscles relax, expiration begins as a result of the elastic recoil of the chest wall that squeezes out most of the air from within the lungs. Then the process repeats and occurs 24 hours per day without conscious effort.

There are two lungs. The right lung is divided into three lobes and the left lung is divided into two lobes. The lungs are covered by a membrane

called the visceral pleura. There is an airtight space between the lining of the lungs, or visceral pleura, and the lining of the chest wall and mediastinum, or parietal pleura. This space contains a thin sheet of lubricating fluid at any given time. Occasionally, the amount of fluid in the airtight space increases and is called a pleural effusion. This can be a sign of disease. Figure 36–1 shows a diagram of the respiratory system.

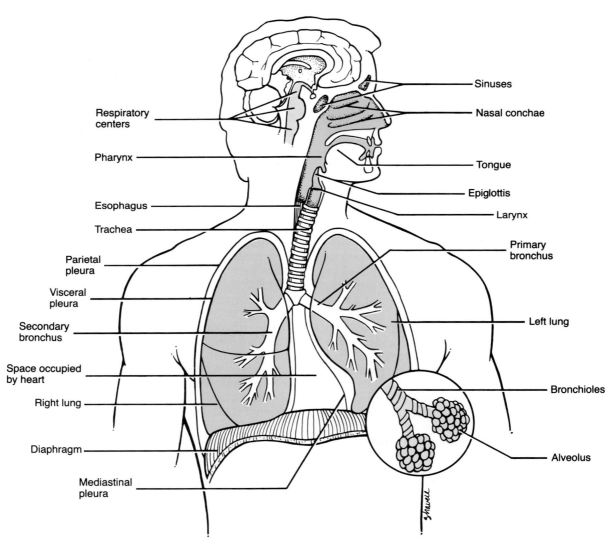

Figure 36–1
Anatomy of the respiratory system.

PHYSIOLOGY

The gas exchange portion of the lungs, or alveoli, receives its blood supply from an extensive network of capillaries within the alveolar walls. Blood in the alveolar capillaries is separated from the alveolar air space by a thin tissue barrier, the alveolar-capillary membrane. The surface of this membrane provides approximately 70 square meters of surface for the exchange of oxygen into the blood and the excretion of carbon dioxide from the blood and subsequently into the environmental air. In disease states, the surface area for gas exchange decreases, sometimes very markedly.

When respiratory disease occurs, it can affect any of the components of the respiratory system such as the airways (asthma, chronic bronchitis, and bronchiectasis), the alveolar capillary membrane (emphysema), or the lung tissue or parenchyma (lung abscess). Some abnormalities affect the chest wall (pectus excavatum and kyphoscoliosis).

REPRESENTATIVE DISEASES

A few common diseases are outlined here, but this is not an inclusive list. A complete description of respiratory diseases can be found in many textbooks on chest medicine. Any generalized ailment will affect the respiratory system. Some of the common abnormalities encountered in respiratory medicine can be divided into the general headings of diseases that affect the airways, diseases that affect the chest wall, and diseases that affect the lung parenchyma. In this section, sleep apnea syndromes will also be presented.

Diseases That Affect the Airways ▪ These include asthma, emphysema, chronic bronchitis, bronchiectasis, cystic fibrosis, and bronchopulmonary aspergillosis.

Diseases That Affect the Chest Wall ▪ Diseases that generally distort the ribs, spine, and/or sternum cause restrictive breathing defects. Examples are kyphoscoliosis, ankylosing spondylitis, pectus excavatum (hollow breast), and pectus carinatum (keeled breast).

Diseases That Affect the Lung Parenchyma ▪ Some of the diseases that affect lung parenchyma include neoplasms, occupational lung diseases, lung abscess, tuberculosis, and in-

fection from *Pneumocystis*. Pneumoconiosis includes diseases that are often work related and occur as the result of significant exposure to agents for which the disease is named: asbestosis, silicosis, talcosis, anthracosis, and others like graphite, alumina, tungsten, and kaolin.

Lung cancer (carcinoma) is a common malignant neoplasm. An estimated 168,000 Americans died of lung cancer in 1992—102,000 men and 66,000 women. The average patient with carcinoma of the lung is a heavy cigarette smoker in the sixth or seventh decade of life. Besides cigarette smoking, atmospheric pollution, occupational factors (radioactive materials, asbestos, and chloromethyl ether), and genetic factors play a role in the development of cancer.[2]

The cancer cell types are grouped into the four general headings of squamous cell carcinoma, small cell carcinoma, adenocarcinoma, and large cell carcinoma. In addition to cancer of the lung, carcinomas can occur in the respiratory tract, larynx (throat), bronchi, and nasal sinuses.

Sleep Apnea Syndromes ▪ The sleep apnea syndromes are divided into obstructive sleep apnea syndrome (OSAS) and central sleep apnea syndrome (CSAS). Many patients with sleep apnea manifest obstructive, central, and mixed apnea. Excessive daytime sleepiness is a frequent patient complaint. Other complaints include memory loss and lack of concentration. The spouses of these individuals complain that their mates snore and periodically stop breathing during the night. To quantify sleep apnea, the patient must be monitored. Detailed monitoring of sleep is called polysomnography.

Many regional sleep disorder centers have sprung up across the nation. They offer testing, diagnosis, evaluation, and treatment. These centers treat sleep-related disorders, such as insomnia, snoring, sleep apnea, excessive daytime sleepiness, narcolepsy, sleep problems in the elderly, oxygenation problems, impotence, and restless leg syndrome.

Some of the known predisposing factors in sleep apnea are male sex, alcohol use, and obesity. Many patients have a short, thick neck. Patients who have increased Pco_2 (carbon dioxide in the blood) were formerly called pickwickian, but are now said to have obesity hypoventilation syndrome (OHS). If a sleep disorder is diagnosed, treatment might consist partly of the use of mask continuous positive airway pressure (CPAP).

SIGNS AND SYMPTOMS

Five signs and symptoms that help in the identification of respiratory disease will be briefly discussed in this section: dyspnea, cough, sputum production, wheezing, and chest pain.

Dyspnea ▪ Healthy persons are unaware of their breathing except during heavy exercise. In contrast, the person with respiratory disease is conscious of air hunger, or labored breathing, even with mild exertion. The term that describes these abnormal breathing sensations is dyspnea. In general, the more intense the sensation of dyspnea, the worse the pulmonary disease.

Cough ▪ Cough protects the lungs from inhaled substances foreign to them and aids in the removal of excess secretions. Cough rarely recurs to any great extent in healthy persons, but persistent cough is the cardinal sign of respiratory disease.[3] Whether or not the person is a smoker is an important consideration in assessing the cough. Additionally, whether the cough is productive or nonproductive is significant. Cough has many causes. Table 36–1 lists categories of diseases and conditions that are associated with cough, along with selected examples.

Although cough is effective in clearing tracheobronchial secretions, there are complications related to coughing. For example, fainting (syncope) associated with uncontrollable coughing can occur, mainly in middle-aged men who have chronic lung disease. They lose consciousness within 10 seconds of cough and regain it in at least 10 seconds.

Cough may cause rib fractures. Associated with rib fractures are problems such as bloody sputum (hemoptysis), pleuritic chest pain, and lung collapse (pneumothorax). Miscellaneous complications of coughing include headache, exhaustion, insomnia, vomiting, depression, anorexia, and a sore, irritated throat.[4]

Sputum ▪ Sputum characteristics often lead to diagnosis. For example, dark yellow or green sputum usually reflects bronchopulmonary infection such as pneumonia, bronchiectasis, or acute bronchitis. On the other hand, mucoid sputum produced early in the morning may signal chronic bronchitis or small airways disease.

Table 36–1 ▪ **Some Causes of Cough**

Exogenous Irritants
Tobacco smoke
Smog
High levels of atmospheric SO_2
Noxious gases in workplace

Mechanical Irritants
Retained bronchopulmonary secretions
Foreign body within airways
Voice strain
Postnasal drip
Aspiration of gastric contents
Abnormally long uvula
Enlarged tonsils

Allergic
Asthma
Airways hyperreactivity
Milk product intolerance
Löffler's pneumonia

Obstructive Airway Disease
Chronic bronchitis
Emphysema
Cystic fibrosis
Bronchiectasis

Restrictive Lung Disease
Pulmonary fibrosis
Congestive heart failure
Pneumoconiosis
Collagen vascular disease
Granulomatous disease

Infectious
Acute laryngitis
Acute bronchitis
Pneumonia
Pleuritis
Pericarditis

Pulmonary Vascular Disease
Pulmonary emboli
Pulmonary hypertension

Neoplastic
Laryngeal tumor
Endobronchial tumor
Extrinsic compression of airway by tumor

Psychogenic

From Sackner, Marvin. Cough. In Murray, J. F., and J. A. Nadel. *Textbook of Respiratory Medicine.* W. B. Saunders Company, Philadelphia, 1988, p. 403.

Also important in evaluating sputum production is the quantity and consistency (thickness) and whether or not odor exists.

Complaints of feeling phlegm or drip at the back of the throat should be considered as postnasal drip, even when secretions are not present on the posterior wall of the upper airway (pharynx) upon physical examination of this area. This problem, which is related to nasal or sinus disease, is often associated with cough.[5]

Wheezing ■ Wheezing is one of many abnormal lung sounds. It is a continuous, high-pitched sound and often has a distinct whistling or squeaking quality. Wheezing is further described by the phase of the breathing cycle in which it is heard, inspiratory or expiratory. Generalized wheezes can be heard in patients with asthma as a result of airway narrowing caused by bronchospasm, mucosal edema, or widespread secretions. In contrast, localized wheezing usually results from a tumor in a bronchus (plural: bronchi) or external squeezing (compression) of the airways.

Chest Pain ■ Chest pain is one of the most frequent of the symptoms causing patients to seek medical advice. The lungs and the membrane that covers them (visceral pleura) are insensitive to painful stimuli. Pain often accompanies involvement of any of the structures in the chest, such as the lining of the chest wall (parietal pleura), the major airways, the chest wall, the diaphragm or other structures in the center of the chest (mediastinum), including the heart muscle and lining of the heart (pericardium).

The nature and location of chest pain help the physician identify its cause. As an example, sudden (acute) inflammation of the lining of the chest wall causes pleuritic chest pain that is localized, is nearly always on one side, and is described as sharp, burning, achy, or a "catch." Pleuritic chest pain usually worsens by deep breathing, sneezing, coughing, bending, stooping, or turning in bed.

DIAGNOSTIC PROCEDURES AND TESTS

Pulmonary Function Testing ■ In the practice of pulmonary medicine, pulmonary function tests are essential for the detection of chronic obstructive pulmonary disease, objective documentation of occupational lung disease (such as asbestosis), quantifying the severity of lung disease, and the response to treatment. Precise and reproducible assessment of the functional state of the respiratory system is available in most hospitals and offices of pulmonary specialists, known as pulmonologists.

The specific breathing tests that fall under the heading of pulmonary function testing include spirometry: pre- and postbronchodilator, lung volumes, diffusion studies, distribution of inspired gas, and bronchial provocation testing. For a total picture of the patient's status, a complete history and physical examination along with a chest x-ray film and evaluation of arterial blood gases (pH, Pco_2 and Po_2) should accompany the pulmonary function tests.

Bronchoscopy ■ This procedure is used to diagnose a wide variety of lung diseases. There are only two major types of bronchoscopes, rigid and flexible.

The rigid bronchoscopy procedure calls for a larger open, stiff tube. Developed in the 1930s, this was the first instrument for looking into the trachea and main stem airways. Its use today is limited to removal of large foreign bodies and occasionally laser therapy of cancers of the major airways.

The flexible fiberoptic bronchoscopes were developed in the 1970s. They have been a major advance in pulmonary medicine. Their diameter varies between 3 and 6 centimeters. They easily slip into the nose (transnasal approach), as shown in Figure 36–2, or throat (transoral) and then are directed into the lower airway. Since the instrument is small, more distal airways can be visualized with much more patient comfort. Local anesthesia (lidocaine) and sometimes sedation or narcotics are used to depress the cough reflex and relax the patient.

Currently, most bronchoscopic procedures are carried out with the flexible fiberoptic bronchoscope, enabling pieces of tissue (biopsy) to be extracted. These pieces of tissue can be obtained by closed lung forceps biopsy, protected brush catheter biopsy, or transbronchial needle biopsy.

To be certain that the forceps used with the bronchoscope open properly and to avoid the complication of a pneumothorax, the technique is performed under fluoroscopy (x-ray visualization). Fluoroscopic imaging is absolutely necessary to biopsy localized lung disease.

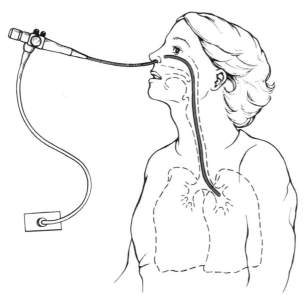

Figure 36–2
Examination with a fiberoptic bronchoscope.

Bronchoalveolar lavage, or washing out of a lung segment with saline solution, is especially useful in patients with undiagnosed infection of the lung. The flexible fiberoptic bronchoscope is essential to make this possible.

Metabolic Cart Study or Indirect Calorimetry ▪ The metabolic cart plays an important role in assessing the nutritional status of the critically ill patient and in identifying the nutritional needs. The goal of nutritional therapy for these patients is to prevent further decline in nutritional status and to replenish any nutritional deficit.

When food is metabolized, oxygen is consumed, and heat in the form of calories is produced. The metabolic rate then can be determined by measuring the heat lost or the oxygen consumed. Measuring the amount of heat (calories) produced via the amount of food ingested (direct calorimetry) is impractical and still a research technique. Measuring the amount of oxygen consumed (indirect calorimetry) has become a major clinical advance in the treatment of patients with respiratory diseases and critical illness.

The metabolic cart is a portable computerized gas collection system that takes expired air from the patient and precisely measures its volume and concentration of oxygen and carbon dioxide. In using the metabolic cart to obtain oxygen uptake (Vo_2) and carbon dioxide produced (Vco_2) with the patient at rest, the resting energy expenditure (REE) can be calculated. From this information, a proper nutritional formula, including the number of calories and proportion of fat, carbohydrates, and protein, can then be given to the patient.

The oxygen consumption measurement (Vo_2) helps quantify the oxygen needs and delivery (cardiac output) of oxygen to the critically ill patient. The respiratory quotient is calculated from the amount of CO_2 produced (Vco_2) divided by the O_2 consumed (Vo_2). The normal value is 0.8. A high value can indicate overfeeding with carbohydrates, which leads to the patient requiring prolonged treatment (with mechanical ventilation).

The oxygen consumption can also be measured during exercise. Combining the amount of exercise using a treadmill or bicycle and the amount of force (watts) expended, the oxygen consumption, and the maximum minute ventilation (total amount of air breathed per minute) is an accurate measure of cardiac and pulmonary fitness.

The metabolic cart can be used for cardiopulmonary stress testing, cardiac output determinations, and work of breathing measurements. Some systems have the capability for pulmonary function testing.

Thoracentesis and Pleural Biopsy ▪ In abnormal conditions, the pleural space can fill with air (pneumothorax), blood (hemothorax), plasma, serum or lymph (hydrothorax or pleural effusion), or pus (pyothorax or empyema). Fluid in the pleural space causes the underlying lung to collapse and can be a source for infection. The process of removing fluid from the pleural space is called thoracentesis (Figure 36–3).

MEDICAL AND SURGICAL TREATMENTS

General Treatment of Respiratory Disease ▪ The medical treatment regimen for each patient largely depends upon the results of tests, the clinical picture, and the patient's symptoms. Six categories of medications will be discussed: beta-adrenergic drugs, anticholinergic drugs,

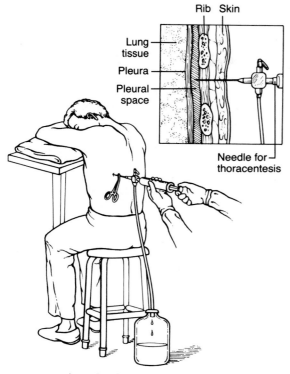

Rib   Skin

Lung tissue

Pleura

Pleural space

Needle for thoracentesis

Figure 36–3
The technique for a thoracentesis.

cromolyn sodium, methylxanthines, corticosteroids, and oxygen.

Beta-Adrenergic Drugs ■ These are the most frequently used pulmonary medications. Their major therapeutic action is bronchodilation (relaxation of the smooth muscle in the airways). The list of widely prescribed beta-agonists includes metaproterenol, albuterol, terbutaline, bitolterol, and fenoterol. These drugs are most commonly prescribed in metered dose inhalers.

Volume reservoirs and spacer attachments are often advantageous. Gas-powered aerosols are sometimes used to deliver the medications. Recent studies suggest that supervised metered-dose inhaler aerosol delivery is as efficacious as gas-powered nebulizer delivery.

Anticholinergic Agents ■ Ipratropium bromide is available as a metered-dose inhaler. This drug is less effective than beta-agonists in treating patients with asthma; however, it appears useful in patients with chronic obstructive pulmonary disease (COPD).

Cromolyn Sodium ■ This drug is not a bronchodilator. It inhibits the release of chemical substances (mediators) from mast cells in the airway. Cromolyn sodium protects against exercise-induced asthma, antigen-induced asthma, and certain occupational asthmas. The clinical response to cromolyn sodium is unpredictable.

Methylxanthines ■ Theophylline, a close relative to caffeine, has been the time-honored drug in the treatment of obstructive lung disease. However, recent evidence, including studies of side effects, has made this drug less favored for use. Therapeutic levels (10 to 20 mg./mL.) are very close to toxic levels. Side effects of nausea, anorexia, diarrhea, insomnia, tachycardia, or tremor are common. The major side effects of seizures and ventricular arrhythmia are life threatening but fortunately rare.

Corticosteroids ■ These drugs have been widely used in the treatment of asthma and asthmatic bronchitis since their discovery in 1950. Corticosteroids are the most effective agents available for the treatment of reversible airways obstruction. They are available as oral, intravenous, or topical (inhaled) preparations. Prednisone is the most common and is used for acute exacerbations in large doses for a few days, then tapered off.

Inhaled corticosteroid preparations are assuming a major role in the maintenance treatment of asthma. Preparations most commonly prescribed are beclomethasone (Beclovent), triamcinolone (Azmacort), and flunisolide (Aerobid). The inhaled agents do not cause the side effects associated with systemic corticosteroid treatment.

Oxygen ■ Patients with acute worsening (exacerbations) of COPD should have measurement of arterial blood gases. Oxygen should be prescribed to keep the arterial blood oxygen (Pao_2) level at 60 mm. Hg or better.

In patients with stable COPD who normally have low arterial oxygen levels ($Pao_2 = 55$ mm. Hg), long-term use of oxygen improves neuropsychiatric function and decreases mortality. Oxygen is usually given by nasal cannula. Rarely, it is given by transtracheal technique. The oxygen can be provided via three systems: gas, liquid, and oxygen concentrator. For ambulatory patients, the liquid source is preferred.

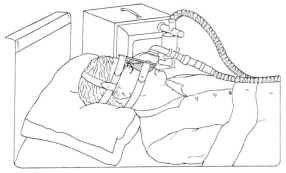

Figure 36–4
Diagram of a nasal continuous positive airway pressure (CPAP) machine in use. (From George, Ronald B. *Chest Medicine: Essentials of Pulmonary and Critical Care Medicine*, 2nd ed. Williams & Wilkins Company, Baltimore, 1990, p. 135.)

Some patients may need other therapies, such as chest percussion and postural drainage, when pulmonary secretions are resistant to expectoration with spontaneous coughing.

Sleep Apnea ▪ The medical treatment of sleep apnea syndromes centers on weight loss for the obese patient, elevation of the head to prevent closure of the airway, drug therapy, and the use of nasal continuous positive airway pressure (CPAP). Figure 36–4 shows a nasal CPAP device in use.

Neoplasms ▪ After proper staging regarding the extent of the lung cancer, a treatment plan is developed. Localized cancers are treated with surgical excision. More advanced cancers are treated with radiation therapy, chemotherapy, or laser therapy.

The most widely accepted staging system for nonsmall cell carcinoma is the tumor-node-metastasis (TNM) classification.

T1   lesion is less than 3 cm.
T2   lesion is greater than 3 cm.
T3   tumor invasion of the chest wall, mediastinum, or diaphragm
T4   invasion of the heart or great vessels, malignant pleural effusion

N0   no lymph node involvement
N1   tracheobronchial or hilar lymph node involvement
N2   ipsilateral mediastinal node involvement
N3   contralateral mediastinal node or supraclavicular lymph node involvement

M0   no metastasis
M1   presumed or systemic metastasis

Small cell carcinoma is usually staged as limited (confined to the thorax) or extensive (metastasis outside the thorax). Patients with nonsmall cell cancer, who have the best 5-year survival (50 per cent), are in surgical-pathologic Stage 1 without metastasis to regional lymph node (T1N0M0 or T2N0M0). Patients with Stage II (T1N1M0 or T2N1M0), with at least one hilar or tracheobronchial lymph node involved, have a postsurgical 5-year survival of 30 per cent.

Patients with Stage IIIa have lesions that involve the chest wall or diaphragm, or are located within 2 cm. of the carina but do not invade it (T3N0M0), or involve a solitary mediastinal lymph node (T1 or T2N2M0). These lesions are still considered resectable for cure (approximately 17 per cent have a 5-year survival). In Stage IIIb, a tumor is present in the supraclavicular or contralateral lymph nodes.

Any T, N3M0 tumor has invaded the carina, heart, great vessels, esophagus (T4, any N, M0). In Stage IV, distant metastasis is present, and patients have no 5-year survival. In Stage IIIb or IV, the tumor is not resectable for cure. These more advanced cancers are treated with radiation therapy, chemotherapy, laser therapy, or a combination.

SURGICAL PROCEDURES

In general, pulmonary physicians do not perform surgical procedures. Surgical techniques such as open lung biopsy, mediastinoscopy, thoracotomy, and thoracoscopy are referred to a thoracic surgeon and are performed in the operating room under general anesthesia.

The surgical treatment of sleep apnea is to bypass the upper airway by tracheostomy. In some cases, the uvula and portions of the soft palate are removed as well as redundant pharyngeal tissue (uvulopharyngopalatoplasty or UPPP). Any nasal obstruction is also repaired.

Some of the procedures performed by the pulmonary physician include transthoracic needle biospy (under fluoroscopy) to diagnose infectious and malignant diseases; transbronchial needle biopsy (aspiration) to diagnose and stage bronchogenic carcinoma; thoracentesis (surgical puncture of the chest wall to remove pleural fluid), sometimes with closed pleural biopsy; and removal of adhesions or scarring between the parietal and visceral pleura (pleurodesis) to prevent recurrent fluid.

INSTRUMENTS

Different biopsy needles are used for closed pleural biopsy (extraction of tissue). Either Cope's or Abrams' pleural biopsy needle is currently most widely used. Which needle the physician uses is a matter of personal preference.

The equipment needed to perform flexible fiberoptic bronchoscopies is a light source, the flexible scope, an anesthetic agent such as lidocaine, brushes, forceps, specimen containers, slides, and other accessories.

The metabolic cart requires calibration gases in addition to an electrocardiographic monitor, treadmill or cycle ergometer (for cardiopulmonary stress testing), a pulse oximeter, and a blood pressure cuff. The treadmill and cycle ergometer are not necessary for nutritional assessments using the metabolic cart.

Pulmonary function testing is accomplished using a calibrated pulmonary function spirometer for simple spirometry. A copy of the tracing should be available for physician interpretation. To perform lung volumes, a device called a body plethysmograph (or body box) is needed. To diagnose asthma, bronchial provocation testing is done, which requires the drug methacholine chloride.

FORMATS

Letters ▪ A pulmonary specialist will dictate three types of letters. (1) The first is the consultation letter, which includes the report of a comprehensive medical history, physical examination, and interpretation of chest roentgenograms and other imaging tests. These other imaging tests can include CT (computed tomography) scan, nuclear scans such as perfusion scans and ventilation scans, pulmonary function tests,

study of pathologic or histologic material, microbiologic and immunologic tests, and bronchoscopy. The pulmonary specialist then will formulate a differential diagnosis, a prognosis, and the therapeutic option for the patient (Figure 36–5).

(2) A follow-up letter is shorter and includes a brief interim history and physical examination, report of appropriate tests, such as spirometry in a patient with asthma, and then further treatment recommendations.

(3) A pulmonary specialist may dictate a letter to an attorney or insurance company for a patient who has suffered an occupational lung disease, such as pneumoconiosis, asbestosis-related lung disease, or exposure to chemical fumes.

Chart Notes ▪ These contain untranscribed pertinent historical and physical findings and treatment adjustments. They include comments about the complexity of the case, the difficulty in making decisions, and most important, the amount of time spent with each patient. These notes form the basis for reimbursement under the Medicare payment system.

Special Pulmonary Medical Reports

Pulmonary Function Study ▪ This special technical report (Figure 36–6) analyzes the results of a "breathing test." This study includes spirometry, lung volumes, a diffusing capacity, and arterial blood gases. Often a description of the type of abnormality is possible, such as obstructive lung impairment or chronic obstructive pulmonary disease (COPD), restrictive impairment (pulmonary fibrosis), the amount of impairment, and the response or lack of response to bronchodilator aerosols.

Methacholine Challenge Test ▪ This test measures the response to the inhalation of a special drug that will bring out bronchospasm, or asthma. This study measures the degree of irritability of the patient's airways.

Cardiopulmonary Stress Test ▪ This test measures the response of the heart and lungs to exercise. The report (Figure 36–7) contains the amount of exercise, the cardiac response including electrocardiographic analysis, the amount of oxygen utilized, and the amount of carbon dioxide produced. It is used in evaluating a patient who has shortness of breath, or dyspnea, to separate the cardiac and the respiratory components. It also forms the basis for pulmonary rehabilitation programs and disability evaluations.

Text continued on page 707

THE LANKENAU HOSPITAL
100 Lancaster Avenue west of City Line
Wynnewood, PA 19096-0000

January 29, 1994

Frederick Blake, M.D.
111 Shore Road
Philadelphia, PA 19104-0000

RE: Susan Rothman

Dear Dr. Blake:

I saw Susan Rothman for a second pulmonary opinion on January 23, 1994. She is a 62-year-old secretary at Jackson University who was found to have an abnormal chest x-ray.

Mrs. Rothman tells me that she was in fairly good health until this past October, 1993 when she developed paroxysms of coughing and wheezing. She was initially treated by Dr. Brownstone with antibiotics and also received Theo-Dur, prednisone, and a bronchodilator in the form of an inhaler. She improved, but when the prednisone was tapered, she again started to have coughing and wheezing and was referred to Dr. Smith. She was seen by Dr. Smith on December 2, 1993 and at that time she had pulmonary function studies done and a chest x-ray. The chest x-ray was within normal limits except for some mild overinflation. She again had an episode of coughing and wheezing and was seen on December 20, 1993 in an urgent visit at the Lankenau emergency room. A chest x-ray now showed a left upper lobe nodule approximately 0.7 cm. A CT scan confirmed the presence of this nodule in the left upper lobe.

SOCIAL HISTORY: Her social history reveals that she unfortunately smokes cigarettes, about one and one-half packs per day. She has been smoking since age 15 and is having a difficult time with smoking cessation.

REVIEW OF SYSTEMS: Her review of systems reveals that she has some heartburn and has been seen by her gastroenterologist, Dr. Brown. She has been treated off and on with antacids over the years. She usually uses Rolaids because she is fearful of taking any chronic medications. She also has some mild arthritic symptoms and some back pains.

(continued)

Figure 36–5
An example of a consultation letter on a patient seen for a pulmonary second opinion.

RE: Susan Rothman   Page two
January 29, 1994

PAST MEDICAL HISTORY: Her past medical history is quite complicated in
that she had a tonsillectomy as a child. She had an appendectomy in 1946,
a cholecystectomy in 1954, a hysterectomy in 1962 , and a laminectomy in
1983.

Her family history reveals that her mother died of heart disease at age 71. Her
father died of Hodgkin's disease at age 57. She has one brother and one
sister, both living and well. She has an uncle who has asthma and she has
five children who are all in good health.

CURRENT MEDICATIONS: Her medications at this time include Theo-Dur
200 mg. in the morning and 100 mg. in the evening, and a Proventil inhaler
used as needed.   She is allergic to codeine which causes gastrointestinal
upset.

PHYSICAL EXAMINATION: On physical examination, she was an anxious
woman in no acute distress. Her vital signs were within normal limits. Her
pulse was 72. Blood pressure was 110/80. The neck veins were flat. The
thyroid was within normal limits. There was no cervical adenopathy. The
oropharynx was within normal limits. Her chest showed some rhonchi on
forced expiration.   The cardiac examination was within normal limits. The
extremities showed no clubbing or edema.

DIAGNOSIS: Left upper lobe pulmonary nodule; chronic obstructive
pulmonary disease.

DISCUSSION: I reviewed the chest x-rays that were taken recently and
compared them with some older films. The films dated 1981, 1985 and 1991
are all within normal limits. The chest x-ray on December 2, 1993 is within
normal limits except for some mild overinflation. Another film taken on
December 20, 1993 shows a small nodule in the left upper lobe. A CT scan
dated January 6, 1994 confirms the left upper lobe nodule. A repeat CT scan
on January 20, 1994 shows the nodule has persisted and is exactly the same.
I also performed screening spirometry which shows that her FEV1 is 1.60 L
with a predicted normal of 2.60 L. This is a mild to moderate obstructive

(continued)

Figure 36–5 Continued

Mrs. Susan Rothman   Page three
January 29, 1994

impairment. There was no significant change following the inhalation of a
bronchodilator. I compared this study with the one taken on December 2,
1993 and at that time her FEV1 was 1.45L, so this represents some
improvement.

This patient has a solitary pulmonary nodule. I discussed the approach to this
problem with her and her son who took copious notes. There are three
approaches. The first is to go forward with an open or excisional biopsy with
all of the problems of a thoracotomy in a patient who is 62-years-old with mild
to moderate chronic obstructive pulmonary disease.

The second option is to perform a percutaneous needle aspiration biopsy under
fluoroscopy or CT scanning guidance, or to perform a fiberoptic bronchoscopy
and brushing under fluoroscopy. Since this lesion is less than 1.0 cm. in
diameter and rather difficult to see on routine chest x-ray, the percutaneous
needle aspiration technique will be a low yield and have a high incidence of a
pneumothorax. This is particularly true in patients who have abnormal
pulmonary function studies. From my experience of 33 cases of pulmonary
nodules of 2 cm. or less, fiberoptic brushing and transbronchial biopsy have a
very, very low yield for establishing a diagnosis. Therefore, I feel at this time,
invasive diagnostic procedures will be of a very limited benefit.

The third option is to treat the patient and not the chest x-ray and simply
follow her along for the next several months with serial chest x-rays. We know
that the doubling time of lung cancer on the average is approximately three
months for rapid growers and much longer for the slow growing type. This is
the work of Dr. William Weiss of the Philadelphia Neoplasm Research Project.
In view of the fact that the chest x-ray on December 2, 1993 did not show this
nodule, I believe that it is possible that this could be an inflammatory lesion.
During this period of observation, other non-invasive procedures such as a
density measurement by Rob Steiner at the Jefferson University Hospital or
Dr. Stanley Siegelman at Johns Hopkins could be performed since a high
density lesion would indicate a benign lesion.

(continued)

Figure 36–5 Continued

Mrs. Susan Rothman   Page four
January 29, 1994

As far as her chronic obstructive pulmonary disease is concerned, she does
need a comprehensive program. This would include a battery of pulmonary
function studies, particularly a diffusing capacity measurement, to see just
how much is emphysema, how much is bronchitis, and how much is possibly
asthma. She then needs to develop a bronchodilator regimen which probably
would be inhaled beta agonists followed by an inhaled corticosteroid and/or
Atrovent. During this time, she also should be on a vigorous antismoking
program which might include the use of a nicotine skin patch.

I discussed these options with Mrs. Rothman and she is quite content to sit
back and wait a while before rushing into surgery. Since, as you know, I am a
medical type person, I favor the more conservative option. Enclosed find a
copy of a paper I wrote a few years ago addressing the pulmonary nodule
issue.

Many thanks for referring her for my opinion.

Sincerely,

Lester T. Berkley, M.D.

LTB:ssb

Enclosure

Figure 36–5 Continued

PULMONARY FUNCTION TESTING

Name: CARSON, CHARLES   ID#:608779-CARSON
Age: 68 years   Room:318   Date:16-SEP-94
Sex/Race: Male/Caucasian   Temp/Pres: 22 C / 757 mmHG
Height: 69 in. 175 cm.   Physician:GOLDMAN
Weight: 179 lb. 81 kg.   Tested by:KMH/1300

		PRED	PRE-RX BEST	%PRED	POST-RX BEST	%PRED	%CHG
SPIROMETRY (BTPS)							
FVC	Liters	4.27	3.20	75*	3.97	93	24
FEV1	Liters	2.91?	1.31#	45*	1.67#	57*	27
FEV1/FVC	%	69	41		42		
FEF25–75%	L/sec	2.70	0.31#	11*	0.39#	14*	26
PEF	L/sec	8.10	5.04	62*	5.83	72	16
FET100%	Sec		16.7		20.6		
FIVC	Liters	4.27	2.93	69*	3.37	79*	15
FIV1	Liters		2.51		1.70		
PIF	L/sec		3.34		1.94		

		PRED	PRE-RX AVG	%PRED	POST-RX AVG	%PRED	%CHG
LUNG VOLUMES (BTPS)							
VC	Liters	4.27	3.45	81			
TLC	Liters	6.30	6.67	106			
RV	Liters	2.44	3.22	132			
RV/TLC	%	40	48				
FRC N2	Liters	3.57	4.67	131*			
ERV	Liters		1.45				
IC	Liters		1.99				
DIFFUSION							
DLCO	ml/min/mmHg	21.2	11.3#	53*			
DLCO/VA	1/min/mmHg	3.67	1.89	51*			
VA	Liters		5.98				

= Outside 95% confidence interval; * = Outside normal range

Figure 36–6
A sample form for pulmonary function testing.

```
ARTERIAL BLOOD GASES
                %FIO2    pH    PCO2    PO2    %HbO2    P(A-a)O2
Predicted                               69-81   93-95
Resting          .21    7.41    37      77     94.7        27
CALIBRATION:    PRED: 2.26        ACTUAL: EXP 2.26    INSP 2.25
IPS-0L01-05 IPS-0L02-05 N-1804-3
```

SUPPLEMENTARY INTERPRETATION:

The vital capacity is mild to moderately decreased. The forced expiratory volumes are markedly decreased. The flow rates at mid and low lung volumes are severely decreased. Following an aerosol of Albuterol there is greater than 15% improvement in the FEV1. The lung volumes show an increase in RV and RV/TLC%. The diffusing capacity is mildly to moderately decreased. Arterial blood gases show a slight increase in the A-a gradient with a normal PCO_2 and pH. CONCLUSION: This study shows a moderately severe obstructive impairment which is somewhat responsive to bronchodilators. There is airtrapping and loss of surface area for the transfer of carbon monoxide, all consistent with chronic bronchitis and emphysema. In comparison with the studies of July 11, 1991, there has been a marked improvement; his FEV1 has gone from .96 up to 1.3 liters. His diffusing capacity remains the same. This patient is at some increased risk for respiratory complications post op CABG but there is adequate reserve. He will need a careful pre- and postoperative pulmonary regimen.

WGF/bs
9/17/94   1300

William G. Figueroa, M.D.

Figure 36-6 Continued

The Lankenau Hospital
Cardiopulmonary Stress Testing Lab
100 Lancaster Avenue west of City Line
Wynnewood, PA 19096

Any Info: T-MILL-CPX-MOD NAUGHTON
Name: KENDRICK, ETHEL
Sex/Race: Female/Caucasian
Weight: 115 lb. 52 kg.
Room: Out/P
Temp/Pres: 23 C/764 mmHg
Tested by: LAB/MBW
HB: 14.7 BSA: 1.53

Age: 84
Height: 63 in., 160 cm.
ID#: 762161-CPX-KENDRICK
Date: 08-MAY-94
Physician: FIGUEROA

Measured FEV1 (L): 1.00
Measured FVC (L): 1.75
Predicted Maximum Exercise Ventilation (FEV1 * 35) (L/min): 35
Predicted Maximum VO2 (mL/min): 750
Predicted Maximum VO2/KG (ml/kg/min): 14
Predicted Maximum Heart Rate (b/min): 141

VOLUME CALIBRATION   Date: 8-MAY-94   Correction Factor 1.01

	Actual	Predicted	% Predicted
	3.30	3.31	100

ANALYZER CALIBRATION: (M.C.) Date: 8-MAY-94

O_2		CO_2	
Pred.	Act.	Pred.	Act.
26.00	26.01	0.00	0.00
16.00	16.01	4.00	4.00

Average of 1 interval(s) in effect.

PULMONARY PROFILE:

Min	Work	Hr	HR %Max	O_2 Puls	VE BTPS	RR	VO2	VO2/KG	VCO2	R	DI	SaO2	RPD
BASELINE													
00:00:20		87	62									97	
00:00:40		86	61									97	
00:01:00		84	60	0.0	3.5	18	1	0.03			0.10	97	
00:01:20		87	61	1.2	9.8	36	108	2.08	74	0.69	0.28	98	
00:01:40		86	61	2.6	8.8	28	223	4.28	155	0.70	0.25	98	
00:02:00		86	61	2.2	8.7	29	193	3.71	143	0.74	0.25	97	

Figure 36-7
An example of a cardiopulmonary stress testing laboratory report.

Min	Work	Hr	HR %Max	O$_2$ Puls	VE BTPS	RR	VO2	VO2/KG	VCO2	R	DI	SaO2	RPD
ACTIVE WARMUP													
00:02:20		89	63	2.6	10.6	30	229	4.40	168	0.73	0.30	97	
00:02:40		90	64	3.0	11.4	30	273	5.26	196	0.72	0.33	97	
00:03:00		91	64	3.4	12.4	30	312	6.00	222	0.71	0.35	97	
00:03:20		92	65	3.7	13.3	32	341	6.55	239	0.70	0.38	97	
00:03:40		94	66	3.5	12.5	31	332	6.38	226	0.68	0.36	97	
EXERCISE													
00:04:00		95	67	4.5	14.9	30	426	8.19	288	0.68	0.43	96	
00:04:20		95	67	4.3	14.3	30	406	7.81	283	0.70	0.41	96	
00:04:40		96	68	4.4	14.9	30	417	8.02	290	0.70	0.43	97	
00:05:00		96	68	3.2	11.1	27	309	5.95	218	0.70	0.32	96	
00:05:20		97	68	4.5	15.3	33	433	8.33	305	0.70	0.44	96	
00:05:40		98	69	3.9	15.5	33	383	7.37	285	0.74	0.44	97	
00:06:00		100	70	4.1	16.5	33	413	7.94	313	0.76	0.47	97	
00:06:20		101	71	3.8	14.0	36	386	7.43	285	0.74	0.40	96	
00:06:40		108	76	4.0	16.4	33	434	8.34	321	0.74	0.47	97	
00:07:00		99	70	4.5	17.5	35	449	8.64	337	0.75	0.50	97	
00:07:20		100	70	4.6	16.6	31	462	8.88	341	0.74	0.48	96	
00:07:40		100	71	4.6	16.8	33	461	8.86	342	0.74	0.48	97	
00:08:00	13	102	72	4.5	16.4	31	459	8.82	343	0.75	0.47	97	
00:08:20	12	104	74	3.4	13.7	47	351	6.74	262	0.75	0.39	96	0.50
00:08:40	13	103	73	5.5	19.5	35	564	10.85	421	0.75	0.56	96	
00:09:00	13	107	75	4.9	18.6	40	519	9.97	401	0.77	0.53	96	
00:09:20	13	109	77	5.2	21.5	36	571	10.98	449	0.79	0.61	96	
00:09:40	13	109	77	5.0	20.6	28	544	10.47	425	0.78	0.59	96	
00:10:00	31	109	77	5.0	18.9	44	550	10.57	435	0.79	0.54	96	1.00
00:10:20	31	113	80	5.9	23.0	36	668	12.84	513	0.77	0.66	95	
00:10:40	32	114	81	6.0	24.0	36	682	13.11	541	0.79	0.69	95	
00:11:00	31	116	82	5.6	23.7	41	650	12.50	535	0.82	0.68	95	1.00
00:11:20	31	118	83	6.2	25.3	34	726	13.97	591	0.81	0.72	95	
00:11:40	31	121	86	5.2	21.4	39	630	12.11	521	0.83	0.61	95	
00:12:00	48	121	85	4.7	19.2	46	565	10.87	473	0.84	0.55	94	2.00
ACTIVE RECOVERY													
00:12:20	2	122	86	6.0	24.9	43	738	14.19	611	0.83	0.71	94	
00:12:40		120	85	5.6	22.9	36	675	12.98	570	0.84	0.65	94	
00:13:00		120	85	6.3	24.7	34	748	14.39	636	0.85	0.71	94	
00:13:20		116	82	5.0	20.7	34	580	11.15	512	0.88	0.59	95	
00:13:40		113	80	3.2	14.7	42	367	7.06	330	0.90	0.42	95	

Figure 36–7 *Continued*

Figure continued

CARDIOPULMONARY STRESS TEST

COMMENTS:

Patient stopped because she felt she "was ready to stop."

INTERPRETATION:

INDICATION: 84-year-old woman who has severe COPD and wishes to continue at a fairly high level of exercise. This study is therefore to define her limits of exercise tolerance.

The patient reported to the exercise laboratory on 5-8-94. Her exercise program was the Modified Naughton Protocol. She exercised for 8 minutes and 20 seconds and she stopped because of fatigue. Her borg dyspnea index was only mild exertional dyspnea. She achieved almost 100% of her predicted maximum oxygen consumption.

Her cardiopulmonary status was excellent. She reached 85% of her maximum heart rate. Her blood pressure was 118/72 to start and stayed at 120/70 throughout the exercise protocol. She achieved 14 cc/kg/min of oxygen consumption or 103% of her predicted normal. There were occasional PVC's but there were no ST changes.

Respiratory evaluation showed her maximum minute ventilation rose to 25 liters per minute and her predicted was 35 liters per minute or 70% of her predicted maximum ventilation. Her baseline oxygen saturation was 97%, dropped to 94% and rose back up to 98% within 2–3 minutes of recovery.

This patient had a normal-to-excellent exercise performance. The limitation here is pulmonary rather than cardiac and that is only by the 70% of the maximum minute ventilation that was utilized before she stopped exercising. This translated more into fatigue than dyspnea in this patient. This patient has such excellent exercise reserve that she does not need a full pulmonary rehabilitation program. She could benefit from simply teaching her regarding medication and aerosol therapy.

William G. Figueroa, M.D.

1440 5-11-94

IMS-0401-04

Figure 36–7 *Continued*

Metabolic Cart Study ■ The test reports the amount of energy utilized at rest. It also includes the respiratory quotient, or R.Q., which is the amount of oxygen that the patient consumes and the amount of carbon dioxide produced during this observation period. It is used for patients who are receiving special feeding, including hyperalimentation or nutritional supplements.

Bronchoscopy (Figure 36–8) ■ Fiberoptic bronchoscopy was described earlier in this chapter. The test report includes

- indications for the bronchoscopy, such as hemoptysis, unilateral wheeze, or abnormal chest x-ray

- preoperative diagnosis

- postoperative diagnosis

- type and amount of sedation and local anesthetic used

- findings such as endobronchial mass or obstructions — type and amount of secretions

- specimens obtained via brush, needle biopsy, transbronchial biopsy, or bronchoalveolar lavage

- complications such as bleeding

- condition of the patient upon leaving the endoscopy suite

Sleep Disorder Studies ■ Sleep disorders usually require two nights of studies. The first night's study measures the patient's sleep physiology. The report includes the reason for the study, such as snoring, witnessed episodes of not breathing during sleep, and daytime sleepiness or somnolence. It includes the following parameters

- the amount and quality of the patient's sleep

- the number and duration of apneas and hypopneas

- electrocardiographic abnormalities

- oxygen saturation

- body movements, including leg movements

A second study on the following night will often be performed to test the patient's response to treatment. This second report includes all the previous parameters and then the response to treatment, such as nasal continuous positive airway pressure (CPAP) or nasal pressure on inspiration and pressure on exhalation (BiPAP). (See the polysomnogram report in Figure 36–9.)

Discharge Summary ■ This report (Figure 36–10) includes

Name of the hospital
Dates of admission and discharge
Final diagnosis, secondary diagnosis
Procedures, such as bronchoscopy or thoracentesis
Discharge treatment plan:
    activity level
    diet
    medications
    special treatments such as nebulizer, oxygen, or home care
    follow-up appointments: date and names of doctors
Consultants
Reason for admission
History and physical examination
Laboratory reports
Hospital course
Condition at discharge

Bibliography

1. George, R. B., R. W. Light, M. A. Matthay, and R. A. Matthay (Eds.). *Chest Medicine; Essentials of Pulmonary and Critical Care Medicine,* 2nd edition. Williams and Wilkins, Baltimore, 1990.
2. Silverberg, E. Cancer statistics. *CA* 40:9-28, 1990.
3. Loudon, R. G. Cough: A symptom and a sign. *Basics of RD* 9:1-6, 1981.
4. Irwin, R. S., and M. J. Rosen. Cough: A comprehensive review. *Archives of Internal Medicine* 137:1186-1191, 1977.

Text continued on page 714

THE LANKENAU HOSPITAL
100 Lancaster Avenue west of City Line
Wynnewood, PA 19096-0000

FIBEROPTIC BRONCHOSCOPY AND TRANSCARINAL NEEDLE ASPIRATION BIOPSY

NAME: AVA CROWLEY

DATE OF PROCEDURE: 4/24/94

OPERATOR: WILLIAM G. FIGUEROA, M.D.

PREOPERATIVE DIAGNOSIS: Preoperative chest x-ray which showed lobulated nodes and/or mass along the right tracheal and superior mediastinal area of her chest, rule out granuloma, rule out tumor.

POSTOPERATIVE DIAGNOSIS: Same.

PROCEDURE: The patient received Demerol 75 and Vistaril 25. She was then brought to the x-ray department. Her upper airway was anesthetized with 4% Xylocaine and the fiberscope was passed by the transnasal technique. The vocal cords were slightly edematous, particularly the right vocal cord, but they moved equally well. The right tracheal rings were obliterated and there seemed to be some tension or pressure extrinsically along the lateral and posterior portion of the trachea on the right side. The carina was sharp and mobile. The segments and subsegments of the lower lobes, middle lobes, and upper lobes were all virtually within normal limits. There was some mucous material coming out of the right upper lobe and there was some yellow mucous coming from the lingula subsegments, but again no significant inflammation or masses were seen. The fiberscope then was passed to just above the carina on the right lateral tracheal wall about two tracheal rings from the carina. A Wang 319 needle was wedged into this area and three aspiration biopsies were taken. She had some bleeding and I estimate 10 to 15 cc. came from the third puncture site. However, this seemed to be subsiding at the completion of the bronchoscopy. An x-ray was taken to verify the position and a post biopsy x-ray was taken.   Good specimens were obtained.

(continued)

Figure 36–8
A fiberoptic bronchoscopy and transcarinal needle aspiration biopsy report.

AVA CROWLEY   page two

Secretions were also taken for fungus, tuberculosis, and bacteriological culture.

She tolerated this procedure quite well and was discharged in good condition at 3:00 p.m.

_____

WILLIAM G. FIGUEROA, M.D.

WGF:bp
D: 4/24/94
T: 4/27/94

Figure 36–8 Continued

THE LANKENAU HOSPITAL
SLEEP DISORDER CENTER
DIVISION OF PULMONARY DISEASES
DEPARTMENT OF MEDICINE

POLYSOMNOGRAM REPORT

Nasal Continuous Positive Airway Pressure Treatment Trial

NAME: ELIAS RANDALL   DATE: 6/5-6/6/94

DESCRIPTION OF PROCEDURE(S): The patient had one night of polysomnography with nasal continuous positive airway pressure (NCPAP) treatment. The polysomnography consisted of the simultaneous measurement of electroencephalogram (EEG), electrooculogram (EOG). electromyogram (EMG), electrocardiogram (ECG), airflow (right and left nares, and mouth), respiratory effort (abdominal and rib cage movement), SaO2, body position and right and left anterior tibialis EMG. The NCPAP treatment consisted of appropriate fitting and placement of the NCPAP mask prior to sleep and the application of air pressure through the nares using the nasal mask during sleep. Pressure was generated with a Respironics Sleep Eazy III NCPAP machine. Air pressure was started at 5 cm. H_2O and slowly increased until maximum reduction of apneas, hypopneas and snoring were achieved. All data were visually scored and analyzed according to standard criteria.

RESULTS: Sleep and NCPAP Data   Page two
                  Movements parameters and additional findings   Page three

SUMMARY OF FINDINGS AND INTERPRETATION: Administration of NCPAP at a pressure of 7.5 cm. H_2O resulted in a decrease from an apnea index of 94.4/hour of sleep as recorded on 5/24-5/25/94 to an index of 5.0/hour of sleep here. This is consistent with a change from severe obstructive sleep apnea to normal respiration in sleep. The remaining hypopneas were short in duration and resulted in minimal arousal. The quantity and quality of sleep showed significant improvements. Total sleep time increased, although the most significant changes were in Stage One and REM sleep. Stage One sleep decreased from 45.6% of total sleep time to 7.1% of total sleep time, while REM sleep increased from 3.9% of total sleep time to 36.9% of total sleep time. The decrease in Stage One sleep, the lightest stage of sleep, is consistent with the elimination of sleep fragmentation caused by apneas and hypopneas. The increase in REM sleep time is consistent with a REM sleep "rebound" thought to result when an extended period of REM sleep fragmentation and deprivation is ended by successful treatment of sleep apnea. The rebound is hypothesized (continued)

Figure 36-9

A polysomnogram report.

ELIAS RANDALL   Page two

to represent the release of REM sleep "pressure" build up over a long period of time. The patient reported that he slept much better than usual.

In summary, administration of a pressure of 7.5 cm. H_2O resulted in a change from severe obstructive sleep apnea to normal respiration in sleep.

_____   _____
DONALD D. PETERSON, M.D.   MARK R. PRESSMAN, Ph.D
MEDICAL DIRECTOR   ASSOCIATE DIRECTOR

Figure 36–9 Continued

THE LANKENAU HOSPITAL
100 Lancaster Avenue west of City Line
Wynnewood, PA 19096-0000

DISCHARGE SUMMARY

NAME: JENNIFER DOWNINGS   MEDICAL RECORD NO.: 732-596
PHYSICIAN: DR. FIGUEROA   DATE OF ADMISSION: 5/20/94
                                       DATE OF DISCHARGE: 5/28/94

DIAGNOSES:
1) Exacerbation of her chronic obstructive pulmonary disease.
2) Purulent tracheobronchitis.
3) Fractured ribs.
4) Osteoporosis.
5) Cor pulmonale.

DISCHARGE MEDICATIONS AND INSTRUCTIONS:
1) Prednisone, 10 mg. b.i.d. for the next four days and then go back to 15 mg. a day.
2) Theo-Dur, 200 mg. b.i.d.
3) Pepcid, 20 mg. b.i.d.
4) Cipro, 500 mg. b.i.d. for five more days.
5) Verapamil, 80 mg. t.i.d.
6) Xanax, 5 mg. b.i.d.
7) Halcion, 125 mg. h.s.

She is to have her eye drops, skin cream and her oxygen, three liters per minute, and to turn it up to four liters per minute when she does any exercise or walking. She is to see Dr. Figueroa in follow-up in approximately two weeks. Her activity levels are to do graded exercise with a controlled breathing program and to try walking and performing activities of daily living. There are no restrictions on her diet.

HISTORY OF PRESENT ILLNESS: This is one of several Lankenau Hospital admissions for a 59-year-old housewife who was admitted as an emergency on 5/20/94 because of fever, cough and purulent mucus. This patient has advanced chronic obstructive pulmonary disease and has had mechanical ventilation in the past and is on an intensive home care program, including

(continued)

Figure 36–10
Discharge summary for a patient admitted through the emergency room with fever, cough, and purulent mucus.

JENNIFER DOWNINGS   Page two
MEDICAL RECORD NO.: 732-596

oxygen, nebulizer therapy and corticosteroids therapy. She has had
complications on steroids. In review, she has already had compression
fractures of her spine and marked fluid retention, and she has a very limited
level of activity. She has nursing help at home as well as a devoted family.

She recently had an episode of purulent mucus and shortness of breath and
was treated with a short pulse dose of steroid increase and was also given a
course of ampicillin. She called about five days later and continued to have
purulent mucus, coughing and difficulty. She was, therefore, given a course
of Biaxin. She called again and actually came to the emergency room
markedly short of breath and still with purulent sputum. At that time, she
also had some diarrhea and there was concern for a Clostridium difficile
infection.

PHYSICAL EXAMINATION: On physical examination, her respiratory rate was
24 at rest and would go up to 36 or even 40 with any exertion. Her pulse was
120 and regular, blood pressure was 120/70. The neck veins were distended
but this, we felt, was related to use of expiratory muscles and the chest
showed markedly decreased breath sounds. The cardiac examination showed
a diffuse point of maximal impulse (PMI) with a tachycardia. No gallops were
noted. Abdomen was protuberant and extremities showed some puffiness. She
had a generalized eruption of a macular type.

LABORATORY DATA: A chest x-ray showed marked overinflation with
changes of advanced chronic obstructive pulmonary disease. There was no
definite change from previous films except for the marked compression
fractures of the vertebral bodies at 3, 4, 5, 6, 7, 8 and 9. These were
probably old. The bones are generally demineralized.

Her hemoglobin was 14, the white count was 11,000, and the electrolytes were
within normal limits. Her glucose was 128 but that was a random blood
sugar. LDH and alkaline phosphatase were elevated but there was some
question of hemolysis. The electrolytes were within normal limits except for an
elevated bicarbonate of 33. Her arterial blood gases showed a pH of 7.35,
Pco_2 was 66 and her PO_2 was 84 and that was on two liters per minute of nasal
cannula indicating that she has a chronic respiratory acidosis which is
compensated. The sputum was cultured on two occasions and was found to
be normal flora. However, there was noted to be mixed gram positive and
gram negative organisms on the gram stain and there were polys.

(continued)

Figure 36–10 Continued

JENNIFER DOWNINGS   Page three
MEDICAL RECORD NO.: 732-596

HOSPITAL COURSE: The patient was given intravenous Fortaz. She was given an increase in her intravenous Solu-Medrol for a few days and, of course, nebulizer therapy and bronchodilators were continued in the form of Theo-Dur. Her cardiac and anti-anxiety medications were also continued.

She developed severe chest pains on the second or third day of admission and there was an evaluation. We felt that she was not a candidate for cardioversion or intensive cardiac medications since she has refused resuscitation efforts because of her disorder being so end stage. However, follow-up evaluation showed this to be a fractured rib and, therefore, a so called "cough fracture". Once this was diagnosed, she seemed to be somewhat more reassured and less anxious and the program was continued. Purulent sputum cleared, the diarrhea stopped and the patient was able to walk around the room on oxygen. She had a pulse oximetry measurement which showed 89% with four liters of oxygen by nasal cannula when she would walk.

The patient improved and was discharged to home on 5/28/94 with the above program. The prognosis is guarded because she has respiratory failure on a chronic basis and even an acute bronchitis causes her to become decompensated.

WILLIAM G. FIGUEROA ,M.D.

WGF:ssb
D: 5/30/94
T: 5/31/94

Figure 36–10 Continued

5. Irwin, R. S., M. R. Pratter, P. S. Holland, et al. Postnasal drip causes cough and is associated with reversible upper airway obstruction. *Chest* 85:346-352, 1984.

J. B. Lippincott, Philadelphia, 1984.
Murray, J. F. and J. A. Nadel. *Textbook of Respiratory Medicine.* W. B. Saunders Company, Philadelphia, 1988.

Reference Sources

Burton, G. G., and J. E. Hodgekin. *Respiratory Care, A Guide to Clinical Practice,* 2nd edition.

For references of specific application to medical transcription, see Appendix 1.

Patricia A. Fenn, M.D., F.A.C.R.

Rheumatology

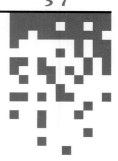

INTRODUCTION

Rheumatology is a subspecialty of the more general field of internal medicine; it is concerned with all types of arthritis and related disorders. The term *rheuma* ("flowing") is derived from the Hippocratic work titled *On Locations in the Human Body* (4th century B.C.) and belongs to the humoral theory of disease. In the 20th century, science has identified that rheumatic disease is in part immunologically mediated — much of which is humoral!

After completing a residency in internal medicine, the rheumatologist continues with a fellowship in order to qualify for treating persons with rheumatic diseases. Most rheumatologists are board-certified or board-eligible in Internal Medicine and in the subspecialty of rheumatology.

There are more than 100 types of rheumatic diseases, and more than 37 million Americans have some type of it. This translates to 1 of 7 persons in this country being significantly affected. These disorders are the leading cause of disability and absence from the workplace.

Rheumatic diseases include arthritis, diseases of the immune system, and other disorders that cause pain and inflammation in joints, muscles, and bones. Metabolic bone disease (osteoporosis, Paget's disease) and soft tissue disorders (tendinitis, bursitis, fibromyalgia) fall within the realm of rheumatology.

The constellation of symptoms and findings often points toward a high element of systemic inflammation, which is characteristic of the connective tissue diseases (formerly referred to as collagen vascular diseases). Examples of these are rheumatoid arthritis, systemic lupus erythematosus, polymyositis, scleroderma, and the various types of vasculitis. Conversely, the signs and symptoms may be more localized without systemic features. Examples of the latter are osteoarthritis, osteoporosis, bursitis, and tendinitis.

Most forms of arthritis and rheumatism are slow to develop and slow to respond to treatment; most require long-term care. Rheumatic diseases can be difficult to diagnose even by specialists because of the subtleties and complexities of symptoms and their overlap with other medical problems. It follows that the association of rheumatologists with their patients is often a protracted one. There are no known causes or cures except for infectious arthritis and gout.

REPRESENTATIVE DISEASES IN RHEUMATOLOGY

Osteoarthritis (Figure 37–1) ▪ Osteoarthritis (OA) is often referred to as degenerative joint disease (DJD), a term used interchangeably with osteoarthritis. Osteoarthritis is extremely common, occurring in nearly 16 million of our population and affecting hands, knees, hips, feet, cervical spine, and lumbar spine. OA or DJD is often referred to as "wear and tear arthritis" as it is much more common in the aging population; women are affected three times more often than men. OA is characterized by stiffness, decreased motion, aching, pain, and usually some degree of swelling and inflammation. These symptoms can result in varying degrees of disability, depending on the severity of involvement.

The diagnosis is based on clinical grounds of history and physical examination plus typical

715

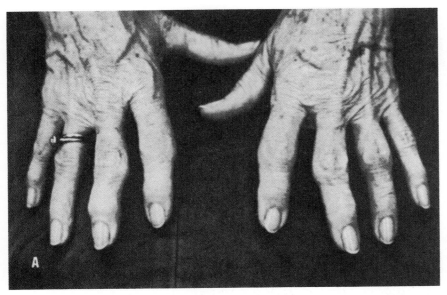

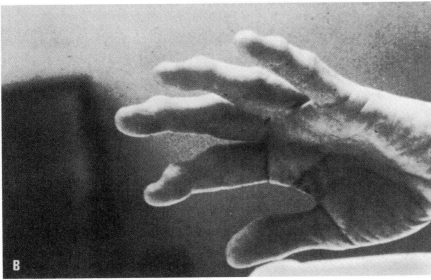

Figure 37–1
The hands of a patient with osteoarthritis, showing A, Bouchard's nodes at the proximal interphalangeal joints, and B, Heberden's nodes at the distal interphalangeal joints. (From Cohen, A. S. *Rheumatology and Immunology*. Grune & Stratton, Orlando, Florida, 1986, p. 351.)

radiologic changes. These changes are quite specific, with x-ray films showing uneven loss of cartilage and bony overgrowth around the joints. The overgrowths are referred to as spurs, or sometimes as arthritic nodes. There is no specific blood test to confirm the diagnosis of osteoarthritis. Generally, a long period of time is involved in the evolution of these changes — years as opposed to months.

The treatments are directed at decreasing pain and stiffness and in some cases attempting to alleviate the inflammation if that symptom is prominent. Treatment includes the use of nonsteroidal anti-inflammatory drugs (NSAIDs), local injections of corticosteroids, specific exercise and rest regimens, and education of the patient about the nature of the disease process. Surgical intervention is indicated in those persons who have marked destruction of joints, with marked reduction in mobility or pain at rest.

Rheumatoid Arthritis ▪ The chief characteristic of rheumatoid arthritis (RA) is diffuse inflammation of joints, often in a symmetric fashion. Many aspects of this disease can be attributed to this inflammatory characteristic. It is the second most common type of arthritis but has the potential to become the most disabling. Rheumatoid arthritis affects more than 2 million persons, and women are affected twice as frequently as men. This disease tends to have its onset during the childbearing years, although the very young and the very old are not exempt. The onset of symptoms is often gradual over months, or it may be explosive.

The symptoms are typically morning stiffness of more than an hour's duration, often symmetric small joint (joints of hands and feet) pain, swelling, and limitation of motion. Rheumatoid arthritis differs from osteoarthritis in that there are accompanying systemic features of fatigue, fever, and weight loss. These latter symptoms may at any time during the course of the disease equal or outweigh the joint difficulties.

Physical examination establishes the presence of warm-to-hot joints, symmetric swelling, joint deformities, decreased painful motion, and a globally ill-appearing patient. Rheumatoid nodules may be present on points of pressure.

Laboratory data include a positive rheumatoid factor in approximately 80 per cent of patients, an elevated erythrocyte sedimentation rate (ESR), anemia, hypoproteinemia, and occasionally a positive antinuclear antibody of a nonspecific type (Table 37–1).

Table 37–1 ▪ **Laboratory Tests in Rheumatology**

Complete blood count (CBC)
Erythrocyte sedimentation rate (ESR)
Uric acid
Antistreptolysin titer
Rheumatoid factor (RF, latex)
Antinuclear antibody (ANA)
Genetic testing
Anti-DNA (double-stranded DNA)
Extractable nuclear antigen (Anti-ENA)
Human lymphocyte antigen (hLA-B27)
Lyme serology
Synovial fluid analysis

Juvenile rheumatoid arthritis (JRA) is a variation of rheumatoid arthritis. It is sometimes referred to as juvenile chronic polyarthritis, and within this category further differentiation is made depending on the constellation of signs and symptoms. Still's disease occurs in infants or young children as an acute febrile illness in association with a recurring salmon-colored rash; usually only one or two large joints are inflamed. The patients characteristically have a very high white blood cell count. The second type of JRA is indistinguishable from the adult variety of RA. A third type is termed *pauciarticular JRA*; only a few joints are involved, but this variety is often associated with eye problems.

Treatment of all forms of rheumatoid arthritis can be as simple as prescribing high-dose aspirin or as complex as several simultaneous systemic medications plus reconstructive surgery of end-stage joints. Treatment, of course, is tailored to the individual.

In general, for the patient with RA rheumatologists employ the simpler strategies first and add more complex or toxic therapies if baseline therapy does not control the disease. These therapies are additive, as depicted by the treatment pyramid in Figure 37–2.

Total joint replacement of the hip and the knee is a frequently exercised option in patients with rheumatoid arthritis. Hand surgery, including repair of tendon rupture and realignment, is also employed.

Systemic Lupus Erythematosus (SLE) ▪ This disease, as the name implies, is a systemic "wolflike" illness that has a myriad of presentations and may literally affect any organ system in the body. Women are afflicted eight times more frequently than men. The disease is characterized by abnormalities of the immune system, which seemingly loses its ability to regulate itself, resulting in attacks on one's own tissues. Especially vulnerable are the skin, kidneys, and brain, but also the lungs, the heart, and the supporting structures of the joints are affected. Approximately 130,000 persons suffer from this disease in the United States today.

The symptoms often have their onset following some kind of physical or emotional insult. For example, some persons come down with the illness after prolonged sun exposure and resultant sunburn. Rashes, characteristically red, scaly plaques, subsequently develop in areas of

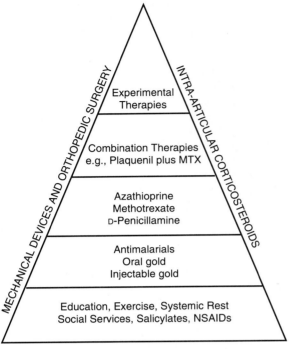

Figure 37–2
Treatment pyramid for rheumatoid arthritis.

exposure and may be accompanied by arthralgias and myalgias. A typical butterfly rash may be obvious over the bridge of the nose and the cheeks, although it may occur anywhere. Oral and nasal ulcerations may be associated. Another common finding is Raynaud's phenomenon, characterized by blanching of the fingers, toes, or nose, followed by a blue or red discoloration in the same distribution upon exposure to cold or emotional stress. Pleurisy, in association with pleural effusions and pericarditis, may be present. In kidney involvement, again there are a number of different presentations, including nephrotic syndrome. Anemia due to destruction of red blood cells, leukopenia due to destruction of white blood cells, and thrombocytopenia secondary to platelet destruction are part of the spectrum. Onset of seizures signals central nervous system involvement.

The laboratory findings are protean with regard to the presence of antinuclear antibodies (ANAs). Almost 100 per cent of patients with SLE are positive for antinuclear antibodies in the serum. The (Sm) anti-Smith pattern of ANA is highly specific for SLE, whereas most of the others are not.

The treatment may range from salicylates to high-dose systemic corticosteroids. Hydroxychloroquine is often very effective for the skin lesions. Corticosteroids are usually required for renal or brain involvement. Cytoxan may be necessary in cases of severe renal involvement or severe systemic vasculitis.

A subset of lupus patients has drug-induced lupus. This may be seen in patients on antihypertensive therapy who take hydralazine or methyldopa, or antiarrhythmic therapy drugs (procaine and quinidine), or anticonvulsant therapy (phenytoin).

Other Connective Tissue Diseases and Vasculitis ■ Scleroderma, or progressive systemic sclerosis, is, as the name implies, a disorder that leads to sclerosis or fibrosis of tissues (Figure 37–3). In addition to characteristic intense tightening of the skin, any of the internal organs may be fibrosed, including kidneys, lungs, heart, and the gastrointestinal tract. These patients have a very high frequency of Raynaud's phenomenon. A subset of patients has a more limited involvement with sclerosis, termed the CREST syndrome (calcinosis, Raynaud's phenomenon, esophageal dysmotility, sclerodactyly, and telangiectasia).

Polymyositis (PM) literally means inflammation of many muscles and if there is skin involvement the descriptive diagnosis of dermatomyositis is used. The hallmark of polymyositis and dermatomyositis is profound weakness, especially of proximal muscles, due to the breakdown of muscle tissue from the inflammation.

Many types of vasculitis occur as distinct entities, such as temporal arteritis, periarteritis nodosa, Wegener's granulomatosis, and Goodpasture's syndrome. However, vasculitis may occur as a complication of any of the connective tissue diseases. Temporal arteritis (TA) or giant cell arteritis is fairly common in persons over 50 years of age, with women being affected twice as often as men. The diagnosis is established by biopsy of the temporal artery showing characteristic giant cell infiltration into the wall of the artery. There is an association of temporal arteritis with polymyalgia rheumatica, but this is not well understood.

Psoriatic Arthritis ■ This disease occurs in a certain percentage of persons who have the

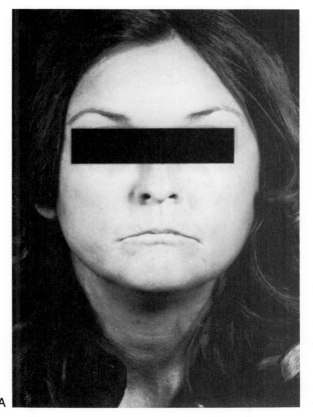

A

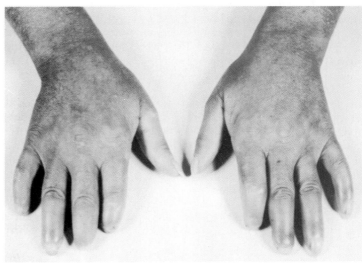

B

Figure 37–3
A, The face of a woman with scleroderma. B,
The hands of a woman with scleroderma.
(From Cohen, A. S. *Rheumatology and Immunology*. Grune & Stratton, Orlando, Florida, 1986,
p. 261.)

chronic skin condition called psoriasis. About 160,000 persons in the United States have this form of arthritis, which in many cases resembles rheumatoid arthritis.

This inflammatory destructive joint disease is often amenable to NSAID therapy and sometimes to gold or methotrexate therapy.

No distinct laboratory test exists, but there are characteristic radiologic changes in many patients. Basically, it is a clinical diagnosis based on the presence of psoriasis and the pattern of involvement. This pattern tends toward arthritis in the small joints of the hands and feet with characteristic fingernail and toenail pitting.

Gout ■ Gout affects about 1 million Americans and four times as many men as women (Figure 37–4).

Podagra is a term used for an acute painful attack of the big toe, although gout may affect any synovial joint. The attack may follow an injury to the affected joint or after a meal containing large amounts of uric acid, or it can start de novo. At the basis of the attack is the precipitation of urate (uric acid) crystals into the joint to which the body responds by very marked inflammation. Generally, this inflammation is of such a magnitude that movement or bearing weight on the affected joint is impossible.

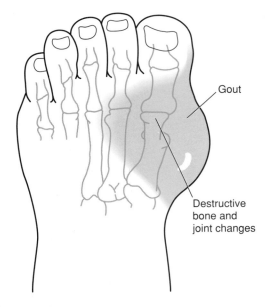

Figure 37–4
Bone and joint changes in a patient with gout.

Gout is often associated with an elevated uric acid as measured in the serum. This is true whether the condition is familial or idiopathic, or secondary to diuretic or chemotherapeutic drugs. Demonstration of sodium biurate crystals in the affected joint establishes a diagnosis.

The treatment of gout is generally twofold. First, the acute attack is treated by high-dose NSAIDs or by colchicine. Second, the high uric acid condition is treated. In the case of an idiopathic condition, probenecid may be employed, allowing the kidney to excrete increased amounts of uric acid, or allopurinol may be used to block the production of uric acid. Both drugs have significant toxicities and need to be monitored.

In the case of cancer chemotherapy, the patient is often put on allopurinol prior to the initiation of chemotherapy in an effort to prevent attacks.

Diuretic agents that cause hyperuricemia may be switched for another type of diuretic or eliminated altogether.

There is a form of chronic gout that is recognized by widespread tophi (gouty deposits) around joints, near the cartilage of the ear, and subcutaneously. Over a long period of time, allopurinol may be effective in eliminating or decreasing the size of the tophi.

In addition to controlling arthritis by keeping uric acid at a near normal level, there is concern for the long-term effect of high uric acid on reducing kidney function.

Pseudogout is a condition very commonly confused with acute gout. In this case, the crystal in the joint is calcium pyrophosphate, which has different characteristics when examined under the polarizing microscope.

Infectious Arthritis ■ This section will deal with those types of arthritis caused by specific microorganisms. It is impossible to address them all, but the principal ones will be discussed. It is very important to diagnose infectious arthritis because appropriate antibiotic therapy can eradicate the process.

Bacterial Arthritis ■ The most common type of bacteria-related arthritis is gonococcal arthritis (GC arthritis). The gonococcal organism is spread as a venereal disease and is most common in urban and suburban areas. Much of the time, the gonococcal organism remains in or around the genitalia, but, especially in women around the time of the menses, the gonococci can become disseminated into the blood. This dissemination results in fever, joint pain and swelling, pain and swelling around the joints (tendons), and occasionally bullous skin lesions. Because the gonococcal organism is very difficult to grow outside the body, cultures of blood and synovial fluid are often negative, although cultures of the genital tract may be positive.

The treatment is with intravenous antibiotics, to which the organism is sensitive.

All the rest of the infectious arthritides are grouped together as "nongonococcal arthritis." The list of organisms that may cause this is legion: most common are *Staphylococcus aureus, S. epidermidis, Haemophilus influenzae,* and *Escherichia coli.* In intravenous drug users in the last several years, *Pseudomonas* and *Serratia* have emerged as etiologic agents. The treatment for nongonococcal arthritis is intravenous antibiotics for at least 6 to 8 weeks.

Lyme Disease ▪ This disorder is named after the town in Connecticut where it was originally described by a group of rheumatologists and epidemiologists.

In addition to the effects the disease has on joints, it can affect the heart and the central and peripheral nervous systems, but most characteristic are the skin manifestations.

Erythema chronicum migrans (ECM) is a rash that usually develops at the site of a specific tick bite (*Ixodes dammini*). The tick bite deposits spirochetes (*Borrelia burgdorferi*) in the skin. After a variable amount of time (3 to 30 days), a red plaque develops that subsequently expands to form a larger, circular lesion with a red border. Often there are similar skin lesions distant from the initial one. These lesions are not painful and disappear with or without treatment.

A second stage, weeks and months later, may be characterized by symmetric arthritis, especially in knees and ankles, that may mimic rheumatoid arthritis. In this stage, the nervous system or cardiac involvement may become manifest. Untreated, these conditions may become chronic.

The diagnosis is suspected in persons living in endemic areas (e.g., Connecticut, Massachusetts, and the Middle Atlantic states), where the white-tailed deer and the white-footed mice are reservoirs for the spirochete that is subsequently transferred to persons by the vector tick. Occa-

sionally, there is no history of rash. The laboratory test confirms the diagnosis of specific antibodies directed against the tick.

Treatment of uncomplicated erythema chronicum migrans rash is 3 weeks of oral tetracycline-type drugs; treatment of the arthritis, nervous system, and cardiac manifestations is with intravenous cephalosporins.

SURGICAL PROCEDURES AND INSTRUMENTS

A mainstay of the rheumatologist is joint aspiration to acquire synovial fluid for analysis. This process is performed with a needle and syringe and is called diagnostic arthrocentesis. It is performed under sterile conditions. The fluid is sent to the laboratory for synovial analysis. The standard tests performed on the fluid include color, clarity, viscosity, white blood cell count, presence or absence of rheumatoid factor, and presence or absence of specific crystals.

On occasion, arthrocentesis is performed solely to instill medications into the joint; this is referred to as a therapeutic arthrocentesis.

Some rheumatologists perform diagnostic and therapeutic arthroscopy using an arthroscope introduced into the joint through a small incision. This allows direct visualization of joint structures; if necessary, a synovial biopsy may be carried out.

FORMATS

Consultation Reports ▪ Figure 37–5 is an example of a new patient consultation.

Chart Notes ▪ Figure 37–6 is a problem list and a record of current medications. These items are usually kept in the same place in the patient's chart so that they can be easily found. The data are reviewed and brought up to date periodically.

A problem-oriented progress note that also becomes part of the patient's chart is seen in Figure 37–7.

Insurance Reports ▪ A medical report to an insurance company regarding disability is seen in Figure 37–8.

Discharge Summary ▪ In this format, the patient's name, admission date, discharge date,

Text continued on page 730

PATRICIA A. FENN, M.D.
933 HAVERFORD ROAD
Bryn Mawr, PA 19010-0000
215/652-3758

July 28, 1994

James Corbin, M.D.
245 Lander Avenue
Bryn Mawr, PA 19010-0000

RE: Katherine B. Lamb
011-56-45-1

Dear Dr. Corbin:

Many thanks for your confidence in having us see Mrs. Lamb for rheumatologic evaluation. She is a 63-year-old widow who has generalized osteoarthritis and erosive osteoarthritis involving her hands and feet. She may have superimposed periodic acute gouty attacks.

Her difficulties date back over 30 years at which time she suffered her first acute attack in her right wrist. She was seen at that time by a rheumatologist at Einstein Northern. She has had infrequent attacks in this joint over the years. When she does have the attacks she is rendered pretty much useless with regard to that joint. At one point, she was told of a diagnosis of rheumatoid arthritis, although she has been repeatedly told that her rheumatoid factor test was negative. She specifically reports disabilities only when there is swelling with an acute attack. She has no morning stiffness. She has no systemic features of chronic fatigue, fever, or weight loss.

Pertinent past medical history includes hypertension for which she takes Zestril, 10 mg. per day. She also takes Triavil 2/25, once daily for chronic depression. Family history: She has one sister with bilateral total hip replacements for the treatment of osteoarthritis.

(continued)

Figure 37–5
A consultation report about a rheumatologic evaluation.

RE: Katherine B. Lamb   Page two
      011-56-45-1

Personal history : She is a full time homemaker and lives with her single daughter. She stopped a three pack-a-day smoking habit 15 years ago at the time of vocal cord polyp removal.

Musculoskeletal examination revealed a normal gait. Examination of her spine revealed a slightly increased dorsal kyphosis. She had good motion of her lumbar spine region. Cervical spine motion had slightly decreased flexion, but was otherwise within normal limits. Examination of her shoulders and elbows was normal. Her right wrist revealed that she had a 2+/4+ dorsal cyst. There was no fluid present, but there was chronic tenosynovial thickening. She had modest tenderness. She had bilateral Heberden's and Bouchard's nodes. There was also slight swelling of the medial aspect of both knees due to fat pad presence, but there was excellent motion of her knees. Likewise, there was excellent motion of both hips. Examination of the ankles revealed normal dorsalis pedis pulses. Her feet revealed bilateral large bunions and bunionettes with a hammertoe on the right side.

X-rays of her hands and feet were consistent with degenerative joint disease, but were not consistent with gout or pseudogout. There were no changes of rheumatoid arthritis noted.

A CBC, Westergren sedimentation rate, rheumatoid factor, and chemistries were within normal limits with the exception of a slightly elevated uric acid at 8 mg. per dilution. She also had a slightly elevated BUN with a normal creatinine.

I asked Mrs. Lamb to continue on her program of aspirin (15 grains b.i.d. PC) and to continue her Triavil 2/25 at bed time and, of course, her Zestril at the same level. Her blood pressure on the day of her visit to me was slightly elevated at 160/92.

She was given a booklet from the Arthritis Foundation on osteoarthritis. She was also advised to get a gynecologic examination, as this is about four years overdue. We discussed the advisability of wearing sensible shoes, especially with any prolonged weight bearing.

(continued)

Figure 37–5 *Continued*   *Figure continued*

RE: Katherine B. Lamb   Page three
     011-56-45-1

We thoroughly discussed her probable diagnoses. I asked to see her urgently if she were to develop an acute arthritis flare.

I do not see the advisability of any chronic uric acid lowering medications at this time. I appreciate the consultation.

Kind personal regards.

                                             Sincerely yours,

                                             Patricia A. Fenn, M.D.

PAF:bp

cc: Joseph McNamara, M.D.

Figure 37–5 Continued

CHART NOTE

Date	Problem	Start Date	Medications	Stop Date
3/82	Rheumatoid Arthritis	5/82	ASA 3200 mg./day	
6/91	Status post left total hip replacement	9/91	Solganal	2/94
4/92	Hypertension	4/92	Diabeta 2.5 mg. b.i.d.	
7/92	Diverticulosis	7/92	Vasotec 10 mg.	
8/93	Adult onset diabetes	9/93	Metamucil Methotrexate	

Figure 37–6
An office chart note for medications.

PROGRESS NOTES - PROBLEM ORIENTED

S - Subjective complaints
O - Objective findings
A - Assessment
P - Plan

Problem: Rheumatoid arthritis (RA). On Methotrexate (MTX).

S: AM stiffness, less than one hour.
Painful, swollen right knee.
One tongue ulcer, after MTX dose.

O: All joints cool except right knee
with 3+/4+ tenderness, swelling,
decreased motion.

A: RA quiescent except right knee.
Minor intolerance of MTX.
Aspiration, right knee. Obtained 40 cc.
of greenish, turbid, poor viscosity fluid.

P: Kenalog, 15 mg. interarticular right knee.
Synovial analysis.
Continue MTX. Watch for further intolerance.
Continue ASA 3200 mg./day.
Review Rx and toxicities.
CBC, expanded chemistries to monitor MTX Rx.
Letter to referring physician.

Figure 37–7
A problem-oriented progress note.

PATRICIA A. FENN, M.D.
933 Haverford Road
Bryn Mawr, PA 19010-0000
215/652-3758

Ms. Jennifer Brownley
Acton Insurance Company
1512 Station Road
Philadelphia, PA 19014-0000

February 3, 1994

RE: June Downing
81-43-67-2

Dear Ms. Brownley:

As you know, the above captioned patient has been unable to work for the past year due to poorly controlled rheumatoid arthritis. I have been seeing her monthly over this period of time and am pleased to tell you that she is ready to return to work as a truck dispatcher at a 50 percent level. If she continues her present rate of improvement, I anticipate she will be able to resume full time work in approximately three months.

If you have any specific questions, please do not hesitate to contact me. June appreciates the support you have given her.

Sincerely yours,

Patricia A. Fenn, M.D.

PAF:ssb

Figure 37–8
A medical report to an insurance company.

BRYN MAWR HOSPITAL
130 South Bryn Mawr Avenue
Bryn Mawr, PA 19010-0000

DISCHARGE SUMMARY

PATIENT'S NAME: JEAN M. STEWART
MEDICAL RECORD NO: 105-42-46-7
ADMISSION: 2/1/94
DISCHARGE: 2/8/94

DISCHARGE DIAGNOSES:

1. Staphylococcal septicemia, secondary to Staphylococcus aureus.
2. Septic arthritis of the right knee, secondary to Staphylococcus aureus.
3. Rheumatoid arthritis.
4. Diabetes mellitus, adult onset.
5. Hypertension.
6. Allergy to sulfa drugs.

DISCHARGE MEDICATIONS:

1. Rocephin, 1 gm. intravenous q. 24 hours.
2. Methotrexate, 7.5 mg., weekly on Wednesdays.
3. Zorprin, 1600 mg. b.i.d. PC breakfast and dinner.
4. Diabeta, 5 mg. b.i.d., 7:00 a.m. and 5:00 p.m.
5. Vasotec, 10 mg. daily in a.m.

CONSULTANT: Brenda Andrews, M.D.

The patient was discharged to her home. The patient and her family were instructed on the care of her intravenous site. Visiting nurses will check the intravenous site twice weekly. The patient was instructed to keep the right leg splint on when ambulatory and to confine ambulation to moving from bed to chair for meals, and to the bathroom. The patient will be seen in the office in one week's time.

(continued)

Figure 37–9
A discharge summary.

Figure continued

JEAN M. STEWART   Page two
105-42-46-7

Mrs. Stewart is a 72-year-old widow who lives with her daughter and family. She was admitted urgently at 10:00 p.m. on 2/1/94, with a history of sudden onset of shaking chills in association with marked pain and swelling of her right knee. There was some question of delirium. Her daughter found her temperature to be 104 degrees Fahrenheit.

When seen in the emergency room, the patient was acutely ill, with a temperature of 104-2/5ths, pulse 110 per minute, blood pressure 110/60, and a respiration rate of 18 per minute. Her skin was warm and dry and her right knee was massively swollen. Aspiration of her right knee revealed 50cc. of thick, tenacious, gross pus. X-ray of the right knee showed moderate changes of rheumatoid arthritis. Two blood cultures were obtained and the synovial fluid was sent for synovial analysis as well as culture and sensitivity. The synovial fluid had a white blood cell count of greater than 100,000 per mm^3. Gram stain showed clusters of gram positive cocci. The peripheral blood cell count showed a normal hemoglobin of 13.0 gm. % with a white cell count of 27,000 with a shift to the left. Blood sugar on admission was 385 mg. per dilution. A chest x-ray and electrocardiogram were normal with the exception of sinus tachycardia.

The diagnosis on admission was acute sepsis with septic arthritis of the right knee. After the cultures were obtained, intravenous Rocephin was begun. Over the next 24 hours, both blood cultures and culture of the right knee grew out Staphylococcus aureus which was sensitive to Rocephin.

Over the next 72 hours, Mrs. Smith's fever defervesced to normal levels. She required daily aspiration of her right knee joint over this 72 hour period. Her white cell count from the fluid diminished to 15,000 on her last aspiration on 2/5/94. Her peripheral white cell count decreased to 7,500 with a normal differential.

She required three days of minimal subcutaneous regular insulin on a sliding scale. Her blood sugar on the day of discharge was 90. Her blood pressure on discharge was 160/90.

(continued)

Figure 37-9 Continued

JEAN M. STEWART   Page three
105-42-46-7

At no time did Mrs. Stewart seem out of touch with her environment as observed by nurses and physicians. She was seen by the physical therapy department for crutch walking instruction.

Dr. Andrews of infectious diseases was consulted and agreed with the present management. She strongly suggested a total of six to eight weeks of intravenous Rocephin.

The patient was discharged in a much improved condition. She was afebrile and had approximately 80% less pain and swelling in her right knee. Her rheumatoid arthritis remained quiet throughout the hospitalization.

                                    PATRICIA A. FENN, M.D.

PAF:bp

D: 2/8/94
T: 2/9/94

Figure 37–9 Continued

and hospital reference number are given first. Then follow:

Discharge diagnoses — list
Discharge medications — list
Consultants
Personal and social issues
Follow-up plans

In the body of the discharge summary is found the following:

Reason(s) for admission (symptoms)
Physical findings on admission
Laboratory findings on admission
X-ray findings on admission
Working diagnoses on admission
Hospital course, including therapy, repeat examinations
Condition on discharge

Figure 37–9 is an example of a discharge summary.

Reference Sources

Consult individual disease pamphlets on osteoarthritis, rheumatoid arthritis, systemic erythematosus, gout, psoriatic arthritis, and so on from the Arthritis Foundation, Atlanta.

Katz, Warren A. (Ed.). *Diagnosis and Management of Rheumatic Diseases,* 2nd edition. J. B. Lippincott, Philadelphia, 1988.
Kelly, William, et al. (Eds.). *Textbook of Rheumatology,* 2nd edition. W. B. Saunders Company, Philadelphia, 1985.
McCarty, Daniel J. (Ed.). *Arthritis and Allied Conditions,* 10th edition. Lea and Febiger, Philadelphia, 1985.
Schumacher, H. Ralph (Ed.). *Primer on Rheumatic Diseases,* 9th edition. Arthritis Foundation, Atlanta, 1988.

For references of specific application to medical transcription, see Appendix 1.

Marty L. Prah, M.D.
Elizabeth Ann Huben, M.T.

CHAPTER
3 8

Urology

INTRODUCTION

Urology, like other disciplines of medicine, is a formally recognized specialty whose administration is entrusted to the American Board of Urology. The Board has many functions, but the two most important are supervising the process of certification of diplomates of the Board of Urology and monitoring the effective practice of urology by those granted certification.

The first is carried out through a required program of education and through successful completion of two qualifying examinations. Each candidate must have been appointed to an accredited residency training program designated as such in the *American Medical Association Directory* of approved residency programs. The program itself must consist of 2 years (preferably in surgical training) of clinical postgraduate education in areas other than urology, followed by a urology residency program of 3 or 4 years approved by the Accreditation Council on Graduate Medical Education and Residency Review Committee for Urology. Following successful completion of required training, the applicant for certification must then take and pass the rigorous written qualifying examination, followed by the equally rigorous but less formal certifying examination, in which the essential feature is assessment by the examiners of the candidate's ability to accurately diagnose and skillfully manage urologic problems. The second is achieved mainly through the programs of continuing education.

Urology, then, is the study of the male and female urinary tracts and of the management of their diseases and disorders. Because of the shared anatomy between the male urinary tract and the male reproductive system, the clinical practitioner deals extensively with diseases and disorders of the male reproductive system as well. To facilitate a better understanding of urology, this chapter first discusses the urinary tract and subsequently the male reproductive system and its implications to the clinical practice of urology.

ANATOMY OF THE URINARY TRACT SYSTEM

The main function of the urinary tract is to remove certain waste products from the body so they do not accrue in levels toxic to the body. Specifically, the urinary tract (kidneys, ureters, bladder, and urethra) removes urea from the human body (Figure 38-1). Urea is nitrogen-based waste material produced in the liver when proteins are consumed and broken down for utilization by the body. The nitrogenous waste material is combined with water and moved out into the bloodstream.

Blood-containing urea and other nitrogenous waste enters the kidneys via the renal arteries at the hilum to begin a highly specialized process of filtration, reabsorption of needed nutrients, and eventual secretion of wastes as it passes through the urinary tract system. Renal arteries branch into very small, numerous arterioles that extend throughout the cortex, or outer portion, of the kidney. These arterioles in turn branch into very small, coiled, and interconnected blood vessels (capillaries). An individual collection of these interconnected capillaries takes on a unique ball shape known as a glomerulus. Thousands of

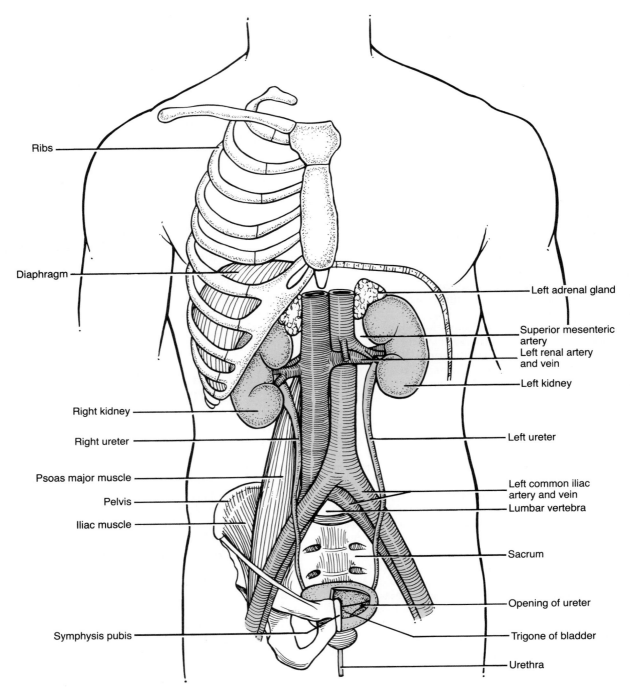

Figure 38–1

The urinary system in anteroposterior view, showing the relationship of the urinary tract, diaphragm, and rib cage.

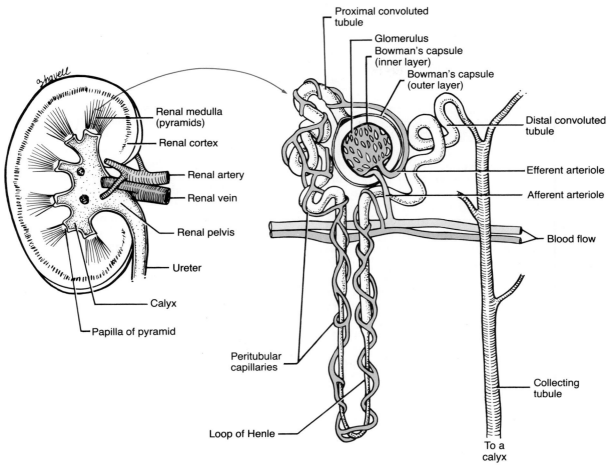

Figure **38–2**
Sagittal view of the kidney, showing detail of one nephron unit.

these glomeruli are located within the cortical region of each kidney. Blood enters the glomerulus via an afferent renal arteriole, and filtered blood exits via the efferent renal arteriole (Figure 38–2).

As blood passes through the glomeruli, very thin, meshlike walls of the glomeruli allow smaller molecules, such as urea, creatinine, and uric acid, to pass out of the bloodstream along with water, various salts, and sugars. This filtrate is collected by a cuplike structure (Bowman's capsule) that surrounds the glomerulus. The filtered material is then directed into a long, tubular structure called the renal tubule. Mate-

rials important to a healthy body are allowed to pass back into the bloodstream by passing through the renal tubule to an associated network of capillaries that are intertwined with the renal tubules. A specialized portion of the renal tubule, the loop of Henle, allows most of the water to be reabsorbed back into the bloodstream, thus conserving the body's water. Concentrated waste then moves to the end of the renal collecting tubule. The entire unit from the glomerulus through the collecting tubule is known as a nephron.

Hundreds of these collecting tubules join to form a cone-shaped structure called the renal papilla. Collecting tubules, the loop of Henle, and the papilla are collectively known as the medulla, or inner kidney. Urine is collected by the calyces, cuplike structures that surround the papilla. Approximately six to eight calyces join to form the renal pelvis at the center of each kidney.

Each renal pelvis narrows down into two long, tubular structures (right and left ureters) that carry urine to the bladder. The funnel-shaped segment connecting the renal pelvis to the ureter is the ureteropelvic junction (UPJ). The ureters enter the bladder at the trigone, a triangular structure at the base of the bladder. Urine is then stored in the bladder until it is passed out of the body via the urethra in the process of urination (voiding or micturition).

In women, the urethra is quite short and terminates at the urethral meatus located anterior to the vaginal orifice. In newborn boys, the glans penis is covered by a retractable foreskin (prepuce). In men, the urethra passes through the penis with the meatus located at the tip or glans penis. The male urethra is divided into four segments: prostatic urethra, membranous urethra, bulbar urethra, and pendulous urethra, the main length of the urethra travelling through the body of the penis. The last inch of the penile urethra is slightly dilated and is referred to as the fossa navicularis.

ANATOMY OF THE MALE REPRODUCTIVE SYSTEM

A study of the anatomy of the male reproductive system logically begins with the testes, or testicles, which are two parenchymatous organs located in the scrotal sac outside the body between the thighs of the male. The testes are organs in which spermatozoa are produced. Inside a single testis is a mass of coiled, very narrow seminiferous tubules. These tubules contain primary germ cells, which yield mature sperm during the process of mitosis and meiosis. This is the process known as spermatogenesis. In addition to sperm, interstitial cells responsible for producing the male hormone testosterone are also found in the testis (Figure 38–3).

As sperm are formed, they move along the seminiferous tubules into a larger duct at the upper portion of the testis (epididymis). Epididymides may be thought of as the holding area where sperm continue to mature and subsequently become motile. At the appropriate time, sperm move up into the body through the vas deferens, which is a long tube that carries sperm into the male pelvic region, around the bladder, and down into the ejaculatory duct. Prior to completion of the route through the vas deferens, sperm are joined by thick fluid produced by the seminal vesicles. Sperm and fluid move from the ejaculatory duct into the prostatic urethra at the utricle, also called the verumontanum or veru, where it mixes with secretions from the prostate gland and the bulbourethral gland (or Cowper's gland) to form the composite fluid known as semen. Contraction of the bulbocavernosus muscle and closure of the bladder neck during orgasm result in propulsion of semen through the urethra and out of the penis. It is interesting to note that, at the point of ejaculation, semen contain only about 1 per cent sperm by volume. Contained within this 1 per cent are some 300,000,000 spermatozoa that are released during ejaculation. Only one of these specialized cells will penetrate the female egg (ova) and result in fertilization and eventual reproduction of a human being.

REPRESENTATIVE DISEASES AND DISORDERS

There are a vast number of representative diseases in the field of urology. Table 38–1 outlines a few of the more common diseases but is not an all-inclusive list.

PROCEDURES

The following glossary represents the most common of the many urologic surgical procedures, with a brief description of their purpose.

Adrenalectomy: Surgical removal of the adrenal gland
Artificial urinary sphincter (AUS): Placement of an artificial urinary sphincter, a silicon mechanism for treatment of incontinence
Corporotomy: Incision of the corpora cavernosa of the penis
Cutaneous ureterostomy: Creation of opening for drainage of urine directly outside the body

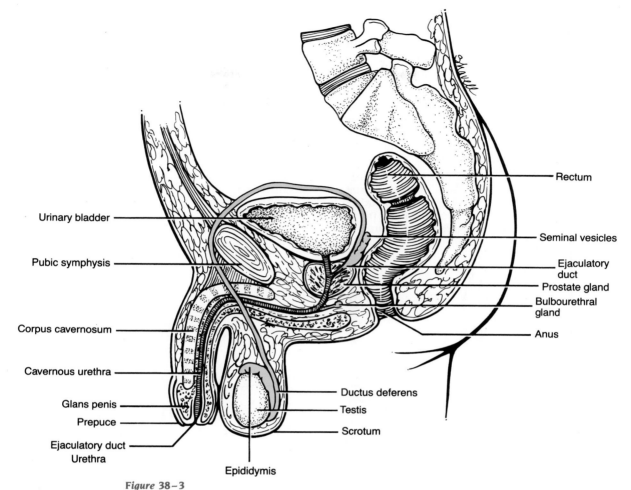

Urinary bladder

Pubic symphysis

Corpus cavernosum

Cavernous urethra

Glans penis

Prepuce

Ejaculatory duct
Urethra

Epididymis

Ductus deferens

Testis

Scrotum

Rectum

Seminal vesicles

Ejaculatory duct

Prostate gland

Bulbourethral gland

Anus

Figure 38–3
The male reproductive system in midsagittal section through the pelvic cavity.

Cystectomy: Surgical removal of all or part of the bladder; radical cystectomy, partial cystectomy

Cystolithectomy (cystolithotomy): Removal of calculus by a cut in the urinary bladder

Cystolitholapaxy: Fragmenting of a bladder calculus via a cystoscope and removal of pieces from the bladder

Cystolithotomy (cystolithectomy): Removal of calculus by a cut in the urinary bladder

Cystopexy: Fixation of bladder to abdominal wall in cystocele repair

Cystoplasty: Plastic/reconstructive surgery of the bladder

Cystoscopy: Endoscopic examination of the bladder and urethra for diagnosis or treatment

Cystostomy (+/− tube): Creation of an opening into the bladder usually with placement of drainage tube

Cystotomy: Surgical incision of the urinary bladder

Cystourethropexy (Pereyra, Stamey, Marshall-Marchetti-Krantz bladder neck suspension): Fixation of the bladder neck and urethra to the abdominal wall for treatment of stress incontinence

Direct internal urethrotomy (DIU): Incision of urethra for treatment of stricture

Text continued on page 744

Table 38-1 ▪ **Representative Urologic Diseases and Disorders**

Diagnosis	Signs and Symptoms	Diagnostic Procedures	Treatment
Adenocarcinoma of prostate (prostate cancer)	Nodule on digital examination; elevated PSA/PAP	Transrectal ultrasound; biopsy of prostate	Observation, hormonal manipulation, radiation, radical prostatectomy
Adrenocortical carcinoma	Adrenogenital syndrome; Cushing's disease	ACTH level; physical characteristics	Surgical excision of tumor
Balanitis	Penile soreness, irritation or discharge due to bacterial or fungal infection of prepuce		Antibiotics; antifungals; sitz baths
Benign prostatic hypertrophy (BPH)	Obstruction of urine from bladder causing frequency, nocturia, pyuria, urinary tract infections (Figure 38-4)	Cystoscopy, uroflow, residual urine	Catheterization, medication, balloon dilation, transurethral prostatectomy, open prostatectomy, laser prostatectomy

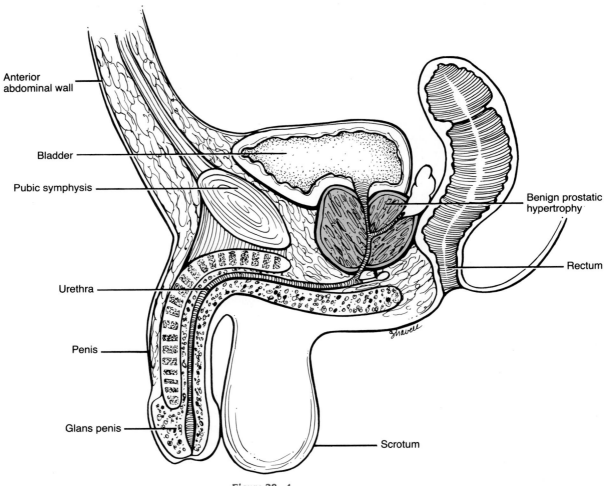

Figure 38-4
Benign prostatic hypertrophy.

Table* 38–1 ▪ Representative Urologic Diseases and Disorders *Continued

Diagnosis	Signs and Symptoms	Diagnostic Procedures	Treatment
Bladder diverticula	Outpouching or herniation of bladder wall; may be congenital (Hutch's diverticula) or secondary to obstruction	Cystogram, cystoscopy	Excision if symptomatic; treat causes, e.g., transurethral resection of prostate (TURP)
Carcinoma of bladder Adenocarcinoma Carcinoma in situ Squamous cell Transitional cell (TCC, most common)	Gross hematuria, rarely dysuria or irritative symptoms	Cystoscopy and biopsy; intravenous pyelogram; cystogram	Transurethral resection of tumor; cystectomy (reserved for invasive disease); and intravesicle chemotherapy
Chronic renal failure	Fatigue, mental confusion, reduced urine output, congestive heart failure, hypertension or anemia, "uremic syndrome"	Serum creatinine level; 24-hr. urine collection for calculation of glomerular filtration rate	Restrict H_2O and protein intake, diuretic therapy; hemodialysis or peritoneal dialysis; transplantation
Cryptorchism (undescended testis)	Nonpalpable testis (Figure 38–5)	Physical examination; scrotal/inguinal sonogram	Hormone manipulation; orchidopexy

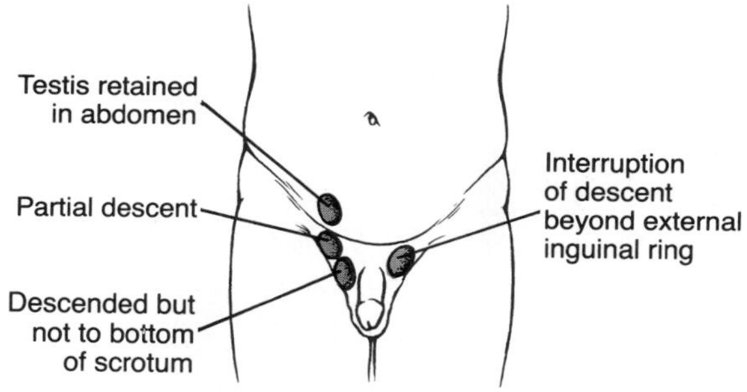

Figure 38–5
Cryptorchidism.

Cystitis	Dysuria with urge and frequency, possibly hematuria	Urinalysis, urine for culture and sensitivity	Antibiotics, antispasmodics, forced fluids
Cystocele	Incomplete voiding or recurrent cystitis	Physical examination and cystoscopy to identify sagging of bladder through vaginal wall	Antibiotics for infections; surgical repair
Fractured kidney	Trauma to flank/abdomen, hematuria, flank tenderness, Grey Turner's sign (flank hematoma)	Intravenous pyelogram, CT scan	Observation with *strict* bed rest and fluids; surgical exploration with repair or nephrectomy

Table **38–1** ▪ **Representative Urologic Diseases and Disorders** *Continued*

Diagnosis	Signs and Symptoms	Diagnostic Procedures	Treatment
Epididymitis	Swelling of epididymis as a result of urinary tract infection, VD, or sepsis (bloodborne infection)	Physical examination, urine for culture and sensitivity, STD testing, scrotal sonogram	Antibiotics, rest, and analgesics
Hematospermia	Blood in the semen	None, other than transrectal ultrasound of prostate	None—almost always a benign condition
Hernia/congenital; hydrocele	Protrusion of organ or peritoneal fluid through muscle wall and into scrotum (Figure 38–6)	Physical examination	Surgical repair

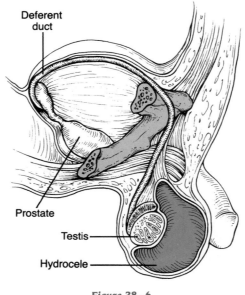

Figure **38–6**
Hydrocele.

Horseshoe kidney	None—in this congenital renal fusion disorder, the lower poles of both kidneys touch or are "fused" (Figure 38–7)	IVP, CT scan, or sonogram to identify horseshoe configuration	No treatment is required unless associated with ureteropelvic junction obstruction

Table 38–1 ▪ Representative Urologic Diseases and Disorders *Continued*

Diagnosis	Signs and Symptoms	Diagnostic Procedures	Treatment

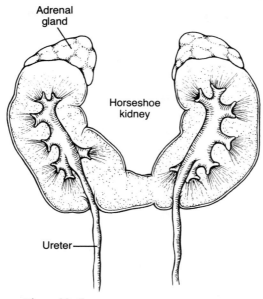

Figure 38–7
Horseshoe kidney, a congenital abnormality.

Diagnosis	Signs and Symptoms	Diagnostic Procedures	Treatment
Hydrocele (can be bilateral)	Accumulation of fluid around the testis with resultant swelling of the ipsilateral scrotum	Transillumination on physical examination, scrotal sonogram	Observation, aspiration, surgical correction
Hypospadias	Congenital defect of penis: spraying or deflection of stream and penile chordee (ventral bend of penis)	Physical examination identifies urethral meatus proximal to normal position	Surgical repair
Infertility (male)	Inability to conceive, low sperm count, decreased motility, pyospermia, low semen volume	Physical examination, laboratory tests, and other tests for infertility and semen analysis	If possible, surgical repair and hormonal manipulation
Incontinence (see also stress urinary incontinence)	Involuntary leakage of urine	History and physical examination	Bladder retraining exercises, medications, corrective surgery
Impotence	Inability to achieve erection; origin may be organic or psychogenic	History and physical examination; nocturnal penile tumescence testing; laboratory investigations	Psychologic counseling, penile implant, vacuum erection device, penile injections

Table 38–1 ▪ **Representative Urologic Diseases and Disorders** *Continued*

Diagnosis	Signs and Symptoms	Diagnostic Procedures	Treatment
Intersex	Presence of both male and female features, i.e., ambiguous genitalia	Physical examination, karyotype, laboratory investigations	Surgery with psychologic and hormonal therapy
Neurogenic bladder: can be congenital (spina bifida) or acquired (spinal trauma)	Incomplete voiding with recurrent UTIs with various associated UTI symptoms	Physical and neurologic examinations, cystoscopy, cystometrogram	Treatment varies greatly depending on severity and level of defect
Oncocytoma	Generally benign tumor of the kidney	IVP, CT scan	Surgical excision
Perinephric abscess	Flank pain, fever, urinary tract infection	Physical examination, sonogram, or CT scan	Antibiotics; surgical drainage
Peyronie's disease	Plaque growth on corpus cavernosum causing bend of phallus, occasionally associated with painful erection	Physical examination	Medication, radiation, surgery; if severe, eventually can lead to impotence.
Pheochromocytoma	Rare type of adrenal tumor causing hypertension, headaches, elevated blood sugar, fainting, sweating, nausea/vomiting	CT scan, MRI scan, serum and urinary laboratory tests	Surgical removal of tumor
Phimosis	Difficult or impossible retraction of foreskin, usually a result of balanitis (Figure 38–8)	Physical examination	Circumcision

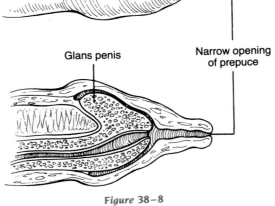

Figure 38–8
Phimosis.

Table **38–1** ▪ **Representative Urologic Diseases and Disorders** *Continued*

Diagnosis	Signs and Symptoms	Diagnostic Procedures	Treatment
Polycystic kidney	Inherited or congenital disease in which kidneys develop mutliple cysts causing hypertension, uremia, kidney failure (Figure 38–9)	Family history, physical examination, CT scan or sonogram	Infantile form is rare and universally fatal; adult form treated with genetic counseling, dialysis, nephrectomy if symptomatic

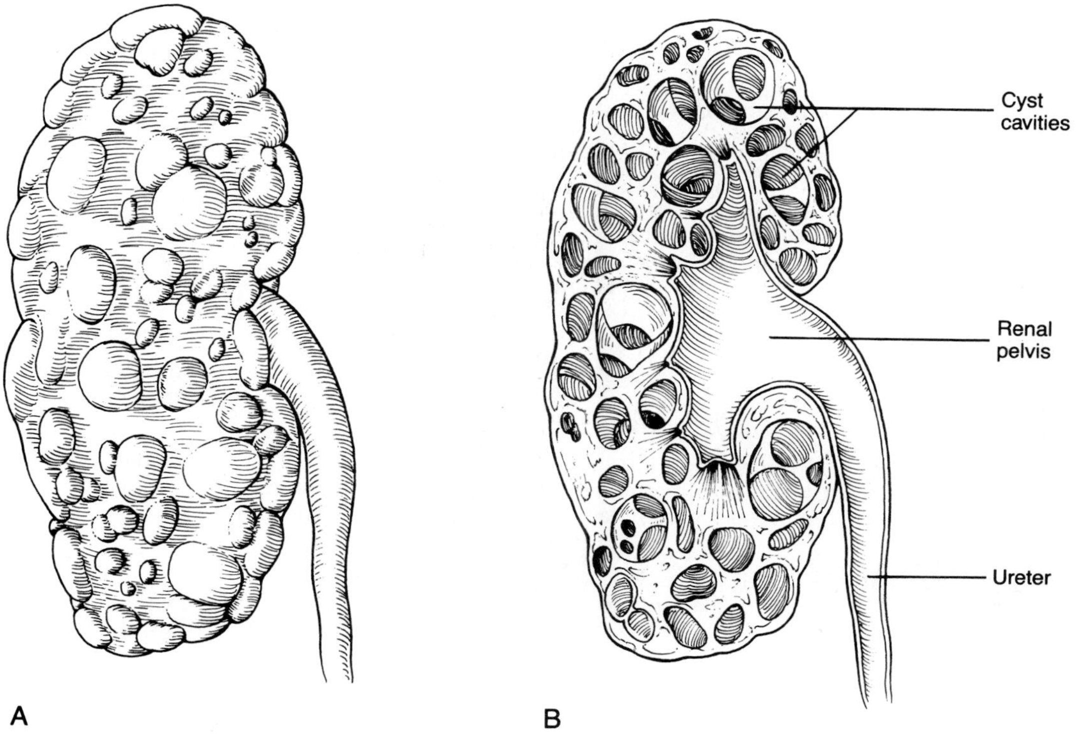

A   B

Figure 38–9
Polycystic kidney. A, Outer view. B, Section through kidney.

Diagnosis	Signs and Symptoms	Diagnostic Procedures	Treatment
Posterior urethral valves of prostate	All the symptoms of urinary obstruction: retention, bladder distention, poor stream, infection, hydronephrosis, vesicoureteral reflux	Physical examination, IVP, voiding cystourethrogram (VCUG), cystoscopy	Catheterization, vesicostomy, transurethral destruction of the valves
Priapism	Painful erection that will not detumesce	Physical examination, evaluate for hematologic or CNS disorder	Based on etiology, includes surgical remediation; review medications
Prostatitis	Acute or chronic inflammation of prostate gland with pain, frequency, urgency, etc.	Physical examination	Antibiotics, sitz baths, increased fluids, prostatic massage

Table 38–1 ▪ Representative Urologic Diseases and Disorders *Continued*

Diagnosis	Signs and Symptoms	Diagnostic Procedures	Treatment
Pyelonephritis	Fevers, chills, flank pain, nausea/vomiting, plus irritative voiding symptoms	Physical examination, urinalysis, urine for culture and sensitivity	Antibiotics, fluids, bed rest
Renal carbuncle (abscess)	Bacterial infection in kidney yielding fevers, chills, flank pain, nausea/vomiting, irritative voiding symptoms	Sonogram, CT scan	Antibiotics, surgical drainage
Renal cell carcinoma (adenocarcinoma)	Kidney tumor causing hematuria, flank pain, palpable mass	IVP, sonogram, CT scan, MRI scan	Radical nephrectomy
Renal contusion or laceration	Please refer to section on fractured kidney		
Renovascular hypertension	Severe hypertension resistant to treatment or of sudden onset; most often caused by stenotic renal artery lesion	History and physical examination (bruit); IVP, angiogram, renin measurement	Medication, percutaneous transluminal angioplasty (PTA), surgical correction of stenotic artery, nephrectomy
Ruptured bladder Intraperitoneal Extraperitoneal	Trauma to abdomen, abdominal pain, hematuria, anuria	Cystogram, IVP, CT scan	Catheterization, surgical repair
Sexually transmitted diseases: AIDS, herpes, syphilis, gonorrhea, others	Various; local irritative voiding symptoms or generalized complaints	History and physical examination, urinalysis, culture, serum and urine laboratory study	Various, depending on diagnosis
Squamous cell carcinoma of penis (Bowen's disease)	Epidermoid tumor on shaft or glans of the penis	Physical examination and biopsy	Radiation, penectomy, lymph node dissection, chemotherapy
Staghorn calculus	Calculus of renal pelvis with extension to the calices; almost always associated with recurrent infections	Plain x-ray film, IVP, retrograde pyelogram, sonogram, CT scan	See *Urolithiasis*
Stress urinary incontinence	Involuntary loss of urinary control, most commonly associated with stress-related activities—coughing, laughing, jogging, sneezing; often associated with cystocele	Physical examination, cystoscopy, cystometrogram	Exercises, medication, surgery (cystourethropexy)
Testis cancer Seminoma Nonseminoma (embryonal, choriocarcinoma, etc.)	Testicular mass noted on examination; may be associated with back pain and abdominal mass if metastatic to retroperitoneal lymph nodes; hemoptysis	Physical examination, sonogram, CT scan, chest x-ray film	Radical orchiectomy plus retroperitoneal lymph node dissection, radiation, chemotherapy

Table* 38–1 ▪ Representative Urologic Diseases and Disorders *Continued

Diagnosis	Signs and Symptoms	Diagnostic Procedures	Treatment
Torsion of testis	Twisting of testis on its cord, resulting in ischemia causing atrophy and eventual necrosis of testis with acute testicular pain and swelling	Physical examination and scrotal sonogram	Orchidopexy for this urologic emergency
Ureteropelvic junction obstruction (UPJ)	Congenital or acquired block of the kidney at the UPJ and resultant flank pain, especially with increased fluids or diuretics such as alcohol	IVP, renal scan, sonogram, CT scan	Pyeloplasty, endoscopic pyelotomy
Urethral caruncle	Erythematous fleshy growth on female urinary meatus	Physical examination	Hormones; surgical resection is performed only if symptomatic
Urolithiasis	Urinary stone formation may cause partial/complete obstruction; may occur from kidney to ureter to bladder	Most stones contain calcium and are radiopaque, thus seen on plain x-ray film; more rare uric acid stones are radiolucent. IVP, retrograde pyelogram, sonogram, CT scan	Observe for passage; extracorporeal shock wave lithotripsy, ureterolithotomy, endoscopic extraction (ureteroscopic or percutaneous nephrolithotomy)
Varicocele	Varicosity of the veins in the spermatic cord, which causes pain or infertility (Figure 38–10)	Physical examination, scrotal sonogram, venogram	Varicocelectomy

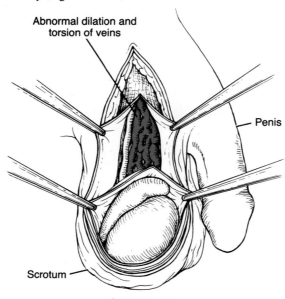

Figure 38–10
Varicocele.

Table 38–1 ▪ **Representative Urologic Diseases and Disorders** *Continued*

Diagnosis	Signs and Symptoms	Diagnostic Procedures	Treatment
Vesicoureteral reflux	Abnormal retrograde passage of urine from bladder into ureter causing UTIs, hydronephrosis, and other symptoms	Voiding cystourethrogram or sonogram	Medical therapy for infections; ureteroneocystotomy
Vesicovaginal fistula	Abnormal channel between bladder and vagina with urinary leakage, incontinence, and recurrent infections	Physical examination, cystoscopy, vesicoureterogram (VCUG)	Surgical repair

Diverticulectomy: Excision of diverticulum of bladder, ureter, etc.

Epididymectomy: Excision of the epididymis without removing its accompanying testis

Extracorporeal shock wave lithotripsy (ESWL): Use of external sound wave to fragment a urinary calculus

Herniorrhaphy: Surgical repair of a hernia

Kock pouch (Indiana pouch): Creation of a neobladder pouch from the small intestine

Lymphadenectomy: Surgical removal of lymph nodes usually specified by location (i.e., pelvic, retroperitoneal, etc.)

Meatotomy: Surgical incision of the urethral meatus

Modified Pereyra's bladder neck suspension: Surgical elevation of bladder neck using Pereyra's needles

Nephrectomy: Excision of a kidney

Nephrocystanastomosis: Surgical opening between the kidney and the urinary bladder

Nephrolithotomy (anatrophic/Boyce): Removal of a calculus via incision of the kidney (renal parenchyma)

Nephropexy: Fixation or suspension of a floating kidney

Nephropyelolithotomy: Removal of a calculus in the renal pelvis via incision through kidney tissues and the renal pelvis

Nephrostomy (percutaneous or open): Placement of a tube into the renal collecting system for temporary drainage of urine

Nephrotomy: Surgical incision into the kidney

Nephroureterectomy: Excision of the kidney and all of the ureter (implies a radical surgery with removal of a cuff of bladder also)

Orchidectomy (orchiectomy): Excision of one or both testes

Orchidoepididymectomy: Excision of testis and epididymis

Orchidopexy (orchiopexy): Surgical fixation of undescended or torsed testis

Orchidotomy (Orchiotomy): Incision and drainage of testis (mostly for biopsy in infertility or cancer)

Orchioplasty: Plastic/reconstructive surgery of the testis

Penectomy: Surgical removal of the penis (radical or partial)

Percutaneous nephrolithotomy (PCNL): Endoscopic removal of kidney stone by placement of nephroscope into the kidney via a nephrostomy site

Placement of penile prosthesis: Surgical placement of a silicon penile prosthesis for artificial erection (can be rigid or inflatable)

Prostatectomy: Surgical removal of part or all of the prostate gland; perineal prostatectomy, radical retropubic prostatectomy, suprapubic transvesical prostatectomy, and transurethral prostatectomy (TURP)

Prostatocystotomy: Incision of bladder and prostate

Prostatolithotomy: Removal of calculus via incision of prostate

Prostatotomy: Incision of the prostate

Pyelocystostomy: Surgical opening between the renal pelvis and urinary bladder

Pyelolithotomy: Removal of calculus from pelvis of kidney

Pyeloplasty: Plastic operation of pelvis of kidney (usually at the UPJ)

Pyelostomy: Formation of opening from renal pelvis to the skin of the back for temporary diversion of urine (usually in infants)

Pyelotomy: Incision into pelvis of kidney

Pyeloureteroplasty: Plastic operation of kidney pelvis and ureter

Radical orchiectomy (for testis cancer): Complete excision of testis, epididymis and spermatic cord via an inguinal incision

Transplantation: Of kidney from one person to another or from one place to another (i.e. autotransplantation)

Transrectal ultrasound (TRUS): Transrectal ultrasound (implies examination of prostate with or without biopsy)

Transurethral resection of bladder tumor (TURBT): Resection of a bladder by means of a special cystoscope, called a resectoscope, passed through the urethra

Subscapular orchiectomy (for prostate cancer): Excision of testicular parenchyma with preservation of epididymis and part of the testicular capsule

Ureterectomy: Surgical excision of ureter

Ureterocalycostomy: Anastomosis between a ureter and a single calyx

Ureterocelectomy: Excision of ureterocele

Ureterocolostomy: Anastomosis of ureter to colon

Ureterocutaneostomy: Creation of opening for drainage of urine directly outside the body

Ureteroileostomy (ileal loop, Bricker loop): Anastomosis of ureter to ileum, drained through stoma on abdominal wall

Ureterolithotomy: Removal of calculus in ureter by surgical incision

Ureteromeatotomy: Incision of ureteral opening in bladder wall

Ureteroneocystostomy (ureterovesicostomy, urethral reimplantation): Implantation of ureter in a new bladder site

Ureteroneopyelostomy (ureteropyeloneostomy): Creation of a new opening for the ureter from the renal pelvis

Ureteropelvioplasty (pyeloplasty): Surgical reconstruction of junction between ureter and renal pelvis

Ureteropyeloneostomy (ureteroneopyelostomy): Creation of a new opening for the ureter from the renal pelvis

Ureteropyelonephrostomy: Anastomosis of ureter and renal pelvis

Ureteropyeloscopy: Endoscopic examination of ureter and renal pelvis

Ureteroscopy: Endoscopic examination of the inside of the ureter (for diagnosis or treatment)

Ureterosigmoidostomy: Anastomosis of the ureter to the sigmoid colon

Ureteroureterostomy: End-to-end anastomosis of transected ureter

Ureterovesicostomy: Implantation of ureter in new bladder wall site

Urethrectomy: Surgical excision of urethra

Urethroplasty: Open surgical repair of urethra for stricture or hypospadia

Urinary diversion: Creation of permanent passageways for urine after injury or removal of the bladder. Usually made from small or large intestine (i.e., ileal loop, Kock pouch, Indiana pouch, Sigmoid conduit, etc.)

Varicocelectomy (varicocele repair): Ligation or excision of varicosities of scrotum

Vasectomy: Surgical ligation of vas deferens

Vasotomy: Incision into the vas deferens

Vasovasostomy: Anastomosis of severed ends of vas deferens as a reversal of the vasectomy procedure

Vasovesiculectomy: Removal of vas deferens and seminal vesicles

Vesicostomy: Formation of opening into bladder (cystostomy); cutaneous vesicostomy

Vesicotomy: Incision of urinary bladder (cystotomy)

FORMATS

Hospital Transcription
History and Physical Examination ■ For specific information and sample reports regarding preparation of this material, refer to previous chapters. In general, a history and physical examination are similar in form and content to the consultation report. The primary goal is to assist a physician in making a diagnosis of the patient's problem(s) which, in turn, will help identify the focus of a treatment plan. Although there is no single, universally utilized format, each hospital or clinic adopts an outline to be followed, and the transcriptionist is encouraged to contact a department supervisor for general guidelines.

Text continued on page 752

HOMETOWN HOSPITAL
4500 Main Street
Ventura, CA 93001-2000

DATE OF PROCEDURE: January 6, 1994

PATIENT: Manual J. Lopez

SURGEON: Hal Griswold, M. D.

ANESTHETIST: John J. Jones, M. D.

ANESTHESIA: General.

PREOPERATIVE DIAGNOSIS: Right cryptorchism.

POSTOPERATIVE DIAGNOSIS: Right cryptorchism.

PROCEDURE PERFORMED: Right orchidopexy.

INDICATIONS: This is a 3-year-old, Hispanic male child
                                      with an undescended testis on the right
side. The physical examination revealed the right testis was palpable just
proximal to the external inguinal ring. He is now undergoing surgical correction
of this.

PROCEDURE: Following successful induction of
                                      general anesthesia and with the patient
in the supine position, the lower abdomen, groin area, genitalia and the upper
thighs were prepped with Betadine and draped in the usual sterile fashion. A
transverse incision was made in the right groin and the incision was deepened
through the fascia down to the level of the aponeurosis of the external oblique.
The external oblique was incised in the direction of its fibers down to and through
the external inguinal ring. The ilioinguinal nerve was identified, isolated, and
retracted from the operative field. The testis was found to be located just
proximal to the external inguinal ring. The testis with its enveloping tunica
vaginalis was carefully separated from the surrounding structures and also the
spermatic cord structures were well elevated from the inguinal canal floor. The
tunica vaginalis was entered near the testis on the anteromedial aspect and the
hernia sac was identified and separated from the rest of the cord structures using
careful sharp and blunt dissection. The hernia sac was ligated with a transfixing
suture of 3-0 silk at the level of the internal inguinal ring. The accessory sac was
then amputated and was sent to the pathologist as a specimen. At this time, the
right testis and epididymis were examined and found to be grossly normal. The
spermatic cord structures were skeletonized and gentle traction was applied in a
downward fashion and the lateral spermatic fascia was visualized and was
sharply incised to gain additional length on the spermatic cord structures. After
determining an adequate length of the cord structures, attention was directed to
(continued)

Figure 38–11

Operative report typed in indented style format.

Page 2
RE: LOPEZ, Manual J.
Hospital No. 0098303
Date: January 6, 1994

the right hemiscrotum where a short transverse incision was made on the inferior aspect. A subductus pouch was created and the testis was brought down into the pouch and anchored into place using 2-0 chromic sutures.

The scrotal incision was carefully inspected and then closed with interrupted simple sutures of 4-0 catgut. The inguinal wound was then irrigated with normal saline. The cyst was reapproximated with interrupted sutures of 3-0 silk and the subcutaneous tissues were reapproximated with continuous running sutures of 4-0 catgut. The skin was then closed with continuous running sutures of 4-0 cat Vicryl. Antibiotic ointment and a sterile dressing was applied and the patient, having tolerated the procedure well, was transferred to the recovery room in satisfactory condition.

SPONGE/NEEDLE COUNTS: Correct.

ESTIMATED BLOOD LOSS: Less than 30 cc.

_____
Hal Griswold, M. D.

mtf
D: 01-06-94
T: 01-07-94

Figure 38–11 *Continued*

HAL GRISWOLD, M. D.
1234 Main Street, Suite 300
Ventura, CA 93003-0101

Telephone: 013-290-4398   **Fax: 013-438-0988**

PATIENT: SMITH, Steve

IDENTIFICATION #   439-99-76-9

DATE OF CONSULTATION: January 2, 1994

REQUESTING PHYSICIAN   John J. Jones, M. D.

CHIEF COMPLAINT: Epididymitis.

HISTORY OF PRESENT ILLNESS: Mr. Smith is a pleasant 56-year-old
                                   gentleman who has had a several-year
history of recurrent epididymitis. He first developed acute epididymitis in 1980.
The patient has had multiple subsequent infections. He specifically relates that
he will develop swelling in the right hemiscrotum and pain along with difficulty
urinating. The patient also complains of a decreased stream with dribbling and
hesitancy. He has nocturia anywhere from six to eight times per night. On a very
good night, this is perhaps two or three times. Although the patient denies any
dysuria, he does complain of an aching sensation in the phallus. He has
moderately severe urgency and some daytime frequency as much as every hour.

The patient denies a prior history of hematuria, urolithiasis, urinary tract infections
or venereal diseases. He has recently completed courses of Floxin and Septra
with no significant improvement.

PAST MEDICAL HISTORY: The patient's past medical history
                                   includes a 10-pound weight loss over
the last two months, hypothyroidism and hay fever. The surgical history is
remarkable for herniorrhaphy in 1983 and 1984. The patient has had several
spontaneous right pneumothoraces. The first of these was 23 years ago, again
five years ago, and the most recent episode required placement of a chest tube.

MEDICATIONS: Synthroid, Proventil, Dimetapp and
                                   Vanceril inhaler.

ALLERGIES: Penicillin.

SOCIAL HISTORY: The patient is married 35 years and has
                                   two children ages 30 and 33. He is an
office products salesman and travels quite frequently. The patient quit smoking
10 years ago. He smoked one pack per day for 38 years prior to that time. On
average, he consumes two beers per week.
(continued)

Figure 38–12
Consultation report typed in indented style format.

Page 2
RE: SMITH, Steve
January 2, 1994

FAMILY HISTORY: The family history is significant for
                                  asthma and ulcer disease.

PHYSICAL EXAMINATION

VITAL SIGNS: Blood pressure is 150/84 mmHg.

ABDOMEN: Abdomen is soft, benign and nontender.
                                  There are no palpable masses and no
CVA tenderness is appreciated. Bilateral herniorrhaphy scars are noted to be
well healed.

GENITALIA: The phallus is unremarkable. The
                                  testes are bilaterally descended. The
left is markedly atrophic and tender. There is a very thick vas deferens on the
left. The right testis is also remarkable for significant tenderness. There is also
an enlarged and firm right epididymis with diffuse induration through the
epididymis and tenderness. Once again, the right cord and vas deferens were
also quite thick. I cannot palpate any specific beading of the vas, however.

RECTAL: The digital rectal examination disclosed
                                  a grade III prostate. It was soft without
                                  nodules or induration.

LABORATORY DATA: PPD and coccidioidomycosis skin tests
                                  are negative. The urine culture is
negative. Urinalysis today demonstrates a specific gravity of 1.025, pH 5.0 with
negative microscopy.

IMPRESSION: 1. Moderate prostatism.
                                  2. Bilateral vasa deferentia thickening
and marked right epididymal induration.

PLAN: I recommend that the patient have an
                                  intravenous pyelogram, chest x-ray, and
return for a flexible cystoscopy. A PSA and renal panel are also ordered today.
The patient's findings and complaints are certainly unusual. Hopefully, our
diagnostic procedures will help me come to a definite conclusion regarding the
patient's pathology.

                                  _____
                                  Hal Griswold, M. D.
mtf

Figure 38–12 Continued

ROLAND, SARA   ID #678-99-08-02

SUBJECTIVE: Mrs. Roland returns today for a followup of her incontinence. A review of the history with the patient today indicates that she has had stress related incontinence for one or two years requiring the use of pads. Interestingly, the patient has had marked urinary frequency of one or two times every hour for at least 15 or possibly 20 to 25 years. She has also had nocturia two or three times per night for a long period of time. This may be somewhat worsened by the diuretics she is currently using, but I suspect that she may have had this even prior to diuretic therapy.

OBJECTIVE: ABDOMEN: The physical exam today demonstrates a massively obese abdomen. There is a well-healed midline infraumbilical incision from prior hysterectomy. PELVIC: The pelvic examination demonstrates a mild cystocele and a moderate to severe rectocele. The speculum exam demonstrates no abnormalities and the bimanual examination is not remarkable for tenderness or mass.

A renal sonogram has been performed and demonstrates normal renal units bilaterally. The remainder of the abdominal sonogram is likewiser unremarkable. Cystoscopy demonstrates slight descensus of the bladder neck. There is diffuse erythema throughout the bladder. Upon distention of the bladder, punctate glomerulations or hemorrhages developed. The remainder of the examination is unremarkable. No tumors or stones are appreciated. The trigone is normal. The cystometrogram demonstrates an increased residual urine of approximately 100 cc. The first sensation, however, is at 75 cc and by 200 to 250 cc, the patient has moderately severe urgency with a maximum volume threshold of only 250 cc which is about half of the normal capacity. A Marshall test was then performed and does demonstrate definite stress-related urinary incontinence. The Bonnie or O-Tip test suggests urethral hypermobility with a resting angulation of 45°. With Valsalva, there is some worsening of this. The patient has definite correction of the stress-related incontinence with elevation of the bladder neck during examination.

ASSESSMENT: Mrs. Roland does definitely have urethral hypermobility with stress-related urinary incontinence and a rectocele which is currently asymptomatic. Unfortunately, the patient also has severe detrusor instability, a decreased volume threshold and changes in the bladder which may indicate a mild form of interstitial cystitis. This would certainly explain her chronic history of frequency and her diminished bladder capacity.

PLAN: I discussed the various treatment alternatives with the patient. Although a bladder neck suspension may correct the incontinence, she would still be left with urgency, frequency and possibly an inability to void successfully and would, therefore, require intermittent catheterizations. For these reasons, I do not feel that this patient is an ideal candidate for a bladder neck suspension. I will, therefore, try to treat her medically. First, I will concentrate on the urgency and frequency. The patient was given a prescription of Ditropan, 5 mg p.o. t.i.d., p.r.n. for one month with refills. I will see her in two months. If she has had some response to this, I could consider adding Ornade to improve her bladder neck tone.

D: 01-02-94   T: 01-03-94   Hal Griswold, M.D./mtf

Figure 38–13
Sample chart entry using the SOAP (Subjective, Objective, Assessment, Plan) method.

HAL GRISWOLD, M. D.
1234 Main Street, Suite 300
Ventura, CA 93003-0101

Telephone: 013-290-4398   **Fax: 013-438-0988**

PATIENT: Alvin B. York

SURGEON: Hal Griswold, M. D.

PROCEDURE: Vasectomy

TECHNIQUE: The patient is placed in the supine
                                            position. His scrotum has been shaved
and prepped and he is draped in the usual sterile fashion. Then, 1 cc of 1% plain
Xylocaine was infiltrated into the scrotal skin and vas deferens for local
anesthesia. Then, utilizing the no-scalpel vasectomy instruments, the right vas
deferens is first mobilized and secured with the vas-grasping instrument. A small
puncture is then made with the vas-dissecting instrument and the vas deferens is
brought up out of the scrotum through the small puncture wound. The vas
deferens is then ligated on both ends and divided. A small segment of the vas is
then sent for pathologic specimen. Following this, the ends of the vas deferens
are cauterized. Following this, the proximal end of the vas deferens is then
closed into the sheath of the vas deferens utilizing a #0000 chromic stitch with
RB1 needle. This effectively separates the two ends of the vas deferens with a
layer of healthy tissue. All hemostasis is excellent at this time. Therefore, the
right vas deferens is now returned to the scrotum.

Then, 1 cc of plain Xylocaine was infiltrated into the left scrotal skin and vas
deferens for local anesthesia. The left vas deferens was then likewise mobilized
and secured with the vas-grasping instrument. The dissecting instrument was
then used to dissect away the sheath of the vas deferens. It was then again
mobilized and brought up out of the scrotal wound and the grasping instrument
was reapplied. The vas deferens was then ligated and a small segment was
removed and sent for pathologic examination. The cut ends were then
cauterized and the proximal end was closed within the sheath of the vas utilizing
a #0000 chromic stitch effectively separating the two ends of the cut vas deferens
with normal healthy tissue. Hemostasis was excellent at this point. I therefore
returned the left vas deferens to the scrotum. Pressure was applied to the small
puncture wound for several minutes. Hemostasis was excellent. No sutures
were required.

I therefore applied Neosporin to the wound, a gauze dressing, and a scrotal
supporter. The patient is again instructed to restrict his activities and apply ice
for 48 hours, to keep the wound dry for 72 hours, and I will see him in one week
for a wound check.

_____
Hal Griswold, M.D.

mtf

Figure 38–14
In-office procedure note typed in indented style format.

Operative Report ▪ Specific formats for operative reports are customarily provided by the hospital's transcription supervisor or director of medical records, and these formats should be strictly adhered to. Transcriptionists who encounter dictations that deviate from formats or introduce new techniques or equipment should always seek the advice of the physician dictating the report or of the medical records supervisor (Figure 38–11).

Consultation Report ▪ Often, in an attempt to provide the best medical care to a patient, the primary care physician seeks the advice of appropriate specialists. The report submitted to the requesting physician is called a consultation report. It may be dictated as part of the patient's hospital chart or as part of a clinical practice setting (Figure 38–12).

Discharge Summary ▪ This one- or two-page report is intended to be a summary of the patient's hospital stay. It customarily includes date of admission, date of discharge, admitting diagnosis, discharge diagnosis, a brief outline of the patient's pertinent medical history, the hospital course including tests and procedures performed during the stay, and disposition on discharge or discharge instructions. Refer to samples of this type of report in other chapters throughout the manual.

Office Transcription

Progress Notes ▪ Progress notes for the practitioner's office follow the subjective, objective, assessment, and plan (SOAP) format with which transcriptionists are familiar. In addition to the four categories of the SOAP, other headings, such as Laboratory and Radiology, may be added when transcribing notes. At times, some headings are not dictated as they may not always be necessary. A representative sampling of such notes is included in Figure 38–13, demonstrating the different aspects of office transcription.

The objective of progress notes is to give a clear and succinct picture of the medical problem and the patient's current status under treatment. Many physicians ask for word processing/computer features, such as bold face, all capital letters, and underlining to highlight diagnoses, allergies, or office tests that are conducted during the patient's visit. Numbering is frequently used in the diagnosis and plan sections, although lists are generally avoided to conserve space in the chart. When in doubt, listen for instructions

from the dictating physician, who will ultimately reread the material.

Letters ▪ Letters commonly transcribed for a urology office include cover letters to be attached to a consultation or sent with a progress note and letters to patients.

Office Consultation ▪ The office consultation report documents for the specialist significant past and present history, physical examination, clinical tests, and suspected diagnoses for patients referred for care. This document must be carefully and meticulously prepared, as it may form the basis of a report to a requesting physician as well as a proposed treatment plan.

In-Office Procedure Notes ▪ In many clinics and offices, selected operative procedures are performed on site. In the urologist's office, one such operation is the vasectomy. Individual physicians differ in their preference for transcribing the procedure. In some cases, it is formatted in the same fashion as an operative report for a hospital chart. In many cases, the report becomes part of the patient's progress note (Figure 38–14).

Reference Sources

Beck, Ernest W., et al. *The Anatomical Chart Series.* The Anatomical Chart Company, Skokie, Illinois, 1988.

Glanze, Walter D., et al. *The Mosby Medical Encyclopedia.* New American Library, New York, 1985.

Golish, Joseph A. (Ed.). *Diagnostic and Procedure Handbook.* Lexi-Comp, Inc., Hudson, Ohio, 1992.

Goss, Charles Mayo. *Gray's Anatomy,* 29th edition. Lea & Febiger, Philadelphia, 1973.

Jacobs, David S. (Ed.). *Laboratory Test Handbook,* 2nd edition. Lexi-Comp, Inc., Hudson, Ohio, 1990.

Kelalis, Panayotes P., et al. *Clinical Pediatric Urology,* 3rd edition. W. B. Saunders Company, Philadelphia, 1992.

Retk, Alan B., Thomas A. Stamey, J. Vaughan, Patrick C. Walsh, et al. *Campbell's Urology,* 6th edition. W. B. Saunders Company, Philadelphia, 1992.

For references of specific application to medical transcription, see Appendix 1.

PART III

Appendices

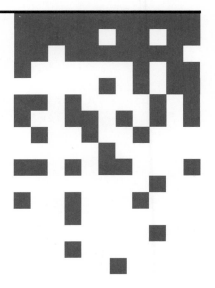

Table of Reference Sources

ABBREVIATIONS DICTIONARY/GENERAL

Crowley, Ellen T., and Helen E. Sheppard (Eds). *Reverse International Acronyms, Initialisms, and Abbreviations Dictionary.* Gale Research Company, Detroit, 1985.

Paxton, John (Ed.). *Everyman's Dictionary of Abbreviations.* B & N Imports, Totowa, New Jersey, 1986.

Spillner, Paul. *World Guide to Abbreviations,* 2nd edition, Vols. 1–3. S.-Z. Bowker, New York, 1973.

ABBREVIATIONS DICTIONARY/MEDICAL

The Charles Press Handbook of Current Medical Abbreviations. The Charles Press Publishers, Philadelphia, 1985.

Davis, Neil M. *Medical Abbreviations: 8600 Conveniences at the Expense of Communications and Safety.* Neil M. Davis Associates, Huntingdon Valley, Pennsylvania, 1992.

Delong, Marilyn Fuller. *Medical Acronyms and Abbreviations.* Medical Economics Books, Oradell, New Jersey, 1985.

Dorland's Medical Abbreviations. W. B. Saunders Company, Philadelphia, 1992.

Garb, Solomon, et al. *Abbreviations and Acronyms in Medicine and Nursing.* Springer Publishing Company, New York, 1976.

Hughes, Harold K. *Dictionary of Abbreviations in Medicine and Health Sciences.* Heath, Lexington, Massachusetts, 1977.

Jablonski, Stanley. *Dictionary of Medical Acronyms and Abbreviations.* Mosby, St. Louis, 1993.

Jenners, Pauline, and Ann Wesson. *Think Metric, U.S.A.* Educulture, Dubuque, Iowa, 1975.

Keller, J. J. *The Modernized Metric System Explained.* J. J. Keller and Associates, Neenah, Wisconsin, 1974.

Kerr, Avice. *Medical Hieroglyphs, Abbreviations and Symbols.* Enterprise Publications, Downey, California, 1970.

Logan, Carolynn, and M. Katherine Rice. *Logan's Medical and Scientific Abbreviations.* J. B. Lippincott, Philadelphia, 1987.

Medical Abbreviations: A Cross Reference Dictionary. The Special Studies Committee of the Michigan Occupational Therapy Association, Lansing, Michigan, 1977.

Medical Abbreviations Handbook. Medical Economics, Oradell, New Jersey, 1983.

Medical Abbreviations, Symbols, and Phrases. Springhouse Publishing Company, Springhouse, Pennsylvania, 1992.

Mitchell-Hatton, Sara Lu. *The Davis Book of Medical Abbreviations.* F. A. Davis, Philadelphia, 1991.

Quick Directory of Medical Abbreviations. Miller and Fink Corporation, Darien, Connecticut, 1977.

Roody, Peter, et al. *Medical Abbreviations and Acronyms.* McGraw-Hill Book Company, New York, 1977.

Schattner, Robert L. *Acronymal Dictionary with Abbreviations.* Springhouse Publishing Company, Springhouse, Pennsylvania, 1988.

Schertel, A. *Abbreviations in Medicine.* S. Karger, New York, 1984.

Sloane, Sheila B. *Medical Abbreviations and*

Eponyms. W. B. Saunders Company, Philadelphia, 1985.

Sloane, Sheila B. *The Medical Word Book.* W. B. Saunders Company, Philadelphia, 1982.

Stedman's Abbreviations, Acronyms and Symbols. Williams and Wilkins, Baltimore, 1992.

Steen, Edwin B. *Bailliere's Abbreviations in Medicine.* Bailliere Tindall, London, Philadelphia, Toronto, 1984.

Stylebook/Editorial Manual of the AMA. Publishing Sciences Group, Littleton, Mississippi, 1976.

Venolia, Jan. *Write Right!* Periwinkle Press, Woodland Hills, California, 1980.

AIDS

(See Specialty References: Immunology/Aids)

ANATOMY AND PHYSIOLOGY

Beck, Ernest W., et al. *The Anatomical Chart Series.* The Anatomical Chart Company, Skokie, Illinois, 1988.

Feneis, Heinz. *Pocket Atlas of Human Anatomy.* Thieme, Inc., New York, 1985.

Goss, Charles Mayo. *Gray's Anatomy.* Lea and Febiger, Philadelphia, 1973.

Grant's Atlas of Anatomy, 9th edition. Williams and Wilkins, Baltimore, 1991.

Shaw, Diane. *Glossary of Anatomy and Physiology.* Springhouse Publishing Company, Springhouse, Pennsylvania, 1991.

Stedman's Anatomy and Physiology Words. Williams and Wilkins, Baltimore, 1992.

ANTONYMS, EPONYMS, HOMONYMS, SYNDROMES, AND SYNONYMS

Chapman, Robert L. *Roget's International Thesaurus,* 4th edition. Harper & Row, New York, 1984.

Fernald, James C. *English Synonyms and Antonyms with Notes on the Correct Use of Prepositions.* Arden Library, Darby, Pennsylvania, 1981.

Firkin, Barry G., and Judith A. Whitworth. *Dic-*
tionary of Medical Eponyms. The Parthenon Publishing Group, Inc., Pearl River, New York, 1987.

Gibson, John, and Olivera Potparic. *A Dictionary of Medical and Surgical Syndromes.* The Parthenon Publishing Group, Inc., Pearl River, New York, 1991.

Jablonski, Stanley. *Jablonski's Dictionary of Syndromes and Eponymic Diseases.* Robert T. Krieger, Malabar, Florida, 1991.

Magalini, Sergio I., et al. *Dictionary of Medical Syndromes,* 2nd edition. J. B. Lippincott, Philadelphia, 1981.

Rodale, J. I. *The Synonym Finder.* Rodale Press, Emmaus, Pennsylvania, 1978.

Sloane, Sheila B. *Medical Abbreviations and Eponyms.* W. B. Saunders Company, Philadelphia, 1985.

Webster's New Dictionary of Synonyms. G & C Merriam Company, Springfield, Massachusetts, 1973.

Webster's Synonyms, Antonyms, and Homonyms. Dennison, Alhambra, California, 1974.

CAREER DEVELOPMENT

American Association for Medical Transcription Journal. American Association for Medical Transcription, Modesto, California, quarterly.

American Association for Medical Transcription Newsletter. American Association for Medical Transcription, Modesto, California, bimonthly.

Analysis: Civil Service Classification of Medical Transcriptionist. American Association for Medical Transcription, Modesto, California, 1981.

Dennis, Robert Lee, and Jean Monty Doyle. *The Complete Handbook for Medical Secretaries and Assistants.* Little, Brown and Company, Boston, 1978.

Fordney, Marilyn T., and Joan J. Follis. *Administrative Medical Assisting.* Delmar Publishers Inc., Albany, New York, 1993.

Gill, Susan. *Communication and Image Skills.* American Association for Medical Transcription, Modesto, California, 1980.

Health Professions Institute. *Perspectives on the Medical Transcription Profession,* Modesto, California, 1988.

Kinn, Mary E. *The Administrative Medical Assistant.* W. B. Saunders Company, Philadelphia, 1988.

CERTIFICATION

The AAMT Test Guide. American Association for Medical Transcription, Modesto, California, 1982.

COMPOSITION

Andrews, William D., and Deborah C. Andrews. *Write for Results.* Little, Brown and Company, Boston, 1982.

Blumenthal, Lassor A. *Successful Business Writing.* Putnam Publishing Group, New York, 1985.

Brogan, John A. *Clear Technical Writing.* McGraw-Hill Book Company, New York, 1973.

Funk and Wagnalls Standard Desk Dictionary. Harper and Row, New York, 1984.

Hodges, John C., and Mary E. Whitten (Eds.). *Harbrace College Handbook*, 8th edition. Harcourt, Brace, Jovanovich, New York, 1984.

Random House Dictionary of the English Language. Random House, New York, 1987.

Ross-Larson, Bruce. *Edit Yourself—A Manual for Everyone Who Works with Words.* W. W. Norton and Company, New York, 1982.

Secretary's Portfolio of Letters Most Often Used in a Physician's Office. Parker Publishing Company, West Nyack, New York, 1968.

Skillin, Marjorie E., and Robert M. Gay. *Words into Type.* Prentice-Hall, Englewood Cliffs, New Jersey, 1974.

COMPUTERIZED DICTIONARIES/MEDICAL SPELL CHECKERS

Brody's Medical Dictionary. MEDICOM, Gaithersburg, Maryland, 1992.

Complete Medical Spell Checker. Sylvan Software, Irvine, California.

CustomMED Computerized Medical Dictionary. Specialized Information Management, Charlotte, North Carolina.

Dorland's Electronic Medical Speller. W. B. Saunders Company, Philadelphia, 1992.

Health Professions Institute. Quick-reference books on disk compatible with WordPerfect: Cardiology, Gastroenterology, Orthopedics, Psychiatry, and Radiology, Modesto, California.

Spellex Medical, Spellex Pharmaceutical. Spellex Development, Tampa, Florida.

Stedman's/25 Plus for WordPerfect. Williams & Wilkins, Baltimore, 1992.

SuperPharmaceutical Spell Checker. Sylvan Software, Irvine, California.

DIAGNOSTIC AND PROCEDURE HANDBOOKS

Golish, Joseph A., (Ed.). *Diagnostic and Procedure Handbook.* Lexi-Comp, Hudson, Ohio, 1992.

The Merck Manual of Diagnosis and Therapy. Merck Sharp and Dohme Research Laboratories, Rahway, New Jersey, 1992.

DICTIONARIES, ENGLISH

American Heritage Dictionary of the English Language. Houghton Mifflin Company, Boston, 1992.

Funk and Wagnalls Standard Desk Dictionary. Harper and Row, New York, 1984.

Random House Dictionary of the English Language, Unabridged. Random House, New York, 1987.

Webster's Ninth New Collegiate Dictionary. Merriam-Webster, Inc., Springfield, Massachusetts, 1983.

DICTIONARIES, FOREIGN

Robb, Louis A. *Diccionario de Terminos Legales.* Editorial LIMUSA, Mexico, 1989. (order from Bernard Hammill, Spanish-English Books, 10977 Santa Monica Boulevard, Los Angeles, California 90025.)

Torres, Ruiz. *Diccionario de Terminos Medicos.*

Madrid, Spain, 1989. (Distributor: Gulf Publishing Company, Book Division, P. O. Box 2608, Houston, Texas 77001).

Unseld, Dieter Werner. *Medical Dictionary of the English and German Languages.* CRC Press, Boca Raton, Florida, 1988.

DICTIONARIES, MEDICAL

Anderson, Kenneth N., Lois E. Anderson, and Walter D. Glanze. *Mosby's Medical, Nursing, and Allied Health Dictionary.* Mosby, St. Louis, 1990.

Blakiston's Gould Medical Dictionary. McGraw-Hill Book Company, New York, 1979.

Churchill's Medical Dictionary. Churchill Livingstone Fulfillment Center, Naperville, Illinois, 1989.

Critchley, Macdonald. *Butterworth's Medical Dictionary.* Butterworth's Publishers, Woburn, Massachusetts, 1980.

Dorland's Illustrated Medical Dictionary, 27th edition. W. B. Saunders Company, Philadelphia, 1988.

Franks, Richard, and H. Swartz. *Simplified Medical Dictionary.* Medical Economics, Oradell, New Jersey, 1977.

Glanze, Walter D., et al. *The Mosby Medical Encyclopedia.* New American Library, New York, 1985.

Glossary of Hospital Terms. American Medical Record Association, Chicago, 1974.

Gomez, Joan. *Dictionary of Symptoms.* Stein & Day, Briarcliff Manor, New York, 1983.

Hinsie, Leland E., and Robert J. Campbell. *Psychiatric Dictionary.* Oxford University Press, New York, 1970.

Isler, Charlotte. *Isler's Pocket Dictionary: A Guide to Disorders and Diagnostic Tests.* Medical Economics, Oradell, New Jersey, 1984.

Melloni, Biagio John, and Gilbert M. Eisner. *Melloni's Illustrated Medical Dictionary.* Williams and Wilkins, Baltimore, 1985.

O'Toole, Marie (Ed.). *Miller-Keane Encyclopedia and Dictionary of Medicine, Nursing and Allied Health,* 5th edition. W. B. Saunders Company, Philadelphia, 1992.

Parker, Sybil. *McGraw-Hill Dictionary of Scientific and Technical Terms.* McGraw-Hill Book Company, New York, 1989.

Pyle, Vera. *Current Medical Terminology.* Prima Vera Publications, Modesto, California, 1992.

Stanaszek, Mary J., Walter F. Stanaszek, Bruce C. Carlstedt, and Steven Strauss. *The Inverted Medical Dictionary.* Technomic Publishing Company, Lancaster, Pennsylvania, 1991.

Stedman's Medical Dictionary. Williams and Wilkins, Baltimore, 1990.

Szycher, Michael. *Szycher's Dictionary of Biomaterials and Medical Devices.* Technomic Publishing Co., Inc., Lancaster, Pennsylvania, 1992.

Thomas, Clayton L. (Ed.). *Taber's Cyclopedic Medical Dictionary.* F. A. Davis, Philadelphia, 1985.

Unseld, Dieter Werner, *Medical Dictionary of the English and German Languages.* CRC Press, Inc., Boca Raton, Florida, 1988.

Wakeley, Cecil. *The Farber Medical Dictionary.* J. B. Lippincott, Philadelphia, 1975.

White, Wallace F. *Language of the Health Sciences.* John Wiley and Sons, New York, 1977.

DRUG REFERENCES

(See Pharmaceutical)

EDITING

Perrin, Porter G. *An Index to English,* 4th edition. Scott Foresman and Company, Glenview, Illinois, 1965.

Plotnik, Arthur. *The Elements of Editing.* Macmillan Publishing Company, New York, 1982.

EPONYMS

(see Antonyms, Eponyms, Homonyms, Syndromes, and Synonyms)

EQUIPMENT

Stedman's Medical Equipment Words. Williams and Wilkins, Baltimore, 1992.

HANDBOOKS (GRAMMAR, PUNCTUATION, AND GENERAL CLERICAL INFORMATION)

Branchaw, Bernadine P., and Bowman, Joel P. *SRA Reference Manual for Office Personnel.* SRA Science Research Associates, Chicago, 1986.

Clark, James L., and Lyn Clark. *How 4: A Handbook for Office Workers.* Kent Publishing Company, Belmont, California, 1985.

Flesch, Rudolf. *Look It up.* Harper and Row, New York, 1977.

Hodges, John C. *Harbrace College Handbook.* Harcourt, Brace, Jovanovich, Orlando, Florida, 1986.

House, Clifford R., and Kathie Sigler. *Reference Manual for Office Personnel.* South Western Publishing Company, Cincinnati, 1981.

Irmscher, W. F. *The Holt Guide to English: A Comprehensive Handbook of Rhetoric, Language, and Literature.* Holt, Rinehart and Winston, New York, 1981.

Johnson, Edward. *Handbook of Good English.* Facts on File Publisher, New York, 1983.

Klein, A. E. *The New World Secretarial Handbook.* William Collins–World Publishing Company, Cleveland, 1973.

Longyear, Marie M. *The McGraw-Hill Style Manual: Concise Guide for Writers and Editors.* McGraw-Hill Book Company, New York, 1982.

Perrin, P. G., and J. W. Corder. *Handbook of Current English.* Scott Foresman and Company, Glenview, Illinois, 1975.

Sabin, William A. *The Gregg Reference Manual.* McGraw-Hill Book Company, New York, 1992.

Shaw, Harry. *Punctuate It Right!* Harper and Row, New York, 1986.

Shertzer, Margaret D. *The Elements of Grammar.* Macmillan Publishing Company, New York, 1986.

Strumpf, Michael, and Auriel Douglas. *Painless Perfect Grammar.* Monarch Press, New York, 1985.

Stylebook/Editorial Manual of the American Medical Association. Publishing Sciences Group, Littleton, Mississippi, 1976.

HOMONYMS

(See Antonyms, Eponyms, Homonyms, Syndromes, and Synonyms.)

HUMOR AND GAMES FOR MEDICAL TYPISTS AND TRANSCRIPTIONISTS

American Association for Medical Transcription. *Dictation PRN.* American Association for Medical Transcription, Modesto, California, 1992.

Pitman, Sally C. (Ed.). *The eMpTy Laugh Book.* American Association for Medical Transcription, Modesto, California, 1981.

Tank, Hazel (Ed.). *The Puzzlement for Medical Transcriptionists.* American Association for Medical Transcription, Modesto, California, 1981.

INSTRUCTION

See Chapter 10 for reference sources for books, video tapes, grading software, and transcription tapes for teachers.

INSURANCE

Fordney, Marilyn T. *Insurance Handbook for the Medical Office,* 3rd edition. W. B. Saunders Company, Philadelphia, 1989.

LAW AND ETHICS

American Medical Association. *Medicolegal Forms with Legal Analysis.* American Medical Association, Chicago, 1991.

Bander, Edward J., and Jeffrey J. Wallach. *Medical Legal Dictionary.* Oceana Publications, Dobbs Ferry, New York, 1970.

Black, Henry Campbell. *Black's Law Dictionary.* West Publishing Company, St. Paul, Minnesota, 1979.

Brody, Howard. *Ethical Decisions in Medicine.* Little, Brown and Company, Boston, 1981.

Council on Ethical and Judicial Affairs of the American Medical Association. *1992 Code of Medical Ethics Current Opinions.* American Medical Association, Chicago, 1992.

Ehrlich, Ann. *Ethics and Jurisprudence.* The Colwell Company, Champaign, Illinois, 1983.

Gifis, Steven H. *Law Dictionary.* Barron's Educational Series, Inc., Hauppauge, New York, 1984.

Hayt, Emanuel. *Medicolegal Aspects of Hospital Records.* Physician's Record Company, Berwyn, Illinois, 1977.

Heller, Marjorie K. *Legal P's and Q's in the Doctor's Office.* Lawyer's Bookshelf, Bayside, New York, 1981.

Holder, Angela Roddey. *Medical Malpractice Law.* John Wiley and Sons, New York, 1978.

Huffman, Edna K. *Medical Record Management.* Physician's Record Company, Berwyn, Illinois, 1985.

Lewis, Marcia A., and Carol D. Warden. *Law and Ethics in the Medical Office, Including Bioethical Issues,* 3rd edition. F. A. Davis, Philadelphia, 1993.

Sloane, Richard. *Sloane-Dorland Annotated Medical-Legal Dictionary; 1992 Supplement.* West Publishing Company, St. Paul, Minnesota, 1987.

Sloane, Sheila B. *The Legal Speller, with Useful Medical Terms,* 2nd edition. West Publishing Company, St. Paul, Minnesota, 1982.

MEDICAL RECORDS

Gordon, B. L. *Simplified Medical Records System.* Publishing Sciences Group, Acton, Massachusetts, 1975.

Hospital Medical Records: Guidelines for Their Use and Release of Medical Information. American Medical Association, Chicago, 1972.

Medical Record Departments in Hospitals: Guide to Organization. American Hospital Association, Chicago, 1972.

Mosier, Alice, and Frank J. Pace. *Medical Records Technology.* Bobbs-Merrill Company, Indianapolis, 1975.

MEDICAL TERMINOLOGY

Austrin, Miriam G. and Harvey R. Austrin. *Learning Medical Terminology: A Worktext.* Mosby, St. Louis, 1991.

Bradbury, Peggy F. *Transcriber's Guide to Medical Terminology.* Medical Examination Publishing Company, Garden City, New York, 1973.

Chabner, Davi-Ellen. *The Language of Medicine; A Write-In Text Explaining Medical Terms.* W. B. Saunders Company, Philadelphia, 1991 (cassettes available).

Cohen, Alan Y. *Medicine/Biology Terminology Cards* (1,000 flash cards). Visual Education Association, Springfield, Ohio, 1978.

DeLorenzo, Barbara, and Doris Fedun. *Medical Terminology,* Vols. I and II. Springhouse Publishing Company, Springhouse, Pennsylvania, 1988.

Dunmore, Charles W., and Rita M. Fleischer. *Medical Terminology: Exercises in Etymology.* F. A. Davis, Philadelphia, 1985.

Fisher, J. Patrick. *Basic Medical Terminology.* Bobbs-Merrill Company, Indianapolis, 1983 (cassettes available).

Frenay, Agnes. *Understanding Medical Terminology.* Catholic Hospital Association, Haverford, Pennsylvania, 1984 (transparencies available).

Gross, Verlee E. *Mastering Medical Terminology: Textbook of Anatomy, Diseases, Anomalies and Surgeries with English Translation and Pronunciation.* Halls of Ivy Press, Simi Valley, California, 1969.

Gross, Verlee E. *The Structure of Medical Terms.* Halls of Ivy Press, Simi Valley, California, 1973.

Gylys, Barbara A., and Mary Ellen Wedding. *Medical Terminology: A Systems Approach.* F. A. Davis Company, Philadelphia, 1988 (software program and user's manual available).

Kinn, Mary E. *Medical Terminology Review Challenge.* Delmar Publishers, Inc. Albany, New York, 1987.

LaFleur-Brooks, Myrna Weber. *Exploring Medical Language.* Mosby, St. Louis, 1993 (computer software available).

Leonard, Peggy. *Building a Medical Vocabulary.* W. B. Saunders Company, Philadelphia, 1993 (cassettes and computer software available).

Prendergast, Alice. *Medical Terminology: A Text/Workbook.* Addison-Wesley Publishing Company, Reading, Massachusetts, 1983.

Smith, Genevieve Love, and Phyllis E. Davis. *Medical Terminology: A Programmed Text.* Delmar Publishers Inc., Albany, New York, 1981 (cassettes available).

Sormunen, Carolee. *Terminology for Allied Health Professionals.* South-Western Publishing Company, Cincinnati, 1985 (cassettes available).

Sorrells, Sally (Ingmire). *Medical Vocabulary from A to Z.* Western Tape, Mountain View, California, 1981 (cassettes available).

Wroble, Eugene M. *Terminology for the Health Professions.* J. B. Lippincott, Philadelphia, 1982.

MEDICAL TERMINOLOGY GUIDES

Current Procedural Terminology. American Medical Association, Chicago, 1977.

Rimer, Evelyn H. *Harbeck's Glossary of Medical Terms.* San Francisco WEB Offset, Brisbane, California, 1967.

Stegeman, Wilson. *Medical Terms Simplified.* West Publishing Company, St. Paul, Minnesota, 1975.

Strand, Helen R. *An Illustrated Guide to Medical Terminology.* Williams and Wilkins, Baltimore, 1968.

Willey, Joy. *Glossary of Medical Terminology.* Springhouse Publishing Company, Springhouse, Pennsylvania, 1992.

PHARMACEUTICAL

Beebe, Judy. *Instant Drug Index.* William Kaufmann, Inc., Los Altos, California, (updates available spring and fall of each year).

Billups, Norman F. *American Drug Index.* J. B. Lippincott, Philadelphia (annual publication).

Compendium of Drug Therapy. Compendium Publishing Group Limited, Hoboken, New Jersey (annual publication).

Deglin, Judith, et al. *Davis's Drug Guide for Nurses.* F. A. Davis Company, Philadelphia, 1992.

DeLorenzo, Barbara. *Pharmaceutical Word Book.* Springhouse Publishing Company, Springhouse, Pennsylvania, 1992.

Drake, Ellen, and Randy Drake. *Saunders Pharmaceutical Word Book.* W. B. Saunders Company, Philadelphia (updated annually).

Griffith, H. Winter. *Complete Guide to Prescription and Nonprescription Drugs.* H. P. Books, Inc., Tucson, Arizona, 1987.

Guide to Drug Names and Classifications, Springhouse Publishing Company, Springhouse, Pennsylvania, 1992.

Hospital Formulary. American Society of Hospital Pharmacists, Washington, D.C., 1978.

Kastrup, Erwin K., and Bernie R. Olin, III. *Drug Facts and Comparisons.* J. B. Lippincott, Philadelphia (updated monthly and reindexed quarterly).

Lane, Karen. *Medications: A Guide for the Health Professions.* F. A. Davis Company, Philadelphia, 1992.

Lewis, Arthur J. *Modern Drug Encyclopedia and Therapeutic Index.* The Yorke Medical Group, The Dun-Donnelly Publishing Corporation, New York, 1973.

Medi-Spell Transcriber's Bulletin. P. O. Box 2546, Mission Viejo, California 92690 (publishes quarterly list of current drugs).

National Drug Code Directory, Vols. 1 and 2. U.S. Government Printing Office, Washington, D.C., 1980.

National Formulary XIV (N.F.). American Pharmaceutical Association, Washington, D.C., 1975.

Patterson, H. Robert, Edward A. Gustafson, and Eleanor Sheridan. *Falconer's Current Drug Handbook.* W. B. Saunders Company, Philadelphia, 1984–1986.

Physicians' Desk Reference for Nonprescription Drugs. Medical Economics, Oradell, New Jersey (annual publication).

Physicians' Desk Reference for Ophthalmology. Medical Economics, Oradell, New Jersey (annual publication).

Physicians' Desk Reference for Radiology and Nuclear Medicine. Medical Economics, Oradell, New Jersey (annual publication).

Physicians' Desk Reference: The Indices. Medical Economics, Oradell, New Jersey (annual publication).

Physicians' Desk Reference (PDR). Medical Economics, Oradell, New Jersey (annual publication).

Quick Look Drug Book. Williams and Wilkins, Baltimore, 1991.

Quick Reference to Discontinued Drugs. Facts and Comparisons, Division of J. B. Lippincott Company, St. Louis, 1976 through 1990.

Shirkey, Harry C. *Pediatric Dosage Handbook.* American Pharmaceutical Association, Washington, D.C., 1980.

Smithwick, Kathryn, and Brenda Hurley. *The Pharmacology Word Book.* F. A. Davis, Philadelphia, 1992.

Squire, Jessie E., and Jean M. Welch. *Basic Pharmacology for Nurses.* Mosby, St. Louis, 1977.

Stedman's Pharmaceutical Words. Williams and Wilkins, Baltimore, 1993.

Turley, Susan M. *Understanding Pharmacology.* Health Professions Institute, Modesto, California, 1988.

The United States Pharmacopoeia (U.S.P.). The Pharmacopoeia of the United States of America, Rockville, Maryland, 1984 (annual supplements).

PROFESSIONAL IMAGE

Communication and Image Skills. American Association for Medical Transcription, Modesto, California, 1992.

PROOFREADING

Dewar, Thadys J., and H. Frances Daniels. *Programmed Proofreading.* South-Western Publishing Company, Cincinnati, 1982.

Preston, Sharon. *Proofreading.* Western Tape, Mountain View, California, 1977.

REFERENCES FOR THE PHYSICALLY CHALLENGED

(also see Computerized Dictionaries/Medical Spell Checkers)

American Association for Medical Transcription, Visually-Impaired MT Committee, c/o Frances Holland, 635 West Grade, Apt. 306, Chicago, 60613.

American Association of Medical Assistants, Inc. *AAMA Guided Study Course: Anatomy, Terminology and Physiology* (cassettes), 20 North Wacker Drive, Chicago, 60606.

American Drug Index (Braille). American Red Cross Braille Service, 707 N. Main, Wichita, KS 67203.

American Foundation for the Blind, 15 West 16th Street, New York, 10011 (annual catalog of publications).

American Printing House for the Blind, P. O. Box 6085, Louisville, Kentucky 40206 (large-print books, books on tape, books put into Braille).

Austrin, Miriam. *Young's Learning Medical Terminology Step by Step.* National Braille Assn., 1290 University Ave., Rochester, NY 14607.

Birmingham, Jacqueline J. *Medical Terminology: A Self-Learning Module* (Braille). Bureau of Library Services for the Blind and Physically Handicapped, 420 Platt Street, Daytona Beach, FL 32114.

Bowe, Frank G. Personal Computers and Special Needs. Sybex, Inc., 2021 Challenger Dr., No. 100, Alameda, California 94501.

Chabner, Davi-Ellen. Audio tapes to *The Language of Medicine.* W. B. Saunders Company, Independence Square West, Philadelphia, 19106-3399; (Braille) Peninsula Braille Transcribers Guild, 340 N. Elsworth Avenue, San Mateo, California 94401.

Clearinghouse-Depository for the Handicapped Student, State Department of Education, 721 Capitol Mall, Sacramento, California 95814 (for information on large-print books, books on tape, and books put into Braille).

DeLorenzo, Barbara. *Pharmaceutical Terminology* (Braille). Iowa Dept. for the Blind, 524 4th Street, Des Moines, Iowa 50309.

Diehl, Marcy O., and Marilyn T. Fordney. *Medical Transcribing Techniques and Procedures,* first edition on cassettes from Recording for the Blind, Inc., 5022 Hollywood Boulevard, Los Angeles, 90027.

Dorland's Illustrated Medical Dictionary (Braille). National Library Service for the Blind and Physically Handicapped, Washington, DC, telephone (202)707-5000.

Fisher, J. Patrick. *Basic Medical Terminology* (cassettes). The Bobbs-Merrill Educational Publishing Company, 4300 West 62nd Street, Indianapolis, Indiana 46268.

Frenay, Agnes. *Understanding Medical Termi-*

nology (Braille). National Braille Assn., 1290 University Ave., Rochester, NY 14607.

Gross, Verlee E. *Mastering Medical Terminology* (Braille). Braille Institute, 1150 East Fourth Street, Long Beach, California 90802.

Hollander, Charles S. *Patient's Guide to Vision Rehabilitation for the Partially Sighted.* Sight Improvement Center, Inc., 25 West 43rd Street, New York, 10036.

Johnson, Carrie. *Medical Spelling Guide* (Braille). National Braille Assn., 1290 University Ave., Rochester, NY 14607.

Leonard, Peggy C. Audio tapes for *Building a Medical Vocabulary.* W. B. Saunders Company, Independence Square West, Philadelphia, 19106-3399.

Lewis, Jane. *Perspectives* bimonthly magazine (cassette tapes); *The Student Syllabus* (cassette tapes). Health Professions Institute, Modesto, California.

McWilliams, Peter. *Personal Computers and the Disabled.* New York, Doubleday, 1984.

Pathology Words and Phrases: A Quick-Reference Guide (Braille). National Braille Assn., 1290 University Ave., Rochester, New York 14607.

Physicians' Desk Reference 1990 (Braille). National Braille Assn., 1290 University Ave., Rochester, New York 14607

Pyle, Vera. *Current Medical Terminology* (Braille). Mrs. Gerri Beeson, Volunteer Services Director, Oklahoma Library for the Blind and Physically Handicapped, 1108 N. E. 36th Street, Oklahoma City, Oklahoma 73111.

Raised Dot Computing Newsletter (monthly newsletter). 310 South 7th Street, Lewisburg, Pennsylvania 17837.

Recordings for the Blind (RFB): Books on cassettes are available on anatomy and physiology, medical terminology, and many of the medical specialties. Call (800) 221-4792 or (609) 452-0606 for a complete list of all titles.

Russell, Philip C. *Dynamic Job Interviewing for Women* (Braille). Federally Employed Women, P. O. Box 251, Port Hueneme, California 93041.

Sensory Aids Foundation, 399 Sherman Avenue, Palo Alto, California 94306 (quarterly journal, research sensory aids, job opportunities, information on latest equipment).

Sloane, Sheila B. *Medical Abbreviations and Eponyms* (Braille). National Braille Assn.,

1290 University Ave., Rochester, New York 14607.

Sloane, Sheila B. *The Medical Word Book* (Braille). Ms. Betty Bruno, Midwestern Braille Volunteers, 106 West Madison Avenue, St. Louis, 63122.

Sloane, Sheila B., and John L. Dusseau. *A Word Book in Pathology and Laboratory Medicine* (Braille). Ms. Betty Bruno, Midwestern Braille Volunteers, 106 West Madison Avenue, St. Louis, 63122.

Smith, Genevieve L., and Phyllis E. Davis. Audio cassettes for *Medical Terminology.* John Wiley and Sons, 330 West State Street, Media, Pennsylvania 19063.

Szulec, Jeanette. *A Syllabus for the Surgeon's Secretary* (Braille). National Braille Assn., 1290 University Ave., Rochester, NY 14607.

Tessier, Claudia. *The Surgical Word Book* (Braille). National Braille Assn., 1290 University Ave., Rochester, NY 14607.

Tessier, Claudia, and Sally Pitman. *Style Guide for Medical Transcription* (Braille). Volunteer Braillists and Tapists, 517 N. Segoe Road, Madison, Wisconsin 53705.

SELF-EMPLOYMENT AND FREELANCING

Adams, Paul. *The Complete Legal Guide for Your Small Business.* John Wiley and Sons, New York, 1982.

Avila-Weil, Donna, and Mary Glaccum. *Independent Medical Transcriptionist: A Comprehensive Guide for the Medical Transcription Professional.* Williams and Wilkins, Baltimore, 1991.

Blanchard, Kenneth, and Spencer Johnson. *The One Minute Manager.* William Morrow and Company, New York, 1982.

Bly, Robert W. *Selling Your Services: Proven Strategies for Getting Clients to Hire You (or Your Firm).* Henry Holt and Company, New York, 1990.

Boos, Patricia. *Typing. . . A Way to Your Own Business.* The Seasons Publishing Company, Bowie, Maryland, 1981.

Davidson, Jeffrey P. *Marketing for the Home-Based Business.* Bob Adams, Inc., Publishers, Holbrook, Massachusetts, 1991.

DeMenezes, Ruth. *You Can Type for Doctors at*

Home! Claremont Press, Thousand Oaks, California, 1981.

Edwards, Paul, and Sarah Edwards. *Working From Home.* Jeremy P. Tarcher, Inc., Los Angeles, California, 1990.

Home Office Computing, P. O. Box 51344, Boulder, Colorado 80321-1344 (monthly magazine).

Murray, Jean Wilson. *Starting and Operating a Word Processing Service.* Pilot Books, Babylon, New York, 1983.

The Office Professional, 116 East Main Street, Round Rock, Texas 78664 (monthly newsletter).

Scott, Bill. *The Skills of Negotiating.* John Wiley and Sons, Somerset, New Jersey, 1981.

Small Business Reports, P. O. Box 53140, Boulder, Colorado 80322-3140.

Strickland, Lois. *How to Start a Manuscript Typing Business in Your Home,* 1983. Order from 513 Polk Street, Manchester, Tennessee 37355.

Will-Harris, Daniel. *TypeStyle: How to Choose and Use Type on a Personal Computer.* Peachpit Press, Berkeley, California, 1991.

Wisely, Rae, and Gladys Sanders. *The Independent Woman: How to Start and Succeed in Your Own Business.* Houghton Mifflin Company, Los Angeles, 1981.

SPECIALTY REFERENCES

Cardiology

Cardiology Words and Phrases: A Quick Reference Guide. Health Professions Institute, Modesto, California, 1989.

Cardiopulmonary Words. F. A. Davis, Philadelphia, 1993.

Dorland's Cardiology Speller. W. B. Saunders Company, Philadelphia, 1993.

Littrell, Helen E. *Cardiovascular and Pulmonary Terminology.* Springhouse Publishing Company, Springhouse, Pennsylvania, 1992.

Stedman's Cardiology Words. Williams and Wilkins, Baltimore, 1992.

Dental
(see also Oral and Maxillofacial Surgery)

Fairpo, Jenifer, and Gavin Fairpo. *Heinemann Dental Dictionary.* Butterworth-Heinemann Limited, Stoneham, Massachusetts, 1991.

Stedman's Dentistry Words. Williams and Wilkins, Baltimore, 1993.

Dermatology

Carter, Robert L. *A Dictionary of Dermatologic Terms,* 4th edition. Williams and Wilkins, Baltimore, 1992.

Leider, Morris, and Morris Rosenblum. *A Dictionary of Dermatological Words, Terms, and Phrases.* Dome Laboratories, West Haven, Connecticut, 1976.

Gastroenterology

Dorland's Gastroenterology Speller. W. B. Saunders Company, Philadelphia, 1993.

Gastroenterology Words and Phrases: A Quick Reference Guide. Health Professions Institute, Modesto, California, 1989.

Stedman's Gastrointestinal Words. Williams and Wilkins, Baltimore, 1991.

History and Physical

Dirckx, John H. *A Nonphysician's Guide to the Medical History and Physical Examination.* Prima Vera Publications, Modesto, California, 1987.

Jarvis, Carolyn. *Physical Examination and Health Assessment.* W. B. Saunders Company, Philadelphia, 1992.

Immunology/AIDS

DeLorenzo, Barbara. *Oncologic Terminology with AIDS-Related Terms.* Springhouse Publishing Company, Springhouse, Pennsylvania, 1991.

Littrell, Helen E. *Immunologic and AIDS Word Book.* Springhouse Publishing Company, Springhouse, Pennsylvania, 1992.

McIntyre, Maureen, and Diane K. Cartwright. *AIDS-Related Terminology.* Write to 1484 Old Forest Road, Pickering, Ontario, Canada L1V 1N9.

Sloane, Sheila B. *A Word Book in Oncology and Hematology, Including Terminology of AIDS.* Brian C. Decker, Philadelphia, 1992.

Internal Medicine
(see Cardiology)

Laboratory
(see Pathology)

Neonatology
(see also Obstetrics and Gynecology and Pediatrics)

Hughes, Edward C. *Obstetric-Gynecologic Terminology with Section on Neonatology and Glossary of Congenital Anomalies.* F. A. Davis, Philadelphia, 1972.

Neurology

Health Professions Institute. *Orthopedic/Neurology Words and Phrases.* Modesto, California, 1993.
Littrell, Helen. *Neurologic and Psychiatric Terminology.* Springhouse Publishing Company, Springhouse, Pennsylvania, 1992.
Stedman's Neurosurgery Words. Williams and Wilkins, Baltimore, 1993.

Nuclear Medicine
(see Radiology)

Obstetrics and Gynecology

Hughes, Edward C. *Obstetric-Gynecologic Terminology with Section on Neonatology and Glossary of Congenital Anomalies.* F. A. Davis, Philadelphia, 1972.
Littrell, Helen. *Obstetric and Gynecologic Terminology.* Springhouse Publishing Company, Springhouse, Pennsylvania, 1991.
Stedman's OB/GYN Words. Williams and Wilkins, Baltimore, 1991.

Oncology/Hematology

DeLorenzo, Barbara. *Oncologic Word Book.* Springhouse Publishing Company, Springhouse, Pennsylvania, 1991.
Dorland's Hematology/Oncology Speller. W. B. Saunders Company, Philadelphia, 1993.
Littrell, Helen. *The Oncology Word Book.* F. A. Davis Company, Philadelphia, 1993.
Sloane, Sheila B. *A Word Book in Oncology and Hematology, Including Terminology of AIDS.* Brian C. Decker, Philadelphia, 1992.

Stedman's Oncology Words. Williams and Wilkins, Baltimore, 1991.

Ophthalmology

Adams, Joyce. *Saunders Ophthalmology Word Book.* W. B. Saunders Company, Philadelphia, 1991.
Cassin, Barbara, and Sheila Solomon. *Dictionary of Eye Terminology.* Triad Publishing Company, Gainesville, Florida, 1984.
DeLorenzo, Barbara, and Doris Fedun. *Ophthalmic Word Book.* Springhouse Publishing Company, Springhouse, Pennsylvania, 1991.
Indovina, Theresa, and Wilburta Q. Lindh. *The Ophthalmology Word Book.* F. A. Davis, Philadelphia, 1992.
Millodot, Michael M. *Dictionary of Optometry.* Butterworth and Company, Stoneham, Massachusetts, 1990.
Stedman's Ophthalmology Words. Williams and Wilkins, Baltimore, 1991.
Stein, Harold A., Bernard J. Slatt, and Penny Cook. *Manual of Ophthalmic Terminology.* St. Louis, Mosby, 1992.

Oral and Maxillofacial Surgery
(see also Dental)

American Society of Oral Surgeons: The Oral and Maxillofacial Surgery Procedural Terminology with Glossary. American Society of Oral Surgeons, Chicago, 1975.
Littrell, Helen E. *Dental and Otolaryngology Word Book.* Springhouse Publishing Company, Springhouse, Pennsylvania, 1992.
Nicolosi, Lucille, et al. *Terminology of Communication Disorders: Speech, Language, Hearing.* Williams and Wilkins, Baltimore, 1986.

Orthopaedics

American Association of Electrodiagnostic Medicine. *Glossary of Terms in Clinical Electromyography.* American Association of Electrodiagnostic Medicine, Rochester, Minnesota, 1987.
Apley, A. Graham. *Apley's System of Orthopaedics and Fractures.* Butterworths, Boston, 1982.
Arthritis Foundation. Individual disease pamphlets on osteoarthritis, rheumatoid arthritis,

systemic erythematosus, gout, psoriatic arthritis, and Schumacher, H. Ralph (Ed.). *Primer on Rheumatic Diseases,* 9th edition, 1988. Arthritis Foundation, Atlanta.

Bernstein, Saul, and Deborah Collins. *Dictionary of Orthopedic Terminology.* Triad Publishing Company, Gainesville, Florida, 1993.

Blauvelt, Carolyn T., and Fred R. T. Nelson. *A Manual of Orthopaedic Terminology.* Mosby, St. Louis, 1990.

Cittadine, Thomas J. *Orthopaedic Word Book.* Springhouse Publishing Company, Springhouse, Pennsylvania, 1991.

Dorland's Orthopedic Speller. W. B. Saunders Company, Philadelphia, 1993.

Health Professions Institute. *Orthopedic Words and Phrases: A Quick Reference Guide.* Health Professions Institute, Modesto, California, 1988.

Kilcoyne, Ray F., and Edward L. Farrar. *CRC Handbook of Orthopaedic Terminology.* CRC Press, Inc., Boca Raton, Florida, 1990.

Stedman's Orthopaedic Words. Williams and Wilkins, Baltimore, 1991.

Otorhinolaryngology

(see Oral and Maxillofacial Surgery)

Stedman's ENT Words. Williams and Wilkins, Baltimore, 1993.

Pathology

Atkinson, Kaye. *Pathology Word Book.* D and T Products, Mission Viejo, California, 1992-1993.

Bennington, James L. *Encyclopedia and Dictionary of Laboratory Medicine and Technology.* W. B. Saunders Company, Philadelphia, 1983.

DeLorenzo, Barbara. *Clinical Laboratory Word Book.* Springhouse Publishing Company, Springhouse, Pennsylvania, 1992.

A Guide to Pathology Terminology. Gold Coast Chapter of AAMT, Fort Lauderdale, Florida, 1984.

Dorland's Hematology/Oncology Speller. W. B. Saunders Company, Philadelphia, 1993.

Jacobs, David S. *Laboratory Test Handbook.* Lexi-Comp Inc., Hudson, Ohio, 1990.

Laboratory Medicine: Essentials of Anatomic and Clinical Pathology. Health Professions Institute, Modesto, California, 1991.

Pathology Words and Phrases. Health Professions Institute, Modesto, California, 1988.

Shaw, Diane. *Pathophysiologic Word Book.* Springhouse Publishing Company, Springhouse, Pennsylvania, 1991.

Sloane, Sheila B. *A Word Book in Oncology and Hematology, Including Terminology of AIDS.* Brian C. Decker, Philadelphia, 1992.

Sloane, Sheila B., and John L. Dusseau. *A Word Book in Pathology and Laboratory Medicine.* W. B. Saunders Company, Philadelphia, 1984.

Stedman's ASP Parasite Names. Williams and Wilkins, Baltimore, 1992.

Stedman's ATCC Fungus Words. Williams and Wilkins, Baltimore, 1992.

Stedman's Bergey's Bacteriology Words. Williams and Wilkins, Baltimore, 1992.

Stedman's ICTV Virus Words. Williams and Wilkins, Baltimore, 1992.

Stedman's Pathology and Laboratory Medicine Words. Williams and Wilkins, Baltimore, 1992.

Tietz, Norbert W. (Ed.). *Clinical Guide to Laboratory Tests.* W. B. Saunders Company, Philadelphia, 1990.

Wallach, Jacques B. *Interpretation of Diagnostic Tests: A Handbook Synopsis of Laboratory Medicine.* Little, Brown and Company, Boston, 1986.

Willatt, E. Murden. *Medical Spelling Handbook: Book 1: Pathology.* Medical Spelling Handbooks Publishing Company, Bellaire, Texas, 1970.

Pediatrics

Tank, Hazel, and Catherine Gilliam. *Neonatology Word Book.* American Association for Medical Transcription, Modesto, California, 1992.

Periodicals

Journal of the American Association for Medical Transcription. American Association for Medical Transcription, Modesto, California (bimonthly).

Perspectives on the Medical Transcription Profession. Health Professions Institute, Modesto, California (quarterly).

Transvision. TransCom Resources, Menomonee

Falls, WI (newsletter for medical transcription supervisors).

Physical Therapy
(see Rehabilitation/Physical Therapy)

Plastic Surgery
(see Oral and Maxillofacial Surgery)

Podiatry

Podiatry for the Assistant. Williams and Wilkins, Baltimore, 1988.

Psychiatry

American Psychiatric Association. *Diagnostic and Statistical Manual of Mental Disorders,* 3rd edition (DSM-III-R). American Psychiatric Press, Inc., Washington, D.C., 1987.

D'Onofrio, Mary Ann, and Elizabeth D'Onofrio. *Psychiatric Words and Phrases*. Health Professions Institute, Modesto, California, 1990.

Dorland's Psychiatry and Psychology Speller. W. B. Saunders Company, Philadelphia, 1993.

Drever, James. *A Dictionary of Psychology*. Penguin Books, Harmondsworth, Middlesex, England, 1952.

Forbis, Pat. *The Psychiatric Word Book with Street Talk Terms*. F. A. Davis Company, Philadelphia, 1993.

Goldenson, Robert M. (Ed.) *Longman Dictionary of Psychology and Psychiatry*. Longman, Inc., New York, 1984.

Hinsie, Leland E., and Robert J. Campbell. *Psychiatric Dictionary*. Oxford University Press, New York, 1970.

International Classification of Diseases Adapted, 9th Revision, Clinical Modification. Commission on Professional and Hospital Activities, Ann Arbor, Michigan, 1978.

Kaplan, Harold II, and Benjamin J. Sadock. *Comprehensive Glossary of Psychiatry and Psychology*. Williams and Wilkins, Baltimore, 1991.

Littrell, Helen. *Neurologic and Psychiatric Terminology*. Springhouse Publishing Company, Springhouse, Pennsylvania, 1992.

Pettijohn, Terry F. *Encyclopedic Dictionary of Psychology*. Dushkin Publishing Group, Inc., Guilford, Connecticut, 1991.

Stedman's Psychiatry Words. Williams and Wilkins, Baltimore, 1992.

Stone, Evelyn M. *American Psychiatric Association Glossary*. American Psychiatric Press, Inc., Washington, D.C., 1988.

Pulmonary
(see Cardiology)

Radiology

American College of Radiology Glossary of MR Terms. American College of Radiology, Reston, Virginia, 1991.

Atkinson, Kaye. *Words of Radiology Dictation*. D & T Products, Mission Viejo, California, 1991.

Bachn, Peter. *Anatomical Chart Series*. Anatomical Chart Company, P. O. Box 379, Asbury Park, New Jersey 07712.

Ballinger, Philip W. *Merrill's Atlas of Radiographic Positions and Radiologic Procedures,* Vols. I, II, and III. Mosby, St. Louis, 1991.

Chernok, Normal B. *Radiology Typist's Handbook*. Medical Examination Publishing Company, Flushing, New York, 1970.

DeLorenzo, Barbara. *Radiologic Word Book*. Springhouse Publishing Company, Springhouse, Pennsylvania, 1991.

Ehlert, Theodora. *Handbook for Medical Secretaries*. Picker Corporation, Cleveland.

Etter, Lewis E. *Glossary of Words and Phrases Used in Radiology, Nuclear Medicine and Ultrasound*. Charles C Thomas, Springfield, Illinois, 1970.

Goldman, Myer, and David Cope. *A Radiographic Index*. PSG Publishing Company, Littleton, Massachusetts, 1987.

Indovina, Theresa, and Wilburta W. Lindh. *The Radiology Word Book*. F. A. Davis, Philadelphia, 1990.

Pugh, Janet C. *The Radiology Transcriptionist's Quick Reference Guide*, 1991. Write to 5158 Miller Road, Columbus, Georgia 31907.

Radiology Words and Phrases. Health Professional Institute, Modesto, California, 1990.

Roentgenographic Anatomical Terminology. E. I. DuPont de Nemours and Company, Wilmington, Delaware.

Sloane, Sheila B. *A Word Book in Radiology, with Anatomic Plates and Tables*. W. B. Saunders Company, Philadelphia, 1988.

Stedman's Radiology Words. Williams and Wilkins, Baltimore, 1991.

Words of Radiology Dictation. D and T Products, Mission Viejo, California, 1992.

Rehabilitation/Physical Therapy

Rothstein, Jules. *Rehabilitation Specialist's Handbook.* F. A. Davis, Philadelphia, 1991.

Respiratory and Pulmonary
(see Cardiology).

Rheumatology
(see Orthopaedics).

Speech, Language, Hearing

Nicolosi, Lucille, et al. *Terminology of Communication Disorders: Speech, Language, Hearing.* Williams and Wilkins, Baltimore, 1988.

Surgery

Chernok, Normal B. *Surgical Typist's Handbook.* Medical Examination Publishing Company, Garden City, New York, 1972.

Coleman, Frances. *Guide to Surgical Terminology.* Medical Economics, Oradell, New Jersey, 1978.

Goldman, Maxine A. *Pocket Guide to the Operating Room.* F. A. Davis Company, Philadelphia, 1988.

McMillan, Sam. *Surgical Word Book.* Springhouse Publishing Company, Springhouse, Pennsylvania, 1992.

Smith, E. J., and Y. R. Smith. *Smiths' Reference and Illustrated Guide to Surgical Instruments.* J. B. Lippincott, Philadelphia, 1982.

Szulec, Jeanette, and Z. A. Szulec. *Syllabus for the Surgeon's Secretary.* The Medical Arts Publishing Company, Detroit, 1980.

Tessier, Claudia. *The Surgical Word Book.* W. B. Saunders Company, Philadelphia, 1991.

Willatt, E. Murden. *Medical Spelling Handbook; Book 2: Surgery.* Medical Spelling Handbooks Publishing Company, Bellaire, Texas, 1970.

Yentis, Stephen, Nick Hirsch, and Gary B. Smith. *Anesthesia A-Z.* Butterworth-Heinemann, Stoneham, MA, 1993.

Urology

Beck, Ernest W., et al. *The Anatomical Chart Series.* The Anatomical Chart Company, Skokie, Illinois, 1988.

Stedman's Urology Words. Williams and Wilkins, Baltimore, 1993.

Walsh, Patrick C., et al. *Clinical Pediatric Urology,* 3rd edition. W. B. Saunders Company, Philadelphia, 1992.

SPELLING BOOKS, ENGLISH

Ellis, Kaeth. *The Word Book II.* Houghton Mifflin, Boston, 1983.

Emerich, Joan. *Proper Noun Speller.* Quik Ref Publishing, Los Angeles, 1991.

Flesch, Rudolf. *Look It up: A Deskbook of American Spelling and Style.* Harper and Row, New York, 1977.

Gilman, Mary Louise. *One Word, Two Words, Hyphenated?* National Shorthand Reporters Associations, Vienna, Virginia, 1988.

Horowitz, Edward. *Words Come in Families.* A and W Publishers, New York, 1979.

Leslie, L. A. *20,000 Words.* Gregg Division, McGraw-Hill Book Company, New York, 1981.

Lewis, Norman. *Correct Spelling Made Easy.* Dell Publishing Company, New York, 1987.

Lewis, Norman. *Instant Spelling Power.* Amsco College Publications, New York, 1976.

Rice, Jane. *Spellright.* Appleton and Lange, Norwalk, Connecticut, 1992.

SPELLING BOOKS, MEDICAL

American Medical Association, *Current Medical Information and Terminology,* 5th edition. American Medical Association, Chicago, 1981.

Bolander, Donald O., and Rita Bisdorf. *Instant Spelling Medical Dictionary.* Career Publishing Institute, Mundelein, Illinois, 1970.

Byers, Edward E. *Ten Thousand Medical Words; Spelled and Divided for Quick Reference.* McGraw-Hill Book Company, New York, 1972.

Campbell, Linda C. *The Anatomy Word Book.* PrimaVera Publications, Modesto, California, 1988.

Carlin, Harriette L. *Medical Secretary Medi-Speller: A Transcription Aid.* Charles C Thomas, Springfield, Illinois, 1973.

Churchill Livingstone's Medical Word Guide. Churchill Livingstone, New York, 1991.

Coleman, Frances. *Guide to Surgical Terminology.* Medical Economics, Oradell, New Jersey, 1978.

Cooper, Elsa Swanson. *The Language of Medicine: A Guide for Stenotypists.* Medical Economics, Oradell, New Jersey, 1977.

DDC Medical Speller. Dictation Disc Company, 240 Madison Avenue, New York, New York 10016.

DeLorenzo, Barbara, and Doris Fedun. *Medical Word Book.* Springhouse Publishing Company, Springhouse, Pennsylvania, 1992.

Doyle, John M. and Rita G. Doyle. *Spelling Reference for Business and School.* Reston Publishing Company, Reston, Virginia, 1976.

Drake, Ellen. *Dorland's Medical Speller.* W. B. Saunders Company, Philadelphia, 1992.

Emery, Donald W. *Variant Spellings in Modern American Dictionaries.* National Council of Teachers of English, Urbana, Illinois, 1973.

Franks, Richard, and H. Swartz. *Simplified Medical Dictionary.* Medical Economics/Delmar Publishers, Albany, New York, 1977. (This book can help you locate a word if you know how the word ends and how the beginning is pronounced. The terms are categorized by their prefixes, suffixes, and roots, so you can seek out the word with minimal effort.)

Glossary of Hospital Terms. American Health Information Management Association, Chicago, 1974.

Hafer, Ann. *The Medical and Health Sciences Word Book.* Houghton Mifflin, Boston, 1982.

Johnson, Carrie E. *Medical Spelling Guide.* Charles C Thomas, Springfield, Illinois, 1966.

Kreivsky, Joseph, and Jordon L. Linfield. *The Bad Speller's Dictionary.* Random House, New York, 1974.

Lee, Richard V., and Doris J. Hofer. *How to Divide Medical Words.* Southern Illinois University Press, Carbondale, Illinois, 1972.

Lorenzini, Jean W. *Medical Phrase Index.* Medical Economics, Oradell, New Jersey, 1978.

Magalini, Sergio I., and Euclide Scrascia. *Dictionary of Medical Syndromes.* J. B. Lippincott, Philadelphia, 1981.

Pease, Roger W., Jr. (Ed.). *Webster's Medical Speller.* G & C Merriam Company, Springfield, Illinois, 1987.

Prichard, Robert W., and Robert E. Robinson. *Twenty Thousand Medical Words.* McGraw-Hill Book Company, New York, 1972.

Pyle, Vera. *Current Medical Terminology.* Health Professions Institute, Modesto, California, 1992.

Rice, Elaine P. *Phonetic Dictionary of Medical Terminology: A Spelling Guide.* Williams and Wilkins, Baltimore, 1985.

Rice, Jane. *Spellright.* Appleton and Lange, Norwalk, Connecticut, 1992.

Rimer, Evelyn Harbeck. *Harbeck's Glossary of Medical Terms.* San Francisco WEB Offset, Brisbane, California, 1967.

Shaw, Diane. *Anatomy and Physiology Glossary.* Springhouse Publishing Company, Springhouse, Pennsylvania, 1990.

Sloane, Sheila B. *The Medical Word Book,* 3rd edition. W. B. Saunders Company, Philadelphia, 1991.

Stedman's Medical Speller. Williams and Wilkins, Baltimore, 1992.

Taylor, Donna M., and Patricia A. Collins. *For Your Information.* For Your Information Book Company, Santa Ana, California, 1991.

Tessier, Claudia J. *The Surgical Word Book.* W. B. Saunders Company, Philadelphia, 1981.

Thomas, Clayton L. *Taber's Medical Word Book with Pronunciations.* F. A. Davis, Philadelphia, 1990.

Webster's Medical Desk Dictionary. Merriam-Webster, Inc., Springfield, Illinois, 1986.

Willeford, Jr., George. *Webster's New World Medical Word Finder.* Prentice-Hall, Englewood Cliffs, New Jersey, 1987.

Willey, Joy. *Glossary of Medical Terminology for the Health Professions.* Springhouse Publishing Company, Springhouse, Pennsylvania, 1992.

STYLE MANUALS/MEDICAL AND GENERAL

American Medical Association. *Manual of Style.* Williams and Wilkins, Baltimore, 1989.

American Psychological Association: Publication Manual. American Psychological Association, Washington, D.C., 1974.

Barclay, William R., et al. (compiled for American Medical Association). *Manual for Authors and Editors: Editorial Style and Manuscript Preparation.* Lange Medical Publications, Los Altos, California, 1981.

The Chicago Manual of Style. University of Chicago Press, Chicago, 1982.

Council of Biology Editors Committee on Form and Style: CBE Style Manual. American Institute of Biological Sciences, Washington, D.C., 1974.

Ebbitt, Wilma R., and David Ebbitt. *Writer's Guide and Index to English.* Scott Foresman and Company, Glenview, Illinois, 1982.

Fordney, Marilyn T., and Marcy O. Diehl. *Medical Transcription Guide: Do's and Don'ts.* W. B. Saunders Company, Philadelphia, 1990.

Huth, Edward J. *Medical Style and Format — An International Manual for Authors, Editors, and Publishers.* Institute for Scientific Information Press, Philadelphia, 1987.

Jordan, Lewis. *The New York Times Manual of Style and Usage.* Random House, New York, 1976.

Preston, Sharon. *Proofreading.* Western Tape, Mountain View, California, 1977.

Schramm, Dwane. *Typing Term Papers and Reports.* Western Tape, Mountain View, California, 1974.

Schwager, Edith. *Medical English Usage and Abuse.* Oryx Press, Phoenix, Arizona, 1990.

Strunk, William Jr., and E. B. White. *The Elements of Style: with Index.* Macmillan Publishing Company, New York, 1979.

Tessier, Claudia, and Sally C. Pitman. *Style Guide for Medical Transcription.* American Association for Medical Transcription, Modesto, California, 1985.

Trelease, S. F. *How to Write Scientific and Technical Papers.* MIT Press, Cambridge, Massachusetts, 1969.

Webster's Standard American Style Manual. Merriam-Webster, Springfield, Massachusetts, 1985.

TYPING AND TRANSCRIPTION

Blake, Rachelle S. *The Medical Transcriptionist's Handbook.* South-Western Publishing Company, Cincinnati, 1993.

Diehl, Marcy O., and Marilyn T. Fordney. *Medical Typing and Transcribing; Techniques and Procedures.* W. B. Saunders Company, Philadelphia, 1991.

Also see Chapter 10 for sources for transcription tapes, reference books, video tapes, and grading software for teachers.

VIDEO TAPES

Exploring Transcription Practices: Punctuation and Grammar Video. American Association for Medical Transcription, Modesto, California, 1990.

Exploring Transcription Practices: Self-Assessment Video. American Association for Medical Transcription, Modesto, California, 1988.

Exploring Transcription Practices: Surgery Transcription Video. American Association for Medical Transcription, Modesto, California, 1989.

Health Professions Institute. *Building a Successful Medical Transcription Business. Teaching Medical Transcription: Meeting the Challenges of the 90s!* Modesto, California, 1993.

WORD DIVISION

Byers, Edward E. *Ten Thousand Medical Words, Spelled and Divided for Quick Reference.* McGraw-Hill Book Company, New York, 1972.

Hafer, Ann. *The Medical and Health Sciences Word Book.* Houghton Mifflin, Boston, 1982.

Lee, Richard B., and Doris J. Hofer. *How to Divide Medical Words.* Southern Illinois University Press, Carbondale, Illinois, 1972.

Pease, Roger W., Jr. (Ed.). *Webster's Medical Speller.* G & C Merriam, Springfield, Massachusetts, 1975.

Silverthorn, J. E., and Devern J. Perry. *Word Division Manual.* South-Western Publishing Company, Cincinnati, 1970.

Willeford, George, Jr. *Webster's New World Medical Word Finder.* Prentice-Hall, Englewood Cliffs, New Jersey, 1987.

The Word Book II. Houghton Mifflin, Boston, 1983.

Zoubek, C. E., and G. A. Condon. *Twenty Thousand Words.* McGraw-Hill Book Company, New York, 1985.

WORKING AT HOME/ INDEPENDENT MEDICAL TRANSCRIPTIONISTS

(see Self-Employment and Freelancing)

WRITING, SCIENTIFIC/TECHNICAL

Alvarez, Joseph A. *Elements of Technical Writing.* Academic Press, Albany, New York, 1986.

Brogan, John A. *Clear Technical Writing.* McGraw-Hill Book Company, New York, 1973.

Dagher, Joseph P. *Technical Communication: A Practical Guide.* Prentice-Hall, Englewood Cliffs, New Jersey, 1978.

Ehrlich, Eugene H., and Daniel Murphy. *Art of Technical Writing: A Manual for Scientists, Engineers, and Students.* Apollo Editions, Scranton, Pennsylvania, 1969.

Huth, Edward J. *How to Write and Publish Papers in the Medical Sciences.* Williams and Wilkins, Baltimore, 1990.

Huth, Edward J. *Medical Style and Format: An International Manual for Authors, Editors, and Publishers.* Williams and Wilkins, Baltimore, 1987.

King, Lester S. *Why Not Say It Clearly: A Guide to Scientific Writing.* Little, Brown and Company, Boston, 1978.

Mitchell, John H. *Writing for Technical and Professional Journals.* Books Demand UMI, Ann Arbor, Michigan, 1968.

Skillin, Marjorie, and Robert Gay. *Words into Type.* Prentice-Hall, Englewood Cliffs, New Jersey, 1974.

Trelease, Sam F. *How to Write Scientific and Technical Papers.* MIT Press, Cambridge, Massachusetts, 1969.

Typing Styles for Letters and Reports

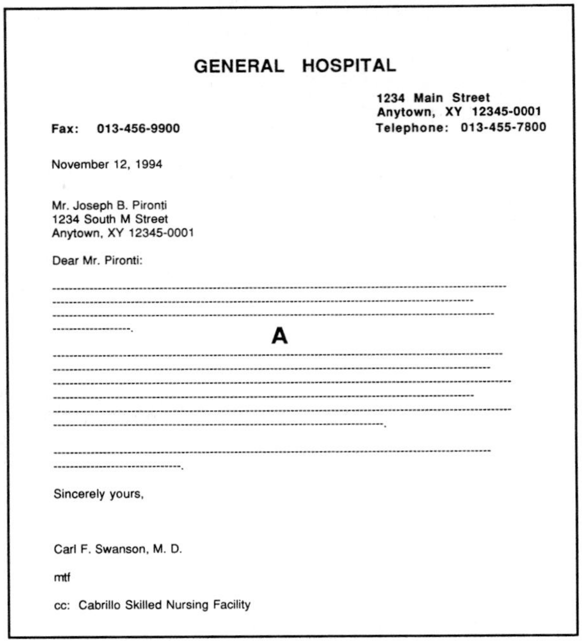

GENERAL HOSPITAL

1234 Main Street
Anytown, XY 12345-0001
Fax: 013-456-9900   Telephone: 013-455-7800

November 12, 1994

Mr. Joseph B. Pironti
1234 South M Street
Anytown, XY 12345-0001

Dear Mr. Pironti:

-------------------.
A

--.

-------------------------------.

Sincerely yours,

Carl F. Swanson, M. D.

mtf

cc: Cabrillo Skilled Nursing Facility

A, Full-block style and mixed punctuation.

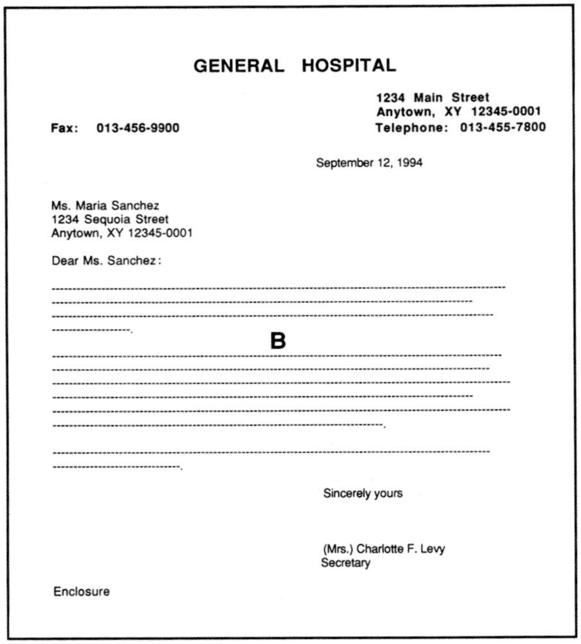

GENERAL HOSPITAL

1234 Main Street
Anytown, XY 12345-0001
Fax: 013-456-9900   Telephone: 013-455-7800

September 12, 1994

Ms. Maria Sanchez
1234 Sequoia Street
Anytown, XY 12345-0001

Dear Ms. Sanchez:

-------------------.
B

--.

-------------------------------.

Sincerely yours

(Mrs.) Charlotte F. Levy
Secretary

Enclosure

B, Modified-block style and open punctuation.

Figure 1
Letters illustrating varying styles and punctuation.

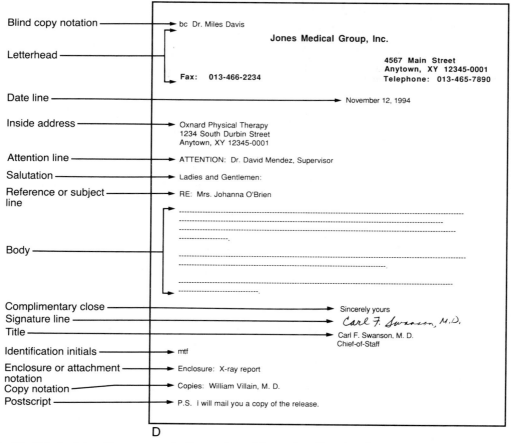

John B. Doe, M. D.
1234 Main Street
Anytown, XY 12345-0001

Fax: 013-456-9900   Telephone: 013-455-7800

October 12, 1994

Miss Daisy F. Chain
1234 Center Street
Anytown, XY 12345-0001

Dear Miss Chain:

C

Sincerely yours,

David P. Bronson, M. D.

mtf

cc: Cabrillo Skilled Nursing Facility

C, Modified-block style with indented paragraphs and mixed punctuation.

Blind copy notation → bc Dr. Miles Davis

Letterhead → **Jones Medical Group, Inc.**

4567 Main Street
Anytown, XY 12345-0001
Fax: 013-466-2234   Telephone: 013-465-7890

Date line → November 12, 1994

Inside address → Oxnard Physical Therapy
1234 South Durbin Street
Anytown, XY 12345-0001

Attention line → ATTENTION: Dr. David Mendez, Supervisor

Salutation → Ladies and Gentlemen:

Reference or subject line → RE: Mrs. Johanna O'Brien

Body →

Complimentary close → Sincerely yours
Signature line → *Carl F. Swanson, M.D.*
Title → Carl F. Swanson, M. D.
Chief-of-Staff

Identification initials → mtf

Enclosure or attachment notation → Enclosure: X-ray report

Copy notation → Copies: William Villain, M. D.

Postscript → P.S. I will mail you a copy of the release.

D

D, Modified-block style with open punctuation and special notations (i.e., the placement of the parts of a letter).

GENERAL HOSPITAL

1234 Main Street
Anytown, XY 12345-0001
Telephone: 013-455-7800

Fax: 013-456-9900

BLAKE, Amanda F.

Charles M. Jones, M. D.

HISTORY

CHIEF COMPLAINT:
Variations: 1) No space below main topic. 2) Main topics underlined

PRESENT ILLNESS:

PAST HISTORY:

ALLERGIES:
Variations: Allergies in all caps and/or
underlined for emphasis.

MEDICATIONS:

OPERATIONS:

SOCIAL:

(continued)

A

BLAKE, Amanda F.
560-39-7690
Room 640-A
History, Page 2

FAMILY HISTORY:

REVIEW OF SYSTEMS:
Variations: Subtopics grouped after main heading in paragraph format.
The subtopic title is typed in full caps or both upper and lower case.
SKIN:
HEENT:
CR:
GI:
OB-GYN:
EXTREMITIES:
NEUROLOGIC:

PHYSICAL EXAMINATION

GENERAL:

HEENT:

CHEST:

ABDOMEN:

GENITALIA:

RECTAL:

(continued)

B

BLAKE, Amanda F.
560-39-7690
Room 640-A
Physical Examination, Page 3

NEUROMUSCULAR:

DIAGNOSIS:
1.
2.

PLAN OF DIRECTION:

Charles M. Jones, M. D.

mtf
D: 11-02-94
T: 11-03-94

C

Figure 2

History and physical examination reports. A, Example of a history typed in full-block format. B and C, Examples of a physical examination typed in full-block format. Variations mentioned within the figure.

GENERAL   HOSPITAL

1234 Main Street
Anytown, XY 12345-0001

Fax: 013-456-9900

Telephone: 013-455-7800

BLAKE, Amanda F.

Date: November 3, 1994

Hospital No.: 560-39-7690

Room No.: 640-A

OPERATIVE REPORT

PREOPERATIVE DIAGNOSIS: 1. ----------------------------.
2. ---------------------------------------.

POSTOPERATIVE DIAGNOSIS: 1. ----------------------------.
2. --.

OPERATION: 1. --------------------------------------.
2. --.

PROCEDURE: ---

---.
---.

---.

Charles M. Jones, M. D.

mtf
D: 11-03-94
T: 11-04-94

Figure 3

Operative report typed in indented format. The data are begun on the same line as the topic or subtopic. First and second lines are tabulated 23 to 27 spaces from the left margin. The third and subsequent lines are brought back to the left margin (as long as they clear the outline—if too brief, block under the first two lines.

GENERAL   HOSPITAL

1234 Main Street
Anytown, XY 12345-0001

Fax: 013-456-9900   **Telephone: 013-455-7800**

Date: November 3, 1994
Patient: Amanda F. Blake   Pathology No. : 450986
Hospital No.: 560-39-7690   Room No.: 640-A
Specimen Submitted: -------------------------

PATHOLOGY REPORT

GROSS DESCRIPTION: --

                            --.

                            ----------------------------.

RFW:mtf

MICROSCOPIC DESCRIPTION: --

                            --.

DIAGNOSIS: --.
                            ---.

                            _____
                            Stanley T. Nason, M. D.

STN:mtf
D: 11-03-94
T: 11-04-94

Figure 4
Pathology report typed in modified-block format. Variations: 1. Underlining topics. 2. Single space between subtopics.

GENERAL   HOSPITAL

Fax: 013-456-9900

1234 Main Street
Anytown, XY 12345-0001
Telephone: 013-455-7800

BLAKE, Amanda F.
Hospital No. 560-39-7690
Charles M. Jones, M. D.

DISCHARGE SUMMARY

ADMISSION DATE: ---------------------------   DISCHARGE DATE: ---------------------
Variations: 1) Single space between topics. 2) Subtopics begun on a separate line and
typed in caps. 3) Main topics underlined.

HISTORY OF PRESENT ILLNESS: ---

-------------------------.

ADMITTING DIAGNOSIS: ---

LABORATORY DATA ON ADMISSION: ---
--.

HOSPITAL COURSE AND TREATMENT: ---
---.

SURGICAL PROCEDURES: ---
---.

DISCHARGE DIAGNOSIS: --.

Surgeon_____
Charles M. Jones, M. D.

mtf
D: 11-09-94
T: 11-09-95

Figure 5
Discharge summary typed in run-on format. Variations mentioned within the figure.

Combining Forms in
Medical Terminology*

The following is a list of combining forms encountered frequently in the vocabulary of medicine. A dash or dashes are appended to indicate whether the form usually precedes (as *ante-*) or follows (as *-agra*) the other elements of the compound or usually appears between the other elements (as *-em-*). Following each combining form, the first item of information is the Greek or Latin word, or both a Greek and a Latin word, from which it is derived. Greek words have been transliterated into Roman characters. Latin words are identified by [L.], Greek words by [Gr.]. Information necessary to an understanding of the form appears next in parentheses. Then the meaning or meanings of the words are given, followed where appropriate by reference to a synonymous combining form. Finally, an example is given to illustrate the use of the combining form in a compound English derivative.

a- a- [L.] (*n* is added before words beginning with a vowel) negative prefix. Cf. in-³. a*metria*

ab- *ab* [L.] away from. Cf. apo-. ab*ducent*

abdomin- *abdomen, abdominis* [L.] abdomen. *abdomin*oscopy

ac- See ad-. *ac*cretion

acet- *acetum* [L.] vinegar. *acet*ometer

acid- *acidus* [L.] sour. *acid*uric

acou- *akouō* [Gr.] hear. *acou*ethesia. (Also spelled acu-)

acr- *akron* [Gr.] extremity, peak. *acr*omegaly

act- *ago, actus* [L.] do, drive, act. *act*ion

actin- *aktis, aktinos* [Gr.] ray, radius. Cf. radi-. *actin*ogenesis

acu- See acou-. osteo*acu*sis

ad- *ad* [L.] (*d* changes to *c, f, g, p, s,* or *t* before words beginning with those consonants) to. *ad*renal

aden- *adēn* [Gr.] gland. Cf. gland-. *aden*oma

adip- *adeps, adipis* [L.] fat. Cf. lip- and stear-. *adip*ocellular

aer- *aēr* [Gr.] air. an*aer*obiosis

aesthe- See esthe-. *aesthe*sioneurosis

af- See ad-. *af*ferent

ag- See ad-. *ag*glutinant

-agogue *agōgos* [Gr.] leading, inducing. galact*agogue*

-agra *agra* [Gr.] catching, seizure. po*dagra*

alb- *albus* [L.] white. Cf. leuk-. *alb*ocinereous

alg- *algos* [Gr.] pain. neur*algia*

all- *allos* [Gr.] other, different. *all*ergy

alve- *alveus* [L.] trough, channel, cavity. *alve*olar

amph- See amphi-. *amph*eclexis

amphi- *amphi* [Gr.] (*i* is dropped before words beginning with a vowel) both, doubly. *amphi*celous

amyl- *amylon* [Gr.] starch. *amyl*osynthesis

an-¹ See ana-. *an*agogic

an-² See a-. *an*omalous

ana- *ana* [Gr.] (final *a* is dropped before words beginning with a vowel) up, positive. *ana*phoresis

ancyl- See ankyl-. *ancyl*ostomiasis

andr- *anēr, andros* [Gr.] man. gyn*andr*oid

angi- *angeion* [Gr.] vessel. Cf. vas-. *angi*emphraxis

ankyl- *ankylos* [Gr.] crooked, looped. *ankyl*odactylia. (Also spelled ancyl-)

*Compiled by Lloyd W. Daly, A.M., Ph.D., Litt. D., Allen Memorial Professor of Greek Emeritus, University of Pennsylvania. In Sloane, S. B. *The Medical Word Book*, 3rd ed. Philadelphia, W. B. Saunders Company, 1991.

ant-	See anti-. *ant*ophthalmic
ante-	*ante* [L.] before. *ante*flexion
anti-	*anti* [Gr.] (*i* is dropped before words beginning with a vowel) against, counter. Cf. contra*anti*pyogenic
antr-	*antron* [Gr.] cavern. *antr*odynia
ap-¹	See apo-. *ap*heter
ap-²	See ad-. *ap*pend
-aph-	*haptō, haph-* [Gr.] touch. dysa*aph*ia. (See also hapt-)
apo-	*apo* [Gr.] (*o* is dropped before words beginning with a vowel) away from, detached. Cf. ab-. *apo*physis
arachn-	*arachnē* [Gr.] spider. *arachno*dactyly
arch-	*archē* [Gr.] beginning, origin. *arch*enteron
arter(i)-	*arteria* [Gr.] windpipe, artery. *arter*iosclerosis, peri*arter*itis
arthr-	*arthron* [Gr.] joint. Cf. articul-. syn*arthr*osis
articul-	*articulus* [L.] joint. Cf. arthr-. dis*articul*ation
as-	See ad-. *as*similation
at-	See ad-. *at*trition
aur-	*auris* [L.] ear. Cf. ot-. *aur*inasal
aux-	*auxō* [Gr.] increase. enter*aux*e
ax-	*axōn* [Gr.] or *axis* [L.] axis. *ax*ofugal
axon-	*axōn* [Gr.] axis. *axon*ometer
ba-	*bainō, ba-* [Gr.] go, walk, stand. hypno*ba*tia
bacill-	*bacillus* [L.] small staff, rod. Cf. bacter-. actino*bacill*osis
bacter-	*bactērion* [Gr.] small staff, rod. Cf. bacill-. *bacter*iophage
ball-	*ballō, bol-* [Gr.] throw. *ball*istics. (See also bol-)
bar-	*baros* [Gr.] weight. pedo*bar*ometer
bi-¹	*bios* [Gr.] life. Cf. vit-. aero*bi*c
bi-²	*bi-* [L.] two (see also di-¹). *bi*lobate
bil-	*bilis* [L.] bile. Cf. chol-. *bil*iary
blast-	*blastos* [Gr.] bud, child, a growing thing in its early stages. Cf. germ-. *blast*oma, zygoto*blast*
blep-	*blepō* [Gr.] look, see. hemia*blep*sia
blephar-	*blepharon* [Gr.] (from *blepō*; see blep-) eyelid. Cf. cili-. *blephar*oncus
bol-	See ball-. em*bol*ism
brachi-	*brachiōn* [Gr.] arm. *brachio*cephalic
brachy-	*brachys* [Gr.] short. *brachy*cephalic
brady-	*bradys* [Gr.] slow. *brady*cardia
brom-	*brōmos* [Gr.] stench. podo*brom*idrosis
bronch-	*bronchos* [Gr.] windpipe. *bron*choscopy
bry-	*bryō* [Gr.] be full of life. em*bry*onic
bucc-	*bucca* [L.] cheek. disto*bucc*al

cac-	*kakos* [Gr.] bad, abnormal. Cf. mal*cac*odontia, arthro*cac*e. (See also dys-)
calc-¹	*calx, calcis* [L.] stone (cf. lith-), limestone, lime. *calc*ipexy
calc-²	*calx, calcis* [L.] heel. *calc*aneotibial
calor-	*calor* [L.] heat. Cf. therm-. *calor*imeter
cancr-	*cancer, cancri* [L.] crab, cancer. Cf. carcin-. *cancr*ology. (Also spelled chancr-)
capit-	*caput, capitis* [L.] head. Cf. cephal-. de*capit*ator
caps-	*capsa* [L.] (from *capio;* see cept-) container. en*caps*ulation
carbo(n)-	*carbo, carbonis* [L.] coal, charcoal. *carbo*hydrate, *carbon*uria
carcin-	*karkinos* [Gr.] crab, cancer. Cf. cancr-. *carcin*oma
cardi-	*kardia* [Gr.] heart. lipo*cardi*ac
cary-	See kary-. *cary*okinesis
cat-	See cata-. *cat*hode
cata-	*kata* [Gr.] (final *a* is dropped before words beginning with a vowel) down, negative. *cat*abatic
caud-	*cauda* [L.] tail. *caud*ad
cav-	*cavus* [L.] hollow. Cf. coel-. con*cav*e
cec-	*caecus* [L.] blind. Cf. typhl-. *cec*opexy
cel-¹	See coel-. amphi*cel*ous
cel-²	See -cele. *cel*ectome
-cele	*kēlē* [Gr.] tumor, hernia. gastro*cele*
cell-	*cella* [L.] room, cell. Cf. cyt-. *cell*iferous
cen-	*koinos* [Gr.] common. *cen*esthesia
cent-	*centum* [L.] hundred. Cf. hect-. Indicates fraction in metric system. [This exemplifies the custom in the metric system of identifying fractions of units by stems from the Latin, as centimeter, decimeter, millimeter, and multiples of units by the similar stems from the Greek, as hectometer, decameter, and kilometer.] *cent*imeter, *cent*ipede
cente-	*kenteō* [Gr.] to puncture. Cf. punct-. entero*cente*sis
centr-	*kentron* [Gr.] or *centrum* [L.] point, center. neuro*centr*al
cephal-	*kephalē* [Gr.] head. Cf. capit-. en*cephal*itis
cept-	*capio, -cipientis, -ceptus* [L.] take, receive. re*cept*or
cer-	*kēros* [Gr.] or *cera* [L.] wax. *cer*oplasty, *cer*omel
cerat-	See kerat-. a*cerat*osis
cerebr-	*cerebrum* [L.] brain. *cerebro*spinal

cervic-   *cervix, cervicis* [L.] neck. Cf. trachel-. *cervicitis*

chancr-   See cancr-. *chancriform*

cheil-   *cheilos* [Gr.] lip. Cf. labi-. *cheiloschisis*

cheir-   *cheir* [Gr.] hand. Cf. man-. *macrocheiria.* (Also spelled chir-)

chir-   See cheir-. *chiromegaly*

chlor-   *chlōros* [Gr.] green. *achloropsia*

chol-   *cholē* [Gr.] bile. Cf. bil-. *hepatocholangeitis*

chondr-   *chondros* [Gr.] cartilage. *chondromalacia*

chord-   *chordē* [Gr.] string, cord. *perichordal*

chori-   *chorion* [Gr.] protective fetal membrane. *endochorion*

chro-   *chrōs* [Gr.] color. *polychromatic*

chron-   *chronos* [Gr.] time. *synchronous*

chy-   *cheō, chy-* [Gr.] pour. *ecchymosis*

-cid(e)   *caedo, -cisus* [L.] cut, kill. *infanticide, germicidal*

cili-   *cilium* [L.] eyelid. Cf. blephar-. *superciliary*

cine-   See kine-. *autocinesis*

-cipient   See cept-. *incipient*

circum-   *circum* [L.] around. Cf. peri-. *circumferential*

-cis-   *caedo, -cisus* [L.] cut, kill. *excision*

clas-   *klaō* [Gr.] break. *cranioclast*

clin-   *klinō* [Gr.] bend, incline, make lie down. *clinometer*

clus-   *claudo, -clusus* [L.] shut. *Malocclusion*

co-   See con-. *cohesion*

cocc-   *kokkos* [Gr.] seed, pill. *gonococcus*

coel-   *koilos* [Gr.] hollow. Cf. cav-. *coelenteron.* (Also spelled cel-)

col-¹   See colon-. *colic*

col-²   See con-. *collapse*

colon-   *kolon* [Gr.] lower intestine. *colonic*

colp-   *kolpos* [Gr.] hollow, vagina. Cf. sin-. *endocolpitis*

com-   See con-. *commasculation*

con-   *con-* [L.] (becomes co- before vowels or *h*; col- before *l*; com- before *b*, *m*, or *p*; cor- before *r*) with, together. Cf. syn-. *contraction*

contra-   *contra* [L.] against, counter. Cf. anti-. *contraindication*

copr-   *kopros* [Gr.] dung. Cf. sterco-. *coproma*

cor-₁   *korē* [Gr.] doll, little image, pupil. *isocoria*

cor-²   See con-. *corrugator*

corpor-   *corpus, corporis* [L.] body. Cf. somat-. *intracorporal*

cortic-   *cortex, corticis* [L.] bark, rind. *corticosterone*

cost-   *costa* [L.] rib. Cf. pleur-. *intercostal*

crani-   *kranion* [Gr.] or *cranium* [L.] skull. *pericranium*

creat-   *kreas, kreato-* [Gr.] meat, flesh. *creatorrhea*

-crescent   *cresco, crescentis, cretus* [L.] grow. *excrescent*

cret-¹   *cerno, cretus* [L.] distinguish, separate off. Cf. crin-. *discrete*

cret-²   See -crescent. *accretion*

crin-   *krinō* [Gr.] distinguish, separate off. Cf. cret-¹. *endocrinology*

crur-   *crus, cruris* [L.] shin, leg. *brachiocrural*

cry-   *kryos* [Gr.] cold. *cryesthesia*

crypt-   *kryptō* [Gr.] hide, conceal. *cryptorchism*

cult-   *colo, cultus* [L.] tend, cultivate. *culture*

cune-   *cuneus* [L.] wedge. Cf. sphen-. *cuneiform*

cut-   *cutis* [L.] skin. Cf. derm(at)-. *subcutaneous*

cyan-   *kyanos* [Gr.] blue. *anthocyanin*

cycl-   *kyklos* [Gr.] circle, cycle. *cyclophoria*

cyst-   *kystis* [Gr.] bladder. Cf. vesic-. *nephrocystitis*

cyt-   *kytos* [Gr.] cell. Cf. cell-. *plasmocytoma*

dacry-   *dakry* [Gr.] tear. *dacryocyst*

dactyl-   *daktylos* [Gr.] finger, toe. Cf. digit-. *hexadactylism*

de-   *de* [L.] down from. *decomposition*

dec-¹   *deka* [Gr.] ten. Indicates multiple in metric system. Cf. dec-². *decagram*

dec-²   *decem* [L.] ten. Indicates fraction in metric system. Cf. dec-¹. *decipara, decimeter*

dendr-   *dendron* [Gr.] tree. *neurodendrite*

dent-   *dens, dentis* [L.] tooth. Cf. odont-. *interdental*

derm(at)-   *derma, dermatos* [Gr.] skin. Cf. cut-. *endoderm, dermatitis*

desm-   *desmos* [Gr.] band, ligament. *syndesmopexy*

dextr-   *dexter, dextr-* [L.] right-hand. *ambidextrous*

di-¹   *di-* [Gr.] two. *dimorphic.* (See also bi-²)

di-²   See dia-. *diuresis*

di-³   See dis-. *divergent*

dia-   *dia* [Gr.] (*a* is dropped before words beginning with a vowel) through, apart. Cf. per-. *diagnosis*

didym-   *didymos* [Gr.] twin. Cf. gemin-. *epididymal*

digit-   *digitus* [L.] finger, toe. Cf. dactyl-. *digitigrade*

diplo-   *diploos* [Gr.] double. *diplomyelia*

dis-   *dis-* [L.] (*s* may be dropped before a word beginning with a consonant) apart, away from. *dislocation*

disc-	*diskos* [Gr.] or *discus* [L.] disk. *disc*oplacenta
dors-	*dorsum* [L.] back. ventro*dors*al
drom-	*dromos* [Gr.] course. hemo*dro*mometer
-ducent	See duct-. ad*ducent*
-duct	*duco, ducentis, ductus* [L.] lead, conduct. ovi*duct*
dur-	*durus* [L.] hard. Cf. scler-. in*dur*ation
dynam(i)-	*dynamis* [Gr.] power. *dynam*oneure, neuro*dynam*ic
dys-	*dys-* [Gr.] bad, improper. Cf. mal-. *dys*trophic. (See also cac-)
e-	*e* [L.] out from. Cf. ec- and ex-. *e*mission
ec-	*ek* [Gr.] out of. Cf. e- *ec*centric
-ech-	*echō* [Gr.] have, hold, be. syn*ech*otomy
ect-	*ektos* [Gr.] outside. Cf. extra-. *ect*oplasm
ede-	*oideō* [Gr.] swell. *ede*matous
ef-	See ex-. *ef*florescent
-elc-	*helkos* [Gr.] sore, ulcer. enter*elc*osis. (See also helc-)
electr-	*ēlectron* [Gr.] amber. *electr*otherapy
em-	See en-. *em*bolism, *em*pathy, *em*physis
-em-	*haima* [Gr.] blood. an*em*ia. (See also hem(at)-)
en-	*en* [Gr.] (*n* changes to *m* before *b, p* or *ph*) in, on. Cf. in-². *en*celitis
end-	*endon* [Gr.] inside. Cf. intra-. *end*angium
enter-	*enteron* [Gr.] intestine. dys*enter*y
ep-	See epi-. *ep*axial
epi-	*epi* [Gr.] (*i* is dropped before words beginning with a vowel) upon, after, in addition. *epi*glottis
erg-	*ergon* [Gr.] work, deed. en*erg*y
erythr-	*erythros* [Gr.] red. Cf. rub(r)-. *erythr*ochromia
eso-	*esō* [Gr.] inside. Cf. intra-. *eso*phylactic
esthe-	*aisthanomai, aisthē-* [Gr.] perceive, feel. Cf. sens-. an*esthe*sia
eu-	*eu* [Gr.] good, normal. *eu*pepsia
ex-	*ex* [Gr.] or *ex* [L.] out of. Cf. e-. *ex*cretion
exo-	*exō* [Gr.] outside. Cf. extra-. *ex*opathic
extra-	*extra* [L.] outside of, beyond. Cf. ect- and exo-. *extra*cellular
faci-	*facies* [L.] face. Cf. prosop-. brachio*faci*olingual
-facient	*facio, facientis, factus, -fectus* [L.] make. Cf. poie-. cale*facient*
-fact-	See facient-. arte*fact*
fasci-	*fascia* [L.] band. *fasci*orrhaphy
febr-	*febris* [L.] fever. Cf. pyr-. *febr*icide
-fect-	See -facient. de*fect*ive
-ferent	*fero, ferentis, latus* [L.] bear, carry. Cf. phor-. ef*ferent*
ferr-	*ferrum* [L.] iron. *ferr*oprotein
fibr-	*fibra* [L.] fiber. Cf. in-¹. chondro*fibr*oma
fil-	*filum* [L.] thread. *fil*iform
fiss-	*findo, fissus* [L.] split. Cf. schis-. *fiss*ion
flagell-	*flagellum* [L.] whip. *flagell*ation
flav-	*flavus* [L.] yellow. Cf. xanth-. ribo*flav*in
-flect-	*flecto, flexus* [L.] bend, divert. de*flect*ion
-flex-	See -flect-. re*flex*ometer
flu-	*fluo, fluxus* [L.] flow. Cf. rhe-. *flu*id
flux-	See flu-. af*flux*ion
for-	*foris* [L.] door, opening. per*for*ated
-form	*forma* [L.] shape. Cf. oid. ossi*form*
fract-	*frango, fractus* [L.] break. re*fract*ive
front-	*frons, frontis* [L.] forehead, front. naso*front*al
-fug(e)	*fugio* [L.] flee, avoid. vermi*fuge*, centri*fug*al
funct-	*fungor, functus* [L.] perform, serve, function. mal*funct*ion
fund-	*fundo, fusus* [L.] pour. in*fund*ibulum
fus-	See fund-. dif*fus*ible
galact-	*gala, galactos* [Gr.] milk. Cf. lact-. dys*galact*ia
gam-	*gamos* [Gr.] marriage, reproductive union. a*gam*ont
gangli-	*ganglion* [Gr.] swelling, plexus. neuro*gangli*itis
gastr-	*gastēr, gastros* [Gr.] stomach. cholangio*gastr*ostomy
gelat-	*gelo, gelatus* [L.] freeze, congeal. *gelat*in
gemin-	*geminus* [L.] twin, double. Cf. didym-. quadri*gemin*al
gen-	*gignomai, gen-, gon-* [Gr.] become, be produced, originate, or *gennaō* [Gr.] produce, originate. cyto*gen*ic
germ-	*germen, germinis* [L.] bud, a growing thing in its early stages. Cf. blast-. *germ*inal, ovi*germ*
gest-	*gero, gerentis, gestus* [L.] bear, carry. con*gest*ion
gland-	*glans, glandis* [L.] acorn. Cf. aden-. intra*gland*ular
-glia	*glia* [Gr.] glue. neuro*glia*
gloss-	*glōssa* [Gr.] tongue. Cf. lingu-. tricho*gloss*ia
glott-	*glōtta* [Gr.] tongue, language. *glott*ic
gluc-	See glyc(y)-. *gluc*ophenetidin
glutin-	*gluten, glutinis* [L.] glue. ag*glutin*ation
glyc(y)-	*glykys* [Gr.] sweet. *glyc*emia, *glycy*rrhizin. (Also spelled gluc-)

gnath-   *gnathos* [Gr.] jaw. ortho*gnath*-ous

gno-   *gignōsiō, gnō-* [Gr.] know, discern. dia*gno*sis

gon-   See gen-. anphi*gon*y

grad-   *gradior* [L.] walk, take steps. retro*grad*e

-gram   *gramma* [Gr.] letter, drawing. cardio*gram*

gran-   *granum* [L.] grain, particle. lipo*gran*uloma

graph-   *graphō* [Gr.] scratch, write, record. histo*graph*y

grav-   *gravis* [L.] heavy. multi*grav*ida

gyn(ec)-   *gynē, gynaikos* [Gr.] woman, wife. andro*gyn*y, *gyn*ecologic

gyr-   *gyros* [Gr.] ring, circle. *gyr*ospasm

haem(at)-   See hem(at)-. *haem*orrhagia, *haemat*oxylon

hapt-   *haptō* [Gr.] touch. *hapt*ometer

hect-   *hekt-* [Gr.] hundred. Cf. cent-. Indicates multiple in metric system. *hect*ometer

helc-   *helkos* [Gr.] sore, ulcer. *helc*osis

hem(at)-   *haima, haimatos* [Gr.] blood. Cf. sanguin-. *hem*angioma, *hemat*ocyturia. (See also -em-)

hemi-   *hēmi-* [Gr.] half. Cf. semi-. *hemi*ageusia

hen-   *heis, henos* [Gr.] one. Cf. un-. *hen*ogenesis

hepat-   *hēpar, hēpatos* [Gr.] liver. gastro*hepat*ic

hept(a)-   *hepta* [Gr.] seven. Cf. sept-[2]. *hept*atomic, *hepta*valent

hered-   *heres, heredis* [L.] heir. *here*doimmunity

hex-[1]   *hex* [Gr.] six. Cf. sex-. *hex*yl-. An *a* is added in some combinations

hex-[2]   *echō, hex-* [Gr.] (added to *s* becomes *hex-*) have, hold, be. ca*chex*ia

hexa-   See hex-[1]. *hexa*chromic

hidr-   *hidros* [Gr.] sweat. hyper*hidr*osis

hist-   *histos* [Gr.] web, tissue. *hist*odialysis

hod-   *hodos* [Gr.] road, path. *hod*oneuromere. (See also od- and -ode[1])

hom-   *homos* [Gr.] common, same. *hom*omorphic

horm-   *ormē* [Gr.] impetus, impulse. *horm*one

hydat-   *hydōr, hydatos* [Gr.] water. *hy*datism

hydr-   *hydōr, hydr-* [Gr.] water. Cf. lymph-. anclor*hydr*ia

hyp-   See hypo-. *hyp*axial

hyper-   *hyper* [Gr.] above, beyond, extreme. Cf. super-. *hyper*trophy

hypn-   *hypnos* [Gr.] sleep. *hypn*otic

hypo-   *hypo* [Gr.] (*o* is dropped before words beginning with a vowel) under, below. Cf. sub-. *hypo*metabolism

hyster-   *hystera* [Gr.] womb. colpo*hyster*opexy

iatr-   *iatros* [Gr.] physician. ped*iatr*ics

idi-   *idios* [Gr.] peculiar, separate, distinct. *idi*osyncrasy

il-   See in-[2, 3]. *il*linition (in, on), *il*legible (negative prefix)

ile-   See ili- [*ile-* is commonly used to refer to the portion of the intestines known as the ileum]. *ile*ostomy

ili-   *ilium (ileum)* [L.] lower abdomen, intestines [*ili-* is commonly used to refer to the flaring part of the hip bone known as the ilium]. *ili*osacral

im-   See in-[2, 3]. *im*mersion (in, on), *im*perforation (negative prefix)

in-[1]   *is, inos* [Gr.] fiber. Cf. fibr-. *in*osteatoma

in-[2]   *in* [L.] (*n* changes to *l, m,* or *r* before words beginning with those consonants) in, on. Cf. en-. *in*sertion

in-[3]   *in-* [L.] (*n* changes to *l, m,* or *r* before words beginning with those consonants) negative prefix. Cf. a-. *in*valid

infra-   *infra* [L.] beneath. *infra*orbital

insul-   *insula* [L.] island. *insul*in

inter-   *inter* [L.] among, between. *inter*carpal

intra-   *intra* [L.] inside. Cf. end- and eso-. *intra*venous

ir-   See in-[2, 3]. *ir*radiation (in, on), *ir*reducible (negative prefix)

irid-   *iris, iridos* [Gr.] rainbow, colored circle. kerato*irid*ocyclitis

is-   *isos* [Gr.] equal. *is*otope

ischi-   *ischion* [Gr.] hip, haunch. *ischi*opubic

jact-   *iacio, iactus* [L.] throw. *jact*itation

-ject   *iacio, -iectus* [L.] throw. in*jec*tion

jejun-   *ieiunus* [L.] hungry, not partaking of food. gastro*jejun*ostomy

jug-   *iugum* [L.] yoke. con*jug*ation

junct-   *iungo, iunctus* [L.] yoke, join. con*junct*iva

kary-   *karyon* [Gr.] nut, kernel, nucleus. Cf. nucle-. mega*kary*ocyte. (Also spelled cary-)

kerat-   *keras, keratos* [Gr.] horn. *kerat*olysis. (Also spelled cerat-)

kil-   *chilioi* [Gr.] one thousand. Cf. mill-. Indicates multiple in metric system. *kil*ogram

kine-   *kineō* [Gr.] move. *kine*matograph. (Also spelled cine-)

labi-   *labium* [L.] lip. Cf. cheil-. gingivo*labi*al

lact-   *lac, lactis* [L.] milk. Cf. galact-. gluco*lact*one

lal-   *laleō* [Gr.] talk, babble. glosso*lal*ia

lapar-   *lapara* [Gr.] flank. *lapar*otomy

laryng-   *larynx, laryngos* [Gr.] windpipe. *laryng*endoscope

lat-   *fero, latus* [L.] bear, carry. See -ferent. trans*lat*ion

later-   *latus, lateris* [L.] side. ventro*later*al

lent-   *lens, lentis* [L.] lentil. Cf. phac-. *lent*iconus

lep-   *lambanō, lēp-* [Gr.] take, seize. cata*lep*tic

leuc-   See leuk-. *leuc*inuria

leuk-   *leukos* [Gr.] white. Cf. alb-. *leu*korrhea. (Also spelled leuc-)

lien-   *lien* [L.] spleen. Cf. splen-. *lien*ocele

lig-   *ligo* [L.] tie, bind. *lig*ate

lingu-   *lingua* [L.] tongue. Cf. gloss-. sub*lingu*al

lip-   *lipos* [Gr.] fat. Cf. adip-. glyco*lip*in

lith-   *lithos* [Gr.] stone. Cf. calc-[1]. nephro*lith*otomy

loc-   *locus* [L.] place. Cf. top-. *loc*omotion

log-   *legō, log-* [Gr.] speak, give an account. *log*orrhea, embryo*logy*

lumb-   *lumbus* [L.] loin. dorso*lumb*ar

lute-   *luteus* [L.] yellow. Cf. xanth-. *lute*oma

ly-   *lyō* [Gr.] loose, dissolve. Cf. solut-. kerato*ly*sis

lymph-   *lympha* [Gr.] water. Cf. hydr-. *lymph*adenosis

macr-   *makros* [Gr.] long, large. *macr*omyeloblast

mal-   *malus* [L.] bad, abnormal. Cf. cac- and dys-. *mal*function

malac-   *malakos* [Gr.] soft. osteo*malac*ia

mamm-   *mamma* [L.] breast. Cf. mast-. sub*mamm*ary

man-   *manus* [L.] hand. Cf. cheir-. *man*iphalanx

mani-   *mania* [Gr.] mental aberration. *mani*graphy, klepto*mani*a

mast-   *mastos* [Gr.] breast. Cf. mamm-. hyper*mast*ia

medi-   *medius* [L.] middle. Cf. mes-. *medi*frontal

mega-   *megas* [Gr.] great, large. Also indicates multiple (1,000,000) in metric system. *mega*colon, *mega*dyne. (See also megal-)

megal-   *megas, megalou* [Gr.] great, large. acro*megal*y

mel-   *melos* [Gr.] limb, member. sym*mel*ia

melan-   *melas, melanos* [Gr.] black. hippo*melan*in

men-   *mēn* [Gr.] month. dys*men*orrhea

mening-   *mēninx, mēningos* [Gr.] membrane. encephalo*mening*itis

ment-   *mens, mentis* [L.] mind. Cf. phren-, psych- and thym-. de*ment*ia

mer-   *meros* [Gr.] part. poly*mer*ic

mes-   *mesos* [Gr.] middle. Cf. medi-. *mes*oderm

met-   See meta-. *met*allergy

meta-   *meta* [Gr.] (a is dropped before words beginning with a vowel) after, beyond, accompanying. *meta*carpal

metr-[1]   *metron* [Gr.] measure. stereo*metr*y

metr-[2]   *metra* [Gr.] womb. endo*metr*itis

micr-   *mikros* [Gr.] small. photo*micr*ograph

mill-   *mille* [L.] one thousand. Cf. kil-. Indicates fraction in metric system. *mill*igram, *mill*ipede

miss-   See -mittent. intro*miss*ion

-mittent   *mitto, mittentis, missus* [L.] send. inter*mittent*

mne-   *mimnērcō, mnē-* [Gr.] remember. pseudo*mne*sia

mon-   *monos* [Gr.] only, sole. *mon*oplegia

morph-   *morphē* [Gr.] form, shape. poly*morph*onuclear

mot-   *moveo, motus* [L.] move. vaso*mot*or

my-   *mys, myos* [Gr.] muscle. ino*leiomy*oma

-myces   *mykēs, mykētos* [Gr.] fungus. myelo*myces*

myc(et)-   See -myces. asco*mycet*es, strepto*myc*in

myel-   *myelos* [Gr.] marrow. polio*myel*itis

myx-   *myxa* [Gr.] mucus. *myx*edema

narc-   *narkē* [Gr.] numbness. topo*narc*osis

nas-   *nasus* [L.] nose. Cf. rhin-. palato*nas*al

ne-   *neos* [Gr.] new, young. *ne*ocyte

necr-   *nekros* [Gr.] corpse. *necr*ocytosis

nephr-   *nephros* [Gr.] kidney. Cf. ren-. para*nephr*ic

neur-   *neuron* [Gr.] nerve. esthesio*neur*e

nod-   *nodus* [L] knot. *nod*osity

nom-   *nomos* [Gr.] (from *nemō* deal out, distribute) law, custom. taxo*nom*y

non-   *nona* [L.] nine. *non*acosane

nos-   *nosos* [Gr.] disease. *nos*ology

nucle-   *nucleus* [L.] (from *nux, nucis* nut) kernel. Cf. kary-. *nucle*ide

nutri-   *nutrio* [L.] nourish. mal*nutri*tion

ob-   *ob* [L.] (*b* changes to *c* before words beginning with that

	consonant) against, toward, etc. *obtuse*
oc-	See ob-. *occlude*
ocul-	*oculus* [L.] eye. Cf. ophthalm-. *oculomotor*
-od-	See -ode¹. *periodic*
-ode¹	*hodos* [Gr.] road, path. *cathode*. (See also hod-)
-ode²	See -oid. *nematode*
odont-	*odous, odontos* [Gr.] tooth. Cf. dent-. *orthodontia*
-odyn-	*odynē* [Gr.] pain, distress. *gastrodynia*
-oid	*eidos* [Gr.] form. Cf. -form. *hyoid*
-ol	See ole-. *cholesterol*
ole-	*oleum* [L.] oil. *oleoresin*
olig-	*oligos* [Gr.] few, small. *oligospermia*
omphal-	*omphalos* [Gr.] navel. *periomphalic*
onc-	*onkos* [Gr.] bulk, mass. *hematoncometry*
onych-	*onyx, onychos* [Gr.] claw, nail. *anonychia*
oo-	*ōon* [Gr.] egg. Cf. ov-. *perioothecitis*
op-	*horaō, op-* [Gr.] see. *erythropsia*
ophthalm-	*ophthalmos* [Gr.] eye. Cf. ocul-. *exophthalmic*
or-	*os, oris* [L.] mouth. Cf. stom(at)-. *intraoral*
orb-	*orbis* [L.] circle. *suborbital*
orchi-	*orchis* [Gr.] testicle. Cf. test-. *orchiopathy*
organ-	*organon* [Gr.] implement, instrument. *organoleptic*
orth-	*orthos* [Gr.] straight, right, normal. *orthopedics*
oss-	*os, ossis* [L.] bone. Cf. ost(e)-. *ossiphone*
ost(e)-	*osteon* [Gr.] bone. Cf. oss-. *enostosis, osteanaphysis*
ot-	*ous, ōtos* [Gr.] ear. Cf. aur-. *parotid*
ov-	*ovum* [L.] egg. Cf. oo-. *synovia*
oxy-	*oxys* [Gr.] sharp. *oxycephalic*
pachy(n)-	*pachynō* [Gr.] thicken. *pachyderma, myopachynsis*
pag-	*pēgnymi, pag-* [Gr.] fix, make fast. *thoracopagus*
par-¹	*pario* [L.] bear, give birth to. *primiparous*
par-²	See para-. *parepigastric*
para-	*para* [Gr.] (final *a* is dropped before words beginning with a vowel) beside, beyond. *paramastoid*
part-	*pario, partus* [L.] bear, give birth to. *parturition*
path-	*pathos* [Gr.] that which one undergoes, sickness. *psychopathic*
pec-	*pēgnymi, pēg-* [Gr.] (*pēk-* before *t*) fix, make fast. *sympectothiene*. (See also pex-)
ped-	*pais, paidos* [Gr.] child. *orthopedic*

pell-	*pellis* [L.] skin, hide. *pellagra*
-pellent	*pello, pellentis, pulsus* [L.] drive. *repellent*
pen-	*penomai* [Gr.] need, lack. *erythrocytopenia*
pend-	*pendeo* [L.] hang down. *appendix*
pent(a)-	*pente* [Gr.] five. Cf. quinque-. *pentose, pentaploid*
peps-	*peptō, peps-* [Gr.] digest. *bradypepsia*
pept-	*peptō* [Gr.] digest. *dyspeptic*
per-	*per* [L.] through. Cf. dia-. *pernasal*
peri-	*peri* [Gr.] around. Cf. circum-. *periphery*
pet-	*peto* [L.] seek, tend toward. *centripetal*
pex-	*pēgnumi, pēg-* [Gr.] (added to *s* becomes *pēx*) fix, make fast. *hepatopexy*
pha-	*phēmi, pha-* [Gr.] say, speak. *dysphasia*
phac-	*phakos* [Gr.] lentil, lens. Cf. lent-. *phacosclerosis*. (Also spelled phak-)
phag-	*phagein* [Gr.] eat. *lipophagic*
phak-	See phac-. *phakitis*
phan-	See phen-. *diaphanoscopy*
pharmac-	*pharmakon* [Gr.] drug. *pharmacognosy*
pharyng-	*pharynx, pharyng-* [Gr.] throat, *glossopharyngeal*
phen-	*phainō, phan-* [Gr.] show, be seen. *phosphene*
pher-	*pherō, phor-* [Gr.] bear, support. *periphery*
phil-	*phileō* [Gr.] like, have affinity for. *eosinophilia*
phleb-	*phleps, phlebos* [Gr.] vein. *periphlebitis*
phleg-	*phlogō, phlog-* [Gr.] burn, inflame. *adenophlegmon*
phlog-	See phleg-. *antiphlogistic*
phob-	*phobos* [Gr.] fear, dread. *claustrophobia*
phon-	*phōne* [Gr.] sound. *echophony*
phor-	See pher-. Cf. -ferent. *exophoria*
phos-	See phot-. *phosphorus*
phot-	*phōs, phōtos* [Gr.] light. *photerythrous*
phrag-	*phrassō, phrag-* [Gr.] fence, wall off, stop up. Cf. sept-¹. *diaphragm*
phrax-	*phrassō, phrag-* [Gr.] (added to *s* becomes *phrax-*) fence, wall off, stop up. *emphraxis*
phren-	*phrēn* [Gr.] mind, midriff. Cf. ment-. *metaphrenia, metaphrenon*
phthi-	*phthinō* [Gr.] decay, waste away. *phthisis*
phy-	*phyō* [Gr.] beget, bring forth, produce, be by nature. *nosophyte*
phyl-	*phylon* [Gr.] tribe, kind. *phylogeny*

-phyll	*phyllon* [Gr.] leaf. xantho*phyll*
phylac-	*phylax* [Gr.] guard. pro*phylactic*
phys(a)-	*physaō* [Gr.] blow, inflate. *physocele, physalis*
physe-	*physaō, physē-* [Gr.] blow, inflate. em*physema*
pil-	*pilus* [L.] hair. e*pilation*
pituit-	*pituita* [L.] phlegm, rheum. *pituitous*
placent-	*placenta* [L.] (from *plakous* [Gr.]) cake. extra*placental*
plas-	*plassō* [Gr.] mold, shape. ci*neplasty*
platy-	*platys* [Gr.] broad, flat. *platyrrhine*
pleg-	*plēssō* [Gr.] strike. di*plegia*
plet-	*pleo, -pletus* [L.] fill. de*pletion*
pleur-	*pleura* [Gr.] rib, side. Cf. cost-. peri*pleural*
plex-	*plēssō, plēg-* (added to *s* becomes *plēx-*) strike. apo*plexy*
plic-	*plico* [L.] fold. compli*cation*
pne-	*pneuma, pneumatos* [Gr.] breathing. traumato*pnea*
pneum(at)-	*pneuma, pneumatos* [Gr.] breath, air. *pneumodynamics, pneumatothorax*
pneumo(n)-	*pneumōn* [Gr.] lung. Cf. pulmo(n)-. *pneumocentesis, pneumonotomy*
pod-	*pous, podos* [Gr.] foot. *podiatry*
poie-	*poieō* [Gr.] make, produce. Cf. -facient. sarco*poietic*
pol-	*polos* [Gr.] axis of a sphere. peri*polar*
poly-	*polys* [Gr.] much, many. *polyspermia*
pont-	*pons, pontis* [L.] bridge. *pontocerebellar*
por-[1]	*poros* [Gr.] passage. myelo*pore*
por-[2]	*pŏros* [Gr.] callus. *porocele*
posit-	*pono, positus* [L.] put, place. re*positor*
post-	*post* [L.] after, behind in time or place. *postnatal, postoral*
pre-	*prae* [L.] before in time or place. *prenatal, prevesical*
press-	*premo, pressus* [L.] press. *pressoreceptive*
pro-	*pro* [Gr.] or *pro* [L.] before in time or place. *progamous, procheilon, prolapse*
proct-	*prōktos* [Gr.] anus. entero*proctia*
prosop-	*prosōpon* [Gr.] face. Cf. faci-. di*prosopus*
pseud-	*pseudēs* [Gr.] false. *pseudoparaplegia*
psych-	*psychē* [Gr.] soul, mind. Cf. ment-. *psychosomatic*
pto-	*piptō, ptō-* [Gr.] fall. nephro*ptosis*
pub-	*pubes* and *puber, puberis* [L.] adult. ischio*pubic*. (See also puber-)
puber-	*puber* [L.] adult. *puberty*
pulmo(n)-	*pulmo, pulmonis* [L.] lung. Cf. pneumo(n)-. *pulmolith, cardiopulmonary*
puls-	*pello, pellentis, pulsus* [L.] drive. pro*pulsion*
punct-	*pungo, punctus* [L.] prick, pierce. Cf. cente-. *punctiform*
pur-	*pus, puris* [L.] pus. Cf. py-. sup*puration*
py-	*pyon* [Gr.] pus. Cf. pur-. nephro*pyosis*
pyel-	*pyelos* [Gr.] trough, basin, pelvis. nephro*pyelitis*
pyl-	*pylē* [Gr.] door, orifice. *pylephlebitis*
pyr-	*pyr* [Gr.] fire. Cf. febr-. galacto*pyra*
quadr-	*quadr-* [L.] four. Cf. tetra-. *quadrigeminal*
quinque-	*quinque* [L.] five. Cf. pent(a)-. *quinquecuspid*
rachi-	*rachis* [Gr.] spine. Cf. spin-. encephalo*rachidian*
radi-	*radius* [L.] ray. Cf. actin-. ir*radiation*
re-	*re-* [L.] back, again. *retraction*
ren-	*renes* [L.] kidneys. Cf. nephr-. ad*renal*
ret-	*rete* [L.] net. *retothelium*
retro-	*retro* [L.] backwards. *retrodeviation*
rhag-	*rhēgnymi, rhag-* [Gr.] break, burst. hemor*rhagic*
rhaph-	*rhaphē* [Gr.] suture. gastror*rhaphy*
rhe-	*rhaphē* [Gr.] flow. Cf. flu-. diar*rheal*
rhex-	*rhegnymi, rhēg-* [Gr.] (added to *s* becomes *rhēx*) break, burst. metror*rhexis*
rhin-	*rhis, rhinos* [Gr.] nose. Cf. nas-. basi*rhinal*
rot-	*rota* [L.] wheel. *rotator*
rub(r)-	*ruber, rubri* [L.] red. Cf. erythr-. bili*rubin, rubrospinal*
salping-	*salpinx, salpingos* [Gr.] tube, trumpet. *salpingitis*
sanguin-	*sanguis, sanguinis* [L.] blood. Cf. hem(at)-. *sanguineous*
sarc-	*sarx, sarkos* [Gr.] flesh. *sarcoma*
schis-	*schizō, schid-* [Gr.] (before *t* or added to *s* becomes *schis-*) split. Cf. fiss-. *schistorachis, rachischisis*
scler-	*sklēros* [Gr.] hard. Cf. dur-. *sclerosis*
scop-	*skopeō* [Gr.] look at, observe. endo*scope*
sect-	*seco, sectus* [L.] cut. Cf. tom-. *sectile*
semi-	*semi* [L.] half. Cf. hemi-. *semiflexion*
sens-	*sentio, sensus* [L.] perceive, feel. Cf. esthe-. *sensory*

sep-   *sepō* [Gr.] rot, decay. *sep*sis

sept-¹   *saepio, saeptus* [L.] fence, wall off, stop up. Cf. phrag-. naso*sept*al

sept-²   *septem* [L.] seven. Cf. hept(a)-. *sept*an

ser-   *serum* [L.] whey, watery substance. *ser*osynovitis

sex-   *sex* [L.] six. Cf. hex-¹. *sex*digitate

sial-   *sialon* [Gr.] saliva. poly*sial*ia

sin-   *sinus* [L.] hollow, fold. Cf. colp-. *sin*obronchitis

sit-   *sitos* [Gr.] food. para*sit*ic

solut-   *solvo, solventis, solutus* [L.] loose, dissolve, set free. Cf. ly-. dis*solut*ion

-solvent   See solut-. dis*solvent*

somat-   *sōma, somatos* [Gr.] body. Cf. corpor-. psycho*somat*ic

-some   See somat-. dictyo*some*

spas-   *spaō, spas-* [Gr.] draw, pull. *spas*m, *spas*tic

spectr-   *spectrum* [L.] appearance, what is seen. micro*spectr*oscope

sperm(at)-   *sperma, spermatos* [Gr.] seed. *sperm*acrasia, *spermat*ozoon

spers-   *spargo, -spersus* [L.] scatter. di*spers*ion

sphen-   *sphēn* [Gr.] wedge. Cf. cune-. *sphen*oid

spher-   *sphaira* [Gr.] ball. hemi*spher*e

sphygm-   *sphygmos* [Gr.] pulsation. *sphygm*omanometer

spin-   *spina* [L.] spine. Cf. rachi-. cerebro*spin*al

spirat-   *spiro, spiratus* [L.] breathe. in*spirat*ory

splanchn-   *splanchna* [Gr.] entrails, viscera. neuro*splanchn*ic

splen-   *splēn* [Gr.] spleen. Cf. lien-. *splen*omegaly

spor-   *sporos* [Gr.] seed. *spor*ophyte, zygo*spor*e

squam-   *squama* [L.] scale. de*squam*ation

sta-   *histēmi, sta-* [Gr.] make stand, stop. genesi*sta*sis

stal-   *stellō, stal-* [Gr.] send. peri*stal*sis. (See also stol-)

staphyl-   *staphylē* [Gr.] bunch of grapes, uvula. *staphyl*ococcus, *staphyl*ectomy

stear-   *stear, steatos* [Gr.] fat. Cf. adip-. *stear*odermia

steat-   See stear-. *steat*opygous

sten-   *stenos* [Gr.] narrow, compressed. *sten*ocardia

ster-   *stereos* [Gr.] solid. chole*ster*ol

sterc-   *stercus* [L.] dung. Cf. copr-. *sterc*oporphyrin

sthen-   *sthenos* [Gr.] strength. a*sthen*ia

stol-   *stellō, stol-* [Gr.] send. dia*stol*e

stom(at)-   *stoma, stomatos* [Gr.] mouth, orifice. Cf. or-. ana*stom*osis, *stomat*ogastric

strep(h)-   *strephō, strep-* (before *t*) [Gr.] twist. Cf. tors-. *streph*osymbolia, *strep*tomycin. (See also stroph-)

strict-   *stringo, stringentis, strictus* [L.] draw tight, compress, cause pain. con*strict*ion

-stringent   See strict-. a*stringent*

stroph-   *strephō, stroph-* [Gr.] twist. ana*stroph*ic. (See also strep(h)-)

struct-   *struo, structus* [L.] pile up (against). ob*struct*ion

sub-   *sub* [L.] (*b* changes to *f* or *p* before words beginning with those consonants) under, below. Cf. hypo-. *sub*lumbar

suf-   See sub-. *suf*fusion

sup-   See sub-. *sup*pository

super-   *super* [L.] above, beyond, extreme. Cf. hyper-. *super*motility

sy-   See syn-. *sy*stole

syl-   See syn-. *syl*lepsiology

sym-   See syn-. *sym*biosis, *sym*metry, *sym*pathetic, *sym*physis

syn-   *syn* [Gr.] (*n* disappears before *s*, changes to *l* before *l*, and changes to *m* before *b*, *m*, *p*, and *ph*) with, together. Cf. con-. myo*syn*izesis

ta-   See ton-. *ta*ctasis

tac-   *tassō, tag-* [Gr.] (*tak-* before *t*) order, arrange. a*tac*tic

tact-   *tango, tactus* [L.] touch. con*tact*

tax-   *tassō, tag-* [Gr.] (added to *s* becomes *tax-*) order, arrange. a*tax*ia

tect-   See teg-. pro*tect*ive

teg-   *tego, tectus* [L.] cover. in*teg*ument

tel-   *telos* [Gr.] end. *tel*osynapsis

tele-   *tēle* [Gr.] at a distance. *tele*ceptor

tempor-   *tempus, temporis* [L.] time, timely or fatal spot, temple. *tempor*omalar

ten(ont)-   *tenōn, tenontos* [Gr.] (from *teinō* stretch) tight stretched band. *ten*odynia, *ten*onitis, *tenont*agra

tens-   *tendo, tensus* [L.] stretch. Cf. ton-. ex*tens*or

test-   *testis* [L.] testicle. Cf. orchi-. *test*itis

tetra-   *tetra-* [Gr.] four. Cf. quadr-. *tetra*genous

the-   *tithēmi, thē-* [Gr.] put, place. syn*the*sis

thec-   *thēkē* [Gr.] repository, case. *thec*ostegnosis

thel-   *thēlē* [Gr.] teat, nipple. *thel*erethism

therap-	*therapeia* [Gr.] treatment. hy-dro*therapy*
therm-	*thermē* [Gr.] heat. Cf. calor-. dia*thermy*
thi-	*theion* [Gr.] sulfur. *thiogenic*
thorac-	*thōrax, thōrakos* [Gr.] chest. *thoracoplasty*
thromb-	*thrombos* [Gr.] lump, clot. *thrombopenia*
thym-	*thymos* [Gr.] spirit. Cf. ment-. dys*thymia*
thyr-	*thyreos* [Gr.] shield (shaped like a door *thyra*). *thyroid*
tme-	*temnō, tmē-* [Gr.] cut. axon-*otmesis*
toc-	*tokos* [Gr.] childbirth. dys*tocia*
tom-	*temnō, tom-* [Gr.] cut. Cf. sect-. appendec*tomy*
ton-	*teino, ton-* [Gr.] stretch, put under tension. Cf. tens-. peri*toneum*
top-	*topos* [Gr.] place. Cf. loc-. *topesthesia*
tors-	*torqueo, torsus* [L.] twist. Cf. strep-. ec*torsion*
tox-	*toxicon* [Gr.] (from *toxon* bow) arrow poison, poison. *toxemia*
trache-	*tracheia* [Gr.] windpipe. *tracheotomy*
trachel-	*trachēlos* [Gr.] neck. Cf. cervic-. *trachelopexy*
tract-	*traho, tractus* [L.] draw, drag. pro*traction*
traumat-	*trauma, traumatos* [Gr.] wound. *traumatic*
tri-	*treis, tria* [Gr.] or *tri-* [L.] three. *trigonid*
trich-	*thrix, trichos* [Gr.] hair. *trichoid*

trip-	*tribō* [Gr.] rub. en*tripsis*
trop-	*trepō, trop-* [Gr.] turn, react. sito*tropism*
troph-	*trepō, troph-* [Gr.] nurture. a*trophy*
tuber-	*tuber* [L.] swelling, node. *tubercle*
typ-	*typos* [Gr.] (from *typto* strike) type. a*typical*
typh-	*typhos* [Gr.] fog, stupor. adeno*typhus*
typhl-	*typhlos* [Gr.] blind. Cf. cec-. *typhlectasis*
un-	*unus* [L.] one. Cf. hen-. *unioval*
ur-	*ouron* [Gr.] urine. poly*uria*
vacc-	*vacca* [L.] cow. *vaccine*
vagin-	*vagina* [L.] sheath. in*vaginated*
vas-	*vas* [L.] vessel. Cf. angi-. *vascular*
vers-	See vert-. in*version*
vert-	*verto, versus* [L.] turn. di*verticulum*
vesic-	*vesica* [L.] bladder. Cf. cyst-. *vesicovaginal*
vit-	*vita* [L.] life. Cf. bi-¹. de*vitalize*
vuls-	*vello, vulsus* [L.] pull, twitch. con*vulsion*
xanth-	*xanthos* [Gr.] yellow, blond. Cf. flav- and lute-. *xanthophyll*
-yl-	*hyte* [Gr.] substance. cacod*yl*
zo-	*zoē* [Gr.] life, *zōon* [Gr.] animal. micro*zoaria*
zyg-	*zygon* [Gr.] yoke, union. *zygodactyly*
zym-	*zymē* [Gr.] ferment. en*zyme*

*Medically Significant Prefixes and Suffixes**

A hyphen appears following a prefix (as in ante-) and precedes a suffix (as in -agra).

a-	not, without: *atypical*, *anodontia* (*n* is added to the prefix before words beginning with a vowel)	blasto-	formation of cells: *blasto*derm
		-blast	an immature cell: histio*blast*
ab-	away from: *abducent*	blephar(o)-	eyelid or eyelash: *blephar*edema,
abdomin(o)-	abdomen: *abdomin*algia, *abdomino*cystic		*blepharo*adenoma
		brachy-	short: *brachy*cephalic
		brady-	slow: *brady*cardia
actino-	ray, radium: *actino*genesis	bronch-, bronchi-,	windpipe: *bronch*itis, *bronchi*ectasis,
ad-	toward: *adduct*	broncho-	*broncho*malacia
aden(o)-	gland: *aden*itis, *adeno*pharyngitis	calor-	heat: *calor*imeter
		carbo-	coal, charcoal: *carbo*hydrate
aer(o)-	air: *aer*emia, *aero*cele	cardi(o)-	heart: *cardi*asthenia, *cardio*cele
-agogue	leading, inducing: galact*agogue*	cata-	down, lower: *cata*crotism
alb-	white: *alb*umin	caud(o)-	tail: *caud*ate, *caudo*cephalad
-algia	pain: neur*algia*		
ambi-	both: *ambi*lateral	-cele	tumor, hernia: cysto*cele*
an-	see *a*	centi-	hundred; hundredth
ante-	before: *ante*flexion		part: *centi*meter
anti-	against: *anti*pyogenic	cephal(o)-	cranium, head: *cephal*hydrocele, *cephalo*thoracic
antro-	cavern: *antro*dynia		
arachn(o)-	spider: *arachn*idism, *arachno*dactyly	cerebro-	brain: *cerebro*spinal
arteri(o)-	artery: *arteri*ectasis, *arterio*sclerosis	cervic(o)-	neck: *cervic*itis, *cervico*vesical
arthr(o)-	joint: *arthr*ectomy, *arthro*cele	chol-, chole-, cholo-	bile: *chol*angitis, *chole*cystitis, *cholo*lith
-asis, -esis, -iasis, -osis	state or condition: metast*asis*, metath*esis*, cholelith*iasis*, trichin*osis*	chondro-	cartilage: *chondro*malacia
auri-	ear: *auri*nasal	cili-	eyelid: *cili*ary;
auto-	self: *auto*intoxication	circum-	around: *circum*ferential
bi-	twice: *bi*lateral	cleid(o)-	hook, clavicle:
bili-	bile: *bili*ary		
bio-	life: *bio*genous		
			*cleid*arthritis, *cleido*mastoid
colp(o)-	bosom or fold; vagina: *colp*ectomy, *colpo*dynia
contra-	against: *contra*indication
cortico-	bark, rind: *cortico*steroid
costo-	rib: *costo*chondral
cox(o)-	hip, hip joint: *cox*algia, *coxo*dynia
crani(o)-	cranium: *crani*ectomy, *cranio*cele
cry(o)-	cold: *cry*esthesia, *cryo*pathy
crypt(o)-	hidden, obscure: *crypt*esthesia, *crypto*empyema
cut-	skin: *cut*aneous
cyst-, cysti-, cystido-, cysto-	bladder: *cyst*itis, *cysti*cercoid, *cystido*laparotomy, *cysto*myxoma
cyt(o)-	cell: *cyt*ase, *cyto*clasis
dacry(o)-	tears: *dacry*adenitis, *dacryo*lith
derma-, dermat-, dermato-, dermo-	skin: *derma*brasion, *dermat*algia, *dermato*phytosis, *dermo*blast
dextr(o)-	right side: *dextr*al, *dextro*cardia
di-	two: *di*morphic
dia-	throughout, completely: *dia*kinesis
digit-	finger, toe: *digit*ate
diplo-	double: *diplo*pia
dis-	absence, reversal,

*From Sloane, S. B. *A Word Book in Radiology*. W. B. Saunders Company, Philadelphia, 1988, pp. 430–437.

	separation: *dis*location	gymno-	naked: *gymno*cyte
dolicho-	long: *dolicho*cephaly	gyn-, gyne-,	woman, female sex:
dorsi-,	back: *dorsi*spinal,	gyneco-,	*gyn*atresia,
dorso-	*dorso*lumbar	gyno-	*gyne*phobia,
-duct	draw, lead: ovi*duct*		*gyneco*mastia,
dys-	difficult, painful, bad,		*gyno*pathy
	disordered: *dys*trophy	gyro-	round, ring, circle:
ec-	out of: *ec*centric		*gyro*spasm
ect(o)-	out of, away from:	hema-,	blood: *hema*pheresis,
	*ect*iris, *ecto*pic	hemo-,	*hemo*globin,
-ectomy	surgical removal of:	hemato-	*hemato*cele
	cholecyst*ectomy*	hemi-	one half: *hemi*plegia
em-, en-	in: *em*bolism,	hepat(o)-	liver: *hepat*itis,
	*en*capsulated		*hepato*megaly
end(o)-	inward, within:	heter(o)-	other, different:
	*end*aural, *endo*carditis		*heter*adenia,
enter(o)-	intestines: *enter*itis,		*hetero*genous
	*entero*cele	hex(a)-	six: *hex*ose,
ep-, epi-	on, upon, above, over:		*hexa*chromic
	*ep*axial, *epi*dermis	hidr(o)-	sweat: *hidr*adenitis,
eso-	inside, within:		*hidro*cystoma
	*eso*phoria	histio-,	web, tissue:
eu-	well, good, easily:	histo-	*histio*cytoma,
	*eu*crasia		*histo*genesis
ex-	out, away from:	homo-,	same, common, similar:
	*ex*cretion	homeo-,	*homo*geneous,
exo-	outside, extra: *exo*toxin	homoio-	*homeo*pathic,
extra-	beyond, in addition:		*homoio*thermy
	*extra*cellular	hydr(o)-	water or hydrogen:
-facient	making: cale*facient*		*hydr*amnios,
fasci-	band: *fasci*culus		*hydro*cephalus
febr-	fever: *febr*ile	hyper-	above, beyond,
fil-	thread: *fil*iform		extreme: *hyper*trophy
-flect	bend, divert: de*flect*	hypno-	sleep: *hypno*tic
-form	shape: ossi*form*	hypo-	beneath, under
galact(o)-	milk: *galact*emia,		deficient:
	*galacto*phoritis		*hypo*chondrium
gam(o)-	marriage or sexual	hypso-	height: *hypso*kinesis
	union: *gam*etophyte,	hyster(o)-	womb: *hyster*ectomy,
	*gamo*genesis		*hystero*salpingostomy
gangli(o)-	ganglion, knot: *gangli*al,	-iasis	morbid or diseased
	*ganglio*neuroma		condition: elephant*iasis*
gastr(o)-	stomach:	iatro-	relation to physician or
	*gastr*itis,		to medicine:
	*gastro*duodenal		*iatro*physics
gelat-	freeze, congeal:	-id	having the shape of,
	*gelat*inous		resembling:
-genic	producing, productive		dermatophyt*id*
	of: osteo*genic*	-ide	a binary chemical
genio-	chin: *genio*plasty		compound: chlor*ide*
genito-	relationship to	idio-	self: *idio*pathic
	organs of	ileo-	ileum: *ileo*cecal
	reproduction:	ilio-	ilium or flank: *ilio*pubic
	*genito*crural	im- or in-	in, within, into:
geno-	reproduction or sex:		*im*mersion,
	*geno*type		*in*jection
-glia	glue: neuro*glia*	infra-	beneath, below:
gloss(o)-	tongue: *gloss*itis,		*infra*clavicular
	*glosso*dynia	inter-	occurring between:
glyc-	sweet: *glyc*emia		*inter*capillary
-gram	write, record:	intra-	occurring within:
	encephalo*gram*		*intra*nasal
-graph	scratch, write, record:	ischio-	hip, haunch:
	cardio*graph*		*ischio*pubic

ischo-	suppressed: *ischo*gyria		
-ism	state, condition, or fact		
	of being: magnet*ism*		
-ites	dropsy: tympan*ites*		
-itis	inflammation: arthr*itis*		
jejuno-	jejunum: *jejuno*ileal		
juxta-	near, close by,		
	adjoining: *juxta*position		
labio-	lip: *labio*gingival		
laparo-	flank, loin:		
	*laparo*gastroscopy		
laryng(o)-	larynx, windpipe:		
	*laryng*itis, *laryngo*cele		
leuc(o)- or	white: *leuk*emia,		
leuk(o)-	*leuko*blast		
levo-	left: *levo*cardia		
lien(o)-	spleen: *lien*ectomy,		
	*lieno*pancreatic		
lig-	tie, bind: *lig*ation		
linguo-	tongue: *linguo*cervical		
lipo-	relationship to fat or		
	lipids: *lipo*adenoma		
litho-	stone or calculus:		
	*litho*nephritis		
-lith	concretion or calculus:		
	phlebo*lith*		
loco-	place: *loco*motor		
logo-	speech, words:		
	*logo*rrhea		
lymph(o)-	water: *lymph*adenosis,		
	*lympho*matosis		
lyso-	dissolution, lysis:		
	*lyso*staphin		
lysso-	rabies: *lysso*dexis		
macro-	large, long, of abnormal		
	size: *macro*blast		
mal-	ill, bad: *mal*adjustment		
mammo-	breast, mammary gland:		
	*mammo*gram		
mast(o)-	breast or mastoid		
	process: *mast*adenoma,		
	*masto*plasia		
mega-	big, great:		
	*mega*cephalic		
megal(o)-	great size:		
	*megal*erythema,		
	*megalo*blast		
-megaly	enlargement:		
	spleno*megaly*		
meio-	small, decreasing:		
	*meio*sis		
meningo-	membrane: *meningo*cele		
meno-	menses: *meno*rrhagia		
mento-	chin: *mento*labial		
mero-	part, one of similar		
	parts: *mero*diastolic		
meso-	middle, medium,		
	moderate: *meso*cardium		
meta-	change or		
	transformation, beyond,		
	over: *meta*basis		
metra-,	uterus: *metra*tonia,		
metro-	*metro*malacia		
micr(o)-	small size:		

	*micr*encephalon, *micro*biology
mio-	smaller, less: *mio*pragia
mogi-	difficult: *mogi*phonia
mono-	one or single, limited to one part: *mono*clonal
-morph	form or shape: *meso*morph
muco-	mucus: *muco*lipidosis
multi-	many: *multi*cellular
myc-, mycet-, myco- -myces	fungus: *myc*elium, *myce*toma, *myco*phage, fungus: myelo*myces*
myel(o)-	marrow: *myel*itis, *myelo*cyte
my(o)-	muscle: *my*itis, *myo*blast
myria-	a great number: *myria*pod
myx(o)-	mucus or slime: *myx*adenoma, *myxo*cystitis
naso-	nose: *naso*lacrimal
necro-	death: *necro*lysis
neo-	new or strange: *neo*genesis
nephelo-	cloudiness or mistiness: *nephelo*pia
nephr(o)-	kidney: *nephr*itis, *nephro*megaly
neur(o)-	a nerve or the nervous system: *neur*algia, *neuro*cytoma
nitro-	presence of the group —NO_2: *nitro*benzene
noto-	the back: *noto*chord
ob-	against, in front of, toward: *ob*elion
octa-, octi-, octo-	eight: *octa*decanoate, *octi*para, *octo*genarian
oculo-	the eye: *oculo*facial
odonto-	tooth or teeth: *odonto*genesis
-ology	a science or branch of knowledge: radi*ology*
-oma	tumor or neoplasm: carcin*oma*
onco-	tumor, swelling, or mass: *onco*lysis
oophor(o)-	ovary: *oophor*algia, *oophoro*salpingitis
ophthalm(o)-	the eye: *ophthalm*algia, *ophthalmo*plegia
orchi-, orchido-, orchio-	the testes: *orchi*dic, *orchido*ptosis, *orchio*cele
oro-	mouth: *oro*lingual
orrho-	serum: *orrho*meningitis
ortho-	straight, normal, correct: *ortho*gnathia
-osis	a disease or morbid process: scler*osis*

osteo-	bone or bones: *osteo*arthritis
-ostomy	mouth or opening: gastroenter*ostomy*
ot(o)-	ear: *ot*itis, *oto*laryngology
-otomy	surgical incision: cholecyst*otomy*
ovi-, ovo-	egg or ova: *ovi*gerous, *ovo*testis
oxy-	sharp, quick, or sour: *oxy*chloride
pachy-	thick: *pachy*onychia
pan-	all: *pan*arthritis
para-	beside, beyond, accessory to: *para*thyroid
patho-	disease: *patho*genesis
-pathy	morbid condition or disease: cardio*pathy*
-penia	poverty, need, reduction in number: leuko*penia*
peri-	around, near: *peri*cystitis
-petal	directed, moving toward a center: cortici*petal*
-pexy	fixing, putting together: entero*pexy*
phaco-	lentil-shaped object: *phaco*glaucoma
-phagia, phagy	perversion of appetite: aero*phagia*, aero*phagy*
pharmaco-	relation to drug or medicine: *pharmaco*logic
phleb(o)-	vein or veins: *phleb*itis, *phlebo*pexy
phon(o)-	voice, sound: *phon*ation, *phono*cardiogram
phot(o)-	relationship to light: *phot*esthesis, *photo*allergic
phren(o)-	diaphragm or mind: *phren*algia, *phreno*hepatic
physio-	nature: *physio*nomy
physo-	air or gas: *physo*cephaly
phyto-	plant or plants: *phyto*chrome
picro-	bitter: *picro*geusia
-piesis	pressure: oto*piesis*
plasmo-	plasma or substance of a cell: *plasmo*cyte
-plasty	shaping or surgical formation: peritoneo*plasty*
platy-	broad or flat: *platy*coria
-plegia	paralysis, stroke: para*plegia*
pleur(o)-	pleura, rib: *pleur*isy, *pleuro*dynia

-plexy	stroke or seizure: apo*plexy*
pluri-	several, more: *pluri*visceral
-pnea	breathing: ortho*pnea*
pneuma-, pneumato-	air, gas, or respiration: *pneuma*tic, *pneumato*dyspnea
pod-, podo-	foot: *pod*iatry, *podo*dynia
polio-	relationship to gray matter: *polio*dystrophy
poly-	many, much: *poly*articular
post-	after: *post*partum
pre-	before: *pre*natal
pro-	forward, in front of, or precursor: *pro*collagen
proct(o)-	rectum: *proct*itis, *procto*scope
proso-	forward, anterior: *proso*palgia
prosopo-	relationship to the face: *prosopo*plegic
prostat(o)-	prostate: *prostat*ic, *prostato*cystitis
psammo-	sand or sandlike: *psammo*sarcoma
pseud(o)-	false or spurious: *pseud*albuminuria, *pseudo*bulbar
psych(o)-	psyche, mind: *psych*iatric, *psycho*motor
-ptosis	downward displacement: cardio*ptosis*
pyel(o)-	pelvis, usually the renal pelves: *pyel*itis, *pyelo*nephritis
pyloro-	pylorus: *pyloro*plasty
py(o)-	pus: *py*uria, *pyo*nephrosis
quadri-	four, fourfold: *quadri*plegia
rachi(o)-	spine: *rachi*algia, *rachio*myelitis
radio-	ray or radiation: *radio*plastic
re-	back, again: *re*activation
retro-	backward, located behind: *retro*sternal
-rhage	breaking, bursting forth: hemor*rhage*
-rhaphy	joining in a seam, suture of a part: blepharor*rhaphy*
-rhea	flow: gonor*rhea*
rheo-	relationship to electric current, flow: *rheo*stat

rhin(o)-	nose: *rhin*encephalon, *rhino*plasty	spondyl(o)-	vertebra, or spinal column: *spondyl*algia, *spondylo*desis
rhizo-	root: *rhizo*meningomyelitis	staphyl(o)-	resemblance to a bunch of grapes: *staphyl*edema, *staphylo*coccus
rhodo-	red: *rhodo*phylaxis		
sacro-	sacrum: *sacro*iliac		
salpingo-	relationship to a tube, uterine or auditory: *salpingo*cele	stearo-, steato-	fat: *stearo*pten, *steato*lytic
sangui-	blood: *sangui*neous	stereo-	solid, three dimensional: *stereo*cineflurography
sarco-	flesh: *sarco*matoid		
scapho-	boat-shaped: *scapho*cephalic	steth(o)-	chest: *steth*algia, *stetho*scope
scato-	fecal matter: *scato*scopy	stomato-	mouth or ostium uteri: *stomato*gastric
schizo-	divided, division: *schizo*phrenia		
scirrho-	hard cancer or scirrhous carcinoma: *scirrho*phthalmia	-stomy	surgical creation of an artifical opening: gastroentero*stomy*
sclero-	hard: *sclero*derma	streph(o)-	twisted: *streph*enopodia, *strepho*symbolia
scolio-	twisted, crooked: *scolio*sis		
-scope	instrument for examining: sigmoido*scope*	strepto-	twisted: *strepto*coccus
		stylo-	stake, pole: *stylo*mastoid
-scopy	act of examining: procto*scopy*	sub-	under, near, almost: *sub*dural
semi-	one half, partly: *semi*membranous	sulfo-	indicating presence of a divalent sulfur: *sulfo*namide
sial(o)-	saliva, salivary glands: *sial*adenosis, *sialo*lithiasis	super-	above or in excess: *super*genual, *super*numerary
sidero-	iron: *sidero*blast	syndesmo-	connective tissue or ligaments: *syndesmo*rrhaphy
sinistro-	left, left side: *sinistro*cerebral		
skia-	shadows by roentgen rays: *skia*scopy	tachy-	swift, rapid: *tachy*cardia
spasmo-	spasm: *spasmo*lysant	tarso-	edge of eyelid; instep of the foot: *tarso*cheiloplasty, *tarso*clasis
spermato-, spermo-	seed, specifically male: *spermato*cele, *spermo*lith		
		tauto-	same: *tauto*meral
spheno-	wedge-shaped: *spheno*temporal	tele-	end, distance, far away: *tele*fluoroscopy
spir(o)-	coil, spiral; breath or breathing: *spir*adenoma, *spiro*graphy	telo-	end: *telo*dendron
		teno-, tenonto-	tendon: *teno*nitis, *tenonto*plasty
splen(o)-	spleen: *splen*emia, *spleno*renal	tera-	three, threefold: *tera*curie

tetra-	four: *tetra*chirus
therm(o)-	heat: *therm*algia, *thermo*dynamics
thio-	sulfur: *thio*cyanate
thoraco-	chest: *thoraco*stenosis
-thrix	hair: endo*thrix*
thyro-	thyroid gland: *thyro*cele
toco-	childbirth or labor: *toco*graphy
tomo-	cutting, slicing: *tomo*graphy
-tomy	cutting, incising: colo*tomy*
tono-	tone, tension: *tono*graphy
toxo-	toxin, poison: *toxo*plasmosis
tracheo-	trachea: *tracheo*bronchitis
trans-	through, across, beyond: *trans*duction
tri-	three, thrice: *tri*angular
tropho-	food or nourishment: *tropho*chromidia
-tropin	affinity for structure or thing denoted by stem: gonado*tropin*
typhlo-	cecum: *typhlo*colitis
ulo-	gingivae: *ulo*rrhagia
ultra-	excess, beyond: *ultra*sonogram
uni-	one: *uni*locular
urethro-	urethra: *urethro*cele
-uria	urine: olig*uria*
ur-, uro-, urono-	urine, urinary tract, urination: *ur*inate, *uro*bilinuria, *urono*phile
varico-	twisted and swollen: *varico*cele
ventro-	pertaining to the belly or located anteriorly: *ventro*inguinal, *ventro*dorsal
vivi-	life: *vivi*fication
xeno-	strange, foreign: *xeno*phthalmia
xero-	dryness: *xero*derma

Laboratory Values of Clinical Importance*

*From Rakel, R. E. (ed.). *Conn's Current Therapy 1992.* W. B. Saunders Company, Philadelphia, 1992.

method of
REX B. CONN, M.D.
Thomas Jefferson University
Philadelphia, Pennsylvania

Reference values for laboratory tests serve as indispensible benchmarks when evaluating laboratory data on an individual patient. However, reference values should not be considered equivalent to normal values, because in medicine it is a logical impossibility to define normality. There can be no sharp dividing line between normal and abnormal values, and there is a gradual transition during any pathologic process from what is clearly normal to a value that is clearly abnormal.

Reference values are derived from statistical studies on subjects believed to have no condition that might affect the measurement being evaluated. An important consideration is that the reference ranges derived by these statistical methods encompass only 95% of the reference population. Thus, a value slightly outside the range might be due to a chance distribution or to an underlying pathologic process.

A single reference range for all individuals may be inadequate for some measurements. Values obtained on presumably normal persons may vary because of age, sex, body build, race, environment, and state of gastrointestinal absorption. Another consideration is that values for some constituents found in a "normal" population may reflect a general disorder in the population rather than normality. Thus, reference values for serum cholesterol level now indicate the "desirable" range rather than that actually found in the reference population.

Tables of reference values must be revised and updated frequently to reflect the addition of new tests, the deletion of obsolete tests, and changes in techniques used in the clinical laboratory. As with many other aspects of medicine, widespread use of computers has both simplified and complicated application of reference ranges. Most laboratory computer systems permit use of as many as one or two dozen age- and sex-corrected ranges for each constituent, and the appropriate range is indicated on each patient's report. Serum alkaline phosphatase determination is an example of a test in which the values change dramatically with age and differ between sexes. The computer handles this well, but one can imagine how the following tables would appear if up to a dozen ranges were included for each test listed.

THE INTERNATIONAL SYSTEM OF UNITS FOR LABORATORY MEASUREMENTS (LE SYSTÈME INTERNATIONAL D'UNITÉS)

The United States is the only major industrialized country that has not adopted the International System of Units (abbreviated SI units) for expressing measurements in all areas of science and industry. The medical profession in the United States has been remarkably firm in its opposition to introduction of SI units, even though many American medical journals express laboratory data only in SI units. A much more significant change occurred some 35 years ago when the apothecaries' system was abandoned in favor of the metric system for expressing drug dosages, and it appears to be only a matter of time until the International System is adopted. Because of this, the following information on SI units is being reprinted from *Current Therapy 1991.*

The International System is a coherent approach to all types of measurement that uses seven dimensionally independent basic quantities: mass, length, time, thermodynamic temperature, electrical current, luminous intensity, and amount of substance. Each of these quantities is expressed in a clearly defined *base unit* (Table 1).

Two or more base units may be combined to provide *derived units* (Table 2) for expressing other measurements such as mass concentration (kilograms per cubic meter) and velocity (meters per second). Standardized prefixes (Table 3) for base and derived units are used to express fractions or multiples of the base units so that any measurement can be expressed in a value between 0.001 and 1000.

Medical Applications

The most profound change in laboratory reports will result from expressing concentration as amount per volume (moles per liter) rather than mass per volume (milligrams per 100 mil-

TABLE 1. BASE UNITS

PROPERTY	BASE UNIT	SYMBOL
Length	meter	m
Mass	kilogram	kg
Amount of substance	mole	mol
Time	second	s
Thermodynamic temperature	kelvin	K
Electrical current	ampere	A
Luminous intensity	candela	cd

TABLE 2. DERIVED UNITS

DERIVED PROPERTY	DERIVED UNIT	SYMBOL
Area	square meter	m^2
Volume	cubic meter	m^3
	liter	L
Mass concentration	kilogram/cubic meter	kg/m^3
	gram/liter	g/L
Substance concentration	mole/cubic meter	mol/m^3
	mole/liter	mol/L
Temperature	degree Celsius	C = K − 273.15

liliters). The advantages of the former expression can be seen in the following:

Conventional Units

1.0 gram of hemoglobin
Combines with 1.37 ml of oxygen
Contains 3.4 mg of iron
Forms 34.9 mg of bilirubin

SI Units

1.0 mmol of hemoglobin
Combines with 4.0 mmol of oxygen
Contains 4.0 mmol of iron
Forms 4.0 mmol of bilirubin

Chemical relationships between lactic acid and pyruvic acid and the glucose from which both are derived, as well as the relationship between bilirubin and the binding capacity of albumin, are other examples of chemical relationships that will be clarified by using the new system.

There are a number of laboratory and other medical measurements for which the SI units appear to offer little advantage, and some that are disadvantageous because the change would require replacement or revision of instruments such as the sphygmomanometer. The cubic meter is the derived unit for volume; however it is inappropriately large for medical measure-

TABLE 3. STANDARD PREFIXES

PREFIX	MULTIPLICATION FACTOR	SYMBOL
atto	10^{-13}	a
femto	10^{-15}	f
pico	10^{-12}	p
nano	10^{-9}	n
micro	10^{-6}	μ
milli	10^{-3}	m
centi	10^{-2}	c
deci	10^{-1}	d
deca	10^{1}	da
hecto	10^{2}	h
kilo	10^{3}	k
mega	10^{6}	M
giga	10^{9}	G
tera	10^{12}	T

ments, and the liter has been retained. Thermodynamic temperature expressed in kelvins is not more informative for medical measurements. Since the Celsius degree is the same as the Kelvin degree, the Celsius scale is used. Celsius rather than centigrade is the preferred term.

Selection of units for expressing enzyme activity presents certain difficulties. Literally dozens of different units have been used in expressing enzyme activity, and interlaboratory comparison of enzyme results is impossible unless the assay system is precisely defined. In 1964, the International Union of Biochemistry attempted to remedy the situation by proposing the International Unit for enzymes. This unit was defined as the amount of enzyme that will catalyze the conversion of 1 μmol of substrate per minute under standard conditions. Difficulties remain, however, as enzyme activity is affected by temperature, pH, the type and amount of substrate, the presence of inhibitors, and other factors. Enzyme activity can be expressed in SI units, and the katal has been proposed to express activities of all catalysts, including enzymes. The katal is that amount of enzyme that catalyzes a reaction rate of 1 mol per second. Thus, adoption of the katal as the unit of enzyme activity would provide no more information than is obtained when results are expressed in International Units.

Hydrogen ion concentration in blood is customarily expressed as pH, but in SI units it would be expressed in nanomoles per liter. It appears unlikely that the very useful pH scale will be discarded.

Pressure measures, such as blood pressure and partial pressures of blood gases, would be expressed in SI units using the pascal, a unit that can be derived from the base units for mass, length, and time. This change probably will not be adopted in the early phases of the conversion to SI units. Similarly, a proposed change in expressing osmolality in terms of the depression of freezing point is inappropriate, because osmolality may be calculated from vapor pressure as well as freezing point measurement.

In the following tables, reference ranges for the most commonly used diagnostic tests are given in conventional units and in SI units. The conversion of weight per volume (conventional units) to amount per volume (SI units) is based on the molecular weight of the analyte. For heterogeneous analytes, for example, gamma globulins, weight per volume must be retained as the unit; however, volume is expressed as the liter rather than as the deciliter as in conventional units. Weight per volume is retained for albumin, to be consistent with the other serum proteins. Hemoglobin is expressed here in SI units as the tetramer; in some countries it is expressed as the monomer, in which case the numerical values in SI units are four times as great as those shown. Plasma drug concentrations for therapeutic monitoring are not given in SI units, since it is unlikely that pharmaceutical manufacturers will change to molar quantities for expressing drug dosages.

Reference Values in Hematology

		Conventional Units	SI Units
Acid hemolysis test (Ham)		No hemolysis	No hemolysis
Alkaline phosphatase, leukocyte		Total score 14–100	Total score 14–100
Cell counts			
Erythrocytes			
Males		4.6–6.2 million/mm³	4.6–6.2×10^{12}/L
Females		4.2–5.4 million/mm³	4.2–5.4×10^{12}/L
Children (varies with age)		4.5–5.1 million/mm³	4.5–5.1×10^{12}/L
Leukocytes			
Total		4500–11,000 mm³	4.5–11.0×10^{9}/L
Differential	*Percentage*	*Absolute*	*Absolute*
Myelocytes	0	0/mm³	0/L
Band neutrophils	3–5	150–400/mm³	150–400×10^{6}/L
Segmented neutrophils	54–62	3000–5800/mm³	3000–5800×10^{6}/L
Lymphocytes	25–33	1500–3000/mm³	1500–3000×10^{6}/L
Monocytes	3–7	300–500/mm³	300–500×10^{6}/L
Eosinophils	1–3	50–250/mm³	50–250×10^{6}/L
Basophils	0–0.75	15–50/mm³	15–50×10^{6}/L
Platelets		150,000–350,000/mm³	150–350×10^{9}/L
Reticulocytes		25,000–75,000/mm³	25–75×10^{9}/L
		0.5–1.5% of erythrocytes	
Coagulation tests			
Bleeding time (template)		2.75–8.0 min	2.75–8.0 min
Coagulation time (glass tubes)		5–15 min	5–15 min
Factor VIII and other coagulation factors		50–150% of normal	0.5–1.5 of normal
Fibrin split products (Thrombo-Welco test)		<10 µg/mL	<10 mg/L
Fibrinogen		200–400 mg/dL	2.0–4.0 g/L
Partial thromboplastin time (PTT)		20–35 sec	20–35 s
Prothrombin time (PT)		12.0–14.0 sec	12.0–14.0 s
Coombs' test			
Direct		Negative	Negative
Indirect		Negative	Negative
Corpuscular values of erythrocytes			
Mean corpuscular hemoglobin (MCH)		26–34 pg	0.40–0.53 fmol
Mean corpuscular volume (MCV)		80–96 µm³	80–96 fL
Mean corpuscular hemoglobin concentration (MCHC)		32–36%	0.32–0.36
Haptoglobin		26–185 mg/dL	260–1850 mg/L
Hematocrit			
Males		40–54 mL/dL	0.40–0.54 volume fraction
Females		37–47 mL/dL	0.37–0.47 volume fraction
Newborns		49–54 mL/dL	0.49–0.54 volume fraction
Children (varies with age)		35–49 mL/dL	0.35–0.49 volume fraction
Hemoglobin			
Males		14.0–18.0 gm/dL	2.17–2.79 mmol/L
Females		12.0–16.0 gm/dL	1.86–2.48 mmol/L
Newborns		16.5–19.5 gm/dL	2.56–3.02 mmol/L
Children (varies with age)		11.2–16.5 gm/dL	1.74–2.56 mmol/L
Hemoglobin, fetal		<1.0% of total	<0.01 of total
Hemoglobin A_{1C}		3–5% of total	0.03–0.05 of total
Hemoglobin A_2		1.5–3.0% of total	0.015–0.03 of total
Hemoglobin, plasma		0–5.0 mg/dL	0–0.8 µmol/L
Methemoglobin		30–130 mg/dL	4.7–20 µmol/L
Sedimentation rate (ESR)			
Wintrobe: Males		0–5 mm/hr	0–5 mm/h
Females		0–15 mm/hr	0–15 mm/h
Westergren: Males		0–15 mm/hr	0–15 mm/h
Females		0–20 mm/hr	0–20 mm/h

Reference Values for Blood, Plasma, and Serum
(For some procedures the reference values may vary depending on the method used)

	Conventional Units	SI Units
Acetoacetate plus acetone, serum		
Qualitative	Negative	Negative
Quantitative	0.3–2.0 mg/dL	3–20 mg/L
Acid phosphatase (thymolphthalein monophosphate substrate), serum	0.11–0.60 U/L	0.11–0.60 U/L
Adrenocorticotropin (ACTH), plasma		
6 a.m.	10–80 pg/mL	10–80 ng/L
6 p.m.	<50 pg/mL	<50 ng/L
Alanine aminotransferase (ALT, SGPT), serum	5–30 U/L	5–30 U/L
Albumin, serum	3.5–5.5 gm/dL	35–55 g/L
Aldolase, serum	1.5–12.0 U/L	1.5–12.0 U/L
Aldosterone, plasma		
Supine	3–10 ng/dL	0.08–0.30 nmol/L
Standing		
Males	6–22 ng/dL	0.17–0.61 nmol/L
Females	5–30 ng/dL	0.14–0.83 nmol/L
Alkaline phosphatase (ALP), serum	20–90 U/L (30° C)	20–90 U/L (30° C)
Ammonia nitrogen, plasma	15–49 μg/dL	11–35 μmol/L
Amylase, serum	25–125 U/L	25–125 U/L
Anion gap	8–16 mEq/L	8–16 mmol/L
Ascorbic acid, blood	0.4–1.5 mg/dL	23–85 μmol/L
Aspartate aminotransferase (AST, SGOT), serum	10–30 U/L	10–30 U/L
Base excess, blood	0 ± 2 mEq/L	0 ± 2 mmol/L
Bicarbonate		
Venous plasma	23–29 mEq/L	23–29 mmol/L
Arterial blood	18–23 mEq/L	18–23 mmol/L
Bile acids, serum	0.3–3.0 mg/dL	3–30 mg/L
Bilirubin, serum		
Conjugated	0.1–0.4 mg/dL	1.7–6.8 μmol/L
Unconjugated	0.2–0.7 mg/dL	3.4–12 μmol/L
Total	0.3–1.1 mg/dL	5.1–19 μmol/L
Calcium, serum	9.0–11.0 mg/dL	2.25–2.75 mmol/L
Calcium, ionized, serum	4.25–5.25 mg/dL	1.05–1.30 mmol/L
Carbon dioxide, total, serum or plasma	24–30 mEq/L	24–30 mmol/L
Carbon dioxide tension (P_{CO_2}), blood	35–45 mmHg	35–45 mmHg
β-Carotene, serum	40–200 μg/dL	0.74–3.72 μmol/L
Ceruloplasmin, serum	23–44 mg/dL	230–44 mg/L
Chloride, serum or plasma	96–106 mEq/L	96–106 mmol/L
Cholesterol, serum or EDTA plasma		
Desirable range	<200 mg/dL	<5.18 mmol/L
LDL cholesterol	60–180 mg/dL	600–1800 mg/L
HDL cholesterol	30–80 mg/dL	300–800 mg/L
Copper		
Males	70–140 μg/dL	11–22 μmol/L
Females	85–155 μg/dL	13–24 μmol/L
Cortisol, plasma		
8 A.M.	6–23 μg/dL	170–635 nmol/L
4 P.M.	3–15 μg/dL	82–413 nmol/L
10 P.M.	<50% of 8 A.M. value	<0.5 of 8 A.M. value
Creatine, serum	0.2–0.8 mg/dL	15–61 μmol/L
Creatine kinase (CK, CPK), serum		
Males	55–170 U/L	55–170 U/L
Females	30–135 U/L	30–135 U/L
Creatine kinase MB isozyme, serum	0.0–4.7 ng/mL	0.0–4.7 μg/L
Creatinine, serum	0.6–1.2 mg/dL	53–106 μmol/L
Ferritin, serum	20–200 ng/mL	20–200 μg/L
Fibrinogen, plasma	200–400 mg/dL	2.0–4.0 g/L
Folate, serum	1.8–9.0 ng/mL	4.1–20.4 nmol/L
Erythrocytes	150–450 ng/mL	340–1020 nmol/L
Follicle-stimulating hormone (FSH), plasma		
Males	4–25 mU/mL	4–25 U/L
Females	4–30 mU/mL	4–30 U/L
Postmenopausal	40–250 mU/mL	40–250 U/L
γ-Glutamyltransferase, serum		
Males	5–38 U/L	5–38 U/L
Females	5–29 U/L	5–29 U/L
Gastrin, serum	0–200 pg/mL	0–200 ng/L

Reference Values for Blood, Plasma, and Serum *Continued*
(For some procedures the reference values may vary depending on the method used)

	Conventional Units	SI Units
Glucose (fasting), plasma or serum	70–115 mg/dL	3.89–6.38 mmol/L
Growth hormone (hGH), plasma	0–10 ng/mL	0–10 µg/L
Haptoglobin, serum	26–185 mg/dL	260–1850 mg/L
Immunoglobulins, serum		
IgG	550–1900 mg/dL	5.5–19.0 g/L
IgA	60–333 mg/dL	0.60–3.3 g/L
IgM	45–145 mg/dL	0.45–1.5 g/L
IgD	0.5–3.0 mg/dL	5–30 mg/L
IgE	<500 ng/mL	<500 µg/L
Insulin (fasting), plasma	5–25 µU/mL	36–179 pmol/L
Iron, serum	75–175 µg/dL	13–31 µmol/L
Iron binding capacity, serum		
Total	250–410 µg/dL	45–73 µmol/L
Saturation	20–55%	0.20–0.55
Lactate		
Venous blood	4.5–19.8 mg/dL	0.50–2.2 mmol/L
Arterial blood	4.5–14.4 mg/dL	0.50–1.6 mmol/L
Lactate dehydrogenase (LD, LDH), serum	100–190 U/L	100–190 U/L
Lipase, serum	10–140 U/L	10–140 U/L
Lipids, total, serum	450–850 mg/dL	4.5–8.5 g/L
Luteinizing (LH), serum		
Males	6–18 IU/L	6–18 U/L
Females		
Premenopausal	5–22 IU/L	5–22 U/L
Mid-cycle	3 times baseline	3 times baseline
Postmenopausal	>30 IU/L	>30 U/L
Magnesium, serum	1.8–3.0 mg/dL	0.75–1.25 mmol/L
Osmolality	286–295 mOsm/kg water	285–295 mmol/kg water
Oxygen, blood		
Capacity (varies with hemoglobin)	16–24 vol %	7.14–10.7 mmol/L
Content, arterial	15–23 vol %	6.69–10.3 mmol/L
Saturation, arterial	94–100 %	0.94–1.00
Oxygen tension (P_{O_2}), blood	75–100 mmHg	75–100 mmHg
P_{50}	26–27 mmHg	26–27 mmHg
pH, arterial blood	7.35–7.45	7.35–7.45
Phenylalanine, serum	<3 mg/dL	<0.18 mmol/L
Phosphate, inorganic, serum	3.0–4.5 mg/dL	1.0–1.5 mmol/L
Potassium, serum or plasma	3.5–5.0 mEq/L	3.5–5.0 mmol/L
Prolactin		
Males	1–20 ng/mL	1–20 µg/L
Females	1–25 ng/mL	1–25 µg/L
Protein, serum		
Total	6.0–8.0 gm/dL	60–80 g/L
Albumin	3.5–5.5 gm/dL	35–55 g/L
Alpha$_1$ globulin	0.2–0.4 gm/dL	2–4 g/L
Alpha$_2$ globulin	0.5–0.9 gm/dL	5–9 g/L
Beta globulin	0.6–1.1 gm/dL	6–11 g/L
Gamma globulin	0.7–1.7 gm/dL	7–17 g/L
Pyruvate, blood	0.3–0.9 mg/dL	0.03–0.10 mmol/L
Sodium, serum or plasma	136–145 mEq/L	136–145 mmol/L
Testosterone, plasma		
Males	275–875 ng/dL	9.5–30 nmol/L
Females	23–75 ng/dL	0.8–2.6 nmol/L
Pregnant	38–190 ng/dL	1.3–6.6 nmol/L
Thyroid-stimulating hormone (TSH), serum	0–7 µU/mL	0–7 mU/L
Thyroxine, free (FT), serum	1.0–2.1 ng/dL	13–27 pmol/L
Thyroxine (T_4), serum	4.4–9.9 µg/dL	57–128 nmol/L
Triglycerides, serum	40–150 mg/dL	0.4–1.5 g/L
Triiodothyronine (T_3), serum	150–250 ng/dL	2.3–3.9 nmol/L
Triiodothyronine uptake, resin (T_3RU)	25–38% uptake	0.25–0.38 uptake
Urate, serum		
Males	2.5–8.0 mg/dL	0.15–0.48 mmol/L
Females	1.5–7.0 mg/dL	0.09–0.42 mmol/L

Reference Values for Blood, Plasma, and Serum *Continued*
(For some procedures the reference values may vary depending on the method used)

	Conventional Units	SI Units
Urea, serum or plasma	24–49 mg/dL	4.0–8.2 mmol/L
Urea nitrogen, serum or plasma	11–23 mg/dL	3.9–8.2 mmol/L
Viscosity, serum	1.4–1.8 times water	1.4–1.8 times water
Vitamin A, serum	20–80 μg/dL	0.70–2.80 μmol/L
Vitamin B_{12}, serum	180–900 pg/mL	133–664 pmol/L

Reference Values for Urine
(For some procedures the reference values may vary depending on the method used)

	Conventional Units	SI Units
Acetone and acetoacetate, qualitative	Negative	Negative
Albumin		
Qualitative	Negative	Negative
Quantitive	10–100 mg/24 hr	0.15–1.5 μmol/24 h
Aldosterone	3–20 μg/24 hr	8.3–55 nmol/24 h
δ-Aminolevulinic acid	1.3–7.0 mg/24 hr	10–53 μmol/24 h
Amylase	3–20 U/hr	3–20 U/h
Amylase/creatinine clearance ratio	1–4%	0.01–0.04
Bilirubin, qualitative	Negative	Negative
Calcium (usual diet)	<250 mg/24 hr	<6.3 mmol/24 h
Catecholamines		
Epinephrine	<10 μg/24 hr	<55 nmol/24 h
Norepinephrine	<100 μg/24 hr	<590 nmol/24 h
Total free catecholamines	4–126 μg/24 hr	24–745 nmol/24 h
Total metanephrines	0.1–1.6 mg/24 hr	0.5–8.1 μmol/24 h
Chloride (varies with intake)	110–250 mEq/24 hr	110–250 mmol/24 h
Copper	0–50 μg/24 hr	0–0.80 μmol/24 h
Cortisol, free	10–100 μg/24 hr	27.6–276 nmol/24 h
Creatinine	15–25 mg/kg body weight/24 hr	0.13–0.22 mmol/kg body weight/24 h
Creatinine clearance (corrected to 1.73 m² body surface area)		
Males	110–150 mL/min	110–150 ml/min
Females	105–132 mL/min	105–132 ml/min
Dehydroepiandrosterone		
Males	0.2–2.0 mg/24 hr	0.7–6.9 μmol/24 h
Females	0.2–1.8 mg/24 hr	0.7–6.2 μmol/24 h
Estrogens, total		
Males	4–25 μg/24 hr	14–90 nmol/24 h
Females	5–100 μg/24 hr	18–360 nmol/24 h
Glucose (as reducing substance)	<250 mg/24 hr	<250 mg/24 h
Hemoglobin and myoglobin, qualitative	Negative	Negative
17-Hydroxycorticosteroids		
Males	3–9 mg/24 hr	8.3–25 μmol/24 h
Females	2–8 mg/24 hr	5.5–22 μmol/24 h
5-Hydroxyindoleacetic acid		
Qualitative	Negative	Negative
Quantitative	<9 mg/24 hr	<47 μmol/24 h
17-Ketosteroids		
Males	6–18 mg/24 hr	21–62 μmol/24 h
Females	4–13 mg/24 hr	14–45 μmol/24 h
Magnesium	6.0–8.5 mEq/24 hr	3.0–4.2 mmol/24 h
Metanephrines (see Catecholamines)		
Osmolality	38–1400 mOsm/kg water	38–1400 mmol/kg water
pH	4.6–8.0	4.6–8.0
Phenylpyruvic acid, qualitative	Negative	Negative
Phosphate	0.9–1.3 grams/24 hr	29–42 mmol/24 h
Porphobilinogen		
Qualitative	Negative	Negative
Quantitative	<2.0 mg/24 hr	<9 μmol/24 h
Porphyrins		
Coproporphyrin	50–250 μg/24 hr	77–380 nmol/24 h
Uroporphyrin	10–30 μg/24 hr	12–36 nmol/24 h
Potassium	25–100 mEq/24 hr	25–100 mmol/24 h

Reference Values for Urine *Continued*
(For some procedures the reference values may vary depending on the method used)

	Conventional Units	SI Units
Pregnanediol		
Males	0.4–1.4 mg/24 hr	1.2–4.4 μmol/24 h
Females		
Proliferative phase	0.5–1.5 mg/24 hr	1.6–4.7 μmol/24 h
Luteal phase	2.0–7.0 mg/24 hr	6.2–22 μmol/24 h
Postmenopausal	0.2–1.0 mg/24 hr	0.6–3.1 μmol/24 h
Pregnanetriol	<2.5 mg/24 hr	<7.4 μmol/24 h
Protein		
Qualitative	Negative	Negative
Quantitative	10–150 mg/24 hr	10–150 mg/24 h
Sodium	130–260 mEq/24 hr	130–260 mmol/24 h
Specific gravity	1.003–1.030	1.003–1.030
Urate	200–500 mg/24 hr	1.2–3.0 mmol/24 h
Urobilinogen	<4.0 mg/24 hr	<6.8 μmol/24 h
Vanillylmandelic acid (VMA, 4-hydroxy-3-methoxymandelic acid)	1–8 mg/24 hr	5–40 μmol/24 h

Reference Values for Therapeutic Drug Monitoring

	Therapeutic Range	Toxic Levels	Proprietary Names
Antibiotics			
Amikacin, serum	25–30 μg/mL	Peak: >35 μg/mL Trough: >5–7 μg/mL	Amikin
Chloramphenicol, serum	10–20 μg/mL	>25 μg/mL	Chloromycetin
Gentamicin, serum	5–10 μg/mL	Peak: >12 μg/mL Trough: >2 μg/mL	Garamycin
Tobramycin, serum	5–10 μg/mL	Peak: >12 μg/mL Trough: >2 μg/mL	Nebcin
Anticonvulsants			
Carbamazepine, serum	5–12 μg/mL	>12 μg/mL	Tegretol
Ethosuximide, serum	40–100 μg/mL	>100 μg/mL	Zarontin
Phenobarbital, serum	10–30 μg/mL	Vary widely because of developed tolerance	
Phenytoin, serum	10–20 μg/mL	>20 μg/mL	Dilantin
Primidone, serum	5–12 μg/mL	>15 μg/mL	Mysoline
Valproic acid, serum	50–100 μg/mL	>100 μg/mL	Depakene
Analgesics			
Acetaminophen, serum	10–20 μg/mL	>250 μg/mL	Tylenol
Salicylate, serum	100–250 μg/mL	>300 μg/mL	Disalcid
Bronchodilator			
Theophylline (aminophylline), serum	10–20 μg/mL	>20 μg/mL	
Cardiovascular Drugs			
Digitoxin, serum (specimen must be obtained 12–24 hr after last dose)	15–25 ng/mL	>25 ng/ml	Crystodigin
Digoxin, serum (specimen must be obtained 12–24 hr after last dose)	0.8–2.0 ng/mL	>2.4 ng/mL	Lanoxin
Disopyramide, serum	2–5 μg/mL	>5 μg/mL	Norpace
Lidocaine, serum	1.5–5.0 μg/mL	>6–8 μg/mL	Xylocaine
Procainamide, serum (measured as procainamide + *N*-acetylprocainamide)	4–10 μg/mL	>16 μg/mL	Pronestyl
Propranolol, serum	50–100 ng/mL	Variable	Inderal
Quinidine, serum	2–5 μg/mL	>10 μg/mL	Cardioquin Quinaglute Quinidex Quinora
Psychopharmacologic Drugs			
Amitriptyline, serum (measured as amitriptyline + nortriptyline)	120–150 ng/mL	>500 ng/mL	Amitril Elavil Endep Limbitrol Triavil

Reference Values for Therapeutic Drug Monitoring *Continued*

	Therapeutic Range	Toxic Levels	Proprietary Names
Desipramine, serum (measured as desipramine + imipramine)	150–300 ng/mL	>500 ng/mL	Norpramin Pertofrane
Imipramine, serum (measured as imipramine + desipramine)	150–300 ng/mL	>500 ng/mL	Antipress Imavate Janimine Presamine Tofranil
Lithium, serum (obtain specimen 12 hr after last dose)	0.8–1.2 mEq/L	>2.0 mEq/L	Lithobid
Nortriptyline, serum	50–150 ng/mL	>500 ng/mL	Aventyl Pamelor

Reference Values in Toxicology

	Conventional Units	SI Units
Arsenic		
Blood	3.5–7.2 µg/dL	0.47–0.96 µmol/L
Urine	<100 µg/24 hr	<1.3 µmol/24 h
Bromides, serum	0	0
	Toxic: >17 mEq/L	Toxic: >17 mmol/L
Carboxyhemoglobin, blood	<5% saturation	<0.05 saturation
Symptoms occur	>20% saturation	>0.20 saturation
Ethanol, blood	<0.05 mg/dL (<0.005%)	<1.0 mmol/L
Marked intoxication	300–400 mg/dL (0.3–0.4%)	65–87 mmol/L
Alcoholic stupor	400–500 mg/dL (0.4–0.5%)	87–109 mmol/L
Coma	>500 mg/dL (0.5%)	>109 mmol/L
Lead		
Blood	0–40 µg/dL	0–2 µmol/L
Urine	<100 µg/24 hr	<0.48 µmol/24 h
Mercury, urine	<100 µg/24 hr	<50 nmol/24 h

Reference Values for Cerebrospinal Fluid

	Conventional Units	SI Units
Cells	<5/mm³; all mononuclear	<5 × 10⁶/L, all mononuclear
Electrophoresis	Predominantly albumin	Predominantly albumin
Glucose	50–75 mg/dL	2.8–4.2 mmol/L
	(20 mg/dL less than serum)	(1.1 mmol less than serum)
IgG		
Children under 14	<8% of total protein	<0.08 of total protein
Adults	<14% of total protein	<0.14 of total protein
IgG index $\left(\dfrac{\text{CSF/serum IgG ratio}}{\text{CSF/serum albumin ratio}} \right)$	0.3–0.6	0.3–0.6
Oligoclonal banding on electrophoresis	Absent	Absent
Pressure	70–180 mm water	70–180 mm water
Protein, total	15–45 mg/dL	150–450 mg/L

Reference Values for Semen

	Conventional Units	SI Units
Volume	2–5 mL	2–5 mL
Liquefaction	Complete in 15 min	Complete in 15 min
Leukocytes	Occasional or absent	Occasional or absent
Count	60–150 million/mL	60–150 × 10⁶/mL
Motility	>80% motile	>0.80 motile
Morphology	80–90% normal forms	0.80–0.90 normal forms
Fructose	>150 mg/dL	>8.33 mmol/L

Reference Values for Feces

	Conventional Units	SI Units
Bulk	100–200 gm/24 hr	100–200 g/24 h
Dry matter	23–32 gm/24 hr	23–32 g/24 h
Fat, total	<6.0 gm/24 hr	<6.0 g/24 h
Nitrogen, total	<2.0 gm/24 hr	<2.0 g/24 h
Water	Approximately 65%	Approximately 0.65

REFERENCES

1. Brown SS, Mitchell FL, and Young DS (eds): Chemical Diagnosis of Disease. Amsterdam, Elsevier/North-Holland Biomedical Press, 1979.
2. Conn RB (ed): Current Diagnosis. 8th ed. Philadelphia, WB Saunders Co, 1991.
3. Goodman AG, Gilman LS, Rall TW, and Murad F: Goodman and Gilman's The Pharmacological Basis of Therapeutics. 7th ed. New York, Macmillan Co, 1985.
4. Henry JB (ed): Clinical Diagnosis and Management by Laboratory Methods. 18th ed. Philadelphia, WB Saunders Co, 1991.
5. Lundberg GD, Iverson C, and Radulescu G: JAMA *255*:2247, 1986.
6. Miale JB: Laboratory Medicine-Hematology. 6th ed. St. Louis, CV Mosby, 1982.
7. Physicians' Desk Reference. 45th ed. Oradell, NJ, Medical Economics Co, 1991.
8. Tietz NW: Clinical Guide to Laboratory Tests. 2nd ed. Philadelphia, WB Saunders Co, 1990.
9. Tietz NW: Textbook of Clinical Chemistry. Philadelphia, WB Saunders Co, 1986.
10. Williams WJ, Beutler E, Erslev AJ, and Lichtman MA: Hematology. 3rd ed. New York, McGraw-Hill Book Co, 1983.

Some of these values have been established by the Clinical Laboratories at Thomas Jefferson University Hospital, Philadelphia, PA, and have not been published elsewhere.

Tables of Weights and Measures*

MEASURES OF MASS

AVOIRDUPOIS WEIGHT

Grains	Drams	Ounces	Pounds	Metric Equivalents, Grams
1	0.0366	0.0023	0.00014	0.0647989
27.34	1	0.0625	0.0039	1.772
437.5	16	1	0.0625	28.350
7000	256	16	1	453.5924277

APOTHECARIES' WEIGHT

Grains	Scruples ($\ni$)	Drams ($\mathfrak{Z}$)	Ounces ($\mathfrak{Z}$)	Pounds (lb.)	Metric Equivalents, Grams
1	0.05	0.0167	0.0021	0.00017	0.0647989
20	1	0.333	0.042	0.0035	1.296
60	3	1	0.125	0.0104	3.888
480	24	8	1	0.0833	31.103
5760	288	96	12	1	373.24177

TROY WEIGHT

Grains	Pennyweights	Ounces	Pounds	Metric Equivalents, Grams
1	0.042	0.002	0.00017	0.0647989
24	1	0.05	0.0042	1.555
480	20	1	0.083	31.103
5760	240	12	1	373.24177

*From Miller, B. F., and C. B. Keane. *Encyclopedia and Dictionary of Medicine, Nursing, and Allied Health,* 5th edition. W. B. Saunders Company, Philadelphia, 1992, pp. 1664-1668.

METRIC WEIGHT

Micro-gram	Milli-gram	Centi-gram	Deci-gram	Gram	Deka-gram	Hecto-gram	Kilo-gram	Equivalents	
								Avoirdupois	Apothecaries'
1	—	—	—	—	—	—	—	0.000015 grains	
10^3	1	—	—	—	—	—	—	0.015432 grains	
10^4	10	1	—	—	—	—	—	0.154323 grains	
10^5	10^2	10	1	—	—	—	—	1.543235 grains	
10^6	10^3	10^2	10	1	—	—	—	15.432356 grains	
10^7	10^4	10^3	10^2	10	1	—	—	5.6438 dr.	7.7162 scr.
10^8	10^5	10^4	10^3	10^2	10	1	—	3.527 oz.	3.215 oz.
10^9	10^6	10^5	10^4	10^3	10^2	10	1	2.2046 lb.	2.6792 lb.
10^{12}	10^9	10^8	10^7	10^6	10^5	10^4	10^3	2204.6223 lb.	2679.2285 lb.

MEASURES OF CAPACITY

APOTHECARIES' (WINE) MEASURE

Min-ims	Fluid Drams	Fluid Ounces	Gills	Pints	Quarts	Gal-lons	Cubic Inches	Milliliters	Cubic Centimeters
1	0.0166	0.002	0.0005	0.00013	—	—	0.00376	0.06161	0.06161
60	1	0.125	0.0312	0.0078	0.0039	—	0.22558	3.6967	3.6967
480	8	1	0.25	0.0625	0.0312	0.0078	1.80468	29.5737	29.5737
1920	32	4	1	0.25	0.125	0.0312	7.21875	118.2948	118.2948
7680	128	16	4	1	0.5	0.125	28.875	473.179	473.179
15360	256	32	8	2	1	0.25	57.75	946.358	946.358
61440	1024	128	32	8	4	1	231	3785.434	3785.434

METRIC MEASURE

Microliter	Milliliter	Centiliter	Deciliter	Liter	Dekaliter	Hectoliter	Kiloliter	Myrialiter	Equivalents (Apothecaries' Fluid)	
1	—	—	—	—	—	—	—	—	0.01623108	minim
10^3	1	—	—	—	—	—	—	—	16.23	minims
10^4	10	1	—	—	—	—	—	—	2.7	fluid drams
10^5	10^2	10	1	—	—	—	—	—	3.38	fluid ounces
10^6	10^3	10^2	10	1	—	—	—	—	2.11	pints
10^7	10^4	10^3	10^2	10	1	—	—	—	2.64	gallons
10^8	10^5	10^4	10^3	10^2	10	1	—	—	26.418	gallons
10^9	10^6	10^5	10^4	10^3	10^2	10	1	—	264.18	gallons
10^{10}	10^7	10^6	10^5	10^4	10^3	10^2	10	1	2641.8	gallons

1 liter = 2.113363738 pints (Apothecaries').

MEASURES OF LENGTH

METRIC MEASURE

Micrometer	Millimeter	Centimeter	Decimeter	Meter	Dekameter	Hectometer	Kilometer	Myriameter	Megameter	Equivalents	
1	0.001	10^{-4}	—	—	—	—	—	—	—	0.000039	inch
10^3	1	10^{-1}	—	—	—	—	—	—	—	0.03937	inch
10^4	10	1	—	—	—	—	—	—	—	0.3937	inch
10^5	10^2	10	1	—	—	—	—	—	—	3.937	inches
10^6	10^3	10^2	10	1	—	—	—	—	—	39.37	inches
10^7	10^4	10^3	10^2	10	1	—	—	—	—	10.9361	yards
10^8	10^5	10^4	10^3	10^2	10	1	—	—	—	109.3612	yards
10^9	10^6	10^5	10^4	10^3	10^2	10	1	—	—	1093.6121	yards
10^{10}	10^7	10^6	10^5	10^4	10^3	10^2	10	1	—	6.2137	miles
10^{12}	10^9	10^8	10^7	10^6	10^5	10^4	10^3	10^2	1	621.37	miles

CONVERSION TABLES

AVOIRDUPOIS—METRIC WEIGHT	
Ounces	*Grams*
1/16	1.772
1/8	3.544
1/4	7.088
1/2	14.175
1	28.350
2	56.699
3	85.049
4	113.398
5	141.748
6	170.097
7	198.447
8	226.796
9	255.146
10	283.495
11	311.845
12	340.194
13	368.544
14	396.893
15	425.243
16 (1 lb.)	453.59

Pounds		
1 (16 oz.)	453.69	
2	907.18	
3	1360.78	(1.36 kg.)
4	1814.37	(1.81 kg.)
5	2267.96	(2.27 kg.)
6	2721.55	(2.72 kg.)
7	3175.15	(3.18 kg.)
8	3628.74	(3.63 kg.)
9	4082.33	(4.08 kg.)
10	4535.92	(4.54 kg.)

METRIC—AVOIRDUPOIS WEIGHT	
Grams	*Ounces*
0.001 (1 mg.)	0.000035274
1	0.035274
1000 (kg.)	35.274 (2.2046 lb.)

APOTHECARIES'—METRIC LIQUID MEASURE	
Minims	*Milliliters*
1	0.06
2	0.12
3	0.19
4	0.25
5	0.31
10	0.62
15	0.92
20	1.23
25	1.54
30	1.85
35	2.16
40	2.46
45	2.77
50	3.08
55	3.39
60 (1 fl. dr.)	3.70
Fluid Drams	
1	3.70
2	7.39
3	11.09
4	14.79
5	18.48
6	22.18
7	25.88
8 (1 fl. oz.)	29.57
Fluid Ounces	
1	29.57
2	59.15
3	88.72
4	118.29
5	147.87
6	177.44
7	207.01
8	236.58
9	266.16
10	295.73
11	325.30
12	354.88
13	384.45
14	414.02
15	443.59
16 (1 pt.)	473.18
32 (1 qt.)	946.36
128 (1 gal.)	3785.43

METRIC—APOTHECARIES' LIQUID MEASURE

Milliliters	*Minims*	*Milliliters*	*Fluid Drams*	*Milliliters*	*Fluid Ounces*
1	16.231	5	1.35	30	1.01
2	32.5	10	2.71	40	1.35
3	48.7	15	4.06	50	1.69
4	64.9	20	5.4	500	16.91
5	81.1	25	6.76	1000 (1 L.)	33.815
		30	7.1		

APOTHECARIES'—METRIC WEIGHT		METRIC—APOTHECARIES' WEIGHT	
Grains	*Grams*	*Milli-grams*	*Grains*
1/150	0.0004	1	0.015432
1/120	0.0005	2	0.030864
1/100	0.0006	3	0.046296
1/80	0.0008	4	0.061728
1/64	0.001	5	0.077160
1/50	0.0013	6	0.092592
1/48	0.0014	7	0.108024
1/30	0.0022	8	0.123456
1/25	0.0026	9	0.138888
1/16	0.004	10	0.154320
1/12	0.005	15	0.231480
1/10	0.006	20	0.308640
1/9	0.007	25	0.385800
1/8	0.008	30	0.462960
1/7	0.009	35	0.540120
1/6	0.01	40	0.617280
1/5	0.013	45	0.694440
1/4	0.016	50	0.771600
1/3	0.02	100	1.543240
1/2	0.032		
1	0.065	*Grams*	
1 1/2	0.097 (0.1)	0.1	1.5432
2	0.125	0.2	3.0864
3	0.20	0.3	4.6296
4	0.25	0.4	6.1728
5	0.30	0.5	7.7160
6	0.40	0.6	9.2592
7	0.45	0.7	10.8024
8	0.50	0.8	12.3456
9	0.60	0.9	13.8888
10	0.65	1.0	15.4320
15	1.00	1.5	23.1480
20 (1 Э)	1.30	2.0	30.8640
30	2.00	2.5	38.5800
Scruples		3.0	46.2960
1	1.296 (1.3)	3.5	54.0120
2	2.592 (2.6)	4.0	61.728
3 (1Э)	3.888 (3.9)	4.5	69.444
Drams		5.0	77.162
1	3.888	10.0	154.324
2	7.776		
3	11.664		*Equivalents*
4	15.552	10	2.572 drams
5	19.440	15	3.858 drams
6	23.328	20	5.144 drams
7	27.216	25	6.430 drams
8 (1 ℥)	31.103	30	7.716 drams
Ounces		40	1.286 oz.
1	31.103	45	1.447 oz.
2	62.207	50	1.607 oz.
3	93.310	100	3.215 oz.
4	124.414	200	6.430 oz.
5	155.517	300	9.644 oz.
6	186.621	400	12.859 oz.
7	217.724	500	1.34 lb.
8	248.828	600	1.61 lb.
9	279.931	700	1.88 lb.
10	311.035	800	2.14 lb.
11	342.138	900	2.41 lb.
12 (1 lb.)	373.242	1000	2.68 lb.

METRIC DOSES WITH APPROXIMATE APOTHECARY EQUIVALENTS*

These *approximate* dose equivalents represent the quantities usually prescribed, under identical conditions, by physicians trained, respectively, in the metric or in the apothecary system of weights and measures. In labeling dosage forms in both the metric and the apothecary systems, if one is the approximate equivalent of the other, the approximate figure shall be enclosed in parentheses.

When prepared dosage forms such as tablets, capsules, pills, etc., are prescribed in the metric system, the pharmacist may dispense the corresponding *approximate* equivalent in the apothecary system, and vice versa, as indicated in the following table.

Caution—For the conversion of specific quantities in a prescription which requires compounding, or in converting a pharmaceutical formula from one system of weights or measures to the other, *exact* equivalents must be used.

LIQUID MEASURE		LIQUID MEASURE	
Metric	*Approx. Apothecary Equivalents*	*Metric*	*Approx. Apothecary Equivalents*
1000 ml.	1 quart	3 ml.	45 minims
750 ml.	1 1/2 pints	2 ml.	30 minims
500 ml.	1 pint	1 ml.	15 minims
250 ml.	8 fluid ounces	0.75 ml.	12 minims
200 ml.	7 fluid ounces	0.6 ml.	10 minims
100 ml.	3 1/2 fluid ounces	0.5 ml.	8 minims
50 ml.	1 3/4 fluid ounces	0.3 ml.	5 minims
30 ml.	1 fluid ounce	0.25 ml.	4 minims
15 ml.	4 fluid drams	0.2 ml.	3 minims
10 ml.	2 1/2 fluid drams	0.1 ml.	1 1/2 minims
8 ml.	2 fluid drams	0.06 ml.	1 minim
5 ml.	1 1/4 fluid drams	0.05 ml.	3/4 minim
4 ml.	1 fluid dram	0.03 ml.	1/2 minim

WEIGHT		WEIGHT	
Metric	*Approx. Apothecary Equivalents*	*Metric*	*Approx. Apothecary Equivalents*
30 gm.	1 ounce	30 mg.	1/2 grain
15 gm.	4 drams	25 mg.	3/8 grain
10 gm.	2 1/2 drams	20 mg.	1/3 grain
7.5 gm.	2 drams	15 mg.	1/4 grain
6 gm.	90 grains	12 mg.	1/5 grain
5 gm.	75 grains	10 mg.	1/6 grain
4 gm.	60 grains (1 dram)	8 mg.	1/8 grain
3 gm.	45 grains	6 mg.	1/10 grain
2 gm.	30 grains (1/2 dram)	5 mg.	1/12 grain
1.5 gm.	22 grains	4 mg.	1/15 grain
1 gm.	15 grains	3 mg.	1/20 grain
0.75 gm.	12 grains	2 mg.	1/30 grain
0.6 gm.	10 grains	1.5 mg.	1/40 grain
0.5 gm.	7 1/2 grains	1.2 mg.	1/50 grain
0.4 gm.	6 grains	1 mg.	1/60 grain
0.3 gm.	5 grains	0.8 mg.	1/80 grain
0.25 gm.	4 grains	0.6 mg.	1/100 grain
0.2 gm.	3 grains	0.5 mg.	1/120 grain
0.15 gm.	2 1/2 grains	0.4 mg.	1/150 grain
0.12 gm.	2 grains	0.3 mg.	1/200 grain
0.1 gm.	1 1/2 grains	0.25 mg.	1/250 grain
75 mg.	1 1/4 grains	0.2 mg.	1/300 grain
60 mg.	1 grain	0.15 mg.	1/400 grain
50 mg.	3/4 grain	0.12 mg.	1/500 grain
40 mg.	2/3 grain	0.1 mg.	1/600 grain

Note: A milliliter (ml.) is the approximate equivalent of a cubic centimeter (cc.).

*Adopted by the latest Pharmacopeia, National Formulary, and New and Nonofficial Remedies, and approved by the Federal Food and Drug Administration.

Table of Chemical Elements*

*From Miller, B. F., and C. B. Keane. *Encyclopedia and Dictionary of Medicine, Nursing, and Allied Health,* 5th edition. W. B. Saunders Company, Philadelphia, 1992, pp. 1659-1663.

Element (Date of Discovery)	Symbol	Atomic Number	Atomic Weight	Valence	Specific Gravity or Density (*Grams/Liter*)	Descriptive Comment
Actinium (1899)	Ac	89	[227]	3	10.07	radioactive element associated with uranium
Aluminum (1827)	Al	13	26.9815	3	2.6989	silvery-white metal, abundant in earth's crust, but not in free form
Americium (1944)	Am	95	[243]	3, 4, 5, 6	13.67	fourth transuranium element discovered
Antimony (prehistoric)	Sb	51	121.75	3, 5	6.691	exists in 4 allotropic forms
Argon (1894)	Ar	18	39.948	0?	1.7837 g/l	colorless, odorless gas
Arsenic (1250)	As	33	74.9216	3, 5	5.73 / 4.73 / 1.97	(gray) semimetallic solid / (black) / (yellow)
Astatine (1940)	At	85	[210]	1, 3, 5, 7		radioactive halogen
Barium (1808)	Ba	56	137.34	2	3.5	silvery-white, alkaline earth metal
Berkelium (1949)	Bk	97	[247]	3, 4		fifth transuranium element discovered
Beryllium (1798)	Be	4	9.0122	2	1.848	light, steel-gray metal
Bismuth (1753)	Bi	83	208.980	3, 5	9.747	pinkish-white, crystalline, brittle metal
Boron (1808)	B	5	10.811	3	2.34, 2.37	crystalline or amorphous element, not occurring free in nature
Bromine (1826)	Br	35	79.909	1, 3, 5, 7	3.12 / 7.59 g/l	mobile, reddish brown liquid, volatilizing readily / red vapor with disagreeable odor
Cadmium (1817)	Cd	48	112.40	2	8.65	soft, bluish-white metal
Calcium (1808)	Ca	20	40.08	2	1.55	metallic element, forming more than 3 per cent of earth's crust
Californium (1950)	Cf	98	[251]	2, 3		sixth transuranium element discovered
Carbon (prehistoric)	C	6	12.01115	2, 3, 4	1.8–2.1 / 1.9–2.3 / 3.15–3.53	(amorphous) element widely distributed in nature / (graphite) / (diamond)
Cerium (1803)	Ce	58	140.12	3, 4	6.67–8.23	most abundant rare earth metal
Cesium (1869)	Cs	55	132.905	1	1.873	silvery-white, soft, alkaline metal
Chlorine (1774)	Cl	17	35.453	1, 3, 5, 7	3.214 g/l	greenish-yellow gas of the halogen group
Chromium (1797)	Cr	24	51.996	2, 3, 6	7.18–7.20	steel-gray, lustrous, hard metal
Cobalt (1735)	Co	27	58.9332	2, 3	8.9	brittle, hard metal
Copper (prehistoric)	Cu	29	63.54	1, 2	8.96	reddish, lustrous, malleable metal
Curium (1944)	Cm	96	[247]	3, 4	13.51	third transuranium element discovered
Dysprosium (1886)	Dy	66	162.50	3	8.536	rare earth metal with metallic bright silver luster
Einsteinium (1952)	Es	99	[252]	2, 3		seventh transuranium element discovered

ELEMENT (DATE OF DISCOVERY)	SYMBOL	ATOMIC NUMBER	ATOMIC WEIGHT	VALENCE	SPECIFIC GRAVITY OR DENSITY (Grams/Liter)	DESCRIPTIVE COMMENT
Element 106 (1974)		106	[263]			thirteenth transuranium element discovered; no name yet proposed
Erbium (1843)	Er	68	167.26	3	9.051	soft, malleable rare earth metal
Europium (1896)	Eu	63	151.96	2, 3	5.259	lustrous, silvery-white rare earth metal
Fermium (1953)	Fm	100	[257]	2, 3		eighth transuranium element discovered
Fluorine (1771)	F	9	18.9984	1	1.696 g/l	pale yellow, corrosive gas of the halogen group
Francium (1939)	Fr	87	[223]	1		product of alpha disintegration of actinium
Gadolinium (1880)	Gd	64	157.25	3	7.8, 7.895	lustrous, silvery-white rare earth metal
Gallium (1875)	Ga	31	69.72	2, 3	5.907	beautiful, silvery-appearing metal
Germanium (1886)	Ge	32	72.59	2, 4	5.323	grayish-white, brittle metal
Gold (prehistoric)	Au	79	196.967	1, 3	19.32	malleable yellow metal
Hafnium (1923)	Hf	72	178.49	4	13.29	gray metal associated with zirconium
Hahnium (1970) (*Element 105*)	Ha	105	[260]			twelfth transuranium element discovered
Helium (1895)	He	2	4.0026	0	0.177 g/l	inert gas
Holmium (1879)	Ho	67	164.930	3	8.803	relatively soft malleable rare earth metal
Hydrogen (1766)	H	1	1.00797	1	0.08988 g/l 0.070 (liquid)	(gas) most abundant element in the universe
Indium (1863)	In	49	114.82	1, 2?, 3	7.31	soft, silvery-white metal
Iodine (1811)	I	53	126.9044	1, 3, 5, 7	4.93, 11.27 g/l	grayish-black, lustrous solid or violet-blue gas
Iridium (1803)	Ir	77	192.2	3, 4	22.42	white, brittle metal of platinum family
Iron (prehistoric)	Fe	26	55.847	2, 3, 4, 6	7.874	fourth most abundant element in earth's crust
Krypton (1898)	Kr	36	83.80	0	3.733 g/l	inert gas
Lanthanum (1839)	La	57	138.91	3	5.98–6.186	silvery-white, ductile, rare earth metal
Lawrencium (1961)	Lr	103	[260]	3		tenth transuranium element discovered
Lead (prehistoric)	Pb	82	207.19	2, 4	11.35	bluish-white, lustrous, malleable metal
Lithium (1817)	Li	3	6.939	1	0.534	lightest of all metals
Lutetium (1907)	Lu	71	174.97	3	9.872	rare earth metal
Magnesium (1808)	Mg	12	24.312	2	1.738	silvery-white metallic element, eighth in abundance in earth's crust
Manganese (1774)	Mn	25	54.9380	1, 2, 3, 4, 6, 7	7.21–7.44	exists in 4 allotropic forms
Mendelevium (1955)	Md	101	[258]	2, 3		ninth transuranium element discovered
Mercury (prehistoric)	Hg	80	200.59	1, 2	13.546	heavy, silvery-white metal, liquid at ordinary temperatures
Molybdenum (1782)	Mo	42	95.94	2, 3, 4?, 5?, 6	10.22	silvery-white, very hard metal
Neodymium (1885)	Nd	60	144.24	3	6.80, 7.004	exists in 2 allotropic forms
Neon (1898)	Ne	10	20.183	0?	0.89990 g/l	inert gas

Element (Date of Discovery)	Symbol	Atomic Number	Atomic Weight	Valence	Specific Gravity or Density (Grams/Liter)	Descriptive Comment
Neptunium (1940)	Np	93	237.0482	3, 4, 5, 6	20.45	first transuranium element discovered
Nickel (1751)	Ni	28	58.71	0, 1, 2, 3	8.902	silvery-white, malleable metal
Niobium (1801)	Nb	41	92.906	2, 3, 4?, 5	8.57	shiny white, soft ductile metal
Nitrogen (1772)	N	7	14.0067	3, 5	1.2506 g/l	colorless, odorless, inert element, making up 78 per cent of the air
Nobelium (1958)	No	102	[259]	2, 3		acceptance of this element considered premature
Osmium (1803)	Os	76	190.2	2, 3, 4, 8	22.57	bluish-white, hard metal of platinum family
Oxygen (1774)	O	8	15.9994	2	1.429 g/l	colorless, odorless gas, third most abundant element in the universe
Palladium (1803)	Pd	46	106.4	2, 3, 4	12.02	steel-white metal of the platinum family
Phosphorus (1669)	P	15	30.9738	3, 5	1.82 2.20 2.25–2.69	(white) waxy solid, transparent when pure (red) (black)
Platinum (1735)	Pt	78	195.09	1?, 2, 3, 4	21.45	silvery-white, malleable metal
Plutonium (1940)	Pu	94	[244]	3, 4, 5, 6, 7	19.84	second transuranium element discovered
Polonium (1898)	Po	84	[210]	2, 4, 6	9.32	very rare natural element
Potassium (1807)	K	19	39.102	1	0.862	soft, silvery, alkali metal, seventh in abundance in earth's crust
Praseodymium (1885)	Pr	59	140.907	3, 4	6.782, 6.64	soft, silvery rare earth metal
Promethium (1941)	Pm	61	[145]	3	7.22 ± 0.02	produced by irradiation of neodymium and praseodymium; identity established in 1945
Protactinium (1917)	Pa	91	231.0359	4, 5	15.37	bright lustrous metal
Radium (1898)	Ra	88	226.0254	2	5.5	brilliant white, radioactive metal
Radon (1900)	Rn	86	[222]	0	9.73 g/l	heaviest known gas
Rhenium (1925)	Re	75	186.2	−1, 2, 3, 4, 5, 6, 7	21.02	silvery-white lustrous metal
Rhodium (1803)	Rh	45	102.905	−2, 3, 4, 5	12.41	silvery-white metal of platinum family
Rubidium (1861)	Rb	37	85.47	1, 2, 3, 4	1.532	soft, silvery-white, alkali metal
Ruthenium (1844)	Ru	44	101.07	0, 1, 2, 3, 4, 5, 6, 7, 8	12.41	hard white metal of platinum family
Rutherfordium (1969) (*Element 104*)	Rf	104	[261]			eleventh transuranium element discovered
Samarium (1879)	Sm	62	150.35	2, 3	7.52, 7.40	bright silver lustrous metal
Scandium (1879)	Sc	21	44.956	3	2.992	soft, silvery-white metal
Selenium (1817)	Se	34	78.96	2, 4, 6	4.79, 4.28	exists in several allotropic forms
Silicon (1823)	Si	14	28.086	4	2.33	a relatively inert element, second in abundance in earth's crust
Silver (prehistoric)	Ag	47	107.870	1, 2	10.50	malleable, ductile metal with brilliant white luster

Table continued on following page

Element (Date of Discovery)	Symbol	Atomic Number	Atomic Weight	Valence	Specific Gravity or Density (Grams/Liter)	Descriptive Comment
Sodium (1807)	Na	11	22.9898	1	0.971	most abundant of alkali metals, sixth in abundance in earth's crust
Strontium (1808)	Sr	38	87.62	2	2.54	exists in 3 allotropic forms
Sulfur (prehistoric)	S	16	32.064	2, 4, 6	1.957, 2.07	exists in several isotopic and many allotropic forms
Tantalum (1802)	Ta	73	180.948	2?, 3, 4?, 5	16.6	gray, heavy, very hard metal
Technetium (1937)	Tc	43	98.9062	3?, 4, 6, 7	11.50	first element produced artificially
Tellurium (1782)	Te	52	127.60	2, 4, 6	6.24	silvery-white, lustrous element
Terbium (1843)	Tb	65	158.924	3, 4	8.272	silvery-gray, malleable, ductile rare earth metal
Thallium (1861)	Tl	81	204.37	1, 3	11.85	very soft, malleable metal
Thorium (1828)	Th	90	232.038	4	11.66	silvery-white, lustrous metal
Thulium (1879)	Tm	69	168.934	2, 3		least abundant rare earth metal
Tin (prehistoric)	Sn	50	118.69	2, 4	5.75 ... 7.31	(gray) malleable metal existing in 2 or 3 allotropic forms, changing from white to gray on cooling and back to white on warming (white)
Titanium (1791)	Ti	22	47.90	2, 3, 4	4.54	lustrous white metal
Tungsten (1783)	W	74	183.85	2, 3, 4, 5, 6	19.3	steel-gray to tin-white metal
Uranium (1789)	U	92	238.03	3, 4, 5, 6	18.95	heavy, silvery-white metal
Vanadium (1801)	V	23	50.942	2, 3, 4, 5	6.11	bright, white metal
Xenon (1898)	Xe	54	131.30	0?	5.887 g/l	one of the so-called rare or inert gases
Ytterbium (1878)	Yb	70	173.04	2, 3	6.977, 6.54	exists in 2 allotropic forms
Yttrium (1794)	Y	39	88.905	3	4.45	rare earth metal with silvery metallic luster
Zinc (1746)	Zn	30	65.37	2	7.133	bluish-white, lustrous metal, malleable at 100–150°C
Zirconium (1789)	Zr	40	91.22	4	6.4	grayish-white, lustrous metal

*Figures in brackets represent mass number of most stable isotope.

TABLE OF ELEMENTS BY ATOMIC NUMBERS

1 hydrogen	16 sulfur	31 gallium	46 palladium
2 helium	17 chlorine	32 germanium	47 silver
3 lithium	18 argon	33 arsenic	48 cadmium
4 beryllium	19 potassium	34 selenium	49 indium
5 boron	20 calcium	35 bromine	50 tin
6 carbon	21 scandium	36 krypton	51 antimony
7 nitrogen	22 titanium	37 rubidium	52 tellurium
8 oxygen	23 vanadium	38 strontium	53 iodine
9 fluorine	24 chromium	39 yttrium	54 xenon
10 neon	25 manganese	40 zirconium	55 cesium
11 sodium	26 iron	41 niobium	56 barium
12 magnesium	27 cobalt	42 molybdenum	57 lanthanum
13 aluminum	28 nickel	43 technetium	58 cerium
14 silicon	29 copper	44 ruthenium	59 praseodymium
15 phosphorus	30 zinc	45 rhodium	60 neodymium

61 promethium	76 osmium	91 protactinium
62 samarium	77 iridium	92 uranium
63 europium	78 plantinum	93 neptunium
64 gadolinium	79 gold	94 plutonium
65 terbium	80 mercury	95 americium
66 dysprosium	81 thallium	96 curium
67 holmium	82 lead	97 berkelium
68 erbium	83 bismuth	98 californium
69 thulium	84 polonium	99 einsteinium
70 ytterbium	85 astatine	100 fermium
71 lutetium	86 radon	101 mendelevium
72 hafnium	87 francium	102 nobelium
73 tantalum	88 radium	103 lawrencium
74 tungsten	89 actinium	104 rutherfordium
75 rhenium	90 thorium	105 hahnium
		106 element 106

Acronyms for Selected Health Care Organizations, Associations, and Agencies*

AAAA	American Academy of Anesthesiologist's Assistants
AAATP	Association for Anesthesiologist's Assistants Training Program
AAB	American Association of Bioanalysts
AABB	American Association of Blood Banks
AACAHPO	American Association of Certified Allied Health Personnel in Ophthalmology
AACC	American Association for Clinical Chemistry
AACCN	American Association of Critical Care Nurses
AACN	American Association of Colleges of Nursing
AADS	American Association of Dental Schools
AAFP	American Academy of Family Physicians
AAHA	American Academy of Health Administration
AAHC	Association of Academic Health Centers
AAHE	Association for the Advancement of Health Education
AAHP	American Association of Hospital Planners
AAHPER	American Association for Health, Physical Education, and Recreation
AAMA	American Association of Medical Assistants
AAMC	Association of American Medical Colleges
AAMI	Association for the Advancement of Medical Instrumentation
AAMT	American Association for Music Therapy
AAN	American Academy of Neurology
AANA	American Association of Nurse Anesthetists
AAO	American Association of Ophthalmology
AAO	American Association of Orthodontists
AAOHN	American Association of Occupational Health Nurses
AAP	American Academy of Pediatrics
AAPA	American Academy of Physicians Assistants
AAPMR	American Academy of Physical Medicine and Rehabilitation
AARC	American Association for Respiratory Care
AART	American Association for Rehabilitation Therapy
AATA	American Art Therapy Association
AATS	American Association for Thoracic Surgery
ABCP	American Board of Cardiovascular Perfusion
ABNF	Association of Black Nursing Faculty in Higher Education
ACC	American College of Cardiology
ACCP	American College of Chest Physicians
ACEP	American College of Emergency Physicians
ACHA	American College of Hospital Administrators
ACNM	American College of Nurse-Midwives
ACP	American College of Physicians

---

*From Miller, B. F., and C. B. Keane. *Encyclopedia and Dictionary of Medicine, Nursing, and Allied Health*, 5th edition. W. B. Saunders Company, Philadelphia, 1992, pp. 1754–1756.

ACR	American College of Radiology
ACS	American College of Surgeons
ACTA	American Cardiovascular Technologists Association
ACTA	American Corrective Therapy Association
ADA	American Dental Association
ADA	American Dietetic Association
ADAA	American Dental Assistants Association
ADHA	American Dental Hygienists' Association
ADTA	American Dance Therapy Association
AES	American Electroencephalographic Society
AHA	American Hospital Association
AHPA	American Health Planning Association
AIBS	American Institute of Biological Sciences
AIHA	American Industrial Hygiene Association
AIUM	American Institute of Ultrasound in Medicine
AMA	American Medical Association
AMEA	American Medical Electroencephalographic Association
AMI	Association of Medical Illustrators
AmSECT	American Society of Extra-Corporeal Technology
AMT	American Medical Technologists
ANA	American Nurses Association
ANF	American Nurses Foundation
ANRC	American National Red Cross
AOA	American Optometric Association
AOA	American Osteopathic Association
AONE	American Organization of Nurse Executives
AORN	Association of Operating Room Nurses
AOTA	American Occupational Therapy Association
APA	American Podiatry Association
APA	American Psychiatric Association
APA	American Psychological Association
APAP	Association of Physician Assistants Programs
APHA	American Public Health Association
APIC	Association of Practitioners in Infection Control
APTA	American Physical Therapy Association
ARCA	American Rehabilitation Counseling Association
ARN	Association of Rehabilitation Nurses
ASA	American Society of Anesthesiologists
ASAHP	American Society of Allied Health Professionals
ASC	American Society of Cytotechnology
ASCP	American Society of Clinical Pathologists
ASE	American Society of Echocardiography
ASET	American Society of Electroencephalographic Technologists
ASHA	American Speech and Hearing Association
ASIA	American Spinal Injury Association
ASIM	American Society of Internal Medicine
ASM	American Society of Microbiology
ASMT	American Society for Medical Technology
ASNSA	American Society of Nursing Service Administrators
ASPAN	American Association of Post Anesthesia Nurses
ASPH	Association of Schools of Public Health
ASRT	American Society of Radiologic Technologists
AST	Association of Surgical Technologists
ASUTS	American Society of Ultrasound Technical Specialists
ATS	American Thoracic Society
AUPHA	Association of University Programs in Health Administration
AVA	American Vocational Association
AVMA	American Veterinary Medical Association
CAP	College of American Pathologists
CAHEA (AMA)	Committee on Allied Health Education and Accreditation
CDC	Centers for Disease Control
CGFNS	Commission on Graduates of Foreign Nursing Schools
CGNA	Canadian Gerontological Nursing Association
CME(AMA)	Council on Medical Education of the American Medical Association
CNA	Canadian Nurses Association
COEAMRA	Council on Education of the American Medical Record Association
DHHS	Department of Health and Human Services
ENA	Emergency Nurses Association
FDA	Food and Drug Administration
HCFA	Health Care Financing Administration

HRA	Health Resources Administration
HSCA	Health Sciences Communications Association
HSRA	Health Services and Resources Administration
IAET	International Association for Enterostomal Therapy
ISCV	International Society for Cardiovascular Surgery
JCAHO	Joint Commission on the Accreditation of Healthcare Organizations
JCAHPO	Joint Commission on Allied Health Personnel in Ophthalmology
MLA	Medical Library Association
NAACLS	National Accrediting Agency for Clinical Laboratory Science
NAACOG	Nurses Association of the American Association of Obstetrics and Gynecology
NACA	National Advisory Council on Aging—Canadian
NACT	National Alliance of Cardiovascular Technologists
NADONA/LTC	National Association of Directors of Nursing Administration in Long Term Care
NAEMT	National Association of Emergency Medical Technicians
NAHC	National Association of Home Care
NAHM	National Association for Mental Health
NAHSR	National Association of Human Services Technologists
NAMT	National Association for Music Therapy
NANDA	North American Nursing Diagnosis Association
NANPHR	National Association of Nurse Practitioners in Reproductive Health
NAPNES	National Association for Practical Nurse Education and Services
NARF	National Association of Rehabilitation Facilities
NASW	National Association of Social Workers
NATTS	National Association of Trade and Technical Schools
NCEHPHP	National Council on the Education of Health Professionals in Health Promotion
NCRE	National Council on Rehabilitation Education
NEHA	National Environmental Health Education
NFLPN	National Federation of Licensed Practical Nurses
NHC	National Health Council
NIH	National Institutes of Health
NIOSH	National Institute of Occupational Safety and Health
NLN	National League for Nursing
NNBA	National Nurses in Business Association
NRCA	National Rehabilitation Counseling Association
NREMT	National Registry of Emergency Medical Technicians
NSCPT	National Society for Cardiopulmonary Technology
NSH	National Society for Histotechnology
NSNA	National Student Nurses Association
NTRS	National Therapeutic Recreation Society
OAA	Opticians Association of America
ONS	Oncology Nurses Association
SAAABB	Subcommittee on Accreditation of the American Association of Blood Banks
SDMS	Society of Diagnostic Medical Sonographers
SNIVT	Society of Non-Invasive Vascular Technology
SNM	Society of Nuclear Medicine
SNM-TS	Society for Nuclear Medicine—Technologists Section
SPHE	Society of Public Health Educators
STS	Society of Thoracic Surgeons
SVS	Society for Vascular Surgery
TAANA	American Association of Nurse Attorneys
USPHS	United States Public Health Services
VA	Veterans Administration
WHO	World Health Organization

Voluntary Health and Welfare Agencies and Associations*

There are a wide variety of agencies and associations that contribute to the well being of individuals with health care problems. These agencies can be sponsored by governmental agencies or they may be voluntary. A *voluntary agency* is nongovernmental and nonprofit in nature; the term voluntary is used to denote that a major source of support is contributed. Regardless of the nature of the sponsoring group, health and welfare agencies provide many services such as development of educational programs, sponsorship of research, increasing public awareness of a specific disease or disorder, and support services. The agencies listed below will help the physician, nurse, and allied health professional to improve patient care and services. The listing of agencies is current at the time of publication of the *Miller-Keane Encyclopedia and Dictionary of Medicine, Nursing, and Allied Health;* users are cautioned that these addresses change frequently.

ACTION (programs for older adults)
806 Connecticut Ave. NW
Washington, DC 20525
202-254-7310

Administration on Aging
Department of Health and Human Services
200 Independence Ave. SW
Washington, DC 20201
202-245-0724

Alcoholics Anonymous
475 Riverside Drive
New York, NY 10015
212-686-1100

Alzheimer's Disease and Related Disorders
  Association
70 E. Lake St.
Chicago, IL 60601
800-621-0379

American Academy of Allergy and Immunology
611 E. Wells St.
Milwaukee, WI 53202
414-272-6071

American Anorexia/Bulimia Association, Inc.
133 Cedar Ln.
Teaneck, NJ 07666
201-836-1800

American Association on Mental Deficiency
PO Box 96
Willimantic, CT 06226

American Association of Retired Persons (AARP)
1909 K St. NW
Washington, DC 20005

American Burn Association
Shriner's Burn Institute
University of Cincinnati
202 Goodman St.
Cincinnati, OH 45219
513-751-3900

American Cancer Society
1599 Clifton Rd. NE
Atlanta, GA 30329
404-320-3333

American Dental Association
Council on Dental Care Programs
211 E. Chicago Ave.
17th Floor
Chicago, IL 60611
312-440-2500

*From Miller, B. F., and C. B. Keane. *Encyclopedia and Dictionary of Medicine, Nursing, and Allied Health,* 5th edition. W. B. Saunders Company, Philadelphia, 1992, pp. 1745-1747.

American Diabetes Association
National Center
1660 Duke St.
Alexandria, VA 22314
800-232-3472

American Foundation for the Blind
15 W. 16th St.
New York, NY 10016
212-620-2000

American Liver Foundation
1425 Pompton Ave.
Cedar Grove, NJ 07009
800-223-0179

American Lung Association
1740 Broadway
New York, NY 10019
215-315-8700

American Pain Society
PO Box 186
Skokie, IL 60076
312-475-7300

American Parkinson's Disease Association, Inc.
116 John St.
New York, NY 10038
212-732-9550

American Speech-Language-Hearing Association
10801 Rockville Pike
Department AP
Rockville, MD 20852
301-897-5700

American Spinal Injury Association
2020 Peachtree Rd. NW
Atlanta, GA 30309

American Tinnitus Association
PO Box 5
Portland, OR 97207
503-248-9985

Arthritis Foundation
1314 Spring St. NW
Atlanta, GA 30309
404-872-7100

Asthma and Allergy Foundation of America
1717 Massachusetts Ave. NW
No. 305
Washington, DC 20036
800-7ASTHMA

Centers for Disease Control
Department of Health and Human Services
U.S. Public Health Service
Atlanta, GA 30333
404-639-3534

Concern for Dying
250 W. 57th St.
New York, NY 10107
215-246-6962

Cystic Fibrosis Foundation
6931 Arlington Rd.
Bethesda, MD 20814
800-FIGHT-CF

Epilepsy Foundation of America
815 15th St. NW, Suite 528
Washington, DC 20005
202-638-5229

Guide for Infant Survival (sudden infant death
  syndrome)
PO Box 17432
Irvine, CA 92713-7432

Guillain-Barré Foundation
129 North Carolina Ave. SE
Washington, DC 20003
202-387-2216

HELP (Herpes Resource Center)
PO Box 100
Palo Alto, CA 94302
919-361-2120

La Leche League International
9616 Minneapolis Ave.
Franklin Park, IL 60131
800-LA-LECHE

Leukemia Society of America
31 St. James Ave.
Boston, MA 02116
617-482-2256

Muscular Dystrophy Association
3561 E. Sunrise Ave.
Tucson, AZ 85718
602-529-2000

Myasthenia Gravis Foundation
61 Gramercy Park North
New York, NY 10010
212-533-7005

National Association to Control Epilepsy
22 E. 67th St.
New York, NY 10012

National Association of Patients on Hemodialysis
and Transplantation
211 E. 43rd St.
New York, NY 10017
212-867-4486

National Association for Retarded Citizens
2501 Ave. J
Arlington, TX 76011

National Association for Sickle Cell Disease
4221 Wilshire Blvd., Suite 360
Los Angeles, CA 90010
213-936-7205

National Cancer Institute
Office of Cancer Communications
Building 31, Room 10A24
National Institutes of Health
Bethesda, MD 20892
800-4-CANCER

National Center for the American Heart Association
7320 Greenville Ave.
Dallas, TX 75231
214-373-6300

National Easter Seal Society
2023 W. Ogden Ave.
Chicago, IL 60612
312-243-8400

National Foundation for Ileitis and Colitis
444 Park Ave. South
New York, NY 10016
212-685-3440

National Head Injury Foundation
333 Turnpike Rd.
Southborough, MA 01722
508-485-9950

National Hemophilia Foundation
110 Greene St., Suite 406
New York, NY 10012
212-219-8180

National Institute of Allergy and Infectious Diseases
Building 10, National Institutes of Health
Bethesda, MD 20892
301-496-4000

National Institute of Arthritis and Musculoskeletal
and Skin Diseases
National Institutes of Health
Bethesda, MD 20892
301-496-4000

National Jewish Center for Immunology and
Respiratory Medicine
1400 Jackson St.
Denver, CO 80206
800-222-LUNG

National Kidney Foundation
30 E. 33rd St.
New York, NY 10016
212-889-2210

National Multiple Sclerosis Society
205 E. 42nd St.
New York, NY 10017
212-532-3060

National Parkinson's Foundation
1501 NW 9th Ave.
Miami, FL 33136
305-547-6666

National Psoriasis Foundation
6443 Southwest Beaverton Hwy., Suite 210
Portland, OR 97221
503-297-1545

National Safety Council
444 N. Michigan Ave.
Chicago, IL 60611
800-621-7619

National SIDS Alliance (sudden infant death
syndrome)
10500 Little Patuxent Pkwy., Suite 420
Columbia, MD 21044
800-221-SIDS

National Society to Prevent Blindness
500 E. Remington Rd.
Schaumburg, IL 60173
312-843-2020

National Spinal Cord Injury Association
600 W. Cumming Park, #3200
Woburn, MA 01801
800-962-9629

Office for Handicapped Individuals
Department of Education
Room 3106, Switzer Building
400 Maryland Ave. SW
Washington, DC 20202
202-245-0080

Orton Dyslexia Society
Chester Building
Suite 382
8600 LaSalle Road
Baltimore, MD 21286-2044
800-ABCD-123

Osteoporosis Foundation
612 N. Michigan Ave., Suite 510
Chicago, IL 60611

Paget's Disease Foundation
PO Box 2772
Brooklyn, NY 11202
718-596-1043

Parkinson Disease Foundation
Medical Center
William Black Medical Research Bldg.
640 W. 168th St.
New York, NY 10032
212-923-4700

Phoenix Society (assistance following burn injuries)
11 Rust Hill Rd.
Levittown, PA 19056
215-946-BURN
800-888-BURN

Scoliosis Association
PO Box 51353
Raleigh, NC 27609
919-846-2639

Self Help for Hard of Hearing People (Shhh)
4848 Battery Ln.
Department E
Bethesda, MD 20814
301-657-2248

Sex Information and Education Council of the
   United States (SIECUS)
130 W. 42nd St., Suite 2500
New York, NY 10036
212-819-9770

United Cerebral Palsy Association (UCPA)
1522 K St. NW
Washington, DC 20005
800-872-5827

United Network for Organ Sharing
3001 Hungary Spring Rd.
Richmond, VA 23228
804-289-5380

Forms of Address*

Forms of address should not always follow set rules, for the relationship of and degree of friendliness between correspondents will often suggest informal salutations. The forms given hereunder are formal and imply a conventional rather than casual or intimate relationship. When the addressee is a woman, Madam may be substituted for Sir and, less formally, Mrs., Miss, or Ms. may be substituted for Mr.

Academic and Other University Titles	Form of Address	Salutation
assistant professor, college or university	Dr. (or Mr., Mrs.) John Day Assistant Professor Department of	Dear Professor Day:
associate professor, college or university	Dr. (or Mr., Mrs.) John Day Associate Professor Department of	Dear Professor Day:
chancellor, university	Chancellor John Day	Dear Chancellor Day:
dean, college or university	Dean John Day or Dr. (or Mr., Mrs.) John Day Dean, School of	Dear Dean Day: Dear Dr. (or Mr., Mrs.) Day:
president, college or university	President John Day Dr. (or Mr., Mrs.) John Day President, ...	Dear President Day: Dear Dr. (or Mr., Mrs.) Day:
professor, college or university	Professor John Day or Dr. (or Mr., Mrs.) John Day Department of	Dear Professor Day: Dear Dr. (or Mr., Mrs.) Day:

Clerical and Religious Titles	Form of Address	Salutation
abbot	The Right Reverend John Day, O.S.B. (or other initials of an order) Abbot of	Right Reverend Abbot:
archbishop, Armenian Church	His Eminence the Archbishop of	Your Eminence: or Your Excellency:
archbishop, Greek Orthodox	His Eminence Archbishop John Day	Your Eminence:
archbishop, Roman Catholic	The Most Reverend John Day Archbishop of	Your Excellency:
archbishop, Russian Orthodox	His Eminence the Archbishop of ...... or The Most Reverend Archbishop of	Your Grace:
archdeacon, Episcopal	The Venerable John Day Archdeacon of	Venerable Sir: Dear Archdeacon Day: Dear Father Day:
archpriest, Russian Orthodox	Very Reverend Father John Day	Very Reverend Father: Very Reverend Father Day:
bishop, Episcopal	The Right Reverend John Day Bishop of	Right Reverend Sir: Dear Bishop Day:
bishop, Greek Orthodox	The Right Reverend John Day	Your Grace:
bishop, Methodist	Bishop John Day The Reverend John Day	Dear Bishop Day: Dear Reverend Day:
bishop, Mormon	Mr. John Day	Dear Mr. Day:
bishop, Roman Catholic	The Most Reverend John Day Bishop of	Your Excellency:
brother, Roman Catholic	Brother John Day (initials of appropriate order)	Dear Brother: Dear Brother John:
canon, Episcopal	The Reverend Canon John Day	Dear Canon Day:
cantor	Cantor John Day	Dear Cantor Day:
cardinal	His Eminence John Cardinal Day	Your Eminence:
clergyman, Protestant	The Reverend John or Susan Day or The Reverend John or Susan Day, D.D.	Dear Mr. Day: Dear Mrs. (or Dr.) Day: Dear Dr. Day:

Clerical and Religious Titles	Form of Address	Salutation
elder, Presbyterian	Elder John Day	Dear Elder Day:
dean of a cathedral, Episcopal	The Very Reverend John Day Dean of	Very Reverend Sir: Dear Dean Day:
metropolitan, Russian Orthodox	His Eminence the Metropolitan of ...... or The Most Reverend Metropolitan of	Your Grace:
monsignor, Roman Catholic	Reverend Monsignor John Day	Reverend Monsignor: Dear Monsignor: Dear Monsignor Day:
patriarch, Armenian Church	His Beatitude the Patriarch of	Your Beatitude:
patriarch, Greek Orthodox	His All Holiness Patriarch Demetrios	Your All Holiness:
patriarch, Russian Orthodox	His Beatitude the Patriarch of	Your Beatitude:
pope	His Holiness Pope John Paul II or His Holiness, The Pope	Your Holiness:
priest, Greek Orthodox	Reverend Father John Day	Dear Reverend Day: Dear Reverend Father:
priest, Roman Catholic	The Reverend John Day, S.J. (or other initials of order)	Dear Reverend Father: Dear Father: Dear Father Day:
priest, Russian Orthodox	The Reverend John Day	Reverend Father: Reverend Father Day:
rabbi	Rabbi John Day or John Day, D.D.	Dear Rabbi (or Dr.) Day:
sister, Roman Catholic	Sister Joanna Day, S.C.J. (or other initials of an order)	Dear Sister: Dear Sister Joanna:
supreme patriarch, Armenian Church	His Holiness the Supreme Patriarch and Catholicos of all Armenians	Your Holiness:

Diplomatic Titles	Form of Address	Salutation
ambassador, U.S.	The Honorable John Day The Ambassador of the United States	Sir: Dear Mr. (or Mrs.) Ambassador:

ambassador to the U.S.	His Excellency John Day The Ambassador of	Excellency: Dear Mr. (or Mrs.) Ambassador:
chargé d'affaires, U.S.	John Day, Esq. American Chargé d'Affaires	Dear Sir: Dear Madam:
chargé d'affaires to the U.S.	John Day, Esq. Chargé d'Affaires of	Dear Sir: Dear Madam:
consul, U.S.	Mr. John Day American Consul	Sir: Dear Mr. (or Mrs.) Consul:
minister, U.S.	The Honorable John Day The Minister of the United States	Sir: Dear Mr. (or Mrs.) Minister:
minister to the U.S.	The Honorable John Day The Minister of	Sir: Dear Mr. (or Mrs.) Minister:
secretary general, United Nations	His Excellency John Day Secretary General of the United Nations	Excellency: Dear Mr. (or Mrs.) Secretary General:
U.S. representative to the United Nations	The Honorable John Day United States Representative to the United Nations	Sir: Dear Mr. (or Mrs.) Day:

Federal, State, and Other Official Titles	**Form of Address**	**Salutation**
alderman	The Honorable John Day	Dear Mr. (or Mrs.) Day:
assistant to the President	The Honorable John Day Assistant to the President The White House	Dear Mr. (or Mrs.) Day:
Attorney General, U.S.	The Honorable John Day Attorney General of the United States	Dear Mr. (or Mrs.) Attorney General:
attorney general, state	The Honorable John Day Attorney General State of	Dear Mr. (or Mrs.) Attorney General:
assemblyman, state	The Honorable John Day ...... Assembly State Capitol	Dear Mr. (or Mrs.) Day:
cabinet member	The Honorable John Day Secretary of	Dear Mr. (or Mrs.) Secretary:
assistant secretary of a department	The Honorable John Day Assistant Secretary of	Dear Mr. (or Mrs.) Day:
undersecretary of a department	The Honorable John Day Undersecretary of	Dear Mr. (or Mrs.) Day:

Federal, State, and Other Official Titles	Form of Address	Salutation
deputy secretary of a department	The Honorable John Day Deputy Secretary of	Dear Mr. (or Mrs.) Day:
chairman, House Committee	The Honorable John Day Chairman, Committee on ...... United States House of Representatives	Dear Mr. (or Mrs.) Chairman:
chairman, joint committee of Congress	The Honorable John Day Chairman, Joint Comittee on ...... Congress of the United States	Dear Mr. (or Mrs.) Chairman:
chairman, Senate Committee	The Honorable John Day Chairman, Committee on ...... United States Senate	Dear Mr. (or Mrs.) Chairman:
chief justice, U.S. Supreme Court	The Chief Justice of the United States The Supreme Court of the United States	Dear Mr. (or Mrs.) Chief Justice:
associate justice, U.S. Supreme Court	Mr. Justice Day The Supreme Court of the United States	Dear Mr. (or Mrs.) Justice:
commissioner (federal, state, or local)	The Honorable John Day	Dear Mr. (or Mrs.) Day:
delegate, state	The Honorable John Day ...... House of Delegates State Capitol	Dear Mr. (or Mrs.) Day:
governor	The Honorable John Day Governor of	Dear Governor Day: Dear Governor:
judge, federal	The Honorable John Day Judge of the United States Tax Court	Dear Judge Day:
judge, state or local	The Honorable John Day Judge of the Superior Court of	Dear Judge Day:
lieutenant governor	The Honorable John Day Lieutenant Governor of	Dear Mr. (or Mrs.) Day:
mayor	The Honorable John Day Mayor of	Dear Mayor Day:
Postmaster General	The Honorable John Day Postmaster General of the United States	Dear Mr. (or Mrs.) Postmaster General:

Federal, State, and Other Official Titles	Form of Address	Salutation
President, U.S.	The President The White House	Dear Mr. President: Dear Madam President:
representative, state	The Honorable John Day House of Representatives State Capitol	Dear Mr. (or Mrs.) Day: Dear Representative Day:
representative, U.S.	The Honorable John Day United States House of Representatives	Dear Mr. (or Mrs.) Day: Dear Representative Day:
secretary of state, state	The Honorable John Day Secretary of State State Capitol	Dear Mr. (or Mrs.) Secretary:
senator, state	The Honorable John Day The State Senate State Capitol	Dear Senator Day: Dear Mr. (or Mrs.) Day:
senator, U.S.	The Honorable John Day United States Senate	Dear Senator Day:
Speaker, U.S. House of Representatives	The Honorable John Day Speaker of the House of Representatives	Dear Mr. Speaker: Dear Madam Speaker:
Vice President, U.S.	The Vice President United States Senate	Dear Mr. Vice President: Dear Madam Vice President:

Professional Titles	Form of Address	Salutation
attorney	Mr. John Day Attorney at Law or John Day, Esq.	Dear Mr. (or Mrs.) Day:
chiropractor	John Day, D.C. (office) or Dr. John Day (residence)	Dear Dr. Day:
dentist	John Day, D.D.S. (office) or Dr. John Day (residence)	Dear Dr. Day:
physician	John Day, M.D. (office) or Dr. John Day (residence)	Dear Dr. Day:
veterinarian	John Day, D.V.M. (office) or Dr. John Day (residence)	Dear Dr. Day:

Military Titles	Form of Address	Salutation
admiral vice admiral rear admiral	Full rank, full name abbreviation of service branch	Dear Admiral Day:
airman first class airman	Full rank, full name, abbreviation of service branch	Dear Airman Day:
cadet (air force, army)	Cadet John Day United States Air Force Academy or United States Military Academy	Dear Cadet Day: or Dear Mr. (or Ms.) Day:
captain, (air force, army, coast guard, marine corps, navy)	Full rank, full name, abbreviation of service branch	Dear Captain Day:
chief petty officer (coast guard, navy)	Full rank, full name, abbreviation of service branch	Dear Mr. (or Ms.) Day: or Dear Chief Day:
chief warrant officer, warrant officer (air force, army, marine corps, navy)	Full rank, full name, abbreviation of service branch	Dear Mr. (or Ms.) Day:
colonel, lieutenant colonel (air force, army, marine corps)	Full rank, full name, abbreviation of service branch	Dear Colonel Day:
commander (coast guard, navy)	Full rank, full name, abbreviation of service branch	Dear Commander Day:
commodore (navy)	Full rank, full name, abbreviation of service branch	Dear Commodore Day:
corporal (army) lance corporal (marine corps)	Full rank, full name, abbreviation of service branch	Dear Corporal Day:
ensign (coast guard, navy)	Full rank, full name, abbreviation of service branch	Dear Mr. (or Ms.) Day: or Dear Ensign Day:
first lieutenant, second lieutenant (air force, army, marine corps)	Full rank, full name, abbreviation of service branch	Dear Lieutenant Day:

Military Titles	Form of Address	Salutation
general, lieutenant general, major general, brigadier general (air force, army, marine corps)	Full rank, full name, abbreviation of service branch	Dear General Day:
lieutenant commander, lieutenant, lieutenant (jg) (coast guard, navy)	Full rank, full name, abbreviation of service branch	Dear Mr. (or Ms.) Day: or Dear Commander Day: Dear Lieutenant Day:
major (air force, army, marine corps)	Full rank, full name, abbreviation of service branch	Dear Major Day:
midshipman	Midshipman John Day United States Coast Guard Academy of United States Naval Academy	Dear Midshipman Day:
petty officer (coast guard, navy)	Full rank, full name, abbreviation of service branch	Dear Mr. (or Ms.) Day:
private first class, private (air force, army, marine corps)	Full rank, full name, abbreviation of service branch	Dear Private Day:
seaman, seaman apprentice, seaman recruit (coast guard, navy)	Full rank, full name, abbreviation of service branch	Dear Seaman Day:
master sergeant (air force, army, marine corps)	Full rank, full name, abbreviation of service branch	Dear Sergeant Day:

Noble Titles	Form of Address	Salutation
Baron	The Right Honourable Lord ...... or The Lord	My Lord:
Baroness	The Right Honourable the Baroness ...... or The Lady	Madam:
Baronet	Sir John ......, Bt. (or Bart.)	Sir;
Baronet's wife (see Lady)		
Countess	The Right Honourable the Countess of	Madam:
Dame	Dame	Madam:

Noble Titles	Form of Address	Salutation
Duchess	Her Grace the Duchess of ...... or The Most Noble the Duchess of	Madam: or Your Grace:
Duchess of the Blood Royal	Her Royal Highness The Duchess of	Madam: or May it please Your Royal Highness:
Duke	His Grace the Duke of ...... or The Most Noble The Duke of	My Lord Duke: or Your Grace:
Duke of the Blood Royal	His Royal Highness The Duke of	Sir: or May it please Your Royal Highness:
Earl	The Right Honourable The Earl of ...... or The Earl of	My Lord:
Earl's wife (see Countess)		
King	The King's Most Excellent Majesty or His Most Gracious Majesty King	Sir: or May it please Your Majesty:
Knight	Sir .... (initials of his order such as K.C.B.)	Sir:
Knight's wife (See Lady)		
Lady	Lady ...... or Hon. Lady (if daughter of Baron or Viscount) or Lady .... (if the daughter of an Earl, Marquis or Duke)	Madam: or My Lady: or Your Ladyship:
Marchioness	The Most Honourable the Marchioness of	Madam:

Noble Titles	Form of Address	Salutation
Marquis	The Most Honourable the Marquis of ...... or Marquis of	My Lord Marquis:
Prince of the Blood Royal	His Royal Highness Prince	Sir:
Prince of Wales	His Royal Highness The Prince of Wales	Sir: or May it please Your Royal Highness:
Princess of the Blood Royal	Her Royal Highness the Princess	Madam:
Queen	The Queen's Most Excellent Majesty or Her Gracious Majesty, The Queen	Madam: or May it please Your Majesty:
Queen Mother	Her Gracious Majesty Queen	Madam: or May it please Your Majesty:
Viscount	The Right Honourable the Viscount ...... or The Viscount	My Lord:
Viscountess	The Right Honourable the Viscountess ...... or The Viscountess	Madam:

Other Titles	Form of Address	Salutation
Divorced Woman	Mrs. Joanna Day	Dear Mrs. Day:
Doctor of Philosophy or Laws	John Day, Ph.D. or L.L.D.	Dear Sir: or Dear Mr. or Dr. Day:
Known Man	Mr. Day	Dear Mr. Day:

Other Titles	Form of Address	Salutation
Known Woman	Mrs. Day	Dear Mrs. Day:
	Miss Day	Dear Miss Day:
	Ms. Day	Dear Ms. Day:
	Misses Smith and Day	Dear Mses. or Mss. Smith and Day:
	Mrs. Smith and Mrs. Day	Dear Mrs. Smith and Mrs. Day:
	Dr. Dorn and Dr. Phillips	Dear Drs. Dorn and Phillips:
Unknown men		Gentlemen:
Unknown Recipient		To Whom It May Concern:
		Dear Sir or Madam:
		Ladies and Gentlemen:
Unknown Women		Ladies:
		Mesdames:
Widow	Mrs. John Day	Dear Mrs. Day:

Postal Abbreviations for States

Two-Letter Abbreviations for the United States and Its Dependencies

Alabama	AL	Kentucky	KY	Oklahoma	OK
Alaska	AK	Louisiana	LA	Oregon	OR
Arizona	AZ	Maine	ME	Pennsylvania	PA
Arkansas	AR	Maryland	MD	Puerto Rico	PR
California	CA	Massachusetts	MA	Rhode Island	RI
Canal Zone	CZ	Michigan	MI	South Carolina	SC
Colorado	CO	Minnesota	MN	South Dakota	SD
Connecticut	CT	Mississippi	MS	Tennessee	TN
Delaware	DE	Missouri	MO	Texas	TX
District of Columbia	DC	Montana	MT	Utah	UT
Florida	FL	Nebraska	NE	Vermont	VT
Georgia	GA	Nevada	NV	Virginia	VA
Guam	GU	New Hampshire	NH	Virgin Islands	VI
Hawaii	HI	New Jersey	NJ	Washington	WA
Idaho	ID	New Mexico	NM	West Virginia	WV
Illinois	IL	New York	NY	Wisconsin	WI
Indiana	IN	North Carolina	NC	Wyoming	WY
Iowa	IA	North Dakota	ND		
Kansas	KS	Ohio	OH		

Two-Letter Abbreviations for Canadian Provinces and Territories

Alberta	AB	Newfoundland	NF	Quebec	PQ
British Columbia	BC	Northwest Territories	NT	Saskatchewan	SK
Labrador	LB	Nova Scotia	NS	Yukon Territory	YT
Manitoba	MB	Ontario	ON		
New Brunswick	NB	Prince Edward Island	PE		

*Common Prescription Abbreviations**

a̅a̅	of each	garg.	gargle
a.c.	before meals	gm. or g.	gram
ad	up to	gr.	grain
adde	add; let it be added	gt.	drop
ad lib.	as much as needed	gtt.	drops
agit.	shake; stir	guttat.	drop by drop
alt. dieb.	alternate days	h.	hour
alt. hor	alternate hours	h.s.	before bedtime (hour of sleep)
alt. noc.	alternate nights		
a.m.	morning	inj.	injection; to be injected
ante	before	kg.	kilogram
aq.	water	M. or m.	mix
aq. bull.	boiling water	mcgm.	microgram
aq. com.	common water; tap water	M. et f. pil.	mix and make into pill
aq. dest.	distilled water	M. et f. pulv.	mix and make into powder
aq. ferv.	hot water	M. et sig	mix and label
aq. frig.	cold water	mg. or mgm.	milligram
aq. susp.	water suspension	ml.	milliliter
b.i.d.	two times a day	noct.	night
c̄	with	o.h.	every hour
caps.	capsule	o.m.	every morning
comp.	compound	o.n.	every night
contra	against	p.c.	after meals
coq.	boil	pil.	pill
dil.	dilute	p.o.	by mouth
div.	to be divided	p.r.n.	whenever necessary
dos.	doses	pulv.	powder
DSD	double starting dose	q.	every
elix.	elixir	q. a.m.	every morning
emul.	emulsion	q.d.	one time daily; every day
et	and	q. 4 h.	every 4 hours
ext.	extract	q.h.	every hour
f. or ft.	make; let there be made	q.i.d.	four times a day (not at night)
fl.	fluid		

---

*Many of these abbreviations are derived from Latin; they are usually typed in lowercase and with periods. Periods are especially important if without periods an abbreviation would spell a word; for example, b.i.d. without periods is bid.

q. noc.	every night	ss	one-half
q.n.s.	quantity not sufficient	stat.	immediately
q.o.d.	every other day	syr.	syrup
q. p.m.	every night	tab.	tablet
q.s.	quantity sufficient	tr. or tinct.	tincture
q. 2 h.	every 2 hours	troc.	lozenge
Rx	take (recipe) prescription	tsp.	teaspoon
rep	let it be repeated	u.	unit
s̄	without	i, ii, iv, viii, etc.	1, 2, 4, 8, etc.
sat.	saturated	5", 10", 15", etc.	5 minutes, 10 minutes, 15 minutes, etc.
sig.	write on label; give directions on prescription	5', 10', 15', etc.	5 hours, 10 hours, 15 hours, etc.
sol.	solution		

Symbols and Metric Prefixes

□, ♂	male		←	is due to, transfer to, secondary to, to the left
o, ♀	female		⇌	reversible reaction
*	birth		↑↑	extensor response, Babinski sign (neurologic examination)
†	death		↓↓	plantar response, Babinski sign (neurologic examination)
Ⓛ	left			
®	right, trademark		↓↓	testes descended
⊖	normal		↑↑	testes undescended
@	at		∨	systolic blood pressure
⌣	combined with		∧	diastolic blood pressure
#	gauge, number, weight, pound(s), fracture		>	greater than, from which is derived
			≯	not greater than
φ	none		≥	greater than or equal to
%	per cent		<	less than, derived from
○	pint		≮	not less than
?	question of, questionable, possible		≤	less than or equal to
℞	*recipe* (L) take		°	degree
↑ or ↗	increase, increases, above, elevated, rising, greater than		24°	24 hours
			1°	primary, first degree
↓ or ↘	decrease, decreases, below, falling, less than		2°	secondary, second degree
			3°	third degree
→ or ←	direction of reaction		°F	degrees Fahrenheit
⇡	up		°C	degrees Centigrade
↑V	increase due to *in vivo* effect		2d	second
↓V	decrease due to *in vivo* effect		2ndry	secondary
↑C	increase due to chemical interference during the assay		1×	once
			2×	twice
↓C	decrease due to chemical interference during the assay		×2	twice
→	to the right, causes, no change, transfer to, yields, leads to, approaches limit of			

Symbol	Meaning	Symbol	Meaning
′	foot, minute, primary accent, univalent	$\pm$	plus or minus; either positive or negative; indefinite
″	inch, second, secondary accent, bivalent	$\div$	divided by
ⅱ	two	$\times$	multiplied by; magnification
/	of, per	$\sqrt{}$	root, square root, radical
:	ratio (is to)	$\sqrt[2]{}$	square root
::	equality between ratios, "as," proportionate to	$\sqrt[3]{}$	cube root
∴	therefore	$\sqrt{c}$	check with
∼	approximate	$\overline{X}$	average of all X's
=	equals	⊙	start of operation
≠	does not equal, not equal to, unequal	⊗	end of operation
≅	approximately equals	X	start of anesthesia (on anesthesia records)
≡	identical with	Ⓧ	end of anesthesia (on anesthesia records)
≢	not identical with	○	respirations (on anesthesia records)
≐	approaches	●	pulse rate (on anesthesia records)
≈ or ≑	is approximately equal to	△	temperature (on anesthesia records)
≠ or ∓	is unequal to	S	suction (on anesthesia records)
∼	is similar to, difference, cycle	⌢, or Ⓜ	murmur
≅	is congruent to	α	alpha, particle, is proportional to
≎	equivalent	Δ	prism diopter, change
∫	integral (sign also called a "fluent")	Δt	time interval
∞	infinity, indefinitely great	ΔA	change in absorbance
0	infinitesimal, indefinitely small; zero	$\Delta \mathrm{pH}$	change in pH
$\pm$	not definite, plus/minus, very slight trace	Ω	ohm
(+)	significant	π	pi, 3.1416—ratio of circumference of a circle to its diameter
(−)	insignificant	λ	wavelength
(±)	possibly significant	Σ	sum of

Symbols used in recording results of qualitative tests:

Symbol	Meaning	Symbol	Meaning
−	negative	σ	1/100 of a second, standard deviation
±	very slight trace or reaction	χ^2	chi square (test)
+	slight trace or reaction	τ	life (time)
++	trace or noticeable reaction	$\tau^{1/2}$	half-life (time)
+++	moderate amount of reaction	μ	micron
++++	large amount or pronounced reaction	$\mu\mu$	micromicron
+	plus; excess; acid reaction; positive	μc	microcurie
−	minus; deficiency; alkaline reaction; negative	μEq	microequivalent
		μf	microfarad

μg	microgram	mμg	millimicrogram (nanogram)
μl	microliter	mμ	millimicron
$\mu\mu$c	micromicrocurie (picocurie)	$\bar{\text{p}}$	after
$\mu\mu$g	micromicrogram (picogram)	$\bar{\text{a}}$	before
μm	micrometer	$\bar{\text{c}}$	with
μM	micromolar	$\bar{\text{s}}$	without
μr	microroentgen	℥	ounce
μsec	microsecond	f℥	fluid ounce
μu	microunit	℈	scruple, apothecaries'; ℈ i, one scruple
μv	microvolt	♍	minim
μw	microwatt	ℨ	drachm, dram
$\mu\gamma$	milligamma (nanogram)	f℈	fluidrachm, fluidram
mμc	millimicrocurie (nanocurie)		

METRIC PREFIXES

Prefixes for Metric System Multiples and Submultiples

Symbol	Name	Value
T	tera	10^{12}
G	giga	10^9
M	mega	10^6
my	myria	10^4
k	kilo	10^3
h	hecto	10^2
dk	deka	10
d	deci	10^{-1}
c	centi	10^{-2}
m	milli	10^{-3}
μ	micro	10^{-6}
n	nano	10^{-9}
p	pico	10^{-12}
f	femto	10^{-15}
a	atto	10^{-18}

The Greek Alphabet

Character		Greek Name	Names of Letters	Pronunciation
Capital	**Small**			
A	α α	alpha	"Αλφα	ăl'fà
B	β ϐ	beta	Βῆτα	bā'tà, or bē'tà
Γ	γ	gamma	Γἀμμα	găm'à
Δ	δ	delta	Δἐλτα	dĕl'tà
E	ε	epsilon	"Εψιλον	ĕp'sĭ-lŏn (Br. ĕp-sil'on)
Z	ζ	zeta	Ζῆτα	zā'tà, or zē'tà
H	η	eta	'Ητα	ā'tà, or ē'tà
Θ	θ ϑ	theta	Θῆτα	thā'tà, or thē'tà
I	ι	iota	'Ιῶτα	ī-ō'tà
K	κ	kappa	Κἀππα	kăp'à
Λ	λ	lambda	Λἀμϐδα	lăm'dà
M	μ	mu	Μῦ	mū, or moo
N	ν	nu	Νῦ	nū, or noo
Ξ	ξ	xi	Ξῦ	zī, or ksē
O	ο	omicron	"Ομικρον	ŏm'ĭ-krŏn (Br. ō-mĭk'rŭn)
Π	π	pi	Πῖ	pī
P	ρ	rho	Ρῶ	rō
Σ	σ ς	sigma	Σῖγμα	sĭg'mà
T	τ	tau	Ταῦ	ta, or tou
Υ	υ	upsilon	"Υψιλον	ŭp'sĭ-lŏn (Br. ūp-sīl'on)
Φ	φ φ	phi	Φῖ	fī
X	χ	chi (Br. Khi)	Χῖ	kī, or kē
Ψ	ψ	psi	Ψῖ	sī, or psē
Ω	ω	omega	'Ωμἐγα	ō-mē'gà, or ōmĕg'à

Index

Note: Page numbers in *italics* refer to illustrations; page numbers followed by t refer to tables.

Abbé flap, 601, *604*
Abbreviations, for chemotherapeutic regimens, 466t
  in medical records, 28, 99
    references on, 755–756
  postal, 832
  prescription, 833–834
Abdomen, CT of, *670–671*
    report on, *672–673*
  quadrants of, *245*
  wall defects of, neonatal, 579
Abdominoplasty, 619
Abducens, 398
Abduction, *497*
Abductor hallucis flap, 607–608
ABO grouping, 337, 340, 341t
Abortion, *497–428*
Abruptio placentae, 429
Abscess, kidney, 742t
  perinephric, 740t
Academics, forms of address for, 821
Acanthocytosis, *316*
Accommodation-convergence synkinesis, 398
Accounts, 58
  overdue, 60
Accuracy, 20–22, 97–99
Acetaminophen, monitoring of, 360t
Achilles tendon lengthening, 643
Acid-base disturbances, 390, 390t
Acidosis, 390, 390t
Acinic cell adenocarcinoma, salivary gland, 539
Acne, 195
Acne keloidalis, 195–196
Acquired immunodeficiency syndrome (AIDS), 291. See also *Human immunodeficiency virus (HIV).*
  confidentiality and, 24, 34, 37
  discharge summary in, *296–297*

Acquired immunodeficiency syndrome (AIDS) *(Continued)*
  opportunistic infections in, 344, 351–352
  terminology of, 4, 764
Acrochordon, 196
Acrodermatitis chronica atrophicans, 190
Acronyms, Appendix 8
Actinic keratosis, 197
Activated partial prothrombin time (PTT), 317
Acute tubular necrosis, urinalysis findings in, 327t
Adam's apple, 526, *530*
Addenda reports, in pathology, 562
Adduction, *497*
Adenocarcinoma, 454
  lung, 265–266
Adenocystic carcinoma, salivary gland, 539
Adenoids, 539
  surgery on, 545
Adenoviruses, 353
Adiadokokinesia, 398
Adjustment disorders, 650
Adjuvant therapy, 462. See also *Chemotherapy.*
Admission of observers, consent form for, *31*
Adrenal glands, 219, *220*
  abnormal conditions of, 222t
  hormones produced by, 221t
  cancer treatment and, 465
Adrenalectomy, 734
Adrenocortical carcinoma, 736t
Adrenocorticotropic hormone, 221t
Adson's maneuver, 398
Advances, publishers', 112
Advertising, 62–63, *64*, 80, *81*, 82

Aerosols, 695
Aerotitis, 532
A/G ratio, 307
AIDS. See *Acquired immunodeficiency syndrome (AIDS).*
Airways, 689
  disorders of, 691
Alanine aminotransferase (ALT), 307
  monitoring of, 360t
Albumin, globulin, and total protein, 307
  monitoring of, 360t
Albumin:globulin ratio, 307
Alcohol, blood, monitoring of, 360t
Aldosterone, 221t
Alert and critical laboratory values, 359, 360t–368t, 368–369
Alkaline phosphatase (ALP), 307
Alkalosis, 390, 390t
Allergens, 287
Allergies, 292t
  dermatitis and, 187
  patch testing in, 200
  emphasis on, in medical record, 21–22
Allograft, 597
Alloplastic materials, in plastic surgery, 597
Allopurinol, 720
ALP (alkaline phosphatase), 307
Alphabet, Greek, 838
ALT (alanine aminotransferase), 307
  monitoring of, 360t
Alveolus(i), *690*, 691
American Association for Medical Transcription, 10
  Code of Ethics of, 13–20, *19*
  competency profile of (COMPRO), 123, *124–127*
  model job description of, *6–9*, 93
  problem solving by, 140–141

American Association of Medical Assistants, 10
American Board of Family Practice, 230–231
American College of Radiology, 686–687
American Health Information Management Association, Code of Ethics of, *18*
American Medical Association, Principles of Medical Ethics of, *16*
American Medical Technologists, 10
Amikacin, monitoring of, 360t
Amitriptyline, monitoring of, 360t
Amobarbital, monitoring of, 360t
Amoxapine, monitoring of, 360t
Ampicillin, urinary sediments and, 338t
Amputation, 510
Amylase, monitoring of, 360t
ANA (antinuclear antibodies) test, 357, 718
Anaphylactic shock, urticaria and, 187–188
Anasarca, 303
Anatomic pathology. See *Pathology.*
Anatomy. See also specific discipline.
    references on, 756
Androgens, 221t
Anemia, 304–305
    pediatric, 582
    red cell evaluation in, 311, *312–317*
Anesthesia, 259–260, 260t, 261t
    in cardiovascular surgery, 170
    in podiatry, 645
Aneurysm, brain, 395–396
    ventricular, surgery for, 171
Angina pectoris, 155
Angiofibroma, nasopharyngeal, 540
Angiography, coronary, *166–168*
    in kidney disorders, 374
Angioma, cherry, 197
Angioplasty, 156
    balloon, 663
Angiotensin-converting enzyme inhibitors, 154t
Anisocytosis, *314, 315*
Ankle, 498–499, *498*
    disorders of, 643
    fracture of, 509–510
    reconstruction of, 607–608
    trauma to, 632, *632*
Ankyloglossia, 537
Answering machines, 49, 68
Antacids, in gastroesophageal reflux disease, 243, 304
Antiarrhythmics, 154t
Antibodies, 290
Anticholinergics, 695
Anticoagulants, 154t
Antidiuretic hormone, 221t
Anti-dsDNA, 357
Antigens, 287
Antiglobulin tests, 341

Antihypertensives, 154t, 389t
Anti-La (SSB), 357
Antinuclear antibodies (ANA) test, 357, 718
Anti-Ro (SSA), 357
Antonyms, references on, 756
Anxiety disorders, 650, 653
    consultation report in, *656, 659*
Aorta, coarctation of, 574, *575*
    diseases of, 157
Apert's syndrome, 610
Apgar score, 573, 574t
Apnea, pediatric, 581
    sleep, 691–692
    treatment of, 696, *696*
Apolipoprotein, 309
Appendicitis, 284
    history and physical examination format in, *285–286*
    in children, 588, 591
Apposition, 398
Apraxia, 398
Arboviruses, 354
Arm, 494, 496, *496*
    fracture of, 504–505
    range of motion of, *497*
    reconstruction of, 605, 607
        cosmetic, 619, 622
Arm flaps, 605, 607
Arrhythmias, agents against, 154t
    classification of, 159t
    diagnosis of, 158
Arteriography, coronary, 161, *166–169*, 169
    in neurology, 397
Arteriosclerosis, *161*
    in diabetes, 226–227
Arteritis, temporal, 718
Artery(ies), coronary, *152*
    occlusion of, *161*
    diseases of, 157
Arthritis, 302
    degenerative, 302, 715–717, *716*
        hip, 500–501
            surgery in, 501–502
    infectious, 720–721
    psoriatic, 718, 720
    rheumatoid, 195, 717
        juvenile, 584
    treatment of, *718*
Arthrocentesis, 721
Arthrodesis, 510
Arthroplasty, 510
Arthropods, 352
Arthroscopy, 510, 721
    record of, *515–516*
Arthrotomy, 510
Artificial urinary sphincter, 734
Artists, medical, 114
Arytenoidectomy, 543
Aspartate aminotransferase (AST), 308
    monitoring of, 361t
Aspiration, 510

AST (aspartate aminotransferase), 308
    monitoring of, 361t
Asthma, diagnosis of, 697
    pediatric, 580–581
    treatment of, 697
Ataxia, 398
Athlete's foot, 192, 627
Atopic dermatitis, 186
Atrial arrhythmias, 159t
Atrial septal defect, 574
Atrophy, skin, *184*
Attention deficit disorder, 585
Audiometry, in family medicine, 233
Audiovisual aids, 131–132
Auditory canal, disorders of, 528–531
Augmentation mammaplasty, 614
Auricle, 521, *522*
    congenital malformation of, 528
Authorship. See *Publication.*
Autoantibodies, 341
Autograft, 597
Autoimmune disorders, 292t
    laboratory studies in, 356–359
Autoimmune hemolytic anemia, red cells in, *315*
Autonomic nervous system, 393–394. See also *Nervous system.*
Autopsy reports, 564, 566
    deadlines for, 28
AV junctional arrhythmias, 159t
Avulsion, nail, 638, 640

B cell, 290, *290*
Babinski's sign, 399, 631, *631*
Bacterial infections. See also specific infection.
    arthritis and, 720–721
    laboratory studies in, 344, 350–351
        critical and alert values in, 367t
    respiratory tract, 581
    urinalysis in, 337
Bacteriuria, 337, 350–351
Balanitis, 736t
Balloon angioplasty, 663
Banking, 60–61
Barium contrast, 661
    studies with, 662, *668*
        report on, 666, *669*
Barré's position, 399
Barrett's esophagus, 244, 304
Basal cell carcinoma, skin, 197
Basophil, 311, *324*
Basophilic stippling, *316*
Batch sheet, *59*
Bed sore, 199
Bedbugs, 352
Bell's palsy, 533
Benign prostatic hypertrophy, *736*, 736t
Beta-adrenergics, 695
Beta-blockers, 154t
Bethesda System, for reporting Papanicolaou smears, 564, 565t

Bibliographies, 115
Biceps brachii flap, 605
Bile, 247
Bilirubin, 308
    in urine, 331
    monitoring of, 361t
    urinary sediments and, 338t
Billing, 50, *51*, 57–58
Bing's sign, 400
Bioethics, 24. See also *Ethics.*
Biologic response modifiers, 465, 466t
Biopsy, 457–458
    bronchoscopic, 693
    cone, 434, *435*
    CT-guided, *674*
        report on, *675*
    kidney, 374
    lymph node, neck, 542
    muscle, 397
    needle aspiration, *458*
        pathology report on, *468*
    nerve, 397
    pathology report on, 562, *563*
    pleural, 694
        instruments for, 697
    punch, 200
    shave, 200
Biopsy and resection report, 569
Bipolar disorder, 653
Birth, 430
Birth defects, breast, reconstruction in, *611*
    of central nervous system, 584
    of ear, 528
    of esophagus, 575
    of foot, *634*
    of heart, 151–152, 574, *575*
        surgery on, 170
    of kidney, 381–382, 738t, *739*
    of nose, 534
    of oral cavity, 537
    reconstructive surgery in, *604*, 608, *609*, 610
    urologic, *738*, 738t
Bladder, urinary, *735*
    cancer of, 737t
        transurethral resection of, 745
    diverticula of, 737t
    neurogenic, 740t
    ruptured, 742t
    surgery on, 735
Bleeding, from nose, 535–536
    from stomach, 244
    from ulcer, 304
    in pregnancy, 427, 429
    pediatric, 579–580
    vaginal, 434–435
Blepharoplasty, 544
    record of, *620–621*
Blood. See also *Hematology.*
    cultures of, 344
    in urine, 331, 332–333, 332t, 333t

Blood circulation, 151–152
    disorders of, 156t
    extracorporeal, 170
    through heart, *152*
Blood count. See *Complete blood count.*
Blood grouping, 337, 340, 341t, 342t, 343
Blood urea nitrogen (BUN), 308
    monitoring of, 361t
Body contouring, 615, 619
Boil, 188
Bone, 492–493, *494*
    growth of, 491–492
    instruments used on, 512
    nuclear studies of, 421t, 663
        reports on, *422*, *474*
Bone grafting, 510, 597
Bone marrow reports, 564
Bonuses, 87–88, 87t
Bookkeeping, 58, *59*
Borrelia burgdorferi, 356
Bouchard's nodes, *716*
Bowen's disease, 742t
Brachioplasty, 619, 622
Brachioradialis flap, 607
Brachymetatarsia, *635*
Brachytherapy, 683–684, *684*
Brain, 391–392, *392*
    MRI of, *676*
        report on, *677*
    surgery on, 397, 398t
    symptoms referable to, 396
    tumors of, 395
Branchial arch syndromes, 608
Branchial cleft cyst, removal of, 543
Breach of contract, physician-patient, 30
Breast, cancer of, 268–269, 273–274
    classification of, 268
    diagnosis of, 273–274, *458*, 662, *666*
    discharge summary in, *472–473*
    history and physical examination in, 273
    incidence of, 268
    pathology reports in, 277, *468*, *470–471*
    radiology reports in, *467*, *475*
    recurrence of, 269, 273
    spread of, 268–269
    treatment of, 462
        chemotherapeutic, 464–465
        consultation report in, *476*
        hormonal, 465
        operative reports on, *275–276*, *469*
        surgical, 274
    gynecologist and, 449
    reconstruction of, 610–614, *611–613*
        pedicle flaps in, 601
        record of, *616–617*
Breast implants, 610–611
Breast self-examination, 273
Brochures, 80, *81*
Bromide, monitoring of, 361t

Bronchitis, 303–304
Bronchoalveolar lavage, 694
Bronchodilators, 695
Bronchogenic carcinoma. See *Lung.*
Bronchopulmonary dysplasia, 574
Bronchoscopy, *459*, 545, 693–694, *694*, 697, 707
    in lung cancer, 267–268
    report on, *708–709*
Brow lift, 615
Bulla, skin, *183*
Bulldog sign, 400
Bulletin boards, 132
    electronic, 65
Bullous pemphigoid, 186–187
BUN (blood urea nitrogen), 308
    monitoring of, 361t
Bunion, 633, *639*
    treatment of, 638, 641–642
Burns, red cells in, *315*
    surgery in, 610
Burrow, skin, *184*
Business cards, 61, *62*
Butabarbital, monitoring of, 361t
Butalbital, monitoring of, 361t

CA 125, 322
Calcium, 308
    monitoring of, 361t
    regulation of, 390
Calcium carbonate, urinary sediments and, 338t
Calcium channel blockers, 154t
Calcium oxalate, urinary sediments and, 338t
Caldwell-Luc operation, 546
Callus, 625
Calorimetry, indirect, 694, 707
    equipment for, 697
Canada, postal abbreviations for, 832
Cancer, 292t, 453–454, *454*, *455*, 682. See also *Oncology/hematology; Tumors.*
    defined, 259
    diagnosis of, 457–459, *458*, *459*
        tumor markers in, 321–323, 326, 459t
    head and neck surgery in, 541–543
    immune system and, 291
    incidence of, *456*
    mortality from, *456*
    screening for, 454–457
        guidelines for, 457t
    staging of, 459–460, *460–461*, 462
    treatment of, 462–466, 477
        biologic response modifier, 465, 466t
        chemotherapeutic, 463–465, 464t–466t
        clinical trials of, 466, 477
        hormonal, 465, 466t

Cancer *(Continued)*
  radiation, 463, 682–686. *See also*
    Radiation therapy.
  surgical, 462–463
Candidiasis, skin, 192–193
  urinary, *336*
Capsulectomy, 510
Capsulotomy, 510
Carbamazepine, monitoring of, 361t
Carbon, radioactive, 416t, 418t
Carbon dioxide, monitoring of, 362t
Carbon monoxide, monitoring of, 361t
Carbuncle, 188
Carcinoembryonic antigen (CEA),
    322–323
Carcinoma. *See also Cancer.*
  defined, 259, 454, 682
Cardiac. *See also Heart.*
Cardiac catheterization, 161, *166–169*,
    169
  neonatal, 574
    procedure note on, *576–578*
Cardiac transplantation, 170–171
Cardiac tumors, 157
Cardiology, 151–178. *See also*
    Cardiovascular disorders.
  anatomy and physiology in, 151–153,
    152, 153
  history and physical examination in,
    153, 155, 155t
    format for, 171, *172–175*
  invasive, 161, *166–169*, 169
  neonatal, 574
  noninvasive, 158–161, *158, 160,*
    162–165
  references on, 178, 764
Cardiomyopathies, 157
Cardiopulmonary stress test, 697
  report on, *706*
Cardiotonics, 154t
Cardiovascular disorders, 155–158,
    156t, *161*, 303
  diagnosis of, 158–169
    invasive procedures in, 161,
      166–169, 169
    noninvasive procedures in,
      158–161, *158, 160, 162–165*
    nuclear medicine in, 421t
  drugs for, 154t
  history and physical examination in,
    153, 155, 155t
    format for, 171, *172–175*
  in diabetes, 226–227
  renal diseases with, 158
  risk factors for, 153, 302
  surgery for, 169–171, 178
    record of, 171, *176–178*, 179
Cardiovascular system, 151–153
Career development. *See also*
    Employment.
  references on, 65, 756–757
Carpal tunnel syndrome, 503–504, *503*
  history and physical examination in,
    506–507

Cassettes, 49, 50, 67
Cast, instruments used for, 512, 513
  materials used for, 512, 513, 645
Casts, urinary, 333, 333t, *335*
Cataract surgery, 483–484, *483*
  operative report on, *487–488*
Catheterization, cardiac, 161, *166–169*,
    169
  neonatal, 574
    procedure note on, *576–578*
CEA (carcinoembryonic antigen),
    322–323
Cell(s). *See also specific cell.*
  immunologic, 287–290, *288–290*
  lung cancer, 261, 265–266
  skin, 179–180
Cell cycle, 453, *454*
Cellulitis, 189, 304
Central nervous system, 391–392,
    392–394. See also Nervous system.
  nuclear studies of, 421t
  tumors of, 395
Cerebellopontine angle, tumor of, 544
Cerebral palsy, 584
Cerebrospinal fluid (CSF), examination
    of, 344, 350
Cerebrovascular disease, 394–395
Certification, 10
  reference on, 757
Cerumen, impacted, 528
Cervical visor flap, 604
Cervix, uterine, biopsy of, 434, *435*
  cancer of, 434
  dysplasia of. *See Papanicolaou*
    (Pap) smear.
Cesarean section, 430
  record of, *432–433*
Chaddock's sign, 400
Chancroid, 193–194, 350
Charitable organizations, Appendix 9
Chart notes. *See also Medical records.*
  in gastroenterology, 250
  in podiatry, 645, *646*
  in psychiatry, 654, *655*
  in rheumatology, *724, 725*
  in urology, *750–751*, 752
Checking accounts, 61
Chemical elements table, Appendix 7
Chemistry tests, 307–311
Chemotherapy, 463–465. *See also*
    Drugs; specific agent.
  agents used in, 464t
  combination, 464–465
    abbreviations for, 466t
  consultation report on, *476*
  tumor response to, 465t
  white cell count and, *322–323*
Cherry angioma, 197
Chest, examination of, 155t
  x-ray, 661–662, *664*
    report on, 664, *665*, 666
Chest pain, 693
  pleuritic, 689, 693
Chest wall, disorders of, 691

Chickenpox, 353
Childbirth, 430
Children. *See also Neonatology;*
    Pediatrics.
  bone growth in, 491–492
  family medicine and, 232
  gait treatment in, 638
  slipped capital femoral epiphysis in,
    499–500
  supracondylar fracture of humerus
    in, 504–505
Chin, augmentation of, 614
Chinese flap, 605
Chlamydia trachomatis, cultures of, 350
Chlamydial infections, 355
Chloramphenicol, monitoring of, 361t
Chlorazepate, monitoring of, 362t
Chlordiazepoxide, monitoring of, 362t
Chloride, 311
  monitoring of, 362t
Chlorpromazine, monitoring of, 362t
Choanal atresia repair, 545
Cholecystectomy, 249
Cholesteatoma, 531
Cholesterol, 302, 308–309
  LDH, monitoring of, 364t
  urinary sediments and, 338t
Cholesterol-reducing agents, 154t
Chronic obstructive pulmonary disease
    (COPD), treatment of, 695
Chvostek's sign, 399
Circulation, blood, 151–152
  disorders of, 156t
  through heart, *152*
  extracorporeal, 170
Circumduction, *497*
Cirrhosis, 247
Cleft palate, 537
  repair of, 545, *604*, 608, *609*
Clergy, forms of address for, 822–823
Clinical trials, 466, 477
Clonazepam, monitoring of, 362t
Closed reduction, 510
Coagulation, disorders of, pediatric, 580
  evaluation of, 317
Coarctation of aorta, 574, *575*
Coauthorship, 119
Codes, in pathology reports, 566
Codes of ethics, 13, *14–19*
Coitus, pain in, 435
Cold, common, 303
Colitis, ulcerative, 246
Collagen vascular disorders, 715, 718
  laboratory studies in, 356–359
  skin in, 194–195
Collection, 60
Colles' fracture, 508–509
Colon, cancer of, 279–281, 284
  diagnosis of, 281
  obstruction in, 281
  risk factors for, 280–281
  surgery for, 281, 284, *284*
    record of, *282–283*
  decompression of, 281

Colon (Continued)
  disorders of, 246
  surgery on, 249
  visualization of, 250
Colonoscopy, 246, 250
Colporrhaphy, 442, *451*
Colposcopy, 434
  in family medicine, 233
Coma, diabetic, 224, 225
Combining forms, in medical
    terminology, Appendix 3
Comedo, skin, *184*
Common cold, 303
Competency profile (COMPRO), of
    American Association for Medical
    Transcription, 123, *124–127*
Complete blood count, 311–313, *312–
    326*, 317
  platelet evaluation in, 312–313, 317,
    326
  red cell evaluation in, 311, *312–317*
  water artifact in, *316*
  white cell evaluation in, 311–312,
    318, 320–326
Completeness, of medical records,
    28–29
Composition. See also *Publication.*
  references on, 757
Computed tomography (CT), 662,
    670–671
  biopsy guided by, *674*
  report on, *675*
  in kidney disorders, 374
  in neurology, 396
  report on, 666, *672–673*
Computers, 45, 68
  comfort and safety considerations
    with, 71–72, *71, 73*, 74t
  confidentiality and, 23
  in pathology, 566, *567–568*, 569
  Macintosh, 70
  networking through, 65
  printers for, 45, 68–69
  setup of, 69
Condylomata acuminata, 192
Cone biopsy, 434, *435*
Confidentiality, 5, 22–24, 29–30
  AIDS and, 34, 37
  American Association for Medical
    Transcription Code of Ethics on, 19
  computer access and, 23
  court orders and, 30
  disclosure and, 30, 32–34, 37
    consent forms for, *31–33, 35*
  electronic transmission devices and,
    23, 37–38, *39*
  employer's statements on, *20, 21*
  exceptions to, 32–34
  of Association determinations, 18
  of patient's name, 34
  of psychiatric documents, 38, 654
  privilege and, 23–24, 29–30
  right to privacy and, 23–24
Congenital defects. See *Birth defects.*

Conjugate gaze, 399
Conjunctiva, 399
Connective tissue diseases, 715, 718
  laboratory studies in, 356–359
  skin in, 194–195
Consent forms, for admission of
    observers, *31*
  for disclosure of information by
    physician, *32*
  for examination of physicians'
    records, *33*
  for furnishing information, *33, 35*
  for HIV testing, *36*
Consultation reports, in dermatology,
    203
  in family medicine, *236–237*, 240
  in immunology, 291–292, *293–295*
  in nephrology, *375–376, 379, 380*
  in neurology, *404*
  in oncology, *476*
  in ophthalmology, 489
  in orthopaedics, *517–518*, 519
  in otorhinolaryngology, 546, *549*
  in pathology, 569, *570*
  in pediatrics, *589*
  in psychiatry, *656*, 659
  in pulmonary medicine, 697, *698–701*
  in rheumatology, *722–724*
  in urology, *748–749*, 752
Contact dermatitis, 187
Continuing education, 10–11
Continuous ambulatory peritoneal
    dialysis, 381, *384*
Continuous positive airway pressure
    (CPAP), 696, *696*
Contraception, 424–425
Contractors, independent, agreement
    form for, *46–48*
  characterization of, 55, 56t, 57
Contracts, with publishers, 111–112
Contrast media, 661
Convergence, 399
Convulsions, 584–585
COPD (chronic obstructive pulmonary
    disease), treatment of, 695
Copy editors, 116
Copy machines, 49, 72
Copyright, 118–119
Cor pulmonale, 158
Corn, 625, *626*
  treatment of, 636, 640, 641
Cornea, 399
Corneal reflex, 399
Coronary arteries, 152, *152*
  occlusion of, *161*
Coronary arteriography, 161, *166–169*,
    169
Coronaviruses, 354
Corporations, 57
Corporotomy, 734
Correction, of author's proof, 116, *117*
  of medical records, 22, 29, 97–98,
    102–104
  emergency, *218*

Correction (Continued)
  in pathology, 562
Cortisol, 221t
Cosmetic surgery, 595. See also *Plastic
    surgery.*
Cost containment, medical
    documentation and, 4
Course evaluation, 137, *138*
Court orders, confidentiality and, 30
Cover letters, for publication proposals,
    10
Coxsackie virus, 354
CPAP (continuous positive airway
    pressure), 696, *696*
CPK, monitoring of, 362t
Cramps, menstrual, 435
Cranial nerve, 392
  surgery on, 544
Cranial sutures, 403
  premature fusion of, consultation
    letter on, *589*
Craniostenosis, 399
Craniosynostosis, 399
Craniotomy, 397
C-reactive protein, 307
Creatinine, 308
  monitoring of, 362t
Credit, 60
Crenated cell, *316*
CREST syndrome, 718
Critical and alert laboratory values,
    359, 360t–368t, 368–369. See also
    Appendix 5.
Crohn's disease, 244–246
Cromolyn sodium, 695
Cross-leg flap, 607
Croup, 540
Crouzon's syndrome, 610
Crust, skin, *183*
Cryoglobulins, 357–358
Cryosurgery, in dermatology, 200
Cryptorchism, *737*, 737t
Crystals, in urine, 333, *336, 337,
    338t–340t*
CSF (cerebrospinal fluid), examination
    of, 344, 350
CT. See *Computed tomography (CT).*
Cultures, in bacterial infections, 344,
    350
Curettage, 200, 510
Curette, 512
  ear, 546
Curie, 416–417
Current Procedural Terminology, 566
Cutaneous T-cell lymphoma, 198
Cutaneous ureterostomy, 734–735
Cyanide, blood, monitoring of, 362t
Cyst, branchial cleft, removal of, 543
  epidermal inclusion, 196
  foot, 642
  laryngeal, 541
  ovarian, 442
  pilar, 196
  preauricular, 526, 528

Cyst *(Continued)*
　skin, *182*
　　Thornwaldt's, 540
　　thyroglossal duct, 540
　　　removal of, 543
Cystectomy, 735
Cystic fibrosis, 580
Cystine, urinary sediments and, 338t
Cystitis, 737t
　urinalysis findings in, 327t
Cystocele, 737t
Cystography, voiding, consultation
　　report on, *380*
Cystolithectomy, 735
Cystolitholapaxy, 735
Cystolithotomy, 735
Cystopexy, 735
Cystoplasty, 735
Cystoscopy, 735
Cystotomy, 735
Cystourethroplexy, 735
Cytology, report forms in, 562, 564
　request forms in, 555–557, *558–561*
Cytology-tissue report correlation, 569

Dataforms, 4
Deadlines, for medical reports, 28,
　　87–88
Debridement, 510
Debulking, 463
Decerebrate posturing, 399
Decorticate posturing, 399
Decubitus ulcer, 199
Deep venous thrombosis, 303
Defamation, 30
Degenerative disk disease, 396, 502–503
Dehydration, in diabetes, 223, 225
Delivery services, 44
Deltoid flap, 605
Deltopectoral flap, 599, *599*, 604
Demyelinating disease, 395
Dentistry, references on, 764
Dermatitis, allergic contact, 187
　atopic, 186
　seborrheic, 185
Dermatitis herpetiformis, 187
Dermatofibroma, 197
Dermatology, 179–206. See also *Skin.*
　anatomy and physiology in, 179–181,
　　180, 181
　consultation report in, *203*
　diagnosis in, 199–200
　discharge summary in, *204–205*
　history and physical examination in,
　　format for, *201*
　references on, 206, 764
　surgery in, 200
　　record of, *202*
　terms used in, *182–184*
Dermatomyositis, 195, 718
Dermatophytosis, 192

Dermis, 180
Design, publication, 116
Desipramine, monitoring of, 362t
Desks, 50
Developmental disorders, 650
Deviated nasal septum, 536
Diabetes, 222–228, 302
　clinical picture of, 223
　complications of, 223, 224t, 226–228,
　　377–378
　emergencies in, 224–225
　foot in, 627–628
　gestational, 429
　in children, 585–586
　pathophysiology of, 222–223
　treatment of, 225–226, 225t, 226t
　　home monitoring in, 226
　types of, 223, 224t
Diagnosis. See also specific discipline
　　or technique.
　degree of certainty in, 414–415
　handbooks on, 757
*Diagnostic and Statistical Manual III,
　　Revised* (DSM-III-R), 650, 652
Dialysis, 381, *383, 384*
　discharge summary for, *385–387*
　review report on, *388*
Diarrhea, cultures in, 351
　pediatric, 581–582
Diazepam, monitoring of, 362t
Dictation, discrepancies in, 22
　equipment for, 67
　foreign, 101–102
　interrupted, 208
　omissions from, 21
　transcription skills and, 4, 5
Dictionaries, 143–146
　computerized, 757
　English, 143, 144–145, 757
　foreign, 757–758
　medical, 145–146, 758
Diet, 241
　in diabetes, 225
　kidney disease and, 384, 389
Dietician, radiation therapy and, 686
Digestive system, 241, *242.* See also
　　Gastroenterology.
　disorders of, 242–248, *242*
　surgery on, 248–250
Digital systems, 67
Digitoxin, monitoring of, 362t
Digoxin, monitoring of, 362t
Dilation and curettage, 428, *428*
Diplomatic personnel, forms of address
　　for, 823–824
Direct internal urethrotomy, 735
Disability insurance, 53–54
Disabled persons, equipment for, 70
　references for, 762–763
　teaching of, 140
Disarticulation, 510
Discharge summaries, in dermatology,
　　204–205

Discharge summaries *(Continued)*
　in emergency medicine, 209
　in family medicine, *238–239*, 240
　in gastroenterology, 250–251
　in immunology, 292, *296–297*
　in nephrology, *385–387*
　in neurology, *405–406*
　in oncology, *472–473*
　in ophthalmology, 489
　in orthopaedics, 519
　in otorhinolaryngology, 546,
　　551–552, 553
　in pediatrics, *590–591*, 591, 593
　in psychiatry, *657–658*, 659
　in pulmonary medicine, 707, *712–714*
　in rheumatology, 721, *727–729*, 730
　in urology, 752
　typing style for, 777
Disclosure, 30, 32–34, 37
　consent forms for, *31–33, 35*
　required, 32–34
　subpoenas for, 38, *40, 41*
Discoid lupus erythematosus, 194–195
Disk, intervertebral, disorders of, 396,
　　502–503
Diskettes, 68
Disopyramide, monitoring of, 363t
Displacement osteotomy, 510
Dissociative disorders, 650
Distribution channels, 80
Diuretics, 154t
Diverticulectomy, 744
Diverticulitis, 246
Diverticulosis, 246
Dizziness, 534
Dolichocephaly, 399
Dorsalis pedis flap, 608
Dosimetrist, 685, *685*
Doxepin, monitoring of, 363t
Drugs. See also specific drug or category.
　abused, 651–652t
　chemotherapeutic. See *Chemotherapy.*
　for cardiovascular disorders, 154t
　for respiratory disorders, 695
　in diabetes, 225–226, 225t, 226t
　in psychiatry, 654
　kidney failure and, 378, 379, 381, 381t
　lupus and, 718
　monitoring of, 359, 360t–368t,
　　368–369
　positive antiglobulin test and, 341
　prescription abbreviations for,
　　833–834
　references on, 143–144, 761–762
　urine color changes with, 330t
DSM-III-R *(Diagnostic and Statistical
　　Manual III, Revised)*, 650, 652
Duodenal ulcer, 244
Dysmenorrhea, 435
Dyspareunia, 435
Dysphagia, 243
Dyspnea, 692
　in cardiovascular disorders, 153, 155

Dystocia, 430
Dysuria-pyuria syndrome, urinalysis
    findings in, 327t

Ear, anatomy of, 521–522, *522–525*
    bacterial infections of, 350
    external, 521, *522*
        disorders of, 526, 528–531
    inner, 522, *525*
        disorders of, 533–534
        instruments used on, 546
    middle, 521–522, *523, 524*
        disorders of, 531–533, 581
    surgery on, 542, 543–544
        cosmetic, 614
Earwax, impacted, 528
ECG. See *Electrocardiography.*
Echocardiography, 159–160, *163*
Echo-Doppler studies, 159–160
Echoviruses, 354
ECT (electroconvulsive therapy), 654
Ecthyma, 188–189
Ectopic pregnancy, 427–428
Eczema, external ear, 528
Edema, 303
    of foot, 627–627
Editing, 97–105
    guidelines for, 97–99
    levels of, 101
    of foreign dictation, 101–102
    of substandard language, 101
    page makeup and, 100–101
    proofreading and, 90–91, 102
    reference materials for, 104–105,
        758. See also *Reference materials.*
    types of errors in, 99–101
Editors, 108, 110, 116
    correspondence with, 111
Education, 44
    careers in. See *Teaching.*
    competency profile for, 123, *124–127*
    continuing, 10–11
    general medical, 229–231
    in medical transcription, 5
    in podiatry, 623–624
    in radiology, 661, 684–686
Ejaculation, 734
Elbow, 494
    supracondylar fracture of humerus
        and, 504–505
Electrocardiography, 158–159, *158, 160*
    Holter, 161, *165*
    in family medicine, 233
    stress, 159, *162*
Electroconvulsive therapy (ECT), 654
Electroencephalography, 396–397
Electrolytes, 311
Electromyography, 397
Electronic bulletin boards, 65
Electronystagmography, 534

Electrophoresis, CSF immunoglobulin,
    358
    lipoprotein, 309
Electrosurgery, in dermatology, 200
ELISA (enzyme-linked immunosorbent
    assay) testing, for HIV, 343
Elliptic scalpel excision, 200
Elliptocytosis, *315*
E-mail, confidentiality and, 23
Embolism, pulmonary, nuclear studies
    of, 415, *415, 416*
Embryo, implantation of, *426*
Emergency medicine, 207–218
    ancillary studies in, 209
    diabetes and, 224–225
    discharge instructions in, 209
    prehospital treatment in, 209
    procedures in, 208–209
    record transcription in, 207–209,
        210–217, 218
        stat, 208, 218
        turn-around time for, 207–208
    referrals in, 209
    timekeeping in, 209
Emphasis, in medical record, 1–22
Employees, benefits for, 91–92
    dismissal of, 92–93
    foulmouthed, 90
    grievances of, 90
    hiring of, 92
    production by, 88–89
    recruitment of, 92
    salaries of, 90
    slow, 89
    socializing by, 90
    supervision of. See *Management.*
    training of, 90
    untidy, 89–90
Employment. See also *Self-employment.*
    as manager. See *Management.*
    confidentiality agreements for, *20, 21*
    job description for, *6–9*, 93
        as pathology secretary, 571–572
    opportunities for, 5, 10, 43–65
    references on, 65, 756–757
    vs. independent contractor status,
        55, 56t, 57
Encephalocele, 534
Endocarditis, infective, surgery for, 171
Endocrinology, 219–228
    abnormal conditions in, 222t. See
        also *Diabetes.*
    anatomy and physiology in, 219, *220,*
        221, 221t
Endolymphatic sac, surgery on, 544
Endometriosis, 435–436, *436*
    history and physical examination
        format in, *437–439*
    operative report in, *440–441*
Endoscopy, 241–242, 249–250
    in cancer diagnosis, 458–459, *459*
    in otorhinolaryngology, 545
    upper gastrointestinal, 243

Endoscopy *(Continued)*
    video, 250, *251*
English dictionaries, 143, 144–145, 757
Enteritis, regional, 244–246
Enterocolitis, necrotizing, 575, 579
Enteroviruses, 353–354
Enzyme-linked immunosorbent assay
    testing (ELISA), for HIV, 343
Eosinophil, 289, 311, 312, *324*
Epidermal inclusion cyst, 196
Epidermal necrolysis, toxic, 188
Epidermis, 179–180, *180*
Epidermoid carcinoma, lung, 261, 265
Epididymectomy, 744
Epididymis, 734
Epididymitis, 738t
Epiglottis, 526
Epiglottitis, acute, 540
Epilepsy, 584–585
Epinephrine, 221t
Epiphysiodesis, 510
Epistaxis, 535–536
    surgery for, 546
Eponyms, references on, 756
Epstein-Barr virus, 353, 354t
Equipment, 45, 49–50, 67–75. See also
    Instruments.
    comfort and safety of, 71–72, *71, 73,*
        74t
    for physically challenged, 70
    leasing of, 49, 69
    maintenance of, 69–70
    new, 94
    problems with, 72, 74
Ergonomics, 71–72, *73,* 74t
    adjustments for, *71*
Erosion, skin, *184*
Erysipelas, 189
Erythema chronicum migrans, 721
Erythema multiforme, 188
Erythrasma, 189
Erythrocyte. See *Red blood cell.*
Esophagoscopy, 545
Esophagostomy, 543
Esophagus, disorders of, 242–244, 304
    congenital, 575
    surgery on, 249, 543
Estlander flap, 601
Estradiol, 221t
Estrogen replacement therapy, 441
Estrogens, 221t
Ethchlorvynol, monitoring of, 363t
Ethics, 13–26
    codes of, 13, *14–19*
    in medical transcription, accuracy
        and, 17–18, 20–22
    confidentiality and, 19
        of Association determinations, 18
    elected Association positions and,
        18
    knowledge enhancement and,
        19–20
    priority of goals and, 15–16

Ethics (Continued)
    professional attitude and, 14–15
    representation of committees and,
        18–19
    standards of conduct and, 13–14
    unethical procedures and, 16–17
    of service owners, 24–25
    problem solving in, 25–26
    references on, 26, 759–760
    transcriptionist's moral code and, 24
Ethmoidectomy, 546
Ethosuximide, monitoring of, 363t
Eustachian tube, disorders of, 532–533
Evoked potentials, 397
Excision, 510
    elliptic scalpel, 200
Extension, 497
Extensor digitorum longus anterior
        flap, 607
Extensor toe signs, 399–400
External ear, 521, 522
    disorders of, 526, 528–531
Extracorporeal circulation, 170
Extracorporeal shock wave lithotripsy,
        744
Eye, anatomy of, 480, 480–482, 481
    cultures of, in bacterial infections, 350
    disorders of, 482
        diagnosis in, 482–483
        medical treatment of, 483
        surgical treatment of, 483–485, 483
    trauma to, 485
Eye strain, 72
Eyelid, 482
    reconstruction of, donor sites for, 596
        record of, 620–621

FABER test, 400
Facelift, 544, 614–615, 618–619
    record of, 620–621
Facial diplegia, 400
Facial nerve, paralysis of, 533
    surgery on, 544
Facial spasm, 400
Facsimile machines, 49, 72
    confidentiality and, 23, 37–38, 39
    transmittal sheet for, 39
Factitious disorders, 650
Failure to thrive, 582
    evaluation of, 583
Fajersztajn's sign, 402
Family medicine, 229–240
    consultation report in, 236–237, 240
    discharge summary in, 238–239, 240
    history and physical examination in,
        format for, 234–235, 240
    history of, 229–231
    instruments used in, 233
    obstetrics in, 232
    practice setting of, 231–232
    records in, 233, 234–239, 235, 237, 240

Family medicine (Continued)
    residency training in, 232
    surgery in, 232–233
Fascial sling procedures, 545
Fasciocutaneous flap, 601, 602–603
Fax machines. See Facsimile machines.
Feces, cultures of, 351
Fees, 57–58, 79
Feet. See Foot.
Felon, 626–627, 628
Female reproductive system, anatomy
        of, 424–425
    disorders of, 433–436, 441
    examination of, 431, 434
Femoral stretch test, 400
Femur, fracture of, 505, 508, 508
Ferritin, 310
Fetus, monitoring of, 429–430
Fibrinogen, monitoring of, 363t
Fibroids, 436, 439, 442
    operative report in, 443–444
Fibula, 498
Fibula flap, 608
Figures, preparation of, 114
File cabinets, 50
File clerks, 44–45
Finger-to-nose test, 400
Firing, 92–93
Fissure, skin, 184
Flagging, 102, 103
Flaps, 544, 545, 598–608
    arm, 605, 607
    deltopectoral, 599, 599, 604
    forehead, 598–599, 598, 603–604
    free, 601
        head and neck, 605
    head and neck, 601, 603–605, 604
    in breast reconstruction, 611
    Indian, 598, 598
    leg, 607–608
    scalping, 599, 601, 603
    terminology for, 598–599, 601
    trunk, 605, 606
Flashcards, 132
Fleas, 352
Flexion, 497
    foot, 632, 633
Flexor carpi ulnaris flap, 607
Flies, 352
Floppy disks, 68
Flurazepam, monitoring of, 363t
Fluorine, radioactive, 416t
Fluoroscopy, 662
    bronchoscopy with, 693
Folliculitis, 188
Foot, 499, 499. See also Podiatry.
    anatomy of, 624–625, 624
    disorders of, 625–636
        integumentary, 625–627, 626–628
        surgery in, 638, 640
        musculoskeletal, 631–636, 632–636
        surgery in, 641–643
        neurologic, 628, 631, 631

Foot (Continued)
    surgery in, 640–641, 640
        peripheral vascular, 627–628
            evaluation of, 629, 630
            surgery in, 641
            treatment of, 636–643
    fracture of, 633–634, 635
    gout of, 720, 720
    orthotic devices for, 636, 637
    range of motion of, 633
    reconstruction of, 607–608
Footnotes, 115
Foramen closure test, 400
Forceps, 511
    bone-cutting, 644
    ear, 546
    nasal, 546
    obstetric, 430
Forearm, 494, 496
Forehead flaps, 598–599, 598, 603–604
Forehead lift, 615
Foreign body obstruction, of ear,
        528–529
    of esophagus, 244
    of nose, 536
    removal of, 545
Foreign dictionaries, 757–758
Formats. See specific discipline.
Forms of address, Appendix 10
Fractures, 504–505, 508–510
    ankle, 509–510
    facial, 544
    foot, 633–634, 635
    hip, 505, 508, 508
    kidney, 737t
    nasal, 535
    supracondylar, of humerus, 504–505
    wrist, 508–509
Free flaps, 601
    head and neck, 605
Freelancing. See Self-employment.
Frontal lobe release signs, 400
Frontal sinus, surgery on, 546
Frontoethmoidectomy, 546
Frozen section–final report correlation,
        569
Fungal infections. See also specific
        infection.
    critical and alert values in, 367t
    deep, 193
Furniture, 50
    adjustable, 71, 71
Furuncle, 188
    nasal, 534–535
Fusion, 510
Fusospirochetal infections, 356

Gait, analysis of, 632
    correction of, 638, 643
Gallbladder, disorders of, 247–248
    surgery on, 249

Gallbladder *(Continued)*
  ultrasonography of, *678*
    report on, *679*
Galley proofs, 116
Gallium, radioactive, 416t–417t, 418t
Gallstones, 247–248
Games, 759
Gamma-glutamyltransferase (GGT), 309
Ganslen's test, 400
Gas exchange, 691
Gastric ulcer, 244
Gastritis, 244
Gastrocnemius flap, 607
Gastroenterology, 241–257
  anatomy in, 241, *242*
  barium studies in, 661, 662, *668*
    report on, *669*
  chart notes in, 250
  discharge summary in, 250–251
  endoscopy in, 241–242
  history and physical examination in, 250
    format for, *252–255*
  instruments used in, 249–250, *251*
  nutrition in, 241
  pain location in, *245*
  references on, 257, 764
  representative disorders in, 242–248, *242*, 304
    of colon, 246, 248
    of duodenum, 244
    of esophagus, 242–244, 304
    of gallbladder, 247–248
    of liver, 246–247
    of mouth, 242
    of pancreas, 248
    of rectum, 246
    of small intestine, 244–246
    of stomach, 244
  surgery in, 248–250
    record of, 250, *256*
Gastroesophageal reflux, 243, 304
Gastrointestinal obstruction, neonatal, 579
Gastrointestinal tract, 241, *242*. See also *Gastroenterology.*
  disorders of, 242–248, *242*
  nuclear studies in, 421t
  surgery on, 248–250
General practice. See also *Family medicine.*
  vs. specialization, 229–231
General surgery, 259–286. See also *Surgery.*
Gentamicin, monitoring of, 363t
Geographic tongue, 537
German measles, skin in, 191–192
Gestational diabetes, 429
Gestational trophoblastic disease, 310
GGT (gamma-glutamyltransferase), 309
Gingivitis, 537
Glabellar sign, 400

Glaucoma, *484*
  surgery for, 484–485
Glioma, 395
  defined, 682
Glomerular filtration rate, 374
Glomerulonephritis, 374, 376
  causes of, 377t
  lupus, 378
  rapidly progressive, 376, 378t
  urinalysis findings in, 327t
Glomerulus, 372–373, *373*, 731, 733, *733*
Glomus jugulare, 532
Glossitis, 537
Glucagon, 221t
Glucose, 309
Glucose monitoring, 226
  alert and critical values in, 363t
Glucosuria, 331
Gluten enteropathy, 246
Glutethimide, monitoring of, 363t
Gluteus maximus flap, 607
Gonadotropins, 221t
Gonads, 219, *220*
Gonda's sign, 400
Gonococcemia, skin in, 190
Gonorrhea, arthritis in, 720–721
  cultures in, 350
Gordon's sign, 400
Gout, 720, *720*
Governmental officials, forms of address for, 824–826
Gracilis flap, 607
Grading, of medical transcription student, 127, *129*, 132–133
  point system in, 133, *134*, *135*
  software for, 142
Grafts, 597–598
  bone, 510, 597
  compound, 597–598
  skin, 545, 597–598
  tendon, 511
Grammar, references on, 759
Granulocyte, 311
Granuloma, ear, 532
Granuloma inguinale, 194
Greek alphabet, 838
Grievances, employee, 90
Groin flap, 605, *606*
Growth hormone, 221t
Guillain-Barré syndrome, 400–401
Gynecology, 423, 431–452
  breast disorders and, 449
  disorders in, 433–436, 439, 441
  family practitioner and, 232
  history and physical examination in, 431, 433–434
    format for, *437–439*
  pathology report in, 564, 565t
  references on, 452, 765
  surgery in, 442, 449, *450*
    records of, *440–441*, *443–449*, *451*
  tissue request form in, 556, 557, *560–561*

Hair, 180–181
Hairy tongue, 537
Half-life, radionuclide, 418, 418t
Hallux valgus, 633, *635*, *639*
  treatment of, 638, 641–642
Haloperidol, monitoring of, 363t
Hammertoe, 633
  treatment of, 641
Hand, 496, *496*
  osteoarthritis of, *716*
  reconstruction of, 601, *602–603*, 607
Handbooks, diagnostic and procedure, 757
  grammar, 759
Handouts, educational, 132
hCG (human chorionic gonadotropin), 309–310
Head and neck surgery, 541–542
  reconstructive, *599*, 601, 603–605, *604*
    in congenital deformities, *604*, 608, *609*, 610
Headache, pediatric, 585
Health and welfare agencies, Appendix 9
Hearing loss, otosclerosis and, 531–532, *532*, 533
  presbycusis and, 533
  sensorineural, 533
Heart, anatomy and physiology of, 151–153, *152*, *153*
  blood supply to, 152, *152*
  congenital defects of, 151–152, 574, *575*
    surgery on, 170
  disorders of. See *Cardiovascular disorders.*
  innervation of, 152–153, *153*
  physical examination of, 155, 155t
  SPECT of, 663, *680*
    report on, *681*
  tumors of, 157
  valves of, 151
    disorders of, 156
    surgery in, 171
Heart failure, 155–156
Heart transplantation, 170–171
Heartburn, 242–243, 304
Heart-lung transplantation, 171
Heberden's nodes, *716*
Heel, disorders of, 642–643
Heel-shin maneuver, 401
Hematin, urinary sediments and, 338t
Hematocrit, monitoring of, 363t
Hematology. See also *Oncology/hematology.*
  laboratory studies in, 311–313, *312–326*, 317, 319
  immunologic, 337, 340–344
  in kidney disorders, 374
Hematoma, external ear, 528
Hematopoietic system, disorders of, nuclear studies in, 421t
Hematospermia, 738t

Hematuria. See also *Urinalysis.*
  vs. hemoglobinuria and
    myoglobinuria, 333t
Hemifacial atrophy, 610
Hemifacial microsomia, 608
Hemilaminectomy, 510
Hemochromatosis, 247
Hemodialysis, 381, *383*
  discharge summary for, *385–387*
  review report on, *388*
Hemoglobin, evaluation of, 311
  monitoring of, 363t–364t
Hemoglobinuria, vs. myoglobinuria and
    hematuria, 333t
Hemolytic anemia, red cells in,
    315, 316
Hemoptysis, in lung cancer, 266
Hemorrhage. See *Bleeding.*
Hemorrhagic telangiectasia, 535–536
Hemorrhoids, 246
  treatment of, 249
Hemosiderin, urinary sediments and,
    338t
Hemostat, 511, 644
Hepatitis, 247
  A, 317, 319
  B, 319
  C, 319–320
  D, 320–321
  E, 321
  lupoid, 358
  pediatric, 579
  serodiagnosis of, 317, 319–321
Hepatorenal syndrome, 247
Hernia, congenital, *738*, 738t
  hiatal, 243, 244
Herniated intervertebral disc, 396,
    502–503
Herniorrhaphy, 744
Herpes simplex virus, 353
  skin in, 190–191, 535
Hiatal hernia, 243, 244
Hidradenitis suppurativa, 196
Highlighting, in medical record, 21–22
Hip, 496
  fracture of, 505, 508, *508*
  osteoarthritis of, 500–501
    surgery in, 501–502
  slipped capital femoral epiphysis of,
    499–500
Hippocratic oath, *14*
Hippuric acid, urinary sediments and,
    338t
Hiring, 92
History, psychiatric, 654–655, 659
History and physical examination,
    format for, in appendicitis,
    285–286
  in cardiology, 171, *172–175*
  in dermatology, *201*
  in family medicine, *234–235*, 240
  in gastroenterology, *252–255*
  in gynecology, *437–438*

History and physical examination
    (Continued)
  in orthopaedics, *506–507*
  in otorhinolaryngology, *548*
  in urology, 745, 752
  typing style for, *774*
  references on, 764
Hitchhiker sign, 401
HIV. See *Human immunodeficiency
    virus (HIV).*
Hives, 187–188
Hoarseness, in lung cancer, 266
Holter monitoring, 161, *165*
Home glucose monitoring, 226
Home office, 45
Homeostasis, immunologic, 290–291
Homonyms, references on, 756
Hormones, 219, 221t
  cancer treatment with, 465, 466t
Horner's syndrome, 401
Horseshoe kidney, 381, 738t, *739*
Hospitals, family practice in, 232
  market segmentation and, 77–78
  training programs in, 130
Howell-Jolly bodies, *317*
HTLV (human T-cell lymphotropic
    viruses), 355
Human chorionic gonadotropin (hCG),
    309–310
Human immunodeficiency virus (HIV),
    291, 355. See also *Acquired
    immunodeficiency syndrome
    (AIDS).*
  testing for, 343–344, 344t, *345–349*
    consent form for, *36*
Human retroviruses, 355
Human T-cell lymphotropic viruses
    (HTLV), 355
Humor and games, 759
Hydrocele, *738*, 738t, 739t
Hydrocephaly, 399
Hyperabduction test, 401
Hyperactivity, 585
Hyperbaric oxygen, in dermatology, 200
Hypercholesterolemia, 302
Hyperosmolar coma, 225
Hypertension, 303
  of pregnancy, 429
  pulmonary, neonatal, 574
  renovascular, 742t
Hypertrophic scar, 196–197
Hypertrophy, benign prostatic, *736*, 736t
Hyphenation, 99
  references on, 770
Hypoglycemic agents, 225–226, 225t,
    226t
Hypolipemics, 154t
Hyponychium, 181, *181*
Hypophysectomy, 546
Hypopituitarism, 586
Hypospadias, 739t
Hysterectomy, 442, *450*
Hysteroscopy, 434

Illustrations, preparation of, 114
Imipramine, monitoring of, 364t
Immune complexes, assays for, 358
Immune system, 287–291, *288–290*
  disorders of, 292t
  environment and, 287, *288*, 289t, *290*
  functions of, 290–291, 291t
  interrelationships with, *288*
Immunohematology, 337, 340–344
Immunology, 287–297
  anatomy and physiology in, 287–291,
    288–290, 291t
  discharge summary in, 292, *296–297*
  references on, 292, 764
  referral letter in, 291–292, *293–295*
  representative diseases in, 292t
Immunotherapy, 466
  radiation, 686
Impetigo contagiosa, 188
  nasal, 534
Implant materials, in plastic surgery,
    597
  breast, 610–611
Impotence, 739t
Impulse control disorders, 650
Incentive programs, 87–88, 87t
Income tax, 55
Incoming dictating equipment, 49
Inconsistencies, 99–100
  in emergency records, 208
  in teaching materials, 140–141
Incontinence. See *Urinary incontinence.*
Independent contractors, agreement
    form for, *46–48*
  characterization of, 55, 56t, 57
Indexing, 115
Indian flap, 598, *598*
Indiana pouch, 744
Indigotin, urinary sediments and, 338t
Indirect calorimetry, 694, 707
  equipment for, 697
Indium, radioactive, 416t–417t, 418t
Induration, skin, *183*
Infant, newborn. See *Neonatology.*
Infantile hypertrophic pyloric stenosis.
    See *Pyloric stenosis.*
Infections, 292t. See also specific type
    or infection.
  opportunistic, 344, 351–352
Infectious mononucleosis, diagnosis of,
    353, 354t
  lymphocytes in, *318*
  pharynx in, 540
Infective endocarditis, surgery for, 171
Infertility, male, 739t
Inflammation, 289–290
Inflammatory bowel disease, 244–246
Influenza, 303, 354
Informed consent, forms for. See
    Consent forms.
Ingrown toenail, 626–627, *628*
  treatment of, 638, 640
Inhalers, 695

Inner ear, 522, *525*
  disorders of, 533, 534
Insects, 352
Instruments, general surgical, 511–513
  in family medicine, 233
  in gastroenterology, 249–250, *251*
  in neurosurgery, 398t
  in ophthalmology, 485
  in orthopaedics, 511–513
  in otorhinolaryngology, 546
  in plastic surgery, 622
  in podiatry, 643–645
  in pulmonary medicine, 697
  in rheumatology, 721
  references on, 758
Insulin, 221t
  resistance to, 222
  treatment with, 225–226, 226t
Insurance, 53–54
  codes used for, 566
  references on, 759
  report for, in podiatry, 645, 648
    in rheumatology, *726*
  workers' compensation, 55
Intermittent claudication, in diabetes,
  226
Internal fixation, 510
  device for, 512
Internal medicine, 299–305
  history and physical examination in,
    301–302
  history of, 299–300
  practice of, 300
  references on, 305
  representative disorders in, 302–305
Internal Revenue Service, on
  employment vs. independent
  contractor status, 55, *56*, 57
  publications of, 65
International Classification of Diseases,
  566
Intersex, 740t
Interstitial nephritis, 382
  causes of, 389t
Intertrigo, 189
Intervertebral disk, disorders of, 396,
  502–503
Intramedullary fixation device, 512
Intranasal antrotomy, 545
Intravascular erythrocyte destruction,
  urine and plasma findings in,
  332t
Intravenous pyelography, 374
  report of, *375–376*
Intussusception, 586, 588, *588*
Iodine, radioactive, 416t–417t, 418t
Iron, measurement of, 310
Iron deficiency anemia, pediatric, 582
  red cells in, *314*
Irritable bowel syndrome, 248
Ischemic ulcer, 198–199
Island flap, 601, *602–603*
Isopropanol, monitoring of, 364t

Jaundice, 247
  pediatric, 579
  red cells in, *316*
Jaw jerk, 400
Job description, *6–9*, 93
  of pathology secretary, 571–572
Joint. See also *Arthritis*.
  aspiration of, 721
  replacement of, 511
    hip, 501–502
Joint Commission on Accreditation of
  Healthcare Organizations, medical
  record standards of, 27
*Journal of the American Association for
  Medical Transcription*, 94–95
Journals, 104
Juvenile rheumatoid arthritis, 584, 717

Kaposi's sarcoma, 198
Keloid, 196–197
  external ear, 528
Keratitis obturans, 531
Keratoma, plantar, treatment of, 641
Keratosis, actinic, 198
  seborrheic, 196
Ketoacidosis, diabetic, 224–225
Ketones, in urine, 331
Ketosis, monitoring of, 364t
Keyboards, comfort and, 71–72
Kidney, abscess of, 742t
  anatomy of, 371–373, *372, 373*, 731,
    733–734, *733*
  biopsy of, 374
  cancer of, 742t
  dialysis and, 381, *383, 384*
    discharge summary for, *385–387*
    review report on, *388*
  disorders of, 373–381, 738t–742t
    cardiovascular disorders with, 158
    congenital, 381–382, 738t, *739*
    consultation reports in, *375–376,
      379, 380*
    glomerular, 374, 376, 377t, 378t
    laboratory studies in, 327t, 373–374
    nuclear studies in, 421t
    signs and symptoms in, 382, 384,
      389
    systemic diseases and, 277, 377–378
    treatment of, 389–390, 389t, 390t,
      744–745
  failure of, acute, 378–379, 381, 381t
    chronic, 381, *382*, 737t
  fracture of, 737t
  polycystic, *741*, 741t
Kidney transplantation, 381
  rejection of, urinalysis findings in,
    327t
Knee, 497–498, *498*
Kocher's clamp, 511
Kock pouch, 744
KOH (potassium hydroxide)
  examination, 199–200

LA (lupus anticoagulant), 357
Labor, 430
Labor laws, 55
Laboratory medicine, 301–302, 307–369
  blood grouping in, 337, 340, 341t
  blood tests in, 311–313, *312–326*,
    317, 319
  chemical elements table in, Appendix
    7
  chemistry tests in, 307–311
  clinically important values in,
    Appendix 5
    critical and alert, 359, 360t–368t,
      368–369
  HIV testing in, 343–344, *345–349*
  in autoimmune disorders, 356–359
  in bacterial infections, 344, 350–351
  in hepatitis diagnosis, 317, 319–321
  in insect-borne diseases, 352
  in kidney disorders, 373–374
  in mycologic infections, 351
  in parasitic infections, 351–352
  in rheumatology, 717t
  in syphilis diagnosis, 355–356, 356t
  in viral infections, 352–355
  references on, 369
  therapeutic drug monitoring in, 359
  tumor markers in, 321–323, 326,
    459t
  urinalysis in. See *Urinalysis*.
  weights and measures in, Appendix 6
Labyrinthectomy, 544
Lactate, monitoring of, 364t
Lactic dehydrogenase (LD), 310
Laminectomy, 397, 503, 510
Laparoscopy, 245, 442, 449
Large cell carcinoma, lung, 266
Laryngectomy, 542–543
Laryngitis, 540
Laryngopharyngectomy, 543
Laryngoplasty, 544
Laryngoscopy, 545
Larynx, 524, 526, *529, 530*
  disorders of, 540–541
  surgery on, 542–543, 544
Lasagna Professional Oath, *15*
Lasègue's sign, 402
Laser surgery, in dermatology, 200
  in podiatry, 645
  laparoscopic, 442
Lateral arm flap, 605
Latissimus dorsi flap, 604, 605
Lavage, 510–511
Law, 27–42
  copyright, 118–119
  labor, 55
  references on, 42, 759–760
  self-employment and, 54–55
  tax, 55
LD (lactic dehydrogenase), 310
Le Fort fractures, 544
Lead, blood, monitoring of, 364t
Leasing, of equipment, 49, 69

Leg, 496–499, *498, 499*
  range of motion of, *497*
  reconstruction of, 607–608
Leg flaps, 607–608
Leptospirosis, 356
Leri's sign, 400
Letters, forms of address for, Appendix 10
  in family medicine, 233, 235
  in gastroenterology, 250
  in immunology, 291–292, *293–295*
  in neurology, 403
  in ophthalmology, 485, *486*
  in orthopaedics, 513
  in otorhinolaryngology, 546, *547*
  in pediatrics, *589*
  in psychiatry, 654
  in pulmonary medicine, 697
  in urology, 752
  typing style for, *772–773*
Leukemia, defined, 682
  in children, 582
  white cell evaluation in, *322–323, 325*
Leukocyte esterase, in urine, 332
Leukoplakia, 537–538, 540
Libel, 30
Lice, 352
  pubic, 194
Lichen planus, 185, 538
Lichenification, skin, *183*
Lidocaine, monitoring of, 364t
Life insurance, 54
Lip, cleft, 537
  repair of, *604*, 608, *609*
  reconstruction of, 601, *604*
  surgery on, 542
Lipase, monitoring of, 364t
Lipids, 308–309
Lipoma, 196
Lipoprotein electrophoresis, 309
Liposuction, 615, 619
Lithium, monitoring of, 364t
Lithotripsy, extracorporeal shock wave, 744
Liver, CT-guided biopsy of, *674*
  report on, *675*
  disorders of, 246–247
  autoimmune, 358
Logos, 61, *62*
Lower extremity, 496–499, *498, 499*
  range of motion of, *497*
  reconstruction of, 607–608
Lumbar puncture, 396
Lumpectomy, operative report on, *469*
  pathology report on, *470–471*
Lung, anatomy and physiology of, 689–691, *690*
  cancer of, 260–261, 265–268, 691, 696
  cell types in, 261, 265–266
  diagnosis of, 267–268
  pathology report in, *272*
  screening for, 267
  staging of, 696

Lung *(Continued)*
  surgery for, 268
  record of, *270–271*
  symptoms of, 266–267
  disorders of, 691
  nuclear medicine studies of, 415, *415, 416*
Lupoid hepatitis, 358
Lupus anticoagulant (LA), 357
Lupus erythematosus, discoid, 194–195
  systemic, 717–718
  kidney in, 378
  laboratory studies in, 357
  skin in, 194–195
Lyme disease, 356, 721
  skin in, 190
Lymph nodes, in cancer staging, 459–460, *460–461*, 462
Lymphadenectomy, 744
Lymphocyte, 311, 312, *324*
  in infectious mononucleosis, *318*
Lymphogranuloma venereum, 194, 355
Lymphoma, cutaneous T-cell, 198
  defined, 682

Macrocytic anemia, red cells in, *312–313*
Macrocytosis, *314, 315*
Macroglossia, 537
Macrophage, 289
Macule, skin, *182*
Magnesium, 310–311
  monitoring of, 364t
Magnetic resonance imaging (MRI), 662, 666
  in cardiovascular disorders, 160–161
  in kidney disorders, 374
  in neurology, 396, *676*
  report on, *677*
Malabsorption, 246
Malaria, monitoring of, 364t
Male reproductive system, anatomy of, 734, *735*
  representative disorders of, 736t–744t
  surgery on, 734–735, 744–745
Malignancies. See *Cancer.*
Malignant hypertension, 303
Malignant melanoma, 197–198
Mallet, 512, 644
Mammaplasty, augmentation, 614
  reduction, 611–612, *613*
Mammography, 274, 458, 662, *666*
  radiology report on, *467, 667*
Management, 83–95
  constructive criticism and, 86–87
  delegation of responsibility and, 83–86
  incentive programs and, 87–88, 87t
  interpersonal relationships and, 85
  job description and, *6–9*, 93
  motivation and, 85–86

Management *(Continued)*
  new technology and, 94
  of deadlines, 87–88
  of employee benefits, 91–92
  of employee performance, 86–91
  rating scale for, 89t
  of employee training, 90
  of employment status, 92–93
  of student intern programs, 83, *84*
  of word processing, 88
  of work schedules, 84–85
  procedural manual for, 93–94
  quality assurance and, 86, 86t, 90–91
  reference materials for, 50, 94–95. See also *Reference materials.*
  salaries and, 90
Mandible, fracture of, 544
  surgery on, 542
Manuscript preparation, for publication, 112–114
Maprotiline, monitoring of, 364t
Marketing, 61, *62, 63,* 77–82
  distribution channels and, 80
  of publications, 116, 118
  price setting and, 57–58, 79
  promotion and, 61–63, *62–64,* 80, *81, 82*
  research in, 77
  segment analysis in, 77–78, *78*
  targeting of, 78–79
Mastoidectomy, 543
Mastopexy, 613–614
Matricectomy, 638, 640
Maxilla, fracture of, 544
  surgery on, 542
Measles, 354
  skin in, 191
Meatotomy, 744
Meconium aspiration syndrome, 574
Medial arm flap, 605
Median rhomboid glossitis, 537
Mediastinoscopy, 545
  in lung cancer, 268
Mediators, 289–290, *289*
Medical artists, 114
Medical dictionaries, 145–146, 758
Medical ethics. See *Ethics.*
Medical history, formats for. See *History and physical examination, format for.*
Medical journals, 104
Medical physicist, 684–685, *685*
Medical records, abbreviations in, 28, 99
  references on, 755–756
  accuracy of, 20–22, 97–99
  completeness of, 28–29
  confidentiality of. See *Confidentiality.*
  correction of, 22, 29, 97–98, 102–104, *218*
  emergency, *218*
  in pathology, 562
  deadlines for, 28, 87–88
  destruction of, 22, 72

Medical records *(Continued)*
  disclosure of. See *Disclosure.*
  emergency, 207–209, *210–217,* 218
  in family medicine, 233, 235, 237, 240
  in gastroenterology, 250–251
  in ophthalmology, 485, 488–489
  in orthopaedics, 513–514, 519
  in otorhinolaryngology, 546, 553
  in psychiatry, 38, 654–655, 659
  in pulmonary medicine, 697, 707
  in radiology, 664, 666
  in urology, 745, 752
  information in, 27–28
  legal status of, 27–42
  of surgery. See *Operative reports.*
  ownership of, 29
  references on, 760
  retention of, 38
  tagging or flagging of, 102, *103*
  typing styles for, Appendix 2
Medical staff, relations with, 85
Medical terminology, combining forms
  in, Appendix 3
  prefixes and suffixes in, Appendix 4
  references on, 760–761
Medical transcription, as profession, 3
  certification programs in, 10
  cost containment and, 4
  current practice of, 4–5
  editing of, 96–105
  education for, 5
  employment opportunities in, 5, 10
  ethics and. See *Ethics.*
  Greek in, 838
  in emergency medicine, 207–209,
    218. See also *Emergency medicine.*
  job description for, *6–9,* 93
  publishers of materials on, 108t–
    109t, 110
  references for, Appendix 1. See also
    specific subject or discipline.
  skills for, 4–5
  spacing of, 100–101
  symbols in, 835–837
  teaching of. See *Teaching.*
  writing on. See *Publication.*
Medical Transcription Service Owners,
  Code of Ethics and Standards of,
  17, 24–25
Medical word books, 143, 146–147,
  768–769
Medications. See *Drugs.*
Medullary sponge kidney, 382
Megaloblastic anemia, red cells in, *314,*
  316, 317
Melanocyte-stimulating hormone, 221t
Melanoma, malignant, 197–198
Ménière's disease, 533
Meningeal irritation signs, 401
Meningioma, 395
Meningitis, bacterial, CSF examination
  in, 344, 350
  pediatric, 581

Meningococcemia, skin in, 189–190
Menopause, 441
Menstrual cycle, 424–425, 433, *434*
  pain in, 435
Mental retardation, 584
Mentoplasty, 544
Meprobamate, monitoring of, 364t
Metabolic cart study, 694, 707
  equipment for, 697
Metastasis, 454, *455*
Methacholine challenge, 697
Methanol, monitoring of, 365t
Methotrexate, monitoring of, 365t
Methylxanthines, 695
Metric prefixes, 837
Microalbuminuria, in diabetes, 227
Microcassettes, 48, 67
Microsurgery, instruments used in,
  512
Microsurgical free flap, 545
Middle ear, 521–522, *523, 524*
  disorders of, 531–533
Milia, 196
Military personnel, forms of address
  for, 827–828
Millard II rotation-advancement
  repair, *609*
Modems, confidentiality and, 23
Moh's surgery, 200
Molluscum contagiosum, 191
Moniliasis, 539
Mono test, 354t
Monocyte, 311, *324*
Mononucleosis, infectious. See
  Infectious mononucleosis.
Mood disorders, 650
Mosquitoes, 352
Motivation, of employees, 85–86
Mouth, 523, *528*
  disorders of, 537–538
  gastroenterology and, 242
  reconstruction of, 603–604
  surgery on, 542
MRI. See *Magnetic resonance imaging
  (MRI).*
Mucoepidermal tumor, 539
Multiple myeloma, red cells in, *317*
Multiple sclerosis, 395
  diagnosis of, 358
Multitape systems, 49
Mumps, 354, 538
Muscle, biopsy of, 397
Musculocutaneous flap, 599, *600*
Musculoskeletal system, trauma to, 492
Mycobacteriology, 351
Mycosis fungoides, 198
Myeloblastic leukemia, acute, white
  cell evaluation in, *322–323, 325*
Myelofibrosis, red cells in, *315*
Myelography, in neurology, 396
Myocardial infarction, 156
Myocutaneous flaps, 544, 599, *600,*
  604–605

Myoglobinuria, vs. hemoglobinuria and
  hematuria, 333t
Myringoplasty, 543
Myringotomy, 543
  report on, *550*

Naffziger's test, 402
Nails, 181, *181,* 626–627, *627, 628.* See
  also *Toenails.*
Nasal septum, deviated, 536
  surgery on, 545
Nasolabial flaps, 604
Nasopharynx, angiofibroma of, 540
  bacterial infections of, 350
Neck, surgery on, 542
  reconstructive, *599*
Necrotizing enterocolitis, 575, 579
Necrotizing gingivitis, 537
Needles, surgical, 265t, 511–512, 644
  holder for, 512, 644
Negotiation, 55
Neisseria gonorrhoeae, cultures of, 350
Neonatology, 573–575, 579. See also
  Pediatrics.
  Apgar score in, 573, 574t
  cardiac catheterization in, 574
    procedure note on, 574, *576–578*
  congenital heart disease in, 574, *575*
  jaundice in, 579
  references in, 593, 765
  sepsis in, 574
  surgical disorders in, 574–575, 579
  weight for age chart in, *583*
Nephrectomy, 744
Nephritis, causes of, 389t
  hereditary, 381–382
  systemic lupus erythematosus, 378
Nephrocystanastomosis, 744
Nephrolithotomy, 744
Nephrology, 370–390. See also *Kidney.*
  anatomy in, 371–373, *372, 373*
  consultation reports in, *375–376,*
    379, 380
  discharge summaries in, *385–387*
  representative diseases in, 373–381
    congenital, 381–382
    treatment of, 389–390, 389t, 390t
  signs and symptoms in, 382, 384, 389
Nephron, 373, *373,* 733, *733*
Nephropathy, diabetic, 227, 377–378
Nephropexy, 744
Nephropyelolithotomy, 744
Nephrostomy, 744
Nephrotic syndrome, causes of, 377t
  urinalysis findings in, 327t
Nephrotomy, 744
Nephroureterectomy, 744
Nerve. See also *Nervous system.*
  biopsy of, 397
  decompression of, 398
Nerve root, instruments used on, 512

Nervous system, 391–394, *392–394*
  diabetes and, 227–228
  glossary of terms for examination of,
    398–403
  heart and, 152–153, *153*
  representative diseases of, 394–396
    signs and symptoms of, 396
  surgery on, 397–398
    instruments used in, 398t
  records of, *407–411*
Networking, 10, 20, 65, 80
  by students, 130
Neurectomy, 511
Neurofibroma, 196, 534
Neurogenic bladder, 740t
Neurology, 391–411. See also
    Neurosurgery.
  anatomy in, 391–394, *392–394*
  consultation report in, *404*
  diagnosis in, 396–397
  discharge summary in, *405–406*
  glossary for, 398–403
  references on, 411, 765
  representative diseases in, 394–396
  signs and symptoms in, 396
Neurolysis, 511
Neuroma, digital, 635–636, *636*
  excision of, 640, *640*
    record of, *647–648*
  treatment of, 638
Neuropathic ulcer, 199
Neuropathy, in diabetes, 227–228
Neurosurgery, 391–411. See also
    Neurology.
  anatomy in, 391–394, *392–394*
  instruments used in, 398t
  operative reports in, *407–411*
  procedures in, 397–398
  representative diseases in, 394–396
Neutrophil, 311–312, *324*
Newborn. See *Neonatology.*
Nipple, in reduction mammaplasty,
    611–612
  reconstruction of, 611
Nitrite, in urine, 332
Nitrogen, radioactive, 416t
Nobility, forms of address for, 828–830
Nodule, skin, *182*
  vocal cord, 541
Nonprivileged information, 24
Norepinephrine, 221t
Normocephaly, 399
Nortriptyline, monitoring of, 360t
Nose, 522–523, *526, 527*
  bleeding from, 535–536
  disorders of, 534–536
  foreign bodies in, 536
  fracture of, 535
  instruments used on, 546
  reconstruction of, 598–599, *598*
  surgery on, 542, 545–546, 614
Nuclear medicine, 413–422, 663
  diagnostic process in, 414–415

Nuclear medicine *(Continued)*
  heart studies in, 160–161, 663, *680*
    reports on, *164, 681*
  lung studies in, 415, *415, 416*
  radiation detection in, 418–419,
    418
  radiopharmaceuticals for, 415–418,
    416t–417t, 418t
  references on, 421, 687, 767–768
  reports on, 413–414, *420, 422, 474,
    681*
  requisitions for, 413
  technique for, 415–418
  types of studies in, 419, 421t
Nurse, radiation therapy, 686, *686*
Nutrition, 241
  evaluation of, 694
Nystagmus, vertigo and, 534

Oath of Hippocrates, *14*
Obstetrics, 423–431. See also
    Pregnancy.
  anatomy in, *424–425*
  family practitioner and, 232
  operative, 430
    record of, *432–433*
  references on, 452, 765
Obstruction, eustachian tube, 532
  foreign body, of ear, 528–529
    of esophagus, 244
    of nose, 536
  gastrointestinal, neonatal, 579
  in colorectal cancer, 281
  ureteropelvic junction, 743t
  urinary tract, 378–379
Office copy machines, 49, 72
Oncocytoma, 538, 740t
Oncogenes, 453–454
Oncology/hematology, 453–477. See
    also *Cancer.*
  diagnosis in, 457–459, *458, 459*
    tumor markers in, 321–323, 326,
      459t
  discharge summary in, *472–473*
  pathology reports in, *272, 277, 468,
    470–471*
  radiology reports in, *467, 474, 475*
  references on, 489, 765
  screening in, 454–457
    guidelines for, 457t
  staging in, 459–460, *460–461*, 462
  treatment in, 462–466, 477
    chemotherapeutic, 463–465,
      464t–466t
      consultation report on, *476*
    clinical trials of, 466, 477
    hormonal, 465, 466t
    radiation, 463, 682–686. See also
      Radiation therapy.
    surgical, 462–463
      records of, *275–276, 469*

Onychomycosis, 192, 626–627, *627*
  treatment of, 638, 640
Oophorectomy, 442
Open reduction, 511
Operative reports, in breast cancer
    surgery, *275–276, 469*
  in cardiology, 171, *176–178*, 179
  in colorectal cancer surgery, *282–283*
  in dermatology, *202*
  in gastroenterology, 250, *256*
  in gynecology, *440–441, 443–449, 451*
  in lung cancer surgery, *270–271*
  in neurosurgery, *407–411*
  in obstetrics, *432–433*
  in oncology, *469*
  in ophthalmology, *487–488*, 488–489
  in orthopaedics, 514, *515–516*, 519
  in otorhinolaryngology, 546, *550*
  in pediatrics, *592–593*, 593
  in podiatry, *647–648*, 648
  in pyloric stenosis surgery, *278–279*
  in reduction mammaplasty, *616–617*
  in urology, *746–747*, 752
  typing style for, *775*
Ophthalmologist, 479
Ophthalmology, 479–489. See also *Eye.*
  anatomy in, *480*, 480–482, *481*
  consultation report in, 489
  diagnosis in, 482–483
  discharge summary in, 489
  history and physical examination in,
    488–489
  instruments used in, 485
  references on, 489, 765
  referral letter in, 485, *486*, 488
  representative diseases in, 482
    medical treatment of, 483
    surgical treatment of, 483–485, *483*
      record of, *487–488*, 488–489
  subspecialties in, 479–480
Oppenheim's sign, 400
Opportunistic infections, 344, 351–352
Opposition, 401
Optician, 479
Optometrist, 479
Oral and maxillofacial surgery,
    references on, 553, 765
Oral cavity, 523, *528*
  disorders of, 537–538
Orbit, 482
  fracture of, 544
  surgery on, 542
Orchidopexy, 744
  record of, *746–747*
Orchidotomy, 744
Orchiectomy, 745
Orchioplasty, 744
Organic mental disorders, 650, 653
Oroantral fistula repair, 545
Orthopaedics, 491–519
  anatomy in, 492–494, *494–499*,
    496–499
  of bone, 492–493, *494*

Orthopaedics *(Continued)*
    of lower extremity, 496–499, *498,*
        499
    of spine and pelvis, 493–494, *495*
    of upper extremity, 494, 496, *496*
    carpal tunnel syndrome in, 503–504,
        503
    consultation reports in, *517–518,* 519
    discharge summary in, 519
    fractures in, 504–505, 508–510
        ankle, 509–510
        hip, 505, 508, *508*
        supracondylar, of humerus,
            504–505
        wrist, 508–509
    glossary for, 510–511
    hip disorders in, 499–502
    history and physical examination in,
        514
        format for, *506–507*
    instruments used in, 511–513
    intervertebral disk disorders in, 396,
        502–503
    medical records in, 513–514, 519
    operative reports in, 514, *515–516,*
        519
    pediatric, 491–492
    references on, 519, 765–766
Orthotic devices, 636, *637*
Osmolality, monitoring of, 365t
Ossiculoplasty, 544
Ostectomy, 511
Osteoarthritis, 302, 715–717, *716*
    hip, 500–501
    surgery in, 501–502
Osteoma, external canal, 530
Osteotome, 512, 644
Osteotomy, 511
    displacement, 510
    hip, 501
Otitis, externa, 529
Otitis media, 529, 581
    serous, 532–533
Otoplasty, 544, 614
Otorhinolaryngology, 521–553
    anatomy in, 521–524, *522–530,* 526
    consultation report in, 546, *549*
    discharge summary in, 546, *551–552,*
        553
    history and physical examination in,
        546
        format for, *548*
    instruments used in, 546
    records in, 546, 553
    references on, 553, 765, 766
    referral letter in, 546, *547*
    representative diseases in, 526,
        528–541
        of ear, 526, 528–534
            external, 526, 528–531
            inner, 533–534
            middle, 531–533
        of larynx, 540–541

Otorhinolaryngology *(Continued)*
        of nose, 534–536
        of pharynx, 539–541
        of salivary glands, 538–539
        of throat, 537–538
    surgery in, 541–546
        endoscopic, 545
        general, 545–546
        on head and neck, 541–542
        otologic, 543–544
        plastic, 544–545
        record of, 546, *550*
Otosclerosis, 531–532, *532,* 533
    discharge summary in, *551–552*
Otoscope, 546
Oval window, surgery on, 544
Ovary(ies), 219, *220*
    cancer of, 439, 442
        marker for, 322
    cysts of, 442
    function of, 431, 433
        abnormal, 433
    hormones produced by, 221t
    tumors of, 439
        operative report in, *445–446*
Ovulation, 433
Ownership, of medical records, 29
Oxygen, consumption of, 694
    hyperbaric, in dermatology, 200
    in respiratory disease therapy,
        695–696
Oxytocin, 221t

Pacemaker implantation, 170
Pain, abdominal, location of, *245*
    chest, 693
    foot, 634–636
    hip, 501
    lower back, 502
    pelvic, 435–436
    pleuritic, 689, 693
Palate, 524, *528*
    cleft, 537
        repair of, 545, *604,* 608, *609*
Palliation, 462
    surgical, 463
Palmomental sign, 400
Pancreas, 219, *220,* 221
    abnormal conditions of, 222t, 248.
        See also *Diabetes.*
    CT-guided biopsy of, *674*
        report on, *675*
    hormones produced by, 221t
    surgery on, 249
Panendoscopy, 545
PAP (prostatic acid phosphatase), 323,
    326
Papanicolaou (Pap) smear, 433–434
    pathology report on, 564
        Bethesda System for, 565t
        request form for, 556, 557, *560–561*

Paper shredders, 72
Papilloma, laryngeal, 541
    oral cavity, 537
Papillomaviruses, 355
Papule, skin, *182*
Papulosquamous skin disorders, 181,
    185–186
Paranasal sinuses, 522–523, *527*
    infection of, 536–537
    tumors of, 537
Parapharyngeal space, tumor of,
    541–542
Parasitic infections. See also specific
        infection.
    diagnosis of, 351–352
    urinalysis in, 337
Parathyroid glands, 219, *220*
    abnormal conditions of, 222t
    hormone produced by, 221t
    surgery on, 543
Paresis, 401
Paronychia, 626–627, *628*
    treatment of, 638, 640
Parotid gland, 524, *530*
    benign mixed tumor of, 538
    surgery on, 541
Partial thromboplastin time (PTT), 317
    monitoring of, 366t
Partnerships, 57
Past due accounts, 60
Patch, skin, *182*
Patch testing, 200
Patent ductus arteriosus, 574, *575*
Pathology, 555–572
    administrative reports in, 569
    consultation report in, 569, *570*
    job description for secretary in,
        571–572
    quality assurance reports in, 569, *570*
    references on, 572, 766
    tissue reports in, 458, 557, 559, 562,
        564, 566
        addenda, 562
        autopsy, 564, 566
        bone marrow, 564
        codes in, 566
        computerization of, 566, *567–568,*
            569
        cytologic, 562, 564, 565t
        gross description in, 557
        in breast cancer, *277, 468, 470–471*
        in lung cancer, *272*
        microscopic description in, 557, 559
        preliminary, 559, 562
        signatures on, 566
        surgical, 562
        typing style for, *776*
        UPIN on, 566
    tissue request forms in, 555–557,
        558–561
    work flow in, 555, *556*
Payroll management, 50–51
    summary sheet for, *52*

Payroll tax, 55
Pectoralis major flap, 604, 605
Pediatrics, 573–593. See also *Children;*
 Neonatology.
 consultation letter in, *589*
 discharge summary in, *590–591*, 591,
 593
 neonatal, 573–575, 579
 references on, 593, 766
 representative diseases in, 579–591
 stature for age chart in, *587*
 surgical disorders in, 586, 588, 588t,
 591
 record of, *592–593*, 593
 weight for age chart in, *583*
Pedicle flap, 544, 601
Pediculosis pubis, 194
Peer review, of publications, 115–116
Pelvic examination, 431
Pelvic inflammatory disease (PID), 435
Pelvis, 494
 CT of, *670–671*
 report on, *672–673*
Pemphigus, 186, 538
Penectomy, 744
Penis, 734, *735*
 cancer of, 742t
 prosthesis for, 744
Pension plans, 61
Pentobarbital, monitoring of, 365t
Peptic ulcer, 304
Percutaneous transluminal coronary
 angioplasty (PTCA), 156
Pereyra's bladder neck suspension, 744
Pericarditis, 157
Perichondritis, 528
Perinephric abscess, 740t
Periodicals, 766–767
Periosteal elevator, 512
Peripheral nervous system, 393. See
 also *Nervous system.*
 disorders of, 395
 surgery on, 397–398
 symptoms referable to, 396
Peripheral vascular system, foot and,
 627–628
 in diabetes, 226
Peroneus flaps, 607
Personality disorders, 650
Pes cavus, 632–633, *634*
Pes planus, 632
PET (positron emission tomography),
 419, 663
Peyronie's disease, 740t
pH, urinary, 328, 331
Phacoemulsification, 484
Phagocytosis, 288–289, *289*
Phalen's test, 401
Pharmaceuticals. See *Drugs;*
 Radiopharmaceuticals.
Pharyngeal flap, 545
Pharyngitis, acute, 539
 chronic, 539–540
 cultures in, 350

Pharyngoesophagectomy, 543
Pharynx, 524, *529*
 disorders of, 539–541
 gastroenterology and, 242
 surgery on, 543
Phencyclidine, monitoring of, 365t
Phenobarbital, monitoring of, 365t
Phenytoin, monitoring of, 365t
Pheochromocytoma, 740t
Phimosis, *740*, 740t
Phosphate, 308
 urinary sediments and, 339t
Phosphorus, monitoring of, 365t
 regulation of, 390
Photocopy equipment, 49, 72
Photographs, consent form for taking
 and publication of, *31*
Photophoresis, in dermatology, 200
Physical examination, emergency, 208
 formats for. See *History and physical*
 examination, format for.
 routine, 301–302
 typing style for, *774*
Physical therapy, reference on, 768
Physically challenged, equipment for, 70
 references for, 762–763
 teaching of, 140
Physicist, medical, 684–685, *685*
Physiology, references on, 756
PID (pelvic inflammatory disease), 435
Pilar cyst, 196
Pinch test, 401
Pineal gland, 219, *220*
Pituitary gland, 219, *220*
 abnormal conditions of, 222t
 hormones produced by, 221t
Pityriasis rosea, 185–186
Placenta, *427*
 abruption of, 429
Placenta previa, 429, *429*
Plantar keratoma, treatment of, 641
Plantar warts, 626, *626*
 treatment of, 640
Plaque, skin, *182*
Plaster of Paris bandages, 512
Plastic surgery, 544–545, 595–622
 congenital deformity reconstruction
 in, *604*, 608, *609*, 610
 cosmetic, 614–615, *618–619*, 619, 622
 donor sites in, 596
 flaps in, 598–608
 arm, 605, 607
 head and neck, 601, 603–605, *604*
 Indian, 598, *598*
 leg, 607–608
 terminology for, 598–599, 601
 trunk, 605, *606*
 for burns, 610
 grafts in, 597–598
 implant materials in, 597
 instruments used in, 622
 of breast, 610–614, *611–613*
 record of, *616–617*
 reconstruction principles in, 595–596

Plastic surgery *(Continued)*
 references on, 553, 622, 765
Platelet, evaluation of, 312–313, 317,
 326
 specimen handling for, 313, 317
 monitoring of, 365t
Platysma myocutaneous flap, 604
Plegias, 401
Pleura, 689, 690, 693
 biopsy of, 694
 instruments for, 697
PMS (premenstrual tension syndrome),
 435
Pneumoconiosis, 691
Pneumonia, 303–304
 pediatric, 581
 pneumocystic, 351
Pneumothorax, neonatal, 574–575
Podagra, 720
Podiatry, 623–648
 anatomy in, 624–625, *624*
 anesthesia in, 645
 chart notes in, 645, *646*
 disability reports in, 645, 648
 instruments used in, 643–645
 references on, 648, 767
 representative diseases in, 625–636
 integumentary, 625–627, *626–628*
 surgery in, 638, 640
 musculoskeletal, 631–636, *632–636*
 surgery in, 641–643
 neurologic, 628, 631, *631*
 surgery in, 640–641, *640*
 peripheral vascular, 627–628
 evaluation of, *629*, *630*
 surgery in, 641
 treatment in, 636–643
 nonsurgical, 636, *637*, 638
 surgical, 638, 640–643
 record of, *647–648*, 648
Poland's syndrome, 614
Polycystic kidney, 382, *741*, 741t
Polydipsia, 223
Polymorphonuclear cell, 289
Polymyositis, 718
Polyp, colon, 246
 vocal cord, 541
Polyphagia, 223
Polysomnography, 691
 report on, 707, *710–711*
Polyuria, 223
Porphyria cutanea tarda, 187
Positron emission tomography (PET),
 419, 663
Possessives, 100
Postage meters, 49–50
Postal abbreviations, 832
Posterior nasal pack, 535
Postnasal drip, 693
Potassium, 311
 monitoring of, 365t
 regulation of, 390
Potassium hydroxide (KOH)
 examination, 199–200

Pott's fracture, *635*
Preauricular fistula, 526, 528
Pre-excitation syndromes, 159t
Prefixes, Appendix 4
  metric, 837
Pregnancy, 425–426, *426–428*
  disorders of, 426–429, *429*
  ectopic, 427–428
  hCG testing in, 310
  Rh typing in, 340–341
Premenstrual tension syndrome
  (PMS), 435
Presbycusis, 533
Prescriptions, abbreviations in,
  833–834
Priapism, 741t
Pricing, 57–58, 79
Primary gaze, 401
Primidone, monitoring of, 365t
Printers, 45, 68–69
Privacy, invasion of, 30
  right to, 23–24, 29
Privileged communication, 24
Privileged information, 23–24, 29–30,
  34
Privileges, clinical, 229
Procainamide, monitoring of, 365t–366t
Procedural manuals, 994
Procedure notes, in urology, *751, 752*
Profession, associations in, 10
  characteristics of, 3
  forms of address in, 826
  image and, reference on, 762
Professional liability insurance, 54
Progesterone, 221t
Progestins, 221t
Progress notes, in rheumatology, *725*
  in urology, *750, 752*
Prolactin, 221t
Promotion, 61–63, *62–64*, 80, *81*, 82
Pronation, 494, *497*
Proofreaders' marks, *117*
Proofreading, 90–91, 102
  of author's proof, 116
  references on, 762
Proofs, 116
Property insurance, 53
Proposals, for publication, 110–111
Prostate gland, benign hypertrophy of,
  736, 736t
  cancer of, 736t
    markers for, 323, 326
    treatment of, hormonal, 465
  posterior urethral valves of, 741t
  surgery on, 744
Prostatectomy, 744
Prostate-specific antigen (PSA), 323,
  326
Prostatic acid phosphatase (PAP), 323,
  326
Prostatitis, 741t
Prostatocystotomy, 744
Prostatolithotomy, 744
Prostatomy, 744

Prosthesis, 512
  penile, 744
Prosthetic replacement, 511
  materials for, 597
Protein, albumin and globulin
  and, 307
  C-reactive, 307
  monitoring of, 366t
Proteinuria, 331
  in diabetes, 227
Prothrombin time (PT), 317
  monitoring of, 366t
Protriptyline, monitoring of, 366t
PSA (prostate-specific antigen), 323,
  326
Pseudogout, 720
Psoriasis, 181, 185
  arthritis in, 718, 720
Psychiatric documents, confidentiality
  of, 38, 654
Psychiatry, 649–660
  chart notes in, 654, *655*
  confidentiality in, 38, 654
  consultation report in, *656*, 659
  diagnosis in, 652–653
  discharge summary in, *657–658*, 659
  history in, 654–655, 659
  letters in, 654
  references on, 660, 767
  reports in, 654
  representative diseases in, 650, 652
  treatment in, 653–654
Psychoanalysis, 649
Psychologic tests, 653
Psychologist, 649
Psychotherapy, 649
PT (prothrombin time), 317
  monitoring of, 366t
PTCA (percutaneous transluminal
  coronary angioplasty), 156
PTT (partial thromboplastin time),
  317
  monitoring of, 366t
Puberty, female, 424
Publication, 107–119
  coauthored, 119
  contracts for, 111–112
  copyright of, 118–119
  design for, 116
  figure preparation for, 114
  index for, 115
  manuscript preparation for, 112–114
    electronic, 114
  marketing of, 116, 118
  production schedule for, 115–116
  proposal submission for, 110–111
  rejection of, 111
  publishers for, 108t–109t, 110
  references on, 757, 759, 769–770, 771
  source citation for, 115
  table preparation for, 14
  teacher's guides for, 115
  topic selection for, 107–108
Publicity, 61–63, *62–64*, 80, *81*, 82

Publishers, of medical transcription
  materials, 108t–109t, 110
  contracts with, 111–112
  manuscript guidelines for, 113–114
  marketing by, 116, 118
  production schedule of, 115–116
Puerperium, 431
Pulmonary embolism, nuclear medicine
  studies of, 415, *415*, *416*
Pulmonary function testing, 693
  equipment for, 697
  report on, 697, *702–705*
Pulmonary hypertension, neonatal, 574
Pulmonary medicine, 689–714. See
  also *Respiratory system.*
  anatomy in, 689–691, *690*
  chart notes in, 697
  consultation in, 697, *698–701*
  diagnosis in, *459*, 693–694, *694, 695*
  discharge summary in, 707, *712–714*
  instruments in, 697
  physiology in, 691
  records in, 697, 707
  references on, 714, 764
  reports in, 697, *702–706*, 707,
    708–711
  representative diseases in, 691–692
    signs and symptoms of, 692–693,
    692t
  treatment in, medical, 694–696, *696*
    surgical, 696–697
Pulmonary stenosis, 574, *575*
Punch biopsy, 200
Punctuation, 91, 99, 100
  references on, 759
Purpura, pediatric, 579–580
Pustule, skin, *183*
Pyelocystostomy, 744
Pyelolithotomy, 744
Pyelonephritis, 382, 742t
  urinalysis findings in, 327t
Pyeloplasty, 744
Pyelostomy, 745
Pyelotomy, 745
Pyeloureteroplasty, 745
Pyloric stenosis, 274, 276–277, 279, 588
  diagnosis of, 276
  symptoms of, 274, 276
  treatment of, 276–277, 279
    surgical, 277, 279, *280*
      record of, *278–279*
Pyloromyotomy, 277, 279, *280*
Pyoderma gangrenosum, 199
Pyrosis, 242–243

Quadrantectomy, operative report on,
  275–276
Quadrants, of abdomen, *245*
Quality assurance, 86, 86t, 90–91
  checklist for, *129*
  in pathology, 569, *570*
Quinidine, monitoring of, 366t
Quotations, 119

Radial forearm flap, 605
Radiation oncologist, 684
Radiation therapy, 463, 682–686
  brachytherapy in, 683–684, *684*
  external beam, 683, *683, 684*
  future applications of, 686
  in dermatology, 200
  references on, 686–687
  team for, 684–686, *685, 686*
Radiation therapy technologist, 685
Radical orchiectomy, 745
Radioactive isotopes, 415–416
Radioimmunotherapy, 686
Radiology, 661–682. See also *Radiation therapy.*
  contrast media for, 661
    urinary sediments and, 339t
  diagnostic techniques in, 661–663.
    See also specific technique, e.g.,
    Computed tomography (CT).
  in family medicine, 233
  in lung cancer, 267
  in podiatry, 645
  in psychiatry, 653
  interventional, 663
  references on, 687, 767–768
  reports in, 664
  safety in, 663–664
Radiopharmaceuticals, 415–418,
    416t–417t
  half-life of, 418, 418t
Range of motion, 514
  of extremities, *497*
  of foot, *633*
Ranula, 537
Raynaud's phenomenon, 718
Reamers, 513
Reconstructive surgery, 544–545. See
    also *Plastic surgery.*
  principles of, 595–596
Records. See *Medical records.*
Rectocele, repair of, 442
  record of, *451*
Rectum, cancer of, 279–281, 284
  disorders of, 246
Rectus abdominis myocutaneous flap,
    599, 601, 605
Rectus femoris flap, 607
Red blood cell, evaluation of, 311,
    312–317
  grouping of, 337, 340, 341t, 342t, 344
  in urine, 332–334
  intravascular destruction of, urine
    and plasma findings in, 332t
  Rh typing of, 340–341
Reduction, 510, 511
Reduction mammaplasty, 611–612, *613*
Redundancies, 99–100
Reference materials, 50, 94–95,
    104–105, 143–148, Appendix 1.
    See also specific subject or
    discipline.
  dictionaries as, 144–146, 757–758

Reference materials *(Continued)*
  for teaching, 141–142
    inconsistencies in, 140–141
  on spelling, 144–148, 768–769
  word books as, 143, 146–147, 768–769
Referrals, emergency, 209
  in gastroenterology, 250
  in immunology, 291–292, *293–295*
  in ophthalmology, 485, *486*, 488
  in orthopaedics, 513
  in otorhinolaryngology, 546, *547*
  in psychiatry, 654
Reflexes, 401–402, 631, *631*
Rehabilitation, reference on, 768
Rejection, of publication proposal, 111
Release forms. See *Consent forms.*
Renal. See also *Kidney.*
Renal cell carcinoma, 742t
Renal tubular epithelial cell, in urine,
    332, *334, 335*
Renal tubule, 373, *373*, 733–734, *733*
Renal venography, consultation report
    on, *379*
Rendu-Osler-Weber disease, 535–536
Renovascular hypertension, 742t
Reports. See *Medical records; Operative
    reports;* and specific discipline.
Reproductive system, female, anatomy
    of, *424–425*
  disorders of, 433–436, 439, 441
  examination of, 431, 434
  male, anatomy of, 734, *735*
    representative disorders of,
      736t–744t
    surgery on, 734–735, 744–745
Request forms, in pathology, 555–557,
    558–561
Resection, 511
  pathology report on, 562
    correlation with biopsy report, 569
Respiration, 689–690
Respiratory distress, neonatal, 573–574
Respiratory system. See also
    Pulmonary medicine.
  bacterial infections of, cultures in, 350
  disorders of, 691–692. See also *Lung.*
    diagnosis of, *459*, 693–694, *694, 695*
    in newborn, 573–574
    pediatric, 580–581
    signs and symptoms of, 692, 692t
    treatment of, 694–697
      medical, 694–696, *696*
      surgical, 696–697
  nuclear studies of, 421t
  physiology of, 691
Respiratory-syncytial virus, 354
Retina, in diabetes, 227
  surgery on, 485
Retirement plans, 61
Retractor, 512, 513, 644
  nerve root, 512
Revision, 511
RF (rheumatoid factor), 357

Rh typing, 340–341
Rhabdomyolysis, causes of, 332t
Rheumatoid arthritis, 195, 717
  juvenile, 584
  treatment of, *718*
Rheumatoid factor (RF), 357
Rheumatology, 715–730
  chart notes in, *724, 725*
  consultation report in, 722–724
  discharge summary in, 721, 727–729,
    730
  insurance report in, *726*
  laboratory studies in, 717t
  progress note in, *725*
  references on, 730, 765–766
  representative diseases in, 715–721
  surgery in, 721
Rhinectomy, 542
Rhinitis, 536
Rhinophyma, 535
Rhinoplasty, 544, 614
Rhinotomy, 542
Rhinoviruses, 354
Rhytidectomy, 544, 614–615, *618–619*
  record of, *620–621*
Rickettsial infections, 355
Ringworm, 192
Rinne's test, 402
Risk factors, for breast cancer, 268
  for cardiovascular disorders, 153, 302
  for colorectal cancer, 280–281
  for lung cancer, 261
Rocky Mountain spotted fever, 355
  skin in, 190
Romberg's disease, 610
Romberg's test, 402
Rosacea, 195
Rotation, *497*
Rouleaux, *317*
Royalties, 111–112
Rubella, 354–355
  skin in, 191–192
Rural family practice, 231–231

Safety, radiation, 63–664
Sagittal synostosis, operative report in,
    592–593
Salaries, 90
Sales tax, 55
Salicylate, monitoring of, 366t
Salivary glands, 524, *530*
  disorders of, 538–539
  surgery on, 541–542
Salpingectomy, 442
Salpingitis, acute, 435
Sarcoma. See also *Cancer.*
  defined, 259, 454, 682
  Kaposi's, 198
Sartorius flap, 607
Saws, surgical, 644
Scalded skin syndrome, 189

Scale, skin, *183*
Scalpel, 512
Scalping flap, 599, 601, 603
Scar, hypertrophic, 196–197
Schaefer's sign, 400
Schirmer's test, 402
Schizophrenia, 650, 653
Sciatic nerve tests, 402
Sciatica, 502
Scissors, surgical, 512, 644
Sclera, 402
Scleroderma, 195, 718, *719*
Scotoma, 402
Screening, for cancer, 454–457
  breast, 274
  guidelines for, 457t
  lung, 267
Screwdriver, 513
Scribes, 3
Seborrheic dermatitis, 185
Seborrheic keratosis, 196
Secobarbital, monitoring of, 366t
Secretary, pathology, 571–572
Seizures, 584–585
Self-blood glucose monitoring, 226
Self-employment. See also *Management.*
  advertising in, 62–63, *64*, 80, *81*, 82
  as corporation, 57
  as partnership member, 57
  as sole proprietor, 57
  auxiliary personnel for, 44–45
  banking and, 60–61
  billing management in, 50, *51*, 57–58
  bookkeeping in, 58, *59*, 60
  equipment for, 45, 49–50, 67–75
    lease vs. purchase of, 49, 69
  fee setting in, 57–58, 79
  financial planning in, 51, 53
  home-based, 45
    preparation for, 130
  independent contractors and, 55, 56t, 57
    agreement form for, *46–48*
  insurance for, 53–54
  legal issues in, 54–55
  marketing in, 61, *62*, *63*, 77–82
  negotiation and contracts in, 55, 57
  networking in, 65, 80
  obtaining credit in, 60
  payroll management in, 50–51
    summary sheet for, *52*
  preparation for, 44
  references on, 65, 763–764
  retirement plans in, 61
  supplies for, 70
  tax management in, 50–51, 55
Self-evaluation, by teacher, 137, *139*
Semen, 734
  blood in, 738t
Semicolons, 100
Sensorineural hearing loss, 533
Sepsis, neonatal, 574
Septal hematoma, nasal, 536

Septicemia, 304
Serratus anterior flap, 605
Service Core of Retired Executives, 65
Sexual disorders, 650
Sexually transmitted diseases, 742t
  confidentiality and, 24
  laboratory studies in, 350, 355–356, 356t
  skin in, 193–194
Shave biopsy, 200
Sheet wadding, 513
Shingles, 353
Shock, anaphylactic, urticaria and, 187–188
  toxic, 189
Shoe, molded, 638
Shortness, 586, *587*
Shoulder, 494, *496*
Shoulder depression test, 402
Shoulder flap, 605
Shredders, 72
Sialadenitis, acute suppurative, 538
Sialoadenopathy, benign lymphoepithelial, 538
Sialolithotomy, 542
Sideroblastic anemia, red cells in, *315*
Sigmoidoscopy, 233, 250
Silastic, 597
Single photon emission tomography (SPECT), 419, 663, 666
  in cardiovascular disorders, 160, *164*, *680*
  report on, 666, *681*
Sinus node arrhythmias, 159t
Sinuses, 522–523, *527*
  infection of, 536–537
  surgery on, 546
  tumors of, 537
Sinusitis, 536–537
Skin, anatomy and physiology of, 179–181, *180*, *181*
  disorders of, 185–199, 304
    acneiform, 195–196
    bacterial, 188–190, 534–535
    benign, 196–197
    collagen vascular, 194–195
    consultation report on, *203*
    diagnosis of, 199–200
    discharge summary in, *204–205*
    erythematous, 187–188
    fungal and yeast, 192–193
    history and physical examination format for, *201*
    papulosquamous, 181, 185–186
    premalignant and malignant, 197–198, 535
    radiation therapy for, *682*
    surgery for, 200
      record of, *202*
    terms describing, *182–184*
    treatment of, 200
    ulcerous, 198–199
    venereal, 193–194

Skin *(Continued)*
  vesiculobullous, 186–187
  viral, 190–192, 535
  specialized functions of, 596
Skin grafts, 545, 597–598
Skin peels, 615
Skin tag, 196
Slander, 30
Sleep apnea syndromes, 691–692
  treatment of, 696, *696*
Sleep disorders, 650, 691
  report on, 707, *710–711*
Slides, 132
Slipped capital femoral epiphysis, 499–500
Small cell carcinoma, lung, 265
Small intestine, disorders of, 244–246
Smith's sign, 402
Smoking, lung cancer and, 261
SNOMED (Standardized Nomenclature of Medicine) code, 566
Snouting, 400
SOAP format, in podiatry, 645, *646*
  in urology, *750*, 752
Social worker, radiation therapy and, 686
Sodium, 311
  monitoring of, 366t
  regulation of, 390
Sodoku, 356
Sole proprietorship, 57
Soleus flap, 607
Somatiform disorders, 650
  discharge summary in, *590–591*
Sore throat, 539
Spacing, 100–101
Specialization, vs. general practice, 229–230
Specific gravity, urinary, 328, 331t
SPECT. See *Single photon emission tomography (SPECT).*
Speculum, nasal, 546
Speech, language, hearing, reference on, 768
Spelling, 91, 100
  electronic correction of, 99, 147–148, 757
  of possessives, 100
  reference materials on, 144–148, 768–769
Spermatogenesis, 734
Sphenoidotomy, 546
Spherocytosis, *314*, *315*
Spinal cord, 392, *393*, *394*
  degenerative disk disease and, 396, 502–503
  surgery on, 397
  symptoms referable to, 396
  tumors of, 395
Spinal fusion, 511
Spine, 493–494, *495*
Spirochetal infections, 355–356, 356t

Spirometry, 693, 697
  in family medicine, 233
Springing test, 402
Spur, heel, 642
Sputum, 692–693
  culture of, 350
Squamous cell carcinoma, oral cavity, 538
  penis, 742t
  salivary gland, 538–539
  skin, 197
Staghorn calculus, 742t
Staging, cancer, 459–460, *460–461*, 462, 696
Staining, of white blood cells, *325*
Standardized Nomenclature of Medicine (SNOMED) code, 566
Stapedectomy, 531–532, *532*, 544
Staphylococcal scalded skin syndrome, 189
Stat transcription, 208, 218
States, postal abbreviations for, 832
Stationery, 61, *63*
Stature, 586, *587*
Steel sutures, 263t
Stenosis, pyloric. See *Pyloric stenosis.*
Stereognosis, 402
Sternocleidomastoid myocutaneous flap, 604
Sternomastoid muscle, 402–403
Stevens-Johnson syndrome, 188
Still's disease, 717
Stockinette, 513
Stomach, disorders of, 244
  surgery on, 249
Stratum corneum, 179, *180*
Stress electrocardiography, 159, *162*
  Cardiolite, *164*
Stress testing, cardiopulmonary, 697
  report on, *706*
Stress urinary incontinence, 439–441, 442, 742t
  operative report in, *447–449, 451*
Stroke, 394–395
Strumpell's sign, 400
Student intern programs, 83, *84*
Sturge-Weber syndrome, 403
Style manuals, 104–105, 144, 759, 769–770
Subcontractors, agreement form for, *46–48*
  characterization of, 55, 56t, 57
Submandibular gland, excision of, 541
Subpoenas, 38, *40, 41*
Substance abuse, 650, 651–652t
Sucking, 400
Sudden infant death syndrome, 581
Suffixes, Appendix 4
Suicide attempt, discharge summary in, *657–658, 659*
Sulfonamides, urinary sediments and, 339t
Supervisory positions. See *Management.*

Supination, 494, *497*
Supplies, 70
Support groups, Appendix 9
Surgery. See also *Operative reports*; and specific discipline or disorder.
  anesthesia for, 259–260, 260t, 261t
  family practitioner and, 232–233
  glossary for, 510–511
  instruments used in, 511–513
  references on, 768
  sutures for, 260, *262*, 263t–265t
Surgical speech fistula, 543
Sutures, cranial, 403
  premature fusion of, consultation letter on, *589*
  surgical, 260, *262*, 263t–265t
Sweat glands, 180
Syllabus, *128*
Symbols, 835–837
Syndromes, references on, 756
Synonyms, references on, 756
Synostosis, sagittal, operative report in, *592–593*
Synovectomy, 511
Syphilis, diagnosis of, 355–356, 356t
  skin in, 193
Systemic lupus erythematosus, 717–718
  kidney in, 378
  laboratory studies in, 357
  skin in, 194–195

T cell, 290, *290*
  evaluation of, 343–344
Table of chemical elements, Appendix 7
Tables, preparation of, 114
Tables of weights and measures, Appendix 6
Tagging, 102, *103*
Tagliacozzi flap, 598–599
Tamponade, pericardial, 157
  surgery for, 171
Tandem stance, 403
Tarsal tunnel syndrome, 631
  treatment of, 640–641
Taxes, management of, 50–51, 55
  publications on, 65
Teacher's guides, 115
Teaching, 121–142
  audiovisual aids for, 131–132, 142
  community needs and, 122–123
  competency profile for, 123, *124–127*
  course description for, 123, *124–127*, 127
  course evaluation in, 137, *138*
  curriculum for, 131, *131*
  environments for, 123
  grading in, 127, *129*, 132–133
    point system for, 133, *134, 135*
    software for, 142
  objectives of, 127–130
  of multicultural students, 140

Teaching *(Continued)*
  of physically challenged students, 140
  of slow learners, 140
  qualifications for, 121–122
  reference materials for, 141–142
    inconsistencies in, 140–141
  self-evaluation in, 137, *139*
  syllabus for, *128*
  testing in, 133–134, *136*, 137
  textbooks for, 131
  tips for, 141
Technetium, radioactive, 416t–417t, 418t
Telangiectasia, skin, *184*
Telephone lines, 49, 67–68
Television, continuing education by, 11
Temporal arteritis, 718
Temporalis muscle flap, 604
Tendon graft, 511
Tendon lengthening, 511
Tendon repair, flexor, 511
Tendon retriever, 513
Tendon stripper, 513
Tendon transfer, 511
Tenotomy, 511
Tensor fasciae latae flap, *600*, 607
Terminology, medical, combining forms in, Appendix 3
  prefixes and suffixes in, Appendix 4
  references on, 760–761
Testing, of medical transcription student, 133–134, *136*, 137
Testis(es), 219, *220*, 734, *735*
  cancer of, 742t
  hormone produced by, 221t
  surgery on, 744
  torsion of, 743t
  undescended, 737, 737t
Testosterone, 221t
Tetralogy of Fallot, 574, *575*
Textbooks, 131
Thallium, radioactive, 416t, 418t
Theophylline, 695
  monitoring of, 366t
Thigh, 496
  cosmetic surgery on, 619
Thiothixene, monitoring of, 366t
Thoracentesis, 694, *695*
Thornwaldt's cyst, 540
Throat, 523–524, 526, *528–530*
  disorders of, 537–541
  instruments used on, 546
Thrombin time (TT), 317
Thrombocytopenia, 313
  pediatric, 580
Thrombocytosis, 312–313
Thrombolytics, 154t, 156
  monitoring of, 317
Thrombosis, deep venous, 303
Thrush, 539
Thumb, reconstruction of, 608
Thymus gland, 219

Thyroglossal duct cyst, 540
  removal of, 543
Thyroid cartilage, 526, *530*
Thyroid gland, 219, *220*
  abnormal conditions of, 222t
  autoimmune, 358
  hormones produced by, 221t
  nuclear medicine report on, *420*
  surgery on, 543
Thyroid-stimulating hormone, 221t
Thyrotomy, 542
Thyroxine, 221t, 311
TIBC (total iron-binding capacity), 310
Tibia, 498
Tibialis anterior flap, 607
Ticks, 352
Tinea infections, 192, 193
Tinel's sign, 403
Tinnitus, 533–534
Tissue culture, 350
Tissue reports. See *Pathology.*
Tissue request forms, 555–557, *558–561*
Titubation, 403
TNM system, in cancer staging,
  459–460, *460–461*, 462
Tobramycin, monitoring of, 366t
Toe, disorders of, 633, *635*
  extensor signs of, 399–400
Toenails, disorders of, 626–627, *627,
  628*
  treatment of, 638, 640
Toe-to-thumb flap, 608
Tongue, 523
  disorders of, 537–538
  surgery on, 542
Tongue depressor, 546
Tonsillectomy, 545
Tonsillitis, 539
Torsion, testicular, 743t
Total iron-binding capacity (TIBC),
  310
Total joint replacement, 511
  hip, 501–502
Toxic epidermal necrolysis, 188
Toxic shock syndrome, 189
Toxoplasmosis, diagnosis of, 351
Trachea, 689, *690*
  surgery on, 543, 544
Tracheoplasty, 544
TRAM (transverse rectus abdominis
  myocutaneous) flap, 599, 601
  in breast reconstruction, *612, 613*
Transcribers, 45, 49, 67
Transcription. See *Medical
  transcription.*
Transferrin, 310
Transparencies, 132
Transplantation, 292t
  heart, 170–171
  heart-lung, 171
  kidney, 381
    rejection of, urinalysis findings in,
    327t

Transverse rectus abdominis
  myocutaneous (TRAM) flap, 599,
  601
  in breast reconstruction, *612, 613*
Trapezius myocutaneous flap, 604–605
Trauma. See also *Fractures.*
  bladder, 742t
  eye, 485
  facial nerve, 533
  foot, 631–632
  musculoskeletal, 492
  tympanic membrane, 529–530
Trazodone, monitoring of, 366t
Treacher Collins syndrome, 608, 610
Trendelenburg's sign, 403
Treponema pallidum, 355–356
Triglycerides, 308
Triiodothyronine, 221t
TT (thrombin time), 317
Tubular necrosis, acute, urinalysis
  findings in, 327t
Tubule, renal, 373, *373*, 733–734, *733*
  function tests of, 374
Tumor markers, 321–323, 326, 459t
Tumors. See also *Cancer.*
  external auditory canal, 530–531
  heart, 157
  laryngeal, 541
  nasal, 534, 535
  nervous system, 395
  oral cavity, 538
  ovarian, 439
  paranasal sinus, 537
  salivary gland, 538–539
  skin, 196–198
  small intestine, 244
  uterine, 436, 439, *442*
Tuning fork, 546
Turbinectomy, 545
Two point discrimination, 403
Tympanic membrane, traumatic
  perforation of, 529–530
Tympanoplasty, 543
Tympanosclerosis, 531
Typewriters, 69
  corrections on, 103–104
Typing, references on, 770
Typing styles, Appendix 2
Tyrosine, urinary sediments and, 339t
Tzanck's preparation, 200

Ulcer, duodenal, 244
  foot, 628
    treatment of, 636, 638
    surgical, 641
  gastric, 244
    surgery for, 249
  peptic, 304
  skin, *184*
    decubitus, 199
    ischemic, 198–199

Ulcer *(Continued)*
  neuropathic, 199
  venous stasis, 198
Ulcerative colitis, 246
Ultrasonography, 662–663, 666
  arterial evaluation report in, *630*
  in cancer diagnosis, 458
  in kidney disorders, 374
  in pregnancy, 425–426
  of gallbladder, *678*
    report on, *679*
  transrectal, 745
Ultraviolet light, in dermatology, 200
Understature, 586, *587*
Unique Physician Identifier Number
  (UPIN), 566
UPIN (Unique Physician Identifier
  Number), 566
Upper extremity, 494, 496, *496*
  fracture of, 504–505
  range of motion of, *497*
  reconstruction of, 605, 607
    cosmetic, 619, 622
Urates, urinary sediments and,
  339t–340t
Uremia, 381, *382*
Ureter, 734
  surgery on, 745
Ureterectomy, 745
Ureterocalycostomy, 745
Ureterocelectomy, 745
Ureterocolostomy, 745
Ureterocutaneostomy, 745
Ureteroileostomy, 745
Ureterolithotomy, 745
Ureteromeatotomy, 745
Ureteroneocystostomy, 745
Ureteroneopyelostomy, 745
Ureteropelvic junction obstruction, 743t
Ureteropelvioplasty, 745
Ureteropyeloneostomy, 745
Ureteropyelonephrostomy, 745
Ureteropyeloscopy, 745
Ureteroscopy, 745
Ureterosigmoidostomy, 745
Ureterostomy, cutaneous, 734–735
Ureteroureterostomy, 745
Ureterovesicostomy, 745
Urethra, 734
  caruncle of, 743t
  surgery on, 735, 745
Urethrectomy, 745
Urethroplasty, 745
Urethrotomy, direct internal, 735
Uric acid, 311
  gout and, 720
  monitoring of, 367t
  urinary sediments and, 339t–340t
Urinalysis, 326–337
  disease markers in, 327t–328t
  in kidney disorders, 373–374
  in pediatric urinary tract infections,
    583–584

Urinalysis *(Continued)*
  macroscopic, 326, 328, 331–332
    appearance and color in, 328, 329t, 330t
    bilirubin in, 331
    blood in, 331, 332t, 333t
    glucose in, 331
    ketones in, 331
    leukocyte esterase in, 332
    nitrite in, 332
    pH in, 328, 331
    protein in, 331
    specific gravity in, 331t, 338
    urobilinogen in, 331–332
  microscopic, 332–333, 337
    bacteria in, 337, 350–351
    casts in, 333, 333t, *335*
    crystals in, 333, *336*, *337*, 338t–340t
    parasites in, 337
    red cells in, 333–334
    renal tubular epithelial cells in, 332, *334*, *335*
Urinary bladder, *735*
  cancer of, 737t
    transurethral resection of, 745
  diverticula of, 737t
  neurogenic, 740t
  ruptured, 742t
  surgery on, 735
Urinary diversion, 745
Urinary incontinence, 439–441, 442, 739t
  stress, *447–449*, *451*, 742t
  operative report in, *447–449*, *451*
Urinary sphincter, artificial, 734
Urinary tract, anatomy of, *372*, 731, *732*, *733–734*, *733*
  cancer of, urinalysis findings in, 327t
  infection of, pediatric, 582–584
  obstruction of, 378–379
  representative disorders of, 736t–744t
  surgery on, 734–735, 744–745
Urine, color of, 329t, 330t
Urobilinogen, 331–332
Urography, 374
  report of, *375–376*
Urolithiasis, 743t
Urology, 731–752
  anatomy in, 731, *732*, *733–734*, *733*
  consultation report in, *748–749*, 752
  discharge summary in, 752
  history and physical examination in, 745, 752
  references on, 752, 768
  representative disorders in, 736t–744t
  surgical procedures in, 734–735, 744–745
    record of, *746–747*, 752
Urticaria, 187–188
Uterus, surgery on, 442
  tumors of, 436, 439, *442*
Uvulopharyngopalatoplasty, 696

Vagina, repair of, 442, *451*
Vaginal smear. See *Papanicolaou (Pap) smear.*
Vaginitis, 435
Vaginosis, bacterial, 350
Vagotomy, 249
Valproic acid, monitoring of, 367t
Valvular heart disease, 156
  surgery in, 171
Vancomycin, monitoring of, 367t
Vanillylmandelic acid, monitoring of, 367t
Varicella infection, skin in, 191
Varicella-zoster, 353
Varicocele, *743*, 743t
Varicocelectomy, 745
Vascular evaluation form, *629*
Vascular malformations, 395–396
Vasculitis, 718
Vasectomy, 745
  procedure note on, *751*
Vasodilators, coronary, 154t
Vasopressors, 154t
Vasotomy, 745
Vasovesiculectomy, 745
Vastus lateralis flap, 607
Velopharyngeal incompetence, 608
Vena cavography, consultation report on, *379*
Venereal diseases. See *Sexually transmitted diseases.*
Venous stasis ulcer, 198
Ventricular arrhythmias, 159t
Ventricular septal defect, 574
Verrucae, 192, 625–626, *626*
  treatment of, 640
Vertebrae, 493–494, *495*
Vertex compression, 403
Vertigo, 534
Vesicle, skin, *183*
Vesicostomy, 745
Vesicotomy, 745
Vesicoureteral reflux, 744t
Vesicovaginal fistula, 744t
Vesiculobullous disorders, 186–187
Video endoscopy, 250, *251*
Video tapes, 132, 142, 770
Viets' test, 402
Viral infections. See also specific infection.
  laboratory studies in, 352–355
    critical and alert values in, 368t
  urinalysis findings in, 328t
Vision, disorders of, 482
  tests of, 482–483
  in family medicine, 233
Vocal cords, 526, *530*
  disorders of, 540–541
  injection of, 545
  paralysis of, 541
Voiding cystography, consultation report on, *380*

Voluntary health and welfare agencies, Appendix 9
Vulvitis, 435

Warthin's tumor, 538
Warts, 192
  plantar, 626, *626*
    treatment of, 640
Washio flap, 603
Weber's test, 403
Weight for age chart, *583*
Weights and measures tables, Appendix 6
Western blot testing, for HIV, 343, 344t, *345–349*
Wheal, skin, *184*
Wheezing, 693
White blood cell, evaluation of, 311–312, *318*, *320–326*, 367t
Wire instruments, 513
Wolff-Parkinson-White syndrome, 159t
Wood's light examination, 200
Word books, medical, 143, 146–147, 768–769
Word division, 99
  references on, 770
Word processing, equipment for, 45
  in pathology, 566
  management of, 88
  spell check feature of, 99, 757
Work hours, 45, 80
Work schedules, 84–85
Workers' Compensation Insurance, 55
Wrist, 494, 496
  carpal tunnel syndrome of, 503–504, *503*
    history and physical examination in, *506–507*
  fracture of, 508–509
Writing. See also *Publication.*
  references on, 757
  scientific and technical, references on, 771

Xanthine, urinary sediments and, 339–340t
Xanthoma, 196
Xenograft, 597
Xenon, radioactive, 417t, 418t
X-ray studies, 661–662, *664*
  report on, *65*, 664, 666

Zenker's diverticulum, 540
Zip codes, 832
Zoopsia, 403